Vascular and Endovascular Surgery: Clinical Diagnosis and Management

a LANGE medical book

Vascular and Endovascular Surgery: Clinical Diagnosis and Management

Editors

Munier Nazzal, MD, MBA
Professor of Surgery
Department of Surgery
Department of Medical Education
College of Medicine and Life Sciences
University of Toledo
Toledo, Ohio

John Blebea, MD, MBA
Clinical Professor of Vascular Surgery
Department of Surgery
College of Medicine
Central Michigan University
Saginaw, Michigan

Mohamed F. Osman, MD, MBA
Associate Professor of Surgery,
Department of Surgery
College of Medicine and Life Sciences
University of Toledo
Toledo, Ohio

Mc Graw Hill

New York Chicago San Francisco Athens London Madrid Mexico City
Milan New Delhi Singapore Sydney Toronto

Vascular and Endovascular Surgery: Clinical Diagnosis and Management

1 2 3 4 5 6 7 8 9 DSS 28 27 26 25 24 23

ISBN 978-1-260-46271-5
MHID 1-260-46271-4

This book was set in minion pro by MPS Limited.
The editors were Sydney Keen Vitale and Kim J. Davis.
The production supervisor was Catherine Saggese.
Project management was provided by Poonam Bisht, MPS Limited.

This book is printed on acid-free paper

Library of Congress Cataloging-in-Publication Data

Names: Nazzal, Munier, editor. | Blebea, John, editor. | Osman, Mohamed F., editor.
Title: Vascular and endovascular surgery : clinical diagnosis and management / [edited by] Munier Nazzal, John Blebea, Mohamed F. Osman.
Other titles: Vascular and endovascular surgery | Lange medical book. 1549-5736
Description: New York : McGraw Hill, [2023] | Series: Lange medical book | Includes bibliographical references and index. | Summary: "This book will provide a problem-oriented approach to vascular and endovascular surgery that includes history, clinical findings, differential diagnosis, and management of clinical problems"—Provided by publisher.
Identifiers: LCCN 2022038611 (print) | LCCN 2022038612 (ebook) | ISBN 9781260462715 (paperback; alk. paper) | ISBN 9781260462722 (ebook)
Subjects: MESH: Vascular Diseases—surgery | Vascular Surgical Procedures—methods
Classification: LCC RD594.2 (print) | LCC RD594.2 (ebook) | NLM WG 505 | DDC 617.4/13—dc23/eng/20221103
LC record available at https://lccn.loc.gov/2022038611
LC ebook record available at https://lccn.loc.gov/2022038612

Contents

Contributors vii | Preface xv

SECTION I

GENERAL VASCULAR 1

1. Vascular Biology
Shaunak Roy, Camilla Ferreira Wenceslau **2**
2. Vascular Hemodynamics
Abdul Kader Natour, Loay Kabbani **18**
3. Thrombosis and Hemostasis
Deepak Ravindranathan, Manila Gaddh **34**
4. Radiation Safety and the Vascular Specialist
Drew J. Braet, Todd R. Vogel **44**
5. Wound Healing for the Vascular Specialist
Christina J. Camick, Munier Nazzal **68**
6. Cardiac Evaluation of the Vascular Patient
Lindsay Ahmed, Ramdas G. Pai **92**
7. Noninvasive Evaluation of Venous Disease
Abdullah Nasif, Samih W. Bittar **109**
8. Noninvasive Evaluation of Arterial Disease
Karem C. Harth, Vikram S. Kashyap **126**
9. Physics for the Vascular Specialist
Motaz Al Yafi, Munier Nazzal **144**
10. Vascular Surgical Techniques: Open Surgical Exposure of Arteries, Veins, and Other Open Techniques for Occlusive Disease and Anterior Spine Exposure
Rebecca Kelso **159**
11. Techniques of Amputation in Vascular Disease
Jeff M. Cross, Nabil A. Ebraheim **170**
12. Basics on Endovascular Diagnosis and Treatment
J. Ignacio Torrealba, Mohamed F. Osman **202**
13. Vascular Graft Conduits: Types and Patency
Heitham Albeshri, Daniel Katz **217**
14. Complex Regional Pain Syndrome
Ahmed Bosaily, Munier Nazzal **226**

SECTION II

VENOUS DISEASE 237

15. Venous Anatomy and Physiology
Eric Goldschmidt, John Blebea **238**
16. Deep Venous Thromboembolism
Sriganesh B. Sharma, Andrea Obi **258**
17. Pulmonary Embolism
Emily A. Malgor, Rafael D. Malgor **270**
18. Chronic Venous Disease
Pamela S. Kim, Antonios P. Gasparis **285**
19. Superficial Venous Insufficiency and Varicose Veins
Anastasiya Shchatsko, John Blebea **298**
20. Chronic Venous Disease of the Upper Extremities and Central Veins
Leah Gober, Karl A. Illig **321**
21. Arteriovenous Malformations
Byung-Boong Lee, James Laredo **337**
22. Lymphedema
Stanley G. Rockson **353**
23. Lower Extremity Swelling and Differential Diagnosis
Thomas F. O'Donnell, Jr. **364**

SECTION III
ARTERIAL DISEASE 379

24. Arterial Anatomy and Pathophysiology
Amy Felsted, Peter Henke **380**

25. Abdominal Aortic Aneurysmal Disease
Richard A. Meena, Yazan Duwayri **391**

26. Aortic Dissection
Charles DeCarlo, Matthew J. Eagleton **404**

27. Penetrating Aortic Ulcerations and Intramural Hematomas
Matthew B. Schneck, Behzad S. Farivar **430**

28. Visceral Aneurysms
Rachael Nicholson **438**

29. Thoracoabdominal Aortic Aneurysms
Tanvi Subramanian, Ross Milner **453**

30. Peripheral Arterial Aneurysms
Ahmed A. Sorour, Levester Kirksey **461**

31. Acute Limb Ischemia
Nicolas J. Mouawad, Abdullah Nasif **487**

32. Chronic Lower Extremity Ischemia (CLI)
Steven Scoville, Timur Sarac **504**

33. Chronic Upper Extremity Ischemia (CUI
Joseph P. Hart, Mark G. Davies **516**

34. Atherosclerotic Carotid Disease
Rebecca A. Marmor, Mahmoud Malas **526**

35. Vertebrobasilar Insufficiency
Mouhammad Jumaa, Diana Slawski **547**

36. Chronic Mesenteric Ischemia
Tania A. Torres-Ruiz, Mohamed F. Osman **568**

37. Acute Mesenteric Ischemia
Susan Natalie Eisert, Michael R. Go **578**

38. Renal Artery Stenosis
Christopher J. Cooper, Kristin Schafer **595**

SECTION IV
SPECIAL VASCULAR CONDITIONS 611

39. Thoracic Outlet Syndrome and Supraclavicular Decompression
Francis J. Caputo, John W. Perry **612**

40. Portal Hypertension
Nizar Hariri, Munier Nazzal **622**

41. Hemodialysis Access
Amin Mohamed Ahmed, Ayman Ahmed **650**

42. Peripheral Vascular Trauma
Sarah Hill, Mallory Williams **673**

43. Neck Vascular Trauma
Ahmad Zeineddin, Mallory Williams **693**

44. Central Vascular Trauma
Mallory Williams, Mohamed F. Osman **703**

45. Thoracic Vascular Trauma
Mallory Williams, Abraham Lebenthal **719**

46. Resuscitative Endovascular Balloon Occlusion of the Aorta for Vascular Trauma
Maaz Zuberi, Mallory Williams **729**

47. Compartment Syndrome
Nabil A. Ebraheim, David Yatsonsky, II **740**

48. Native Arterial Infections
Lindsey M. Korepta, Carlos F. Bechara **761**

49. Vasculitis and Other Arteriopathies
Erica Leigh Benvenutti, Nezam Altorok **769**

50. Prosthetic Graft Infections
Mohamad A. Chahrour, Jamal J. Hoballah **784**

51. Vascular Tumors and Vascular Oncosurgery
Mamoun A. Al-Basheer, Samer Alharthi **796**

52. Erectile Dysfunction
Jonathan H. Demeter, Ahmed El-Zawahry **820**

53. Chronic Lower Extremity Ulcers Management and Evaluation
Munier Nazzal, Karen Bauer **839**

54. Business Aspects of a Cardiovascular Center
Bhagwan Satiani, Christopher McQuinn **863**

55. Leadership and Physicians as Leaders in Health Care Organizations
Jack W. Sample, Charles Brunicardi **880**

56. Pediatric Vascular Surgery
Heitham Albeshri, Alexandre d'Audiffret **896**

57. Artificial Intelligence and Vascular Surgery
Qiong Qiu, Munier Nazzal **906**

Index 919

Contributors

Amin Mohamed Ahmed, MBBS
Vascular Surgery Fellow
St. Louis University
St. Louis , Missouri

Ayman Ahmed, MBBS, RPVI
Assistant Professor of Vascular and Endovascular Surgery
University of Toledo
Toledo, Ohio

Lindsay Ahmed, MD
Cardiologist
Beaver Medical Group
Gorgonio Memorial Hospital
Banning, California

Motaz Al Yafi, MD
General Surgery Resident
Department of Surgery
University of Toledo
Toledo, Ohio

Mamoun A. Al-Basheer, MBBS(Lond), FRCSI, FRCSEd, JBS, JBVS, FICA, ASTS
Consultant Vascular and Transplant Surgeon
Director of Vasocare Vascular Center
Amman, Jordan

Heitham Albeshri, MD
Surgery Residency Training Program Director
King Faisal Specialist Hospital and Research Center
Riyadh, Saudi Arabia

Samer Alharthi, MD, MPH
Vascular Surgery Fellow
East Virginia Medical School
Norfolk, Virginia

Nezam Altorok, MD
Associate Professor
Division of Rheumatology
Department of Internal Medicine
University of Toledo
Toledo, Ohio

Karen Bauer, DNP, CWS, FAACWS
Director of Wound Services
Division of Vascular, Endovascular and Wound Surgery
University of Toledo
Toledo, Ohio

Carlos F. Bechara, MD, FACS, RPVI
Professor of Surgery
Loyola University Medical Center
Maywood, Illinois

Erica Leigh Benvenutti, MD
Family Health West Arthritis & Rheumatology
Fruita, Colorado

Samih W. Bittar, MD, FACP, FSVM, RPVI
OhioHealth Heart and Vascular Institute
Riverside Methodist Hospital
Columbus, Ohio

John Blebea, MD, MBA
Professor and Chair
Department of Surgery
Central Michigan University College of Medicine
Saginaw, Michigan

Ahmed Bosaily, MD
General Surgery Resident
Department of Surgery
University of Toledo
Toledo, Ohio

Drew J. Braet, MD
Vascular Surgery Resident
University of Michigan
Ann Arbor, Michigan

Charles Brunicardi, MD, FACS
Dean
SUNY Downstate Medical School
Brooklyn, New York

Christina J. Camick, MD
General Surgery Resident
Department of Surgery
University of Toledo
Toledo, Ohio

Francis J. Caputo, MD
Program Director, Aortic Center Director
Department of Vascular Surgery,
Heart Vascular and Thoracic Institute
Cleveland Clinic
Cleveland, Ohio

Mohamad A. Chahrour, MD
Vascular Surgery Resident
Division of Vascular Surgery
University of Iowa Hospitals and Clinics
Iowa City, Iowa

Christopher J. Cooper, MD
Professor and Dean
College of Medicine and Life Sciences
University of Toledo
Toledo, Ohio

Jeff M. Cross, MD
Orthopedic Surgery Resident
Department of Orthopaedic Surgery
College of Medicine and Life Sciences
University of Toledo
Toledo, Ohio

Alexandre d'Audiffret, MD
Chief of Vascular Surgery
Division of Vascular Surgery
Rush University Medical Center
Chicago, Illinois

Mark G. Davies, MD, PhD, MBA, FRCSI, FRCS, FACS
Professor and Chief
Vascular and Endovascular Surgery
UT Health San Antonio
Medical Director, South Texas Center for Vascular Care
South Texas Medical Center
Joe R. and Teresa Lozano Long School of Medicine
University of Texas Health Sciences Center
San Antonio, Texas

Charles DeCarlo, MD
General Surgery Resident
Division of Vascular and Endovascular Surgery
Massachusetts General Hospital
Boston, Massachusetts

Jonathan H. Demeter, MD
Urology Resident
Department of Urology
College of Medicine and Life Sciences
University of Toledo
Toledo, Ohio

Yazan Duwayri, MD
Associate Professor of Surgery
Vascular Surgery
Emory University School of Medicine
Atlanta, Georgia

Matthew J. Eagleton, MD
Chief
Division of Vascular and Endovascular Surgery
Massachusetts General Hospital
Boston, Massachusetts

Nabil A. Ebraheim, MD
Professor and Chair
Department of Orthopaedic Surgery
University of Toledo Medical Center
College of Medicine and Life Sciences
University of Toledo
Toledo, Ohio

Susan Natalie Eisert, MD, MS
Chief Resident, General Surgery
Department of Surgery
Wexner Medical Center
The Ohio State University
Columbus, Ohio

Ahmed El-Zawahry, MD
Assistant Professor
Department of Urology
College of Medicine and Life Sciences
University of Toledo
Toledo, Ohio

Behzad S. Farivar, MD, FACS
Assistant Professor of Surgery, Division of Vascular Surgery
Director, University of Virginia Aortic Center
University of Virginia
Charlottesville, Virginia

Amy Felsted, MD
Resident in Surgery
University of Michigan Hospitals
Ann Arbor, Michigan

Manila Gaddh, MD
Associate Professor
Department of Hematology and Medical Oncology
Emory University School of Medicine
Atlanta, Georgia

Antonios P. Gasparis, MD
Professor of Vascular Surgery
Department of Surgery
Renaissance School of Medicine
Stony Brook University
Stony Brook, New York

Michael R. Go, MD, MS
Associate Professor of Surgery
Division of Vascular Diseases and Surgery
Department of General Surgery
The Ohio State University
Columbus, Ohio

Leah Gober, MS
Vascular Surgery Resident
University of Wisconsin Hospitals and Clinics
Madison, Wisconsin

Eric Goldschmidt, MD, MS
Resident in General Surgery
Department of Surgery
College of Medicine and Life Sciences
University of Toledo
Toledo, Ohio

Nizar Hariri, MD
Attending Vascular Surgeon
Sentara Medical Group
Hampton, Virginia

Joseph P. Hart, MD, MHL, FACS, DFSVS
Associate Professor of Surgery and Radiology
Division of Vascular and Endovascular Surgery
Department of Surgery
Medical College of Wisconsin
Milwaukee, Wisconsin

Karem C. Harth, MD, MHS, RPVI
Assistant Professor of Surgery
Harrington Heart and Vascular Institute
University Hospitals Cleveland Medical Center
Cleveland, Ohio

Peter Henke, MD
Professor of Surgery
Chief, Section of Vascular Surgery
University of Michigan Hospitals
Ann Arbor, Michigan

Sarah Hill, MD
General Surgery Resident
Department of Surgery
College of Medicine and Life Sciences
University of Toledo
Toledo, Ohio

Jamal J. Hoballah, MD, MBA, FACS
Professor and Chairman
Department of Surgery
American University of Beirut Medical Center
Emeritus Professor of Surgery
University of Iowa Hospitals and Clinics
Beirut, Lebanon

Karl A. Illig, MD
Director of Research and Education
FLOW Vascular Institute
Houston, Texas

Mouhammad Jumaa, MD
Program Director for Vascular Neurology Fellowship
Professor, Department of Neurology
College of Medicine and Life Sciences
University of Toledo
Toledo, Ohio

Loay Kabbani, MD, MHSA
Program Director, Vascular Surgery Fellowship
Vice Chair of Surgery
Henry Ford Hospital
Detroit, Michigan

Vikram S. Kashyap, MD, FACS, RVT, RPVI
Professor of Surgery
Chief, Division of Vascular Surgery and Endovascular Therapy
Harrington Heart and Vascular Institute
University Hospitals Cleveland Medical Center
Cleveland, Ohio

Daniel Katz, MD
Vascular Surgery Assistant Professor
Division of Vascular and Endovascular Surgery
Rush University Medical Center
Chicago, Illinois

Rebecca Kelso, MD
Attending Vascular Surgeon
Novant Health Heart and Vascular Institute
Presbyterian Medical Center
Charlotte, North Carolina

Pamela S. Kim, MD
General Vascular Surgeon
Center for Vein Restoration and Center for Vascular Medicine
Framingham, Massachusetts

Levester Kirksey, MD, MBA
Vice Chairman, Department of Vascular Surgery
Co-Direcrtor of the Peripheral Artery Disease (PAD) Center
The Cleveland Clinic
Cleveland, Ohio

Lindsey M. Korepta, MD, FACS, RPVI
Assistant Professor of Surgery
Loyola University Medical Center
Maywood, Illinois

James Laredo, MD, PhD
Associate Professor of Surgery
Department of Surgery
George Washington University Medical School
Washington, DC

Abraham Lebenthal, MD, MHA
Assistant Professor of Surgery
Division of Thoracic Surgery
Brigham and Women's Hospital
Harvard Medical School
Boston, Massachusetts

Byung-Boong Lee, MD, PhD
Professor of Surgery
Center for the Lymphedema and Vascular Malformations
George Washington University Medical School
Washington, DC

Mahmoud Malas, MD, MHS, RPVI, FACS
Chief of Vascular and Endovascular Surgery
Professor of Surgery
University of California San Diego
La Jolla, California

Emily A. Malgor, MD, FSVS, FACS
Assistant Professor of Surgery
Department of Surgery
University of Colorado
Anschutz Medical Center
Aurora, Colorado

Rafael D. Malgor, MD, FSVS, FACS
Associate Professor of Surgery
Department of Surgery
University of Colorado
Anschutz Medical Center
Aurora, Colorado

Rebecca A. Marmor, MD, MAS
Assistant Professor of Surgery
Department of Surgery
Johns Hopkins University School of Medicine
Baltimore, Maryland

Christopher McQuinn, MD
Vascular Surgery Fellow
Department of Surgery
Division of Vascular Diseases and Surgery
Wexner Medical Center
The Ohio State University
Columbus, Ohio

Richard A. Meena, MD
Resident, Integrated Vascular Surgery
Vascular Surgery
Emory University School of Medicine
Atlanta, Georgia

Ross Milner, MD
Professor of Surgery
Section of Vascular Surgery
University of Chicago
Chicago, Illinois

Nicolas J. Mouawad, MD, MPH, MBA, FSVS, FRCS, FACS, RPVI
Chief and Medical Director
Vascular and Endovascular Surgery
McLaren Health System – Bay Region
Bay City, Michigan

Abdullah Nasif, MD
Research Fellow
Division of Vascular, Endovascular and Wound Surgery
Department of Surgery
University of Toledo Medical Center
Toledo, Ohio

Abdul Kader Natour, MD
General Surgery Resident
Department of Surgery
Henry Ford Hospital
Detroit, Michigan

Munier Nazzal, MD, MBA
Professor of Surgery
Department of Surgery
Department of Medical Education
College of Medicine and Life Sciences
University of Toledo
Toledo, Ohio

Rachael Nicholson, MD
Clinical Associate Professor
Department of Surgery
University of Iowa
Iowa City, Iowa

Thomas F. O'Donnell, Jr., MD
Benjamin Andrews Chair of Surgery
The Cardiovascular Center
Tufts University School of Medicine
Boston, Massachusetts

Andrea Obi, MD
Assistant Professor of Vascular Surgery
Department of Surgery
University of Michigan College of Medicine
Ann Arbor, Michigan

Mohamed F. Osman, MD, MBA
Associate Professor
Division of Vascular, Endovascular and Wound Surgery
Department of Surgery
College of Medicine and Life Sciences
University of Toledo
Toledo, Ohio

Ramdas G. Pai, MD
Riverside School of Medicine
University of California Riverside
Riverside, California

John W. Perry, MD
Vascular Surgery Resident
Department of Vascular Surgery, Heart Vascular and Thoracic Institute
Cleveland Clinic
Cleveland, Ohio

Qiong Qiu, MD
General Surgery Resident
Department of Surgery
University of Toledo
Toledo, Ohio

Deepak Ravindranathan, MD, MS
Assistant Professor
Department of Hematology and Medical Oncology
Emory University School of Medicine
Atlanta, Georgia

Stanley G. Rockson, MD
Allan and Tina Neill Professor of Lymphatic Research and Medicine
Director, Stanford Center for Lymphatic and Venous Disorders
Division of Cardiovascular Medicine
Stanford University School of Medicine
Stanford, California

Shaunak Roy, MS
Medical Student
College of Medicine and Life Sciences
University of Toledo
Toledo, Ohio

Jack W. Sample
General Surgery Resident
Mayo Clinic
Rochester, Minnesota

Timur Sarac, MD
Director Division of Vascular Diseases and Surgery
Department of Surgery
The Ohio State University Wexner Medical Center
Columbus, Ohio

Bhagwan Satiani, MD, MBA, FACHE, FACS
Professor Emeritus and Academy Professor
Wexner Medical Center
The Ohio State University
Columbus, Ohio

Kristin Schafer, MD
General Surgery Resident
Department of Surgery
College of Medicine and Life Sciences
University of Toledo
Toledo, Ohio

Matthew B. Schneck, MD
Vascular Surgery Integrated-Resident
Division of Vascular Surgery
University of California, Davis
Sacramento, California

Steven Scoville, MD, PhD
General Surgery Resident
Department of Surgery
The Ohio State University Wexner Medical Center
Columbus, Ohio

Sriganesh B. Sharma, MD, PhD
General Surgery Resident
Department of Surgery
University of Michigan College of Medicine
Ann Arbor, Michigan

Anastasiya Shchatsko, MD
Geneal Surgery Resident
Department of Surgery
Central Michigan University College of Medicine
Saginaw, Michigan

Diana Slawski, MD
General Neurologist
Palo Alto, California

Ahmed A. Sorour, MD
Vascular Surgery Resident
Department of Vascular Surgery
The Cleveland Clinic
Cleveland, Ohio

Tanvi Subramanian, MD
General Surgery Resident
University of Chicago
Chicago, Illinois

J. Ignacio Torrealba, MD
Assistant Professor in Vascular Surgery
Universidad Católica de Chile
Santiago, Chile

Tania A. Torres-Ruiz
General Surgery Resident
Department of Surgery
College of Medicine and Life Sciences
University of Toledo
Toledo, Ohio

Todd R. Vogel, MD, MPH
Associate Professor of Surgery
Chief of Vascular and Endovascular Surgery
University of Missouri-Columbia
Columbia, Missouri

Camilla Ferreira Wenceslau, PhD
Associate Professor
Laboratory of Vascular Biology
Cardiovascular Translational Research Center
Department of Cell Biology and Anatomy
School of Medicine Columbia
University of South Carolina
Columbia, South Carolina

Mallory Williams, MD, MPH, FACS, FICS, FCCP, FCCM
Professor of Surgery and Chief
Division of Trauma, Critical Care, and Surgical Nutrition
Department of Surgery
Howard University College of Medicine
Trauma Medical Director
Director of the Surgical ICU
Howard University Hospital Level I Trauma Center
Washington, DC

David Yatsonsky, II, MD
Orthopedic Surgery Resident
College of Medicine and Life Sciences
University of Toledo
Toledo, Ohio

Ahmad Zeineddin, MD
General Surgery Resident
Howard University
Washington, DC

Maaz Zuberi, MBBS
General Surgery Resident
Howard University College of Medicine
Washington, DC

Preface

Vascular surgery goes back to the days of medicine giants Hinter brothers and Astley Cooper; however, most of the advancements in the diagnosis and management of vascular disease took place in the last few decades. The recognition of vascular surgery as a specialty occurred in the twentieth century with the explosion of technology and advancement of interventions in vascular disease. The modern field of vascular surgery was led by innovations in the field of endovascular interventions that were influenced by the involvement of both interventional radiology and interventional cardiology which added to the complexity and diversity of vascular interventions. This book was written to guide learners and clinicians in the diagnosis and management of vascular disease including medical therapy, endovascular interventions, and open surgery that transformed vascular disease management and continuously modified treatment guidelines.

The evolution in vascular disease management was complemented by advances in the noninvasive diagnosis of vascular disease. Noninvasive evaluation of vascular disease was revolutionized by advances and improvements in ultrasound and Duplex technology that helped early detection and tried to prevent complications of vascular disease. Other advances in noninvasive vascular diagnosis discussed in this book include magnetic resonance imaging, computed tomography, positron emission tomography and scintigraphy, optical coherence tomography, and intravascular ultrasound.

Vascular disease is a manifestation of systemic disease that has the potential to be treated and modified by lifestyle changes such as smoking cessation and optimal medical therapy. However, in patients who have advanced disease, a more advanced therapy is needed which includes endovascular and open surgery. The pendulum shifts between open and endovascular interventions based on technological innovations and experience of the interventionalists. Endovascular interventions were embraced by a wider variety of health providers including radiologists, cardiologists, and vascular surgeons. The real breakthrough in the diagnostic and later endovascular intervention happened after the introduction of selective arteriography and selective evaluation of vascular beds by Sven-Ivar Selinger of Sweden and later Dotter's accidental recanalization of the iliac artery. Since then, there has been exponential growth in endovascular innovations for arterial and venous occlusive diseases. Endovascular treatment of aneurysmal disease started later with Juan Parodi's conception in 1976 that made clinical application possible using a Palmaz stent in the first patient in Argentina in 1990. Endovascular management of aortic aneurysm changed the direction of surgical interventions in aortic disease. Since their initial introduction, dramatic technological advances in both occlusive and aneurysmal disease, including balloon angioplasty, stents of different types, drug-coated balloons and stents, atherectomy, vena cava filters, embolization, thrombolytic therapy, and mechanical thrombectomy devices for both arterial and venous disease, have transformed vascular disease treatment. Such advances are applied to a different extent in different vascular beds with variable degrees of success, and sometimes without class 1 evidence, but lead by convenience to the patient and operator. Although technology changes continuously, we have tried to include many of the latest treatment options in this book.

The chapters of *Vascular and Endovascular Surgery: Clinical Diagnosis and Management* follow a format that covers all aspects of disease diagnosis and management. Each chapter starts with an overview of the disease process followed by symptoms and signs of disease, then diagnosis and therapy that includes both endovascular and open surgery with comparison between both, when appropriate. A unique part of the clinical chapters is a flowchart to summarize the management of the clinical problem. A set of multiple-choice questions with answers are included in each chapter to augment the learning process.

The book is divided into four sections. Section I: General Vascular contains chapters on vascular biology, hemodynamics, thrombosis and hemostasis, cardiac evaluation, radiation safety, noninvasive evaluation of arterial and venous disease, and surgical techniques in vascular surgery. Section II: Venous Disease covers a continuum of venous disease topics. Section III: Arterial Disease deals with arterial diseases including acute ischemia and chronic occlusive diseases of lower extremities, mesenteric, renal arteries, aneurysmal disease, and cerebrovascular disease. The last section, Section IV: Special Vascular Conditions, contains miscellaneous subjects such as vasculitis, thoracic outlet syndrome, hemodialysis access, portal hypertension, lower extremity ulcers, vascular infections, and vascular disease in pediatric patients in addition to newer subjects of interest to the vascular specialists such as the business of the vascular centers, leadership in medicine, artificial intelligence.

We are dedicating this book to all those who are interested in vascular disease in an easy format to read by the whole continuum of learners from medical students, general surgery residents, vascular surgery residents/fellows, vascular surgeons, general surgeons in addition to nurses, nurse practitioners, and physicians assistants. The efforts of the editors and contributors are complemented by the professional support of the staff at McGraw Hill to ensure a final product that is accurate, of high quality, and follows the intended format.

Finally, we hope that this first edition will gain the satisfaction of the readers and learners. Their support by criticism and suggestions for future editions is greatly appreciated.

Munier Nazzal, MD, MBA, Toledo, Ohio
John Blebea, MD, MBA, Saginaw, Michigan
Mohamed F. Osman, MD, MBA, Toledo, Ohio

SECTION I General Vascular

CHAPTER

1 Vascular Biology

Shaunak Roy and Camilla Ferreira Wenceslau

OUTLINE

OVERVIEW OF BLOOD VESSELS

BLOOD VESSELS' STRUCTURE AND FUNCTION

The Endothelium (*Tunica Intima*)

The Smooth Muscle Layer (*Tunica Media*)

ADVENTITIA AND PERIVASCULAR ADIPOSE TISSUE (TUNICA EXTERNA)

Capillaries

Pericytes

Venous System

BASIC PRINCIPLES OF CIRCULATORY FUNCTION

OVERVIEW OF BLOOD VESSELS

Blood vessels are the structural conduits of the circulatory system which allow for the metabolic needs of our bodily tissues to be met. The circulatory system has two divisions: systemic and pulmonary (supplying the lungs) (Figure 1-1). From the heart, oxygenated blood travels through the aorta, arteries, and arterioles and ends in the capillaries with the uptake of oxygen into the tissues and the transfer of deoxygenated blood and metabolic waste out. Deoxygenated blood is then taken up into venules and carried into veins and the venae cavae to return to the heart to again be oxygenated in the lungs.[1]

Different parts of the circulatory system have distinct macro and micro anatomy to support their roles. Conductance or large vessels are capable of pulsating and propagating blood flow, but do not directly contribute to the regulation of blood pressure. Generally, the wall of a vessel is multilayered and is frequently surrounded by perivascular adipose tissue (PVAT). This can be seen in Figure 1-2. Larger arteries have a lumen higher than 300 μm in diameter, their tunica media, or middle, layer is thicker and more elastic than small arteries, and consequently, they accommodate higher pressures. On the other hand, small arteries present a less elastic, but more muscular tunica media layer. As described in detail in the section "Basic Principles of Circulatory Function," blood flow varies inversely with the total cross-sectional area of the blood vessels (Table 1-1); consequently, small arteries, which present a greater total cross-sectional area compared to larger arteries, present slowest blood flow and lower blood pressure. However, each small artery, arteriole, and capillary are extremely small compared to conductance vessels. Therefore, each small artery and arteriole offer, individually, higher resistance to the flow. As a result, these arteries constrict and dilate to exert local blood flow and, directly, control blood pressure. Taken together, although the resistance of an individual small artery is higher when compared to a larger artery, the flow and blood pressure are lower in small arteries and arterioles because of the higher total cross-sectional area.

The aorta, the largest blood vessel in the body, is an elastic artery and has walls that stretch to

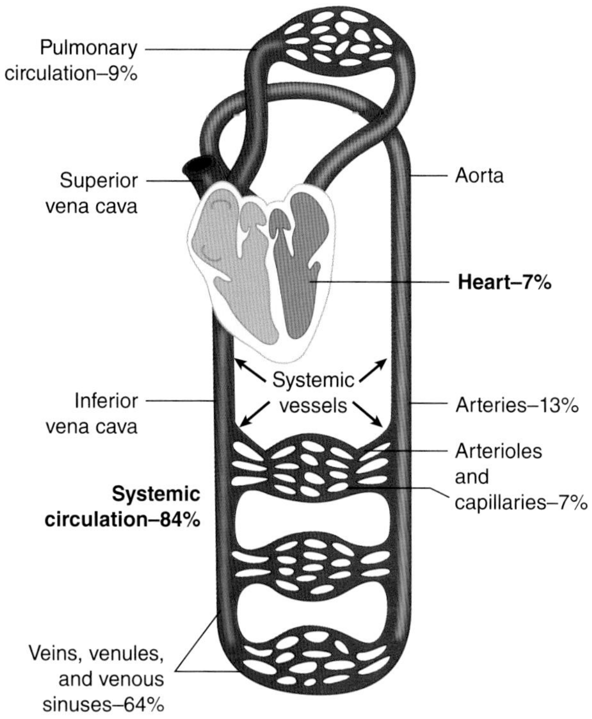

FIGURE 1-1 Schematic of the circulatory system and its components as a percentage of total blood.

TABLE 1-1 Breakdown of Approximate Collective Cross-Sectional Area in the Whole Body (70-kg Male)

Vessel	Cross-Sectional Area (cm^2)
Aorta	2.5
Small Arteries	20
Arterioles	40
Capillaries	2500
Venules	250
Small Veins	80
Venae Cavae	8

accommodate the pulsatile pressure surge coming from the heart. It has three main layers that account for its elasticity: tunica adventitia, tunica media, and tunica intima (Figure 1-3). The outermost layer, tunica adventitia, contains its own small vessel network to support its function (vasa vasorum). The broad middle layer, tunica media, contains fenestrated elastin sheets, collagen, and a few smooth muscle fibers. The innermost layer, the tunica intima,

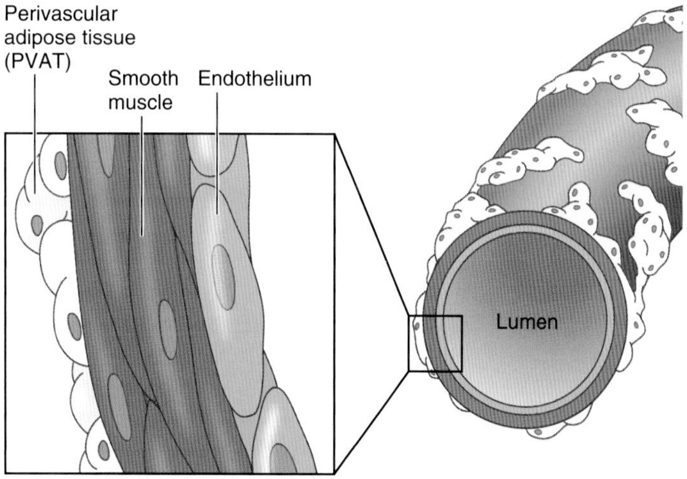

FIGURE 1-2 Representative schematic of a blood vessel with labelled layers and the surrounding perivascular adipose tissue.

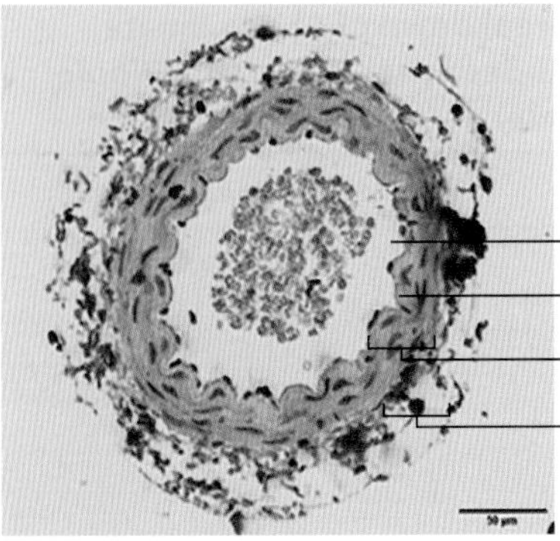

FIGURE 1-3 Cross-sectional histological stain of a representative artery and its various layers.

is a single, flattened layer of endothelial cells (the endothelium) combined with a supporting layer of elastin rich collagen.

Small arteries (lumen diameter between 100 and 300 μm) are characteristically muscular and contract and dilate to change the amount of the blood delivered. The tunica media of these vessels consist primarily of several layers of smooth muscle and is in between the internal elastic layer (the border of the tunica intima and tunica media) and the external elastic layer (the border of the tunica media and tunica adventitia). The tunica adventitia of these vessels is very broad and mostly contains collagen and elastin.

Arterioles (lumen diameter smaller than 100 μm) also contract and dilate their lumen to control blood flow. The tunica intima is thin with a single layer of squamous endothelium. The tunica media of these vessels typically contain one to two layers of smooth muscle with the encompassing tunica adventitia merging with the surrounding tissue. Note that arterioles still contain an internal elastic layer but do not contain an external elastic layer.

Capillaries, the smallest blood vessels, facilitate the exchange of fluid, nutrients, electrolytes, hormones, and other substances between blood and the interstitial fluid. The capillaries are porous and thin given that they only consist of a single layer of flattened endothelial cells and its basal lamina. There are three types of capillary: continuous, fenestrated, and discontinuous (Figure 1-4). Continuous capillaries have a tight endothelial lining, which limits the movement of cells and large molecules between the blood and the interstitial fluid. This type of capillary is found in the nervous system. The fenestrated

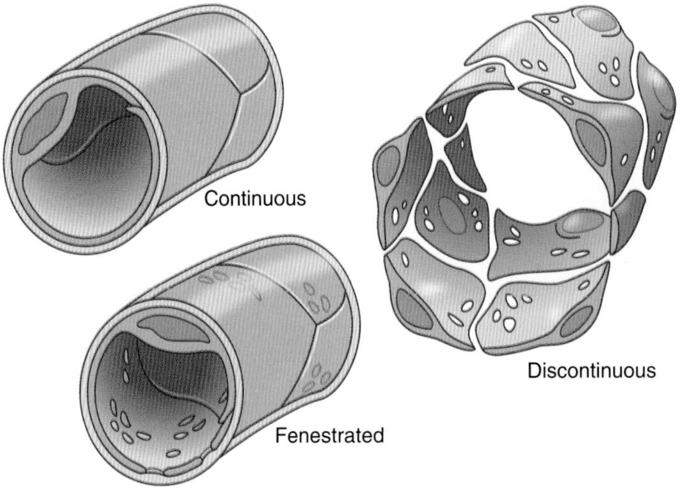

FIGURE 1-4 The physical appearance of the three types of capillaries.

capillaries present small openings or pores in their endothelium called fenestra. The fenestra facilitates movement of macromolecules in and out of the capillary. This type of capillary is found in the kidneys, small intestine, and endocrine glands. The discontinuous capillaries or sinusoidal capillaries are found in the liver, spleen, and bone marrow. They have open spaces between endothelial cells. These type of capillaries present high permeability and, in some cases, allow the passage of blood cells between them.

Venules collect the blood from the capillaries and flow into successively larger veins. Small veins and ultimately the venae cavae, the largest veins, doubly function as pathways back to the heart and as a major reservoir of extra blood. The walls of these vessels are thin and their high capacitance serves as a reservoir for the circulatory system. Venous valves work in conjunction with the musculoskeletal system to propagate blood to flow back toward the heart.

BLOOD VESSELS' STRUCTURE AND FUNCTION

THE ENDOTHELIUM (*TUNICA INTIMA*)

The innermost layer of a vessel, the tunica intima, is a single, flattened layer of endothelial cells: the endothelium. As the major interface between the vascular wall and blood, the endothelium regulates vascular tone, permeability, and hemostasis via its sensitivity to physical and chemical influences. These influences include shear stress induced by the flowing blood, and chemical signals that affect vascular tone, cell adhesion, platelet function, vascular smooth muscle cell (VSMC) phenotype, and vessel wall inflammation.

The endothelium has three major functions: secretion of vasoactive factors, physical barrier properties, and metabolism. In the 1980s, Furchgott and Zawadzki demonstrated that the endothelium plays an obligatory role in acetylcholine (ACh)–mediated relaxation of arterial smooth muscle.[2] They went on to surmise that ACh acts on muscarinic receptors of endothelial cells and stimulates the secretion of a factor that resulted in the relaxation of the smooth muscle cells. At the time, this factor was termed the endothelium-derived relaxing factor or EDRF. Today, the EDRF has been firmly established to be nitric oxide (NO). Other vasorelaxant factors that have been found since then include prostacyclin and endothelium-derived hyperpolarizing factor (EDH), an unknown factor that acts on smooth muscle-localized potassium channels to stimulate hyperpolarization. To this day, several factors have been proposed to be EDH, including potassium itself. Nonetheless, the precise identity of EDH remains to be confirmed. Pro-contractile factors are collectively termed endothelium-derived contractile factors (EDCF) and include endothelin-1 (ET-1), angiotensin-2 (AT-II), and various prostaglandins. In healthy conditions, the endothelium regulates the variety of vasoactive molecules and factors that regulate blood flow. In pathologic conditions, there is a shift in the balance of these factors that promotes a hyper- or hypo-contractile state.

Physically, there are junction structures that link together endothelial cells to create a barrier. In pathologic conditions, these structures are impaired. This endothelial barrier dysfunction enables greater permeability of solutes and immune cells from the blood stream leading to edema and inflammation.

Metabolically, the endothelium contains enzymes and transporters that uptake and process circulating molecules.

THE SMOOTH MUSCLE LAYER (*TUNICA MEDIA*)

As noted above, resistance vessels such as small arteries and arterioles are characterized by their ability to control blood flow. Among the primary determinants of blood flow resistance, the most significant variable is the lumen diameter. As defined by Poiseuille's law, vessel resistance is inversely proportional to the radius to the fourth power (r^4). Thus, alterations in the morphology and/or function of VSMCs impact the luminal radius and consequentially the flow of blood through the vessel.

Contraction of smooth muscle cells is regulated by either receptor activation, stretch, or a change in membrane potential and results in the activation of myosin and actin contractile proteins (Figure 1-5). Contraction is initiated by an increase in the intracellular concentration of Ca^{2+} that combines with calmodulin. This complex activates the myosin light

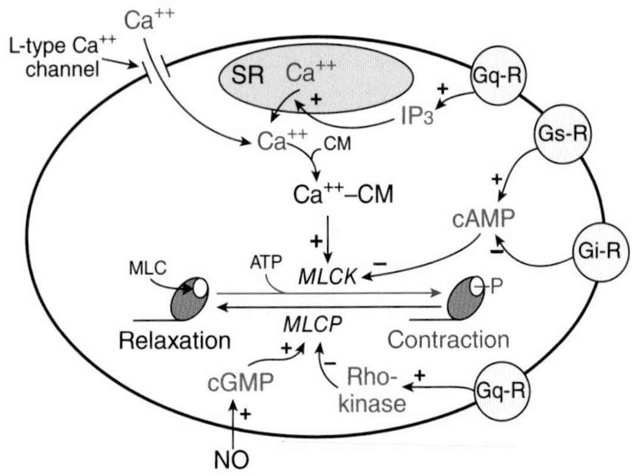

FIGURE 1-5 The smooth muscle contraction and relaxation mechanisms.

chain kinase (MLCK) to phosphorylate the light chain of myosin and facilitates the interaction of myosin with actin. For example, when agonists such as endothelin bind to receptors and couple to a G protein, this stimulates the activity of phospholipase C. This enzyme catalyzes the formation of the powerful second messengers, inositol triphosphate (IP_3) and diacylglycerol (DAG). When IP_3 binds to receptors on the sarcoplasmic reticulum, Ca^{2+} is released from the intracellular stores. This Ca^{2+} along with DAG activates another important enzyme, protein kinase C (PKC). Voltage-operated Ca^{2+} channels (L-type) also open in response to membrane depolarization. These channels are highly expressed in VSMCs and as a result are key mediators of Ca^{2+} concentration. The phosphorylation of the myosin light chain by MLCK is countered by MLC phosphatase, the enzyme which removes the phosphate to promote smooth muscle relaxation. The small G protein RhoA targets Rho kinase and together help regulate MLC phosphatase. When Rho kinase phosphorylates the myosin-binding subunit of MLC phosphatase, the phosphatase's activity is inhibited. This promotes the phosphorylated state of the myosin light chain and therefore the contractile state of the vessel.[3]

Relaxation of vascular smooth muscle can occur either by removing the contractile stimulus or when a substance directly stimulates inhibition of the contractile machinery. As mentioned above, the interaction of myosin with actin is dependent on the intracellular concentration of Ca^{2+} and the activity of MLC phosphatase. As such, a decreased intracellular concentration of Ca^{2+} and increased activity MLC phosphatase promotes relaxation. The process of removing available Ca^{2+} inside of the vascular smooth muscle cells involves the sarcoplasmic reticulum and the plasma membrane. The sarcoplasmic reticulum uses the sarco/endoplasmic reticulum Ca^{2+}-ATPase (SERCA) pump to bind two Ca^{2+} ions and translocate them to the luminal side (of the reticulum). SERCA is endogenously inhibited by phospholamban, but when phospholamban is phosphorylated, this inhibition is released and Ca^{2+} uptake is able to proceed. The plasma membrane also presents a Ca^{2+}ATPase similar to SERCA, as well as Na^{+}/Ca^{2+} exchanger, to help decrease the intracellular concentration of Ca^{2+} and promote relaxation. The closing of receptor-operated and voltage-operated Ca^{2+} channels in the plasma membrane also assists in this function.

Of particular importance to vasodilation is the synthesis of endothelium-derived relaxing factors, including NO. The enzyme that synthesizes NO from arginine, NO synthase (NOS) is present in two forms, constitutive and inducible. The constitutive form is found in endothelial cells and neurons and is activated by an increase in cytosolic calcium. The inducible form is calcium-independent and induced by inflammatory cytokines. Once NO is synthesized, it activates the enzyme guanylate cyclase to produce cGMP. The rise in cGMP leads to the activation of protein kinase G (PKG) which can inhibit L-type calcium channels, RhoA, and phospholamban, activate myosin light chain phosphatase, and promote potassium-induced hyperpolarization. Collectively, this results in decreased Ca^{2+} and relaxation of the vascular smooth muscle.

ADVENTITIA AND PERIVASCULAR ADIPOSE TISSUE (TUNICA EXTERNA)

The adventitia or tunica externa contains connective tissue with collagen and elastic fibers, adrenergic nerves, and lymphatic vessels. Different than tunica intima and media, the contribution of the adventitia to vascular homeostasis and disease has largely been ignored. Growing evidence shows that, rather than being just a structural support to the vessels, the adventitia also functions as a dynamic compartment for immune surveillance and inflammatory cell trafficking, and harbors the vasa vasorum, a dynamic microvasculature that maintains the tunica media and provides an important gateway for macrophage and leukocyte migration into the tunica intima. Recent studies have shown that progenitor cells, with the potential to produce cell types commonly found in blood vessel walls, normally reside within the adventitia of large arteries and veins.[4,5] A combined adventitial fibroblast and inflammatory cell-derived reactive oxygen species are crucial for vascular homeostasis, inflammation, resolution of inflammation, and repair. The initial proliferative response to vascular injury may also occur in the peripheral adventitial layer, and this response declines over days as proliferation in the medial layer is initiated. For this, there are several molecules involved in the adventitia-derived paracrine signaling across the vessel wall, including hydrogen peroxide and fibroblast–derived cytokines.

Adipose tissue is usually classified as either white or brown where white is less vascularized, less innervated, and less metabolically active compared to brown (Figure 1-6).[6] This classification scheme is a spectrum rather than binary categories as tissues can be a mix of the two. PVAT surrounds most systemic blood vessels and can be anywhere from white to beige to brown adipose tissue. It contains adipocytes, cells, penetrating vasa vasorum, infiltrating macrophages, and T lymphocytes. The makeup of PVAT appears to be different in different locations of the body, and the adipocyte type is dynamic. It is important to note that PVAT is a functionally distinct type of adipose tissue with secretory properties. PVAT releases a wide range of biologically active molecules and can act in an endocrine or paracrine manner (Table 1-2).

Initially, PVAT was thought to only serve as structural support and did not functionally interact with the vessel. In a landmark finding, Soltis and Cassis demonstrated in 1991 that PVAT mediated a decrease in the contractile responses to norepinephrine in rat aorta, indicating the potential role of PVAT in vascular function. Since then, in physiological conditions, PVAT has an anticontractile effect on vessel tone. Like the hunt for the EDRF and eventual identification as NO, PVAT has brought upon a new search into PVAT-derived relaxing factors (PVRFs). Key PVRF candidates include Ang (1-7), adipokines such as the leptin, adiponectin, and resistin. The

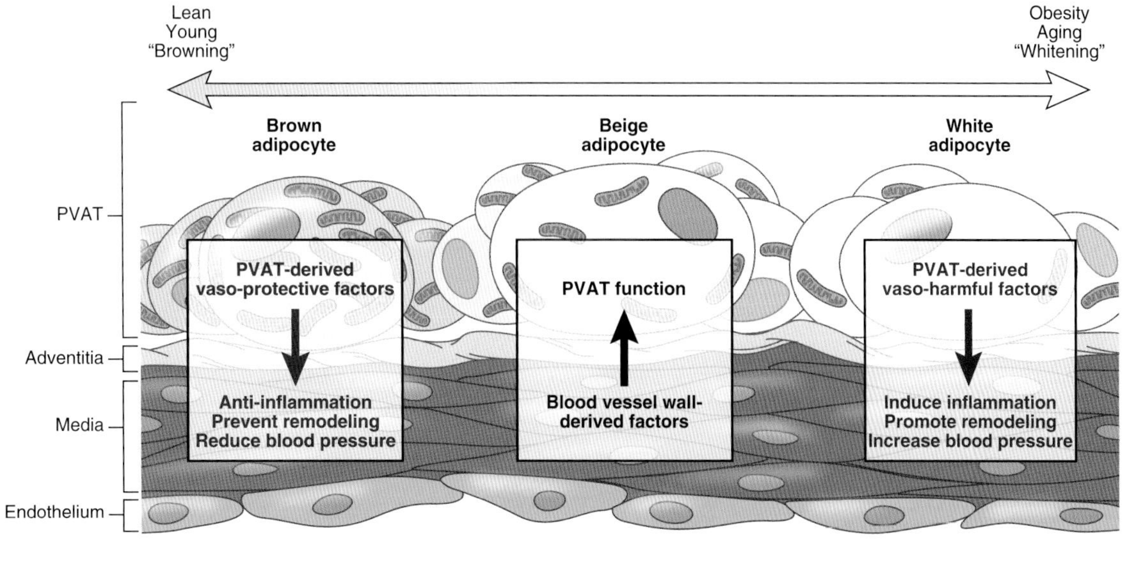

FIGURE 1-6 Figure depicting various stages of PVAT.

TABLE 1-2 The Potential Mechanisms of PVAT Action

Mechanism/Substance	Effect on Vessel	Condition	Vessel Bed and Species	Reference
K_{ATP}	Anticontractile	Physiological	Rat aorta	7
				8
K_{Ca}	Anticontractile	Physiological	Rat aorta	9
			Human internal thoracic	10
K_V	Anticontractile	Physiological	Rat mesenteric	11
Adiponectin	Anticontractile	Physiological	Rat aorta	12
Leptin	Vasodilatory	Physiological	Rat aorta	13
				14
				15
Superoxide	Contractile	Physiological	Rat aorta	16
Hydrogen peroxide	Anticontractile	Physiological	Rat aorta	10
Oxidative stress	Blocks anticontractile effect	Obesity	Human subcutaneous fat arterioles	17
Inflammation	Blocks anticontractile effect	Obesity	Human subcutaneous fat arterioles	17
Hydrogen sulfide	Anticontractile	Physiological hypertension	Rat aorta	18
				19
NO	Anticontractile	Early diet-induced obesity	Mouse mesenteric	20
Angiotensin II	Contractile	Physiological	Rat aorta	21
Ang (1-7)	Anticontractile	Physiological	Rat aorta	21
Mineralocorticoid receptor	Blocks anticontractile effect		Mouse mesenteric	22
AMPK	Endothelial dysfunction	Obesity	Rat mesenteric	23
Infiltrating macrophages	Blocks anticontractile effect		Mouse mesenteric	22
Changes in fatty acid composition	Blocks anticontractile effect	Metabolic syndrome	Rat aorta	24
Hypoxia	Blocks anticontractile effect		Rat aorta	22

potential mechanisms of PVAT action on vascular contraction and PVRFs in both human and animal models are summarized in Table 1-2.

It is important to note that these mechanisms may not be the same in humans and rodent models and human vessel research continues to be an important frontier within the field of PVAT research. For example, in humans, saphenous vein graft function is improved when caution is taken to keep the PVAT layer intact in isolated veins before grafting. A key pathophysiological finding that has been replicated is that in cardiovascular diseases PVAT loses its anticontractile effect and has been specifically demonstrated in low—exercise capacity individuals, high-fat diets, atherosclerosis, metabolic syndrome, and other nonatherosclerotic vascular diseases.[25] It appears that alterations in PVAT function in diseases such as obesity and metabolic syndrome are linked with the release of adipokines, inflammation, and oxidative stress. Most studies that examine the link between PVAT and hypertension note that there is decreased PVAT mass and decreased PVAT anticontractile effect.[26] A similar phenomenon is observed in studies that examine the link between PVAT and intrinsic exercise capacity differences as shown in Figure 1-7.[27] Specifically, it is possible to visualize the gross morphology change between the PVAT from a naïve rat (A), a rat born with low-intrinsic exercise capacity (B) or high-intrinsic exercise capacity (C). Importantly, these changes observed in PVAT morphology are direct associated with changes in function or PVAT-derived paracrine signals as described in Table 1-2.

Most diagrams of vessels that emphasize vascular structure and function still only depict the endothelium, smooth muscle, and adventitia as the layers of the blood vessel. With PVAT lying on the outside of the adventitia without any structure or barrier separating the two, it is critical to recognize PVAT as a key modulator of vascular function.

CAPILLARIES

The peripheral circulation of the body has nearly 10 billion capillaries. The walls of capillaries are composed of a single layer of highly permeable endothelial cells. As a result, water, cell nutrients, and cell waste products can all interchange quickly and easily between the tissues and circulating blood. The precapillary sphincter is the point where each true capillary originates from the terminal arteriole. Here, a smooth muscle fiber encircles the capillary to open and close the entrance to the capillary. The internal diameter of the capillary is just large enough for red blood cells and other blood cells to squeeze through at 4 to 9 μm.

There are two types of "pores" in the capillary membrane. The first is an intracellular cleft, a thin

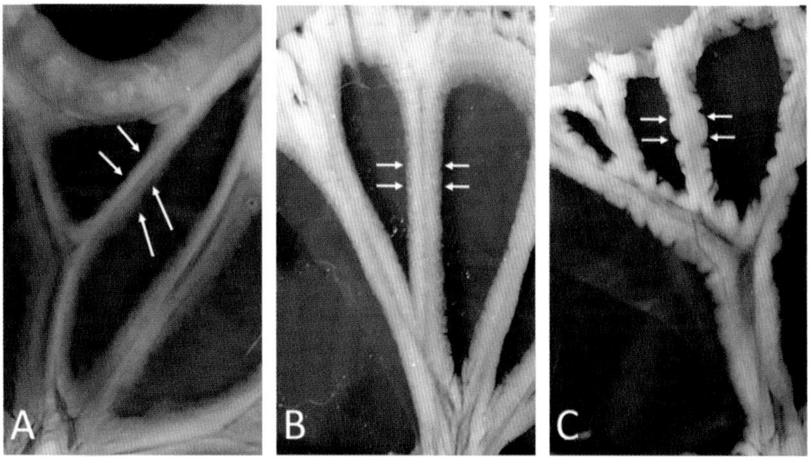

FIGURE 1-7 Images of mesenteric PVAT.

slit, curving channel that has gapped ridges to enable fluid to traverse freely. The second are plasmalemmal vesicles or caveolae. These are oligomers of caveolin proteins that imbibe small packets of plasma or extracellular fluid that contain plasma proteins via endocytosis. These vesicles are what move slowly through the endothelial cell. The "pores" of capillaries differ in different organs in order to meet the specific needs of each organ. For example, in the brain, "tight" junctions exist between the capillary endothelial cells such that only extremely small molecules such as water, oxygen, and CO_2 can pass into or out of the brain tissue. On the other hand, in the liver, the clefts between the capillary endothelial cells are quite large so as to enable all dissolved substances in the plasma to pass from the blood into the liver tissue.

As blood flows along the lumen of the capillary from the arterial end to the venous end, continuous mixing occurs between the interstitial fluid and the plasma due to the thermal motion of water molecules and dissolved substances in the fluid (Figure 1-8). Substances such as oxygen and carbon dioxide can permeate all areas of the capillary membrane since they are lipid-soluble with high rates of transport. Substances that are water-soluble and non-lipid-soluble must diffuse through the intercellular pores of the capillary membrane. These include water molecules, sodium ions, chloride ions, and glucose. The permeability of the capillary pores for different substances varies based on their molecular diameters. Note that the sum rate of diffusion of a substance through any membrane, the capillary membrane in this case, is proportional to the concentration difference of the substance between the two sides of the membrane. Hydrostatic and colloid osmotic forces are what determine the fluid movement through the capillary membrane, also known as Starling forces.

PERICYTES

Hand in hand with the capillaries are a category of cells known as pericytes. These are associated with the external side of vascular capillaries and postcapillary venules (Figure 1-9). Pericytes are thought to play a role in the regulation of blood flow with their contraction, as well as their ability to differentiate into adipocytes, osteoblasts, and phagocytes. Crosstalk between the endothelial cells of capillaries and the surrounding pericytes can be chemically through soluble factors such as platelet-derived growth factor (PDGF)

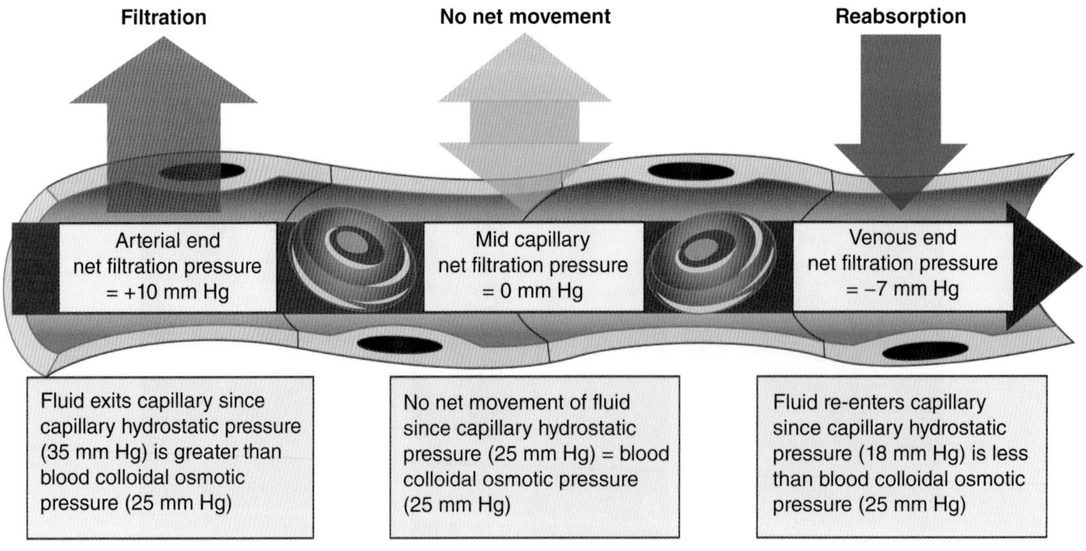
Filtration
No net movement
Reabsorption
Arterial end
net filtration pressure
= +10 mm Hg
Mid capillary
net filtration pressure
= 0 mm Hg
Venous end
net filtration pressure
= −7 mm Hg
Fluid exits capillary since capillary hydrostatic pressure (35 mm Hg) is greater than blood colloidal osmotic pressure (25 mm Hg)
No net movement of fluid since capillary hydrostatic pressure (25 mm Hg) = blood colloidal osmotic pressure (25 mm Hg)
Fluid re-enters capillary since capillary hydrostatic pressure (18 mm Hg) is less than blood colloidal osmotic pressure (25 mm Hg)

FIGURE 1-8 Figure of blood moving through capillaries.

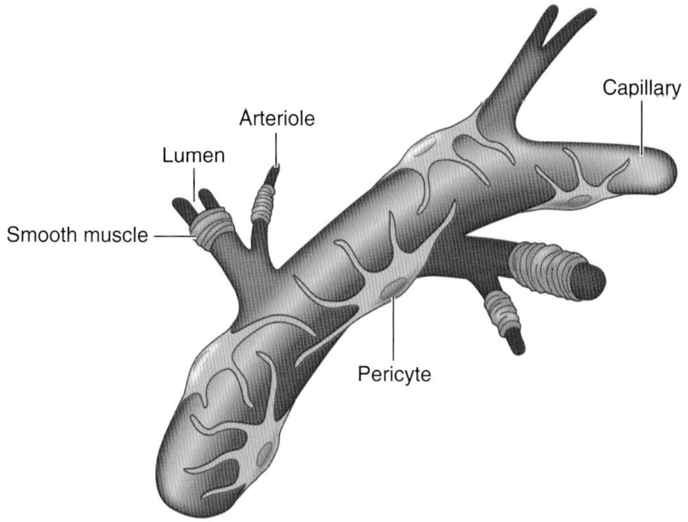

FIGURE 1-9 **Relationship of pericyte to other components of the vasculature.**

and transforming growth-factor-beta (TGF-β), as well as physically through cell adhesion molecules, integrins, and gap junctions. Pericyte dysfunction has been implicated in the development of pathologies such as hypertension, multiple sclerosis, diabetic microangiopathy, and tumor vascularization.[28]

VENOUS SYSTEM

In addition to being the vessels through which blood returns to the heart, veins also perform distinct functions that are necessary for operation of the circulation. By constricting and enlarging, they can store varying quantities of blood that will be made available as required by the circulation. Peripheral veins can also propel blood forward using a venous pump mechanism and can help regulate cardiac output.

The various functions of veins are all contingent upon venous pressure. Recall that all blood from all of the systemic veins will flow into the right atrium of the heart. The pressure at this point is termed the central venous pressure. Large veins typically have some resistance to the flow of blood because they are often compressed by several organs; as a result, the pressure within small peripheral veins can be a few mmHg greater than the central venous pressure. When intra-abdominal pressure rises due to pregnancy, large tumors, or obesity, the pressure in the veins of the legs must rise above the abdominal pressure to enable the abdominal veins to open and allow blood flow to go from the legs to the heart. Gravitational pressure or hydrostatic pressure occurs in the vascular system because of the weight of the blood in vessels. At the point of central venous pressure, it is equal to zero when a person is standing. In an adult who is standing still, the pressure in the veins of the feet is around +90 mmHg solely because of the gravitational pressure between the heart and the feet. Since the veins inside the skull are in the skull cavity, they cannot collapse and as a result negative pressure can exist in the dural sinuses of the head. Note that if the sagittal sinus is opened during surgery, the negative pressure would result in air being sucked immediately into the venous system and could cause air embolism in the heart.

A critical component of the venous system is its valves, arranged in such a way that the venous blood flow is solely directed toward the heart. Every time an individual moves or activates muscles, a certain amount of venous blood is pushed toward the heart. This mechanism is what is known as the venous pump. If a person is standing still, the venous pump

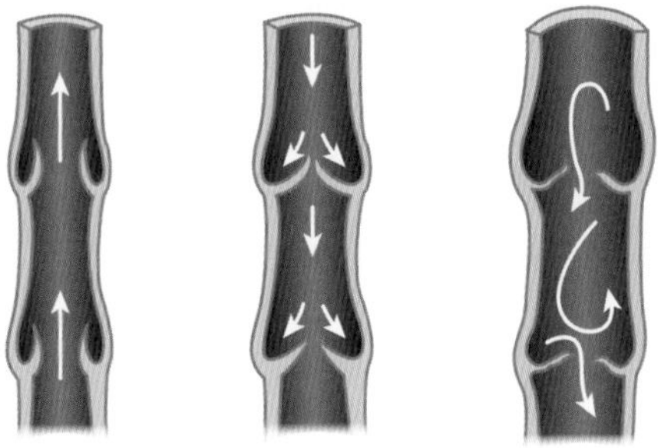
Blood moves
up toward
the heart
Healthy valve
prevents blood
backflow
Damaged valves
allow back flow

FIGURE 1-10 The importance of valves in the venous system.

is inactive and causes increased pressure in the capillaries and fluid leakage into the tissue spaces. When these valves become "incompetent" due to being overstretched by excess venous pressure for weeks or months (e.g. pregnancy), the leaflets no longer close completely (Figure 1-10). This results in the development of varicose veins—large protrusions of the veins beneath the skin of the leg, especially prevalent in the lower leg.

The blood reservoir function of the veins enables them to hold more than 60% of all blood in the circulatory system. When blood is lost from the body and there is a drop in the arterial pressure, nervous signal cascades from the carotid sinuses lead the veins to constrict to replenish the system. Additionally, specific portions of the circulatory system that are extensive and compliant, such as the spleen, can decrease in size to release hundreds of milliliters of blood.

BASIC PRINCIPLES OF CIRCULATORY FUNCTION

Now that we are equipped with an understanding of the individual components of the circulatory system, let's understand how they all connect and function in concert. After the heart pumps blood into the aorta, it flows to arteries, then arterioles, and then capillaries. After oxygen and nutrient exchange in the capillaries, the blood flows back to the heart via venules, then veins, and finally into the venae cava.

Since the heart pumps blood continuously into the aorta, the mean pressure in the aorta averages around 100 mmHg. The pulsatile nature of this pumping results in an alternating arterial pressure between 120 mmHg (systolic) and 80 mmHg (diastolic). As shown in Figure 1-11, note the variation of the blood pressures in the different portions of the circulatory system as we travel through the circulation. In the pulmonary circulation, the pressure is pulsatile in the arteries but at a lower value. The low pressure of the pulmonary system aligns with the needs of the lungs because the sole function is oxygenation.

The rate of blood flow to each bodily tissue is controlled in relation to what each tissue needs. Since it is not possible for blood flow to increase globally when a particular tissue needs increased flow, the micro vessels of each tissue are continuously monitoring and modulating the flow by dilating and constricting. Cardiac output dynamically responds to the demands of the tissues via changes on the heart rate, contractility, preload, and afterload. Arterial blood pressure is tightly regulated via local metabolites, shear stress, mechanical stretch on the arteries, and via nervous signals that respond to blood pressure changes by changing the force of the heart pumping, contractility of the arteries and accessing venous reservoirs, and shifting blood from arterioles to arteries.[29]

Pressure, flow, and resistance are deeply intertwined. Blood flow through a vessel is determined by the pressure gradient traversing the vessel and the resistance to flow through the vessel. This is mathematically represented as Ohm's Law:

$$F = \frac{\Delta P}{R}$$

where F is blood flow, ΔP is the pressure difference between the two ends of the vessel, and R is the resistance between those two points. It is important to note that a difference in pressure determines the rate of flow, not the absolute pressure. Blood flow, or the amount of blood that crosses a certain point in the circulation in a period of time, is normally expressed in milliliters per minute or liters per minute. The overall blood flow is known as the cardiac output as it is the amount of blood pumped into the

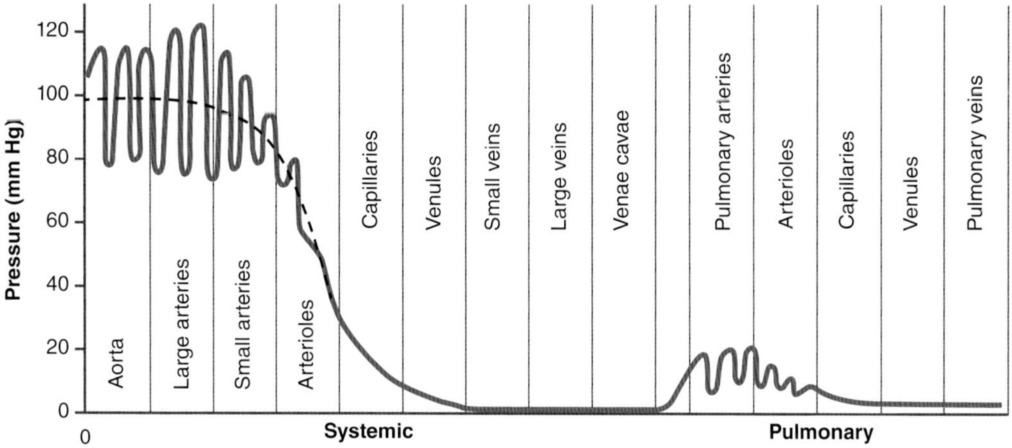

FIGURE 1-11 Representative chart of normal blood pressures in the various portions of the circulatory system when laying horizontal.

aorta by the heart each minute. Blood pressure, or the force exerted by the blood against a unit area of the vessel wall, is normally expressed in millimeters of mercury (mmHg). Resistance, or the impediment of blood flow in a vessel, must be calculated; it cannot be measured. Conductance is the exact reciprocal of resistance and is greatly influenced by small changes in the diameter of a vessel. In fact, the conductance increases in proportion to the fourth power of the diameter (Poiseuille's law). This begins to shed light on how vessels with strong vascular walls, such as arterioles, can respond with small changes in diameter to greatly modulate blood flow. The arrangement of blood vessels throughout the systemic circulation can be arranged in series and parallel. Similar to electrical circuits, in series, the total resistance to blood flow is equal to the sum of the resistances of each vessel and can be represented as follows:

$$R_{tot} = R_1 + R_2 + R_3 + \ldots$$

where R_{tot} is equal to the sum of the resistances of each vessel. In parallel, each tissue is able to regulate its own flow independently of the flow to other tissues and the total resistance to blood flow can be represented as follows:

$$\frac{1}{R_{tot}} = \frac{1}{R_1} + \frac{1}{R_2} + \frac{1}{R_3} + \ldots$$

where again R_{tot} is equal to the sum of the resistances of each vessel. Parallel arrangements enable greater amounts of blood to flow through because adding more parallel vessels reduces the total vascular resistance.

It is important to recognize that the effect of arterial pressure on the blood flow in tissues is dynamically counteracted by local control mechanisms. For this reason, an increase in arterial pressure does not automatically cause an increase in blood flow globally. This phenomenon is known as autoregulation and enables each tissue to adjust its vascular resistance and maintain normal blood flow independent of the changes in arterial pressure. There are two prevailing theories to understand the short-term autoregulation mechanism: *metabolic theory* and *myogenic tone theory*.

The first theory is known as the metabolic theory whereby when the arterial pressure increases above a threshold, the excess flow provides too much oxygen and nutrients and washes out vasodilators released by the tissues. This leads to vasoconstriction and enables the flow to return to normal. While the second theory centers around myogenic tone, an observation that a sudden stretch of small blood vessels causes the vascular smooth muscle cells to spontaneously contract within the vascular wall. This response can occur in the absence of electrical/chemical signals and is most pronounced in the strong, muscular walled arterioles. As a result, when high arterial pressure stretches the vessel, the myogenic tone response causes vasoconstriction in response to reduce the blood flow back to normal.[1-3]

In addition to the stretch forces that oppose the vascular distention that occurs because of blood pressure, the frictional force of the blood on the endothelial layer, known as *shear stress*, also plays a role in vascular mechanobiology. It is well established that shear stress acutely causes vessel dilation. This dilation is dependent on the magnitude and direction of the blood flow and the activity of several enzymes such as NOS, which produces NO, and NADPH oxidase. Under shear stress, endothelial NOS is activated while vascular NADPH oxidase is quickly inactivated, leading to an increase in NO and reduction of superoxide production. As a result, the artery will relax and the resistance to the flow will decrease.[29,30]

REFERENCES

1. Guyton AC, Hall JE. *Textbook of Medical Physiology*. Vol. 369. 12th ed. Elsevier Ltd.; 2013.
2. Zawadski JV, Furchgott RF, Cherry P. The obligatory role of endothelial cells in the relaxation of arterial smooth muscle by substance P. *Fed Proc*. 1981 (abstract);40:689.
3. Webb RC. Smooth muscle contraction and relaxation. *Am J Physiol*. 2003;27(1-4):201-206.
4. Majesky MW, Dong XR, Hoglund V, Mahoney WM, Daum G. The adventitia. *Arterioscler Thromb Vasc Biol*. 2011;31(7):1530-1539.
5. Meijles DN, Pagano PJ. Nox and inflammation in the vascular adventitia. *Hypertension*. 2016;67(1):14-19.
6. Hildebrand S, Stümer J, Pfeifer A. PVAT and its relation to brown, beige, and white adipose tissue in development and function. *Front Physiol*. 2018;9:70.
7. Löhn M, Dubrovska G, Lauterbach B, Luft FC, Gollasch M, Sharma AM. Periadventitial fat releases a vascular relaxing factor. *FASEB J Off Publ Fed Am Soc Exp Biol*. 2002;16(9):1057-1063.
8. Dubrovska G, Verlohren S, Luft FC, Gollasch M. Mechanisms of ADRF release from rat aortic adventitial adipose tissue. *Am J Physiol Heart Circ Physiol*. 2004;286(3):H1107-1113.
9. Gao Y-J, Lu C, Su L-Y, Sharma AM, Lee RMKW. Modulation of vascular function by perivascular adipose tissue: the role of endothelium and hydrogen peroxide. *Br J Pharmacol*. 2007;151(3):323-331.
10. Gao Y-J, Zeng Z, Teoh K, et al. Perivascular adipose tissue modulates vascular function in the human internal thoracic artery. *J Thorac Cardiovasc Surg*. 2005;130(4):1130-1136.
11. Verlohren S, Dubrovska G, Tsang S-Y, et al. Visceral periadventitial adipose tissue regulates arterial tone of mesenteric arteries. *Hypertens (Dallas, Tex 1979)*. 2004;44(3):271-276.
12. Fésüs G, Dubrovska G, Gorzelniak K, et al. Adiponectin is a novel humoral vasodilator. *Cardiovasc Res*. 2007;75(4):719-727.
13. Mohammed MMJ, Myers DS, Sofola OA, Hainsworth R, Drinkhill MJ. Vasodilator effects of leptin on canine isolated mesenteric arteries and veins. *Clin Exp Pharmacol Physiol*. 2007;34(8):771-774.
14. Sahin AS, Bariskaner H. The mechanisms of vasorelaxant effect of leptin on isolated rabbit aorta. *Fundam Clin Pharmacol*. 2007;21(6):595-600.
15. Nakagawa K, Higashi Y, Sasaki S, Oshima T, Matsuura H, Chayama K. Leptin causes vasodilation in humans. *Hypertens Res*. 2002;25(2):161-165.
16. Gao Y-J, Takemori K, Su L-Y, et al. Perivascular adipose tissue promotes vasoconstriction: the role of superoxide anion. *Cardiovasc Res*. 2006;71(2):363-373.
17. Greenstein AS, Khavandi K, Withers SB, et al. Local inflammation and hypoxia abolish the protective anticontractile properties of perivascular fat in obese patients. *Circulation*. 2009;119(12):1661-1670.
18. Fang L, Zhao J, Chen Y, et al. Hydrogen sulfide derived from periadventitial adipose tissue is a vasodilator. *J Hypertens*. 2009;27(11):2174-2185.
19. Schleifenbaum J, Köhn C, Voblova N, et al. Systemic peripheral artery relaxation by KCNQ channel openers and hydrogen sulfide. *J Hypertens*. 2010;28(9):1875-1882.
20. Gil-Ortega M, Stucchi P, Guzmán-Ruiz R, et al. Adaptative nitric oxide overproduction in perivascular adipose tissue during early diet-induced obesity. *Endocrinology*. 2010;151(7):3299-3306.
21. Lee RMKW, Lu C, Su L-Y, Gao Y-J. Endothelium-dependent relaxation factor released by perivascular adipose tissue. *J Hypertens*. 2009;27(4):782-790.
22. Withers SB, Agabiti-Rosei C, Livingstone DM, et al. Macrophage activation is responsible for loss of anticontractile function in inflamed perivascular fat. *Arterioscler Thromb Vasc Biol*. 2011;31(4):908-913.
23. Ma L, Ma S, He H, et al. Perivascular fat-mediated vascular dysfunction and remodeling through the AMPK/mTOR pathway in high-fat diet-induced obese rats. *Hypertens Res*. 2010;33(5):446-453.
24. Rebolledo A, Rebolledo OR, Marra CA, et al. Early alterations in vascular contractility associated to

changes in fatty acid composition and oxidative stress markers in perivascular adipose tissue. *Cardiovasc Diabetol.* 2010;9:65.
25. Watts SW, Gollasch M. Editorial: perivascular adipose tissue (pvat) in health and disease. *Fron Physiol.* 2018;9:1004.
26. Szasz T, Bomfim GF, Webb RC. The influence of perivascular adipose tissue on vascular homeostasis. *Vasc Health Risk Manag.* 2013;9:105-116.
27. Roy S, Edwards JM, Tomcho JC, et al. Intrinsic exercise capacity and mitochondrial DNA lead to opposing vascular-associated risks. *Funct (Oxford, England).* 2021;2(1): zqaa029.
28. Armulik A, Abramsson A, Betsholtz C. Endothelial/pericyte interactions. *Circ Res.* 2005;97(6):512-523.
29. Lu D, Kassab GS. Role of shear stress and stretch in vascular mechanobiology. *J R Soc Interface.* 2011;8(63):1379-1385.
30. Martinez-Quinones P, McCarthy CG, Watts SW, et al. Hypertension induced morphological and physiological changes in cells of the arterial wall. *Am J Hypertens.* 2018;31(10):1067-1078.

SELF-ASSESSMENT STUDY QUESTIONS AND ANSWERS

Questions

1. Which blood vessel facilitates the exchange of fluid, nutrients, electrolytes, hormones, and other substances between blood and the interstitial fluid?
   A. Aorta
   B. Arterioles
   C. Capillaries
   D. Small Arteries
   E. Venules

2. Which substance has been established to be an endothelium-derived relaxing factor (EDRF)?
   A. Angiotensin-2
   B. Diacylgycerol
   C. Endothelin-1
   D. Nitric Oxide
   E. Superoxide

3. Which amino acid is used to synthesize nitric oxide?
   A. Arginine
   B. Glycine
   C. Histidine
   D. Phenylalanine
   E. Tryptophan

4. In physiological conditions, what kind of effect does PVAT have on vessel tone?
   A. Anticontractile
   B. Contractile
   C. No effect

5. At the point of central venous pressure, what is the hydrostatic pressure in the vascular system equal to when a person is standing still?
   A. −45 mmHg
   B. 0 mmHg
   C. +45 mmHg
   D. +90 mmHg

6. Conductance is the exact reciprocal of which of the following parameters?
   A. Diameter
   B. Flow
   C. Length
   D. Pressure
   E. Resistance

7. Shear stress, or the frictional force of blood on the endothelium, acutely causes which of the following?
   A. Vessel aneurysm
   B. Vessel constriction
   C. Vessel dilation
   D. Vessel dissection
   E. Vessel perforation

8. Continuous capillaries are generally found in which of the following?
   A. Bone marrow
   B. Nervous system
   C. Liver
   D. Small intestine
   E. Spleen

9. Which of the following vessels will have the thickest tunica media?
   A. Aorta
   B. Arterioles
   C. Capillaries
   D. Small arteries
   E. Venules

10. Which of the following molecules will induce vascular contraction?
    A. Prostacyclin
    B. Endothelin-1
    C. Hydrogen peroxide
    D. Endothelium-dependent hyperpolarization (EDH)

SELF-ASSESSMENT STUDY QUESTIONS AND ANSWERS

Answers

1. C.
2. D.
3. A.
4. A.
5. B.
6. E.
7. C.
8. B.
9. A.
10. B.

CHAPTER

2 Vascular Hemodynamics

Abdul Kader Natour and Loay Kabbani

OUTLINE

OVERVIEW AND HISTORICAL BACKGROUND
PHYSICS
Velocity of Blood Flow
Ohm's Law
Poiseuille's Law
Types of Resistance
Series
Parallel
Types of Flow
Laminar Flow
Shear
Turbulent Flow
Transitional Flow
Plug Flow
Reynolds Number
Wall Tension
Compliance
VASCULAR CIRCULATION
Type and Characteristics of Blood Vessels
Arteries
Veins
Respiratory Pump
Muscular Pump
Microcirculation
Flow Regulation
Pressures in the Cardiovascular System
Pulse Pressure
Mean Arterial Pressure
Cardiac Output
CLINICAL TWIST: ABI AND SEGMENTAL PRESSURES
Introduction and Pad
Definition and Measurement of ABI
Physiology of ABI
Clinical Correlate of ABI
Segmental Pressures
Treadmill Exercise Testing
Clinical Case
Case 1

OVERVIEW AND HISTORICAL BACKGROUND

Vascular Hemodynamics is the study of the flow of blood and physiology of the cardiovascular system.[1]

The understanding of hemodynamics started in the late 1950s, with William Harvey's quantitative reasoning leading to the idea that blood continuously circulates in our body.[1] This was followed in the late 1960s and mid-1970s by experimental studies run by philosophers and scientists on animal models that led to a clearer understanding of the circulatory pathways and to the direct measurement of arterial pressure.[2] Principles of physics were then integrated in the study of hemodynamics and, with the contribution of Thomas Young and J.L.M Poiseuille, led to an understanding of the elastic properties of the vessels, the pulse speed, and establishing the relationship between flow rate and diameter for a long cylindrical tube subject to a fixed pressure gradient along its length.[3,4]

Pierre Laplace then described the forces regulating the circulation of blood explaining aneurysm development.[5] The standard reference used nowadays in the field of hemodynamics is inspired by the work of Donald A. McDonald in the mid-1990s, where he analyzed the motion of blood in arteries in a time-dependent manner with a fluctuating pressure gradient.[6,7]

PHYSICS

VELOCITY OF BLOOD FLOW

The velocity of blood flow is the rate of displacement of blood at a given time interval.[8] Its basic equation is as follows:

$$v = \frac{Q}{A}$$

where

v = velocity of blood flow (cm/sec)

Q = Flow (mL/sec)

A = Cross-sectional area (cm^2)

Flow (Q) is the volume of blood displaced per unit time. In our circulatory system, blood flow is the same and equal to the cardiac output. This is for the simple reason that in a normal state, the volume of blood that is pumped out of the heart is approximately the same as the one returning to the heart.[8] The area is calculated as $A = \pi r^2$, where π is a constant and r is the radius of a single blood vessel or group of vessels. The cross-sectional area is determined by the area of interest through which the blood flows, that is, if we are interested in the blood flow through the aorta, we would use the cross-sectional area of the aorta. However, if we are interested in the blood flow at the level of a capillary bed, we would need to use the total cross-sectional area of all the capillaries within this bed.[8]

A simple illustration of the inverse relationship between velocity and cross-sectional area is illustrated in Figure 2-1. Assuming the flow is the same throughout the cylinder, as the area of the cylinder decreases, the velocity of blood flow increases, and vice-versa. The aorta has the smallest cross-sectional area (2.5 cm^2) with a flow velocity of 300 mm/sec, as the arteries branch the cumulative area increases, ending in the capillaries (2500 cm^2) with a flow velocity of (0.5 mm/sec). This is advantageous as blood is distributed rapidly through the larger arteries, then slows down at the level needed for nutritional exchange.[9]

It's worth mentioning that although the velocity increases with decreased radius, there is a critical point at which a lot of pressure is lost from the high turbulent flow and reduction in lumen diameter, resulting in an overall loss of blood velocity. This phenomenon usually happens with a greater than 95% decrease in diameter of the blood vessel.[18]

OHM'S LAW

In electricity, the relationship between current (I), voltage (V), and resistance (R) was first elucidated by Georg Ohm's in 1781, where he hypothesized a direct relationship between current and voltage, and an indirect one with the resistance: $I = \Delta V/R^4$. Translating this observation into hemodynamics, blood flow would be equivalent to the current flow (Q), the pressure difference between two ends of a

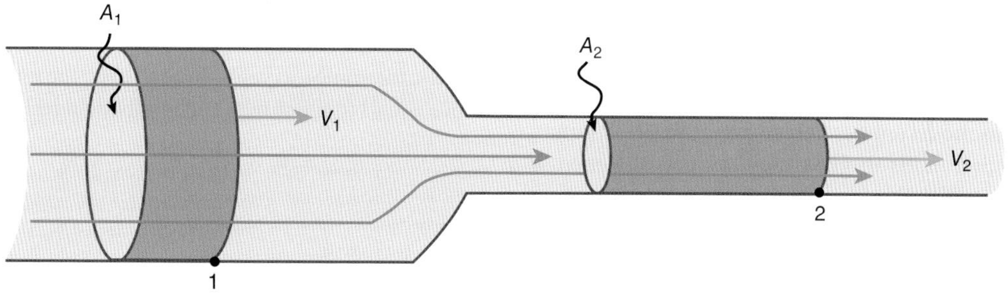

FIGURE 2-1 The relationship between velocity and cross-sectional area. (Reproduced with permission from Urone PP, Hinrichs R. *College Physics*. Iowa Pressbooks. Open Stax; 2016.)

vessel would be equivalent to the voltage difference in a circuit (ΔP), and the hydrodynamic resistance is equivalent to the electrical resistance (R). The equation for blood flow is expressed as follows:

$$Q = \frac{\Delta P}{R}$$

where

Q = flow of blood (mL/min)

ΔP = pressure difference (mmHg)

R = Resistance (mmHg/mL/min)

Note that the above equation can be rearranged to determine the resistance or change in pressure as well.

An important concept to understand is that the direction of the pressure gradient governs the direction of blood flow, and it is always from high to low pressure.[8] Normally, the larger the pressure gradient, the faster the blood flows between two points.[16]

POISEUILLE'S LAW

The resistance to fluid flowing in a long cylinder tube with rigid walls was further elaborated by Jean Léonard Marie Poiseuille and Gotthilf Heinrich Ludwig Hagen in 1940s, with their work leading to Hagen-Poiseuille law[4]:

$$R = \frac{8\mu l}{\pi r^4}$$

where

R = resistance

μ = fluid viscosity (e.g., thickness)

l = length of the tube

r = radius of the tube

This model applies only to nonpulsatile, laminar, Newtonian fluids in glass capillary tubes. Hence, it was extrapolated by scientists to the vascular system just as a model to explain blood flow.

As illustrated from the above equation, the radius plays a massive role in determining resistance to blood flow. Resistance to flow is inversely proportional to the fourth power of the radius. This means that if the radius of a vessel is doubled (e.g., from 2 cm to 4 cm), the resistance decreases by 16-fold and the blood flow increases by 16-fold. Adding to this important rule is the fact that vessel length and viscosity are relatively constant in a given healthy patient. Thus, changes in resistance, and subsequently the blood flow, occur mainly as a result of changes in the radius.[17]

Viscosity plays an important role in the delivery of blood to the organs. It can be understood as the thickness of blood, with an increase in viscosity leading to adherence of red blood cells (RBCs) to each other and to the vessel wall.[16] Viscosity can be inferred from the Hematocrit percentage. An increase in hematocrit due to an increase in the number of RBCs (e.g., polycythemia vera) or to a relative increase (e.g., states of dehydration) increases blood viscosity; on the other hand, anemia or fluid overload decreases the hematocrit and subsequently the viscosity. Moreover, viscosity varies with temperature: the lower the temperature, the higher the viscosity.[9]

TYPES OF RESISTANCE

Resistance type is based on the organization of the resistors in the circulation in relation to each other. Based on that, resistance is divided into two types: series and parallel.

Series

Figure 2-2a illustrates a circuit with a battery and three resistors connected end to end in a long chain from one terminal of the battery to the other. The resistance across such circuit would be three times the resistance if the circuit is made up of only one resistor.

This can be extrapolated to blood vessels within a given organ, flowing from a major artery supplying that organ, passing through smaller arteries, arterioles, capillaries, to venules, to veins. In such case, the total resistance equals to the sum of each individual resistance:

$$R_{\text{total}} = R_1 + R_2 + R_3 + \ldots + R_n$$

where

R_{total} = Total resistance

R_1 = Resistance in a main artery

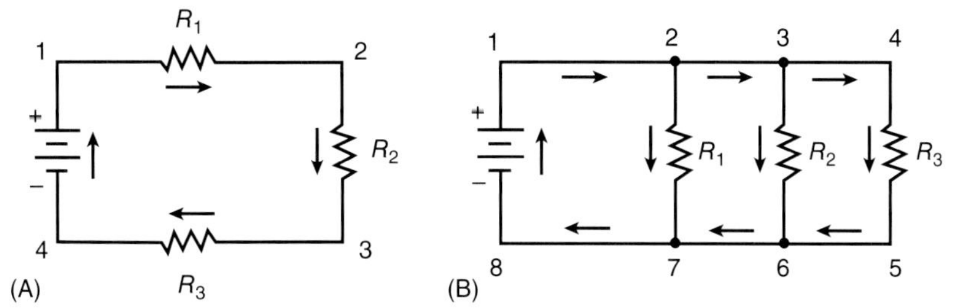

FIGURE 2-2 Resistance. (**A**) Resistance in series. (**B**) Resistance in parallel.

R_2 = Resistance in the first branch of the main artery

R_3 = Resistance in the second branch of the main artery

R_n = Resistance in the final branch of the main artery

To note that the arteriolar resistance is by far the greatest; hence, it largely approximates the total resistance in a given vascular bed.[9]

Parallel

Let's consider now a parallel configuration for the above three resistors as illustrated in Figure 2-2b. As we can notice, all components are connected across each other's leads, forming more than one continuous path for current to flow: There's one path from 1 to 2 to 7 to 8 and back to 1 again, another from 1 to 3 to 6 to 8 and back to 1 again, and a third from 1 to 4 to 5 to 8 to 1 again.

This can be extrapolated to flow of blood among the various major arteries branching off the aorta: Cerebral, Coronary, Renal, Skin, Skeletal muscle, etc. In such a case, the total resistance would be equal to the sum of the reciprocals of each resistance. This means that the total resistance in a parallel circuit is less than any of the individual resistances:

$$\frac{1}{R_{\text{total}}} = \frac{1}{R_1} + \frac{1}{R_2} + \frac{1}{R_3} \ldots + \frac{1}{R_n}$$

The clinical implication of this arrangement is that the mean pressure in each major artery will be approximately equal to the one in the aorta since there's no or very minimal loss of pressure.

TYPES OF FLOW

Laminar Flow

In ideal circumstances, the blood flows in our body in a streamlined, or in a laminar motion.[8] The RBCs are assumed to be moving in parallel layers, at different speeds at different locations within the vessel, forming a bell-shaped curve as illustrated in Figure 2-3a. The differential in speed observed can be explained by the friction that RBC molecules experience the closer they get to the walls of the blood vessel and essentially do not move at all at the surface. The further away they get from the wall, the faster they get. Thus, in a laminar flow, the velocity of blood flow is

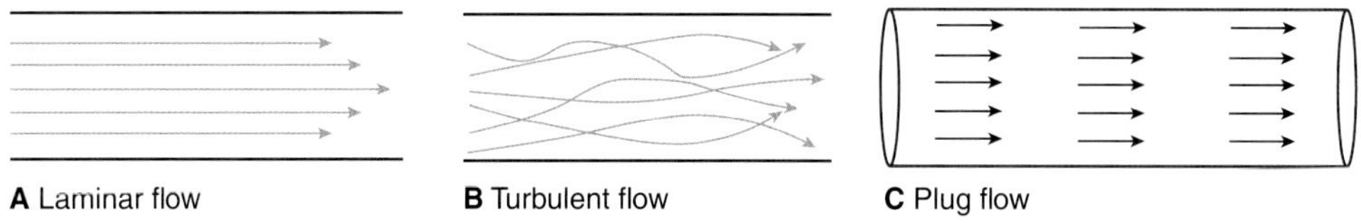

FIGURE 2-3 Flow patterns.

lowest near the vessel walls and highest at the center of the vessel.[15]

Shear

The differential in speed illustrated above allows us to define an important concept in hemodynamics: Shear. In simple terms, shear is the tangential force exerted on the endothelium by the moving blood and is proportional to the difference in velocity of adjacent layers of blood.[8] Thus, shear is highest near the blood vessel walls since the speed of molecules near the walls is almost zero and the layer just after it is moving. Shear is lowest at the center of blood vessel, where adjacent blood layers are moving almost at the same speed. This is physiologically important, since shear breaks down aggregate of RBCs, thus preventing stasis of molecules near the arterial walls and subsequently arterial disease from happening.

Turbulent Flow

In normal arteries, disruption in the smooth, linear structure of blood vessels, such as when they curve or branch, would cause disruption of the laminar flow,[30] as illustrated in Figure 2-3b. This causes axial and radial movement of the molecules, disrupting the parabolic profile of the laminar flow by forming eddies, resulting in loss of energy for the propagation of blood due to the increased resistance.[9] In fluid dynamics, eddy is the swirling of fluid and the reverse current that is created when the fluid is in a turbulent flow, producing low flow near the arterial wall[30,31] (Figure 2-4). This increases stasis of molecules near the arterial walls, thus increasing the risk of plaque formation and atherosclerotic disease.[14] Moreover, turbulent flow generates sound waves that can be heard with a stethoscope, and often mistaken for pathological murmurs (e.g., valve damage, stenotic vessels).[48]

Transitional Flow

This type of flow is a combination of both laminar and turbulent flow and occurs mainly at transitional points: areas of branching, partial obstruction, or near valves[8] (Figure 2-4).

Plug Flow

Plug flow is a type of laminar flow where multiple layers of blood travel at the same speed near the middle of the vessel (Figure 2-3c). This type of flow is usually seen in major arteries, such as the aorta and common carotids, as well as at the entrance of diseased, stenotic blood vessels.[16]

Reynolds Number

In 1980, Sir Osborne Reynolds run a series of experiments by injecting a stream of dye into a fluid moving within a tube and observed the location of the stream of dye.[10] The stream stayed at the middle of the tube and became turbulent when a critical rate of flow was reached. Reynolds number is a dimensionless number and is said to be the critical rate of flow to produce turbulence. Its equation is as follows:

$$R_e = \frac{\rho v d}{n}$$

where

R_e = Reynolds number

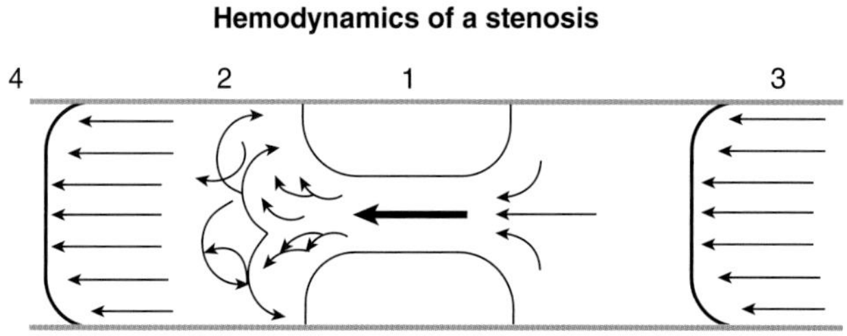

FIGURE 2-4 Hemodynamically significant stenosis. Zone 1: area of maximal stenosis; Zone 2: poststenotic turbulence with Eddie currents at the exit of the stenosis; Zone 3: pe-stenosis resistance; and Zone 4: return to laminar flow decreased velocity.

ρ = density of blood (slugs/ft^2)

v = velocity of blood flow (ft/sec)

d = diameter of the blood vessel (ft)

n = viscosity of blood (lb-s/ft^2)

R_e below 2000 indicates laminar flow. R_e above 4000 indicates turbulent flow, and R_e between 2000 and 4000 indicates an increasing likelihood of turbulent flow.[10]

As illustrated in the above equation, Reynolds number increases with increased velocity, density, and diameter of the vessel, and decreases with increased viscosity. An important note to consider is the variation of Reynolds number with change in radius of the vessel (e.g., vasoconstriction). Looking at the above equation, one would naturally deduce that the viscosity would decrease as the radius decreases due to the direct relationship between the two parameters. However, experimental observations inferred a paradoxical increase in viscosity. This can be explained by the inverse relationship of blood velocity and the radius to the second power (e.g., $V = Q/A = Q/\pi r^2$). Thus, a decrease in radius would lead to a significant increase in velocity, subsequently giving more weight to the change in Reynolds number compared to the direct effect of decreasing the radius as seen in the equation above. Thus, the dependence of Reynolds number on velocity is more powerful than the dependence on diameter.

WALL TENSION

Understanding the mechanics behind wall tension in a sphere was of interest for the French scientist Pierre Simon de Laplace. His work in the late 1970s led to the discovery of Laplace's law, which describes the pressure–volume relationships of spheres.[11] Laplace's formula is as follows:

$$T = \frac{PR}{2W}$$

where

T = Wall tension of the sphere

P = Transmural pressure of the sphere

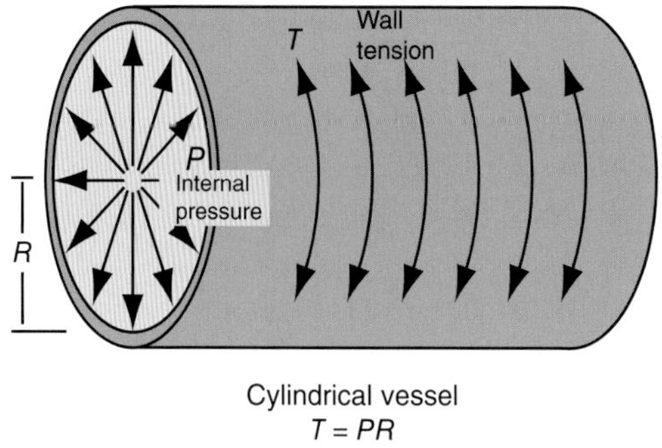

FIGURE 2-5 Wall tension. (Reproduced with permission from HyperPhysics by Rod Nave, Georgia State University.)

R = Radius of the sphere

W = Thickness of the sphere's wall

Extrapolating this equation to a cylindrical vessel with relatively negligible wall thickness, the equation can be simplified as follows:

$$T = PR$$

The equation is illustrated in Figure 2-5. It demonstrates the direct relationship between blood pressure and radius with wall tension: as blood pressure and radius increase, so does wall tension. Laplace's law helps us explain why aneurysms tend to rupture as they increase in diameter.[9]

COMPLIANCE

Compliance or capacitance of a blood vessel is defined as the ability of a vessel to distend and increase its volume with increasing transmural pressure.[12] Wall tension is a product of the elasticity of the blood vessel and it opposes the distending pressure. Thus, wall tension is intrinsically related to the compliance, with the more compliant the vessel is, the less the wall tension. The formula for compliance is as follows:

$$C = \frac{\Delta V}{\Delta P}$$

where

C = Compliance (mL/mmHg)

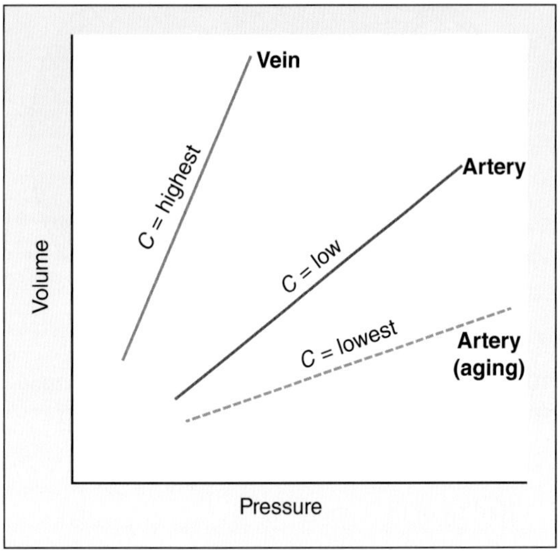

FIGURE 2-6 Compliance. (Reproduced with permission from Costanzo LS. *Physiology*, 7th ed. Philadelphia, PA: Wolters Kluwer; 2018.)

$\Delta V =$ Change in volume (mL)

$\Delta P =$ Change in pressure (mmHg)

As the above equation illustrates, the higher the compliance of a blood vessel, the more volume it can hold at a given pressure.

The above formula can be modified as $\Delta V = C \times \Delta P$, which is a linear equation of the form $y = ax + b$. Compliance of a blood vessel can thus be determined easily by plotting ΔV as a function of ΔP, with the slope of the straight line being the Compliance. Figure 2-6 represents two such lines for a vein and an artery.

The graph illustrates a steeper line for the vein relative to the artery, hence the slope is higher, and the compliance is much greater than that of the artery. This translates physiologically into veins having the ability to store a greater volume of blood at lower pressures.[13] This variation in compliance underlies the concept of stressed and unstressed volume. The arteries are much less compliant and contain the stressed volume, whereas veins are much more compliant and contains the unstressed volume. In fact, more than 2/3 of our blood is stored in our veins at any moment. The redistribution of blood between stressed and unstressed volume has important consequences on the overall body arterial pressure.[8]

VASCULAR CIRCULATION

TYPE AND CHARACTERISTICS OF BLOOD VESSELS

Arteries

Arteries are responsible to deliver the oxygenated blood to all the organs in our body. They are composed of three layers: tunica intima, media, and adventitia. Each of these layers provides important anatomical properties that determine the function of arteries. Most important of which is the tunica media as it constitutes the bulk of the arterial wall.[9] The tunica media is composed of mainly smooth muscles, elastic tissue, and collagen. The elastic fibers are most prevalent in the major arteries, especially those emanating from the heart, as it allows them to withstand the high cardiac pressures. In smaller arteries, smooth muscles predominate that help in the contraction and relaxation, as well as forming the site of highest resistance to blood flow.[8]

Arteries can also be divided into communicating and end arteries. Communicating arteries are the ones that branch and communicate with other arteries, forming the so-called arterio-arterial anastomosis. This is important to prevent ischemia of organs: if one of the arteries is blocked, the blood can flow through the other ones. End arteries, as their name implies, do not have this property.[19] Most commonly, end arteries supply blood to a portion of a tissue or organ, blockage of which would lead to ischemia of the supplied territory.[20]

Arteries regulate the amount of blood reaching a specific organ/tissue depending on its need. For example, at rest, the arteries supplying the muscles of the lower extremities contract. Thus, the amount of blood reaching the muscles of the lower extremities is low since the metabolic demand is low. Upon exercise, the demand increases and in response the arterioles dilate, subsequently increasing the blood flow.[21]

Veins

The venous system is responsible to deliver back the blood from the organs to the heart, completing the cardiovascular circulation. Veins are also composed of three layers: tunica intima, media, and adventitia. However, the amount of elastic fibers and smooth muscles is much lower as compared to the arteries, making their walls very thin and easily collapsible.[9] This explains the low-pressure profile of veins, earning them the name of "capacitance vessels," and making them an important storage area for blood.[22]

To secure return of blood to the heart, most veins, especially those in the lower extremities, are equipped with valves that prevent retrograde flow.[22] Moreover, muscle contraction and respiration help the blood to flow against gravity by compressing the lower extremity as well as the major veins in our abdomen.[23]

Respiratory Pump As the thoracic cavity expands during inspiration, the contraction of the diaphragm compresses the abdominal cavity, squeezing the abdominal vessels, thus propelling blood upward. During expiration, the relaxation of the diaphragm decreases the pressure in the intra-abdominal cavity, thus relieves the pressure on the vessels, and consequently drawing blood into abdominal organs.[23]

Muscular Pump Since most blood vessels and their branches course through muscles, muscle contraction and relaxation can push and pull blood in blood vessels. When muscles are relaxed, blood tends to pool in the veins. However, when muscles contract, the veins are compressed and the blood is propelled upward toward the heart, with the valves ensuring no retrograde flow from happening.[23] Dysfunction of the calf pump contributes to venous hypertension and lower extremity ulcers.

Microcirculation

The microcirculation is composed of arterioles, precapillary sphincters, capillaries, venules, and arteriovenous anastomoses.[24] Capillaries form a hub where nutrients, gases, solutes, and water are exchanged between tissues and blood, and in the lungs, between the alveoli and the blood.[9] Each capillary has a venous end and an arterial end, and the flow of blood going through it is regulated by the pre-capillary sphincter. Depending on the tissue need, the precapillary sphincter 0.+6, contracts or dilates, regulating the amount of exchange depending on tissue metabolic activity.[25] The arteriovenous anastomosis shunts blood directly from the arterioles to the venules, bypassing the capillary bed. This is important in many instances, such as episodes of decreased vascular volume, where blood is shunted to vital organs.[26]

Flow Regulation

Vessels contraction and relaxation is regulated by the autonomic nervous system, which is composed of sympathetic and parasympathetic fibers.[27] The smooth muscles of the arteries and veins are generally innervated by sympathetic fibers through two receptors: α1-adrenergic receptors that are responsible for the contraction of the vascular smooth muscle, and less commonly, β2 receptors that causes relaxation of the vascular smooth muscle.[27] At baseline, the vascular smooth muscles are continuously weakly contracted due to a basal discharge by the vasomotor center in the brainstem.[9] To note, the relaxation of the vascular smooth muscle is mainly regulated by the absence of α1-adrenergic receptor stimulation, rather than activation of the β2 receptors. In response to the autonomic nervous system stimulation, the endothelium of the vessels produces many substances that regulate contraction and relaxation.[9] For example, prostacyclin, prostaglandin, and endothelium-derived relaxing factor nitric oxide causes relaxation of vascular smooth muscle, whereas endothelin promotes constriction of blood vessels.[9,27]

Autoregulation of blood flow is the tendency for blood flow to remain constant despite changes in arterial perfusion pressure.[28] There are two popular philosophies that explain the autoregulation phenomenon: the myogenic and metabolic theories. The myogenic theory states that as vascular smooth muscle is extended, the vascular tone increases. Thus, increase in blood pressure causes vascular constriction. The metabolic theory suggests that as blood flow decreases in a certain tissue, metabolic by-products such as lactic acid and carbon monoxide start to build up, leading to vasodilation and subsequent increase in blood flow.[28,29]

PRESSURES IN THE CARDIOVASCULAR SYSTEM

Pressure is the amount of force applied to the surface of an object per unit area at right angles,[32] as

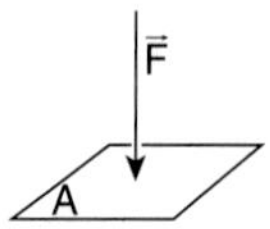

FIGURE 2-7 Pressure.

illustrated in Figure 2-7. Mathematically, it has the following formula:

$$P = \frac{F}{A}$$

where

P = Pressure (N/m^2 or Pa)

F = Force magnitude (N)

A = Area of the surface of contact (m^2)

In hemodynamics, pressure is created by the force of the flowing blood that is exerted on the walls of the blood vessels.[33] Two pressures are formed by the beating heart: systolic and diastolic pressures. Systolic pressure is the highest arterial pressure formed after blood has been expelled from the left ventricle during systole. Diastolic pressure is the lowest arterial pressure formed when no blood is being ejected during ventricular relaxation.[8]

Pulse Pressure Pulse pressure is the difference between systolic and diastolic pressure. Pulse pressure reflects the stroke volume under normal circumstances and has the following formula:

$$PP = SBP - DBP$$

where

PP = Pulse pressure (mmHg)

SBP = Systolic blood pressure (mmHg)

DBP = Diastolic blood pressure (mmHg)

Mean Arterial Pressure Mean arterial Pressure is the average pressure in a cardiac cycle and has the following formula:

$$MAP = \frac{1}{3}PP + DBP$$

Diastole lasts longer than systole, hence earning a greater contribution to the mean arterial pressure, which is reflected in the above formula.

Cardiac Output Cardiac output (CO) is the amount of blood the heart pumps in a minute through the circulatory system.[34] Total peripheral resistance (TPR) is the total resistance of the circulatory system. Blood flow into the arteries is determined by the cardiac output CO and the TPR, with their formula as follows:

$$CO \times TPR = MAP - P(VC)$$

where

$P(VC)$ = Pressure in the vena cava (mmHg)

Note that, because the pressure in the vena cava is relatively negligible, the equation becomes as follows:

$$CO \times TPR = MAP \text{ or } CO = \frac{MAP}{TPR}$$

An overview of the pressures during one cardiac cycle is illustrated in Figure 2-8. The large volume of blood ejected from the left ventricle, along with the low compliance of the aorta, explains why the mean arterial pressure is highest in the aorta. High pressures are preserved in large arteries due to their innate high elastic recoil, preventing them from losing a lot of energy. Once fluid flow pasts the large arteries, resistance in the vasculature starts to increase, subsequently decreasing the mean arterial pressure. The highest drop in MAP happens at the level of arterioles as they constitute the major resistances in the vasculature. At the level of the capillaries, their small diameter, property of filtering the blood along with their precapillary sphincter, decreases further the pressure. The pressure declines further when blood reaches the venules and veins, due to their high capacitance and their ability to hold onto blood at very low pressures. By the time blood reaches the vena cava and right atrium, the pressure can reach as low as 0 to 4 mmHg.

The oscillations in Figure 2-8 represent the pulsatile activity of the heart, with each pulsation cycle overlapping one cardiac cycle. Note that, except for

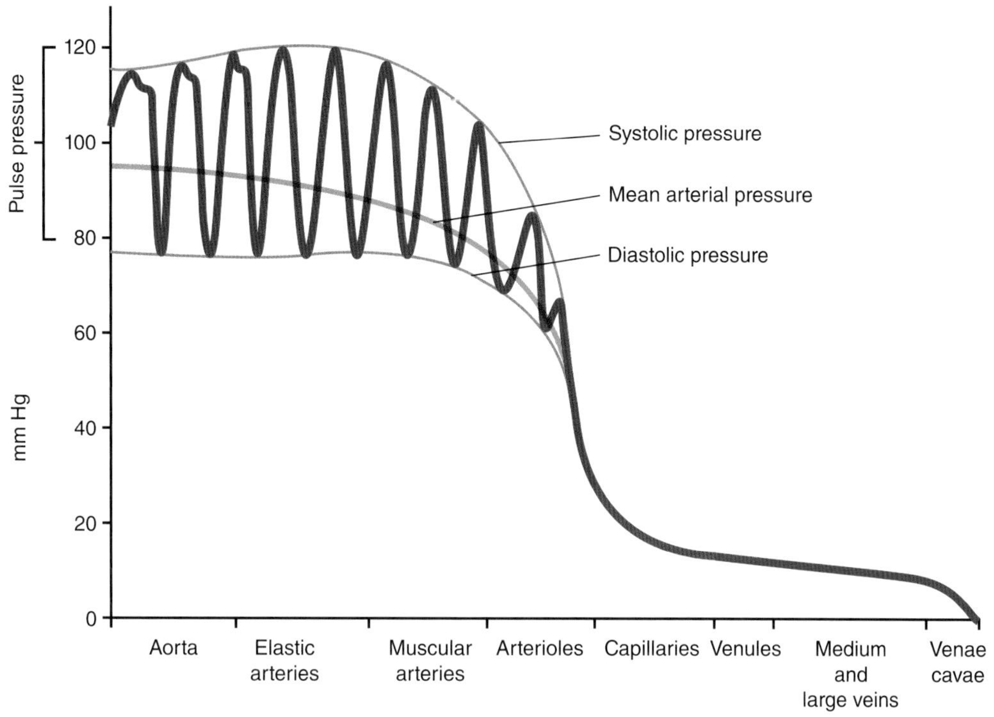

FIGURE 2-8 **Pulsatility activity of the heart, pulse pressure in different arterial segments.**

large arteries, the pulse pressure decreases hand in hand with the mean arterial pressure. The explanation for the increased in pulse pressure in large arteries is the fact that the pressure wave travels at a higher velocity than the blood itself due to the inertia of the blood, and the branch points causes backward reflection of the blood flow, thereby augmenting the downstream pulse pressure.[9] Pulse pressure decreases thereafter due to the increased resistance of the smaller arteries, especially the arterioles, and the high compliance of the veins.

CLINICAL TWIST: ABI AND SEGMENTAL PRESSURES

INTRODUCTION AND PAD

Peripheral artery disease (PAD) is characterized by a decrease in blood flow to the limbs due to obstruction or narrowing of the blood vessels that supply them.[35] Lower extremity PAD is common and affects approximately 10% of the population in the United States, with incidence increasing with age, smoking, diabetes, and inactivity.[36] The most common cause of PAD is atherosclerosis of the arteries.[37] The presence of PAD is associated with higher cardiovascular morbidity, and is considered an independent predictor for cardiovascular mortality, regardless of the form of presentation (asymptomatic or symptomatic) or gender.[38] The presence of PAD is indicative of widespread atherosclerosis, especially among coronary, carotids, and cerebral arteries.[39] The ankle brachial index (ABI) is a simple, noninvasive, cost-effective, and sensitive screening test for patients at risk for PAD, and diagnostic tool for those that present with symptoms of PAD.[38]

DEFINITION AND MEASUREMENT OF ABI

The ABI is a method of measuring the difference between the blood pressure in the arm and that in the ankle. Calculating the ABI involves measuring the systolic blood pressure in the posterior tibial and

TABLE 2-1 Ankle Brachial Index (ABI Test)

ABI Value	Interpretation
Greater than 1.4	Calcification/vessel hardening
1-1.4	Normal
0.9-1	Acceptable
0.8-0.9	Some arterial disease
0.4-0.8	Moderate arterial disease
Less than 0.4	Severe arterial disease

dorsalis pedis artery of each ankle, and the brachial artery of each arm.[40] ABI is defined as the ratio of the higher systolic blood pressure of the two ankles over the higher systolic blood pressure of the two arms.[38] The ABI is calculated separately for each leg, and the higher of the two values is considered the ABI of the patient.[40] The corresponding formula of ABI is as follows:

$$\text{ABI} = \frac{\text{Highest SBP of the two ankles}}{\text{Highest SBP of the two arms}}$$

As illustrated in Table 2-1, PAD is diagnosed when ABI is ≤ 0.9. When ABI is between 0.5 and 0.8, PAD is referred to as mild-to-moderate, whereas an ABI of less than 0.5 is suggestive of severe PAD. ABI value of more than 1.4 is suggestive of a calcified, noncompressible vessel with a falsely increased ABI value, and is commonly seen among diabetics.[40]

PHYSIOLOGY OF ABI

In healthy individuals, systolic blood pressure in the ankle is higher than that measured in the arm.[41] This observation can be explained by two factors: the first is related to the retrograde wave reflections that arise from the bifurcations of the arteries and arterioles and have an additive effect. The second is the increased hydrostatic pressure in the lower limbs as compared to the upper limbs due to gravity, which induces a physiologic thickening of the arterial wall without changing the diameter, subsequently decreasing its compliance and thus relatively increasing the intraluminal pressure.[42]

CLINICAL CORRELATE OF ABI

Claudication is the phenomenon of lower extremity pain that is felt upon exercise.[40] Patients with mild-to-moderate ABI are likely to experience claudication, whereas those who have ABI below 0.5 are likely to experience lower extremity pain at rest.[43] An ABI below 0.5 increases the risk for ulceration, delayed wound healing, gangrene, and eventual limb loss.[44,45] On the other hand, each increase of 0.4 in ABI correlates with a 6-minutes prolongation of walking distance and maximal walking speed.[46]

SEGMENTAL PRESSURES

A closely related technique to ABI for assessing PAD is segmental blood pressure measurements, where systolic blood pressure is measured in multiple segments of the lower extremity.[47] Using this method, a blood pressure cuff is placed around the upper thigh, lower thigh, calf, and ankle.[48] Segmental Doppler pressures are subsequently obtained bilaterally (one leg at a time) at each of the four leg cuff sites using a handheld sphygmomanometer with manual inflation, photoplethysmography, or a computerized system with automatic inflation and digital display.[49] It's important to start at the ankle level and then move proximally to eliminate the possibility of underestimating the systolic blood pressure measurement. Complete cessation of blood flow should be attained by inflating the cuff 20 to 30 mmHg beyond the last audible Doppler signal.[49] The pressures obtained are compared to the higher of the two upper extremities brachial pressures, which is typically 30 mmHg lower than the high thigh pressures.[50]

In healthy people, the pressure difference in the lower extremities between two adjacent levels should be 20 mmHg or less, with some sources raising this cutoff level to 30 mmHg.[49,50] Typically, a pressure difference of more than 20 to 30 mmHg is representative of an obstruction/occlusion at or above the level in the leg with the lower pressure. A horizontal difference of 20 to 30 mmHg also indicates arterial occlusion.[49,51,52]

In addition, thigh pressure indices (thigh pressure/higher of the brachial pressure) are normally >1.2, with <1.0 indicating a likely proximal occlusion.[49]

Treadmill Exercise Testing

Treadmill exercise testing and postexercise measurement of ankle/brachial indices may be used in addition to resting measurements of lower-extremity arterial pressures and pulse volume recordings. The length of time it takes to recover, combined with the duration of exercise, symptoms, and pressure changes, forms the basis of the interpretation. Ankle pressures that drop to low levels immediately after exercise and then increase to resting levels in 2 to 6 minutes suggest obstruction at a single level, while pressures unrecordable for more than 6 minutes indicate multilevel obstructions are likely.[49]

CLINICAL CASE

Case 1

A 79-year-old lady presented to the vascular surgery clinics for bilateral lower extremity pain upon ambulation. Patient states that she gets pain in her calves after standing for a couple of minutes and after walking half a block. She denies pain at rest. She denies any history of chest pain or neurologic problem. She has a past medical history of rheumatoid arthritis, chronic obstructive pulmonary disease (COPD), osteopenia, chronic low back pain, type 2 diabetes, PAD, and atrial flutter. She has a past surgical history of laparoscopic cholecystectomy, adenoidectomy, and cataract extraction with lens implant in her right eye. Her current medications are atorvastatin, albuterol inhaler, losartan, hydrochlorothiazide, metoprolol, warfarin, and methotrexate. She has allergy to ampicillin and lisinopril. She smokes one pack of cigarette a day for the past 50 years. She drinks alcohol on social occasions and denies any drug use. She has family history of allergic rhinitis and melanoma in her brother.

Her pulse is 109, BP is 160/90, temperature is 36.5°C, and respiratory rate is 18. Her saturated partial pressure of Oxygen (SpO_2) is 94% on room air. Her height is 1.6 m and weighs 74.4 kg with a BMI of 29.5. On physical exam, she's alert and oriented, appears well-developed and well-nourished. Her lungs are clear on auscultation and has a regular heart rate and rhythm. Her abdomen is soft and nontender. Legs showing no palpable artererial segment with possible arterial occlusive disease in legs.

Lower extremity segmental pressures were done, as shown in Figure 2-9:

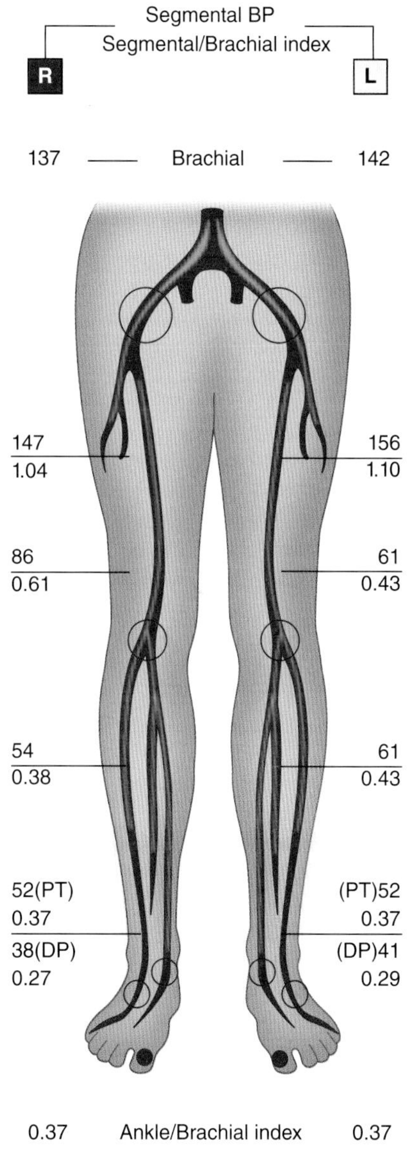

FIGURE 2-9 Ankle Brachial Index (ABI) and segmental pressures.

The ABI is <0.5 bilaterally, suggestive of severe peripheral arterial disease. The pressure indices drop between the upper and lower thigh level (from 1 to 0.6 on the right and 1.1 to 0.4 on the left); this suggests bilateral femoral-popliteal occlusive disease.

A CT scan done was concerning for common femoral as well as Superificial Femoral Artery occlusive disease.

Patient was scheduled for right common femoral endarterectomy with superficial femoral artery angioplasty and stenting. She did well and her postoperative course was uncomplicated.

REFERENCES

1. Secomb TW. Hemodynamics. *Compr Physiol.* 2016;6(2):975-1003.
2. Lewis O. Stephen Hales and the measurement of blood pressure. *J Hum Hypertens.* 1994;8(12):865-871.
3. Young T. XIII. Hydraulic investigations, subservient to an intended Croonian Lecture on the motion of the blood. *Philos Trans R Soc Lon.* 1808;98:164-186.
4. Antonialli L, Silveira-Neto A. Theoretical study of fully developed turbulent flow in a channel, using Prandtl's mixing length model. *J Appl Math Phys.* 2018;6:677-692.
5. Rajkumar JS, Chopra P, Chintamani. Basic physics revisited for a surgeon. *Indian J Surg.* 2015;77(3):169-175.
6. Taylor DEM. *Blood Flow in Arteries.* 2nd ed. By D. A. McDonald. Edward Arnold, London, 1974. Pp. xviii+496. £12. *Q J Exp Physiol Cogn Med Sci.* 1975;60(1):65-65.
7. McDonald DA. The relation of pulsatile pressure to flow in arteries. *J Physiol.* 1955;127(3):533-552.
8. Costanzo LS. Chapter 4: Cardiovascular physiology. In: *Physiology*. Philadelphia, PA: Wolters Kluwer; 2019:117-188.
9. Gavaghan M. Vascular hemodynamics. *AORN Journal.* 1998;68(2):211-226.
10. Menon ES. Chapter Five: Fluid flow in pipes. In: ES Menon (ed). *Transmission Pipeline Calculations and Simulations Manual.* Waltham, MA: Elsevier/Gulf Professional; 2015:149-234.
11. Basford JR. The Law of Laplace and its relevance to contemporary medicine and rehabilitation. *Arch Phys Med Rehabil.* 2002;83(8):1165-1170. doi:10.1053/apmr.2002.3398.
12. Klabunde RE. *Cardiovascular Physiology Concepts.* Philadelphia, PA: Lippincott Williams & Wilkins/Wolters Kluwer; 2012.
13. Classification & Structure of Blood Vessels. *Classification & Structure of Blood Vessels | SEER Training.* https://training.seer.cancer.gov/anatomy/cardiovascular/blood/classification.html. Accessed October 2, 2020.
14. Kushner A, West WP, Pillarisetty LS. *Virchow Triad.* Treasure Island, FL: StatPearls Publishing; September 13, 2020.
15. Kundu PK, Cohen IM, Dowling DR. Chapter 9: Laminar flow. In: *Fluid Mechanics.* Waltham, MA: Academic Press; 2016:409-467.
16. Owen CA, Roberts M. Arterial vascular hemodynamics. *J Diagn Med Sonogr.* 2007;23(3):129-140.
17. Hedrick WR, Hykes DL, Starchman DE. *Ultrasound Physics and Instrumentation.* St. Louis, MO: Elsevier Mosby; 2005.
18. Rumwell C, McPharlin M. *Vascular Technology: An Illustrated Review.* 2nd ed. Pasadena, CA: Davies, 2000.
19. Libretexts. 18.2D: Anastomoses. Medicine LibreTexts. https://med.libretexts.org/Bookshelves/Anatomy_and_Physiology/Book:_Anatomy_and_Physiology_(Boundless)/18:_Cardiovascular_System:_Blood_Vessels/18.2:_Arteries/18.2D:_Anastomoses. Published August 14, 2020. Accessed October 2, 2020.
20. Hyman C. The concept of end arteries and diversion of blood flow. *Invest Ophthalmol Vis Sci.* 1965;4(6):1000-1003.
21. AbuRahma AF, Bandyk DF, Sillesen H. Vascular Hemodynamics. In: *Noninvasive Vascular Diagnosis a Practical Guide to Therapy.* London: Springer, 2013:45-53.
22. Copstead LC. *Perspectives on Pathophysiology.* Philadelphia, PA: W B Saunders Co; 1995:309.
23. Cheng CP. Chapter 2: Deciding what vascular motions you need. In: CP Cheng. *Handbook of Vascular Motion.* London: Academic Press; 2019:7-22.
24. Webster, MW, Ramadan F. Vascular physiology. In Simmons RL, Steed D (eds). *Basic Science Review for Surgeons.* Philadelphia, PA: WB Saunders Co, 1992. 209.
25. Burrell LO. Overview of the anatomy, physiology, and pathophysiology of the hepatobiliary system. In: LO Burrell (ed), *Adult Nursing in Hospital and Community Settings.* Norwalk, CT: Appleton & Lange; 1992.
26. C N Rosenmitt. *Course Manual for Biology 201: Human Physiology.* Salt Lake City: University of Utah Division of Continuing Education Correspondence Study; 1992: 85.
27. Sheng Y, Zhu L. The crosstalk between autonomic nervous system and blood vessels. *Int J Physiol Pathophysiol Pharmacol.* 2018;10(1):17-28.
28. Johnson PC. Autoregulation of blood flow. *Circ Res.* 1986;59(5):483-495.
29. Copstead LE. *Perspectives on Pathophysiology.* Philadelphia, PA: W.B. Saunders; 1995.

30. Chiu JJ, Chien S. Effects of disturbed flow on vascular endothelium: pathophysiological basis and clinical perspectives. *Physiol Rev.* 2011;91(1):327-387.
31. Scher AM. Absence of atherosclerosis in human intramyocardial coronary arteries: a neglected phenomenon. *Atherosclerosis.* 2000;149(1):1-3.
32. Giancoli DC. *Physics Principles with Applications.* Boston, MA: Pearson; 2016.
33. Jakoi E. *Introductory Human Physiology.* https://web.duke.edu/histology/MBS/Videos/Phys/Phys%204.4%20CV%20Pressure%20Vol%20Flow/Phys%204.4%20CV%20Pressure%20Vol%20Flow%20NOTES.pdf. Accessed October 2, 2020.
34. Vincent JL. Understanding cardiac output. *Crit Care.* 2008;12(4):174.
35. Hiatt WR, Goldstone J, Smith SC Jr, et al. Atherosclerotic peripheral vascular disease symposium II: Nomenclature for vascular diseases. *Circulation.* 2008;118:2826.
36. Dhaliwal G, Mukherjee D. Peripheral arterial disease: epidemiology, natural history, diagnosis and treatment. *Int J Angiol.* 2007;16(2):36-44.
37. Weitz JI, Byrne J, Clagett GP, et al. Diagnosis and treatment of chronic arterial insufficiency of the lower extremities: a critical review. *Circulation.* 1996;94:3026-3049.
38. Rac-Albu M, Iliuta L, Guberna SM et al. The role of ankle-brachial index for predicting peripheral arterial disease. *Maedica (Bucur).* 2014;9(3):295-302.
39. Doobay AV, Anand SS. Sensitivity and specificity of the ankle-brachial index to predict future cardiovascular outcomes: a systematic review. *Arterioscler Thromb Vasc Biol.* 2005;25(7):1463-1469.
40. Khan TH, Farooqui FA, Niazi K. Critical review of the ankle brachial index. *Curr Cardiol Rev.* 2008;4(2):101-106.
41. Sutton-Tyrrell K, Venkitachalam L, Kanaya AM, et al. Relationship of ankle blood pressures to cardiovascular events in older adults. *Stroke.* 2008;39(3):863-869.
42. Hope SA, Tay DB, Meredith IT, et al. Waveform dispersion, not reflection, may be the major determinant of aortic pressure wave morphology. *Am J Physiol Heart Circ Physiol.* 2005;289:H2497-H2502.
43. Barnes RW. Noninvasive diagnostic assessment of peripheral vascular disease. *Circulation.* 1991;83(Suppl I):I20-I27.
44. Hirsch AT, Haskal ZJ, Hertzer NR, et al. ACC/AHA 2005 guidelines for the management of patients with peripheral arterial disease (lower extremity, renal, mesenteric, and abdominal aortic): a collaborative report from the American Association for Vascular Surgery/Society for Vascular Surgery, Society for Cardiovascular Angiography and Interventions, Society for Vascular Medicine and Biology, Society of Interventional Radiology, and the ACC/AHA Task Force on Practice Guidelines (Writing Committee to Develop Guidelines for the Management of Patients With Peripheral Arterial Disease). *J Am Coll Car.* 2006;47:e1-192.
45. Sacks D, Bakal CW, Beatty PT, et al. Position statement on the use of the ankle-brachial index in the evaluation of patients with peripheral vascular disease: a consensus statement developed by the Standards Division of the Society of Cardiovascular & Interventional Radiology. *J Vasc Interv Radiol.* 2002;13:353.
46. McDermott MM, Liu K, Guralnik JM, et al. The ankle brachial index independently predicts walking velocity and walking endurance in peripheral arterial disease. *J Am Geriatr Soc.* 1998;46:1355-1362.
47. Mittleider D. Noninvasive arterial testing: what and when to use. *Semin Intervent Radiol.* 2018;35(5):384-392.
48. Shabani Varaki E, Gargiulo GD, Penkala S, Breen PP. Peripheral vascular disease assessment in the lower limb: a review of current and emerging non-invasive diagnostic methods. *Biomed Eng Online.* 2018;17(1):61.
49. Rumwell C, McPharlin M. *Vascular Technology: An Illustrated Review.* Pasadena, CA: Davies Publishing, Inc.; 2015.
50. Del Conde I, Benenati JF. Noninvasive testing in peripheral arterial disease. *Interv Cardiol Clin.* 2014;3:469-78.
51. Allan JS, Terry HJ. The evaluation of an ultrasonic flow detector for the assessment of peripheral vascular disease. *Cardiovasc Res.* 1969;3:503-509.
52. Strandness D, Bell J. Peripheral vascular disease: diagnosis and objective evaluation using a mercury strain gauge. *Ann Surg.* 1965;161:4.

SELF-ASSESSMENT STUDY QUESTIONS AND ANSWERS

Questions

1. In a certain blood vessel, decreasing radius by one-half increases the resistance by a factor of ___.
A. 4
B. 8
C. 16
D. Can't be determined from the information given

2. In normal individuals, at rest, the amount of blood stored in veins is approximately ___% of the total blood volume at any given moment.
A. 30%
B. 50%
C. 75%
D. 90%

3. Which of the following laws explains why aneurysms rupture?
A. Ohm's law
B. Laplace's law
C. Poiseuille's law
D. Starling law

4. What happens to the total resistance of a capillary bed if an additional capillary is recruited in parallel?
A. Increases
B. Decreases
C. Stays the same
D. Can't be determined from the information given

5. Which of the following concerning turbulent flow is incorrect?
A. The resistance to laminar flow is lower than turbulent flow.
B. Above a critical velocity, blood flow becomes turbulent.
C. Turbulence can create sound waves that can be detected as murmurs.
D. Turbulence is found normally in the aorta and in branching vessels.
E. Turbulent flow rate is proportional to the cube root of the driving pressure.

6. Pulse pressure is greatest in the ____.
A. Aorta
B. Large arteries
C. Arterioles
D. Veins

7. Which of the following tends to decrease blood vessel compliance?
A. Decreased transmural pressure
B. Decreased wall stiffness
C. Increased sympathetic activation
D. All of the above

8. According to AHA/TASC II, which of the following should be used as denominator to calculate the ankle-brachial index (ABI)?
A. The highest of the two brachial pressures
B. The lowest of the two brachial pressures
C. The average of the two brachial pressures
D. The ipsilateral brachial pressure

9. While determining the ABI, the lower extremity pressure is measured by placing the Doppler probe on which vessels of the lower extremity?
A. Anterior and posterior tibial arteries
B. Femoral and anterior tibial arteries
C. Popliteal and dorsalis pedis arteries
D. Dorsalis pedis and posterior tibial arteries

10. A 73-year-old woman with diabetes and right lower extremity ulcer was found to have an ABI of 1.5. How is the ABI interpreted?
A. Patient has acute limb ischemia.
B. Patient has peripheral artery disease.
C. Patient has calcified vessels.
D. Patient has normal circulation

SELF-ASSESSMENT STUDY QUESTIONS AND ANSWERS

Answers

1. C.
2. C.
3. B.
4. B.
5. E.
6. B.
7. C.
8. A.
9. D.
10. C.

CHAPTER

3 Thrombosis and Hemostasis

Deepak Ravindranathan and Manila Gaddh

OUTLINE

INTRODUCTION
HEMOSTASIS
APPROACH TO A PATIENT WITH BLEEDING
PT and aPTT
PT and aPTT Mixing Study
Thrombin Time
PFA-100
vWD Profile
Factor XIII Deficiency
APPROACH TO A PATIENT WITH THROMBOSIS
Factor V Leiden
Prothrombin G20210A Mutation or Factor II Mutation
Protein C Deficiency
Protein S Deficiency
Antithrombin Deficiency
Antiphospholipid Syndrome
General Considerations for Thrombophilia Testing
Treatment

INTRODUCTION

The coagulation system is comprised of both procoagulant and anticoagulant factors and serves an important function of maintaining the integrity of the circulatory system in the body. Under normal homoeostatic conditions, the balance between the body's coagulation pathway and natural anticoagulants maintains blood in a state to allow unobstructed flow through the blood vessels. When there is a breach in the vasculature, the coagulation pathway is activated and fibrin clot is formed through a physiological process called hemostasis. Disorders of hemostasis can result in excessive or abnormal bleeding. On the other hand, activation of the coagulation pathway within intact blood vessels leads to pathological (as opposed to physiological) clotting or thrombosis. Thrombi can form in veins and/or arteries with possibly different mechanisms leading to thrombosis in these different vascular settings.

In this chapter, we will discuss the process of hemostasis and the approach to patients with bleeding and thrombotic disorders.

HEMOSTASIS

The basic components of hemostasis include vessel wall, platelets, von Willebrand factor (VWF), and the coagulation cascade. The process starts with injury to the vessel walls and includes the following three steps: (1) vascular constriction, (2) platelet plug formation (primary hemostasis), and (3) fibrin clot formation by the coagulation cascade, which stabilizes the platelet plug (secondary hemostasis). The coagulation cascade in step 3 above goes through phases of initiation, amplification, and propagation, which ultimately leads to formation of a fibrin clot. In the initiation phase, the blood vessels that are injured expose Tissue Factor (TF) on the subendothelial cells to the coagulation factors in the blood. Factor VII binds with TF to activate Factors X and XI and generate a small amount of thrombin from prothrombin. In the amplification phase, the thrombin generated in the initiation phase then interacts with the platelets at the site of injury to "activate" them. Clotting factors such as Factor V and Factor XI are also activated. The activated platelets release Factor V which cleaves Factor VIII from VWF to activate VWF. Also, Factor XI binds to activated platelets' surfaces. Through this phase, the platelets are coated in activated coagulation factors. In propagation, eventually the factors come into play to lead to production of large amount of thrombin which converts fibrinogen into fibrin, thus stabilizing the clot along with Factor XIII.[1,2]

APPROACH TO A PATIENT WITH BLEEDING

Taking a detailed and comprehensive history helps elucidate a clinical bleeding problem. The patient should be asked about bleeding events in their childhood such as umbilical stump bleeding, bleeding with loss of deciduous teeth, or bleeding with childhood trauma and surgeries. Bleeding with dental procedures should be inquired. The patient should be asked about the type of bleeding, severity of bleeding episodes, and sites where bleeding occurred. Presence of petechiae, purpura, epistaxis, gingival bleeding, menorrhagia, and/or hematuria would suggest a disorder of primary hemostasis including platelet and/or vascular abnormalities. Bleeding into joints or muscles would suggest an issue with the secondary hemostasis process. The initiation of bleeding should also be investigated. For example, bruising or bleeding excessively after a minor injury is suggestive of an inherited bleeding problem. Any history of blood or blood product transfusion in relation to surgical procedures or bleeding episodes should be noted, and a thorough review of medications should be done. Physical examination is also a key component of the evaluation. The skin should be thoroughly examined for petechiae or ecchymosis.[2] A standardized bleeding assessment tool such as the ISTH-SSC Bleeding Assessment Tool can be utilized (available online at bleedingscore.certe.nl) which can complement the bleeding history with a scoring system. This bleeding assessment tool has been shown to help discriminate between patients with and without inherited platelet function disorders.[3]

A thorough history and physical examination should be followed by laboratory investigation in patients in whom a bleeding disorder is suspected. However, it must be noted that the results from this part of the investigation should not serve as diagnostic by itself, but should rather supplement the history and physical examination in the diagnostic process. Although there is no set panel of screening first-line tests, most practitioners will include a complete blood count that includes the platelet count, peripheral blood smear examination, comprehensive metabolic profile to review renal and liver functions, and screening tests of the coagulation system including prothrombin time (PT), activated partial thromboplastin time (aPTT), thrombin time (TT), platelet function assay (PFA-100), von Willebrand disease (vWD) profile, and Factor XIII level.[2] Further testing with more definitive tests is based on the results of the screening panel and is usually pursued by a specialized hematology consult service. Details of definitive diagnostic tests and treatment of specific bleeding disorders are outside the scope of this chapter. A brief description of the screening tests of the coagulation system is provided below and summarized as a diagram in Figure 3-1.

PT AND aPTT

The two most commonly used assays for assessment of hemostasis are the PT and aPTT, which measure the time it takes to form a fibrin clot. The process of clot formation in vitro and interpretation of elevated PT and aPTT assays is better understood in terms of intrinsic and extrinsic pathways of coagulation cascade. As shown in Figure 3-2, PT assesses the extrinsic and common pathway comprising TF, Factors VII, V, X, II, and fibrinogen.[4] Because PT can vary based on the source of TF that may be used in the particular assay, a standardized value called the international normalized ratio, or INR, has been developed for monitoring anticoagulation with vitamin K antagonists.[5] The aPTT tests the components of the intrinsic and common pathways comprising Factors XII, XI, IX, VIII, X, V, II, fibrinogen, high-molecular

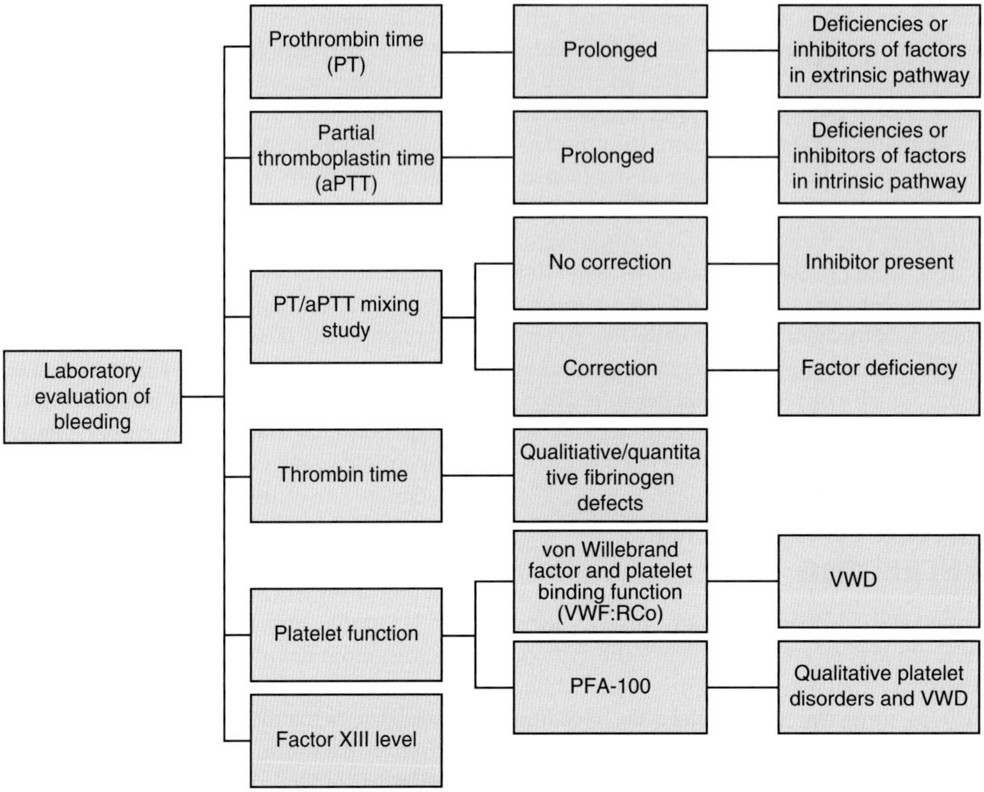

FIGURE 3-1 Laboratory evaluation of bleeding disorder.

weight kininogen, and prekallkrein.[6] Prolonged PT and aPTT can be seen in deficiencies or inhibitors of clotting factors. Isolated elevation of PT results from deficiency or inhibitors of Factor VII, while isolated elevation of aPTT results pertains to high molecular weight kininogen, or Factors XII, XI, VIII, or IX. Elevation of both PT and aPTT indicates deficiency or inhibitors of factors in the common pathway comprising of Factors V, X, II, and fibrinogen. Of note, deficiency of Factor XIII is not detected by measuring either PT or aPTT.[4]

PT AND aPTT MIXING STUDY

A mixing study is the next step in evaluation of elevated PT and/or aPTT. In this study, the patient's plasma is mixed 1:1 with normal control plasma and the abnormal assay is repeated. This study helps with distinguishing between an inhibitor and a clotting factor deficiency. Correction of the clotting test suggests a factor deficiency. If the clotting test does not correct after mixing, then an inhibitor is present. Other reasons of incomplete correction can be the presence of a lupus anticoagulant, elevated fibrin split products, or paraprotein.[7]

THROMBIN TIME

The thrombin time, or thrombin clotting time (TCT), measures the time needed for clot formation after thrombin is added to the citrated plasma. Paraproteinemia or hypofibrinogenemia can lead to TCT prolongation. This is also prolonged in the presence of a thrombin inhibitor like heparin, lepirudin, or argatroban. Laboratories have to neutralize the effect of the thrombin inhibitors using cleaving enzymes like reptilase or the test has to be repeated after the anticoagulant is discontinued.[8]

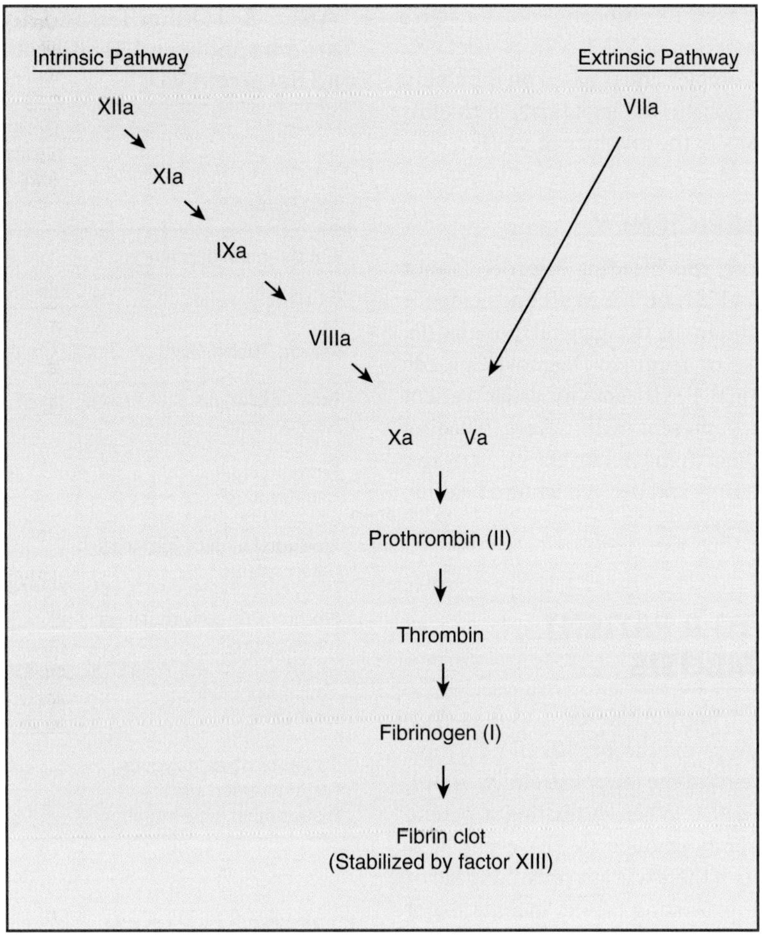

FIGURE 3-2 Coagulation cascade.

PFA-100

The PFA-100 is a screening test for primary hemostasis disorders and is performed on whole citrated blood. The test has essentially replaced the traditional bleeding time which is operator-dependent and has low sensitivity for mild forms of disorders of primary hemostasis. In this test, citrated whole blood is aspirated into a cartridge where it comes into contact with a membrane impregnated with either a mixture of collagen and epinephrine (Col/Epi) or collagen and adenosine diphosphate (Col/ADP). When the blood comes in contact with these membranes, it leads to platelet adhesion, aggregation, and activation. Closure time is the measurement unit for the test and can be prolonged in severe platelet dysfunction and vWD. Prolongation of closure time with Col/Epi, but not Col/ADP, usually indicates aspirin ingestion.[9]

vWD PROFILE

von Willebrand disease is a congenital bleeding disorder. vWD can result from either decreased (type 1) or absent (Type 3) antigen, or decreased activity (type2).[10] The diagnostic tests for this disease are quantitative measurement of von Willebrand Factor(VWF: ag), the platelet-binding function (VWF: RCo) where platelet agglutination in response to patient plasma is measured in the presence of ristocetin, and F VIII level (FVIII:C). The assay for ristocetin cofactor activity looks at the interaction of VWF with platelet glycoprotein Ib/IX/V complex and is based on the ability of the antibiotic ristocetin to agglutinate formalin-fixed normal platelets in the presence of VWF.

FACTOR XIII DEFICIENCY

As mentioned before, this bleeding disorder cannot be detected by PT, aPTT, or TT. With an incidence of one per two million in the general population, this can be inherited or acquired. Diagnosis is made based on a functional F XIII activity assay. Patient with this deficiency present with severe bleeding such as soft tissue hematoma, recurrent miscarriage, umbilical cord bleeding, and delayed wound healing, particularly after surgery.[11]

APPROACH TO A PATIENT WITH THROMBOSIS

Patients with underlying thrombotic disorders typically present with deep vein thrombosis (DVT), most commonly in the veins of the lower extremity, or pulmonary embolism (PE). When evaluating a patient with a venous thromboembolic (VTE) event, it is important to identify if there was any provoking factor for the event. Such provoking factors include major surgical procedures, trauma, hospitalization, infections such as COVID-19, immobility, or pregnancy within 3 months preceding the diagnosis of VTE.[12,13] In addition, enquiry about comorbidities that increase the risk of thrombosis such as autoimmune disorder, neoplasms, nephrotic syndrome, or inflammatory bowel disease should be made. Another important aspect of evaluation is testing for a thrombophilia or hypercoagulable state, which is defined as a tendency, either acquired or hereditary, to develop thrombosis. The common inherited and acquired thrombophilias include Factor V Leiden, Prothrombin G20210A mutation, Protein C deficiency, Protein S deficiency, antithrombin deficiency, and antiphospholipid syndrome (APS).[14] The relative risk of first and recurrent VTE associated with these thrombophilias is listed in Table 3-1, and a brief description of the thrombophilias is provided below.[15–18]

TABLE 3-1 Inherited and Acquired Thrombophilia and Relative Risks for First VTE and Recurrent VTE

Thrombophilia	Relative Risk for First VTE	Relative Risk for Recurrent VTE
Antithrombin deficiency[15]	50	12.5
Protein C deficiency[15]	15	2.5
Protein S deficiency[15]	10	2.5
Factor V Leiden, heterozygous[15]	7	1.5
Factor V Leiden, homozygous[15]	80	-
Prothrombin gene mutation, heterozygous[15]	3-4	1.5
Prothrombin gene mutation, homozygous[15]	30	-
Antiphospholipid syndrome[16]	1.41	1.53
Compound heterozygous Factor V Leiden and Prothrombin gene mutation	20[17]	2.6[18]

FACTOR V LEIDEN

A commonly inherited thrombophilia, Factor V Leiden refers to a point mutation (G1691A) in the Factor V gene which destroys the cleavage site for activated Protein C (APC) and makes Factor Va less susceptible to inactivation by APC, hence predisposing to thrombosis. The inheritance is through an autosomal-dominant manner. It is commonly seen in patients of European ancestry. Prevalence is noted to be about 3% to 8% in Caucasians. The diagnosis of this thrombophilia is made via polymerase chain reaction (PCR) test for the specific mutation.[19]

PROTHROMBIN G20210A MUTATION OR FACTOR II MUTATION

This is the second most commonly inherited risk factor for venous thrombosis and refers to a point mutation in the Factor II gene in the noncoding region in the nucleotide position 20210 (G20210A). This is commonly found in those of southern European ancestry, occurring in 2% of the general population. This test is also detected via PCR, but Factor II levels are not helpful in helping with diagnosis.[20]

PROTEIN C DEFICIENCY

This is a vitamin K–dependent protein that is converted to APC during the coagulation process. The most common type of deficiency is type I, which is a quantitative deficiency with low functional Protein C activity and antigen level. Type II deficiency is less common and is due to functional defects in Protein C. The prevalence is noted to be about 1 in 500 to 600 in the general population. Diagnosis can be started by performing a Protein C functional (activity) test as the screening assay, followed by an antigen test to confirm the type of deficiency if the screening assay is positive. It must be noted that patients with Protein C deficiency who are initiated on warfarin can develop warfarin-induced skin necrosis due to the transient decline in Pprotein C activity right after initiation of anticoagulation. Therefore, overlap with another anticoagulant, usually a form of heparin, for a minimum of 5 days is needed when starting treatment with vitamin K antagonist (VKAs) in patients with Protein C deficiency.[20]

PROTEIN S DEFICIENCY

This is also a vitamin K–dependent protein that serves as a cofactor for APC to inactivate F Va and F VIIIa. It is inherited in an autosomal dominant fashion and prevalence is between 1 in 800 and 1 in 3000. There are three types of Protein S deficiencies. This can be screened and diagnosed by measuring either free Protein S antigen or Protein S activity. Type I is a quantitative deficiency in which both free and total Protein S antigen levels are reduced. Type II is a qualitative defect due to dysfunctional protein in which Protein S activity is low but there are normal free and total antigen levels. Type III is a quantitative deficiency in which free Protein S antigen level is low, but there is a normal total antigen level. Overlap of parenteral anticoagulation when starting a vitamin K antagonist is needed to avoid warfarin-induced skin necrosis.[20]

ANTITHROMBIN DEFICIENCY

Antithrombin is an enzyme that interrupts the coagulation process by inhibiting thrombin, activated Factor X, and activated Factor IXa. This is also inherited in an autosomal-dominant fashion. Prevalence is 1 in 500 to 5000 people and usually of the heterozygous type. In terms of diagnosis, a functional assay to detect both quantitative and qualitative defects should be ordered. Diagnosis should not be made on one single abnormal test result and testing should be repeated.[20]

ANTIPHOSPHOLIPID SYNDROME

This entity refers to acquired autoantibodies against phospholipids and phospholipid-binding proteins that activate the clotting system. Diagnosis requires VTE or arterial thrombosis or unexplained recurrent (three or more) early miscarriages (<10 weeks of gestation) or one or more late pregnancy losses, and laboratory detection of persistently elevated levels of antiphospholipid antibodies (anticardiolipin or beta2-glycoprotein I antibodies, IgM or IgG subtype) or the presence of a lupus anticoagulant on two occasions at least 12 weeks apart.[21]

General Considerations for Thrombophilia Testing

Testing for hypercoagulable disorders should involve a discussion with the patient about potential benefits and limitations of testing, and the potential ramifications of the results. Testing should be offered to patients with unprovoked VTE, in particular those who have a first degree relative with history of VTE. Family history of VTE is a risk factor for first time VTE regardless if a defined thrombophilia is diagnosed in the family. A patient's risk of having a VTE increases two- to fourfold if they have a first degree relative with history of VTE. It is also important to keep in mind factors that can affect the results of the tests so as to determine optimum time for thrombophilia testing. The levels of Protein C, Protein S, and antithrombin can be falsely low in the setting of an acute clot. Therefore, testing for these tests should be done at least a few weeks after an acute episode of VTE. Since Proteins C and S are vitamin K–dependent proteins, VKAs should be held for a week before testing for Proteins C and S deficiency. Heparin can lower the level of antithrombin, whereas direct oral anticoagulants (DOACs) can falsely increase the levels of Protein C, Protein S, and antithrombin. Therefore, these tests should be ordered after the anticoagulants have been held for about four half-lives.[14]

Treatment

Anticoagulation is the mainstay of treatment of VTE. The decision to anticoagulate must be weighed against the risk of bleeding in an individual patient. For patients with active bleeding or contraindications to anticoagulation, a temporary inferior vena cava (IVC) filter should be placed which should be removed as soon as treatment with anticoagulant has been safely established. There are a variety of anticoagulation choices which include DOACs, VKAs, low molecular-weight heparin, and fondaparinux. DOACs are preferred over other anticoagulants given their ease of administration, no associated dietary restrictions or need for monitoring, and lower risk of major bleeding as compared to VKAs.[21,22] However, if high risk (triple positive) APS is noted, then warfarin is preferred given the results of the TRAPS study showing reduced efficacy of DOACs in this patient population.[23]

Duration of anticoagulation takes into account whether or not the VTE event was provoked by a transient risk factor, as well as presence of any other persistent risk factor for recurrence and bleeding. Location of the VTE is also important. Distal DVT or single sub-segmental PE is less likely to recur or progress than proximal VTE. The recommendation for duration of anticoagulation for patients with provoked VTE is 3 months, as long as the provoking factor is resolved at the end of 3 months. For unprovoked VTEs, indefinite anticoagulation with periodic reassessment of risk of bleeding is recommended. The recurrence rate of unprovoked VTE is about 10% in the first year. Some patients prefer not to stay on anticoagulation long-term or may have an intermediate to high risk of bleeding. For those patients, validated models such as the VIENNA score or DASH score, or D-dimer levels, can be utilized in estimating the individual patient's recurrence risk.[24]

REFERENCES

1. Periyah MH, Halim AS, Saad AZM. Mechanism action of platelets and crucial blood coagulation pathways in hemostasis. *Int J Hematol Oncol Stem Cell Res.* 2017;11(4):319-327.
2. Bashawri LAM, Ahmed MA. The approach to a patient a bleeding disorder: for the primary care physician. *J Family Community Med.* 2007;14(2):53-58.
3. Gresele P, Orsini S, Noris P, et al. Validation of ISTH/SSC bleeding assessment tool for inherited platelet disorders: a communication from the platelet physiology SCC. *J Thromb Haemost.* 2020;18(3):732-739.
4. Boender J, Kruip MJHA, Leebeek FWG. A diagnostic approach to mild bleeding disorders. *J Thromb Haemost.* 2016;14(8):1507-1516.
5. Riley RS, Rowe D, Fisher LM. Clinical utilization of the international normalized ratio (INR). *J of Clin Lab Anal.* 2000;14(3):101-114.
6. Hoffman M, Monroe DM. Coagulation 2006: a modern view of hemostasis. *Hematol Oncol Clin North Am.* 2007;21(1):1-11.
7. Choi SH, Rambally S, Shen Y-M. Mixing studying for evaluation of abnormal coagulation testing. *JAMA.* 2016;316(20):2146-2147.
8. Undas A. Determination of fibrinogen and thrombin time (TT). *Methods Mol Biol.* 2017;1646:105-110.
9. Carcao MD, Blanchette VS, Stephens D. Assessment of thrombocytopenic disorders using the platelet function analyzer (PFA-100). *Br J Haematol.* 2002;117(4):961-964.
10. Ng CJ, Paola JK. von Willebrand disease: diagnostic strategies and treatment options. *Pediatr Clin North Am.* 2018;65(3):527-541.
11. Dorgalaleh A, Rashidpanah J. Blood coagulation factor XIII and factor XIII deficiency. *Blood Rev.* 2016;30(6):461-475.
12. Middeldorp S, Coppens M, van Haaps TF, et al. Incidence of venous thromboembolism in hospitalized patients with COVID-19. *J Thromb Haemost.* 2020;18(8):1995-2002.
13. Beckman MG, Hooper WC, Critchley SE, et al. Venous thromboembolism: a public health concern. *Am J Prev Med.* 2010;38(4):S495-S501.
14. Connors JM. Thrombophilia testing and venous thrombosis. *N Engl J Med.* 2017;377:1177-1187.

15. Mannucci PM, Franchini M. Classic thrombophilic gene variants. *Thromb Haemost*. 2015;114(05):885-889.
16. Garcia D, Akl EA, Carr R, et al. Antiphospholipid antibodies and the risk of recurrence after a first episode of venous thromboembolism: a systematic review. *Blood*. 2013;122(5):817-824.
17. Kujovich JL. Factor V Leiden thrombophilia. *Genet Med*. 2011;13(1):1-16.
18. De Stefano V, Martinelli I, Mannucci PM, et al. The risk of recurrent deep venous thrombosis among heterozygous carriers of both Factor V Leiden and G20210A prothrombin mutation. *N Engl J Med*. 1999;341:801-806.
19. Van de Water NS, French JK, Lund M, et al. Prevalence of Factor V Leiden and prothrombin variant G20210A in patients age <50 years with no significant stenoses at angiogaphy three to four weeks after myocardial infarction. *J Am Coll Card*. 2000;36(3):717-722.
20. Khan S, Dickerman JK. Hereditary thrombophilia. *Throm J*. 2006 4(15):1-17.
21. Ghembaza A, Saadoun D. Management of antiphospholipid syndrome. *Biomedicines*. 2020 8(508):1-17.
22. Kearon C, Akl EA, Ornelas J, et al. Antithrombotic therapy for VTE disease. *Chest*. 2016;149 (2):315-352.
23. Pengo V, Denas G, Zoppellaro G, et al. Rivaroxaban vs warfarin in high-risk patients with antiphospholipid syndrome. *Blood*. 2018;132(13):1365-1371.
24. Kearon C, Kahn SR. Long-term treatment of venous thromboembolism. *Blood*. 2020;135 (5):317-325.

SELF-ASSESSMENT STUDY QUESTIONS AND ANSWERS

Questions

1. What is true about the hemostatic system in the body?
   A. It is a part of the body's defense system meant to limit bleeding.
   B. Hemostasis leads to pathologic clots like DVTs and PEs that require treatment with anticoagulation.
   C. Hemostatic system refers to the coagulation factors in the body.
   D. Vessel wall is not a part of the hemostatic system.

2. A 38-year-old patient with history of exercise-induced asthma, depression, and alcohol abuse undergoes breast reconstruction surgery complicated by excessive bleeding at the surgical site. She reports her menstrual periods have become heavier and she has noticed easy bruising over the preceding 4-6 months. She is referred to a hematologist for evaluation of a bleeding disorder. What in her history suggests against a bleeding disorder?
   A. She has undergone wisdom teeth extraction in the past and has had two pregnancies and deliveries without any associated bleeding complications.
   B. She has no family history of bleeding disorders.
   C. Recent menorrhagia.
   D. None of the above.

3. A 38-year-old man with no significant past medical history develops a saddle PE 6 days after undergoing internal fixation for traumatic fracture in his left tibia and fibula. He has no past personal or family history of venous thromboembolism. What should not be included in his management plan?
   A. Anticoagulation for 3 months
   B. Thrombophilia evaluation to determine the etiology of the clot and duration of anticoagulation
   C. Plan for thromboprophylaxis during future high-risk periods for venous thromboembolism
   D. Ultrasound doppler of bilateral lower extremities to look for DVT

4. A 56-year-old man with past medical history of hypertension and dyslipidemia presents to the emergency room with acute shortness of breath and chest pain. He is hypotensive, tachycardic, and hypoxic with O2 saturation of 88% of room air. After tests and imaging, he is diagnosed with massive PE requiring systemic thrombolysis followed by anticoagulation. While planning for thrombophilia evaluation, what factor(s) need to be considered?
   A. Effect of acute clot on the results
   B. Effect of ongoing anticoagulation on the results
   C. Effect of results of evaluation on patient management
   D. All of the above

5. A 75-year-old man is being evaluated for a hip replacement surgery. Which risk factor from his history is associated with the highest risk of thrombosis?
   A. Factor V Leiden heterozygosity
   B. Advanced age
   C. Positive family history of VTE
   D. Obesity

SELF-ASSESSMENT STUDY QUESTIONS AND ANSWERS

Answers

1. A.
2. D.
3. B.
4. D.
5. B.

CHAPTER

4 Radiation Safety and the Vascular Specialist

Drew J. Braet and Todd R. Vogel

OUTLINE

OVERVIEW OF RADIATION, DANGERS, RISKS, AND EXPOSURE
- Basic Definitions of Radiation
  - X-Ray Production
  - Exposure
  - Absorbed Dose
  - Effective Dose
  - Reference Air Kerma (RAK)
  - Substantial Radiation Dose Level (SRDL)
  - Dose Area Product (DAP)
- Radiation Exposure and Biologic Effects
- Radiation Exposure Types

IMPORTANCE OF RADIATION SAFETY EDUCATION AND OCCUPATIONAL EXPOSURE
- Radiation Safety Variation
- The as Low as Reasonably Achievable (ALARA) Principle
- Vascular Procedures and Radiation Exposure
- Occupational Exposure and Health Risk

RADIATION EXPOSURE AND VASCULAR SURGERY PATIENTS

RADIATION EXPOSURE DURING ENDOVASCULAR PROCEDURES

TECHNIQUES TO LOWER RADIATION EXPOSURE DURING PROCEDURES
- Limiting Radiation Exposure to the Patient
- Skin Damage to the Patient
- Imaging Equipment Techniques to Lower Radiation Exposure
- Protective Equipment and Garments
- Fluoroscopy Time and Dosimeters

SPECIAL CONSIDERATIONS
- Pregnancy
- Carbon Dioxide (CO_2) Angiography
- Alternative Imaging
- Patient Radiation Education and Consent

RADIATION EXPOSURE GUIDELINES

CONCLUSIONS

ACKNOWLEDGMENTS

OVERVIEW OF RADIATION, DANGERS, RISKS, AND EXPOSURE

The use of radiation has become essential for the treatment and management of multiple vascular problems. An understanding and systematic implementation of guidelines and techniques to lower radiation exposure is critical for vascular surgeons during their training and throughout their careers. It is well known that radiation exposure is cumulative over time and has long-term effects on the practitioner, the patient, and staff. As such, careful consideration of radiation utilization, in addition to an appreciation of the risks associated with radiation exposure, is crucial to treat patients safely and ensure personal and staff protection.

To begin, we will review the basic terminology used for radiation and fluoroscopy. This will include common terms which were seen and need to be appreciated by practitioners using fluoroscopy on a regular basis. Regarding radiation utilization, the basic principles include optimization as well as radiation dose.

X-rays are composed of high-energy photons within the electromagnetic spectrum.[1] X-rays are notable in that they are powerful enough to break molecular bonds, ionize atoms, and can alter DNA structure.[2] This ionization produces free radicals, which are chemically active compounds that can indirectly damage DNA.[3] DNA damage can occur from radiation exposure resulting in chromosomal aberrations which can lead to genetic mutation and cancer. Ionizing radiation on a human cell has two main effects: direct cellular damage and indirect cellular damage through production of reactive oxidative species.[4]

BASIC DEFINITIONS OF RADIATION

The following are important concepts and terminology to understand prior to reviewing techniques, indications, as well as consequences of radiation exposure.

X-Ray Production

X-rays are formed via interactions of accelerated electrons with electrons of tungsten nuclei within a tube. The flow from the filament to the target is referred to as the tube current and is expressed in milliamperes.[5] The number of x-rays produced at the source of radiation is determined by the tube current and the voltage. The proportion of x-ray production is directly proportional to the tube current.

Exposure

Radiation exposure is defined as the measure of the ionization of air by photons (gamma and X-rays) at a standard temperature and pressure. Measurements of exposure rates for fluoroscopy are typically measured in fluoroscopy output per minute.[1]

Absorbed Dose

The energy imparted per unit mass by ionizing radiation to matter at a specified point. The International System of Units (SI) unit of absorbed dose is the joule per kilogram, which is referred to as gray (Gy).[6] For purposes of radiation protection and assessing dose or risk to humans, the quantity calculated is the mean absorbed dose in an organ or tissue.[6] Absorbed dose is defined as the energy delivered to and deposited in an organ divided by the mass of the organ, in Gy and milligrays (mGy). The equivalent dose is calculated, accounting for the organ-specific radiation exposure, as well as the organ's sensitivity to radiation, and is expressed in millisieverts (mSv).

Effective Dose

The effective dose is the sum over the entire body of the individual organ equivalent doses and is expressed in millisieverts (mSv).[5] This is the risk for potential effects when a part of the body is radiated. This measurement considers the differing radiosensitivity of organs and can be used to estimate the patient's cancer risk. The International Commission on Radiological Protection (ICRP) has produced tissue weighting factors to reflect relative sensitivities of tissues to the carcinogenic effects of radiation.[7]

Reference Air Kerma (RAK)

RAK measures the radiation output at a reference point along a specific fluoroscopic axis. It is a better measure of total dose from a procedure as it includes all the doses that accrue from both fluoroscopy and fluorography acquisitions. Additionally, RAK approximates patient peak skin dose (PSD). Peak skin dose is the highest absorbed dose in any portion of a patient's skin accumulated during a procedure.[1] RAK is the cumulative air kerma at a point in space located at a fixed distance from the focal spot. Therefore, RAK is not a direct measure of PSD, but an approximation.

Substantial Radiation Dose Level (SRDL)

SRDL is a facility-selected radiation value used to trigger follow-up for possible deterministic injury. Although useful for patient dose triggers, the SRDL is not used for occupational exposure. The National Council on Radiation and Protection Measurements has defined a RAK dose of 5 Gy to be an SRDL for which the patient should be informed and monitored for postoperative skin injury.[8]

Dose Area Product (DAP)

The DAP is a quantity used in assessing the radiation risk from diagnostic x-ray examinations and interventional procedures. DAP is absorbed dose multiplied by the area irradiated and is expressed in gray-centimeters squared. DAP reflects not only the dose within the radiation field but also the area of tissue irradiated.[9] It is widely used as a common radiological measure for procedures, and the correlation between DAP and effective dose (*E*) has been established.[10]

RADIATION EXPOSURE AND BIOLOGIC EFFECTS

Ionizing radiation has the potential to cause biological harm either by directly damaging DNA or through the secondary effects of free radicals generated by ionization. The primary health risks to staff exposed to radiation include cancer, cataract formation, and fetal deformities. Risks can be divided into stochastic (random) and deterministic (non-stochastic) effects. These can be somatic in the individual exposed, or hereditary, affecting germ cells. Fortunately, DNA repair mechanisms can help mitigate radiation effects. However, risk of harm increases as exposure cumulates and can ultimately overwhelm repair mechanisms.[7]

Radiation exposure can produce biologic effects as a dose-dependent effect or a dose-dependent probability.[3] X-ray damage is directly proportional to the dose. Radiation exposure is cumulative, and its effects are permanent. Survival rates vary by the dose as well as the cell type affected. The relative biologic effectiveness describes the tissue response to a given dose and increased mitotic activity within the cell, which leads to increased sensitivity to radiation.[4]

A dose-dependent probability is referred to as a stochastic effect and represents an outcome that occurs with a certain probability but without a defined threshold at which these effects are triggered.[4] Stochastic effects can be discovered many years after radiation exposure and include the development of cancer.[11] Deterministic effects are determined by the cumulative amount of radiation exposure an organ or tissue experiences over time (the lifetime equivalent dose).[11] In comparison, there is a chance that a specific x-ray causes DNA damage that later develops into cancer, a stochastic effect.[4] As the number of x-rays a provider or patient is exposed to increases, the chance of a stochastic effect increases. Current literature suggests that medical radiation may result in a modest increase in the risk of cataracts, cancer, and possibly hereditary diseases.[12] Although all areas of the body are susceptible to radiation injury, different tissues have varying tolerances for radiation exposure.

RADIATION EXPOSURE TYPES

When x-rays interact with matter, one of the three things occurs. The incoming x-rays can be completely absorbed, some x-ray beams pass through and continue their path without being absorbed, and others change their direction and scatter as well as change their strength.[13] Scattered x-rays give up part of their energy during the scattering process, and thus energy deposited in tissues from scattered x-rays is lower than directly from the x-ray source. Scatter, the radiation that bounces off the patient, is the primary source of radiation to OR personnel; however, there is also risk of direct exposure via the x-ray beam. Consequently, scatter increases patient dose, degrades the image, and poses the greatest source of radiation exposure to the health care worker.[14] Anything in the path of the x-ray beam may interact with and alter the course of the incoming x-rays including the patient and x-ray table, and are potential sources of scatter. The exact amount of exposure depends on exposure time, distance from the source, and shielding.

The use of good fluoroscopic technique is imperative for physician and patient protection which will be reviewed later in the chapter.[4] Our natural background exposure to radiation is approximately 0.36 rem per year, and the typical c-arm emits an average of 2 rem per minute.[12] Although sometimes medically necessary, experts generally agree that there is no "safe" radiation dose.[15] We do know, however, that the possibility of a biological effect is higher when there is a high exposure in a short time. When exposure occurs intermittently and over a longer period of time, some damaged cells can repair themselves between exposures.

IMPORTANCE OF RADIATION SAFETY EDUCATION AND OCCUPATIONAL EXPOSURE

Radiation education and training are fundamental to creating a safe work environment for the physician, the surrounding staff, and the patient. Radiation emitted during fluoroscopic procedures is responsible for the greatest radiation dose for medical staff and poses the greatest long-term risk. Radiation protection techniques aim to minimize the harmful effects of ionizing radiation by reducing unnecessary radiation exposure.[9]

RADIATION SAFETY VARIATION

Overall, clinicians and medical staff who use fluoroscopic imaging have been shown to have a low adherence to radiation safety guidelines.[9] Enforcing radiation safety guidelines is a difficult process and often lacks formal training. In one evaluation of vascular surgery trainees, 45% had no formal radiation safety training, 74% were unaware of the radiation safety policy for pregnant females, 48% did not know their radiation safety officer's contact information, and 43% were unaware of the yearly acceptable levels of radiation exposure.[16]

There is great variability in radiation safety practices across laboratories, radiation safety courses, use of dosimeters, tracking annual personal radiation exposure, and established patient radiation dose thresholds. There is also significant variability in the use of the fluoro-store function, under-table shields, leaded glasses, ceiling lead glass, disposable radiation shields, and education regarding the adverse effects of radiation. Despite radiation safety being of concern to personnel, there are no agreed upon protection guidelines, highlighting several opportunities for standardization and improvement.[17] Most radiation exposure in medical settings arises from fluoroscopic imaging, which uses x-rays to obtain dynamic and cinematic functional imaging. Formal radiation protection training helps reduce radiation exposure to medical staff and patients. Of interest, it is important to note that individuals with experience remain in the most vulnerable group. This further strengthens the argument that radiological protection should be a subject of periodic training for medical personnel regardless of their position and length of service.[14]

THE AS LOW AS REASONABLY ACHIEVABLE (ALARA) PRINCIPLE

The AS LOW AS REASONABLY ACHIEVABLE (ALARA) principle is a concept that examines the justification, optimization, and limitation of radiation doses and is critical to limit radiation exposure.[18] Often, procedures that expose patients to relatively higher doses of radiation, for example, interventional vascular procedures, are medically necessary, and thus the benefits outweigh the risks. The ALARA principle, defined by the code of federal regulations, was created to ensure that all measures to reduce radiation exposure are taken, while acknowledging that radiation is an integral part of diagnosing and treating patients. Thus, the ALARA principle attempts to reduce both the patient and the operator dose. Any amount of radiation exposure will increase the risk of stochastic effects, and there is no specific threshold to predict whether or not malignancy will develop reliably.[9]

VASCULAR PROCEDURES AND RADIATION EXPOSURE

Different interventional procedures have substantial variability in radiation dose exposure. When evaluating use of fluoroscopy and dosages across multiple disciplines it has been demonstrated that vascular surgery has a high rate of exposure to radiation. Bundy et al. reported,[19] when evaluating the multiple disciplines using fluoroscopy, that vascular surgery had a high DAP by discipline (Figure 4-1). Furthermore, the study evaluated the doses and fluoroscopy time associated with the pocedures performed by vascular interventionalists. It can be seen (Figure 4-2) that arteriography, which is a mainstay of vascular practice, carries

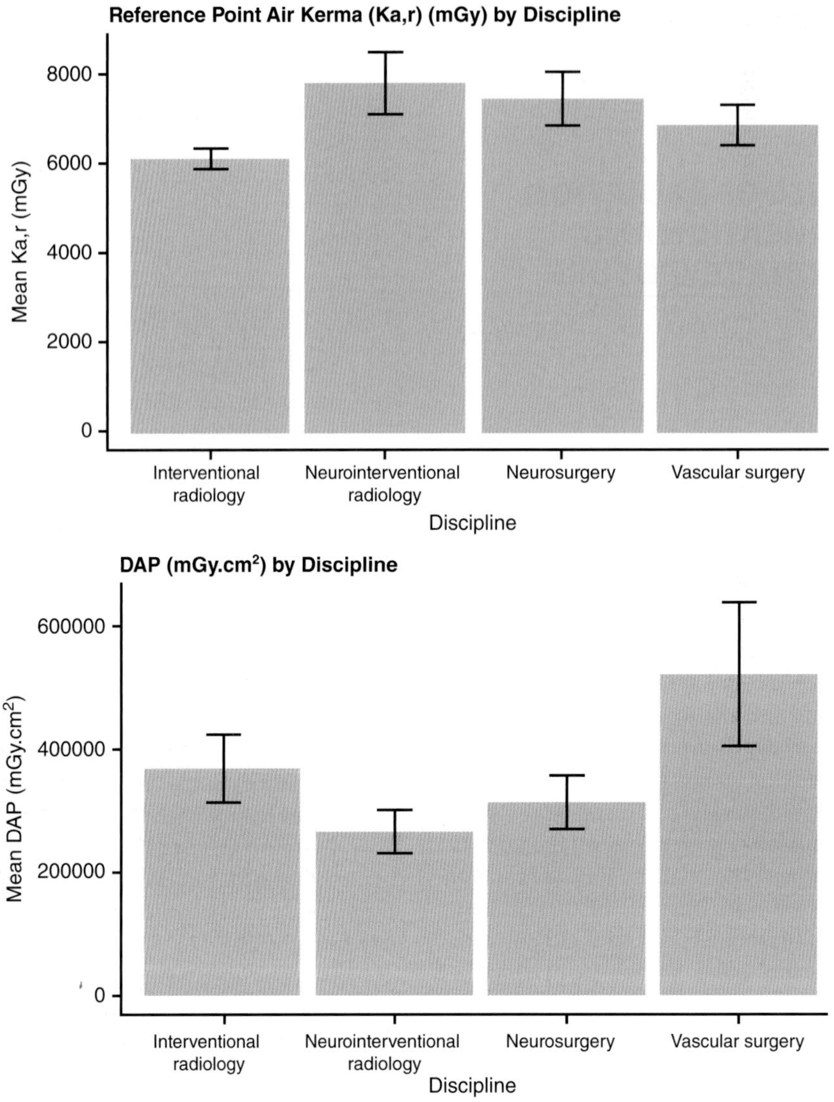

FIGURE 4-1 DAP, and RAK and standard deviation by medical discipline. DAP, dose area product, FT, fluoroscopy time, RAK, reference air kerma. (Adapted with permission from Bundy JJ, McCracken IW, Shin DS, et al. Fluoroscopically guided interventions with radiation doses exceeding 5000 mGy reference point air kerma: a dosimetric analysis of 89,549 interventional radiology, neurointerventional radiology, vascular surgery, and neurosurgery encounters. *CVIR Endovasc.* 2020;3(1):69.)

a large DAP which must be taken into consideration from both a patient and a provider standpoint during interventions for vascular surgery. Furthermore, endovascular aneurysm repair (EVAR) carries a lower DAP, which provides patient benefits, but one needs to be cognizant that the operator is close to the intensifier in each of these procedures and at an increased risk. Therefore, the DAP dose, in addition to the location of the operation, impacts the potential risk of radiation exposure.

Generally, radiation dose is higher on the left side of an operator's body, because the operator's left

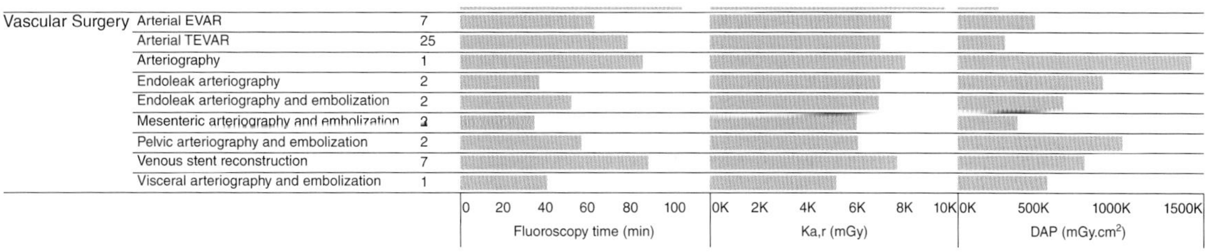

FIGURE 4-2 Mean FT, DAP, and KAR distribution by intervention type. DAP, dose area product, EVAR, endovascular aneurysm repair, FT, fluoroscopy time, KAR, reference point air kerma, TEVAR, thoracic endovascular aortic repair. (Adapted with permission from Bundy JJ, McCracken IW, Shin DS, et al. Fluoroscopically guided interventions with radiation doses exceeding 5000 mGy reference point air kerma: a dosimetric analysis of 89,549 interventional radiology, neurointerventional radiology, vascular surgery, and neurosurgery encounters. *CVIR Endovasc.* 2020;3(1):69.)

side is closer to the primary beam when standing at the patient's right side. The increased complexity of medical procedures appears to have offset dose reductions due to improvements in technology. Better standardization of dosimetric methods will facilitate future analyses aimed at determining how well medical radiation workers are being protected.[20] Stochastic and dose-response effects of radiation make any exposure a concern. Attempts to lessen exposures are worthwhile, with study results identifying a need for greater safety precaution education and adherence.[21] Surgeon education on the appropriate use of fluoroscopy improved operating practice, reduced patient radiation dose, and decreased the number of non-FEVAR cases that exceeded 6 Gy.[22]

OCCUPATIONAL EXPOSURE AND HEALTH RISK

Though there is a generalized understanding of the dangers of radiation regarding occupational exposure, variability of information among staff remains. The first evidence of increased risk of cancer with radiation exposure was a report of a 10-fold increase in leukemia noted in radiologists. Understandably, an entire field of radiation safety has grown out of attempts to reduce the risk of radiation exposure to health care workers.[23] Increased exposure to ionizing radiation is partially due to a lack of awareness to the effects of ionizing radiation, and lack of knowledge on the distribution and behavior of scattered radiation. One analysis evaluated the utility of simulators that incorporated data on scattered ionizing radiation to improve education and training regarding radiation safety, and found this to be an efficacious education method.[24] Simulators can be used to educate trainees in addition to experienced personnel on radiation safety.[24]

Andreassi et al. evaluated the prevalence of health problems among personnel staff working in interventional cardiology and correlated them with the length of occupational radiation exposure. Skin lesions, orthopedic illness, and cataract formation were all significantly higher in exposed versus non-exposed group, with a clear gradient unfavorable for physicians over technicians and nurses and for longer history of work (more than 16 years).[25] Health problems are more frequently observed in workers performing fluoroscopically guided cardiovascular procedures than in unexposed controls, raising the need to spread the culture of safety and decrease occupational exposure.[25] Other studies have demonstrated a higher risk in thyroid cancer formation. Zielinski et al.[26] published registry data for mortality and cancer incidence on a cohort of medical workers in Canada. This study also demonstrated an increase in the risk of all-cause mortality, cancer, thyroid cancer and cardiovascular disease with increasing radiation dose in the medical worker population.[26]

More clearly established are the risks of radiation and the risk of cataracts secondary to occupational radiation exposure. Ocular lens exposure to ionizing radiation can result in posterior lens opacities or cataracts. Data have increasingly indicated that lens sensitivity may be quite variable. Previously, the ICRP recommended an annual exposure limit of 150 (mSv) per year. This recommendation was reduced to an average annual exposure of 20 (mSv) per year averaged over five consecutive years with no one year to exceed 50 (mSv).[5] This was based on accumulating data in the cardiology literature suggesting that posterior cataract formation has a direct correlation with years of exposure. It should be noted that the use of leaded eyewear decreased the incidence of cataracts.[27] Interventionalists can also help mitigate these risks by following established radiation safety practices.[11] Compared with unexposed controls, Cath-lab staff had a higher prevalence of lens changes that may be attributable to ionizing radiation exposure. These findings are important due to the potential to progress to clinical symptoms.[17] Recent epidemiological studies have indicated that the threshold dose for the formation of lens opacities is lower than previously thought at 0.5 Gy for both acute and protracted exposures, again highlighting the need for further investigation of safety guidelines and importance of eye protection for interventionalists.[27]

Conversely, other studies have suggested that there is not a significant increase in risk related to occupational radiation exposure. Jartti et al.[28] examined physicians and radiation exposure, and found no obvious dose–response relationship for the overall cancer incidence; the study concluded that occupational exposure to medical radiation is not a strong risk factor for cancer among physicians.[28]

In summary, it is known that the risk of malignancy after low-dose x-ray exposure is directly proportional to the cumulative dose received.[11] Occupational exposure inherently carries increased risk, although this increase in cancer risk is likely small. Knowledge of specific types of cancer, especially thyroid, as well as inherent risk to the eyes and cataract formation, should be remembered by interventionalists, promoting thyroid shield utilization, lead eye protection, limited radiation exposure by following the ALARA guidelines, and knowledge of techniques to lower radiation exposure for physicians, staff, and patients.

RADIATION EXPOSURE AND VASCULAR SURGERY PATIENTS

Vascular surgery patients are frequently subjected to radiation exposure for preoperative imaging, endovascular procedures, and postoperative monitoring and maintenance. The number of CT scans performed annually in the United States has increased to over 70 million, leading to a large increase in patient radiation exposure.[29,30] As many as 70% of adults less than the age of 65 will undergo at least one imaging procedure associated with radiation within the next 3 years, with nearly one-fifth of the US population receiving a moderate-to-high effective dose of radiation.[31] Moreover, the number of endovascular procedures being performed has been rapidly increasing, leading to further increases in radiation exposure.[32] Many vascular surgery patients undergo numerous x-rays, CT scans, and angiograms during their treatment course. For example, a patient receiving an endovascular intervention may need a nuclear stress test and/or cardiac catheterization for preoperative cardiac optimization, then receive a CT angiogram or diagnostic angiogram for surgical planning, followed by the endovascular procedure, and then multiple CT scans for routine follow-up surveillance. Although medical imaging and endovascular procedures provide valuable diagnostic information and therapeutic outcomes, radiation exposure to vascular surgery patients is not without risks and adverse effects.

As introduced previously, radiation through deterministic and stochastic effects results in cellular damage, mutation, and/or death. High-dose radiation has been shown to be associated with predictable effects such as hematologic disorders, gastrointestinal symptoms, skin injuries, infertility, cataracts, and central nervous system syndrome.[5] Threshold doses for radiation skin injury are 2 Gy for erythema and 3 Gy for hair loss.[33] Chronic, low-dose, radiation exposure has been associated with unpredictable effects such as induction of cancer.[3] In fact, up to 2% of all cancers in the United States may be attributable to the radiation from CT studies alone.[34] Individual patients vary in their sensitivity to radiation based on the presence of coexisting disease such as, obesity, diabetes mellitus, and connective tissue disorders.[35] Complicating these calculations, different imaging and therapeutic modalities have varying levels of radiation exposure to the patient. Thus, the injury risks of radiation must be evaluated on a case-by-case basis.

Plain x-rays are one of the most performed imaging studies. Although a plain x-ray has a low radiation dose, one x-ray is equivalent to the amount of radiation exposure a person experiences from natural surroundings in 10 days.[1] More surprisingly, a CT scan delivers 500 times the radiation than a routine chest x-ray does, while a multiphase abdominal CT angiogram further doubles that amount.[33] The CT scan is one of the most common imaging modalities used for preoperative planning in patients with aortic aneurysms and the most common imaging modality for follow-up postoperatively.[36] Thus, the vascular surgeon needs to be aware of the radiation exposure to the patient from these routine scans. In fact, it is estimated that vascular surgeons are responsible for nearly 30% of CT scans performed that are believed to be unnecessary.[37] In addition to routine imaging, vascular surgery patients, who frequently have many comorbidities such as coronary artery disease, often undergo further invasive imaging for preoperative optimization. Coronary catheterization, a common diagnostic modality frequently required for vascular patients, can deliver radiation doses as high as the amount of radiation exposure one experiences from the natural surroundings in 15 years and equivalent to 3000 times more radiation than a routine AP chest x-ray.[37]

Although radiation exposure during endovascular procedures will be expanded upon later, it is important to consider here that patients who receive endovascular procedures are often committed to long-term follow-up. The invasive and non-invasive imaging needed for follow-up results in the most significant radiation exposure to the patient. For example, during an EVAR the patient is exposed to significant quantities of radiation; however, the preoperative and postoperative surveillance imaging represents the largest percentage of the radiation exposure total.

Imaging modalities are necessary to establish accurate diagnoses, stratify risk, aid in surgical planning, and guide postoperative follow up. While the benefits of imaging seem to greatly outweigh the risks of long-term radiation, concerns remain regarding the burden of radiation exposure to patients. It is imperative that vascular surgeons are aware of and are vigilantly monitoring the radiation exposure to their patients. Furthermore, the vascular surgeon must prudently use alternative imaging modalities and/or strategies to mitigate radiation exposure to their patients throughout their care.

Discussion of the risks of radiation use has taken a back seat to other more obvious and acute risks of procedures; however, with the increasing use of radiation for less invasive procedures, more injuries have been reported. These are most commonly deterministic effects on the skin.[9] Stochastic effects may be more pertinent to consider in children and young adult patients, particularly females.

RADIATION EXPOSURE DURING ENDOVASCULAR PROCEDURES

Although the number of endovascular procedures continues to grow worldwide, there has been no notable progress in the development of standardized guidelines for radiation practices. An abundance of literature outlining the acute and chronic risks posed to patients and surgical teams exists; however, complication rates remain high, while understanding of safety techniques remains low. Exposure dose is variable and dependent partially on patient-related factors such as body size, anatomic complexity but also on operator technique, procedure type, and the equipment used. Effective dosage may vary as much as 20-fold for patients and 200-fold for physicians based on procedure complexity and type.[38] Increasing complexity of the case leads to an increase in total fluoroscopy time, steeper imaging angles, and necessity for repeat procedures.

Angiograms, including coronary, mesenteric, and peripheral, are common diagnostic and therapeutic procedures in vascular surgery. Interventional coronary procedures have one of the highest average doses of radiation at 0.05 mSV per procedure. Radiation for an operator can amount to up to 60 mSV/yr, and the typical exposure of a patient with 10 minute of fluoroscopy time is estimated to be equal to up to 400 chest x-rays.[38] Regarding endovascular lower extremity peripheral interventions, atherectomy has the highest estimated skin doses (nearly 1.5 Gy) of all endovascular interventions.[39] A retrospective review of intraoperative fluoroscopic-guided vascular surgery procedures at a single institution from 2010 to 2017 found the highest doses of radiation were associated with embolization (mean of 932.5 mGy) and highest fluoroscopic time with atherectomies (mean of 44 minutes).[21] In regards to non-extremity endovascular interventions, PSDs are generally highest for renal interventions, followed by visceral interventions and embolization procedures.[35]

Endovascular aortic repair has become increasingly popular in recent years to treat abdominal and thoracic aortic aneurysms. Although it is less invasive compared with traditional open repair and associated with decreased morbidity and mortality in the early setting, it is associated with the risk of re-intervention and exposure to a significant amount of radiation. The most common cause of mortality after EVAR is cardiovascular events, followed by malignancy. However, it is not clear what percentage of patients develop cancer solely as a result of radiation secondary to EVAR.[40] The standard EVAR radiation dose to be up to 0.82 Gy, with median effective dose of 8.7 to 12.6 mSv.[20,41,42] The vascular surgeon must also take into account the type of endovascular intervention when considering radiation exposure. For example, due to the complexity of aortic interventions and frequent need for branched graft devices, endovascular interventions on the thoracic aortic have been shown to have more radiation than cases of the infra-renal aorta.[13,14] In addition to case complexity and risk for re-intervention, special care should be taken to patient positioning. Procedures carried out primarily in the left anterior oblique angulation have higher staff exposures of radiation than those in other angulations; this will be discussed further later in the chapter.[14] Occasionally, oblique views must be used, but the operator should remember that this may also substantially increase their radiation dose due to scatter if they are on the source side of the angled system.[43]

With the introduction and expansion of endovascular treatment methods, the vascular surgeon's responsibilities have expanded to supervising the radiation safety of the patient and surgical team. In addition to the operative procedure itself, the vascular specialist must be aware of the cumulative radiation given to patients as a result of postoperative imaging and follow-up. Follow-up CT imaging may represent up to 87% of the total radiation exposure after 1 year, 92% at 5 years, and 96% in a patient's lifetime.[44] The mean exposure from CTA surveillance one year after EVAR was 15 mSv, which is greater than the effective dose from the procedure itself.[45] Many patients undergoing EVAR require re-intervention for endoleaks, adding additional radiation exposure. It is generally thought that with every Sievert of radiation, there is a 5.5% increase for cancer induction. Thus, the amount of radiation for a patient undergoing EVAR, combined with repeat imaging, and possible re-intervention is substantial and critical for the vascular specialist to consider.

During endovascular procedures, the amount of radiation exposure is dependent on many variables that the vascular surgeon must be acutely aware of. Radiation exposure is determined by the patient's anatomy, safety habits of the surgeon, and the type of case being done. It is germane for the vascular surgeon to be aware of these factors, and specifically aware of cases involving high radiation use. These types of cases can be targeted for future improved dose reduction techniques or staged procedures.

TECHNIQUES TO LOWER RADIATION EXPOSURE DURING PROCEDURES

Reduction and mitigation of radiation exposure must be considered to safely and effectively complete vascular imaging and procedures. Vascular surgeons, trainees, and specialists need to be actively aware and involved in a conscious effort to minimize radiation exposure to their patients, themselves, and other team members. In order to do so, a comprehensive understanding of radiation sources, doses, and effects is essential. In addition, vascular surgeons must deliberately implement techniques and strategies to decrease radiation exposure to themselves and their patients. Special awareness of cases involving high radiation use is imperative. These types of cases can be targeted for future improved dose reduction techniques or staged procedures. Guidelines for safe radiation administration will help providers and patients understand and lessen the risks involved with radiation during imaging and procedures. Further reduction in radiation exposure can be accomplished by careful attention to imaging technique as well.[43]

LIMITING RADIATION EXPOSURE TO THE PATIENT

Limiting radiation exposure to the patient is a primary responsibility of the physician performing any procedure and/or prescribing any imaging study. This begins with proper clinical judgment including a complete patient history, careful patient selection, and meticulous procedural planning. Proper selection of patients should include attention to the patient's weight and age, proposed target of radiation, procedural type, pregnancy status, and prior radiation exposures. In addition, when planning the procedure, the physician should take into consideration all the prior imaging available to him or her. The risks associated with radiation should be included in the procedural consent, and intraprocedural dose monitoring should be included and documented in the medical record.

The benefit of the radiation exposure should outweigh the negative effects. Radiation protection and utilization should be deliberately optimized. When planning radiation exposure, the total dose to an individual should not exceed recommended dose limits. Every effort should be made to limit the exposure to the patient and physician while maintaining the quality of the image and thus the safety and efficiency of the study or intervention.[46] This includes minimizing the exposure pedal and saving images when possible. Although it provides high-quality imaging, digital subtraction angiography (DSA) requires additional radiation when compared with standard fluoroscopy and thus should be limited when possible.[47] In addition, other methods of visualization such as ultrasound should be utilized when appropriate and feasible.

SKIN DAMAGE TO THE PATIENT

The use of fluoroscopy associate with image capture can induce severe skin damage or changes (Table 4-1). Ionizing radiation can cause nonsymptomatic and symptomatic skin reactions that can be the result of lengthy fluoroscopic procedures.[5] Erythema and skin peeling can occur within a week followed by permanent change in skin color or development of tissue necrosis. To minimize the incident of radiation exposure complications, body parts that do not need to be visualized should not be in the radiation beam and moved out of the field. Further reductions can also be achieved by the appropriate use of combination pulse fluoroscopy and minimizing use of magnification. The time to develop these effects after exposure varies from 1 week for skin changes to 20 years for cataract development.

IMAGING EQUIPMENT TECHNIQUES TO LOWER RADIATION EXPOSURE

A complete understanding of the imaging equipment is essential to reduce radiation exposure. Fluoroscopy

TABLE 4-1 Threshold Levels for Deterministic Effects of Radiation.[6,8,27]

Skin Dose (Gy)	Expected Injury Grade	Prompt/Early < 8 weeks	Midterm 6-52 weeks	Long Term >40 weeks
2-5	1	Erythema/Epilation	Recovery	No effects
5-10	1-2	Erythema/Epilation	Prolonged erythema, permanent epilation	Dermal atrophy, induration
>10	2-4	Erythema, epilation, edema, ulceration, desquamation	Epilation, atrophy, necrosis, ulceration	Talangiectasia, induration

Data from Stecker MS, Balter S, Towbin RB, et al. Guidelines for patient radiation dose management. *J Vasc Interv Radiol*. 2009;20(7 Suppl):S263-S273.

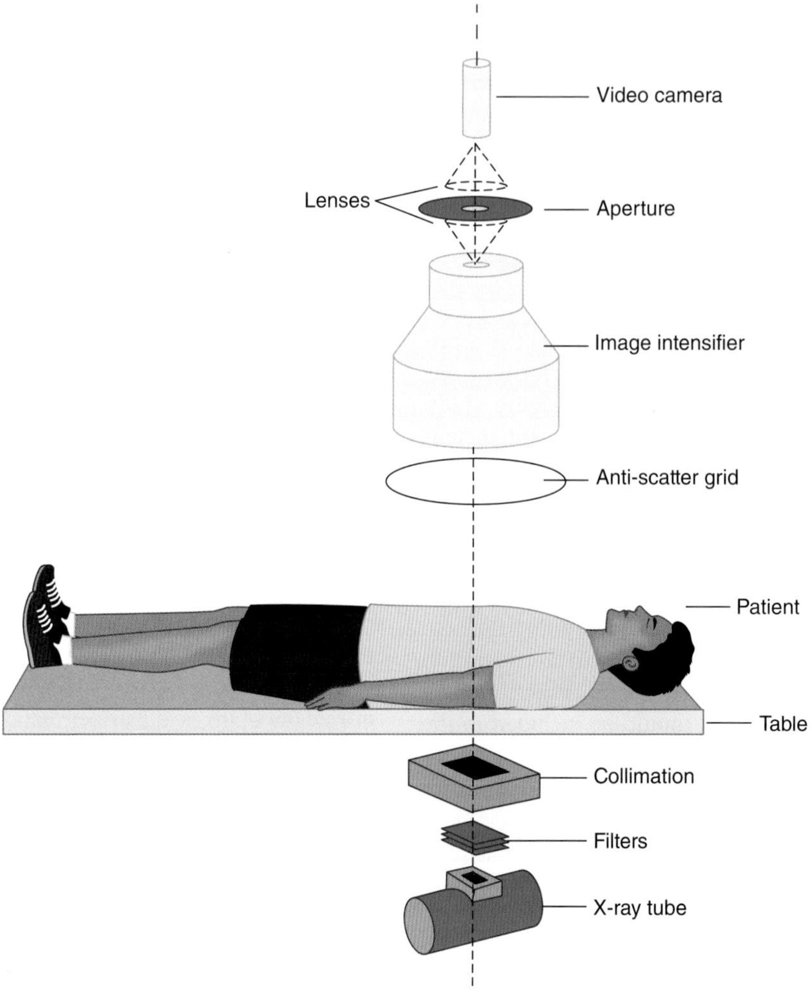

FIGURE 4-3 Components of fluoroscopy equipment.

is most commonly completed with a C-arm, which consists of an x-ray source, collimator, image intensifier, and detector (Figure 4-3). During fluoroscopy, proper positioning of the C-arm, collimation, and pulsed fluoroscopy (PF) can be utilized to decrease radiation exposure. The image intensifier (II) should be positioned as close to the patient as possible, while the x-ray tube should be as far from the patient as possible, lowering exposure and increasing image quality (Figure 4-4).[12] The image intensifier should be as close to the patient as possible to minimize the object–image distance and reduce radiation dose because it reduces beam intensity as well as scatter. Collimation refers to creating parallel radiation rays, resulting in less divergence and minimal dispersion, thus forming the smallest field of view possible. Because the radiation dose is dependent on the x-ray field size, restricting the field allows for lower doses of radiation. Although the disadvantage of collimation is a fractional reduction in the field of view, the exposure doses to surgeons are reduced by approximately 35% while the image quality is maintained.[48] Collimation should be used regularly to avoid large dose of radiation to the patient and operator whenever possible. PF is an additional method to reduce total radiation doses. During PF, the x-ray beam is emitted in short

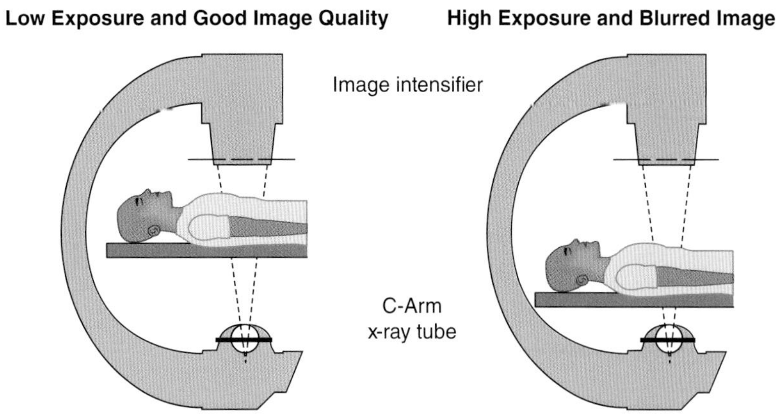

FIGURE 4-4 Positioning of image intensifier (II) to lower exposure. (Reproduced with permission from Mitchell EL, Furey P. Prevention of radiation injury from medical imaging. *J Vasc Surg*. 2011;53(Suppl 1):22S-27S.)

pulses rather than continuously. The digital images can be displayed at a constant frame rate to compensate for loss of resolution and obtain a smooth image. With a frame rate of 7.5 images/s, produced images are reduced by 90% compared with continuous mode, with an equal reduction in the effective dose.[49]

Other simple techniques can also be utilized to decrease radiation and obtain ALARA. Positioning the patient can be done without fluoroscopy, and the pedal can be tapped only to verify positioning. Furthermore, magnification can be reduced. Electronic magnification uses the image intensifier or flat panel detector to enlarge the field of view and is set by the operator to brighten and sharpen the image. Magnification can also be achieved by geometric magnification which is obtained by moving the II away from the patient, but this increases the radiation exposure.[4] Magnification increases image sharpness with increased radiation dose, so magnification should be used sparingly. Radiation exposure can be minimized by limiting magnification and refraining from geometric magnification. Additionally, many of the imaging systems currently used have a low-dose setting designed to reduce skin dose without impairment of the image quality.[50]

Avoiding redundant studies is essential, as repeating studies results in increased total radiation exposure. Additionally, using hybrid angiography suites with ceiling-mounted imaging systems can result in less radiation exposure to the patient and the operator than exposure from portable C-arms. Deliberate attention should be given to the type and number of images acquired during fluoroscopy. Varying imaging techniques results in different radiation exposure to members of an endovascular surgery team. Knowledge of the variable intensity of radiation exposure may allow modification of the technique to minimize radiation exposure to the team while providing suitable imaging.[51] Lead shielding will also decrease the risk to the operator and personnel but not the patient and should be utilized for all interventional procedures using fluoroscopy.[25]

An additional responsibility of the vascular surgeon is to limit the radiation exposure to themselves and the surgical team. By following the ALARA principle, the vascular surgeon must first and foremost minimize radiation amount and time. Additionally, the vascular surgeon must be familiar with and utilize the concepts of the inverse square law. The inverse square law states that radiation exposure is inversely proportional to the square of the distance from the radiation source, meaning that an operator receives more radiation exposure when standing closer to the radiation source. Radiation exposure to the operator is largely due to scattered radiation that results from dispersion of the beam from its intended path. Scatter decreases with the square of the distance from the source as stated by the inverse square law. Thus, it is imperative that the operator increases his or her distance from the source in order to minimize his/her exposure.[12]

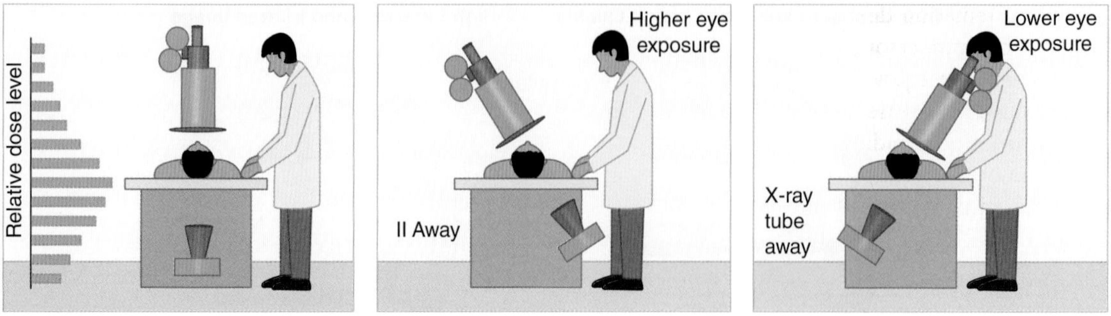

FIGURE 4-5 Positioning of image intensifier (II) and exposure.

Standing two steps behind the c-arm can decrease exposure of the operator by nearly 80%.[15] In fact, an operator positioned three feet from the table will receive 0.1% of the radiation dose emitted to the patient. As stated previously, use of collimation and PF can also reduce radiation exposure to the operator and surgical team by reducing scatter and overall radiation dosage, respectively. Higher scatter results when the II is tilted away from the operator. Thus, the operator should always work on the side of the table ipsilateral to the II (Figure 4-5). Studies comparing imaging angles during fluoroscopy have shown that direct AP shots result in the least exposure to the user, while the 90 degree lateral result in the greatest operator exposure.[52] Thus, attention should be made to have the least amount of obliquity when possible.

The use of oblique views also increases the tissue path for the x-ray beam, ultimately requiring a higher radiation dose to maintain a constant image brightness. The use of steeply angled projections has the same effect as obesity. Cranio-caudal angulation is known for increasing radiation doses due to increased source-to-skin distance. Collimation should always be used with magnification to minimize the skin dose outside the field of interest.[12]

PROTECTIVE EQUIPMENT AND GARMENTS

Protective garments are mandatory for all staff present during fluoroscopic procedures. Lead aprons, which are generally available in 0.5- and 0.25-mm thickness, should be donned by all staff in the fluoroscopy suite. A lead apron with a 0.5-mm thickness will attenuate 98% to 99.5% of radiation dose, while 0.25-mm thickness will attenuate 96% of the dose.[25] Careful consideration of lead apron design should be taken into account when considering complete coverage of the body. Two-part aprons, consisting of a vest and kilt, provide additional coverage of the operators back. Lead aprons must be screened and checked annually to inspect for damage or deterioration which can result with increased use, improper handling, or improper storage.

Current lead aprons are composed of metal alloy to keep them light-weight for user comfort and more efficient in blocking x-rays. Lead apron can crack and break down when handled incorrectly. This includes any action that allows them to fold or crease. Guidelines recommend that they be properly hung on either a rack or a hanger. The Joint Commission recommends annual maintenance with a visual and tactile inspection for wear and tear and, if in question, fluoroscopy to look for holes and cracks. The lead should be discarded based on the size and location of a defect: >15 mm^2 on a critical organ area (chest, pelvis); >670 mm^2 along a seam, overlapped areas, or back; or >11 mm^2 on the thyroid shield.[53] A thyroid collar or shield is currently recommended for staff under the age of 40 and for those with neck radiation exposure of >4 mSv/month, and is mandatory for many institutions.[54]

Leaded glasses are highly recommended and can reduce radiation to the operator's eye by 90%.[55] Lead-lined gloves can help reduce exposure and can reduce radiation doses by up to 30%; however, they may be cumbersome to the operator. The use of leaded or lead equivalent surgical caps have not demonstrated a decrease of operator brain dose since the vast majority of radiation to the operator's head during a fluoroscopically guided intervention is from scatter radiation to the neck and face.[56]

FLUOROSCOPY TIME AND DOSIMETERS

To monitor radiation doses, operators should be constantly aware of fluoroscopy time and should be notified when total fluoroscopy time has approached 30 minutes with regular interval updates thereafter. Fluoroscopy time should be included in the medical record and documented according to state and federal guidelines. Additionally, dosimeters should be donned by all the personnel working in the fluoroscopy unit. Dosimeters include film badges, thermoluminescent dosimetry composed of small lithium fluoride or calcium fluoride crystals, and optically stimulated luminescent dosimeters which utilize laser monitors to record radiation.[57] A dosimeter should be assigned to a single individual and should not be shared. Dosimetry badges should be worn at the level of the waist and on the collar and worn outside of any leaded shielding. Ring badges are also available and can be worn on the hand which is most likely to be exposed (most often the left hand which is used to stabilize sheaths closer to the x-ray beam). Dosimeters can be assigned to monitor a period of up to 3 months, but if exposure reaches 10% of any of the limits, they must be exchanged monthly.[24]

Vascular surgeons must be aware of and formally educated in techniques to reduce radiation doses to themselves and their patients during fluoroscopy. Using as low as reasonably achievable radiation doses should be carefully considered and planned. DSA imaging should be kept to a minimum, all imaging runs should be limited and saved. Proper use of the C-arm, and usage of hybrid rooms if available, can greatly reduce radiation exposure. All operators should be educated on proper use of protective leading, shielding techniques, and dosimeters. Safety checklists (Table 4-2) should be regularly utilized for thoughtful methods to reduce radiation exposure.

TABLE 4-2 Radiation Safety Checklist

- Obtain patient history about previous radiation exposure
- Ensure operators and personnel wear well-fitted lead aprons, thyroid shields, and protective leaded eye wear
- Position hanging table shields and overhead lead shields prior to procedure
- Use ultrasound imaging when possible
- Position the image intensifier as close to the patient as practicable
- For C-arm type fluoroscopy units, maximize distance from the radiation source
- Use the exposure pedal sparingly
- Use pulsed rather than continuous fluoroscopy when possible, and with as low a pulse as possible
- Review and save anatomy with last image hold rather than with live fluoroscopy when possible
- Position and collimate with fluoroscopy off, tapping on the pedal to check position
- Collimate tightly, exclude eyes, thyroid, breast, and gonads, when possible
- Minimize use of electronic magnification; use digital zoom whenever possible
- Adjust acquisition parameters to achieve lowest dose necessary to accomplish procedure: use lowest dose protocol possible for patient size, lower frame rate, minimize magnification, reduce length of run
- Operator and personnel hands out of beam
- Use power injector or extension tubing if hand-injecting
- Move personnel away from table or behind protective shields during acquisitions
- Minimize overlap of fields on subsequent acquisitions
- Plan and communicate in advance the number and timing of acquisitions, contrast parameters, patient positioning, and suspension of respiration with radiology and sedation team to minimize improper or unneeded runs
- Acknowledge fluoroscopy timing alerts during procedure
- After procedure: record and review dose
- Ensure appropriate monitoring of dosimeters
- Arrange for appropriate follow-up and discharge instructions for high-dose procedures

Reproduced with permission from Mitchell EL, Furey P. Prevention of radiation injury from medical imaging. *J Vasc Surg.* 2011;53(Suppl 1): 22S-27S.

SPECIAL CONSIDERATIONS

PREGNANCY

The evolution of endovascular surgery has increased the vascular surgeon's exposure to radiation, raising concern for female vascular interventionalists. There is compelling interest to establish radiation safety guidelines for the pregnant trainee or vascular surgeon.[58] Surveys conducted by Shaw et al. aimed at evaluation of radiation exposure during pregnancy have demonstrated that 68% of trainees and 82% of faculty performed endovascular procedures during pregnancy, but only 42% of trainees and 50% of faculty wore a fetal badge.[58] Consideration should be given at the professional society leadership level to develop and support radiation safety guidelines for all vascular surgeons.[58]

A study evaluating pregnant women in the workplace concerning occupational radiation exposure found that only 3.2% of institutions required that workplace modifications be implemented for the worker.[59] The implementation of a declared pregnancy and fetal assessment program, careful planning, an understanding of the risks, and minimization of radiation dose by employing appropriate radiation safety measures as needed can allow medical staff to perform procedures and normal activities without incurring significant risks to the conceptus, or significant interruptions of job activities for most medical workers.[59]

Radiation risks apply to both the mother and the fetus. They depend on the radiation dose and gestational age. For most x-ray imaging, the dose to the fetus is from scattered radiation, as the fetus can be kept out of the direct x-ray beam. Most pregnant interventionalists continue to practice while pregnant. Pregnancy and fetal outcomes parallel that of the general population when matched for demographics. However, perceptions of impact of pregnancy on work lives of colleagues vary notably.[60,61] The fetus is most sensitive to the effects of radiation between weeks 8 and 15. Steps to reduce radiation exposure to the fetus include: reducing time and increasing distance from the radiation source and the use of wrap-around lead aprons. Pregnant operators and trainees should wear maternity aprons with a lead equivalent of 1.00 mm, with double-lead inserts over the pelvis, which decrease dose by a factor of nearly 100 compared to standard aprons.[62] Consistent radiation protection practices can protect the fetus, allowing pregnant operators and staff to pursue active careers without exposing their offspring to radiation risk. If unavailable, standard lead aprons also provide sufficient shielding to protect the embryo and fetus from typical exposures to operators and staff during fluoroscopically guided interventional procedures.[11] Diligent monitoring and radiation safety practices permit pregnant interventionalists and ancillary staff to maintain fetal doses well below published guidelines.[8] The National Council on Radiation Protection and Measurements (NCRP) recommends that pregnant operators wear two dosimeters, one at the collar outside the apron and one under the apron at the abdomen to estimate fetal exposure. The NCRP recommends a limit of 5 mSv for the entire pregnancy.[8]

Studies have shown that fetal risk is negligible when using appropriate shielding and radiation safety practices.[8] With best radiation safety practices, most pregnant operators have little risk of exposure that will exceed the allowable limits considered safe in pregnancy. The occupational radiation dose limits during the 9 months of pregnancy that are considered safe are 500 mrem during the entire pregnancy or 50 mrem/month. This translates to 100 to 1000 fluoroscopic examinations of 5 minutes each per gestational month.[62]

CARBON DIOXIDE (CO_2) ANGIOGRAPHY

Carbon dioxide (CO_2) is odorless, colorless, and slightly acidic. Its angiography is dependent on forming a bubble of gas which fills the arterial tree and displaces the blood causing a low-density image which contrasts to the surrounding tissue. Injection systems must have one-way valves to ensure that while loading the gas into the syringe, or injecting it into the patient, there is no risk for air contamination after flushing it several times. Intra-arterial CO_2 is contraindicated above the diaphragm due to the risk of stroke related to vapor lock in the cerebrovascular arteries.[63] Generally, single, large gas bubbles are best and preferably done using a single end-hole catheters, rather than many small bubbles when using a multihole catheter.[63]

Vapor lock can occur with injection of an excessive volume of CO_2 or insufficient spacing of repeated large-volume injections. Cardiac or pulmonary artery vapor lock may occur when CO_2 is used in percutaneous venography or venous interventions mimicking pulmonary embolism. Initial management includes placing the patient in the left lateral decubitus and Trendelenburg position. If that does not relieve the symptoms, catheter aspiration of the gas bubble in the pulmonary artery can be considered.[63]

CO_2 imaging requires specific parameters, including a high mA (60-90)/low kV (50-70) technique, pulse width of 60 milliseconds, and digital subtraction.[63] As previously stated, DSA leads to higher radiation exposure. Furthermore, CO_2 angiography is susceptible to motion artifact and often requires multiple injections, thus increasing radiation exposure to both the operator and the patient.[63] However, studies comparing radiation exposure between CO_2 and conventional angiography are limited.

ALTERNATIVE IMAGING

Alternative imaging methods may also be utilized to lower the contrast utilized as well as the radiation during interventional procedures. Several studies have been performed evaluating intravascular ultrasound (IVUS) as well as fusion imaging to lower the contrast as well as radiation dose during vascular procedures. Intraoperatively, the use of IVUS is recommended as an alternative or adjunct to angiography because of its ability to decrease the volume of contrast injected as well as the radiation exposure. Compared with standard angiography-assisted EVAR, IVUS was found to significantly reduce the contrast media, fluoroscopy time, and radiation dose while preserving endograft deployment efficiency.[64] Fusion imaging may also be considered to lower the radiation dose as well as the contrast utilized during endovascular revascularization. It has proved feasible and can significantly reduce radiation and contrast medium exposure during endovascular revascularization.[65] Other imaging modalities to consider are intravenous magnetic resonance imaging, magnetic resonance angiography, vascular positron emission tomography, optical coherence tomography, near infrared spectroscopy, and fractional flow reserve. Further studies are needed to assess the value of alternative imaging modalities in regards to radiation exposure.

PATIENT RADIATION EDUCATION AND CONSENT

Protection of patients from excessive medical radiation has become a high priority in health care.[43] Patients should be counseled regarding the potential for use of significant amounts of radiation when complicated procedures are planned and should be included as part of the process of obtaining informed consent. Stecker et al. stress the concept that radiation reduction begins before the procedure.[43] This includes appropriate preprocedural planning for fluoroscopy to be used and thoughtful planning on ways to lower exposure. If significant radiation is used, patients should be alerted to have appropriate follow-up.[43] Medical radiological exposure is frequently underestimated and rarely explained to patients. For example, only 32% of interventionalists inform patients about the long-term potential risks of ionizing radiation. With a clear understanding of radiological exposure and proper communication, clinicians need to accurately inform patients.[66] Authors have suggested that actions to protect patients include development of appropriateness criteria/referral guidelines by professional societies for patients who require recurrent imaging studies, development of equipment with lower radiation doses, and development of policies by risk management organizations to enhance patient radiation safety.[67]

RADIATION EXPOSURE GUIDELINES

A principal step to optimize safe use of radiation is education of hospital staff, physicians, and administrators on radiation best practices. Each institution, their radiation safety department, and quality assurance personnel are responsible for educating and enforcing safe radiation practices. Simple interventions have been shown to play a large role in decreasing radiation doses. For example, a 20-minute video shown to physicians was found to reduce median fluoroscopy time by 30% to 50%.[68] Following the ALARA principles is critical with deliberate justification, optimization, and adherence to dose limits. Institutional protocols should be developed carefully and should incorporate principles from guideline statements on radiation safety.

Multiple organizations and agencies have been involved in addressing the issue of medical radiation exposure to minimize radiation exposures from medical imaging.[13] Detailed recommendations for institutional protocols and practices aimed at radiation safety have been created.[13] These reports suggest that facilities should first evaluate their own performance with respect to radiation safety, and then ensure health care professionals are optimally trained on radiation safety and utilize dose information in quality assurance programs to identify areas of improvement. It is recommended that facilities use diagnostic reference levels and submit these to national registries. Institutions should ensure that they have hired proper staff including quality assurance officers, purchase proper personal protective equipment and radiation safe barriers, and implement procedures in place to limit doses. Additionally, the report specifies that workers should declare their pregnancy status, in order to ensure safe doses to the fetus, and that all staff working in fluoroscopic procedure and/or operating rooms should wear dosimeters. Furthermore, facility procedures for fluoroscopy and computed tomography should specify that these modalities can deliver significant radiation doses even when used properly during the consent process. Each institution should ensure that every staff member who operates fluoroscopic procedures be trained in safe use and receive additional training for high-risk procedures. Moreover, each facility should establish procedures to avoid inadvertent or unapproved imaging or modification of imaging protocols.

The Society of Interventional Radiology (SIR) has set forth recommendations regarding radiation dose management related to interventional radiologic procedures. These guidelines defined a significant radiation dose threshold for patients as any of the following: PSD > 2000 mGy, DAP > 500 Gy · cm², or fluoroscopy time > 60 minutes (Table 4-3).[6]

TABLE 4-3 Thresholds for Patient Follow-up

Parameter	Threshold
Peak skin dose	3000 mGy
Reference point air kerma	5000 mGy
Kerma-area-product	500 Gy · cm²
Fluoroscopy time	60 min

Reproduced with permission from Stecker MS, Balter S, Towbin RB, et al. Guidelines for patient radiation dose management. *J Vasc Interv Radiol.* 2009;20(Suppl 7):S263-273.

In addition to institutional guidelines, patient- and procedure-specific guidelines have been proposed. The ICRP proposed dose recommendations to limit radiation exposure to general members of the public, with a limitation to 1 mSv per year (Table 4-4).[9] For radiation workers, the dose limit is recommended to be 20 mSv per year on average and is not to exceed 50 mSv in a single year. The FDA has guidelines requiring dose monitoring for fluoroscopy via reporting fluoroscopy times, although some authors suggest that this provides minimal information regarding x-ray field size or position and does not account for differences in equipment, technique, or patient size.[69]

The average background radiation is 2 to 4 mSv per year. The ICRP recommends <20 mSv whole body effective dose per year for radiation workers. Specific organs, such as eyes (<20 mSv) and the pregnant uterus (1 mSv), have separate dose recommendations.[5] For reference, 20 mSv/year roughly equates to 2 to 3 abdominal and pelvic computed tomography (CT) scans or 7 to 9 years of background radiation. Exposure surpassing this threshold averaged over 5 years has been associated with a 1 in 1000 lifetime risk of fatal cancer.[26]

The Joint Commission added that a reviewable sentinel event include any incident with: a cumulative dose exceeding 15 Gy to a single field, any delivery of radiotherapy to the wrong body region, or dose more than 25% above the planned radiotherapy dose. Often, the consequences of increased radiation do not occur until months or years after the event, which can lead to misdiagnosis and delays in care. The Joint

TABLE 4-4 ICRP Dose Recommendations

Type of Dose Limit	Limit on Dose from Occupational Exposure	Limit on Dose from Public Exposure
Effective dose	20 mSv/yr, averaged over defined 5-year periods, with no single year exceeding 50 mSv	1 mSv/yr
Effective dose	Once employee declares pregnancy, the dose to embryo/fetus should not exceed 1 mSv during remainder of pregnancy	-
Equivalent dose: lens of the eye	20 mSv/yr, averaged over defined 5-year periods, with no single year exceeding 50 mSv	15 mSv/yr
Equivalent dose: skin	500 mSv/yr	50 mSv/yr
Equivalent dose: Hands and feet	500 mSv/yr	-

From Frane N, Bitterman A. Radiation Safety and Protection. 2022 May 23. In: StatPearls [Internet]. Treasure Island (FL): StatPearls Publishing; 2022 Jan–. Reproduced with permission from Nicholas Frane, DO.

Commission recommends that doses from previous procedures to the same body area be summed over a 6- to 12-month period. Interventional procedures with a skin dose >15 Gy to a single skin field over a period of 6 months to 1 year is considered a reviewable sentinel event.[5,8]

CONCLUSIONS

Radiation safety is an important concept for the vascular specialist to understand and practice. It is a broad area which includes knowledge of the equipment, understanding of radiation, appreciating the dangers of radiation, and the key concepts to protect the physician, staff, and patient from exposure. Adherence to ALARA principles, as well as understanding methods to lower radiation exposure, while performing procedures is paramount to safety. Being cognizant of which procedures carry the highest rate of radiation exposure is also imperative for the vascular surgical practitioner. With a combination of radiation safety education, planned thoughtfulness of procedures, and critical awareness radiation exposure, procedures requiring radiation can be performed in a safe and effective manner while lowering the overall risk for the operator, the staff, and the patient. Paying attention to these factors must be considered prior to performing a procedure, during the procedure, and follow-up of the patient. Future research is needed on lowering radiation exposure through improved equipment, increased information and education for patients and staff regarding radiation safety, and strict adherence to key technical concepts to lower occupational exposures.

ACKNOWLEDGMENTS

We would like to thank Maraya Camazine for assistance in proofreading the final chapter.

REFERENCES

1. Brix G, Nekolla E, Griebel J. Radiation exposure of patients from diagnostic and interventional X-ray procedures. Facts, assessment and trends. *Radiologe*. 2005;45(4):340-349.
2. Frane N, Megas A, Stapleton E, Ganz M, Bitterman AD. Radiation exposure in orthopaedics. *JBJS Rev*. 2020;8(1):e0060.
3. Hamada N, Fujimichi Y. Classification of radiation effects for dose limitation purposes: history, current situation and future prospects. *J Radiat Res*. 2014;55(4):629-640.
4. Brown KR, Rzucidlo E. Acute and chronic radiation injury. *J Vasc Surg*. 2011;53(Suppl 1):15S-21S.
5. ICRP Publication 105. Radiation protection in medicine. *Ann ICRP*. 2007;37(6):1-63.
6. Stecker MS, Balter S, Towbin RB, et al. Guidelines for patient radiation dose management. *J Vasc Interv Radiol*. 2009;20(Suppl 7):S263-273.
7. Williams MC, Stewart C, Weir NW, Newby DE. Using radiation safely in cardiology: what imagers need to know. *Heart*. 2019;105(10):798-806.
8. National Council on Radiation Protection and Measurements. *Radiation Dose Management for Fluoroscopically Guided Interventional Medical*

Procedures. Bethesda, MD: National Council on Radiation Protection and Measurements; 2011.
9. Frane N, Bitterman A. Radiation safety and protection. In: *StatPearls*. Treasure Island, FL: StatPearls; 2020.
10. Smans K, Struelens L, Hoornaert MT, et al. A study of the correlation between dose area product and effective dose in vascular radiology. *Radiat Prot Dosimetry*. 2008;130(3):300-308.
11. Stahl CM, Meisinger QC, Andre MP, Kinney TB, Newton IG. Radiation risk to the fluoroscopy operator and staff. *AJR Am J Roentgenol*. 2016;207(4):737-744.
12. Mitchell EL, Furey P. Prevention of radiation injury from medical imaging. *J Vasc Surg*. 2011;53(Suppl 1): 22S-27S.
13. Gebrewold B. Assessment of current radiation protection practices to minimize radiation exposures from medical imaging. *J Nucl Med*. 2017:58.
14. Szarmacha A, Piskunowicz M, Swieton D, et al. Radiation safety awareness among medical staff. *Pol J Radiol*. 2015;80:57-61.
15. Chang YJ, Kim AN, Oh IS, Woo NS, Kim HK, Kim JH. The radiation exposure of radiographer related to the location in c-arm fluoroscopy-guided pain interventions. *Korean J Pain*. 2014;27(2):162-167.
16. Bordoli SJ, Carsten CG 3rd, Cull DL, Johnson BL, Taylor SM. Radiation safety education in vascular surgery training. *J Vasc Surg*. 2014;59(3):860-864.
17. Menon R, Karatasakis A, Patel S, et al. Radiation safety in the catheterization laboratory: current perspectives and practices. *J Invasive Cardiol*. 2018;30(8):296-300.
18. Willis CE, Slovis TL. The ALARA concept in radiographic dose reduction. *Radiol Technol*. 2004;76(2): 150-152.
19. Bundy JJ, McCracken IW, Shin DS, et al. Fluoroscopically-guided interventions with radiation doses exceeding 5000 mGy reference point air kerma: a dosimetric analysis of 89,549 interventional radiology, neurointerventional radiology, vascular surgery, and neurosurgery encounters. *CVIR Endovasc*. 2020;3(1):69.
20. Kim KP, Miller DL, Balter S, et al. Occupational radiation doses to operators performing cardiac catheterization procedures. *Health Phys*. 2008;94(3):211-227.
21. Sidwell RA, Smith HL, Halsey JP, McFarlane MJ. Surgical resident radiation knowledge, attitudes, practices, and exposures. *J Surg Educ*. 2016;73(6): 1032-1038.
22. Kirkwood ML, Arbique GM, Guild JB, et al. Surgeon education decreases radiation dose in complex endovascular procedures and improves patient safety. *J Vasc Surg*. 2013;58(3):715-721.
23. Stewart A. Detecting the health risks of radiation. *Med Confl Surviv*. 1999;15(2):138-148.
24. Katz A, Shtub A, Solomonica A, Poliakov A, Roguin A. Simulator training to minimize ionizing radiation exposure in the catheterization laboratory. *Int J Cardiovasc Imaging*. 2017;33(3):303-310.
25. Andreassi MG, Piccaluga E, Guagliumi G, Del Greco M, Gaita F, Picano E. Occupational health risks in cardiac catheterization laboratory workers. *Circ Cardiovasc Interv*. 2016;9(4):e003273.
26. Zielinski JM, Garner MJ, Band PR, et al. Health outcomes of low-dose ionizing radiation exposure among medical workers: a cohort study of the Canadian national dose registry of radiation workers. *Int J Occup Med Environ Health*. 2009;22(2):149-156.
27. Authors on behalf of I, Stewart FA, Akleyev AV, et al. ICRP publication 118: ICRP statement on tissue reactions and early and late effects of radiation in normal tissues and organs—threshold doses for tissue reactions in a radiation protection context. *Ann ICRP*. 2012;41(1-2):1-322.
28. Jartti P, Pukkala E, Uitti J, Auvinen A. Cancer incidence among physicians occupationally exposed to ionizing radiation in Finland. *Scand J Work Environ Health*. 2006;32(5):368-373.
29. Smith-Bindman R, Lipson J, Marcus R, et al. Radiation dose associated with common computed tomography examinations and the associated lifetime attributable risk of cancer. *Arch Intern Med*. 2009;169(22): 2078-2086.
30. Smith-Bindman R, Miglioretti DL, Larson EB. Rising use of diagnostic medical imaging in a large integrated health system. *Health Affair*. 2008;27(6):1491-1502.
31. Fazel R, Krumholz HM, Wang Y, et al. Exposure to low-dose ionizing radiation from medical imaging procedures. *N Engl J Med*. 2009;361(9):849-857.
32. Goodney PP, Beck AW, Nagle J, Welch HG, Zwolak RM. National trends in lower extremity bypass surgery, endovascular interventions, and major amputations. *J Vasc Surg*. 2009;50(1):54-60.
33. Walsh SR, Cousins C, Tang TY, Gaunt ME, Boyle JR. Ionizing radiation in endovascular interventions. *J Endovasc Ther*. 2008;15(6):680-687.
34. Brenner DJ, Hall EJ. Computed tomography: an increasing source of radiation exposure. *N Engl J Med*. 2007;357(22):2277-2284.
35. Miller DL, Balter S, Noonan PT, Georgia JD. Minimizing radiation-induced skin injury in interventional radiology procedures. *Radiology*. 2002;225(2):329-336.
36. Chaikof EL, Dalman RL, Eskandari MK, et al. The Society for vascular surgery practice guidelines on the

care of patients with an abdominal aortic aneurysm. *J Vasc Surg*. 2018;67(1):2-77 e72.
37. Zhou W. Radiation exposure of vascular surgery patients beyond endovascular procedures. *J Vasc Surg*. 2011;53(Suppl 1):39S-43S.
38. Goldsweig AM, Abbott JD, Aronow HD. Physician and patient radiation exposure during endovascular procedures. *Curr Treat Options Cardiovasc Med*. 2017; 19(2):10.
39. Bannazadeh M, Altinel O, Kashyap VS, Sun ZY, Clair D, Sarac TP. Patterns of procedure-specific radiation exposure in the endovascular era: impetus for further innovation. *J Vasc Surg*. 2009;49(6):1520-1524.
40. Wibmer A, Nolz R, Teufelsbauer H, et al. Complete ten-year follow-up after endovascular abdominal aortic aneurysm repair: survival and causes of death. *Eur J Radiol*. 2012;81(6):1203-1206.
41. Kalef-Ezra JA, Karavasilis S, Ziogas D, Dristiliaris D, Michalis LK, Matsagas M. Radiation burden of patients undergoing endovascular abdominal aortic aneurysm repair. *J Vasc Surg*. 2009;49(2):283-287; discussion 287.
42. Geijer H, Larzon T, Popek R, Beckman KW. Radiation exposure in stent-grafting of abdominal aortic aneurysms. *Br J Radiol*. 2005;78(934):906-912.
43. Stecker MS. Patient radiation management and preprocedure planning and consent. *Tech Vasc Interv Radiol*. 2010;13(3):176-182.
44. Zoli S, Trabattoni P, Dainese L, et al. Cumulative radiation exposure during thoracic endovascular aneurysm repair and subsequent follow-up. *Eur J Cardiothorac Surg*. 2012;42(2):254-259; discussion 259-260.
45. Walsh C, O'Callaghan A, Moore D, et al. Measurement and optimization of patient radiation doses in endovascular aneurysm repair. *Eur J Vasc Endovasc Surg*. 2012;43(5):534-539.
46. Hertault A, Maurel B, Midulla M, et al. Editor's choice: minimizing radiation exposure during endovascular procedures: basic knowledge, literature review, and reporting standards. *Eur J Vasc Endovasc Surg*. 2015;50(1):21-36.
47. Bartal G, Vano E, Paulo G, Miller DL. Management of patient and staff radiation dose in interventional radiology: current concepts. *Cardiovasc Intervent Radiol*. 2014;37(2):289-298.
48. Yamashita K, Higashino K, Hayashi H, Hayashi F, Fukui Y, Sairyo K. Pulsation and collimation during fluoroscopy to decrease radiation: a cadaver Study. *JB JS Open Access*. 2017;2(4):e0039.
49. Hertault A, Maurel B, Sobocinski J, et al. Impact of hybrid rooms with image fusion on radiation exposure during endovascular aortic repair. *Eur J Vasc Endovasc Surg*. 2014;48(4):382-390.
50. Lederman HM, Khademian ZP, Felice M, Hurh PJ. Dose reduction fluoroscopy in pediatrics. *Pediatr Radiol*. 2002;32(12):844-848.
51. Haqqani OP, Agarwal PK, Halin NM, Iafrati MD. Minimizing radiation exposure to the vascular surgeon. *J Vasc Surg*. 2012;55(3):799-805.
52. Haqqani OP, Agarwal PK, Halin NM, Iafrati MD. Defining the radiation "scatter cloud" in the interventional suite. *J Vasc Surg*. 2013;58(5):1339-1345.
53. Lopez PO, Dauer LT, Loose R, et al. ICRP Publication 139: occupational radiological protection in interventional procedures. *Ann ICRP*. 2018;47(2):1-118.
54. Schueler BA. Operator shielding: how and why. *Tech Vasc Interv Radiol*. 2010;13(3):167-171.
55. Burns S, Thornton R, Dauer LT, Quinn B, Miodownik D, Hak DJ. Leaded eyeglasses substantially reduce radiation exposure of the surgeon's eyes during acquisition of typical fluoroscopic views of the hip and pelvis. *J Bone Joint Surg Am*. 2013;95(14):1307-1311.
56. Kirkwood ML, Arbique GM, Guild JB, et al. Radiation brain dose to vascular surgeons during fluoroscopically guided interventions is not effectively reduced by wearing lead equivalent surgical caps. *J Vasc Surg*. 2018;68(2):567-571.
57. Buls N, Pages J, de Mey J, Osteaux M. Evaluation of patient and staff doses during various CT fluoroscopy guided interventions. *Health Physics*. 2003;85(2):165-173.
58. Shaw PM, Vouyouka A, Reed A. Time for radiation safety program guidelines for pregnant trainees and vascular surgeons. *J Vasc Surg*. 2012;55(3):862-868 e862.
59. Chu B, Miodownik D, Williamson MJ, Gao YM, Germain JS, Dauer LT. Radiological protection for pregnant women at a large academic medical cancer center. *Phys Medica*. 2017;43:186-189.
60. Ghatan CE, Fassiotto M, Jacobsen JP, Sze DY, Kothary N. Occupational radiation exposure during pregnancy: a survey of attitudes and practices among interventional radiologists. *J Vasc Interv Radiol*. 2016;27(7):1013-1020 e1013.
61. Dauer LT, Miller DL, Schueler B, et al. Occupational radiation protection of pregnant or potentially pregnant workers in IR: a joint guideline of the Society of Interventional Radiology and the Cardiovascular and Interventional Radiological Society of Europe. *J Vasc Interv Radiol*. 2015;26(2):171-181.
62. Shaw P, Duncan A, Vouyouka A, Ozsvath K. Radiation exposure and pregnancy. *J Vasc Surg*. 2011;53(Suppl 1): 28S-34S.
63. Sharafuddin MJ, Marjan AE. Current status of carbon dioxide angiography. *J Vasc Surg*. 2017;66(2):618-637.

64. Illuminati G, Pacile MA, Ceccanei G, Ruggeri M, La Torre G, Ricco JB. Peroperative intravascular ultrasound for endovascular aneurysm repair versus peroperative angiography: a pilot study in fit patients with favorable anatomy. *Ann Vasc Surg.* 2020;64:54-61.
65. Stahlberg E, Sieren M, Anton S, et al. Fusion imaging reduces radiation and contrast medium exposure during endovascular revascularization of iliac steno-occlusive disease. *Cardiovasc Intervent Radiol.* 2019;42(11):1635-1643.
66. Lumbreras B, Vilar J, Gonzalez-Alvarez I, et al. Evaluation of clinicians' knowledge and practices regarding medical radiological exposure: findings from a mixed-methods investigation (survey and qualitative study). *BMJ Open.* 2016;6(10):e012361.
67. Brambilla M, Vassileva J, Kuchcinska A, Rehani MM. Multinational data on cumulative radiation exposure of patients from recurrent radiological procedures: call for action. *Eur Radiol.* 2020;30(5):2493-2501.
68. Barakat MT, Thosani NC, Huang RJ, et al. Effects of a brief educational program on optimization of fluoroscopy to minimize radiation exposure during endoscopic retrograde cholangiopancreatography. *Clin Gastroenterol Hepatol.* 2018;16(4):550-557.
69. Ketteler ER, Brown KR. Radiation exposure in endovascular procedures. *J Vasc Surg.* 2011;53(Suppl 1): 35S-38S.

SELF-ASSESSMENT STUDY QUESTIONS AND ANSWERS

Questions

1. Which of the following statements is NOT true regarding reference air kerma (RAK)?
   A. RAK is a better measure of total radiation dose.
   B. RAK is a facility-selected radiation value used to determine the risk of deterministic injury.
   C. RAK measures the radiation output at a point in space located at a fixed distance from the focal spot.
   D. RAK is an approximation of peak skin dose.

2. A 65-year-old male with a 30-pack year smoking history was seen in clinic with complaints of right foot pain at rest and a poorly healing wound located on his right foot. After a complete history, physical, and review of his ABIs, you elect to offer the patient a diagnostic angiogram for further workup and surgical planning. Which of the following statements is true regarding YOUR radiation exposure during diagnostic angiogram?
   A. Your greatest radiation exposure will be from that to your hands during manipulation of the catheters and wires.
   B. Use of DSA will lead to lower radiation exposure.
   C. Scatter radiation from the patient will be your primary source of radiation exposure.
   D. A dosimeter is not required during routine diagnostic angiography.

3. Which of the following statement regarding radiation dose is NOT true?
   A. Skin damage can occur at radiation doses as low as 2 Gy.
   B. Hair loss can occur at radiation doses as low as 3 Gy.
   C. The substantial radiation dose level (SRDL) is 5 Gy.
   D. Damage to the eyes does not occur under a radiation dose of 2 Gy.

4. A 78-year-old male with mild COPD, well-controlled hypertension, and hyperlipidemia is found to have a 5.6-cm infrarenal AAA. After discussing risks and benefits of open AAA repair and EVAR, the patient elects for endovascular repair. How should the image intensifier and x-ray tube be placed to reduce overall radiation to the patient?
   A. Both the image intensifier and the x-ray tube should be positioned as close to patient as possible.
   B. Both the image intensifier and the x-ray tube should be positioned as far away from the patient as possible.
   C. The image intensifier should be positioned as close to the patient as possible, while the x-ray tube should be positioned as far away from the patient as possible.
   D. The image intensifier should be positioned as far away from the patient as possible, while the x-ray tube should be positioned as close to the patient as possible.

5. A patient is referred to your clinic for possible repair of a thoracoabdominal aortic aneurysm with a maximum diameter of 7 cm. After reviewing the case and imaging, you offer the patient a four-vessel fenestrated EVAR. Which of the following techniques should NOT be used to reduce the patient's radiation exposure?
   A. Regular use of DSA should be utilized to decrease total radiation dosing.
   B. Collimation should be used regularly to minimize radiation to the field of interest.
   C. Avoiding use of oblique views as much as possible can decrease radiation doses.
   D. Save image runs to reduce amount of repeat imaging needed.

SELF-ASSESSMENT STUDY QUESTIONS AND ANSWERS

6. When considering the use of protective gear during fluoroscopic procedures, which of the statements is/are true?
   A. Leaded gloves have been shown to reduce radiation exposure to the hands.
   B. The use of leaded surgical caps has not clearly been shown to decrease overall radiation exposure to the brain.
   C. Thyroid collars are generally recommended for staff during fluoroscopic procedures.
   D. The use of leaded aprons has been shown to attenuate up to 99.5% of radiation dose.
   E. All of the above.
   F. None of the above.

7. A female colleague at your institution is pregnant. Which of the following statements is true regarding radiation and pregnancy.
   A. The occupational radiation dose limit during the 9 months of pregnancy that is considered safe is 500 mrem during the entire pregnancy.
   B. The fetus is most sensitive to the effects of radiation during the third trimester.
   C. Studies have demonstrated that even with the use of appropriate shielding and protective gear the risk of radiation to the fetus is significantly increased.
   D. Pregnant operators and trainees should wear standard aprons and protective gear.

8. With all other factors excluded, tripling your distance from the source of radiation will lead to what change in your radiation exposure?
   A. Decreased by one-third
   B. Decreased by one-ninth
   C. Increased by one-third
   D. Increased by one-ninth
   E. No change

9. A 66-year-old male with history of obesity, diabetes mellitus type II, smoking, and hyperlipidemia underwent an EVAR for a 5.8-cm infrarenal AAA 1 year ago, routine surveillance has revealed that the patient has a stable type II endoleak. After discussing the nature of endoleaks with the patient, the patient elects for continued follow-up. However, the patient is concerned about the risk of radiation and repeat imaging. Which of the following factors is NOT significant when considering his overall radiation exposure.
   A. BMI
   B. Multiple subtracted runs during his index EVAR
   C. History of smoking
   D. Repeat imaging for follow-up type II endoleak

10. A 70-year-old female with a long history of smoking and PAD presents for bilateral kissing iliac stents. The patient is positioned supine on the operating table with the fluoroscopy unit under the table and the imagine intensifier is oriented in a posterior-anterior direction. Without any additional shielding in the place, which of the following locations will contain the highest about of scatter radiation exposure to the operator"
   A. Scatter will be equal at all points of the table without additional shielding.
   B. Scatter will be highest on the right side of the table.
   C. Scatter will be highest on the left side of the table.
   D. Scatter will be highest above the table.
   E. Scatter will be highest below the table.

SELF-ASSESSMENT STUDY QUESTIONS AND ANSWERS

Answers

1. B.
2. C.
3. D.
4. C.
5. A.
6. E.
7. A.
8. B.
9. C.
10. E.

CHAPTER

5 Wound Healing for the Vascular Specialist

Christina J. Camick and Munier Nazzal

OUTLINE

PHASES OF WOUND HEALING
- Hemostasis and Inflammation
- Proliferation
- Matrix Synthesis
- Maturation and Remodeling
- Epithelialization

THE ROLE OF GROWTH FACTORS IN WOUND HEALING

WOUND CONTRACTION

CLASSIFICATION OF WOUNDS

FACTORS AFFECTING WOUND HEALING
- Advanced Age
- Hypoxia, Hypoperfusion, and Anemia
- Drugs, Steroids, and Chemotherapeutic Drugs
- Metabolic Disorders
  - Diabetes Mellitus
  - Uremia
    - *Obesity*
- Nutrition

WOUND INFECTION

SUMMARY

The practice of wound healing dates back many millennia, with the earliest accounts from the Sumerians in 2000 B.C. Their practice consisted of both a spiritual component with incantations and a physical component with application of a poultice-like material to the wound. The Egyptians can be credited with differentiating infected and diseased wounds from noninfected wounds. In the Edwin Smith Surgical Papyrus, a copy of a document dated to 1650 B.C., there are descriptions of over 48 types of wounds. The Ebers Papyrus (1550 B.C.) describes concoctions containing honey for antibacterial purposes, lint for absorbance of moisture, and grease to provide a barrier in the treatment of wounds. The Egyptians recognized properties within these substances that are still fundamental in modern wound management. Building on this knowledge, the Greeks classified wounds as acute or chronic. Galen of Pergamum (120–201 A.D.), who was appointed as physician to the Roman gladiators, was one of most famous Greek physicians who emphasized the importance of maintaining moisture within the wound environment to ensure adequate healing.

A turning point in the history of wound healing was the discovery of antiseptics and their significance in reducing puerperal sepsis by washing hands with soap and hypochlorite by the Hungarian obstetrician Ignaz Philipp Semmelweis (1818–1895), the discovery of existence of microbes in the environment by Louis Pasteur (1822–1895), and the discovery by Joseph Lister (1827–1912) during a visit to Scotland that carbolic acid (phenol) in sewage reduces bacteria. Soaking surgical instruments in phenol and spraying it in the operating rooms resulted in reduction of postoperative mortality rates from 50% to 15%. After attending a lecture by Lister in 1872, Robert Wood Johnson began research and eventually went on to produce an antiseptic dressing in the form of cotton gauze impregnated with iodoform. Since this invention, multiple other materials have been utilized to achieve antiseptic dressing materials.[1,2]

PHASES OF WOUND HEALING

The complex process of wound healing begins with an injury or wound. The normal process of wound healing can be divided into phases defined by cellular populations and biochemical events: hemostasis and inflammation, proliferation, and maturation and remodeling. This sequence of events spans the time from injury to resolution of acute wounds. It is necessary for all wounds to progress through this series of cellular and biochemical events that characterize the phases of healing in order to successfully reestablish tissue integrity (Figure 5-1 A and B).

There are multiple factors, however, that can interfere with these phases and can lead to prolonged length of healing or nonhealing. It is important for the vascular specialist to be familiar with these phases in order to recognize patient factors that may interfere with wound healing.

HEMOSTASIS AND INFLAMMATION

The process of hemostasis precedes and initiates inflammation by a release of chemotactic factors from the wound site. A wound by definition is a disruption of tissue integrity, which leads to the division of blood vessels and direct exposure of extracellular matrix to platelets. Exposure of subendothelial collagen to platelets triggers platelet aggregation, degranulation, and activation of the coagulation cascade. Platelet α granules release a number of wound-active substances, including platelet-derived growth factor (PDGF), transforming growth factor-β (TGF-β), platelet-activating factor (PAF), fibronectin, and serotonin. The fibrin clot achieves hemostasis and also serves as a scaffold for the migration of inflammatory cells such as polymorphonuclear leukocytes (PMNs, neutrophils) and monocytes.

After tissue injury, cellular infiltration follows a characteristic, predetermined sequence (Figure 5-2). PMNs are the first infiltrating cells to enter the wound site, peaking at 24 to 48 hours. Increased vascular permeability, local prostaglandin release, and the presence of chemotactic substances such as complement factors, interleukin-1 (IL-1), tumor necrosis factor-α (TNF-α), TGF-β, platelet factor 4, or bacterial products all stimulate neutrophil migration to the area of injury. The primary role of neutrophils in this phase is thought to be phagocytosis of bacteria and tissue debris. PMNs also are a major source of cytokine production during the early inflammatory phase, especially of TNF-α[3] which may have a significant influence on subsequent angiogenesis and collagen synthesis. In addition, PMNs release proteases such as collagenases, which contribute to matrix and ground substance degradation in the early phase of wound healing. While they play a role in limiting infections, PMNs do not appear to contribute to collagen deposition or acquisition of mechanical wound strength. Rather, the presence of neutrophil factors is implicated in delayed epithelial closure of wounds.[4]

The second population of inflammatory cells to invade the wound consists of macrophages, which are derived from monocytes and are recognized as essential to successful healing.[5] Significant numbers of macrophages appear in the wound 48 to 96 hours postinjury and remain present until completion of wound healing. Like neutrophils, macrophages participate in wound debridement via phagocytosis and contribute to microbial stasis via synthesis of oxygen radicals and nitric oxide. The macrophage's central function is activation and recruitment of other cells via mediators such as cytokines and growth factors, as well as directly by cell cell interaction and intercellular adhesion molecules (ICAM). Macrophages play a significant role in regulating cell proliferation, matrix synthesis, and angiogenesis through release of cell mediators TGF-β, vascular endothelial growth factor (VEGF), insulin-like growth factor (IGF), and epithelial growth factor (EGF).[6,7]

T lymphocytes invade the wound in the first day and peak around 1-week postinjury. While less numerous than macrophages, T lymphocytes bridge the transition from the inflammatory phase of wound healing to the proliferative phase. The role of lymphocytes in healing is recognized as essential but not fully defined.[8] Multiple studies support the hypothesis that T lymphocytes play an active role in the modulation of the wound environment. Depletion of T lymphocytes within the wound environment decreases wound strength and collagen content,[9] while selective depletion of the $CD8^+$ suppressor subset of T lymphocytes has been shown to enhance wound healing. However,

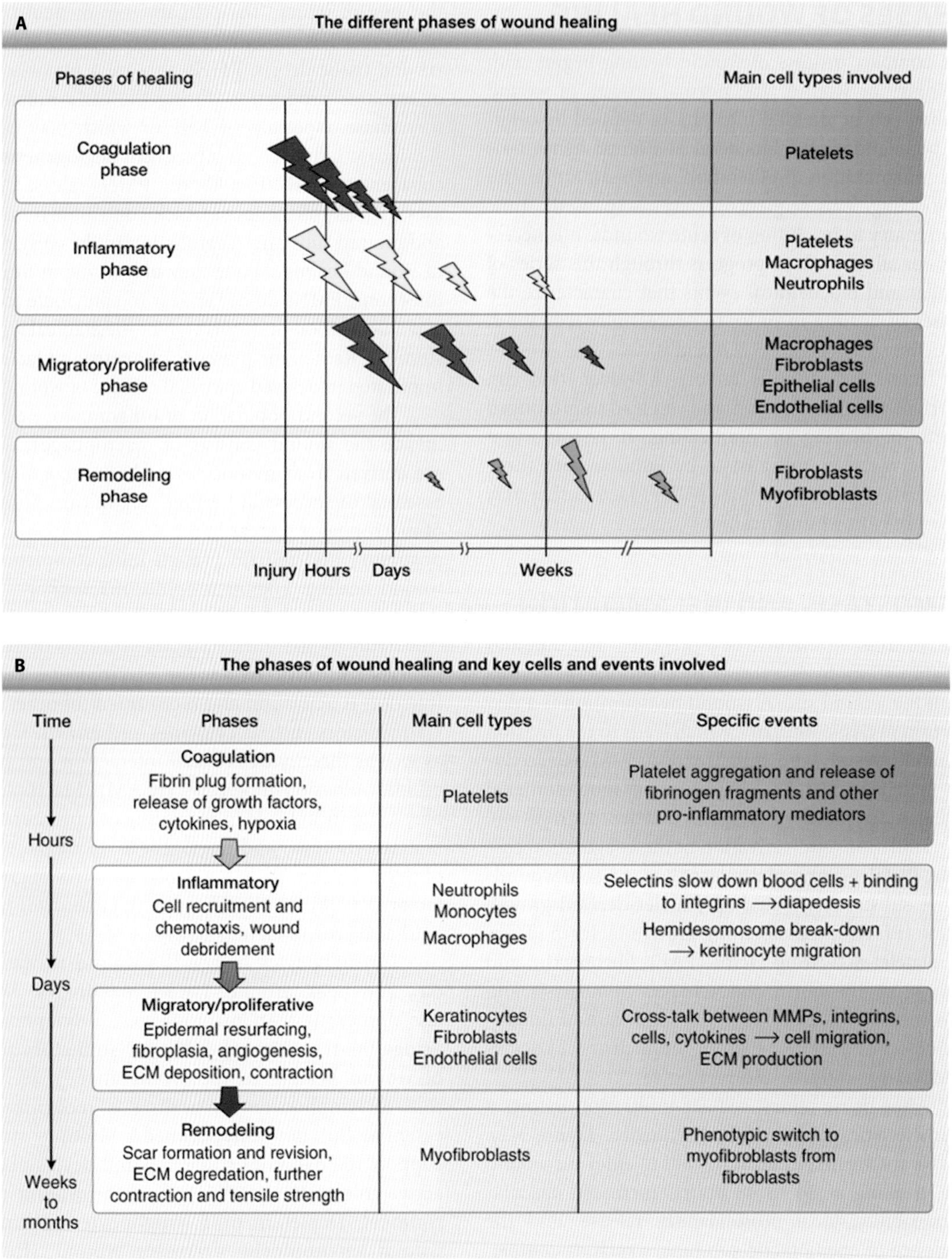

FIGURE 5-1 Phases of wound healing. A. Different phases of wound healing. **B**. The phases of wound healing and key cells and events involved. (Reproduced with permission from Kang S, Amagai M, Bruckner AL, et al. *Fitzpatrick's Dermatology*, 9th ed. New York, NY: McGraw Hill; 2019.)

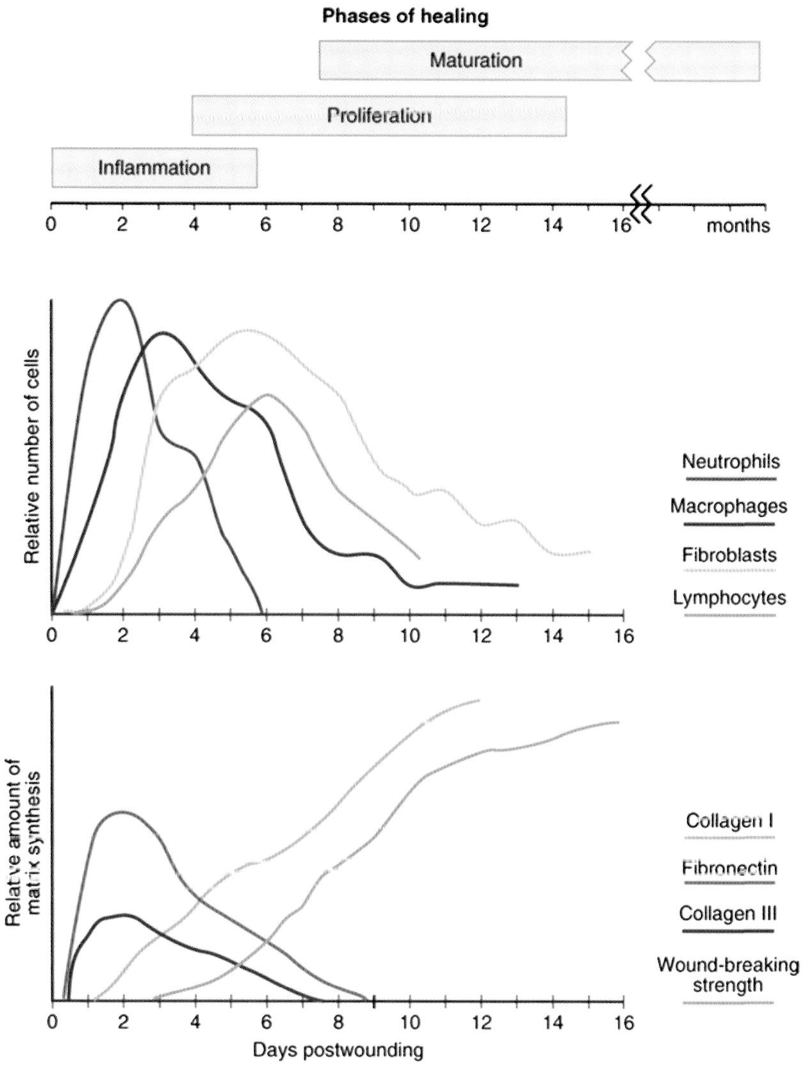

FIGURE 5-2 The cellular, biochemical, and mechanical phases of wound healing. (Reproduced with permission from Brunicardi FC, Andersen DK, Billiar TR, et al. *Schwartz's Principles of Surgery*, 11th ed. New York, NY: McGraw Hill; 2019.)

depletion of the $CD4^+$ helper subset has no effect on wound healing.[10] Lymphocytes can exert a down regulating effect on fibroblast collagen synthesis by cell-associated interferon IFN-γ, TNF-α, and IL-1. However, this effect is lost if the cells are physically separated, suggesting that the regulation of extracellular matrix synthesis involves not only soluble factors but also direct cell–cell contact between lymphocytes and fibroblasts.[11]

PROLIFERATION

The second phase of wound healing is the proliferative phase and occurs over the course of days 4 through 12 postinjury. During this phase, tissue continuity is reestablished and infiltration of the last cell populations to the healing wound, fibroblasts and endothelial cells, occurs. The strongest chemotactic factor for fibroblast migration is PDGF.[12,13] Upon entering the wound environment, recruited fibroblasts must first proliferate, and then become activated to carry out their primary function of matrix synthesis remodeling. Activation of fibroblasts is mediated mainly by the cytokines and growth factors released from wound macrophages.

Fibroblasts isolated from wounds synthesize more collagen than nonwound fibroblasts, proliferate less, and actively carry out matrix contraction. Although it is clear that the cytokine-rich wound environment plays a significant role in this phenotypic alteration and activation, the exact mediators are only partially characterized.[14,15] In addition, lactate, which may accumulate in significant amounts in the wound environment over time (~10 mmol), is a potent regulator of collagen synthesis through a mechanism involving adenosine diphosphate (ADP)-ribosylation.[16,17]

Extensive proliferation of endothelial cells also occurs during this phase. Endothelial cells participate in formation of new capillaries, known as angiogenesis, a process essential to successful wound healing. These cells migrate from intact venules close to the wound, replicate, and form new capillary tubules. This process occurs under the influence of cytokines and growth factors such as TNF-α, TGF-β, and VEGF. Although many cells produce VEGF, macrophages contribute a major source in the healing wound. VEGF receptors are located specifically on endothelial cells.[18,19]

MATRIX SYNTHESIS

The synthesis, deposition, and remodeling of collagen and proteoglycans are essential to the functional integrity of the wound. Collagen, the most abundant protein in the body, plays a critical role in successful completion of adult wound healing. There are at least 18 types of collagen described; however, the main types of interest to wound repair are types I and III. Type I collagen is the major component of the extracellular matrix in skin. Type III, which is also normally present in skin, becomes more prominent and important during the repair process (Figure 5-2.)

Biochemically, each chain of collagen is composed of a glycine residue in every third position and the second position in the triplet is composed of proline or lysine during the translation process. The polypeptide chain that is translated from mRNA contains approximately 1000 amino acid residues and is called *protocollagen*. Release of protocollagen into the endoplasmic reticulum results in the hydroxylation of proline and lysine by specific hydroxylases. Prolyl hydroxylase requires oxygen and iron as cofactors, α-ketoglutarate as a co-substrate, and ascorbic acid (vitamin C) as an electron donor. In the endoplasmic reticulum, the protocollagen chain also undergoes glycosylation by the linking of galactose and glucose at specific hydroxylysine residues. Hydroxylation and glycosylation alter the hydrogen bonding forces within the chain, imposing steric changes that force the protocollagen chain to assume an α-helical configuration. Three α-helical chains entwine to form a right-handed superhelical structure known as *procollagen*. At both ends, this structure contains nonhelical peptide domains called *registration peptides*. Although initially joined by weak, ionic bonds, the procollagen molecule becomes much stronger by the covalent cross-linking of lysine residues.

Extracellularly, the nonhelical registration peptides undergo cleavage by a procollagen peptidase, and the procollagen strands undergo further polymerization and cross-linking. The resulting monomeric collagen is further polymerized and cross-linked by the formation of intra- and intermolecular covalent bonds.

The synthesis and posttranslational modifications of collagen are highly dependent on systemic factors such as an adequate oxygen supply, the presence of sufficient nutrients (amino acids and carbohydrates), cofactors (vitamins and trace metals), and the local wound environment (vascular supply and lack of infection). As a clinician, addressing these factors and reversing nutritional deficiencies can optimize collagen synthesis and deposition necessary for wound healing.

A large portion of the "ground substance" that makes up granulation tissue is composed of glycosaminoglycans. Rarely found free, glycosaminoglycans couple with proteins to form proteoglycans. The polysaccharide chain is made up of repeating disaccharide units composed of glucuronic or iduronic acid and a hexosamine, which is usually sulfated. The disaccharide composition of proteoglycans varies from about 10 units, in the case of heparin sulfate, to as much as 2000 units in the case of hyaluronic acid.

Dermatan and chondroitin sulfate comprise the major glycosaminoglycans present in wounds. Fibroblasts synthesize glycosaminoglycans, increasing their concentration greatly during the first 3 weeks of healing.

Studies are ongoing, examining the interaction between collagen and proteoglycans. It is thought that the assembly of collagen subunits into fibrils and fibers is dependent upon the lattice provided by the sulfated proteoglycans. The extent of sulfation appears to be critical in determining the configuration of the collagen fibrils. As scar collagen is deposited, the proteoglycans are incorporated into the collagen scaffolding. However, with scar maturation and collagen remodeling, the content of proteoglycans gradually diminishes.

MATURATION AND REMODELING

Maturation and remodeling of the scar begins during the fibroblastic phase and is characterized by a reorganization of previously synthesized collagen. Matrix metalloproteinases (MMPs) break down collagen and the net wound collagen content is the result of a balance between collagenolysis and collagen synthesis. With a net shift toward collagen synthesis, eventually the extracellular matrix is composed of a relatively acellular collagen-rich scar.

The quantity and quality of the newly deposited collagen determine wound strength and mechanical integrity in the fresh wound. The deposition of matrix at the wound site follows a characteristic pattern: fibronectin and collagen type III constitute the early matrix scaffolding; glycosaminoglycans and proteoglycans represent the next significant matrix components; and collagen type I is the final matrix. Several weeks postinjury, the amount of collagen in the wound reaches a plateau but the tensile strength continues to increase for several more months.[20] Fibril formation and fibril cross-linking result in decreased collagen solubility, increased strength, and increased resistance to enzymatic degradation of the collagen matrix. Fibroblasts secrete the glycoprotein fibrillin, which is essential for the formation of elastic fibers found in connective tissue. Scar remodeling continues for many (6–12) months postinjury, gradually resulting in a mature, avascular, and acellular scar. The mechanical strength of the scar never achieves that of the uninjured tissue.

Collagen constantly turns over in the extracellular matrix, both in the healing wound and during normal tissue homeostasis. Collagenolysis is the result of collagenase activity, a class of MMPs that require activation. Both collagen synthesis and lysis are strictly controlled by cytokines and growth factors. Some factors affect both aspects of collagen remodeling. For example, TGF-β increases new collagen transcription and also decreases collagen breakdown by stimulating synthesis of tissue inhibitors of metalloproteinase.[21] This balance of collagen deposition and degradation is the ultimate determinant of wound strength and integrity.

EPITHELIALIZATION

The final step in establishing tissue integrity is epithelialization. This process is characterized primarily by proliferation and migration of epithelial cells adjacent to the wound (Figure 5-3). The process begins within 1 day of injury and is seen as thickening of the epidermis at the wound edge. Marginal basal cells at the edge of the wound lose their firm attachment to the underlying dermis, enlarge, and migrate across the surface of the provisional matrix. Fixed basal cells in a zone near the cut edge undergo a series of rapid mitotic divisions, and these cells appear to migrate by moving over one another in a leapfrog fashion until the defect is covered.[22] After the defect is bridged, the migrating epithelial cells lose their flattened appearance, become more columnar in shape, and increase their mitotic activity. The epithelial layer is reestablished, and the surface layer eventually keratinizes.[23]

In less than 48 hours, reepithelialization is complete in the case of approximated incised wounds but may take substantially longer in wounds with significant epidermal/dermal defects. If only the epithelium and superficial dermis are damaged, such as occurs in split-thickness skin graft donor sites or in superficial second-degree burns, then repair consists primarily of reepithelialization with minimal or no fibroplasia and granulation tissue formation. The stimuli for reepithelialization remain incompletely defined;

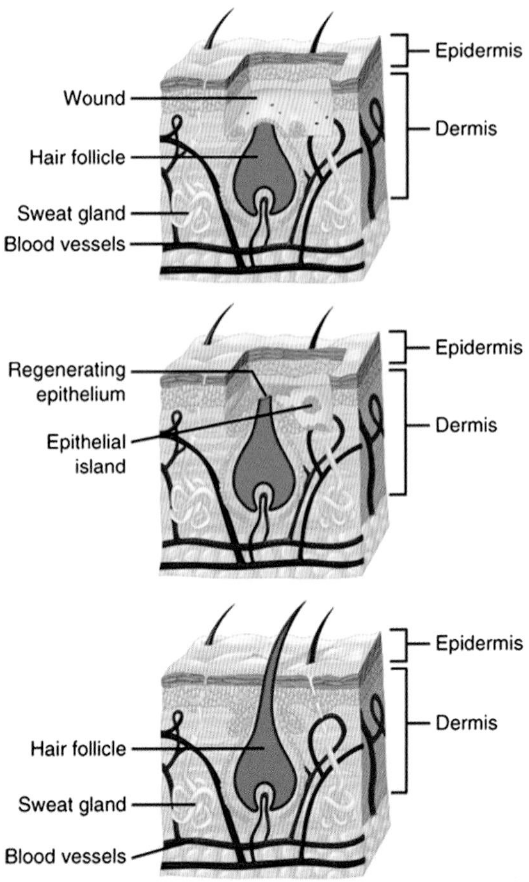

FIGURE 5-3 Epithelialization of superficial wounds. (Reproduced with permission from Brunicardi FC, Andersen DK, Billiar TR, et al. *Schwartz's Principles of Surgery*, 11th ed. New York, NY: McGraw Hill; 2019.)

however, it appears that the process is mediated by a combination of a loss of contact inhibition; exposure to constituents of the extracellular matrix, particularly fibronectin; and cytokines produced by immune mononuclear cells.[24,25] In particular EGF, TGF-β, basic fibroblast growth factor (bFGF), PDGF, and IGF-1 have been shown to promote epithelialization.

THE ROLE OF GROWTH FACTORS IN WOUND HEALING

Growth factors and cytokines are polypeptides produced in normal and wounded tissue that stimulate cellular migration, proliferation, and function. Their names orginate from the cells from which they were first derived (e.g., PDGF), or for their initially identified function (e.g., fibroblast growth factor, FGF). These names are often misleading because growth factors have been demonstrated to have multiple functions. Most growth factors are extremely potent and produce significant effects in nanomolar concentrations (Table 5-1).

Growth factors and cytokines may act in an autocrine manner (where the growth factor acts on the cell producing it), a paracrine manner (by release into the extracellular environment, where it acts on the immediately neighboring cells), or in an endocrine manner (where the effect of the substance is distant to the site of release and the substance is carried to the effector site through the bloodstream). Not only is the concentration of the growth factor important in determining its effectiveness, the timing of release

TABLE 5-1 Growth Factors in Wound Healing

PDGF	Platelets, macrophages, monocytes, smooth muscle cells, endothelial cells	Chemotaxis: fibroblasts, smooth muscles cells, monocytes, neutrophils
		Mitogenesis: fibroblasts, smooth muscle cells
		Stimulation of angiogenesis
		Stimulation of collagen synthesis
		Enhance reepithelization
		Modulate tissue remodeling
FGF	Fibroblasts, endothelial cells, keratinocytes, smooth muscle cells, chondrocytes	Stimulation of angiogenesis (by stimulation of endothelial cell proliferation and migration)
		Mitogenesis: mesoderm and neuroectoderm

TABLE 5-1 Growth Factors in Wound Healing—Continued

HGF	Fibroblasts	Stimulates fibroblasts, keratinocytes, chondrocytes, myoblasts Suppresses inflammation, granulation tissue formation, angiogenesis, re-epithelialization
Keratinocyte growth factor	Keratinocytes, fibroblasts	Significant homology with FGF; stimulates keratinocytes
EGF	Platelets, macrophages, monocytes (also identified in salivary glands, duodenal glands, kidney, and lacrimal glands)	Stimulates proliferation and migration of all epithelial cell types
TGF-α	Keratinocytes, platelets, macrophages	Homology with EGF; binds to EGF receptor Mitogenic and chemotactic for epidermal and endothelial cells
TGF-β (three isoforms: β1, β2, β3)	Platelets, T lymphocytes, macrophages, monocytes, neutrophils, fibroblasts, keratinocytes	Stimulates angiogenesis Stimulates leukocyte chemotaxis TGF-β1 stimulates wound matrix production (fibronectin, collagen glycosaminoglycans); regulation of inflammation TGF-β3 inhibits scar formation
Insulin-like growth factors (IGF-1, IGF-2)	Platelets (IGF-1 in high concentrations in liver; IGF-2 in high concentrations in fetal growth); likely the effector of growth hormone action	Promote protein/extracellular matrix synthesis Increase membrane glucose transport
Vascular endothelial growth factor	Macrophages, fibroblasts, endothelial cells, keratinocytes	Mitogen for endothelial cells (not fibroblasts) Stimulates angiogenesis Proinflammatory
IL-1 IL-4 IL-6 Activin Angiopoitein-1/-2CX3CL1	Macrophages, leukocytes, keratinocytes, fibroblasts Fibroblasts, endothelial cells, macrophages, keratinocytes, fibroblasts Macrophages, endothelial cells	Proinflammatory Stimulates angiogenesis, reepithelialization, tissue remodeling Enhances collagen synthesis Stimulates inflammation, angiogenesis, reepithelialization, collagen deposition, tissue remodeling Stimulates granulation tissue formation, keratinocyte differentiation, reepithelialization Stimulates angiogenesis Stimulates inflammation, angiogenesis, collagen deposition
Granulocyte-macrophage colony-stimulating factor	Macrophage/monocytes, endothelial cells, fibroblasts	Stimulates macrophage differentiation/proliferation

CX3CL1, chemokine (C-X3-C motif) ligand; EGF, epidermal growth factor; FGF, fibroblast growth factor; HGF, hepatocyte growth factor; IL, interleukin; PDGF, platelet-derived growth factor; TGF, transforming growth factor.

Reproduced with permission from Brunicardi FC, Andersen DK, Billiar TR, et al. *Schwartz's Principles of Surgery*, 11th ed. New York, NY: McGraw Hill; 2019.

is also important. As these growth factors exert their effects by cell-surface receptor binding, the appropriate receptor on the responding cells must be present at the time of release in order for the biologic effect to occur. Growth factors result in divergent downstream effects on different cells; they can be chemoattractant to one cell type while stimulating replication of a different cell type. Little is known about the ratio of growth factor concentrations, which may be as important as the absolute concentration of individual growth factors.

Growth factors act on cells via surface receptor binding. Various receptor types have been described, such as ion channels, G-protein linked, or enzyme-linked through phosphorylation or dephosphorylation of second-messenger molecules by phosphatases or kinases, resulting in activation or deactivation of proteins in the cytosol or nucleus of the target cell. Phosphorylation of nuclear proteins is followed by the initiation of transcription of target genes.[26] The signal is stopped by internalization of the receptor-ligand complex.

WOUND CONTRACTION

Some degree of contraction occurs in all wounds. While wounds with approximated edges heal with minimal contraction, in those that do not have surgically approximated edges, contraction is necessary to decrease the area of the wound (healing by secondary intention and tertiary intention) (Figure 5-4). The major cell responsible for contraction is the myofibroblast, which differs from the normal fibroblast in that it possesses a cytoskeletal structure. Typically myofibroblasts contain α-smooth muscle actin in thick bundles called *stress fibers,* which give myofibroblasts contractile capability. Myofibroblasts are undetectable before the 6th day but increase over the subsequent 15 days of wound healing, then undergo apoptosis after 4 weeks.[27,28] Interestingly, contraction starts immediately after injury in the absence of myofibroblasts, possibly by fibroblast cytoskeleton reorganization.[29,30]

CLASSIFICATION OF WOUNDS

Wounds may be classified as either acute or chronic. An acute wound by definition becomes chronic if healing is not achieved after 4 weeks of treatment. Acute wounds heal in a predictable manner and time frame as previously described. This process occurs with few, if any, complications, and the end result is a well-healed wound.

Surgical wounds can heal in multiple ways. An incised wound that is clean and closed by sutures is said to heal by primary intention. In the presence of bacterial contamination or tissue loss, a wound may be left open to heal by granulation tissue formation and contraction; this constitutes healing by secondary intention. Delayed primary closure, or healing by tertiary intention, represents a combination of the first two, consisting of the delayed placement of sutures, allowing the wound to stay open for a few days with subsequent closure.

The healing spectrum of acute wounds is broad. A constant and continual increase in mechanical integrity and strength during healing occurs until a plateau is reached at some point after injury. Maximal wound strength is reached after about 6 weeks of healing in normal wounds. A fully healed wound achieves only 75% to 80% tensile strength of a normal tissue. Conditions discussed above such as nutritional deficiencies, infections, or severe trauma result in delayed healing. However, healing may revert to normal with correction of the underlying pathophysiology. Impaired healing is characterized by a failure to achieve mechanical strength equivalent to normally healed wounds. Patients with diabetes, chronic steroid usage, or tissues damaged by radiotherapy are immunocompromised and are prone to this type of impaired healing. It is imperative that the surgeon be aware of these situations and exercise great care in the placement of incision, suture selection, postoperative care, and adjunctive therapy to maximize the chances of healing without supervening complications (Figure 5-5).

FACTORS AFFECTING WOUND HEALING

As previously discussed, wounds heal by a combination of mechanisms, including connective tissue deposition, contraction, and epithelialization. Surgically closed wounds need mostly

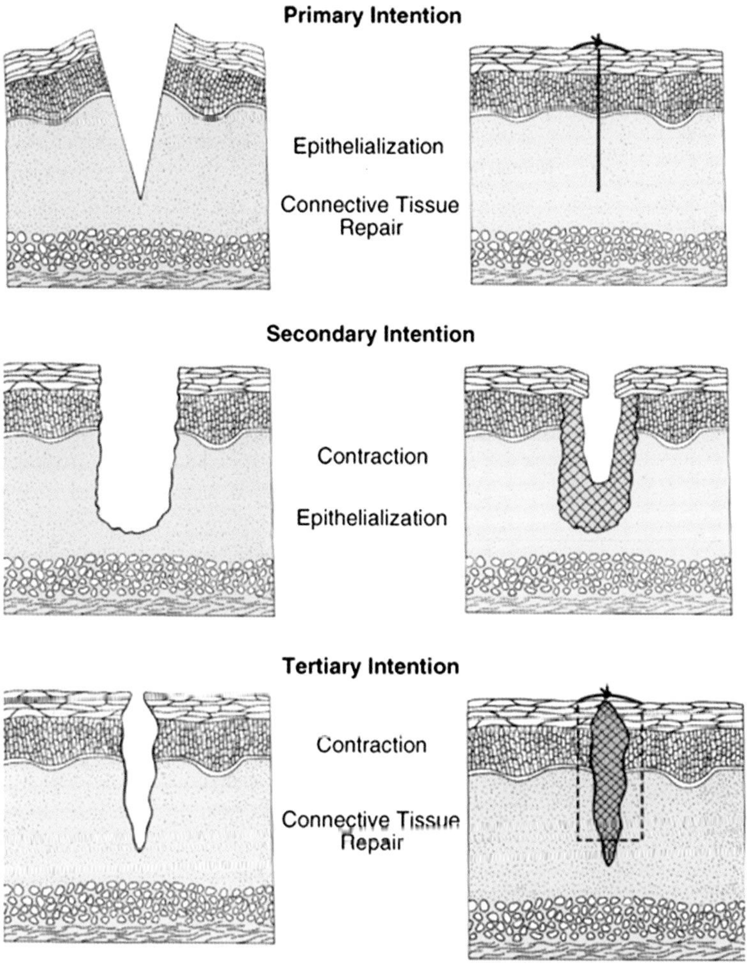

FIGURE 5-4 Epithelialization and contraction in healing different wounds. (Reproduced with permission from Brunicardi FC, Andersen DK, Billiar TR, et al. *Schwartz's Principles of Surgery*, 11th ed. New York, NY: McGraw Hill; 2019.)

epithelialization for healing, while open wounds require a combination of tissue contraction, connective tissue deposition, and epithelialization to a lesser extent. Chronic ulcers heal by secondary intention similar to open wounds.

Normal healing is affected by both systemic and local factors (Table 5-2). The clinician must be familiar with these factors and should attempt to counteract their deleterious effects. Complications occurring in wounds with higher risk can lead to failure of healing or the development of chronic, nonhealing wounds.

ADVANCED AGE

It is a common belief among most surgeons that aging produces intrinsic physiologic changes that result in delayed or impaired wound healing. Clinical experience with elderly patients tends to support this belief. Studies of hospitalized surgical patients demonstrate a direct correlation between older age and wound healing complications such as dehiscence and incisional hernia.[31,32] However, impaired or delayed wound healing in the elderly might be related to comorbid conditions such as cardiovascular disease, medications, nutritional disorders, diabetes, and

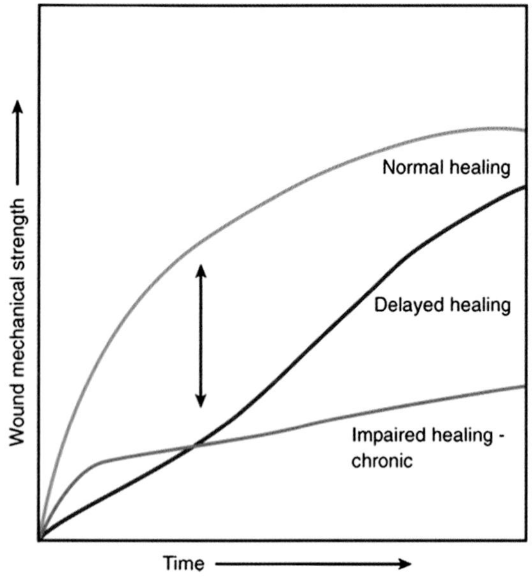

FIGURE 5-5 Acquisition of wound mechanical strength over time in normal, delayed, and impaired healing. (Reproduced with permission from Brunicardi FC, Andersen DK, Billiar TR, et al. *Schwartz's Principles of Surgery*, 11th ed. New York, NY: McGraw Hill; 2019.)

TABLE 5-2 Factors Affecting Wound Healing

Systemic	Local
Age	Infection
Nutrition	Mechanical injury/ tension
Trauma	Edema
Metabolic	Ischemia/necrosis
Drugs	Topical agents
Connective tissue disorders	Radiation
Profound anemia	Low oxygen tension
Smoking	Foreign bodies
Jaundice	Abnormal local skin

others that are more predominant in older patients. More recent clinical experience suggests that major operative interventions can be accomplished safely in the elderly.

The results of animal studies regarding the effects of aging on wound healing have yielded contradictory results. In healthy human volunteers, there was a significant delay of 1.9 days in the epithelialization of superficial skin defects in those older than 70 years of age when compared to younger volunteers.[33] In the same volunteers, using a micro-model of fibroplasia, no difference in DNA or hydroxyproline wound accumulation could be demonstrated between the young and elderly groups; however, the young volunteers had a significantly higher amount of total α-amino nitrogen in their wounds, a reflection of total protein content of the wound. It was concluded that synthesis does not seem to be impaired with advanced age, but noncollagenous protein accumulation at wounded sites is decreased with aging, which may impair the mechanical properties of scarring in elderly patients. In a relatively healthy person, advanced age may cause a delay in wound healing rather than nonhealing.

HYPOXIA, HYPOPERFUSION, AND ANEMIA

There is a profound deleterious effect on all aspects of wound healing with low oxygen tension. Oxygen is necessary in wound healing for migration and proliferation of fibroblasts, although stimulated initially by the hypoxic wound environment, and necessary cofactor for optimal collagen synthesis, particularly in hydroxylation steps. Increased inspired oxygen (FIO_2) results in enhanced collagen deposition and decreased rates of wound infection after elective surgery.[34-36] Hypoperfusion can occur secondary to systemic reasons (low volume or cardiac failure) or local causes (arterial insufficiency, local vasoconstriction, or excessive tissue tension). Optimization of these factors improves capillary circulation and can have a remarkable influence on wound outcome, particularly on decreasing wound infection rates.[35,37] Correction of arterial insufficiency is often the focus of the vascular specialist.

Wound oxygen tension and collagen synthesis do not appear to be adversely affected by mild-to-moderate normovolemic anemia. However, profound anemia with hematocrit less than 15% can interfere with wound healing.[38]

DRUGS, STEROIDS, AND CHEMOTHERAPEUTIC DRUGS

Drugs that interfere with any of the four phases of wound healing are expected to delay wound healing. Cytokines and growth factors are vulnerable to be disrupted by medications. There is a wide range of medications that are expected to interfere with wound healing. The benefits and risks of discontinuing medications should be balanced with the need to improve wound healing.

Steroids, especially those with greater anti-inflammatory effects, inhibit the inflammatory phase of wound healing (angiogenesis, neutrophil and macrophage migration, and fibroblast proliferation), the release of lysosomal enzymes, and Collagen synthesis. When used after the first 3 to 4 days of injury, steroids do not affect wound healing as severely as when they are used in the immediate postoperative period. Whenever possible, steroid use should be delayed or avoided in the beginning of anticipated wound healing, or alternatively, forms with lesser anti-inflammatory effects should be administered.

In addition to their effect on collagen synthesis, steroids inhibit epithelialization and contraction and contribute to increased rates of wound infection, regardless of the time of administration.[39] Collagen synthesis and epithelialization of cutaneous wounds can, however, be stimulated in steroid-delayed healing by topical application of vitamin A[39,40]

Chemotherapeutic drugs impede early cell proliferation, inhibit wound DNA and protein synthesis, attenuate the inflammatory phase, decrease fibrin deposition, and delay wound contraction, all of which are critical to successful healing. The effect is more profound if these agents are given preoperatively. A delay in the use of such drugs for about 2 weeks after injury appears to lessen wound healing impairment.[41] The deleterious effects on wound healing of these drugs are demonstrated by tissue necrosis, marked ulceration, and protracted healing seen in extravasation of chemotherapeutic agents into soft tissue.[42] Generally, all chemotherapeutic antimetabolite drugs adversely affect wound healing.

Commonly used nonsteroidal anti-inflammatory drugs have been reported to delay wound healing. This includes nonselective NSAIDs, cyclooxygenase (COX)-2 inhibitors and disease modifying antirheumatic drugs (DMARDs) (Table 5-3). Other medications that have been reported to interfere with healing include antibiotics, antiseptics, anticoagulants, colchicine, vasoconstrictors, and nicotine (Table 5-4).[42,43]

TABLE 5-3 Commonly Used Anti-Inflammatory Drugs

Nonselective NSAIDs	Cyclooxygenase (COX)-2 Inhibitors	Disease-Modifying Antirheumatic Drugs (DMARDs)
Aspirin	Celecoxib	Azathioprine
Diclofenac (Voltaren)	Parecoxib	Penicillamine
Fenoprofen (Nalfon)	Rofecoxib	Methotrexate
Ibuprofen (Motrin, Rufen)	Valdecoxib	
Indomethacin (Indocin)		
Ketoprofen (Orudis)		
Meclofenamate (Meclofen, Meclomen)		
Naproxen (Anaprox, Naprosyn)		
Piroxicam (Feldene)		
Sulindac (Clinoril)		
Tolmetin (Tolectin)		

Acute healing time is difficult to evaluate and compare between groups of patients. Healing of acute wounds is expected to occur in a linear process following the phases of wound healing. However, chronic wounds do not follow the same pattern and healing follows a nonlinear process. It is difficult to evaluate the effect of individual factors and

TABLE 5-4 Drugs Affecting Wound Healing

Medications	Effect on healing
Antiseptics	
Ethyl alcohol,	Decrease in contraction
Povidone iodine	Inhibition of epithelialization
Acetic acid	Inhibition of epithelialization and contraction
Anticoagulants	
Warfarin	Interfere with fibrin deposition
Rivaroxaban	
Apixaban	
Antibiotics	
Erythromycin	Inhibit WBC chemotaxis
Tetracycline	Inhibit WBC chemotaxis
Bacitracin	Inhibition of contraction
Antiplatelets	
Aspirin	Inhibit inflammatory changes.
Clopidogrel	
Dipyridamole	
Colchicine	Vasoconstriction and decreased blood flow
	Decrease cytokine release
	Decrease fibroblast activity
	Interfere with extracellular transport of collagen
	Decrease granulocyte migration
Nicotine	Vasoconstriction and decreased blood flow
	Decrease oxygenation

medications on acute wound healing without taking into account other factors such as age, obesity, and stress. In a study of 1732 patients with 2089 acute wounds, the average healing time was reported to be 35 days, with only chemotherapeutic agents resulting in a significant increase in healing time by 21 days. All other medications including antibiotics, anticoagulants, NSAIDs, and corticosteroids did not reach statistical significance.[44]

METABOLIC DISORDERS

Diabetes Mellitus

Diabetes Mellitus is the most recognized metabolic disorder contributing to increased rates of wound infection and failure.[45] Uncontrolled diabetes results in reduced inflammation, angiogenesis, and collagen synthesis. One of the hallmarks of advanced diabetes includes large- and small-vessel arterial disease, which further contributes to hypoperfusion and local hypoxemia. Defects in granulocyte function, capillary ingrowth, and fibroblast proliferation all have been described in diabetes. Obesity, insulin resistance, hyperglycemia, and diabetic renal failure contribute significantly and independently to the impaired wound healing observed in diabetics.[46] In wound studies on experimental diabetic animals, insulin restores collagen synthesis and granulation tissue formation to normal levels if administered during the early phases of healing.[47] In clean, noninfected, and well-perfused experimental wounds in human diabetic volunteers, type 1 diabetes mellitus was noted to decrease the accumulation of collagen in the wound, independent of the degree of glycemic control. Type 2 diabetic patients showed no effect on collagen accumulation when compared to healthy, age-matched controls.[48] Furthermore, the diabetic wound appears to be lacking in sufficient growth factor levels, which are necessary for cell signaling in normal healing. It remains unclear whether decreased collagen synthesis or an increased breakdown of collagen due to an abnormally high proteolytic wound environment is responsible. Careful preoperative correction of blood sugar levels improves the outcome of wounds in diabetic patients.[49,50]

Uremia

Uremia is another condition associated with impaired wound healing and defenses for infection. Uremic animal models demonstrate decreased wound collagen synthesis and breaking strength, resulting in delayed healing of intestinal anastomoses and abdominal wounds. [47] The clinical use of dialysis to correct metabolic and nutritional abnormalities may greatly impact the wound outcome of such patients. Abnormal deposition of calcium and phosphate in the tissue of some uremic patients can lead to uremic gangrene syndrome, or calciphylaxis which present itself as a chronic ulcer discussed in another part of this book.

Obesity continues to be a growing public health problem in the United States, and the world with over 60% of Americans found to be overweight or obese. In the absence of other comorbid conditions such as cardiovascular disease, uncomplicated obesity by itself has detrimental effects on wound healing. Adipocytes play a role in metabolism and immunity and, through generation of proinflammatory cytokines and adipokines, contribute to the development of metabolic syndrome. Many of these cytokines and adipokines have effects on cell populations that are necessary for wound healing. In nondiabetic obese rodents, wounds are mechanically weaker, and there is less dermal and reparative scar collagen. Preadipocytes infiltrate the dermis, and although they can evolve into fibroblasts, their regulatory mechanisms appear different from those of dermal or wound fibroblasts. Many studies indicate that obese patients have high rates of perioperative complications, with estimates as high as 30% for wound dehiscence, 17% for surgical site infections, 30% for incisional hernias, 19% for seromas, 13% for hematomas, and 10% for fat necrosis.[51,52] Increased subcutaneous fat was associated with a 10-fold increased risk of surgery-related complications including intestinal anastomotic leaks, abdominal fluid collection, and wound infections.[53] In many studies, obesity is a constant and major risk factor for hernia formation and recurrence after repair. The mechanism by which obesity impairs wound healing awaits complete delineation.

NUTRITION

Poor nutritional intake or lack of individual nutrients significantly alters many aspects of wound healing. It is important for the clinician to consider the nutritional status of patients with wounds, since wound failure or wound infections may be no more than a reflection of poor nutrition (Table 5-5). Although the full interaction of nutrition and wound healing is still not fully understood, efforts are being made to develop wound-specific nutritional interventions and institute the pharmacologic use of individual nutrients as modulators of wound outcomes.

In one experiment, rodents fed either a 0% or 4% protein diet had impaired collagen deposition with a secondary decrease in skin and fascial wound-breaking strength and increased wound infection rates. Induction of energy-deficient states by providing only 50% of the normal caloric requirement lead to decreased granulation tissue formation and matrix protein deposition in rats. Acute fasting in rats markedly impairs collagen synthesis while decreasing procollagen mRNA.[54]

In clinical practice, it is extremely rare to encounter pure energy or protein malnutrition, and the vast majority of patients exhibit combined protein-energy malnutrition. These patients have diminished hydroxyproline accumulation, an index of collagen deposition, into subcutaneously implanted polytetrafluoroethylene tubes when compared to normally nourished patients. Furthermore, malnutrition correlates clinically with increased rates of wound complications and failure following diverse surgical procedures. This is a reflection

TABLE 5-5 Nutritional Requirements for Wound Healing

	Calories*	Protein†
Normal (at rest)	20–25 kcal/kg/day (age dependent)	0.8 g/kg/day 60–70 g
Postoperative/ill/injured	30%–50% above normal	1.2–2 g/kg/day
Large open wounds, burns		2–2.5 g/kg/day
Malnourished	50% above normal	1.5 g/kg/day plus anabolic agent[1]

*Data from Demling RH, Nutrition, anabolism, and the wound healing process: an overview. *ePlasty*. 2009;9:65-94.

†Data from Huckleberry Y. Nutritional support and the surgical patient. *Am J Health Syst Pharm*. 2004;61(7):671-682, by permission of Oxford University Press.

From Hamm R. *Text and Atlas of Wound Diagnosis and Treatment*, 2nd ed. New York, NY: McGraw Hill; 2019, Table 11-7.

of poor healing response as well as reduced cell-mediated immunity, phagocytosis, and intracellular killing of bacteria by macrophages and neutrophils during protein-calorie malnutrition.[55] Two additional nutrition-related factors warrant discussion. First, the degree of nutritional impairment need not be long-standing in humans, as opposed to the experimental situation. Patients with brief preoperative illnesses or reduced nutrient intake in the period immediately preceding the injury or operative intervention will thus demonstrate impaired fibroplasias.[56] Second, brief and not necessarily intensive nutritional intervention, either via the parenteral or enteral route, can reverse or prevent the decreased collagen deposition observed with malnutrition or with postoperative starvation.[57]

The role of single amino acids in enhancing wound healing has been studied. Arginine appears to be the most active in terms of enhancing wound fibroplasia. Deficiency in arginine results in decreased wound strength and wound-collagen accumulation in chow-fed rats. Rats that are given 1% arginine HCl supplementation, and are thus not arginine-deficient, have enhanced wound-breaking strength and collagen synthesis when compared to chow-fed control rats.[58] Studies have been carried out in healthy human volunteers to examine the effect of arginine supplementation on collagen accumulation. Young, healthy, human volunteers (age 25–35 years) were found to have significantly increased wound-collagen deposition following oral supplementation with either 30 g of arginine aspartate (17 g of free arginine) or 30 g of arginine Hall (24.8 g of free arginine) daily for 14 days.[59] In a study of healthy older humans (age 67–82 years), daily supplements of 30 g of arginine aspartate for 14 days resulted in significantly enhanced collagen and total protein deposition at the wound site when compared to controls given placebos. There was no enhanced DNA synthesis present in the wounds of the arginine-supplemented subjects, suggesting that the effect of arginine is not mediated by an inflammatory mode of action.[60] In this and later studies, arginine supplementation, whether administered orally or parenterally, had no effect on the rate of epithelialization of a superficial skin defect. This further suggests that the main effect of arginine on wound healing is to enhance wound collagen deposition. Recently, a supplemental regimen of arginine, β-hydroxy-β-methyl butyrate, and glutamine was found to significantly and specifically enhance collagen deposition in elderly, healthy human volunteers when compared to an isocaloric, isonitrogenous supplement.[61] As increases in breaking strength during the first weeks of healing are directly related to new collagen synthesis, arginine supplementation may result in an improvement in wound strength as a consequence of enhanced collagen deposition.

Vitamin C and vitamin A are two vitamins worthy of discussion in regards to wound healing. Vitamin C deficiency, or scurvy, leads to a defect in wound healing, particularly via a failure in collagen synthesis and cross-linking. Biochemically, vitamin C is required for the conversion of proline and lysine to hydroxyproline and hydroxylysine, respectively. Vitamin C deficiency is also associated with an increased incidence of wound infection, and if wound infection does occur, it tends to be more severe. These effects are believed to be due to an associated impairment in neutrophil function, decreased complement activity, and decreased walling-off of bacteria secondary to insufficient collagen deposition. The recommended dietary allowance of Vitamin C is 60 mg daily, which provides a considerable safety margin for most healthy nonsmokers. In severely injured or extensively burned patients, this requirement may increase to as high as 2 g daily. There is no evidence that excess vitamin C is toxic; however, there is no evidence that supratherapeutic doses of vitamin C are of any benefit.[62]

Vitamin A deficiency impairs wound healing, while supplemental vitamin A benefits wound healing in nondeficient humans and animals. Vitamin A increases the inflammatory response in wound healing, probably by increasing the lability of lysosomal membranes. There is an increased influx of macrophages, with an increase in their activation and increased collagen synthesis. Vitamin A directly increases collagen production and epidermal growth factor receptors when it is added in vitro to cultured fibroblasts. As mentioned before, supplemental vitamin A can reverse the inhibitory effects of corticosteroids on wound healing. Vitamin A also can restore wound healing that has been impaired by diabetes, tumor formation, cyclophosphamide, and radiation. It is important to recognize that serious injury or stress leads to increased vitamin A requirements. In the severely injured patient, supplemental vitamin A has been recommended in doses ranging from 25,000 to 100,000 IU per day.

Multiple minerals and trace elements are recognized as crucial for wound healing. Clinically, deficiencies of these are multiple and often include macronutrient deficiencies. As with some of the vitamins described earlier, the specific trace element may function as a cofactor or part of an enzyme that is essential for homeostasis and wound healing. Generally speaking, preventing deficiencies is often easier to accomplish than diagnosing them.

For centuries, zinc has been a well-known element in wound healing, being used empirically in many dermatologic conditions. Zinc is essential for wound healing in animals and humans. There are over 150 known enzymes for which zinc is either an integral part or an essential cofactor, with many of these enzymes critical to wound healing.[54] In zinc deficiency, there is decreased fibroblast proliferation, decreased collagen synthesis, impaired overall wound strength, and delayed epithelialization. These defects are reversed by zinc supplementation. To date, no study has shown improved wound healing with zinc supplementation in patients who are not zinc deficient.[63,64]

WOUND INFECTION

Infected wounds are a major medical problem, not only affecting the outcome of a surgical procedure, but also the length of hospital stay and medical costs.[65] Infection is particularly problematic in the case of implant use. Infected implants often require removal of the prosthetic material and thereby subject the patient to further operations, further increasing morbidity and mortality risk. Infections weaken tissue integrity, which can result in compromised wound closure and subsequent dehiscence. Cosmetically, the patient with an infected wound may experience disfiguration and unsightly delayed closure.

The mere presence of bacteria in an open wound, either acute or chronic, does not constitute an infection, as large numbers of bacteria may be present in the normal wound bed. In addition, bacteria identified in cultures may not represent the causative infectious organism. Differentiation between contamination, colonization, and infection is important. *Contamination* is the presence of bacteria without multiplication, *colonization* is bacterial multiplication without host response, and *infection* is the presence of host response in reaction to deposition and multiplication of bacteria. The presence of a host response helps to differentiate between infection and colonization in chronic wounds.[66] Cellulitis, abnormal discharge, delayed healing, change in pain, abnormal granulation tissue, bridging, abnormal color, and odor may indicate host response and aids in diagnosis of infection.

To decrease the risk of wound infection, antibiotics are routinely administered prophylactically for operative wounds. In order for prophylaxis to be most effective, adequate concentrations of antibiotic must be present at the time of incision. A significant hospital performance measure is now assurance of adequate dose and timing of antibiotic prophylaxis administration.[67] Administration of antibiotics after operative contamination occurs is not an effective method in preventing postoperative wound infections. Antibiotic selection for prophylaxis is based on the type of surgery to be performed, operative contaminants that could be encountered during the procedure, and the profile of resistant organisms present at the institution where surgery is to be performed. As methicillin-resistant *Staphylococcus aureus* (MRSA) and vancomycin-resistant enterococci (VRE) has become more widespread throughout hospitals, routine use of these agents has become significantly restricted.

It is particularly important to consider antibiotic prophylaxis in the patient with any previously implanted prosthetic material. Patients with an orthopedic prosthesis, prosthetic heart valve, or any implanted vascular prosthesis should receive antibiotic prophylaxis prior to a procedure where significant bacteremia may be anticipated. In the case of dental procedures, prophylaxis should be with broad spectrum penicillins or amoxicillin. Patients undergoing urologic instrumentation should be pretreated with second-generation cephalosporin. In gastrointestinal surgery, pretreatment should include a second-generation cephalosporin with the addition of anaerobic coverage.[68] Furthermore, repeat dosing of antibiotics during long operative cases has been shown to be essential in decreasing postoperative wound infections when duration of the procedure exceeds the biochemical half-life ($t_{1/2}$) of the antibiotic or in which there is large-volume blood loss and fluid replacement.[69,70] In cases with long duration, prosthetic implant use, or unexpected contamination, the surgeon may consider administration of additional doses of prophylactic antibiotics for 24 hours postoperatively.

Hyperglycemia has been shown to be a significant risk factor of postoperative infections.[71] It impairs wound healing via several different mechanisms including impaired functions of neutrophils, macrophages, fibroblasts and decreased function of cytokines, and growth factors. In addition, hypoglycemia contributes to nitric oxide dysfunction, altered homocysteine levels, macrovascular and microvascular impairment, neuropathy, immune function impairment, and biochemical and hormonal impairment. Tight blood glucose control, peri- and postoperatively, has been associated with significant reduction in infectious complications. However, too tight of a glycemic control (80–100 mg/dL) appears to be associated with more complications and is no more effective in reducing infectious complications than moderate control (120–180 mg/dL).[72,73] In addition to glycemic control, maintenance of euvolemia, core temperature above 36°C to 36.5°C, and pain control have all been shown to independently and additively reduce rates of wound infections.[36]

Surgical wounds may be classified by the degree of contamination that occurs during the operation or disease process. Class I wounds are considered clean, class II wounds are considered clean contaminated, class III wounds are considered contaminated, and class IV are considered dirty. The incidence of wound infection has a direct relationship with the degree of contamination during the operation. In a study comparing operations performed with and without appropriate antibiotic prophylaxis, class II, III, and IV procedures have one-third the wound infection rate of previously reported untreated series.[74] The incidence of surgical wound infection is about 5% to 10% nationwide and has not changed during the last few decades. It has been shown that if a wound is contaminated with $>10^5$ microorganisms per gram of tissue, the risk of wound infection is markedly increased. Of note, this quantity may be much lower in the presence of foreign materials. Source of infection is generally from the endogenous flora of the patient's skin, mucous membranes, or from hollow organs. In order of decreasing frequency, the most common organisms responsible for wound infection are *Staphylococcus* species, coagulase-negative *Streptococcus*, enterococci, and *Escherichia coli*.

Surgical wound infections usually become apparent within 7 to 10 days postoperatively, although rarely may manifest years later. With shorter lengths of stays, infections may not be detected until follow-up in the outpatient setting, which may lead to underreporting of the true incidence of wound infections. There is much debate about the actual definition of surgical wound infection. Wounds that drain purulent, culture-positive material are in the strictest sense infected. However, broader definitions include wounds draining purulent material whether culture positive or negative, any wound opened by the surgeon postoperatively, and wounds the surgeon considers infected.[75]

Wound infections may be classified anatomically as superficial incisional, deep incisional, or organ/space wound infections, which involve fascia, muscle, or the abdominal cavity. Around three-fourths of wound infections are classified as superficial, involving skin and subcutaneous tissue only. In the case of an edematous, erythematous, and tender wound, clinical diagnosis of infection is clear. However, wound infections may present in a more subtle manner. Development of low-grade postoperative fever, mild or unexplained leukocytosis, or undue incisional pain should direct attention to the wound. Subtle edema around the suture or staple line, seen as a waxy appearance of the skin, is an early indication of infection. In the case of suspected infection, stitches or staples around the most suspicious areas should be removed and a small segment of the subcutaneous tissue opened with a cotton-tipped applicator. Generally, this causes minimal discomfort to the patient. The skin and subcutaneous tissue should be further opened along the extent of the infected pocket if purulence is encountered. Samples may be taken for aerobic and anaerobic culture. Rarely will patients require antibiotic therapy after source control. In the case of immunosuppressed patients, patients with evidence of tissue penetration or systemic toxicity, or patients with prosthetic devices, systemic antibiotics should be administered.[74]

Deep wound infections arise immediately adjacent to the fascia, either above or below it, and usually present with fever and leukocytosis. The incision may drain pus spontaneously, but pus draining between the fascial sutures will be noted. Sometimes wound dehiscence will occur. The most feared deep infection is necrotizing fasciitis as it carries high mortality, especially within the elderly. Infection involves the fascia and leads to secondary skin necrosis. Pathophysiologically, there is septic thrombosis of the vessels between the skin and the deeper soft tissue layers. On examination, the skin will display hemorrhagic bullae and subsequent frank necrosis, with surrounding areas of inflammation and edema. Often, fascial necrosis is usually wider than the skin involvement or than the surgeon estimates clinically. In the toxic, febrile patient with tachycardia and hypovolemia, progression to cardiovascular collapse is imminent if not quickly recognized and corrected. Microbially, this may be a mixed infection, and samples should be obtained for Gram stain smears and cultures to aid in diagnosis and treatment. Broad spectrum antibiotics with anaerobic coverage should be initiated due to concern over the presence of *Clostridia perfringens* and other related species; and the regimen modified based on culture results. However, definitive treatment is surgical. Cardiovascular resuscitation with electrolyte solutions, blood, and/or plasma is carried out as expeditiously as possible prior to induction of anesthesia. The aim of surgical treatment is complete removal of all necrotic skin and fascia. If viable, skin overlies necrotic fascia, multiple longitudinal skin incisions can be made to allow for excision of the devitalized fascia. While removal of all necrotic tissue is the goal of surgical intervention, differentiation between necrotic and simply edematous tissue is often challenging on initial intervention. Careful inspection of the wound every 12 to 24 hours will reveal new areas of necrosis. These areas must be further debrided and excised. After adequate debridement of necrotic tissue and infection control, the surgeon may consider wound coverage with homo- or xenografts until definitive reconstruction and autografting can take place.

In the case where a wound fails to proceed through the phases that produce satisfactory anatomic and functional integrity, it is said to be *chronic*. Wounds that have not healed within 3 months are generally considered chronic, but a duration as low as 4 weeks has been used to indicate chronicity. A major proportion of chronic wounds are skin ulcers, which occur in traumatized tissue or tissue with vascular compromise. The workup and management for these chronic wounds is discussed in another chapter.

SUMMARY

Wound healing is a complex cascade of processes that start at the same time of injury but at different levels of intensity and magnitude. The processes of wound healing are affected by numerous factors and patient characteristics such as age, diabetes mellitus, and uremia. Other factors affecting wound healing including nutrition, patient body habitus, and local factors such as radiation, skin changes, and ischemia. Most wounds heal by the fourth week, but if they do not show signs of adequate healing they can become chronic. Management of acute wounds focuses on identifying factors that might delay wound healing (Figure 5-6). Another factor that plays less role in acute wounds compared to chronic wounds is biofilm formation which represents an aggregate of bacteria that is tolerant to treatment with antibiotic therapy. Biofilm can start to form within hours of debridement and reach full maturity in 2 to 4 days. Organisms, after adhering to the surface of the wound, secrete a surrounding protective matrix called the extracellular polymeric substance (EPS). Biofilm colonies once formed become a source of other bacterial colonies in the wound. Debridement can help eradicate such biofilms, but they may form again in a short period of time relative to the chronicity of wounds.[76]

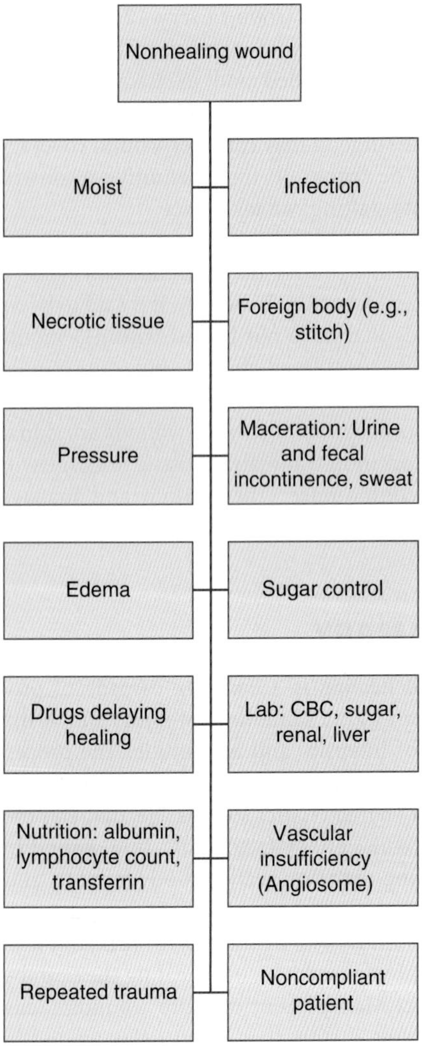

FIGURE 5-6 Checklist for acute wound healing.

REFERENCES

1. Oxford clinical communications. *A Brief History of Wound Healing*. Yardley, PA: OrthoMcNeil Pharmaceuticals and Janssen-Cilog; 1998.
2. Shah JB. The history of wound care. *J Am Col Certif Wound Spec*. 2011;3(3):65-66.
3. Feiken E, Romer J, Eriksen J, et al. Neutrophils express tumor necrosis factor-alpha during mouse skin wound healing. *J Invest Dermatol*. 1995;105(1):120-123.
4. Dovi JV, He L-K, DiPietro LA. Accelerated wound closure in neutrophil-depleted mice. *J Leukoc Biol*. 2003;73(4):448-455.
5. Leibovich SJ, Ross R. The role of the macrophage in wound repair. A study with hydrocortisone and anti-macrophage serum. *Am J Pathol*. 1975;78(1):71-100.
6. DiPietro LA. Wound healing: the role of the macrophage and other immune cells. *Shock*. 1995;4(4):233-240.
7. Zabel DD, Feng JJ, Scheuenstuhl H, et al. Lactate stimulation of macrophage-derived angiogenic activity is associated with inhibition of poly(ADP-ribose) synthesis. *Lab Invest*. 1996;74(4):644-649.
8. Schäffer MR, Barbul A. Lymphocyte function in wound healing and following injury. *Br J Surg*. 1998;85(4):444-460.
9. Efron JE, Frankel HL, Lazarou SA, Wasserkrug HL, Barbul A. Wound healing and T-lymphocytes. *J Surg Res*. 1990;48(5):460-463.
10. Barbul A, Breslin RJ, Woodyard JP, Wasserkrug HL, Efron G. The effect of in vivo T helper and T suppressor lymphocyte depletion on wound healing. *Ann Surg*. 1989;209(4):479-483.
11. Rezzonico R, Burger D, Dayer JM. Direct contact between T lymphocytes and human dermal fibroblasts or synoviocytes down-regulates types I and III collagen production via cell-associated cytokines. *J Biol Chem*. 1998;273(30):18720-18728.
12. Grotendorst GR. Chemoattractants and growth factors. In: Cohen K, Diegelmann RF, Lindblad WJ, eds. *Wound Healing, Biochemical and Clinical Aspects*. Philadelphia, PA: WB Saunders; 1992:237-247.
13. Bonner JC, Osornio-Vargas AR, Badgett A, Brody AR. Differential proliferation of rat lung fibroblasts induced by the platelet-derived growth factor-AA, -AB, and -BB isoforms secreted by rat alveolar macrophages. *Am J Respir Cell Mol Biol*. 1991;5(6):539-547.
14. Pricolo VE, Caldwell MD, Mastrofrancesco B, Mills CD. Modulatory activities of wound fluid on fibroblast proliferation and collagen synthesis. *J Surg Res*. 1990;48(6):534-538.
15. Regan MC, Kirk SJ, Wasserkrug HL, Barbul A. The wound environment as a regulator of fibroblast phenotype. *J Surg Res*. 1991;50(5):442-448.
16. Gimbel ML, Hunt TK, Hussain MZ. Lactate controls collagen gene promoter activity through poly-ADP-ribosylation. *Surg Forum*. 2000;51:26-27.
17. Ghani QP, Hussain MZ, Hunt TK. Control of procollagen gene transcription and prolyl hydroxylase activity by poly(ADP-ribose). In: Poirier G, Moreaer A, eds. *ADP-Ribosylation Reactions*. New York: Springer-Verlag; 1992:111-117.

18. Xiong M, Elson G, Legarda D, Leibovich SJ. Production of vascular endothelial growth factor by murine macrophages: regulation by hypoxia, lactate, and the inducible nitric oxide synthase pathway. *Am J Pathol.* 1998;153(2):587-598.
19. Ferrara N, Davis-Smith T. The biology of vascular endothelial growth factor. *Endocrine Rev.* 1997;18(1):4-25.
20. Levenson SM, Geever EF, Crowley LV, Oates JF III, Berard CW, Rosen H. The healing of rat skin wounds. *Ann Surg.* 1965;161(2):293-308.
21. Zhou LJ, Ono I, Kaneko F. Role of transforming growth factor-beta 1 in fibroblasts derived from normal and hypertrophic scarred skin. *Arch Dermatol Res.* 1997;289(11):646-652.
22. Stenn KS, Depalma L. Re-epithelialization. In: Clark RAF, Hensen PM, eds. *The Molecular and Cellular Biology of Wound Repair.* New York: Plenum; 1988:321-325.
23. Johnson FR, McMinn RMH. The cytology of wound healing of the body surface in mammals. *Biol Rev Camb Philos Soc.* 1960;35:364-412.
24. Woodley DT, Bachman PM, O'Keefe EJ. The role of matrix components in human keratinocyte re-epithelialization. In: Barbul A, Caldwell MD, Eaglstein WH, et al., eds. *Clinical and Experimental Approaches to Dermal and Epidermal Repair. Normal and Chronic Wounds.* New York: Wiley-Liss; 1991:129.
25. Lynch SE. Interaction of growth factors in tissue repair. In: Barbul A, Caldwell MD, Eaglstein WH, et al., eds. *Clinical and Experimental Approaches to Dermal and Epidermal Repair. Normal and Chronic Wounds.* New York. Wiley-Liss; 1991:341.
26. Jans DA, Hassan G. Nuclear targeting by growth factors, cytokines, and their receptors: a role in signaling? *BioEssays.* 1998;20:400-411.
27. Schmitt-Graff A, Desmouliere A, Gabbiani G. Heterogeneity of myofibroblast phenotypic features: an example of fibroblastic cell plasticity. *Virchows Arch.* 1994;425(1):3-24.
28. Darby I, Skalli O, Gabbiani G. Alpha-smooth muscle actin is transiently expressed by myofibroblasts during experimental wound healing. *Lab Invest.* 1990;63(1):21-29.
29. Desmouliere A, Redard M, Darby I, Gabbiani G. Apoptosis mediates the decrease in cellularity during the transition between granulation tissue and scar. *Am J Pathol.* 1995;146(1):56-66.
30. Ehrlich HP. Wound closure: evidence of cooperation between fibroblasts and collagen matrix. *Eye (Lond).* 1988;2(pt 2):149-157.
31. Halasz NA. Dehiscence of laparotomy wounds. *Am J Surg.* 1968;116(2):210-214.
32. Mendoza CB, Postlethwait RW, Johnson WD. Incidence of wound disruption following operation. *Arch Surg.* 1970;101(3):396-398.
33. Holt D, Kirk SJ, Regan MC, Hurson M, Lindblad WJ, Barbul A. Effect of age on wound healing in healthy humans. *Surgery.* 1992;112(2):293-297.
34. Hopf HW, Hunt TK, West JM, et al. Wound tissue oxygen tension predicts the risk of wound infection in surgical patients. *Arch Surg.* 1997;132(9):997-1004.
35. Greif R, Akca O, Horn EP, Kurz A, Sessler DI; Outcomes Research Group. Supplemental perioperative oxygen to reduce the incidence of surgical-wound infection. *N Engl J Med.* 2000;342(3):161-167.
36. Kurz A, Sessler D, Leonhardt R. Perioperative normothermia to reduce the incidence of surgical-wound infection and shorten hospitalization. *N Engl J Med.* 1996;334(19):1209-1215.
37. Hopf HW, Hunt TK, West JM, et al. Wound tissue oxygen tension predicts the risk of wound infection in surgical patients. *Arch Surg.* 1997;132(9):997-1004.
38. Kurz A, Sessler D, Leonhardt R. Perioperative normothermia to reduce the incidence of surgical-wound infection and shorten hospitalization. *N Engl J Med.* 1996;334(19):1209-1215.
39. Ehrlich HP, Hunt TK. Effects of cortisone and vitamin A on wound healing. *Ann Surg.* 1968;167(3):324-328.
40. Anstead GM. Steroids, retinoids, and wound healing. *Adv Wound Care.* 1998;11(6):277-285.
41. Ferguson MK. The effect of antineoplastic agents on wound healing. *Surg Gynecol Obstet.* 1982;154(3):421-429.
42. Smith R. The effects of medications on wound healing. *Podiatry Management.* 2008;(8):195-203.
43. Levine JM. The effect of oral medications on wound healing. *Adv Skin Wound Care.* 2017;30(3):137-142.
44. Khalil H, Cullen M, Chambers H, McGrail M. Medications affecting healing: an evidence-based analysis. *Int Wound J.* 2017;14(6):1340-1345.
45. Larson DL. Alterations in wound healing secondary to infusion injury. *Clin Plast Surg.* 1990;17(3):509-517.
46. Cruse PJE, Foord RA. A prospective study of 23,649 surgical wounds. *Arch Surg.* 1973;107(2):206-210.
47. Yue DK, McLennan S, Marsh M, et al. Effects of experimental diabetes, uremia, and malnutrition on wound healing. *Diabetes.* 1987;36(3):295-299.
48. Goodson WH III, Hunt TK. Studies of wound healing in experimental diabetes mellitus. *J Surg Res.* 1977;22(3):221-227.
49. Black E, Vibe-Petersen J, Jorgensen LN, et al. Decrease in collagen deposition in wound repair in type I diabetes independent of glycemic control. *Arch Surg.* 2003;138(1):34-40.

50. Spiliotis J, Tsiveriotis K, Datsis AD, et al. Wound dehiscence is still a problem in the 21st century: a retrospective study. *World J Emerg Surg.* 2009;4:12.
51. Coon D, Gusenoff JA, Kannan N, et al. Body mass and surgical complications in the postbariatric reconstructive patient: analysis of 511 cases. *Ann Surg.* 2009;249:397-401.
52. Arthurs ZM, Cuadrado D, Sohn V, et al. Post-bariatric panniculectomy: pre-panniculectomy body mass index impacts the complication profile. *Am J Surg.* 2007;193:567-570.
53. Tsukada K, Miyazaki T, Kato H, et al. Body fat accumulation and postoperative complications after abdominal surgery. *Am Surg.* 2004;70:347-351.
54. Williams JZ, Barbul A. Nutrition and wound healing. *Surg Clin North Am.* 2003;83(3):571-596.
55. Goodson WH, Jensen JA, Gramja-Mena L, West J, Granja-Mena L, Chavez-Estrella J. The influence of a brief preoperative illness on postoperative healing. *Ann Surg.* 1987;205(3):250-255.
56. Windsor JA, Knight GS, Hill GL. Wound healing in surgical patients: recent food intake is more important than nutritional status. *Br J Surg.* 1988;75(2):135-137.
57. Haydock DA, Hill GL. Improved wound healing response in surgical patients receiving intravenous nutrition. *Br J Surg.* 1987;74(4):320-323.
58. Seifter E, Rettura G, Barbul A, Levenson SM. Arginine: an essential amino acid for injured rats. *Surgery.* 1978;84(2):224-230.
59. Barbul A, Lazarou S, Efron DT, Wasserkrug HL, Efron G. Arginine enhances wound healing in humans. *Surgery.* 1990;108(2):331-336.
60. Kirk SJ, Regan MC, Holt D, Holt DR, Wasserkrug HL, Barbul A. Arginine stimulates wound healing and immune function in aged humans. *Surgery.* 1993;114(2):155-159.
61. Williams JZ, Abumrad NN, Barbul A. Effect of a specialized amino acid mixture on human collagen deposition. *Ann Surg.* 2002;236(3):369-374.
62. Levenson SM, Seifter E, VanWinkle W. Nutrition. In: Hunt TK, Dunphy JE, eds. *Fundamentals of Wound Management in Surgery.* New York: Appleton-Century-Crofts; 1979:28.
63. Jeejeebhoy KN, Cheong WK. Essential trace metals: deficiencies and requirements. In: Fischer JE, ed. *Nutrition and Metabolism in the Surgical Patient.* Boston, MA: Little, Brown and Company; 1996:295.
64. Wilkinson EAJ, Hawke CI. Oral zinc for arterial and venous ulcers (Cochrane Review), in *The Cochrane Library*, 1:2002. Oxford: Update Software.
65. Strategies for improving surgical quality—should payers reward excellence or effort? *N Engl J Med.* 2006;354(8):864-870.
66. Robson MC. Wound infection: a failure of wound healing caused by an imbalance of bacteria. *Surg Clin North Am.* 1997;77(3):637-650.
67. Anonymous. Antimicrobial prophylaxis for surgery. *Treat Guidel Med Letter.* 2012;10(122):73-78.
68. Gupta N, Kaul-Gupta R, Carstens MM, et al. Analyzing prophylactic antibiotic administration in procedures lasting more than four hours: are published guidelines being followed? *Am Surg.* 2003;69(8):669-673.
69. Ramos M, Khalpey Z, Lipsitz S, et al. Relationship of perioperative hyperglycemia and postoperative infections in patients who undergo general and vascular surgery. *Ann Surg.* 2008;248:585-591.
70. Van den Berghe G, Wouters P, Weekers P, et al. Intensive insulin therapy in critically ill patients. *N Engl J Med.* 2001;345:1359-1367.
71. Lazar HL, Chipkin SR, Fitzgerald CA, et al. Tight glycemic control in diabetic coronary artery bypass graft patients improves perioperative outcomes and decreases recurrent ischemic events. *Circulation.* 2004;109:1497-1502.
72. Gandhi GY, Nuttall GA, Abel MD, et al. Intensive intraoperative insulin therapy versus conventional glucose management during cardiac surgery: a randomized trial. *Ann Int Med.* 2007;146:233-243.
73. Lazar HL, McDonnell MM, Chipkin S, et al. Effects of aggressive versus moderate glycemic control on clinical outcomes in diabetic coronary artery bypass patients. *Ann Surg.* 2011;254:458-463.
74. Classen DC, Evans RS, Pestotnik SL, Horn SD, Menlove RL, Burke JP. The timing of prophylactic administration of antibiotics and the risk of surgical-wound infection. *N Engl J Med.* 1992;326(5):281-286.
75. Arnold MA, Barbul A. Surgical site infections. In: Cameron JL, ed. *Current Surgical Therapy.* 9th ed. St. Louis, MO: Mosby-Elsevier; 2008:1152-1160.
76. Philips PL, Wolcott RD, Fletcher J, Schultz GS. Biofilm made easy. Woundsinternational.com. Accessed 2018.

SELF-ASSESSMENT STUDY QUESTIONS AND ANSWERS

Questions

1. A 36-year-old woman presents to the emergency department after sustaining a laceration to her finger with a cooking knife. The wound is primarily repaired by the on-call surgical resident. Three to five days after repair, cells containing growth factors essential to proliferation and angiogenesis arrive at the site of injury to aid in wound healing. Which of the following cells is necessary for this process to occur?
A. Fibroblasts
B. Neutrophils
C. Macrophages
D. Platelets
E. T lymphocytes

2. A 61-year-old man on daily prednisone for rheumatoid arthritis undergoes urgent femoral thrombectomy for acute limb ischemia. Which of these supplements has been shown to potentially reverse the effects of corticosteroids on wound healing?
A. Vitamin A
B. Vitamin B2
C. Vitamin B6
D. Vitamin C
E. Zinc

3. A 43-year-old man postoperative day 7 from right below the knee amputation for a gangrenous diabetic foot wound presents with erythema, pain, and fluctuance along the medial aspect of the surgical staple line. What is the most appropriate next step in management of the patient?
A. IV fluids and IV antibiotics
B. Application of triple antibiotic ointment to the staple line
C. Removal of staples and opening of the wound
D. Compression and elevation
E. Above the knee amputation

4. A 72-year-old man undergoes open aortobifemoral bypass requiring laparotomy. Which of the following statements regarding the role of collagen in healing of his laparotomy wound is true?
A. Net collagen content increases for up to 24 months after injury.
B. Tensile strength is the force necessary to reopen a wound.
C. Endothelial cells are responsible for collagen synthesis in the initial phase of healing.
D. Tensile strength of the wound increases gradually after injury; however, it reaches a level of only about 80% of that of uninjured tissue.
E. More than 50% of the tensile strength of the wound is restored at 3 weeks after injury.

5. A 45-year-old woman with a history of chemical burn requiring skin grafting to the left calf and shin presents with a nonhealing ulcer on the medial aspect of her lower leg. Despite application of various topical ointments and meticulous wound care, she states the ulcer has never healed. What is the most appropriate next step?
A. Debridement of the ulcer
B. Antibiotic therapy
C. Punch biopsy for pathology
D. Zinc supplementation
E. Hyperbaric therapy

6. An 18-year-old man is seen in clinic with complaints of finger contracture after sustaining a burn to his hand from fireworks. Which of the following statements is true about growth factors?
A. Tumor necrosis factor-α inhibits synthesis of collagen and angiogenesis.
B. Transforming growth factor-β is stored in endothelial cells.
C. Fibroblast growth factor stimulates wound contraction.
D. Vascular endothelial growth factor and platelet-derived growth factor stimulate angiogenesis by binding to a common receptor.
E. Epidermal growth factor stimulates collagen production.

SELF-ASSESSMENT STUDY QUESTIONS AND ANSWERS

7. An 88-year-old nursing home patient has a worsening stage III decubitus ulcer. The ulcer is debrided. Tissue cultures reveal 10^8 organisms per gram of tissue after debridement. Which of the following is the most appropriate next step in management of this patient's wound?

A. Evaluation for muscle flap coverage
B. Intravenous antibiotics
C. Application of wound vacuum assisted closure (VAC) device
D. Repeat debridement
E. Repeat debridement with immediate application of a split-thickness skin graft

8. A 57-year-old man with a history of alcohol abuse and homelessness undergoes right above-the-knee amputation for critical limb ischemia. Before discharge, the patient is started on a multivitamin regimen. Which of the following statements regarding wound healing is true?

A. Iron deficiency is linked to defects in long-term wound remodeling.
B. Zinc deficiency results in delayed early wound healing.
C. High supplementary doses of vitamin C improve wound healing.
D. Vitamin A is required for hydroxylation of lysine and proline in collagen synthesis.
E. Vitamin E stimulates fibroplasia, collagen cross linking, and epithelialization.

9. A 58-year-old man with a history of tobacco abuse presents to the emergency department with a wound on his right foot after stepping on a rusted nail. An x-ray is negative for osteomyelitis. On exam, there is necrotic tissue on the plantar aspect of his foot and pulses in the bilateral lower extremities are not palpable. Tetanus booster is administered. What is the next appropriate step in management?

A. Primary repair of the wound
B. Allow the wound to heal by secondary intention
C. Perform local debridement and irrigation of the wound
D. Obtain noninvasive arterial studies
E. Perform below the knee guillotine amputation

10. A 28-year-old undergoes stab phlebectomy for venous reflux disease. On postoperative day 2, she removes her dressing. There is a large clot with associated erythema at one of her incision sites. Which of the following statements is true regarding the inflammatory phase of wound healing?

A. The presence of neutrophils within the wound is essential for normal wound healing.
B. Platelet-derived growth factor attracts neutrophils to the wound.
C. Initial vasodilation is followed by subsequent vasoconstriction.
D. The inflammatory phase lasts up to 24 hours after the time of tissue injury occurs.
E. Bradykinin causes vasoconstriction, which inhibits migration of neutrophils to the healing wound.

SELF-ASSESSMENT STUDY QUESTIONS AND ANSWERS

Answers

1. C.
2. A.
3. C.
4. D.
5. C.
6. C.
7. D.
8. B.
9. D.
10. B.

CHAPTER

6 Cardiac Evaluation of the Vascular Patient

Lindsay Ahmed and Ramdas G. Pai

OUTLINE

CARDIAC EVALUATION OF THE VASCULAR PATIENT

PREOPERATIVE RISK ASSESSMENT
- Risk Assessment Tools
- Noninvasive Cardiac Evaluation
- Coronary Angiography
- Surgical Timing After Percutaneous Coronary Intervention

PERIOPERATIVE MEDICAL MANAGEMENT
- Antiplatelet Therapy
- Statin Therapy
- Beta-Adrenergic Blockade Therapy

PERIOPERATIVE MYOCARDIAL INJURY AND INFARCTION

CARDIAC SOURCES OF ARTERIAL EMBOLISM
- Atrial Thrombi
- Left Ventricular Thrombi
- Infective Endocarditis
- Cardiac Tumors
  - Myxoma
  - Papillary Fibroelastoma

CARDIAC ARRHYTHMIAS AND CONDUCTION ABNORMALITIES
- Atrial Fibrillation
- Torsades Des Pointes
- Ventricular Arrhythmias
- Atrioventricular Block

CARDIAC EVALUATION OF THE VASCULAR PATIENT

This chapter will explore the approach to assessing the cardiac health of patients with vascular disease, specifically addressing perioperative management in high-risk patients and identifying those who will need further cardiac examination and treatment prior to surgery. It will also offer an overview of cardiac conditions which may provide a source of arterial emboli leading to acute or chronic limb ischemia.

PREOPERATIVE RISK ASSESSMENT

Due to shared risk factors and similarities in underlying pathophysiology, the overlap between coronary artery disease (CAD) and peripheral arterial disease (PAD) is substantial. Patients with known PAD frequently have atherosclerosis of a second vascular bed, and prior studies have demonstrated an incidence of CAD in this population ranging from 46% to 71%.[1,2] Due to the high pretest probability of CAD, cardiac risk assessment in patients planned for vascular surgery is vital in preventing untoward events. In addition, appropriate medical management is essential not only to reduce the perioperative risk but also to improve the long-term outlook.

RISK ASSESSMENT TOOLS

There are numerous tools available for predicting the risk of perioperative major adverse cardiac events (MACE) in patients undergoing noncardiac surgery, with the Revised Cardiac Risk Index (RCRI) being one of the most frequently used (Table 6-1). However, several other scoring systems have been created

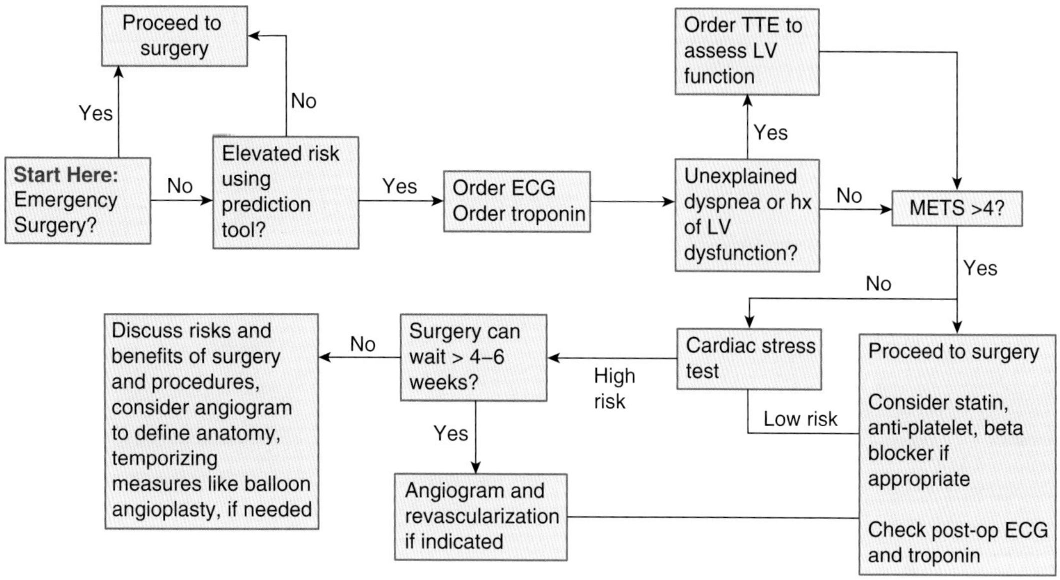

FIGURE 6-1 Preoperative surgical decision-making.

TABLE 6-1 Revised Cardiac Risk Index

Revised Cardiac Risk Index (RCRI)

Each risk predictor is assigned one point:

1. **High-risk surgical procedures**—intraperitoneal, intrathoracic, or suprainguinal vascular
2. **History of ischemic heart disease**—prior myocardial infarction or positive stress test, ECG showing the presence of pathological Q waves, current chest pain felt to be due to cardiac ischemia, or current use of nitrate therapy
3. **Congestive heart failure**—history of congestive heart failure, presence of paroxysmal nocturnal dyspnea, pulmonary edema or S3 gallop on exam, chest radiograph showing pulmonary vascular distribution
4. **History of cerebrovascular disease**—including transient ischemic attack or stroke
5. **Preoperative treatment with insulin**
6. **Preoperative serum creatinine >2.0 mg/dL / 176.8 μmol/L**

Risk of major cardiac event, including myocardial infarction, pulmonary edema, ventricular fibrillation, primary cardiac arrest, and complete heart block:

0 points – 0.4% risk

1 point – 0.9% risk

2 points – 6.6% risk

3 or more points – 11% risk

Data from Lee TH, Marcantonio ER, Mangione CM, et al. Derivation and prospective validation of a simple index for prediction of cardiac risk of major noncardiac surgery. *Circulation*. 1999;100(10):1043-1049.

TABLE 6-2 National Surgical Quality Improvement Program score (NSQIP)

National Surgical Quality Improvement Program score (NSQIP)			
Risk Factors Considered:	Procedure Age category Sex Functional status Urgency of Case ASA classification	Steroid use Presence of ascites Recent sepsis Ventilator dependent Disseminated cancer Diabetes	Hypertension requiring medication Recent CHF Dyspnea Tobacco Use Severe COPD Dialysis BMI
Outcomes Reported as a percentile:	Serious complication Any complication Pneumonia Cardiac complication	Surgical site infection Urinary tract infection Renal failure Readmission Return to OR	Venous thromboembolism Discharge to nursing home/rehab Death Sepsis

Data from American College of Surgeons National Surgical Quality Improvement Program.

such as the American College of Surgeons National Surgical Quality Improvement Program (NSQIP), which appears to outperform the RCRI specifically in patients undergoing vascular surgery (Table 6-2).[3] Guidelines do not support the use of any particular risk calculator over another, but do recommend the use of any validated risk prediction tool to help assess the risk of MACE.[4]

NONINVASIVE CARDIAC EVALUATION

Regardless of risk, it is reasonable for patients who are undergoing a moderate- or high-risk surgery to have a preoperative electrocardiogram (ECG) performed.[4] This can help to identify myocardial ischemia, infarction, chamber hypertrophy, conduction disorders, or rhythm abnormalities, and it provides a baseline by which a postoperative ECG can be compared (Table 6-3). A transthoracic echocardiogram (TTE) should be considered in those who have known left ventricular (LV) dysfunction but have not had assessment of LV function in over a year, and in those who have dyspnea from an unknown cause, or with a known history of heart failure.[4] A TTE is also helpful to evaluate the patients with suspected valvular heart disease on physical examination (Table 6-4). Patients who are determined to be at elevated risk of MACE after using a risk prediction tool should have an assessment of their functional capacity to determine if additional cardiac work-up is needed (Table 6-5). Functional

TABLE 6-3 Indications for Preoperative ECG in Patients Undergoing Vascular Surgery

Indications for 12 lead ECG
IIa Recommendation: Any patient undergoing a moderate- or high-risk procedure with one of the following:
1. Known cardiovascular disease
2. Arrhythmia
3. Significant structural heart disease
4. Peripheral arterial disease
IIb Recommendation: Any patient undergoing a moderate- or high-risk procedure

Data from Fleisher LA, Fleischmann KE, Auerbach AD, et al. 2014 ACC/AHA guideline on perioperative cardiovascular evaluation and management of patients undergoing noncardiac surgery: a report of the American College of Cardiology/American Heart Association Task Force on Practice Guidelines. *Circulation*. 2014;130(24):e278-e333.

TABLE 6-4 Indications for Preoperative Echocardiography in Patients Undergoing Vascular Surgery

Indications for Echocardiogram
IIa Recommendation:
1. Patients with dyspnea of unknown origin
2. Patients with known heart failure and new dyspnea or change in clinical status
IIb Recommendation:
1. Asymptomatic patients with known heart failure and no echocardiogram within the past 1 year

Data from Fleisher LA, Fleischmann KE, Auerbach AD, et al. 2014 ACC/AHA guideline on perioperative cardiovascular evaluation and management of patients undergoing noncardiac surgery: a report of the American College of Cardiology/American Heart Association Task Force on Practice Guidelines. *Circulation*. 2014;130(24):e278-e333.

TABLE 6-5 Indications for Preoperative Stress Testing in Patients Undergoing Vascular Surgery

Indications for Stress Test
Consider stress testing to assess functional status in the following patients if results will change management:
1. Patient has elevated risk and unknown functional capacity
Consider stress testing with cardiac imaging in the following patients if results will change management:
1. Patient has elevated risk and poor functional capacity (METS <4)
2. Patient has elevated risk and unknown functional capacity

Data from Fleisher LA, Fleischmann KE, Auerbach AD, et al. 2014 ACC/AHA guideline on perioperative cardiovascular evaluation and management of patients undergoing noncardiac surgery: a report of the American College of Cardiology/American Heart Association Task Force on Practice Guidelines. *Circulation*. 2014;130(24):e278-e333.

capacity is a reliable predictor of both perioperative and long-term cardiac events in patients undergoing noncardiac surgery.[5] Patients who are able to perform activities requiring four or more metabolic equivalents (METS) without developing symptoms should proceed to surgery without further cardiac testing. For those who have poor functional capacity or who are not able to have functional capacity assessed, cardiac stress testing with imaging should be performed if it will change management related to the planned procedure. Patients may undergo stress testing with echocardiography or myocardial perfusion imaging. Nuclear stress testing with a high summed stress score[6] and stress echocardiography with significant ischemia[7] are predictive of increased perioperative myocardial infarction (PMI) and death.

CORONARY ANGIOGRAPHY

Patients who are actively experiencing an acute coronary syndrome (ACS) at the time of planned surgery should be managed with revascularization,[8] but it is unclear whether those with CAD identified on a positive stress test or through other means benefit from revascularization prior to surgery. The CARP Trial[9] enrolled over 500 patients awaiting surgery for lower extremity PAD or expanding abdominal aortic aneurysms (AAA) who were found to have significant CAD on coronary angiography. Patients were assigned to receive either no revascularization prior to surgery or revascularization prior to surgery with either percutaneous coronary intervention or coronary artery bypass as seen fit. The study found no difference between the study groups when comparing myocardial infarction (MI) at 30 days and mortality at 2.7 years. Of note, patients with severe aortic stenosis (AS), a lesion greater than 50% in the left main coronary artery, or an ejection fraction (EF) less than 20% were excluded. The ACC/AHA has recommended against routine coronary revascularization to reduce perioperative events, except in the case of high-risk coronary anatomy such as significant left main coronary disease, ACS, or life-threatening arrhythmias felt to be due to active ischemia.[4]

SURGICAL TIMING AFTER PERCUTANEOUS CORONARY INTERVENTION

If a patient experiences ACS or is found to have high-risk disease which requires revascularization prior to surgery, shared decision making between the patient and care team should Ensue to determine the appropriate timing and management of each condition. Balloon angioplasty of the culprit vessel can be considered in patients who require an urgent procedure that cannot wait for several weeks, though these patients should still be maintained on aspirin therapy without interruption for at least 14 days. Placement of a bare metal stent (BMS) followed by 4 to 6 weeks of dual antiplatelet therapy (DAPT) is reasonable for those who can delay surgery for a month or two, but will require surgery within the next 12 months.[8] Patients who have placement of a drug eluting stent (DES) should ideally be maintained on DAPT for 12 months before holding the P2Y12 inhibitor for surgery. In circumstances where it is felt the risk of further delaying surgery outweighs the risk of stent thrombosis, the P2Y12 inhibitor can be held for surgery after 6 months, though it should be resumed in the postoperative period.[4]

PERIOPERATIVE MEDICAL MANAGEMENT

ANTIPLATELET THERAPY

Due to overlapping risk factors, patients undergoing vascular surgery may routinely take one or more antiplatelet agents for known CAD, PAD, or cerebral vascular disease. Balancing the risk of bleeding with the benefits of continuing antiplatelet agents in the perioperative period may be difficult, and the decision for administration depends on the indication for antiplatelet therapy, as well as the type and timing of the planned operation. Patients who undergo noncardiac surgery within 6 weeks of PCI have a markedly elevated risk of 30-day MACE[10] and cessation of DAPT during this period is a major risk factor for stent thrombosis.[11] Whenever possible, patients who receive a BMS should have surgery delayed more than 4 to 6 weeks after PCI, and patients with a DES should have surgery delayed for 12 months.[4] Patients who must undergo surgery within 6 weeks of PCI should ideally have dual antiplatelet therapy (DAPT) continued throughout the perioperative period. If the risk of bleeding on DAPT during surgery is felt to be too high, patients should be continued on aspirin with resumption of the P2Y12 inhibitor as soon as possible postoperatively.[4]

Conversely, patients without prior stent placement do not have a strong indication to start or continue an antiplatelet in the perioperative period. The POISE-2 Trial[12] enrolled over 10,000 patients planned for noncardiac surgery who were deemed high-risk for vascular complications, some of whom were already taking aspirin, and placed them on perioperative aspirin versus placebo. No significant difference in the rate of death or MI at 30-days post-procedure was found between the groups, but patients who received aspirin had higher rates of major bleeding. It is not clear if certain high-risk patients may benefit from initiation or continuation of an antiplatelet agent in the perioperative period, and patients should be considered on an individual basis.

STATIN THERAPY

Per the ACC/AHA 2018 guideline on the management of blood cholesterol, all patients with clinical atherosclerotic cardiovascular disease (ASCVD) should adhere to therapy with high-intensity or maximally tolerated statin. Patients deemed to be at very high risk for future ASCVD events include those who have had recent ACS, or who have a history of MI, ischemic stroke, or symptomatic peripheral vascular disease, with the latter defined as claudication symptoms with prior revascularization or amputation, or known ankle brachial index (ABI) <0.85.[13] As many patients undergoing vascular surgery will fall into one of these categories, it is anticipated that the patient may already be taking a statin regularly. Regardless of outpatient statin use, patients undergoing vascular surgery should have a statin initiated or continued in the early perioperative period. In a large retrospective cohort consisting of 180,478 patients, statin use on the day of surgery, or first day after surgery, was associated with decreased all-cause mortality, cardiac arrest, and MI within 30 days.[14]

BETA-ADRENERGIC BLOCKADE THERAPY

Beta blockers are frequently prescribed for mortality benefit in heart failure, rate control in cardiac arrhythmias, and for hypertension, but their use for reduction of perioperative cardiac events has been a topic of dispute. Beta blockers were initially assessed for perioperative benefit in patients undergoing noncardiac surgery, with the rationale that an exaggerated sympathetic response led to an increase in heart rate, and thus myocardial injury and ischemia.[15] Several studies in the 1990s showed favorable results, with findings suggesting a decrease in all-cause mortality which persisted for 2 years after the perioperative administration of atenolol[16] and a reduction in cardiac death and MI in high-risk patients undergoing vascular surgery who were treated with perioperative bisoprolol.[17] However, subsequent trials that employed variable beta blockers and administration methods raised concerns about the safety of beta blockers in the perioperative period. In 2008, the PeriOperative ISchemic Evaluation (POISE) trial assessed the effect of extended release metoprolol on the development of nonfatal MI, nonfatal cardiac arrest, and all-cause mortality when given on the day of surgery and for 30 days thereafter. Although there was a decrease in the number of perioperative MIs, there was an increase in clinically significant hypotension and bradycardia, as well as an increase in the rate of death and stroke when compared to placebo.[18] The ACC/AHA Task Force subsequently performed a systematic review of available data and found results similar to those of the POISE Trial: clinically significant increases in perioperative bradycardia, hypotension, nonfatal stroke, and all-cause mortality, but with a decrease in perioperative MI. The conclusion was drawn that beta blockade started 1 day or less prior to surgery reduced the risk of MIs, but increased the risk of bradycardia, hypotension, stroke, and death. Because of this, it is recommended that beta blockers are not generally started on the day of surgery.[4] No conclusions could be made regarding whether beta blocker started more than 1 day prior to surgery would yield different outcomes, as none of the trials assessed in the meta-analysis studied patients who began beta blockers prior to this time.[19] Separate trials assessing the effect of ambulatory use of beta blockers prior to the day of surgery have shown beneficial effect in reducing all-cause mortality[20] and have led to the recommendation to continue beta blockers in those patients who have already been prescribed them prior to surgery.[4]

PERIOPERATIVE MYOCARDIAL INJURY AND INFARCTION

PMI is a frequent complication of noncardiac surgeries, with the prevalence dependent upon preexisting risk factors and the operation performed. Unlike traditional MI which is marked by ischemic symptoms, patients experiencing PMI are frequently asymptomatic due to the presence of anesthesia and pain medications in the perioperative period.[21] A high index of suspicion and reliance on objective measures are therefore required to make the diagnosis. Patients who are at elevated risk of PMI should have preoperative cardiac troponin (cTn) values measured to assist in the differentiation between chronic and new elevation in those who are found to have rising cTn postoperatively.[22] PMI may occur due to new plaque rupture, which is classified as type 1 MI, or due to increased cardiac oxygen demand in the setting of stable CAD, classified as type 2 MI[23] (see Table 6-6). Patients with a rise in cTn who do not otherwise meet the criteria for MI are most appropriately labeled with myocardial injury.[23] Although this distinction is drawn between myocardial injury and MI in the Fourth Universal Definition of Myocardial Ischemia by the Joint Task Force, the development of either is strongly associated with a higher 30-day mortality.[24,25] In one large study which defined PMI as an absolute increase in cTn T of >14ng/L without requiring additional symptoms or ECG changes, the 30-day mortality rate of those with PMI was 10.4% [95% CI 6.7-15.7] and similar to the 30-day mortality rate of 8.7% (95% CI 4.2-16.7) observed in those who also experienced symptoms or ECG changes consistent with an MI. By comparison, the 30-day mortality rate of those who did not develop a PMI by either definition was only 1.6% [95% CI 1.1–2.4; $P < 0.001$].[24] Patients who develop PMI or myocardial injury should be managed with medications, and those who are not already taking aspirin and a statin should start on these medications.[26] The decision for cardiac revascularization is difficult and should be considered on a case-by-case basis. Unfortunately, patients who undergo revascularization after developing an NSTEMI or STEMI in the postoperative period suffer from high rates of short- and long-term

TABLE 6-6 Definitions of Types of Myocardial Infarctions

Type 1 Myocardial Infarction
Detection of a rise or fall of cardiac troponin values with at least one value above the 99th percentile of the upper limit of normal and with at least one of the following:
1. Symptoms of acute myocardial ischemia
2. New ischemic ECG changes
3. Development of pathologic Q waves
4. Imaging evidence of new loss of viable myocardium or new regional wall motion abnormality in a pattern consistent with an ischemic etiology
5. Identification of a coronary thrombus by angiography including intracoronary imaging or by autopsy
Type 2 Myocardial Infarction
Detection of the rise and/or fall of cardiac troponin values with at least one value above the 99th percentile of the upper limit of normal, and evidence of an imbalance between myocardial oxygen supply and demand unrelated to acute coronary atherothrombosis, requiring at least one of the following:
1. Symptoms of acute myocardial ischemia
2. New ischemic ECG changes
3. Development of pathological Q waves
4. Imaging evidence of new loss of viable myocardium or new regional wall motion abnormality in a pattern consistent with an ischemic etiology

mortality, with the presence of peripheral vascular disease being predictive of both.

CARDIAC SOURCES OF ARTERIAL EMBOLISM

Arterial emboli occur when tissue or other substance travel through the vasculature and ultimately become embedded in a distal artery with resultant obstruction of flow. This may cause a stroke, organ dysfunction, or limb ischemia. In patients who present with evidence of peripheral arterial embolism, identification of the source is vital for treatment and prevention of additional embolic events. The majority of arterial emboli originate from a cardiac source, though other sources include thromboemboli or atheroemboli from the aorta, venous clots that cross a shunt to reach the arterial tree, and rare causes such as tumor fragments, fat, or entrained air.[27] Common cardiac sources of emboli include thrombi arising in the atria or LV, valvular vegetations, and tumor fragments, which will be covered here.

ATRIAL THROMBI

Atrial fibrillation (AF) predisposing to the formation of atrial thrombi is the most common source of arterial emboli.[28] It is a frequently found cardiac arrhythmia, with a prevalence rate ranging from 1% to 4% in the United States, Australia, and Europe, and as high as 18% in adults above 80 years old.[29] The incidence is anticipated to increase globally as risk factors rise in both developed and developing countries. Other atrial arrhythmias such as atrial flutter may increase the risk of atrial thrombi formation, though this risk is less well described and appears to be lower than that seen with AF.[30] While patients with atrial arrhythmias may notice episodes of palpitations, shortness of breath, or fatigue, many are completely asymptomatic. Diagnosis of AF is made with an ECG or telemetry strip showing the arrhythmia, though cardiac imaging can further support the diagnosis. Transthoracic echocardiography (TTE) may identify a large left atrium which can increase suspicion for an atrial arrhythmia, and in some instances, may identify a visible thrombus.[31] Transesophageal echocardiography (TEE) allows for superior assessment of the anatomy and function of the LAA which may contain thrombus or show low emptying velocities.[31] The 5% to 14% of patients who are in AF for more than 2 days have a thrombus in the LAA which may be small or several centimeters in diameter.[32] Patients at increased risk for atrial thrombi formation should receive anticoagulation. Regardless of other risk factors, patients who have moderate-to-severe mitral stenosis and those who have a mechanical valve remain high risk for thrombus formation and should receive warfarin therapy. For all others, risk should be assessed using the CHA2DS2-VASc score (Table 6-4), with initiation of anticoagulation (warfarin or direct oral anticoagulant both acceptable) in men with a score of 2 or greater and women with a score of 3 or greater.[33] Patients who are found to have a peripheral arterial embolism with a concomitant atrial arrhythmia should receive systemic anticoagulation.[34]

LEFT VENTRICULAR THROMBI

Patients with ischemic or nonischemic cardiomyopathies resulting in reduced LV function are at risk of developing LV thrombi due to stagnation of blood, with greater risk in those with markedly reduced LV function and cardiac output. Patients presenting with acute coronary syndromes with LV dysfunction are at increased risk of thrombus formation due to a decline in physiologic anticoagulants and an increase in physiologic procoagulants in the peri-infarct period. The location and extent of infarct, as well as the time lapse prior to hospital presentation, define the risk of developing a thrombus. Patients presenting with anterior ST elevation myocardial infarction (STEMI) are at the greatest risk, with development of LV thrombi in as many as 43% of cases.[35] TTE is a cost-effective and readily available modality for diagnosing LV thrombus, with a sensitivity as high as 95%, and specificity of 85% to 90%, though this is operator-dependent.[34] The use of ultrasound contrast agents can help detect smaller thrombi, those in the apex, and those without a protruding component which are more difficult to localize. Cardiac magnetic resonance (CMR) imaging has the highest sensitivity for detecting LV thrombi[36] and can be considered when contrast-enhanced TTE is still nondiagnostic. Patients who are found to have an LV thrombus should receive warfarin therapy with a goal international normalized ration (INR) 2.0 to 3.0 for 3 to 6 months to prevent embolism.[37,38]

INFECTIVE ENDOCARDITIS

Patients with structural heart disease are predisposed to infective endocarditis (IE), and both native and prosthetic cardiac valves may develop vegetations with embolic potential. Rheumatic heart disease remains the most common risk factor for developing endocarditis in developing countries, whereas degenerative heart disease now accounts for the greatest risk in developed countries. Health care–associated IE has become an important entity with increasing use of dialysis shunts, prosthetic valves, permanent pacemakers, and intravascular catheters which increase the risk for bacteremia and disproportionately affect older adults.[39] Dislodgement of a valvular vegetation may cause septic emboli to any organ system of the body, causing stroke, MI, or infarction of the kidney, spleen, mesentery, or lower extremities. Mycotic aneurysms also may occur from direct bacterial invasion or immune complex deposition in the arterial wall, or through occlusion of the vasa vasorum. They occur most frequently in the cerebral arteries, but on rare occasion may affect the peripheral arteries.[39] Patients who are found to have septic arterial emboli may display overt signs and symptoms of endocarditis. The diagnosis of endocarditis is made utilizing the modified Duke criteria, which take into account infective symptoms, predisposing cardiac conditions, bacteremia, immunologic phenomena, and vascular phenomena including arterial emboli and mycotic aneurysms.[40] All patients in whom IE is considered should receive a TTE, and those who have high-risk findings on the TTE should proceed to TEE for more detailed visualization of the valves. Patients who are felt to have moderate or high risk for IE should have a TTE as well as TEE regardless of the findings on TTE.[41] In some patients, echocardiography may not show endocarditis, but the patient continues to display signs and symptoms concerning for the diagnosis. TEE should be repeated in these patients after 3 to 5 days, or with clinical change in symptoms to assess for new evidence of endocarditis.[41] Patients should be treated with an appropriate antibiotic regimen, and followed by a multidisciplinary team. The team should consist of a cardiologist, infectious disease specialist, and surgeon to determine the appropriate antibiotic regimen, duration of treatment, and approach to surgical management if needed.[41]

CARDIAC TUMORS

Myxoma

Myxomas are the most common primary cardiac neoplasm, and are benign tumors most frequently found in the left atrium attached to the fossa ovalis, though they may be found in other cardiac chambers as well. They may cause constitutional symptoms, and they have the potential to grow to a large size causing obstructive symptoms.[42] Myxomas are frequently friable and susceptible to embolism—a finding that may occur in nearly one-third of patients, and is often the presenting symptom.[43] TTE and TEE are helpful in identifying the mass, stalk, and degree of vascularity if contrast is used. But cardiac MRI offers better tissue characterization which can more confidently differentiate a myxoma from other cardiac masses.[44] Myxomas are treated surgically with excision of the mass and implant site.[45]

Papillary Fibroelastoma

Papillary fibroelastomas (PFE) are the second most common primary cardiac tumor in adults, and they are most frequently found on the aortic and mitral valves.[31] Like myxomas, they are prone to embolization, which may be the initial presentation. They appear as homogenous masses with frond-like extensions which can be very mobile.[46] TTE or TEE can be used to diagnose PFE based on its characteristic appearance. Surgical resection is recommended for all the patients who experience symptoms such as systemic embolization and for those with PFEs larger than 1 cm or with mobile components. However, some data suggests that even small PFEs have embolic potential and should be considered for surgery.[47]

CARDIAC ARRHYTHMIAS AND CONDUCTION ABNORMALITIES

Cardiac arrhythmias in the perioperative period are not uncommon, and the majority of them tend to be asymptomatic.[48] However, even the development of transient arrhythmias has been shown to increase mortality in patients undergoing noncardiac surgery.[49] For this reason, rapid identification, treatment, and, when possible, prevention of arrhythmias is vital.

ATRIAL FIBRILLATION

AF is a frequent finding in the postoperative period, with a rate of development between 3% to 10% of those undergoing noncardiac surgery.[50] Postoperative stress predisposes patients to the development of tachyarrhythmias and may come in the form of hypoxemia, catecholamine excess, instrumentation, and acid-base disorders. AF specifically may be hastened by acute atrial distention, volume shifts, and atrial trauma during surgery. It is identified on ECG or telemetry as an irregular tachyarrhythmia with no discernible P wave.

Patients with postoperative AF lasting 15 or more minutes who are otherwise stable should receive intravenous beta blockers as a first-line choice to slow the ventricular rate, though calcium-channel blockers in patients with a normal ejection fraction and amiodarone are also reasonable choices. Patients who become hemodynamically unstable and select patients who continue to experience symptoms despite ventricular rate control should undergo synchronized direct current cardioversion for restoration to sinus rhythm. In patients who have been in AF for less than 48 hours, the risk of development of left atrial appendage (LAA) thrombus and, therefore, stroke is low. For those who have experienced AF for more than 48 hours, the risk for stroke is increased and the need for anticoagulation should be assessed (see Table 6-7).

TORSADES DES POINTES

Prolongation of the QT interval is an ECG finding which represents prolonged ventricular repolarization, and it is dangerous in that it may cause torsades des pointes (TdP), a type of polymorphic ventricular tachycardia (VT). Patients in the perioperative period may experience QT prolongation due to a combination of administered medications and predisposing factors such as electrolyte abnormalities, bradycardia, and long QT syndrome. Many medications are known to cause QT prolongation, including those frequently administered during the perioperative period such as proton pump inhibitors, certain antibiotics, antipsychotics, and some antiemetics.

The onset of TdP can generally be identified on an ECG with a change in the amplitude and morphology of the QRS complexes around the isoelectric line. The QT interval is generally greater than 500 ms, the typical rate is 160 to 240 beats per minute, and the first few beats of the VT tend to have longer cycle lengths than those which follow.[51] The arrhythmia may terminate spontaneously,

TABLE 6-7 Calculation of CHA2DS2VASc Score and Atrial Fibrillation and Stroke Risk Prediction

CHA2DS2VASc Score	
Risk Factors:	Assigned Points:
Congestive heart failure	1
Hypertension	1
Age > 75 years	2
Diabetes mellitus	1
Stroke/TIA/systemic embolism	2
Vascular disease	1
Age 65–74 years	1
Female sex	1
Annual stroke risk (%) based on score	
1 point – 1.3%	
2 points – 2.2%	
3 points – [illegible]	
4 points – 4.0%	
5 points – 6.7%	
6 points – [illegible]	
7 points – 9.6%	
8 points – [illegible]	
9 points – 15.2%	

but it may also further degenerate to ventricular fibrillation.

Prevention of QT prolongation may be possible by monitoring for electrolyte abnormalities such as hypokalemia and hypomagnesemia, and by avoiding or reducing implicated medications. For those who have developed TdP, magnesium should be administered as magnesium sulfate 2 g intravenously with repeat infusions given as needed regardless of the measured value. Potassium should be repleted with a goal of 4.5 to 5.0 mEq/L.[52] For patients with bradycardia, overdrive pacing or the administration of isoproterenol to increase the heart rate may suppress TdP.[51] Those who do not respond to the above measures or become hemodynamically unstable should receive immediate direct current cardioversion.

VENTRICULAR ARRHYTHMIAS

Perioperative ventricular arrhythmias are rare and occur most frequently in the patients who sustain an MI or have underlying structural heart disease. In the setting of acute ischemia, patients may develop polymorphic ventricular tachycardia, a type of ventricular tachycardia (VT) which arises from multiple ventricular foci. Like other forms of VT, it is characterized by a wide-complex rhythm arising from the ventricles with a rate greater than 100 beats per minute. As the rhythm arises from multiple locations throughout the ventricles, the QRS complexes will display variable axis and amplitude. Alternatively, monomorphic VT most frequently arises in those with underlying structural heart disease and in those who sustained an MI more than 48 hours prior. It arises from a single irritable ventricular focus; therefore, the QRS complexes will have uniform axis and amplitude.

Either form of VT may present with hemodynamic compromise or anginal chest pain, and the development of either should prompt immediate response with direct current cardioversion. For hemodynamically stable patients with sustained VT, treatment with intravenous lidocaine or amiodarone may be initiated, with the latter preferred in those with reduced LV function.

ATRIOVENTRICULAR BLOCK

Atrioventricular (AV) block is a disorder in which electrical signals from the atria experience impaired travel to the ventricles due to disease at the level of the AV node. AV block exists on a spectrum from first to third degree, with first degree characterized by increased time to travel through the AV node, and third degree characterized by a complete block of electrical signals through the AV node. Second degree represents an intermediate level of block which exists in two forms, with type one indicated by a progressive lengthening in the time to travel through the AV node, which is seen as a progressive lengthening of the PR interval. Type two consists of intermittent refractoriness of the AV node, which manifests as occasional "dropped" QRS complexes without an antecedent lengthening of the PR interval. In the perioperative setting, transient AV block may occur due to increased vagal tone from factors such as laryngoscopy or spinal anesthesia.[53] Alternatively, patients who sustain an MI during surgery may experience AV block secondary to ischemia of the AV node.

Transient and asymptomatic AV block does not require any intervention. However, patients who experienced sustained periods of bradycardia or who become symptomatic should receive a beta agonist or antimuscarinic agent, or should undergo temporary transcutaneous or transvenous pacing. In those who experience AV block as a consequence of an MI, coronary revascularization should be considered. As AV block following surgery is best described in patients undergoing cardiac surgery, recommendations related to the management of postoperative block with a permanent pacemaker are gleaned from this population, and extrapolated to those undergoing noncardiac surgery. In patients who develop second-degree type two or third-degree AV block following surgery, a permanent pacemaker should be placed if the block is not expected to resolve, or if 7 days have passed since surgery.[54]

REFERENCES

1. Sukhija R, Aronow WS, Yalamanchili K, Sinha N, Babu S. Prevalence of coronary artery disease, lower extremity peripheral arterial disease, and cerebrovascular disease in 110 men with an abdominal aortic aneurysm. *Am J Cardiol.* 2004;94:1358-1359.
2. Dieter RS, Tomasson J, Gudjonsson T, et al. Lower extremity peripheral arterial disease in hospitalized patients with coronary artery disease. *Vasc Med.* 2003;8:233-236.
3. Gupta PK, Gupta H, Sundaram A, et al. Development and validation of a risk calculator for prediction of cardiac risk after surgery. *Circulation.* 2011;124:381-387.
4. Fleisher LA, Fleischmann KE, Auerbach AD, et al. 2014 ACC/AHA guideline on perioperative cardiovascular evaluation and management of patients undergoing noncardiac surgery: executive summary: a report of the American College of Cardiology/American Heart Association Task Force on practice guidelines. Developed in collaboration with the American College of Surgeons, American Society of Anesthesiologists, American Society of Echocardiography, American Society of Nuclear Cardiology, Heart Rhythm Society, Society for Cardiovascular Angiography and Interventions, Society of Cardiovascular Anesthesiologists, and Society of Vascular Medicine Endorsed by the Society of Hospital Medicine. *J Nucl Cardiol.* 2015;22(1):162-215.
5. Reilly DF, McNeely MJ, Doerner D, et al. Self-reported exercise tolerance and the risk of serious perioperative complications. *Arch Intern Med.* 1999;159:2185-2192.
6. Harafuji K, Chikamori T, Kawaguchi S, et al. Value of pharmacologic stress myocardial perfusion imaging for preoperative risk stratification for aortic surgery. *Circ J.* 2005;69:558-563.
7. van Damme H, Piérard L, Gillain D, et al. Cardiac risk assessment before vascular surgery: a prospective study comparing clinical evaluation, dobutamine stress echocardiography, and dobutamine Tc-99m sestamibi tomoscintigraphy. *Cardiovasc Surg.* 1997; 5:54-64.
8. Levine GN, Bates ER, Blankenship JC, et al. 2011 ACCF/AHA/ SCAI guideline for percutaneous coronary intervention: a report of the American College of Cardiology Foundation/American Heart Association Task Force on Practice Guidelines and the Society for Cardiovascular Angiography and Interventions. *Circulation.* 2011;124:e574-e651.
9. McFalls EO, Ward HB, Moritz TE, et al. Coronary-artery revascularization before elective major vascular surgery. *N Engl J Med.* 2004;351(27):2795-2804.
10. Wijeysundera DN, Wijeysundera HC, Yun L, et al. Risk of elective major noncardiac surgery after coronary stent insertion: a population-based study. *Circulation.* 2012;126(11):1355-1362.
11. van Werkum JW, Heestermans AA, Zomer AC, et al. Predictors of coronary stent thrombosis: the Dutch Stent Thrombosis Registry. *J Am Coll Cardiol.* 2009;53:1399-1409.
12. Devereaux PJ, Mrkobrada M, Sessler DI, et al. Aspirin in patients undergoing noncardiac surgery. *N Engl J Med.* 2014;370:1494-1503.
13. Wilson PWF, Polonsky TS, Miedema MD, Khera A, Kosinski AS, Kuvin JT. Systematic review for the 2018 AHA/ACC/AACVPR/AAPA/ABC/ACPM/ADA/AGS/APhA/ASPC/NLA/PCNA guideline on the management of blood cholesterol: a report of the American College of Cardiology/American Heart Association Task Force on clinical practice guidelines [published correction appears in *J Am Coll Cardiol.* 2019 Jun 25;73(24):3242]. *J Am Coll Cardiol.* 2019;73(24):3210-3227.
14. London MJ, Schwartz GG, Hur K, Henderson WG. Association of perioperative statin use with mortality

and morbidity after major noncardiac surgery. *JAMA Intern Med*. 2017;177(2):231-242.

15. Mangano DT, Wong MG, London MJ, Tubau JF, Rapp JA. Study of perioperative ischemia (SPI) research group. Perioperative myocardial ischemia in patients undergoing noncardiac surgery. II. Incidence and severity during the 1st week after surgery. *J Am Coll Cardiol*. 1991;17:851-857.
16. Mangano DT, Layug EL, Wallace A, et al. Effect of atenolol on mortality and cardiovascular morbidity after non-cardiac surgery. Multicenter study of perioperative ischemia research group. *N Engl J Med*. 1996;335(23):1713-1720.
17. Poldermans D, Boersma E, Bax JJ, et al. The effect of bisoprolol on perioperative mortality and myocardial infarction in high-risk patients undergoing vascular surgery. Dutch echocardiographic cardiac risk evaluation applying stress echocardiography study group. *N Engl J Med*. 1999;341:1789-1794.
18. Devereaux PJ, Yang H, Yusuf S, et al. Effects of extended-release metoprolol succinate in patients undergoing non-cardiac surgery (POISE trial): a randomized controlled trial. *Lancet*. 2008;371:1839-1847.
19. Wijeysundera DN, Duncan D, Nkonde-Price C, et al. Perioperative beta blockade in noncardiac surgery: a systematic review for the 2014 ACC/AHA guideline on perioperative cardiovascular evaluation and management of patients undergoing noncardiac surgery: a report of the American College of Cardiology/American Heart Association Task Force on Practice Guidelines. *Circulation*. 2014;130:2246-2261.
20. Barrett TW, Mori M, De Boer D. Association of ambulatory use of statins and beta-blockers with long-term mortality after vascular surgery. *J Hosp Med*. 2007;2(4):241-252.
21. Magoon R, Makhija N, Das D. Perioperative myocardial injury and infarction following non-cardiac surgery: A review of the eclipsed epidemic. *Saudi J Anaesth*. 2020;14:91-99.
22. Nagele P, Brown F, Gage BF, et al. High-sensitivity cardiac troponin T in prediction and diagnosis of myocardial infarction and long-term mortality after noncardiac surgery. *Am Heart J*. 2013;166:325-332.
23. Thygesen K, Alpert JS, Jaffe AS, et al. Fourth universal definition of myocardial infarction. *Circulation*. 2018;138:e618-e651.
24. Puelacher C, Lurati Buse G, Seeberger D, et al. Perioperative myocardial injury after non-cardiac surgery: incidence, mortality, and characterization. *Circulation*. 2018;137:1221-1232.
25. van Waes JA, Nathoe HM, de Graaff JC, et al. Myocardial injury after noncardiac surgery and its association with short-term mortality. *Circulation*. 2013;127(23):2264-2271.
26. Devereaux PJ, Xavier D, Pogue J, et al. POISE (PeriOperative ISchemic Evaluation) investigators. Characteristics and short-term prognosis of perioperative myocardial infarction in patients undergoing noncardiac surgery. A cohort study. *Ann Intern Med*. 2011;154:523-528.
27. Saric M, Kronzon I. Aortic atherosclerosis and embolic events. *Curr Cardiol Rep*. 2012;14:342-349.
28. Campbell WB, Ridler BM, Szymanska TH. Two-year follow-up after acute thromboembolic limb ischaemia: the importance of anticoagulation. *Eur J Vasc Endovasc Surg*. 2000;19:169-173.
29. Rahman F, Kwan GF, Benjamin EJ. Global epidemiology of atrial fibrillation [published correction appears in *Nat Rev Cardiol*. 2016;13(8):501]. *Nat Rev Cardiol*. 2014;11(11):639-654.
30. Huang JJ, Reddy S, Truong TH, Suryanarayana P, Alpert JS. Atrial appendage thrombosis risk is lower for atrial flutter compared with atrial fibrillation. *Am J Med*. 2018;131(4):442.e13-442.e17.
31. Saric M, Armour AC, Arnaout MS, et al. Guidelines for the use of echocardiography in the evaluation of a cardiac source of embolism. *J Am Soc Echocardiogr*. 2016;29(1):1-42.
32. Menke J, Lüthje L, Kastrup A, Larsen J. Thromboembolism in atrial fibrillation. *Am J Cardiol*. 2012;105:502-510.
33. January CT, Wann LS, Calkins H, et al. 2019 AHA/ACC/HRS focused update of the 2014 AHA/ACC/HRS guideline for the management of patients with atrial fibrillation: a report of the American College of Cardiology/American Heart Association task force on clinical practice guidelines and the Heart Rhythm Society in collaboration with the Society of Thoracic Surgeons. *Circulation*. 2019;140:e125-e151.
34. Lyaker MR, Tulman DB, Dimitrova GT, Pin RH, Papadimos TJ. Arterial embolism. *Int J Crit Illn Inj Sci*. 2013;3(1):77-87.
35. Mir J, Raheel Jahangir J, Asfandyar Q, et al. Left ventricular thrombus in patients with acute anterior wall myocardial infarction. *J Ayub Med Coll Abbottabad*. 2014;26:491-495.
36. Delewi R, Nijveldt R, Hirsch A, et al. Left ventricular thrombus formation after acute myocardial infarction as assessed by cardiovascular magnetic resonance imaging. *Eur J Radiol*. 2012;81:3900-3904.
37. Guyatt GH, Akl EA, Crowther M, et al. Executive summary: antithrombotic therapy and prevention of thrombosis, 9th ed: American College of Chest Physicians evidence-based clinical practice guidelines. *Chest*. 2012;141:7S-47S.

38. van de Werf F, Bax J, Betriu A, et al. Management of acute myocardial infarction in patients presenting with persistent ST-segment elevation: the task force on the management of ST-segment elevation acute myocardial infarction of the European Society of Cardiology. *Eur Heart J*. 2008;29(23):2909-2945.
39. Holland T, Baddour L, Bayer A, et al. Infective endocarditis. *Nat Rev Dis Primer*. 2016;2:16059.
40. Li JS, Sexton DJ, Mick N, et al. Proposed modifications to the Duke criteria for the diagnosis of infective endocarditis. *Clin Infect Dis*. 2000;30:633-638.
41. Baddour LM, Wilson WR, Bayer AS, et al. Infective endocarditis in adults: diagnosis, antimicrobial therapy, and management of complications: A scientific statement for healthcare professionals from the American Heart Association [published correction appears in Circulation. 2015;132(17):e215] [published correction appears in Circulation. 2016 Aug 23;134(8):e113] [published correction appears in Circulation. 2018;138(5):e78-e79]. *Circulation*. 2015;132(15):1435-1486.
42. Wang JG, Li YJ, Liu H, Li NN, Zhao J, Xing XM. Clinicopathologic analysis of cardiac myxomas: seven years'experience with 61 patients. *J Thorac Dis*. 2012;4(3): 272-283.
43. Lee SJ, Kim JH, Na CY, Oh SS. Eleven years' experience with Korean cardiac myxoma patients: focus on embolic complications. *Cerebrovasc Dis*. 2012;33(5):471-479.
44. Abbas A, Garfath-Cox KA, Brown IW, Shambrook JS, Peebles CR, Harden SP. Cardiac MR assessment of cardiac myxomas. *Br J Radiol*. 2015;88(1045):20140599.
45. Garatti A, Nano G, Canziani A, et al. Surgical excision of cardiac myxomas: twenty years experience at a single institution. *Ann Thorac Surg*. 2012;93(3):825-831.
46. Yong MS, Smail H, Saxena P. Management of incidental papillary fibroelastoma: an update. *Int J Cardiol*. 2016;215:338-339.
47. Tamin SS, Maleszewski JJ, Scott CG, et al. Prognostic and bioepidemiologic implications of papillary fibroelastomas *J. Am. Coll. Cardiol*. 2014;65(22):2420-2429.
48. Winkel TA, Schouten O, Hoeks SE, et al. Risk factors and outcome of new-onset cardiac arrhythmias in vascular surgery patients. *Am Heart J*. 2010;159:1108-1115.
49. Winkel TA, Schouten O, Hoeks SE, et al. Prognosis of transient new-onset atrial fibrillation during vascular surgery. *Eur J Vasc Endovasc Surg*. 2009;38:683-688.
50. Bhave PD, Goldman LE, Vittinghoff E, Maselli J, Auerbach A. Incidence, predictors, and outcomes associated with postoperative atrial fibrillation after major noncardiac surgery. *Am Heart J*. 2012;164:918-924.
51. Drew BJ, Ackerman MJ, Funk M, et al. Prevention of torsade de pointes in hospital settings: a scientific statement from the American Heart Association and the American College of Cardiology Foundation. *Circulation*. 2010;121:1047-1060.
52. Zipes DP, Camm AJ, Borggrefe M, et al. ACC/AHA/ESC 2006 guidelines for management of patients with ventricular arrhythmias and the prevention of sudden cardiac death: a report of the American College of Cardiology/American Heart Association Task Force and the European Society of Cardiology Committee for Practice Guidelines (writing committee to develop guidelines for management of patients with ventricular arrhythmias and the prevention of sudden cardiac death). *J Am Coll Cardiol*. 2006;48:e247-e346.
53. Atlee JL. Perioperative cardiac dysrhythmias: diagnosis and management. *Anesthesiology*. 1997;86:1397-1424.
54. Gregoratos G, Cheitlin MD, Conill A, et al. ACC/AHA guidelines for implantation of cardiac pacemakers and antiarrhythmia devices: executive summary. *Circulation*. 1998;97:1325-1335.

SELF-ASSESSMENT STUDY QUESTIONS AND ANSWERS

Questions

1. A 59-year-old man with a history of hypertension, diabetes, and anterior STEMI for which he received two drug eluting stents to the LAD 3 weeks ago presents to the emergency room with sudden onset pain in his left lower extremity at rest. Pulses are inaudible on the affected side. A diagnosis of acute limb ischemia is made, and he undergoes open surgical revascularization. Which test has the highest sensitivity to identify the source of the suspected embolism?
A. TTE
B. TTE with contrast
C. TEE
D. Cardiac MRI

2. A 71-year-old woman with a history of hypertension, diabetes mellitus, and AAA who underwent open repair 6 months prior presents to your office for routine follow-up. She reports some exertional dyspnea and episodes of palpitations. An ECG shows atrial fibrillation at a rate of 84 bpm. She undergoes an echocardiogram which reveals an ejection fraction of 60%, mild left ventricular hypertrophy, moderate enlargement of the left atrium, and moderate mitral stenosis. Which of the following is the best strategy to prevent LA thrombus formation and its embolic complications?
A. Watchful waiting
B. Aspirin therapy
C. warfarin therapy
D. DOAC therapy

3. A 53-year-old man with a history of hypertension, GERD, and bicuspid aortic valve for which he underwent surgical valve replacement 2 years prior presents to the emergency department with fevers and fatigue. He is found to have a fever of 38.4°C. He has no murmur, and no evidence of vascular or immunologic phenomena on exam. He has two sets of blood cultures drawn, and no bacteria are isolated. He is started on broad spectrum antibiotics. He has a TTE and TEE performed, and neither shows evidence of endocarditis. Four days later, he continues to have fevers, and is found to have an II/IV diastolic murmur heard at the right upper sternal border. What is the most appropriate management step to make the diagnosis?
A. Continue antibiotics and do no additional testing at this time
B. Order an ECG to look for new heart block
C. Repeat the TTE
D. Repeat the TEE

4. A 67-year-old man with a history of hypertension, diabetes, diabetic nephropathy and recently diagnosed end-stage renal disease presents to the office for evaluation of surgical AV fistula creation. He had an ECG and TTE performed 6 months ago when he initially presented to the hospital in renal failure appearing hypervolemic. At that time, he was in normal sinus rhythm, and his TTE showed moderate LVH but was otherwise normal with an EF of 60% to 65%. He had a temporary dialysis catheter placed and has been receiving hemodialysis 3 days a week. He currently denies any chest pain or shortness of breath, and he appears euvolemic on exam. He has a treadmill that he jogs on for 30 minutes three times per week without developing symptoms, and he mows his lawn each Sunday. What is the appropriate work-up for preoperative cardiac risk assessment?
A. Order an ECG and troponin level
B. Order an ECG and TTE
C. Arrange for an exercise stress test
D. Arrange for a cardiac catheterization

5. A 79-year-old woman with hypertension, dyslipidemia, CAD with an NSTEMI necessitating placement of 1 BMS in the RCA 6 weeks ago, and PAD presents to discuss surgical planning. Just prior to the NSTEMI, she was evaluated for intermittent claudication of the right lower extremity and a nonhealing ulcer of the right foot. She was found to have a significant right popliteal lesion, and was planned for femoral-popliteal bypass which was subsequently delayed after her MI. She is currently

SELF-ASSESSMENT STUDY QUESTIONS AND ANSWERS

taking aspirin, clopidogrel, atorvastatin, and metoprolol. She continues to report claudication and is starting to notice burning in her toes on the right foot throughout the day and night. What is the most appropriate management strategy regarding surgical timing and antiplatelet use?

A. It has been 6 weeks—stop aspirin and plavix and plan for surgery at the earliest.
B. It has been 6 weeks—continue aspirin but hold plavix and plan for surgery at the earliest.
C. Monitor her symptoms, and explain to the patient that due to her recent PCI she should ideally wait 6 to 12 months before surgery. If she goes for surgery now, she will have a very high risk of stent thrombosis.
D. Explain to the patient that due to her recent PCI she should ideally wait 6 to 12 months before surgery. She will have a very high risk of stent thrombosis if antiplatelet therapy is held, but her symptoms necessitate surgery at the earliest if she is willing.

6. A 71-year-old woman with hypertension, diabetes, dyslipidemia, and AAA measuring 5.4 cm presents to the hospital for planned open AAA repair. Her medication list shows that she takes metoprolol succinate 50 mg a day at home. Your medical student asks if it is ok to continue this medication. How do you respond?

A. Stop the beta blocker to prevent an increase in perioperative MI
B. Stop the beta blocker to prevent an increase in perioperative bradycardia
C. Continue the beta blocker with cautious monitoring
D. Switch to a calcium channel blocker

7. An 81-year-old man with diabetes mellitus, dyslipidemia, and a CVA 2 months prior was found to have a 95% occlusion of the left internal carotid artery which correlated with his stroke symptoms. He is admitted for carotid endarterectomy, and has a preoperative troponin checked which was 0.01, and an ECG which shows normal sinus rhythm without evidence for ischemia. He can perform 9 METs and does not undergo any further testing prior to surgery. His procedure is successful, and the patient feels well. A troponin level is checked on postoperative day 1, and found to be 0.8, which is above the 99th percentile. The level trends down to 0.7 and 0.6 later in the day. His ECG shows no significant change, and a TTE shows a normal EF with no wall motion abnormality. He remains asymptomatic throughout his hospital course and is discharged in good condition. What is the appropriate diagnosis?

A. STEMI
B. Type 1 NSTEMI
C. Type 2 NSTEMI
D. Myocardial Injury

8. The above patient returns to clinic for a postoperative check, and asks you to clarify the significance of the finding. What do you tell him?

A. Since he did not experience an MI and his EF is normal, the finding is of no significance and he should not worry about it.
B. He would benefit from initiating aspirin and a statin, but patients with his condition have a prognosis similar to patients who never had an elevated troponin.
C. He would benefit from initiating aspirin and a statin, and patients with an elevated troponin like his tend to have a worse prognosis compared to those who do not have an elevated troponin.
D. He would benefit from initiation of aspirin and statin, and he should undergo cardiac catheterization.

9. A 69-year-old woman with a history of depression, hypertension and diabetes mellitus complicated by peripheral neuropathy is found to have a AAA measuring 5.6 cm, and is planned for repair. Her surgery is successful, and postoperatively she has her home medications resumed, which consist of citalopram, hydrochlorothiazide, insulin, atorvastatin, and aspirin. While in the hospital, she is also initiated on a PPI and ondansetron for nausea. Overnight in the ICU, the nurse calls you to report that the patient had a change on telemetry, and is

SELF-ASSESSMENT STUDY QUESTIONS AND ANSWERS

now in a wide complex rhythm. You go bedside and notice a ventricular rhythm at 175 bpm with QRS complexes showing variable amplitude and axis. The patient is sitting up in bed and is talking to you calmly. Her blood pressure is 117/81 mmHg. What do you do next?

A. Check serum potassium and magnesium levels, and replace them if low
B. Administer magnesium sulfate 2 g and place the external defibrillator pads on the patient
C. Immediately initiate intravenous lidocaine for treatment of VT
D. Place the external defibrillator pads on the patient and emergently defibrillate the patient

10. A 53-year-old woman with a history of hypertension develops sudden onset right lower extremity pain. She is found to have pain at rest, as well as diminished right popliteal and dorsalis pedis pulses. She has completely normal pulses on the left. She undergoes a peripheral angiogram showing total occlusion of the popliteal artery. She is planned for open surgery and has a TTE performed due to the suspicion of embolic source. She is noted to have a 1-cm mass with multiple projections on its surface attached to the mitral valve, and it is swinging back and forth every time the valve opens. What is the most likely diagnosis?

A. Myxoma
B. Papillary fibroelastoma
C. Valvular vegetation
D. Atrial thrombus in transit

SELF-ASSESSMENT STUDY QUESTIONS AND ANSWERS

Answers

1. D.
2. C.
3. D.
4. A.
5. B.
6. C.
7. D.
8. C.
9. B.
10. B.

CHAPTER

7 Noninvasive Evaluation of Venous Disease

Abdullah Nasif and Samih W. Bittar

OUTLINE

INTRODUCTION
HISTORY AND PHYSICAL EXAMINATION
CLASSIFICATION SYSTEM (CEAP)
REVISED VENOUS CLINICAL SEVERITY SCORE (VCSS)
LABORATORY TESTS
NONINVASIVE IMAGING MODALITIES
Venous Duplex Ultrasound (DUS)
Upper Extremities
Lower Extremity
Intrapelvic/Intra-abdominal
CT Venography
MR Venography
Plethysmography
Air Plethysmography
Photoplethysmography
New Diagnostic Methods (Artificial Intelligence)

INTRODUCTION

The imaging of the vasculature has advanced significantly in recent years and serves as an important tool to assess various types of venous diseases, from monochrome to four-dimensional color images, to the recent implementation of artificial intelligence.

In the early twentieth century, angiography was used to visualize the vascular system by injecting iodine into the bloodstream and viewing it with an X-ray. Ultrasound, CT, and MRI were later developed for more advanced vascular imaging techniques. Novel vascular imaging approaches lead to new discoveries in vascular pathology and more precise diagnosis.

Noninvasive diagnostic modalities have transformed the assessment of vascular diseases. Physicians can reach a diagnosis in a quick and effective way instead of invasive modalities. This chapter describes the current noninvasive diagnostic tools used in evaluating venous disease.

HISTORY AND PHYSICAL EXAMINATION

Obtaining a detailed history and thorough physical examination remains as the basis of venous disease diagnosis. Neglecting this crucial step will result in unnecessary testing and treatment. The onset, course, exacerbating/relieving factors, and related clinical signs and symptoms should all be defined in a thorough history. Recent surgical operations, extensive travel, immobility, history of cancer, trauma, drugs, and other disorders should all be also considered.

It's imperative to determine whether a patient's venous condition is acute or chronic. Early and prompt detection of acute venous illness has a substantial impact on disease progression and patient survival. Pain, swelling, and/or erythema are common symptoms. Upper extremity is less frequently involved with acute venous thrombosis. However, it could be encountered in the setting of venous thoracic outlet syndrome or Paget-Schroetter syndrome. Chronic venous disease, on the other hand, is caused by long-term abnormalities such as venous compression, venous anomaly, or venous insufficiency. The symptoms might range from minor varicose veins to nonhealing venous leg ulcers and incapacitating venous claudication.

Laterality of symptoms (unilateral or bilateral) has a major effect on differential diagnosis and evaluation modalities. In patients with unilateral symptoms, a localized venous cause or trauma is frequently the culprit. Meanwhile, in patients presenting with bilateral symptoms, a systemic condition "such as congestive heart failure, liver cirrhosis, or renal failure" should be suspected.

Risk factors for venous thromboembolism (VTE) should be carefully assessed during history-taking (Table 7-1). Prolonged immobility due to recent hospitalization, air travel, or long car trips increases the risk of deep vein thrombosis (DVT). Trauma is highly linked to DVT, whether to the lower limbs, chest, or abdomen. In addition, central venous catheters, pacemakers, and infusion ports are all linked to the development of DVT at the insertion site. A personal or family history of VTE or spontaneous abortion should raise suspicions of thrombophilia, whether inherited or acquired. DVT is increased by hormone replacement therapy, oral contraceptive pills (OCPs), and selective estrogen receptor modulators. Newer OCPs have a significantly lower amount of estrogen than prescribed decades ago but nonetheless still increase risk of DVT.

Pain, swelling, or discomfort are the most common symptoms of venous diseases. However, many patients with DVTs are asymptomatic, but some still present with various degrees of symptoms. Lower extremity pain that develops toward the end of the day is usually present in patients with chronic venous insufficiency (CVI). In acute exacerbations of CVI, patients may present with acute symptoms, and exclusion of DVT through a duplex ultrasound is recommended. Patients with varicose veins have a different set of local symptoms such as tingling, itching, or burning sensation. Pain is not common in patients with varicose veins. However, evaluation for thrombophlebitis should be performed if pain is present.

TABLE 7-1 Risk Factors for Venous Thrombosis

Acquired
Prior personal history of VTE
Advanced age (>60 years old)
Malignancy
Estrogen therapy
Pregnancy/postpartum
Obesity
Antiphospholipid antibodies
Chronic inflammatory diseases (e.g., rheumatologic disease, inflammatory bowel disease)
Chronic medical conditions (e.g., heart failure, chronic kidney disease, chronic obstructive pulmonary disease, infection, atherosclerosis)
Venous obstructive processes (e.g., May-Thurner syndrome, thoracic outlet syndrome, tumor compression)
Indwelling central venous catheter or pacemaker
Recent hospitalization for medical or surgical issue (within 90 days)
Recent trauma or surgery (within 90 days)
Heparin-induced thrombocytopenia
Inherited
Family history of VTE
Factor V Leiden
Prothrombin gene mutation
Antithrombin deficiency
Protein C deficiency
Protein S deficiency

Swelling is a symptom of venous hypertension, which affects both the superficial and deep veins. It might be unilateral or bilateral. Increased pressure in the deep and connecting veins is caused by venous blockage, reflux, or incompetent valves. Other venous diseases that cause swelling include venous thrombosis and venous compression (e.g., May-Thurner syndrome).

The symptoms and signs of chronic venous insufficiency that occur after a DVT are known as post-thrombotic syndrome. "Post-thrombotic" syndrome has replaced the term "post-phlebitic" syndrome. It develops as a result of long-term venous hypertension. Post-thrombotic syndrome is hypothesized to be caused by a combination of reflux caused by valvular incompetence and venous hypertension caused by thrombotic blockage. An independent predictor of post-thrombotic syndrome is a high peak reflux velocity in the deep proximal veins. Leg pain, leg heaviness, vein dilation, edema, skin discoloration, and venous ulcers are all signs and symptoms of post-thrombotic syndrome.

The physical examination of the patient with suspected venous disease should not be limited to the lower limbs and should include the entire body. Complete examination of the venous system requires adequate understanding of venous anatomy, including the presence of perforating veins. Inspection and palpation should be done with the entire lower extremity exposed. Patients with DVT may present with erythema, pain/tenderness on palpation or ambulation, and swelling (either proximal or distal), or have a normal physical exam requiring further evaluation with imaging modalities. Only phlegmasia and phlebitis can be reliably diagnosed with any degree of a certainty via a clinical examination. Varicose veins are more apparent in the standing position as a result of increased peripheral venous pressure. Patients with chronic venous disease (CVD) presenting with varicose veins should be examined both supine and standing.

CLASSIFICATION SYSTEM (CEAP)

The creation of a standardized clinical classification system for CVD is essential for understanding the disease's natural history and comparing diagnostic and therapeutic techniques. Without reporting standards, clinical scientific communications and practice guidelines for patients with similar pathologies can be difficult to apply. (Figure 7-7)

The Clinical–Etiology–Anatomy–Pathophysiology (CEAP) classification (Table 7-2) is an internationally accepted standard for describing patients with chronic venous disorders, and it has been used for reporting clinical research findings in scientific journals. As the evidence related to these aspects of venous disorders, and specifically of CVDs continues to develop, the CEAP classification needs periodic analysis and revisions.[1]

The venous system of the lower extremities includes *the deep veins*, which lie beneath the muscular fascia and drain the lower extremity muscles; *the superficial veins*, which are above the deep fascia and drain the cutaneous microcirculation; and *the perforating veins* that penetrate the muscular fascia and connect the superficial and deep veins (Figure 7-1). Communicating veins connect veins within the same compartment. The superficial, deep, and most perforating veins contain bicuspid valves that assure unidirectional flow in the normal venous system.[2]

- *C0:* This class represents no diagnosable venous disease.
- *C1: Telangiectasia and reticular veins.* Telangiectasia or "spider veins" can be red or blue and measure 0.1 to 1 mm in diameter. Reticular veins are blue-purple in color, sometimes protruding above the skin, and can measure ≤2 mm in diameter. Reticular or "feeder" veins are flat, blue to blue-green in color, and measuring 2 to 4 mm in diameter.
- *C2: Varicose veins* (Figure 7-2). Varicose veins are dilated, tortuous subcutaneous veins measuring ≥3 mm in diameter with the patient standing.
- *C2r: Recurrent varicose veins.*
- *C3: Edema.* Edema usually begins in the malleolar and distal gaiter regions, where it pits with pressure. As CVI progresses, swelling can ascend into the calf and/or descend into the foot, and nonpitting "woody induration" may ensue.
- *C4a: Hyperpigmentation and/or eczema.* Hemosiderin hyperpigmentation (Figure 7-3) is a brownish hyperpigmentation, typically concentrated on the medial gaiter area. It denotes extravasated intact or fragmented erythrocytes and hemosiderin-laden macrophages. Early red blood cell extravasation appears stippled

TABLE 7-2 The CEAP (Clinical–Etiology–Anatomy–Pathophysiology) Classification

Clinical (C)	
C class	**Description**
C_0	No visible or palpable signs of venous disease
C_1	Telangiectasias or reticular veins
C_2	Varicose veins
C_{2r}	Recurrent varicose veins
C_3	Edema
C_4	Changes in skin and subcutaneous tissue secondary to CVD
C_{4a}	Pigmentation or eczema
C_{4b}	Lipodermatosclerosis or atrophie blanche
C_{4c}	Corona phlebectatica
C_5	Healed
C_6	Active venous ulcer
C_{6r}	Recurrent active venous ulcer

Etiology (E)	
E class	**Description**
E_p	Primary
E_s	Secondary
E_{si}	Secondary-intravenous
E_{se}	Secondary-extravenous
E_c	Congenital
E_n	No cause identified

Pathophysiology (P)	
P class	**Description**
P_r	Reflux
P_o	Obstruction
$P_{r,o}$	Reflux and obstruction
P_n	No pathophysiology identified

Anatomy (A)		
A class		**Description**
A_s		*Superficial*
	Tel	Telangiectasia
	Ret	Reticular veins
	GSVa	Great saphenous vein above knee
	GSVb	Great saphenous vein below knee
	SSV	Small saphenous vein
	AASV	Anterior accessory saphenous vein
	NSV	Nonsaphenous vein
A_d		*Deep*
	IVC	Inferior vena cava
	CIV	Common iliac vein
	IIV	Internal iliac vein
	EIV	External iliac vein
	PELV	Pelvic veins
	CFV	Common femoral vein
	DFV	Deep femoral vein
	FV	Femoral vein
	POPV	Popliteal vein
	TIBV	Crural (tibial) vein
	PRV	Peroneal vein
	ATV	Anterior tibial vein
	PTV	Posterior tibial vein
	MUSV	Muscular veins
	GAV	Gastrocnemius vein
	SOV	Soleal vein

TABLE 7-2 The CEAP (Clinical–Etiology–Anatomy–Pathophysiology) Classification—Continued

Clinical (C)	Anatomy (A)		
	A_p		*Perforator*
		TPV	Thigh perforator vein
		CPV	Calf perforator vein
	A_n		*No venous anatomic location identified*

Data from Eklöf B, Rutherford RB, Bergan JJ, et al. Revision of the CEAP classification for chronic venous disorders: consensus statement. *J Vasc Surg.* 2004;40(6):1248-1252.

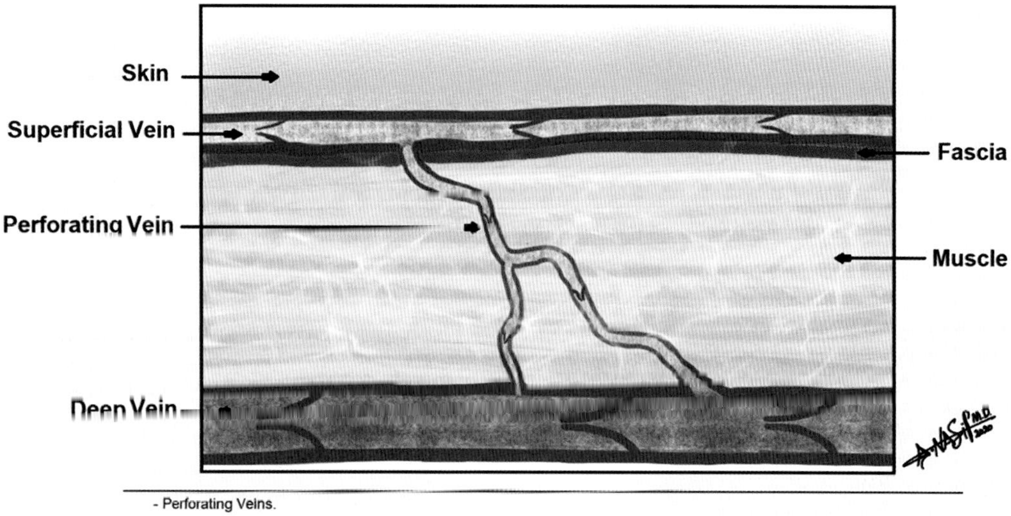

FIGURE 7-1 Perforating veins. (Reproduced with permission from Abdullah Nasif, MD.)

and red. With time, the staining fades to brown and the stippling can change to confluence. In patients with dark skin, those skin changes could be subtle; however, in general with advanced chronic venous changes, the skin of the affected area will appear much darker. Stasis dermatitis is typically well-demarcated, erythematous, dry, and scaly. However, a weeping, blistering transudative eczematous stasis dermatitis may evolve. Chronic pruritus leading to lichenification may ensue. Rarely, stasis dermatitis is complicated by a generalized autosensitization dermatitis or "Id" reaction.

- *C4b: Lipodermatosclerosis (LDS) or* atrophie blanche. LDS (Figure 7-4) reflects localized chronic inflammation and fibrosis of the skin and subcutaneous tissues in late-stage CVI with strikingly "bound down" or sclerotic skin involving the gaiter region of the calf. In the acute phase, a tender erythematous and edematous plaque develops within the distal anteromedial gaiter distribution. When chronic, progressive dermal and subcutaneous atrophy imparts a concave appearance to the mid/distal calf that resembles an "inverted champagne bottle" or "bowling pin."

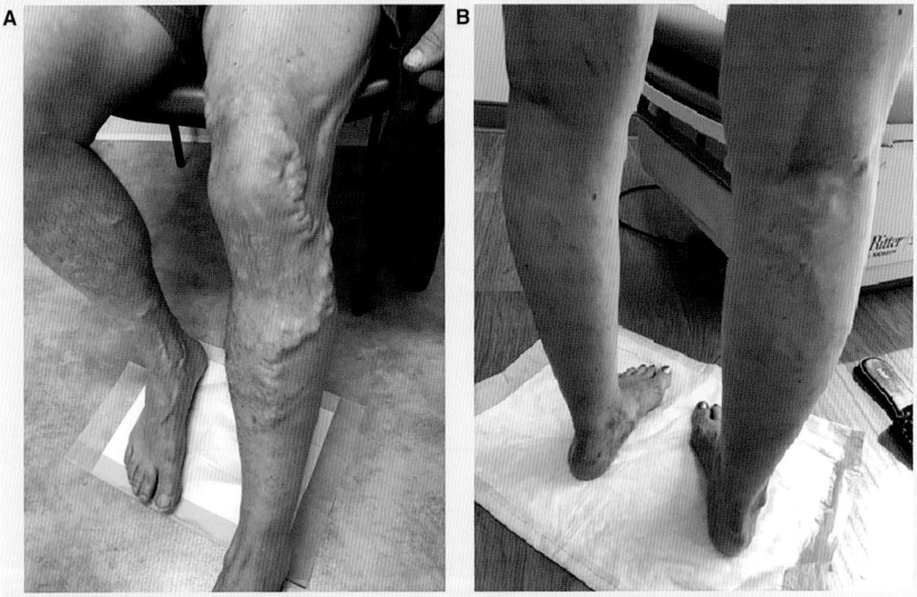

A- Varicose vein path of GSV with tributary originating at mid thigh and courses laterally.
B- Varicose vein path of SSV.

FIGURE 7-2 **Varicose veins.**

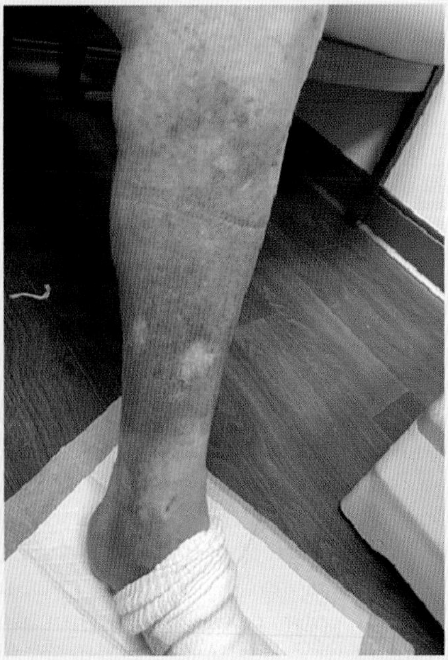

-Healed ulcers with evident hemosiderin hyperpigmentation (C5)

FIGURE 7-3 **Hemosiderin hyperpigmentation.**

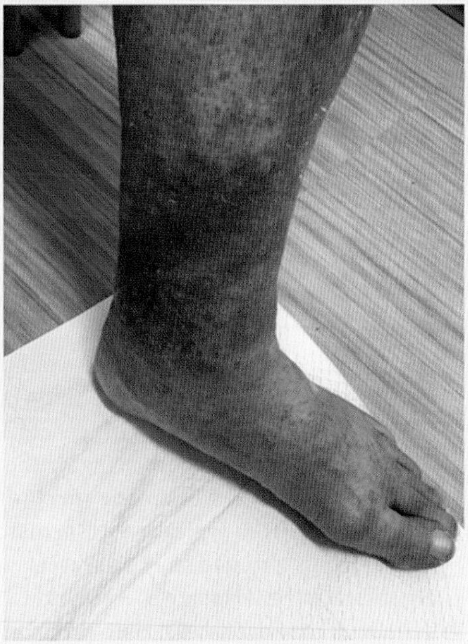

- Early Lipodermatosclerosis (CEAP:C4b)

FIGURE 7-4 **Lipodermatosclerosis.**

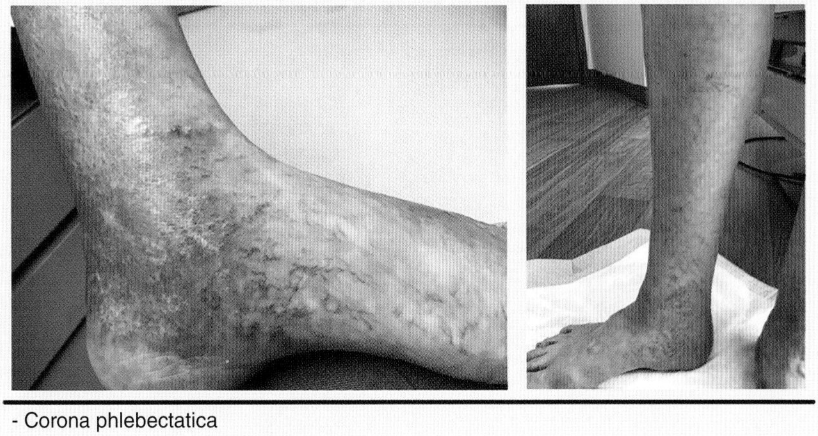

FIGURE 7-5 **Corona phlebectatica.**

- *C4c: Corona phlebectatica* (Figure 7-5). This is defined as a fan-shaped pattern of numerous small intradermal veins on the medial or lateral aspects of the ankle and foot. Synonyms include malleolar flare and ankle flare. Although such lesions would likely be classified as telangiectasias (C1) in the 2004 revision of CEAP, many venous authorities consider corona phlebectatica to be an early sign of advanced venous disease and to warrant inclusion in more advanced C categories. Perhaps most importantly, patients with corona phlebectatica have been demonstrated to be 5.3 times more likely to develop an ulcer, a risk of similar magnitude to other C4 skin changes.
- *C5: Healed ulceration.* The characteristic appearance of *atrophie blanche* should not be confused with healed ulcer scars, as the latter are devoid of capillary stippling.
- *C6: Venous stasis ulceration.* Similar to C4 a/b disease, a venous stasis ulceration usually occurs within the distal medial calf and medial malleolar region. The base is beefy red, shallow, edematous, moist, and friable. The border is mildly irregular and well-defined, with surrounding hyperpigmentation and sometimes eczematous scaling. Granulation tissue and fibrin are often present in the ulcer base. Other findings include lower extremity varicosities, edema, and venous dermatitis associated with LDS or *atrophie blanche*.
- *C6r:* Recurrent venous stasis ulceration.

REVISED VENOUS CLINICAL SEVERITY SCORE (VCSS)

To define the severity of disease or to quantify clinical outcomes, several measures have been developed. In venous disease reporting, condition-specific patient-reported quality-of-life assessments are popular and have excellent sensitivity. Venous disease and its clinically relevant signs/symptoms are evaluated using tools that rely on physician observation. Many of these tools have been validated, and each has advantages and disadvantages. The venous clinical severity score (VCSS) (Table 7-3) was created to complement the CEAP classification and give a means for serial evaluation. It was also created to give more weight to CVD symptoms that were more severe (CEAP clinical class 4 and class 6). It has been found to be responsive and to tolerate variances in intraobserver and interobserver repeatability.[3] A severity scoring system would best be based on data from large

TABLE 7-3 Revised Venous Clinical Severity Score (VCSS)

	Absent = 0	Mild = 1	Moderate = 2	Severe = 3
Pain or other discomfort (aching, heaviness, fatigue, soreness, burning) Presumes venous origin	None	Occasional pain or other discomfort (not restricting regular daily activities)	Daily pain or discomfort (interfering with but not preventing regular daily activities)	Daily pain or discomfort (limits most regular daily activities)
Varicose veins Vein must be >3 mm in diameter to qualify in the standing position	None	Few: scattered (isolated branch varicosities or clusters). Also includes corona phlebatatica (ankle flare)	Confined to calf or thigh	Involves calf and thigh
Venous edema Presumes venous origin	None	Limited to foot and ankle area	Extends above ankle but below knee	Extends to knee and above
Skin pigmentation Presumes venous origin Does not include focal pigmentation over varicose veins or pigmentation due to other chronic diseases	None or focal, low intensity (tan)	Limited to perimalleolar area	Diffuse over lower third of calf	Wider distribution above lower third of calf
Inflammation More than just recent pigmentation (erythema, cellulitis, venous eczema, dermatitis)	None	Limited to perimalleolar area	Diffuse over lower third of calf	Wider distribution above lower third of calf
Induration Presumes venous origin of secondary skin and subcutaneous changes (chronic edema with fibrosis, hypodermitis). Includes white atrophy and lipodermatosclerosis	None	Limited to perimalleolar area	Diffuse over lower third of calf	Wider distribution above lower third of calf
No. of active ulcers	0	1	2	>3
Active ulcer duration	None	<3 months	3 months to 1 year	Not healed >1 year
Active ulcer size	None	<2-cm diameter	2- to 6-cm diameter	>6-cm diameter
Compressive therapy	Not used or not compliant	Intermittent use of stockings	Wears elastic stockings most days	Full compliance: stockings + elevation

Data from Rutherford RB, Padberg FT Jr, Comerota AJ, et al. Venous severity scoring: An adjunct to venous outcome assessment. *J Vasc Surg.* 2000;31(6):1307-1312; and Vasquez MA, Rabe E, McLafferty RB, et al. Revision of the venous clinical severity score: venous outcomes consensus statement: special communication of the American Venous Forum Ad Hoc Outcomes Working Group. *J Vasc Surg.* 2010;52(5):1387-1396.

multicenter studies of patients with venous disease, in whom clinical and duplex scan data were gathered and correlated with CEAP classification, other outcome criteria, and tests of venous function. Such studies are still needed in order to evaluate and modify it.

LABORATORY TESTS

D-dimer is an endogenous fibrinolysis nonspecific marker. It is elevated in VTE, as well as other systemic illnesses and conditions. Outpatients and emergency department patients with suspected VTE benefit the most from D-dimer testing since they are less likely than inpatients to have an alternate explanation for an elevated D-dimer.

Enzyme-linked immunofluorescent assays (ELISA) are the most sensitive testing method. Patients with suspected acute DVT demonstrated that the quantitative D-dimer by ELISA had negative likelihood ratios similar to those for negative venous duplex ultrasonography, with a sensitivity of 96% and a negative predictive value of 99%. Though D-dimer can be utilized on its own, it's preferable when combined with clinical risk scores. D-dimer values increase with age, thus further limiting specificity in older patients. Conventional cutoff values (≤500 ng/mL) demonstrated higher specificity when an age adjusted value (age [years] Å ~ 10 ng/mL for patients over 50) was utilized.

NONINVASIVE IMAGING MODALITIES

Diagnosing diseases through noninvasive modalities was a revolutionary idea. In 1942, Karl Dussik was one of the first physicians to use ultrasound for medical diagnosis. Dr. Ian Donald used ultrasound in his practice to measure the fetal head diameter in 1956. At that time, the device used one-dimensional A-mode (amplitude mode). Two years later, he collaborated with the engineer Tom Brown to design the first medical ultrasound machine that can visualize the density of the tissue. The focus on flow visualization and assessment led to the development of more refined imaging techniques and the use of the Doppler effect as the basis for visualizing blood circulation and flow.[4]

Duplex ultrasonography of the affected limb is the initial imaging testing in the evaluation of suspected upper and lower extremity DVT. Ultrasound offers accurate imaging with no exposure of radiation or iodinated contrast to the patient. Sensitivity and specificity for the evaluation of proximal lower extremity DVT are greater than 95%. Duplex venous ultrasound combines vein compression with B-mode imaging and pulsed Doppler spectrum analysis, with and without color.

CT and MR venography are used for contrast-enhanced evaluation of the proximal veins, including subclavian in the upper extremities, and the iliac and IVC in the pelvis. Concomitant anatomy that may be important in a patient's presentation (e.g., May-Thurner syndrome) can be evaluated using these modalities. CT and MR venography may also be helpful when a mass invading or compressing the veins is suspected. Though rarely performed, invasive contrast venography can still be used if other imaging remains inconclusive.

In the absence of symptoms such as in telangiectasias, reticular veins, and small varicose veins (<6 mm), the patient can generally be treated as desired to improve cosmetic appearance without further diagnostic studies.

VENOUS DUPLEX ULTRASOUND (DUS)

Venous duplex ultrasound (DUS) is the most common tool used in diagnosing venous disease given its noninvasive nature and cost-effectiveness. DUS can be used to evaluate the superficial, deep, and perforator systems, and determine pathology: reflux versus obstruction versus combination.

Normal veins have thin walls and an echo-free lumen. The vein lumen can be obliterated (compressed) with a small amount of extrinsic pressure. However, the walls do not coapt when the lumen contains thrombus, even when enough pressure is applied to distort the shape of an adjacent artery. Vein compressibility is best tested in an image plane transverse to the vein axis. Veins are characterized by anatomical location as deep or superficial and as proximal or distal. The major veins of the thigh and arm are larger in diameter than the corresponding arteries. Extremity veins have valves, which permit only upward unidirectional flow, and these increase in number from proximal to distal. Valve sinuses are widened areas of the lumen that accommodate the valve cusp.

Doppler evaluation of flow in normal veins has four important characteristics: (A) respirophasic variation, (B) augmentation with distal compression, (C) unidirectional flow toward the heart, and (D) and abrogation of flow in the lower extremities by the Valsalva maneuver. Complete analysis of venous spectral waveforms requires comparison of the waveforms from both right and left limbs. The presence of a continuous, unvarying waveform (loss of respirophasic variation in flow) on one side compared with the other suggests the presence of more proximal obstruction of venous return proximal to the site of the Doppler examination.[5]

To stimulate venous engorgement during the study, the patient is placed in a sitting or 15- to 20-degree reverse Trendelenburg position. The legs are turned laterally to make the venous routes more accessible. The examiner begins by using a handheld continuous wave Doppler device to do a Doppler venous study or use the pulsed-wave Doppler device to combine the Doppler and imaging portions of the examination. A standard examination takes 20 to 30 minutes per extremity, but this varies greatly depending on the technician's skill.[6]

Upper Extremities

The internal jugular, subclavian, axillary, brachial, cephalic, and basilic veins can all be assessed during a duplex neck and upper extremity evaluation. Because of their placement within the bony thorax, the innominate veins and superior vena cava cannot be assessed with duplex ultrasonography. The internal jugular and subclavian veins are the first things to look at during the exam. A supraclavicular or subclavicular approach can be used to scan the subclavian vein. The axillary vein, brachial veins, basilic vein, and cephalic vein are all examined with the arm extended in a comfortable position.

The pathognomonic hallmark of venous thrombosis is the loss of venous compressibility. As the thrombus advances from acute to chronic, the thrombus echogenicity increases and the vein's diameter decreases. Elastography can be used to identify the age of a thrombus. The absence of respirophasic variation in the waveform indicates the existence of more proximal venous blockage as a result of thrombosis or extrinsic compression. When flow is absent or echogenic material is observed within the lumen of the vein, venous thrombosis is suspected.

Indwelling venous catheters, pacemaker leads, and hypercoagulability are the most common causes of upper extremity DVTs. Effort thrombosis (Paget-Schroetter syndrome) related to thoracic outlet obstruction or malignancy can also be encountered. Intravascular tumors are uncommon and can be suspected when the echogenic material within the lumen appears to extend through the vessel wall and may contain arterial flow signals.[5]

Lower Extremity

The use of a duplex examination of the extremity veins allows for a noninvasive, reliable diagnosis of DVT. With good interobserver agreement and minimal inconclusive results, whole-leg ultrasonography may be completed in 15 minutes. In most cases with suspected DVT, ultrasound can be used. Additional imaging with CT venography or MR venography is required in rare cases.

The venous ultrasonography examination begins at the inguinal ligament with the identification of the common femoral vein and extends to the calf. The common femoral, femoral, and popliteal veins are among the proximal deep veins studied. The deep calf veins include the posterior tibial, peroneal, gastrocnemius (sural), and soleal veins with special attention to the saphenofemoral and saphenopopliteal junctions. Loss of respirophasic variation in the waveform of the common femoral vein would suggest obstruction proximal to the site of the examination. Augmentation of flow with calf compression is not prevented by proximal venous obstruction. Proximal obstruction may be caused by extrinsic compression or venous thrombosis.[5]

Compressibility along the full course of the veins is determined by using B-mode transverse imaging. With mild pressure, the vein walls normally coapt. The most reliable result for diagnosing venous thrombosis is a lack of compressibility. The thrombus often appears eccentric and adjacent to the vein wall. In acute thrombosis, the intraluminal thrombus has poor echogenicity and the vein is dilated. The thrombus becomes more echogenic and less central within the lumen as it gets older. It is difficult to rule out the presence of small nonocclusive thrombi when severe soft tissue edema is present. The sensitivity for detecting femoral vein thrombosis in the common femoral vein is 91%, and for both the femoral and popliteal veins is 94%.[5]

As long as the calf veins can be visualized clearly, duplex ultrasonography is accurate for diagnosing deep calf vein thrombosis in symptomatic patients. When compared to angiography, it has a sensitivity of 94% and a specificity of 100% for deep calf vein thrombosis. In some cases, the small calf veins are difficult to evaluate; nonetheless, the specificity and positive predictive value remain excellent.

Ultrasonography has its limitations imposed by the ultrasound training of the provider and in the evaluation of recurrent DVT. One year after the initial occurrence, nearly half of patients will show persistent post-thrombotic intravenous fibrous changes and additional imaging may be required. The physician can refer to the previous ultrasound for comparison to detect the presence of a recurrent DVT.

Intrapelvic/intra-abdominal

The purpose of a transabdominal pelvic venous duplex exam is to evaluate irregular blood flow in the abdominal and pelvic veins including inferior vena cava, renal, iliac, uterine/parauterine, and ovarian/gonadal veins with the exclusion of the portal venous system. Abdominal and pelvic venous compressions/venous insufficiency, and the presence or absence of pelvic varicosities can be assessed.

Chronic pelvic pain caused by incompetent pelvic veins is known as pelvic congestion syndrome. Dysfunctional dilatation of ovarian and para-uterine veins, decreased blood flow, retrograde flow, and reflux are indications for incompetent veins. Symptoms include colicky lower abdominal, back or flank pain with accompanying hematuria, dysuria, and urinary frequency. The use of ultrasound allows for a positive identification of pelvic venous involvement as well as classification. The examination begins in the suprapubic region. The typical venous plexus is a straight tubular structure with a normal diameter (<4 mm). In patients with pelvic varicosities, dilated and convoluted veins on either side of the uterus show reversed and decreased flow. Because genital varicose veins might appear as a cluster of small dilated veins, no specific diameter can be used to diagnose them.

Nutcracker syndrome (NCS) is characterized by the stenotic compression of the left renal vein. Several anatomical forms have been identified. The most common compression is the anterior type between the superior mesenteric artery and the abdominal aorta. The less common posterior type described as when the vein is in a retro-aortic position and compressed between the aorta and a lumbar vertebral body. There have been numerous attempts to improve Doppler ultrasound diagnostic criteria. Based on small studies, several quantitative ultrasonography criteria for anterior compression have been identified. The sensitivity and specificity of a Doppler ultrasound ranges from 69% to 89%.

CT VENOGRAPHY

Computerized tomographic venography (CTV) is a diagnostic technique that has transformed vascular disease diagnosis. With the development of the computed tomography (CT) equipment in 1998, adequate imaging of the peripheral venous system during a single acquisition and a single injection of contrast media became possible. As an alternative to duplex ultrasound, CTV is increasingly being utilized to diagnose DVT. A partial or complete intravenous filling defect is the most common finding of a pelvic or proximal lower extremity DVT. There is commonly associated generalized leg and perivenous edema seen on the acquired images.[7] CTV has been shown to have a sensitivity of 89% to 100% and a specificity of 94% to 100% in detecting DVT in the pelvis and lower limbs. However, it exposes the patient to increased radiation and invasive intravenous contrast media.

MR VENOGRAPHY

The advantage of magnetic resonance venography (MRV) is that it eliminates the requirement for

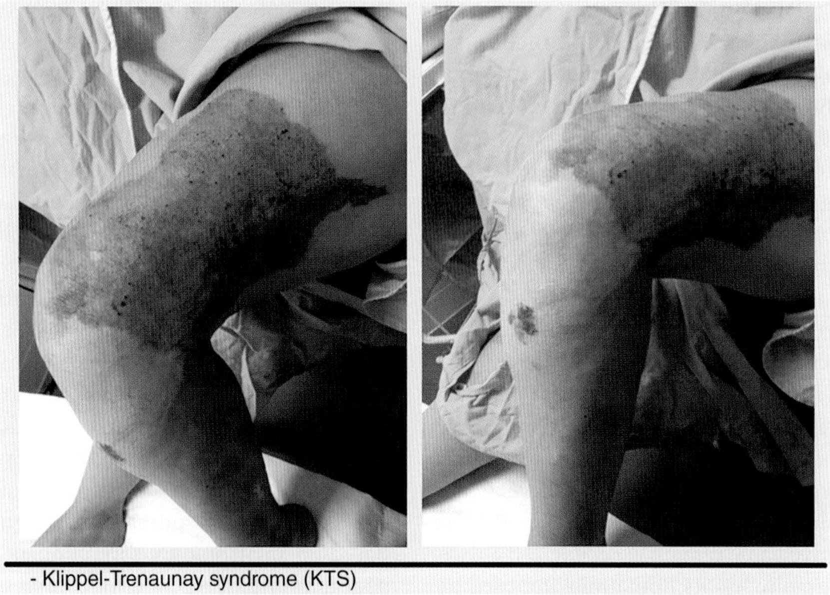

FIGURE 7-6 **Klippel-Trenaunay syndrome.**

nephrotoxic contrast. It clarifies nearby structures and enables for multiple views (sagittal and coronal). The superconducting magnet's radiofrequency can create distinct contrast in the vascular system and nearby structures. Estimating overall thrombus burden in smaller branching veins, establishing a diagnosis of pelvic vein thrombosis, and assessing venous diseases such as Klippel-Trenaunay syndrome (Figure 7-6), MRV may have a distinct advantage over CT or duplex ultrasound. In some cases, duplex ultrasound may not be enough to determine the full degree of thrombus and CT/MR venography may be required. External orthopedic hardware, extensive wounds, morbid obesity, substantial interstitial edema, intestinal gas, or the need to scan surrounding structures are examples of these cases.[2]

PLETHYSMOGRAPHY

Imaging modalities such as ultrasound and venography cannot assess the global severity of reflux or obstruction in a limb. Because of the "segmental" approach, determining the impact of the disease in a single segment compared to an entire venous system in the lower leg can be difficult. Assessment of treatment outcomes and changes in severity over time and after surgery is challenging. These limitations dictate the need for a method of assessing global venous in the lower extremity. Venous pressure measurements can be utilized but are invasive in nature. Plethysmography is the only noninvasive method for assessing the overall physiology of extremity veins. It can be used in conjunction with duplex ultrasound to quantify reflux or obstruction, track the progression of venous disease through time, and assess therapy effects.[2]

Air Plethysmography

By detecting volume changes in the leg, air plethysmography (APG) is a noninvasive diagnostic modality that can quantify venous reflux and blockage. It can test numerous aspects of venous hemodynamics quantitatively, including valvular reflux, calf muscle pump function, and venous obstruction. It has been introduced as an additional technique for venous hemodynamics evaluation. This modality's parameters allow for a quantitative assessment of the severity of chronic venous insufficiency. It can also be utilized to link venous hemodynamic gain and CEAP classification after varicose vein surgery. APG can be technically challenging, despite the fact that it is a noninvasive and reasonably affordable procedure. It is heavily reliant on precise calibration, and as a result, it might be classified as an examiner-dependent test. Minor technical faults during measurements invalidate

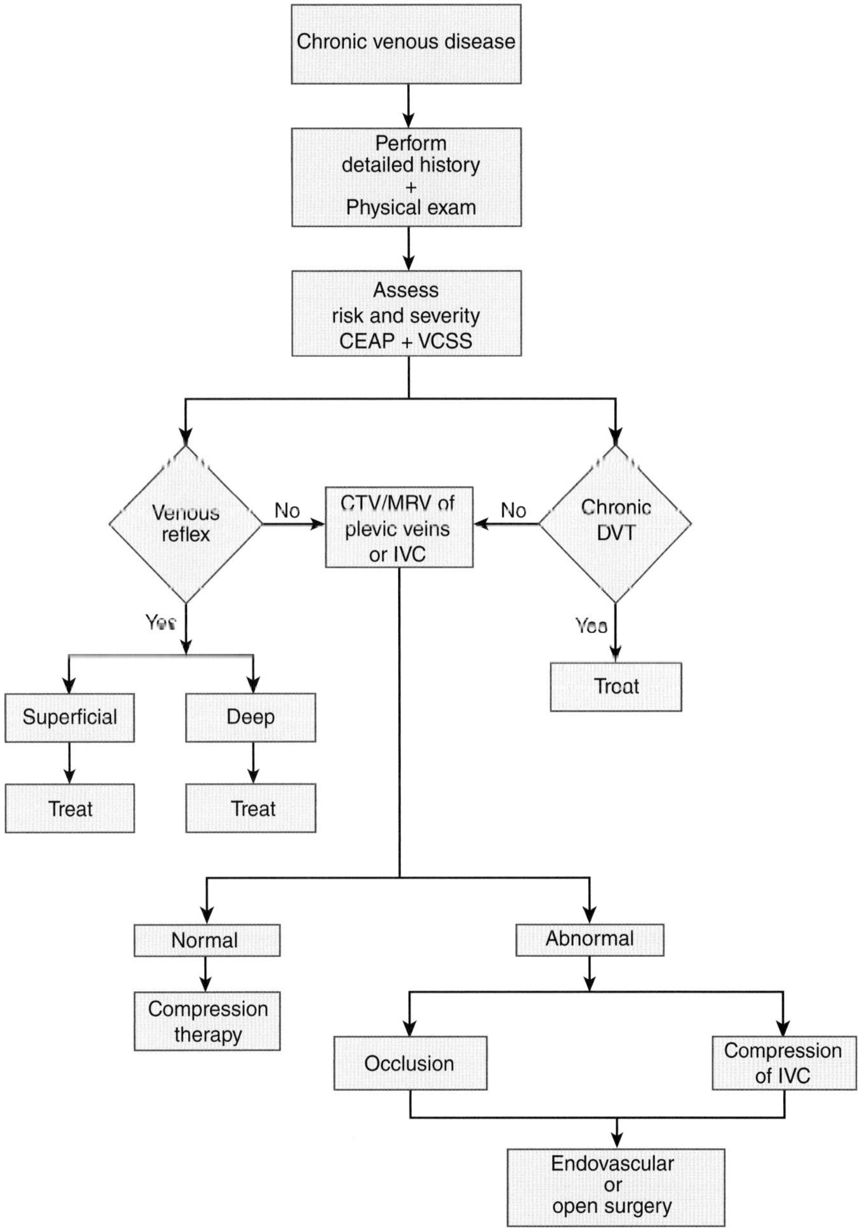

FIGURE 7-7 Chronic venous disease flowchart. CEAP, classification for venous disease (Clinical [C], Etiological [E], Anatomical [A], and Pathophysiological [P]); IVC, inferior vena cava; VCSS, venous clinical severity score.

the test. APG is a time-consuming operation due to calibration and frequent restarting. Obesity can also have an impact on findings, making APG parameters ineffective.[8]

Photoplethysmography

Photoplethysmography (PPG) is a low-cost and easy optical technology for detecting blood volume changes. It is a noninvasive method for taking measurements on the skin's surface. A pulsatile (AC) physiological waveform attributed to changes in blood volume with each heartbeat is superimposed on a slowly varying (DC) baseline with various lower frequency components attributed to respiration, sympathetic nervous system activity, and thermoregulation in the PPG waveform. The DC component of the PPG waveform can be utilized to detect chronic venous insufficiency (CVI) in the lower limbs noninvasively. Because of the related variations in light absorption, PPG can detect changes in limb blood volume with posture. Light reflection rheography (LRR) is a term used to describe this method.

The demand for low-cost, simple, and portable technology in primary care and community-based clinical settings, the wide availability of low-cost and small semiconductor components, and the advancement of computer-based pulse wave analysis techniques have all contributed to a resurgence of interest in the technique in recent years. PPG technology has been employed in a variety of commercially available medical devices to measure oxygen saturation, blood pressure, and cardiac output, as well as to assess autonomic function and diagnose peripheral vascular disease. Pulse oximetry is regarded as one of the most important technological developments in clinical patient monitoring in recent decades. It has a wide range of applications in a variety of clinical contexts.[9]

NEW DIAGNOSTIC METHODS (ARTIFICIAL INTELLIGENCE)

Automated medical imaging classification has become increasingly valuable for disease diagnosis and surgical planning. Although medical image classification algorithms using artificial intelligence (AI) have been used to detect cancer, identify strokes, and diagnose Alzheimer's disease, no AI classification algorithms are available for venous diseases. Low-level image properties such as color, texture, and form are used in traditional medical image categorization algorithms. These low-level features are unable to reflect certain concealed information in medical images, resulting in a "semantic gap" problem between low- and high-level information, which is one of the most difficult problems in medical image classification. The bag of visual word (BoVW) paradigm is used to construct middle-level characteristics for describing high-level semantics in order to close the semantic gap. BoVW has been tested in medical image classification tasks and has shown impressive results. However, some design decisions must be made at various stages of the BoVW model, such as the local feature descriptor, dictionary learning, and middle-level semantic image representation.[10]

REFERENCES

1. Lurie F, Passman M, Meisner M, et al. The 2020 update of the CEAP classification system and reporting standards. *J Vasc Surg Venous Lymphat Disord.* 2020;8(3):342-352. Erratum in: *J Vasc Surg Venous Lymphat Disord.* 2021;9(1):288.
2. Meissner MH, Moneta G, Burnand K, et al. The hemodynamics and diagnosis of venous disease. *J Vasc Surg.* 2007;46(Suppl S):4S-24S.
3. Vasquez MA, Rabe E, McLafferty RB, et al. Revision of the venous clinical severity score: venous outcomes consensus statement: special communication of the American Venous Forum Ad Hoc Outcomes Working Group. *J Vasc Surg.* 2010;52(5):1387-1396.
4. Thomas AMK, Banerjee AK. *The History of Radiology.* Oxford: Oxford University Press; 2013.
5. Gerhard-Herman M, Beckman JA, Creager MA. Vascular laboratory testing. In: Creager MA, Beckman JA, Loscalzo J, eds. *Vascular Medicine: A Companion to Braunwald's Heart Disease.* 2nd ed. Philadelphia, PA: Saunders/Elsevier; 2013:148-165.
6. Stewart JH, Grubb M. Understanding vascular ultrasonography. *Mayo Clinic Proceedings.* 1992;67(12): 1186-1196.
7. Gerhard-Herman M, Beckman JA, Creager MA. Chapter 14: Computed tomographic angiography. In: Creager MA, Beckman JA, Loscalzo J, eds. *Vascular Medicine: A Companion to Braunwald's Heart Disease.* 2nd ed. Philadelphia, PA: Saunders/Elsevier; 2013.

8. Dezotti NRA, Dalio MB, Ribeiro MS, Piccinato CE, Joviliano EE. The clinical importance of air plethysmography in the assessment of chronic venous disease. *J Vasc Bras*. 2016;15(4):287-292.
9. Allen J. Photoplethysmography and its application in clinical physiological measurement. *Physiol Meas*. 2007;28(3):R1-R39.
10. Shi Q, Chen W, Pan Y, et al. An automatic classification method on chronic venous insufficiency images. *Sci Rep*. 2018;8(1):17952.

SELF-ASSESSMENT STUDY QUESTIONS AND ANSWERS

Questions

1. The main advantage of utilizing magnetic resonance venography (MRV) is
   A. Assessing the global severity of reflux or obstruction in a limb
   B. Eliminating the requirement for nephrotoxic contrast
   C. Detecting volume changes in the leg
   D. Evaluating irregular blood flow in the abdominal and pelvic veins

2. Which one of the following statements regarding photoplethysmography is correct:
   A. It is a low-cost and easy optical technology for detecting blood volume changes
   B. Its sensitivity and specificity ranges from 90% to 94%
   C. It can establish a diagnosis of pelvic vein thrombosis
   D. It is the most common tool used in diagnosing venous disease

3. One of the most common causes of upper extremity DVT is
   A. Air travel and long car trips
   B. Multiple pregnancies
   C. Indwelling venous catheters
   D. Diabetes

4. The pathognomonic hallmark of venous thrombosis is
   A. Pain in the legs while walking
   B. Ischemic rest pain
   C. Numbness
   D. Loss of venous compressibility

5. Loss of respirophasic variation in the waveform of the vein during duplex ultrasound suggests
   A. Obstruction proximal to the site of the examination
   B. Obstruction distal to the site of the examination
   C. Obstruction at the site of the examination
   D. None of the above

SELF-ASSESSMENT STUDY QUESTIONS AND ANSWERS

Answers

1. B.
2. A.
3. C.
4. D.
5. A.

CHAPTER

8 Noninvasive Evaluation of Arterial Disease

Karem C. Harth and Vikram S. Kashyap

OUTLINE

OVERVIEW

EXTRACRANIAL CAROTID EVALUATION
- Indication
- Technical
- Interpretation
- Surveillance

RENAL EVALUATION
- Indication
- Technical
- Interpretation
- Surveillance

MESENTERIC EVALUATION
- Indication
- Technical
- Interpretation
- Surveillance

LOWER EXTREMITY EVALUATION
- Indication
- Technical
- Interpretation
- Surveillance

CONCLUSION

OVERVIEW

The natural course of arterial disease is one of the progression and modification via medical and interventional therapies. Peripheral vascular disease has an estimated prevalence of 12% to 20% with risk factors, such as smoking, diabetes, hyperlipidemia, and hypertension exacerbating atherosclerosis. The chronicity of peripheral vascular disease requires testing modalities that are repeatable, easily accessible, low cost, and with low risk to the patient. Vascular laboratory testing offers the ability to provide both anatomic and functional information of multiple vascular beds, in a noninvasive cost-effective manner, that can be serially followed over time and is readily available.

Noninvasive vascular laboratory testing is an integral and universally applied technology across the various vascular beds in contemporary vascular surgery. Despite its broad and deeply rooted application, it is striking to realize how fairly "young" this relationship is and how quickly technology is evolving.[1] Dr. Eugene Strandness, at the University of Washington, pioneered this technology in the 1970s, and by the 1980s, there were commercially available ultrasound scanners being applied to mostly extracranial carotid disease. Fast track to 2020, there are very few vascular beds that are not being evaluated by sophisticated noninvasive ultrasound technologies that continue to evolve (B-mode, spectral analysis, color doppler) and amaze the eyes (power angio, B-flow, 3-d reconstruction). Such advances have allowed us to broaden their clinical application in the areas of screening, intraoperative assessment, surveillance, and procedural guidance.

Current technologies offer the ability to have three-dimensional vessel reconstruction, evaluate plaque morphology, and obtain real-time blood flow characteristics. It is the combination of the anatomic image acquisition (with b-mode imaging) and the blood flow evaluation (using color, pulsed and power Doppler, and spectral analysis) that allows us to make interpretative statements regarding the presence of disease in an arterial bed.

With the rapid expansion of vascular ultrasound, various societies across multiple fields have come together to provide best practice recommendations for indication and interpretation of noninvasive testing.[2–4] The Intersocietal Accreditation Commission maintains and frequently updates its "*IAC Standards and Guidelines for Vascular Testing Accreditation*" document to assure a set of minimum image acquisition standards are met for labs with high-quality accreditation status.[5] This chapter will focus on noninvasive imaging of the extracranial carotid arteries, renal arteries, mesenteric arteries, and evaluation of the lower extremities. Clinical indications, technical considerations, interpretation of noninvasive testing, and the role of surveillance of the various arterial beds affected by atherosclerosis will be highlighted.

EXTRACRANIAL CAROTID EVALUATION

INDICATION

Atherosclerotic disease in the extracranial internal carotid artery accounts for 10% to 20% of causes of ischemic stroke. Noninvasive imaging for the extracranial carotid artery serves various roles depending on where along the spectrum of disease a patient is located. It is endorsed as the primary study in both symptomatic and asymptomatic diseases.[4] Primarily, it is used to screen for the presence of disease and identify patients at risk for stroke. Secondarily, it is used as a surveillance and monitoring tool after initiation of therapies for modifiable risk factors or postprocedurally. Shortly following intervention, such as carotid endarterectomy or stenting, ultrasound is used to document resolution of stenosis, and for long term, it is used to evaluate for any recurrence or progression of disease. This helps guide therapies and need for any reintervention.

TECHNICAL

In general, a linear array transducer between 5 and 12 MHz is used for carotid artery evaluation. Indications for testing are noted in Table 8-1 and should always be consulted when ordering these tests to assure appropriateness. At minimum, components of a good carotid evaluation include the use of b-mode imaging, color and spectral Doppler, and velocity measurements at specified locations (CCA, ECA, ICA, Carotid bifurcation, vertebral, and subclavian artery).[6] Imaging is obtained in both sagittal and transverse views. Descriptors of plaque morphology using b-mode gray scale imaging (location,

TABLE 8-1 Most Common Indications for Noninvasive Vascular Laboratory Testing

Carotid Duplex	Peripheral Imaging	Renal Duplex	Mesenteric Duplex
Carotid Bruit	PVD	Renovascular hypertension	Abdominal bruit
Amaurosis Fugax	Acute limb ischemia	Atherosclerosis of renal artery	CMI
Hemispheric Stroke	CLTI	Primary hypertension	AMI
TIA	Postrevascularization surveillance	Azotemia	Abdominal pain
Carotid stenosis or occlusion	Screening for aneurysm	Atrophic kidney	
Hollenhorst plaque		Flash pulmonary edema without cardiac cause	
Follow-up after intervention (stenting, endarterectomy)		Postintervention surveillance	

AMI, acute mesenteric ischemia; CLTI, critical limb-threatening ischemia; CMI, chronic mesenteric ischemia; PVD, peripheral vascular disease; TIA, transient ischemic attack.

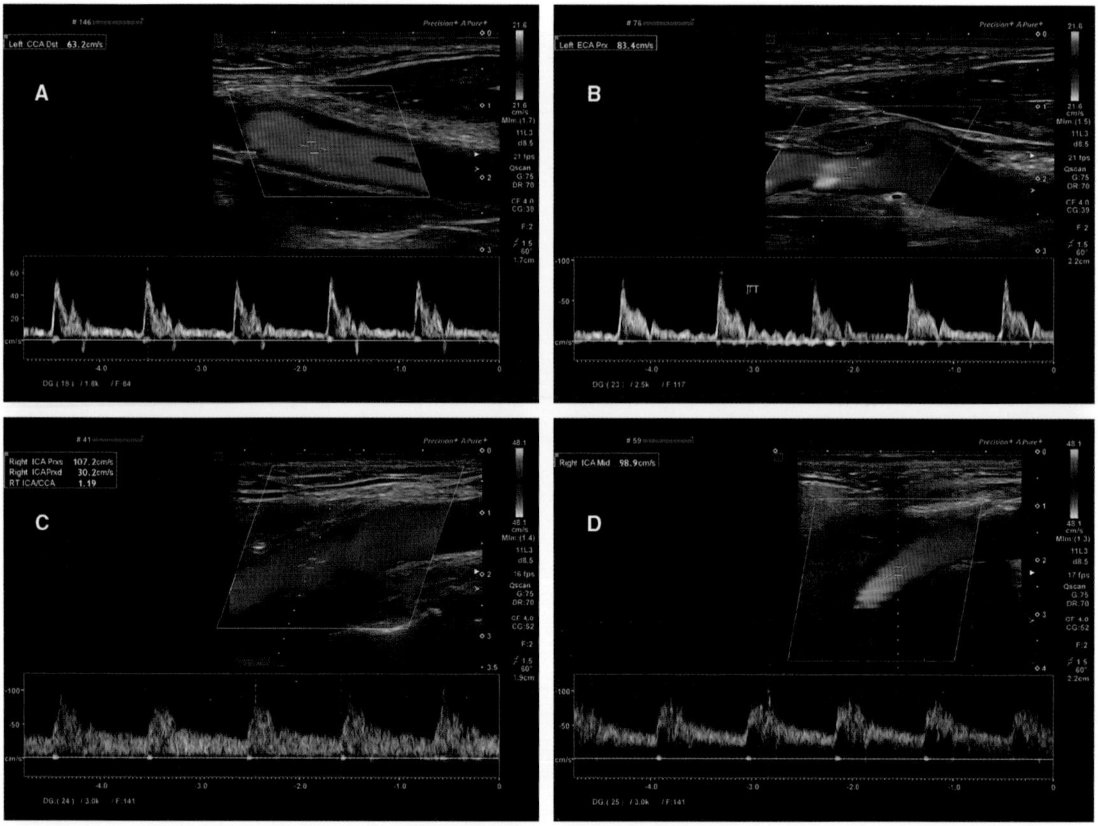

FIGURE 8-1 Representative spectral waveforms for the (A) common carotid artery, (B) external carotid artery, (C) proximal internal carotid artery, and (D) mid-internal carotid artery.

echogenicity, irregularity, ulceration) should be included in the evaluation. Special attention should be given around areas of spectral and color turbulence indicative of stenosis. Spectral broadening and turbulence at the very distal ICA should prompt consideration for nonatherosclerotic-based disease, such as fibromuscular dysplasia (FMD). Switching over to a curvilinear probe may facilitate "deeper" views in the neck toward the skull base. Calcific plaque presents a limitation to vascular ultrasound, and this requires detailed image acquisition of pre and post-plaque spectral waveforms for best interpretation.

In very high-grade stenosis or when there is a question of occlusion, additional supportive techniques such as color power angio (CPA) and b-flow should be applied. Understanding classic waveform patterns based on the outflow vascular bed helps assure that the correct vessel is being interrogated. The ICA is low-resistive with continuous flow during diastole, whereas the ECA is high-resistive and multiphasic (Figure 8-1). The CCA is a hybrid waveform of both ECA and ICA. Certainly, in the setting of occlusion, CCA flow will reflect the vessel that remains patent.

In a postprocedural or postoperative patient, it is important to carefully evaluate both sides. On the intervened side, it is important to document the change in degree of stenosis. The contralateral side should be re-evaluated as velocities may subsequently drop following revascularization. Increased velocities pre-procedurally in the untreated side may be secondary to compensatory collateral flow which will change with revascularization of the opposite side. ECA patency should be evaluated post stenting.

Additionally, it is important to interrogate the inflow native common carotid artery, proximal, mid and distal stent, and the outflow native vessel in stent surveillance imaging.

INTERPRETATION

Several criteria have been published evaluating the presence and degree of internal carotid artery stenosis. The most commonly referenced criteria for categorizing the degree of stenosis are from The Society of Radiologists in Ultrasound (SRU) consensus criteria (Table 8-2).[7] The sensitivity and specificity of carotid ultrasound are very good when compared with invasive angiography when all disease categories are considered and when trying to determine between general presence and absence of disease (99% and 84%, respectively).[3] Similar validation studies have shown a 95% sensitivity and 84% specificity for detecting >70% stenosis when peak systolic velocity (PSV) > 230 cm/s was applied.[8] Criteria for >50% stenosis in the common carotid artery are usually based on a doubling of velocities compared to a more proximal segment. Interpretative waveform consideration should be noted when there is an ICA occlusion or an inflow stenosis or occlusion (such as at the level of the innominate artery or aortic arch). A water hammer-type high resistive/pre occlusive waveform pattern will be noted at the origin of the occluded ICA, whereas a parvus et tardus pattern will be noted in the CCA in the presence of a central lesion.

Following carotid endarterectomy and stenting, native vessel criteria are no longer valid. Studies evaluating post carotid endarterectomy (CEA) and post carotid stent patients have shown increased velocity thresholds to define > 80% stenosis.[9,10] One study in post-CEA patients who underwent carotid duplex surveillance and selective CTA imaging found that a PSV of 274 cm/s correlated with a >70% stenosis with a sensitivity and specificity of 99% and 91%, respectively.[9] Data from the same group evaluated criteria for post carotid stenting surveillance and found that a velocity of >325 cm/s had a sensitivity and specificity of 100% and 99%, respectively, for detecting > 80% in-stent stenosis.[11] A study by Lal et al. found that the optimal threshold for detection of >80% in-stent restenosis was 340 cm/s.[10] In both these settings, criteria for native vessels overestimate stenosis after intervention. While criteria for carotid stenting have been well validated, post-CEA criteria needs further validation.

TABLE 8-2 The Society of Radiologists in Ultrasound Carotid Consensus Criteria

Stenosis Grade	Duplex Criteria
<50%	*PSV < 125 cm/s
	EDV < 40 cm/s; ICA/CCA < 2
50%–69%	*PSV < 125–230 cm/s
	EDV < 40–100 cm/s; ICA/CCA < 2–4
>70%	*PSV > 230 cm/s
	EDV > 100 cm/s; ICA/CCA >4
Occluded	

CCA, common carotid artery; EDV, end-diastolic velocity; ICA, internal carotid artery; PSV, peak systolic velocity.

*Primary criteria.

SURVEILLANCE

Duplex ultrasound is the recommended modality for postintervention surveillance. Recent SVS guidelines following arterial procedures recommend a baseline duplex (usually at <3 months postprocedure) and then every 6 months for 2 years.[4] This is based on the period of highest risk for restenosis or in-stent stenosis. Concerning changes should prompt a modification to this protocol as clinically indicated and particularly in patients who require reintervention. Following a stable clinical pattern, annual surveillance is recommended.

RENAL EVALUATION

INDICATION

The most common indication for renal duplex scanning is in the evaluation of suspected renovascular hypertension or ischemic nephropathy. Atherosclerotic disease is the most common contributor to renovascular disease and accounts for 90% of cases. Often these patients have underlying kidney dysfunction which makes duplex evaluation very appealing as it avoids exposure to nephrotoxic agents associated with axial and angiographic imaging. The second most common condition includes FMD. Other less-common conditions include dissection, thromboembolism, and arteritis.[12] Clinical indications for a renal duplex ultrasound relate to the most common cause of chronic kidney disease – hypertension (sudden worsening of hypertension despite optimal medical therapy, new onset hypertension in a young patient, or malignant hypertension). Other clinical indications include azotemia (after use of ACE-inhibitor or unclear origin), atrophic kidney, and flash pulmonary edema of noncardiac source. From a postprocedural surveillance standpoint, evaluation after renal stenting or bypass surgery is an additional indication for duplex sonography.

TECHNICAL

Given the retroperitoneal location, renal duplex scanning is best performed with a low-frequency curvilinear probe (2.5–3.0 MHz) in the fasting state. The aorta will be scanned in transverse and longitudinal views from the level of the xiphoid to the aortic bifurcation. A typical protocol includes evaluation of the renal arteries (at proximal, mid, and distal), aorta, renal parenchyma (from where a resistive index is measured), renal veins, and length of each kidney. Accessory renal arteries can occur in up to 20% of patients; therefore, when identified during the aortic sweep, they should undergo evaluation. If a stent is present, a similar evaluation should take place with imaging at the proximal, middle, distal, and poststent locations. A renal bypass should ideally be interrogated at the inflow source (iliac, suprarenal aorta, etc.), mid bypass, at the anastomoses, and the native outflow artery. Obtaining prior relevant endovascular or open surgical history will be key to an optimal evaluation. Spectral Doppler velocities are obtained throughout (aorta, renal artery, corticomedullary region) using small sample volumes (1.5–2 mm). At the corticomedullary location, these velocities contribute to the renal resistive index (RI = [peak systolic velocity-end diastolic velocity]/peak systolic velocity) and should be obtained at the upper, mid, and lower poles. A PSV in the aorta at the level of the SMA or the peri-renal level will contribute to the renal-to-aortic ratio (RAR = PSV renal artery origin/PSV of pararenal aorta). Minimal evaluation of the right and left renal veins should include documentation of patency and phasicity of flow. Additional evaluation should include but is not limited to documentation of aberrant anatomy such as a retroaortic renal vein and the presence of acute or chronic thrombus. Measurement of each kidney is relevant as chronic disease, particularly occlusive disease, will lead to renal atrophy. Smaller than normal (<8cm) renal size or asymmetry between right and left kidney (>1.5 cm difference) is indicative of chronic disease.

All Doppler angles should be obtained with a 60-degree angle, and positional maneuvers can aid in achieving this where possible. The exception to this will be at the level of the renal hilum and within the parenchyma where a 0-degree angle can be used. Positional maneuvers are key to achieving the best image, and this includes the use of reverse Trendelenburg, lateral decubitus position, and breath holds. The use of the liver (right) and spleen (left) as an acoustic window can aid in better visualization of the renal hilum.

INTERPRETATION

The kidneys are one of the several low resistive beds in the body, and thereby, in a normal state, will have continuous forward flow throughout diastole. This should be the case from the origin of the renal artery to the corticomedullary parenchyma. When high-resistive waveforms are identified, they are indicative of intrinsic renal disease (Figure 8-2). In a normal kidney, an RI value between 0.5 and 0.7 is expected while higher numbers (>0.8) are associated with parenchymal resistance and a diseased kidney. Based on the University of Washington criteria for evaluation of renal artery stenosis, 180 cm/s or less is considered normal velocities. When performed in experienced vascular laboratories, renal artery duplex has a sensitivity and specificity of 93% and 98% in the identification of renal artery stenosis, respectively.[13,14] Velocities obtained at the pararenal aorta (normal velocities typically range from 40 to 100 cm/s) are combined to achieve an RAR.

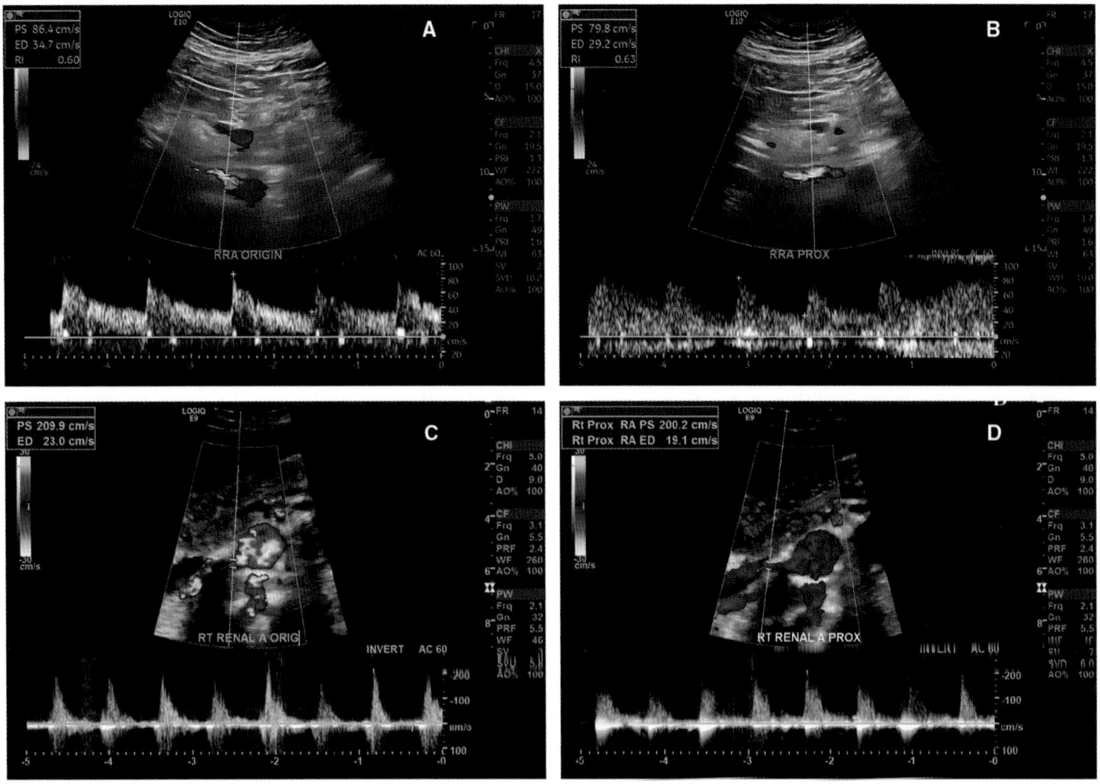

FIGURE 8-2 Renal duplex waveforms in renal artery without stenosis or intrinsic parenchymal disease (A, B) compared to one with evidence of stenosis and intrinsic parenchymal disease (C, D).

An RAR > 3.5 is consistent with > 60% stenosis as is a PSV > 180 cm/s. Interpretive caution should be instituted in the RAR in cases of low or high aortic velocities as they will be inaccurate. In this scenario, the PSV should be used as the main criteria so long as there are concomitant spectral doppler changes such as turbulent flow and delayed upstroke beyond the lesion. In this scenario, a PSV of 200 cm/s or greater can be used.[15] Renal artery occlusion will be accompanied by lack of flow in the artery after visualization and very low-to-absent parenchymal velocities on pulsed or color flow doppler. Patients with FMD will have mid and distal renal artery elevated velocities with increased turbulence, spectral broadening, and may have tortuosity. Criteria for percent stenosis used in patients with atherosclerotic disease cannot be applied to FMD as they have not been developed nor validated for these patients. There is currently no interpretative cut-off for these patients, but when identified, these findings should be reported as suggestive of FMD. Following renal artery stenting, in-stent stenosis criteria cut-off are different than that for native renal arteries. Threshold criteria have been evaluated in both renal stenting for atherosclerotic disease and following fenestrated or branched aortic endovascular repair.[16,17] Based on these and several other studies, PSV > 280 cm/s and RAR > 4.5 can be reasonable applied as a cut-off for > 60% in-stent stenosis.[4]

SURVEILLANCE

The role of surveillance for renal arteries is primarily following endovascular intervention or bypass surveillance. While there is no randomized study evaluating time points of a renal surveillance programs, some general guidelines include obtaining a baseline duplex within 1 month of index procedure, followed by 6-month, 12-month, and annual evaluation thereafter.

MESENTERIC EVALUATION

INDICATION

Commonly associated pathologies of the mesenteric vasculature are similar to those seen in the renal arteries, with atherosclerosis being the most common disease process (Table 8-1). Other nonatherosclerotic and less-common conditions include FMD, dissection, aneurysm, vasculitis, mesenteric venous thrombosis, and median arcuate ligament syndrome. Clinically, atherosclerosis of the mesenteric vessels will present with abdominal pain, and on examination, one may identify a bruit. Under these conditions, indications for this study include concerns for chronic mesenteric ischemia, colonic ischemia, or abdominal bruit. These patients can be quite challenging to diagnose given the various sources of abdominal pain. Duplex evaluation is a good screening test to rule in or out these processes and potentially avoid the use of unnecessary angiography for diagnosis. The use of duplex evaluation for acute mesenteric ischemia is limited due to the acuity, pain, and alternate imaging that is usually chosen for evaluation. Duplex sonography is important in the evaluation of compression disorders (such as MALS) and in postprocedural surveillance following endovascular intervention or after open surgical revascularization.

TECHNICAL

Of primary importance in the sonographic evaluation of the mesenteric vessels is knowledge of anatomy including the multiple described variants. The celiac axis is at the proximal aorta near the hiatus, and classically gives off three main branches: splenic artery, common hepatic, and left gastric artery. The superior mesenteric artery quickly follows the celiac axis. Distally, between the renal arteries and aortic bifurcation and usually at the 2 to 3 o'clock position, the inferior mesenteric artery (IMA) will be located. Standard anatomy is seen in up to 76% of patients.[18] Common variants include an accessory or replaced left hepatic artery originating from the left gastric artery (~10%), accessory or replaced right hepatic artery from the superior mesenteric artery SMA (~10%), or a combination (~4%). Less commonly is a common trunk to both celiac axis and SMA (~1%). Such variants are important to consider and identify for both accurate diagnostic imaging and as it may affect the procedural approach.

This examination is best performed in a fasting state, with a curvilinear low-frequency probe (3–5 MHz) and maintaining a 60-degree or less Doppler angle during spectral imaging with the Doppler cursor parallel to the vessel wall. Consistency in fasting state is important as stenosis criteria were defined in this manner. Initial evaluation should be in the supine position, but oblique position can also be performed. Starting at the level of the xiphoid, a transverse plane gray scale scan is performed to identify vessel anatomy in gray scale. Pulsed Doppler evaluation is then obtained in longitudinal view at the aorta and at the level of each respective mesenteric vessel and spectral waveforms recorded. Sample volumes should be targeted to the center of the vessel and be as focused as possible (1.5 mm) with optimal angle correction. PSV should be obtained at the origin of the celiac artery, SMA, and IMA. Evaluation of the hepatic and splenic artery should be performed if visualized. Beyond this, PSV at the proximal, mid, and distal SMA should be obtained. Positioning is important, and limitations of this study generally relate to body habitus and patient cooperation with position or maneuvers to achieve optimal imaging. Evaluation for MALS requires acquisition of Doppler waveforms and velocities in the celiac and SMA with deep inspiration and expiration. Stent and bypass surveillance requires acquisition of Doppler spectral waveforms at the inflow and outflow vessels as well as within the conduit (stent or bypass). Bypasses should additionally include velocities at the anastomosis.

INTERPRETATION

Interpretation of mesenteric Doppler waveforms should be based on both velocity criteria and spectral waveform analysis. In normal arteries and under fasting conditions, the SMA and IMA will be high-resistive and triphasic, while the celiac axis will have a sharp upstroke but have a low-resistive pattern with forward flow during diastole. Velocities of 125 cm/s or less without turbulence are indicative of a normal vessel. Following a meal, both the SMA and IMA will change to low-resistive waveform patterns. The SMA will also undergo this change in waveform in the setting of a stenosis or if there is a replaced right hepatic artery.

University of Washington criteria developed in the 1980s characterized normal and abnormal criteria for the celiac artery, SMA and IMA. It is generally agreed that PSV is the most accurate value to use for evaluation of the presence of disease. Multiple studies, mostly with small sample sizes, have validated stenosis criteria (Table 8-3). The most recent and largest includes 150 patients by AbuRahma et al. in 2012.[19] In addition to PSV criteria for the celiac artery, the presence of retrograde flow in the celiac, hepatic, or splenic arteries are likely indicative of proximal occlusion/stenosis. In the setting of occlusion, increased abdominal collateral may be seen. If one observes high-resistive waveforms in the celiac artery that persist in the hepatic artery, cirrhosis or parenchymal liver disease should be considered. When PSV in the SMA is >70%, this should also be accompanied by poststenotic turbulence. In the setting of SMA stenosis or occlusion, the IMA waveforms may become low resistive. In general, the IMA waveforms parallel patterns noted for the SMA.

In MALS, expiration will result in elevated PSV at the celiac artery that subsequently drops with deep inspiration. Normalization of velocities with inspiration is considered a positive study and suggestive of MALS. No percent stenosis is assigned in this scenario unless there is a concomitant atherosclerotic disease.

Native vessel criteria for stenosis do not translate into poststenting or bypass evaluation as they overestimate the degree of stenosis. Additionally, of the available data, none has become well established. AbuRahma et al. evaluated stented celiac artery and SMA and identified velocity threshold for >70%

TABLE 8-3 Mesenteric Duplex Criteria and Testing Accuracy for >70% Stenosis in the Celiac, Superior Mesenteric, and Inferior Mesenteric Arteries

	University of Washington	Moneta et al.	Moneta et al.	AbuRahma et al.	AbuRahma et al.
Celiac Artery					
PSV	>200 cm/s	>200 cm/s	SN: 87%	>320 cm/s	SN: 80%
EDV	>55 cm/s		SP: 80%		SP: 89%
			OA: 82%		OA: 85%
SMA					
PSV	>300 cm/s	>275 cm/s	SN: 92%	>400 cm/s	SN: 72%
EDV	>45 cm/s		SP: 96%		SP: 93%
			OA: 96%		OA: 85%
IMA	>200 cm/s			>250 cm/s	
Mesenteric to aortic ratio	>3			>4.5	

EDV, end-diastolic velocity; IMA, inferior mesenteric artery; OA, overall accuracy; PSV, peak systolic velocity; SN, sensitivity; SP, specificity.

stenosis to include PSV > 363 cm/s and 412 cm/s, respectively.[20] Several other studies have evaluated mesenteric stenting for stenosis criteria and published variable criteria, but none exists for postbypass restenosis.[21,22]

SURVEILLANCE

Current surveillance evidence is primarily derived from expert consensus given the lack of quality prospective studies. The combination of clinical evaluation, experience, and use of available vascular laboratory data should drive when additional contrast-based imaging or intervention is needed. Following mesenteric intervention and re-intervention, surveillance with ultrasound early postintervention (within 1 month) is essential to serve as the baseline comparison and by which to interpret future PSV measurements and need for re-intervention. Current SVS recommendations include duplex at one-month post intervention followed by duplex at 6 months, 12 months, and annual thereafter.[4] Suggested velocity criteria for investigation following stenting or bypass, in addition to considering recurrence of symptoms, includes PSV of > 370 cm/s for celiac artery and PSV >420 cm/s for SMA.[4,20] Internal vascular laboratory validation is always encouraged to guide internal protocols.

LOWER EXTREMITY EVALUATION

INDICATION

Noninvasive vascular evaluation of the lower extremities includes a combination of *physiologic* testing (with or without exercise) and *arterial* duplex. The combination of these two tests serves to provide a level of detail that allows identification of the location and extent of the disease.[4] These studies help confirm clinical suspicion, avoid more expensive and invasive testing, and guide therapeutic and surveillance plans. Physiologic testing, in particular, can provide valuable information when a decision is being made about healing potential or the hemodynamic significance of an atherosclerotic lesion in a patient with claudication. The accuracy of these evaluations should be considered in light of some patient-related limitations (obesity, arterial calcification, and limb edema). In general, it is recommended that physiological testing and an arterial duplex be performed at the same setting but not more than 2 weeks apart. A short list of indications for testing is given in Table 8-1.

TECHNICAL

Physiologic testing comprises three main components including the ankle-brachial index (ABI), arterial Doppler waveforms, and plethysmographic waveforms/pulse volume recordings (PVR). Additionally, one may obtain toe pressures (TBI = toe brachial index). The use of either one or both (arterial doppler waveforms and/or PVR) with the ABI is based on local protocol. Minimum IAC standards require performing an ABI with either an arterial Doppler waveforms or PVR, but do not require both. Depending on the indication or suspicion regarding extent of disease, physiologic testing can be limited to the ankle (ABI alone) or be more detailed via segmental limb evaluation (from high thigh to toes). All baseline testing should be performed in supine position, after a brief rest period with appropriately sized blood pressure and digits cuffs with sensors. TBI is generally obtained using photoplethysmography (PPG) technology. Cuffs should be placed at the upper arm, high and low thigh, calf, and ankle. A digit cuff waveforms and pressure can be obtained at the hallux, or in the presence of an amputation, should be placed at the next available digit where feasible and specified in the report. Waveforms should be obtained with Doppler probes that are between 4 and 8 MHz and use continuous Doppler principles.

ABI is obtained with arm and ankle cuffs. Cuffs should ideally be sized 20% larger than limb diameter for that particular level.[23] An undersized cuff will result in a falsely elevated reading while an oversized cuff will result in a falsely lowered pressure reading. In super obese patients, the forearm may be used in order to appropriately size a cuff. After the cuffs are inflated to suprasystemic numbers and loss of signal at the recorded artery occurs, the cuffs are allowed to deflate slowly and when there is return of a Doppler signal, that value is recorded. This is done at the brachial, dorsalis pedis, and posterior tibial artery.

Pressures are taken at both brachial arteries, and the higher of the two is used in calculating the ABI for each extremity. Note should be made of a large difference in blood pressure between right and left brachial pressures as this may be indicative of inflow or subclavian level disease. If full segmental limb pressures are being performed with either the three or four-cuff technique, the Doppler probe should be placed at the loudest audible tibial vessel for recording of all cuff inflations. In the setting of severe disease and inaudible ankle Dopplers, the popliteal signal can be used for thigh cuff measurements. In the setting of noncompressible vessels, a toe pressure provides beneficial information. The most commonly used application is the PPG, which is not based on volume changes but rather detection of light. The digit cuffs consist of an infrared light-emitting diode and a photosensor to detect the light reflected from tissues. Detection of this infrared light, which is proportional to the blood content of the tissue, translates into a waveform much like PVR.

When testing includes exercise ABI, a motor-driven treadmill with an incline is needed, and pre and postexercise ABI (with timed intervals) are recorded. The incline, speed, and time should be predetermined although the ideal protocol is controversial. Examples include (1) a set incline, speed, and time or (2) a set speed and no incline until an endpoint such as absolute claudication is reached (inability to continue walking due to reproducible leg symptoms) If symptoms are reproducible, the technologists need to note timing and location of these symptoms or reasons for stopping the examination prematurely. Following protocol completion, the patient should once again be placed in the supine position and ABI obtained in approximately 1-minute intervals until the ABI returns to the pre-exercise value. In patients with noncompressible and uninterpretable baseline ABI, an exercise ABI should not be performed. Additional exclusions for exercise ABI include critical limb-threatening ischemia (CLTI), shortness of breath at rest, angina, or physical disability.

Pulse volume recordings (PVR) are typically performed with air plethysmography. These cuffs record a change in volume following a change in pressure across the cuff. Similar to ABI, this can be a three or four cuff evaluation. A standard volume of air is injected into the pneumatic cuffs at each level just prior to the beginning of the examination. This will be enough to occlude venous return, but not to occlude arterial flow. Once inflated, the pressure induced by each pulsation will be measured as a volume change in the cuffs and translated into pressure pulse waveform. PVR is less affected by arterial calcification making them useful in providing additional information in the setting of noncompressible vessels.

An arterial duplex of the lower extremities should be performed using a linear array 5 to 7 MHz probe. A curvilinear probe can also be used depending on the depth of the vessel. Image acquisition for lower arterial scanning should include b-mode images, pulsed Doppler spectral waveforms, and color flow imaging. Technique and level of study detail should consider indication for the study (peripheral vascular disease, bypass surveillance, or aneurysmal evaluation). The scan will start at the inguinal ligament and evaluate the arterial tree down to the distal tibial vessels. Long axis grayscale and color/spectral Doppler images with velocities should be obtained at the common femoral artery, superficial femoral artery, proximal profunda artery, popliteal artery, and tibial arteries. Doppler angle correction is important to assure accurate velocity and subsequent interpretation

Lower extremity bypasses should include descriptors if it's a vein or synthetic bypass. A thorough evaluation along the graft (proximal anastomosis, prox/mid/distal bypass, and distal anastomosis) is required. Evaluation of a stent should include proximal, mid, and distal ends of stent. Both scenarios should include the inflow and outflow vessel just beyond the bypass or stent. Peak systolic velocities are recorded along the described segments. Additionally, areas of abnormalities (detected as flow disturbance with color bruit or spectral broadening) should prompt additional images with spectral and velocity measurements to assure accuracy. Aneurysms should be identified when present, and measurements recorded.

INTERPRETATION

Physiologic testing interpretation is based on ipsilateral (across segments) and contralateral (right vs. left

TABLE 8-4 Ankle Brachial Index and Disease Severity Interpretation

ABI	Interpretation
>1.4	Noncompressible
1.0–1.39	Normal
0.91–0.99	Borderline
0.70–0.90	Mild
0.40–0.69	Moderate
0.00–0.39	Severe

ABI, ankle-brachial index.

at same level) comparison in both the segmental pressures and the plethysmographic waveform changes. Generally accepted ABI measurements and interpretation are given in Table 8-4. When a complete segmental evaluation is performed, a drop of 20 mmHg or greater across a segment is considered indicative of a hemodynamically significant lesion. With segmental pressures, the presence of bilateral subclavian or axillary occlusive disease will yield a falsely elevated ABI given a falsely lower brachial pressure. If an ABI > 1.4 is obtained, one should consider the presence of axillary-subclavian disease as a possible contributor. Another scenario producing falsely elevated measurements includes patients with noncompressible lower extremity vessels or when the cuff is not sufficiently upsized to the leg diameter. In this case, the lower extremity pressures will be abnormally elevated, leading to a falsely elevated ABI. Qualitative interpretation of the Doppler waveforms will be necessary for such scenarios which have certainly been shown to have significant inter-rater variability.[24] A TBI can be obtained from the digit waveforms and pressure measurements. Significant disease is present if the TBI is < 0.7 or < 50 mmHg.

Exercise testing results are interpreted based on the extent of the drop in ABI and how long it takes to recover the ABI back to its pre-exercise baseline value. The larger the drop in ABI and the longer the recovery time, the more significant the disease. An exercise treadmill test is considered positive if the following occurs: (1) ankle pressure drops by 20 mmHg or greater from baseline, (2) there is a 20% or greater decrease from baseline ABI, (3) a drop in ABI of 0.2 or more, or (4) failure of ankle pressure to normalize after 3 minutes.[23] If the examination is completed without a drop in ABI and symptoms are reproduced or the patient has to stop due to pain, then their lower extremity symptoms are likely due to a nonvascular source.

PVR waveforms, under normal perfusion, typically have a waveform morphology with a sharp upstroke, a narrow peak, and a downstroke with a dichrotic notch. Their interpretation is qualitative and based on changes to this waveform secondary to the degree of occlusive disease. Progressive changes with dampening of the waveform will occur in the setting of inflow atherosclerotic disease including a dampened upstroke, amplitude, and loss of the dichrotic notch. The reliance on qualitative interpretation of the PVR makes for high inter-rater variability which affects the accuracy of interpretation.[25] When the ABI is uninterpretable due to noncompressible disease, the PVR does provide useful information as it is less affected in this scenario. Both segmental pressures and PVR are indirect evaluations without anatomic detail. This is why the addition of arterial duplex provides relevant anatomic correlation to noninvasive physiologic evaluation.

Interpretative criteria of arterial duplex of the lower extremities are derived from pulsed Doppler spectral waveform analysis. In the absence of disease, lower extremity arterial duplex typically has velocities that are <125 cm/s with waveforms that are high-resistive and triphasic (Figure 8-3). In the setting of disease, expected changes in the waveforms will depend on whether the lesion is on the inflow or the outflow side relative to the probe. In the setting of occlusive disease, waveforms will have blunting of the peak at systole and lose their end-systolic reversal of flow. There will also be a reduction in the flow channel or diameter with b-mode and color Doppler imaging. University of Washington criteria for classification of lower extremity arterial stenosis describe stenosis of > 50% as one with monophasic waveforms and loss of flow reversal with continuous forward flow during diastole. There will be spectral broadening and a doubling in

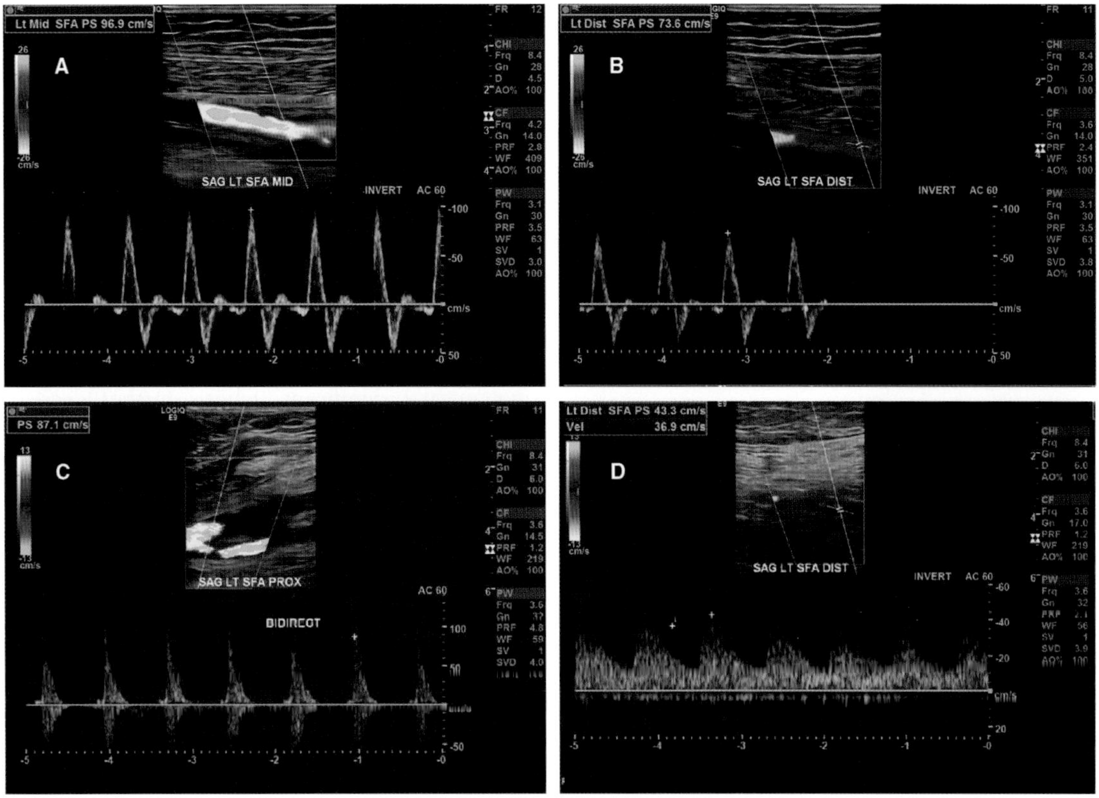

FIGURE 8-3 Lower extremity arterial duplex of SFA with normal triphasic and high-resistive spectral analysis and waveforms (A, B). A pre-occlusive, high-resistive bidirectional waveform proximal to an occluded artery (**C**) and waveforms distal to occlusion showing delayed upstroke, lower overall peak systolic velocities, spectral broadening, and continuous forward flow during diastole (**D**).

the PSV from one segment to the next. Waveforms distal to a significant stenosis will have lower PSV and be monophasic (Figure 8-3). A PSV ratio (max velocity in a stenosis/PSV in the preceding normal segment) of 2 or greater is commonly used as indicative of 50% or greater stenosis.

In the setting of infrainguinal vein bypass, a PSV ratio between 2 and 3.5 and PSV between 180 cm/s and 300 cm/s are associated with increased risk of thrombosis.[4] A PSV ratio of 4 or greater or a PSV of 300 cm/s or greater indicates critical stenosis. A PSV ratio that is between 2 and 4 can be repeated over a shorter surveillance interval or may suffice as a clinically relevant stenosis under the appropriate setting and change in the patient's condition. The highest risk scenarios are when findings on duplex exceed these values, the bypass has low velocities < 45 cm/s or there is a concomitant ABI drop of 0.15 or greater.[26]

Following percutaneous endovascular interventions, it is unclear what velocity criteria should be adopted to define a critical stenosis. Also the significance of postprocedural velocities relative to pre-intervention native vessels velocities is unclear, particularly in the setting of angioplasty and atherectomy. Studies evaluating surveillance program postendovascular intervention for infrainguinal disease have identified similar velocity (PSV >300 cm/s) and ratio criteria (>3.5) with varied sensitivities, specificities, and predictive values that have not translated into any formal stenosis criterion or recommendation.[27,28]

SURVEILLANCE

The primary role of surveillance imaging in the lower extremities has been largely studied in the setting of open revascularization and with mixed benefit from an aggressive surveillance program. Surveillance protocols are considered important in the monitoring of infrainguinal bypasses due to the known failure rates associated with the various types of reconstructions and the relatively noninvasive and low cost associated with these studies. While some studies have shown improvement in patency rates from a formalized surveillance program,[29–31] others have not.[32,33] Consensus recommendations from the SVS based on the currently available evidence align with the known risk for early (within 30 days), mid (1–24 months), and late (>24 months) bypass failures. This includes clinical examination and imaging (ABI and duplex ultrasound) at post revascularization (~1 month), at 3, 6, and 12 months and then (bi)annually based on the stability of studies and interval intervention.[4] This recommendation stems from evidence that 80% of bypass stenosis will occur within the first year. Following the first year, surveillance continues due to the persistent and continued risk of stenosis developing over the life of the bypass (from progressive intimal hyperplasia and later due to progression of disease) and the known overall patency rates of infrainguinal bypasses. Throughout the lifetime of surveillance, adaptations to this algorithm should be made with increased frequency if an abnormality is detected or the clinical status of the patient changes. Knowledge regarding the quality of inflow, conduit, or outflow vessel can also affect the frequency of testing. Plethysmographic evaluation has not been found predictive nor useful in predicting bypass failure. With these considerations, and with the timely intervention of high-grade stenosis, rates of bypass thrombosis can be lowered to less than 5% annually.

The role of a formal surveillance program and the use of duplex ultrasound in detecting high-grade stenosis in at-risk prosthetic bypass grafts are less convincing. Prosthetic bypass grafts with low velocities, however, may be at increased risk of future thrombosis, and anticoagulation has shown some benefit in preventing thrombosis.[34] Certainly, an inflow lesion leading to low flow in any bypass needs to be ruled out. Recommendations for prosthetic bypass surveillance are less frequent with an initial clinical examination and ABI (+/− duplex ultrasound) early postop, followed by one at 6 months, 12 months, and annual thereafter.

The application of surveillance strategies to patients who have undergone endovascular intervention is less established in the literature. The original indication preceding the intervention (claudication vs. CLTI) should be considered as reintervention is not of benefit for all comers. Furthermore, the accuracy of arterial duplex in the ability to detect a hemodynamically significant stenosis further decreases as we approach the tibial vessels. Based on the best available data to date, which is relatively weak, current recommendations include obtaining a postprocedural ABI and arterial duplex to document a new baseline following endovascular intervention and detect any missed lesion. Beyond this, additional surveillance is only suggested for patients with stenting or with CLTI as the indication, at 3 months and every 6 months thereafter.

CONCLUSION

Vascular laboratory testing is a reliable, reproducible, noninvasive, and cost-effective technology that plays a major role in the management of vascular patients. It is applicable across the various stages of care in patients with arterial disease including the detection and/or screening of disease, monitoring for progression of disease, and in the postintervention surveillance stage (Figure 8-4). Certified technologists and readers in accredited vascular laboratories provide imaging and interpretation that plays a critical role in the management of patients afflicted by the growing burden of atherosclerotic disease. With continued advances in ultrasound technology, its application will continue to grow in the areas of imaging and diagnostics. Its application is also being explored beyond diagnostics into the area of therapeutics.[35] With sustained presence and growth of the vascular laboratory in clinical practice, continued investigation and research will be needed to assure fulfillment of appropriate quality standards and protocols.

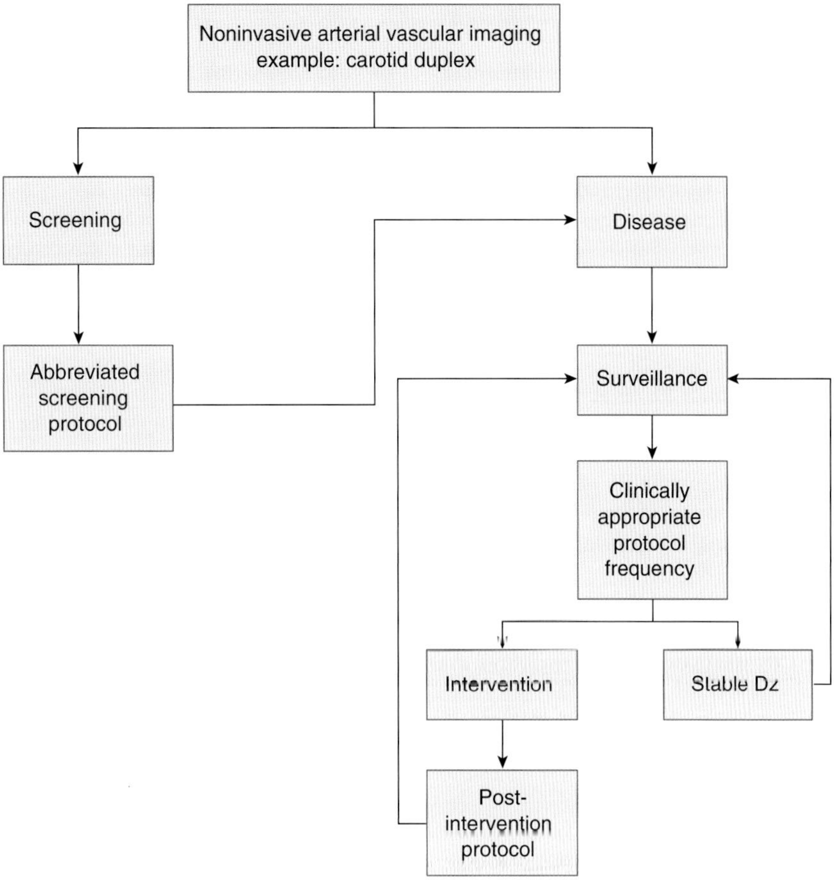

FIGURE 8-4 **Noninvasive vascular laboratory testing algorithm.**

REFERENCES

1. Hamaguchi H. Future of vascular ultrasound. *J Med Ultrasonics*. 2017;44:279.
2. Brott TG, Halperin JL, et al. 2011 ASA/ACCF/AHA/AANN/ACR/ASNR/CNS/SAIP/SCAI/SIR/SNIS/SVM/SVS guideline on the management of patients with extracranial carotid and vertebral artery disease: executive summary. *JACC*. 2011;57(8):1003-1043.
3. Gerhard-Herman M, Gardin JM, Jaff M, et al. Guidelines for noninvasive vascular laboratory testing: a report from the American Society of Echocardiography and the Society for Vascular Medicine and Biology. *Vasc Med*. 2006;11:183-200.
4. Zierler RE, Jordan WD, Lal BK, et al. The Society for Vascular Surgery practice guidelines on follow-up after vascular surgery arterial procedures. *J Vasc Surg*. 2018;68(1):256-284.
5. IAC Standards and Guidelines for Vascular Testing Accreditation. Intersocietal Accreditation Commission website. Updated May 1, 2021. Available at https://www.intersocietal.org/vascular/seeking/vascular_standards.htm. Accessed July 18, 2021.
6. DelBrutto VJ, Gornik HL, Rundek T. Why are we still debating criteria for carotid artery stenosis? *Ann Transl Med*. 2020;8(19):1270-1282.
7. Grant EG, Benson CB, Moneta GL, et al. Carotid artery stenosis: gray-scale and Doppler US diagnosis – Society of Radiologists in Ultrasound Consensus Conference. *Radiology*. 2003;229(2):340-346.
8. AbuRahma AF, Srivastava M, Stone PA, et al. Critical appraisal of the Carotid Duplex Consensus criteria in the diagnosis of carotid artery stenosis. *J Vasc Surg*. 2011;53(1):53-59.
9. AbuRahma AF, Stone P, Deem S, et al. Proposed duplex velocity criteria for carotid restenosis following

carotid endarterectomy with patch closure. *J Vasc Surg.* 2009;50(2):286-291.

10. Lal BK, Hobson RW, Tofighi B, et al. Duplex ultrasound velocity criteria for the stented carotid artery. *J Vasc Surg.* 2008;47:63-73.
11. AbuRahma AF, Abu-Halimah S, Bensenhaver J, et al. Optimal carotid duplex velocity criteria for defining the severity of carotid in-stent restenosis. *J Vasc Surg.* 2008;48:589-594.
12. Zierler RE, Campbell KA. Renal duplex scanning. In: Zierler RE, Dawson DL, eds. *Strandness's Duplex Scanning in Vascular Disorders*. 5th ed. Philadelphia, PA: Wolters Kluwer; 2016:349-378.
13. Hansen KJ, Starr SM, Sands RE, et al. Contemporary surgical management of renovascular disease. *J Vasc Surg.* 1992;16(3):319-330.
14. Olin JW, Piedmonte MR, Young JR, et al. The utility of duplex ultrasound scanning of the renal arteries for diagnosing significant renal artery stenosis. *Ann Intern Med.* 1995;122(11):933-838.
15. Hansen KJ, Tribble RW, Reavis SW, et al. Renal duplex sonograpy: evaluation of clinical utility. *J Vasc Surg.* 1990;12(3):227-236.
16. Mohabbat W, Greenbert RK, Mastracci TM, et al. Revised duplex criteria and outcomes for renal stents and stent grafts following endovascular repair of juxtarenal and thoracoabdominal aneurysms. *J Vasc Surg.* 2009;49(4):827-837.
17. Del Conde I, Galin ID, Trost B, et al. Renal artery duplex ultrasound criteria for the detection of significant in-stent restenosis. *Catheter Cardiovasc Interv.* 2014;83(4):612-618.
18. Kawamoto S. Case 84 – Mesenteric artery anatomic variants. In: Zimmerman SL, Fishman EK, eds. *Pearls and Pitfalls in Cardiovascular Imaging.* Cambridge University Press; 2015:260-262.
19. AbuRahma AF, Stone PA, Srivastava M, et al. Mesenteric/celiac duplex ultrasound interpretation criteria revisited. *J Vasc Surg.* 2012;55(2):428-436.
20. AbuRahma AF, Mousa AY, Stone PA, et al. Duplex velocity criteria for native celiac/superior mesenteric artery stenosis vs in-stent stenosis. *J Vasc Surg.* 2012;55(3):730-738.
21. Soult MC, Wuamett JC, Ahanchi SS, et al. Duplex ultrasound criteria for in-stent restenosis of mesenteric arteries. *J Vasc Surg.* 2016;64(5):1366-1372.
22. Baker AC, Chew V, Li CS, et al. Application of duplex ultrasound imaging in determining in-stent stenosis surveillance after mesenteric artery revascularization. *J Vasc Surg.* 2012;56(5):1364-1371.
23. Moneta GL, Zaccardi MJ. Indirect physiologic assessment of lower extremity arteries. In: Zierler RE, Dawson DL, eds. *Strandness's Duplex Scanning in Vascular Disorders.* 5th ed. Philadelphia, PA: Wolters Kluwer; 2016:164-171.
24. Kim ES, Sharma AM, Scissons R, et al. Interpretation of peripheral arterial and venous Doppler waveforms: a consensus statement from the Society for Vascular Medicine and Society for vascular ultrasound. *Vasc Med.* 2020;25(5):484-506.
25. Eslahpazir BA, Alleman MT, Lakin RO, et al. Pulse volume recording does not enhance segmental pressure readings for peripheral arterial disease stratification. *Ann Vasc Surg.* 2014;28(1):18-27.
26. Bandyk DF, Seabrook GR, Moldenhauer P, et al. Hemodynamics of vein graft stenois. *J Vasc Surg.* 1988; 8(6):688-695.
27. Bui TD, Mills JL, Ihnat DM, et al. The natural history of duplex-detected stenosis after femoropopliteal endovascular therapy suggests questionable clinical utility of routine duplex surveillance. *J Vasc Surg.* 2012;55(2):346-352.
28. Baril DT, Rhee RY, Kim J, et al. Duplex criteria for determination of in-stent stenosis after angioplasty and stenting of the superficial femoral artery. *J Vasc Surg.* 2009;49(1):133-138.
29. Bandyk DF, Schmitt DD, Seabrook GR, et al. Monitoring functional patency of in situ saphenous vein bypasses: the impact of a surveillance protocol and elective revision. *J Vasc Surg.* 1989;9(2):286-296.
30. Lundell A, Lindblad B, Bergqvist D, et al. Femoropopliteal-crural graft patency is improved by an intensive surveillance program: a prospective randomized study. *J Vasc Surg.* 1995;21(1):26-33.
31. Tinder CN, Chavanpun JP, Bandyk DF, et al. Efficacy of duplex ultrasound surveillance after infrainguinal vein bypass may be enhanced by identification of characteristics predictive of graft stenosis development. *J Vasc Surg.* 2008;48(3):613-618.
32. Davies AH, Hawdon AJ, Sydes MR, et al. Is duplex surveillance of value after leg vein bypass grafting? Principal results of the Vein Graft Surveillance Randomised Trial (VGST). *Circulation.* 2005;112(13):1985-1991.
33. Abu Dabrh AM, Mohammed K, Farah W, et al. Systemic review and meta-analysis of duplex ultrasound surveillance for infrainguinal vein bypass grafts. *J Vasc Surg.* 2017;66(6):1885-1891.
34. Brumberg RS, Back MR, Armstrong PA, et al. The relative importance of graft surveillance and warfarin therapy in infrainguinal prosthetic bypass failure. *J Vasc Surg.* 2007;46(6):1160-1166.
35. Yang C, Li Y, Du M, Chen Z. Recent advances in ultrasound – triggered therapy. *J Drug Target.* 2019;27(1):33-50.

SELF-ASSESSMENT STUDY QUESTIONS AND ANSWERS

Questions

1. Minimum standards for image acquisition in accredited vascular laboratories are set by:
   A. Society for Vascular Surgery
   B. Intersocietal Accreditation Commission
   C. Society for Vascular Ultrasound
   D. Society for Diagnostic Medical Sonography

2. As it pertains to imaging of the extracranial carotid arteries, a standard duplex ultrasound examination:
   A. Does not require evaluation with spectral analysis
   B. Only requires a transverse view
   C. Requires plaque morphology description
   D. FMD lesions are typically seen in the proximal ICA

3. Evaluation of the internal carotid artery following carotid endarterectomy (CEA) or carotid artery stenting (CAS)
   A. Should use the same peak systolic velocity criteria as prior to intervention to define stenosis
   B. Only requires imaging of the middle segment of the intervened ICA and the outflow vessel
   C. Should not use native vessel criteria as it overestimates degree of stenosis
   D. Has equally validated data for stenosis criteria in poststenting and post-CEA patients

4. Renal duplex imaging involves:
   A. Only imaging the dominant/main renal artery on either side
   B. Use of a linear array transducer between 5 and 12 MHz for image acquisition
   C. Obtaining a renal to aortic ratio (RAR) even with elevated PSV in the aorta
   D. Obtaining both a renal resistive index (RI) and an RAR

5. Identification of renal artery stenosis using vascular ultrasound
   A. Is associated with a sensitivity and specificity of 93% and 98%, respectively
   B. Can be identified if the PSV is 150 cm/s or greater
   C. Only includes diagnostic criteria of a PSV of >200 cm/s
   D. In FMD patients, includes a PSV of >250 cm/s at the proximal renal artery segment

6. Mesenteric duplex evaluation of the celiac and superior mesenteric artery
   A. Has EDV as the most accurate measure of stenosis
   B. will have a high-resistive SMA in the fasting state
   C. will have a high-resistive celiac axis in the fasting state
   D. can be diagnostic of median arcuate ligament syndrome (MALS) if expiration will result in decreased PSV at the celiac artery that subsequently increases with deep inspiration

7. Regarding postintervention stenosis evaluation for celiac artery or SMA
   A. Established criteria exist to define high-grade stenosis
   B. Native vessel criteria overestimate degree of stenosis post intervention
   C. Surveillance recommendations are derived from level 1 data
   D. Societal recommendations to define stenosis includes a PSV > 200 cm/s

SELF-ASSESSMENT STUDY QUESTIONS AND ANSWERS

8. Evaluation of the lower extremities using noninvasive vascular testing
A. Can generally be done without much limitation
B. Must include all three components (ABI, arterial Doppler, and plethysmographic waveforms) when performing physiologic testing
C. Can include evaluation of alternate digits for the TBI when the hallux has undergone amputation.
D. Should never only include an ABI

9. An exercise ABI
A. Includes resting and postexercise ABI recordings at 5 minutes
B. Must include a predetermined incline and speed to be up to standards
C. Can be performed in patients with noncompressible vessels
D. Is considered positive if the ankle pressure drops by 20 mmHg or greater from baseline

10. Arterial duplex surveillance following peripheral intervention
A. In a patient following peripheral arterial stenting, can use the same criteria for stenosis as established for vein bypass
B. Prosthetic and vein bypass surveillance criteria are equally well established
C. Does not have established criteria for vein bypasses
D. Is not established in the tibial vessels

SELF-ASSESSMENT STUDY QUESTIONS AND ANSWERS

Answers

1. B.
2. C.
3. C.
4. D.
5. A.
6. B.
7. B.
8. C.
9. D.
10. D.

CHAPTER

9 Physics for the Vascular Specialist

Motaz Al Yafi and Munier Nazzal

OUTLINE

ARTERIAL HEMODYNAMICS
- Fluid Pressure and Energy
- Fluid Energy Losses
  - Bernoulli's Principle

POISEUILLE'S LAW AND VASCULAR RESISTANCE

NORMAL PRESSURE AND FLOW

BLOOD FLOW PATTERNS
- Laminar Flow
- Turbulent Flow
- Boundary Layer Separation
- Pulsatile Flow
- Bifurcations and Branches

HEMODYNAMICS OF ARTERIAL STENOSIS
- Energy Losses
- Critical Stenosis
- Stenosis Length and Multiple Stenoses
- Bruits and Poststenotic Dilatation
- Abnormal Pressure and Flow
- Collateral Circulation
- Distribution of Vascular Resistance and Blood Flow
- Vascular Steal

HEMODYNAMIC PRINCIPLES IN THE TREATMENT OF ARTERIAL DISEASE

ANEURYSMS AND ARTERIAL WALL STRESS

Hemodynamic principles describe how blood flows in arteries and veins. This includes the relationship between pressure, flow, and resistance in normal, diseased, and collateral vessels. The clinical significance of arterial disease such as obstruction depends on its location, severity, and duration, as well as on the ability of the circulation to compensate, by changing cardiac output and developing collateral pathways. The aim of this chapter is to describe the principles and laws that are essential to understanding the pathophysiology and the fundamentals of the treatment of vascular disease. There are a few principles that govern flow in tubes including blood vessels; however, blood vessels are more compliant than rigid tubes making blood vessels more complex than rigid tubes. Additionally, blood vessels are affected by biological and hormonal factors that add to the complexity of the flow in blood vessels.

ARTERIAL HEMODYNAMICS

FLUID PRESSURE AND ENERGY

Blood flows through the arterial system in response to differences in total fluid energy. The pressure in a fluid system is defined as force per unit area, which is expressed in units such as dynes per square centimeter (dyn/cm^2) or millimeters of mercury (mmHg). Total fluid energy (E) is made up of potential energy (Ep) and kinetic energy (Ek). The potential energy (Ep) consists of intravascular pressure (P) and gravitational potential energy. Intravascular pressure (P) has three components: (1) dynamic pressure produced by cardiac contraction, (2) hydrostatic pressure, and (3) static filling pressure.[1] The specific gravity of blood and the height of the point of measurement above or below a reference level (usually the right atrium) determine the hydrostatic pressure. The hydrostatic pressure is described by the equation:

$$P(\text{hydrostatic}) = pgh$$

p: the specific gravity of blood (~1.056 g/cm³)

g: the acceleration due to gravity (980 cm/sec²)

h: the distance in centimeters above or below the right atrium

The static filling pressure illustrates the residual pressure that exists in the absence of flow and is determined by the volume of blood and the elastic properties of the vessel wall. In contrast to hydrostatic pressure, static filling pressure is usually low (5–10 mmHg).[2] Gravitational potential energy is the work a volume of blood can do because of its height above a specific reference level. The formula for gravitational potential energy is: +pgh. Since gravitational potential pressure and hydrostatic pressure usually cancel each other out, and static filling pressure is relatively low, the cardiac contraction dynamic pressure is the predominant component of potential energy (E_p). This is expressed as follows:

$$E_p = P + (pgh)$$

Kinetic energy (E_k), on the contrary, is of more biological and physiological significance and is the ability of blood to do work because of its motion. It is proportional to the specific gravity of blood and the square of blood velocity (v):

$$E_k = \frac{1}{2} pv^2$$

Therefore by combining Ep and Ek, the following would describe the total fluid energy per unit volume of blood:

$$E = P + pgh + \frac{1}{2} pv^2$$

FLUID ENERGY LOSSES

Bernoulli's Principle

When fluid flows from one point to another, the total fluid energy (E) remains constant, provided

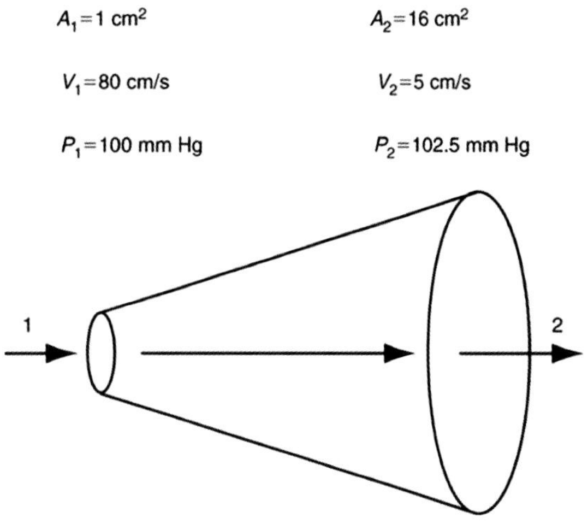

FIGURE 9-1 Conversion of kinetic energy to potential energy. (Reproduced with permission from Rutherford RB. *Vascular Surgery*. Philadelphia, PA: WB Saunders; 1977.)

that flow is steady, and there is no frictional energy loss. This is in line with the law of conservation of energy and constitutes Bernoulli's principle. This is depicted in Figure 9-1 demonstrating how the widening of the tube results in the conversion of kinetic energy (velocity) to potential energy (pressure), and therefore, the total fluid energy remains constant. In human circulation, the fluid energy lost in moving blood through the arterial circulation is dissipated mainly in the form of heat. This loss of energy is not accounted for in Bernoulli's principle.

POISEUILLE'S LAW AND VASCULAR RESISTANCE

Viscosity is described as the resistance to flow that arises due to the intermolecular attractions between fluid layers. Fluids with strong intermolecular attractions offer a high resistance to flow and have high coefficients of viscosity. The coefficient of viscosity (η) is defined as the ratio of shear stress (r) to shear rate (D):

$$\eta = \frac{\tau}{D}$$

Shear stress is proportional to the energy loss resulting from friction between adjacent fluid layers, whereas the shear rate is the relative velocity of adjacent fluid layers.

The viscosity of whole blood is largely due to the concentration of red blood cells; therefore, blood viscosity increases exponentially with increases in hematocrit. Similarly with plasma, the viscosity is mostly determined by the concentration of plasma proteins. These components of blood are also responsible for its non-Newtonian character. In a Newtonian fluid, like water, viscosity is independent of shear rate or flow velocity. On the other hand, the viscosity of blood can vary greatly with the shear rate. Blood viscosity increases rapidly at low shear rates but approaches a constant value at higher shear rates (Figure 9-2).

Energy losses in flowing blood occur either as viscous losses resulting from friction or as inertial losses related to changes in velocity or direction of flow. The viscous energy losses that occur in an idealized flow model are described by Poiseuille's law. The law states that the pressure gradient between two points along a tube (P1-P2) is directly proportional to the mean flow velocity (V) or volume flow (Q), the tube length (L), and the fluid viscosity (η) and is inversely proportional to either the second or the fourth power of the radius (r):

$$P_1 - P_2 = \bar{V}\frac{8L\eta}{r^2} = Q\frac{8L\eta}{\pi r^4}$$

This is often simplified to pressure = flow × resistance, where resistance (R) is

$$R = \frac{8L\eta}{\pi r^4}$$

The hemodynamic resistance of an arterial segment increases as the flow velocity increases provided the lumen size remains constant. The predominant factor influencing hemodynamic resistance is the fourth power of the radius.

The strict application of Poiseuille's law requires a steady (nonpulsatile) laminar flow of Newtonian fluid in a straight, rigid, cylindrical tube. Since these conditions do not exist in the arterial circulation, Poiseuille's law can only estimate the minimum pressure gradient or viscous energy losses that could be expected in arterial flow. Energy losses owing to inertial effects often exceed viscous energy losses, particularly in the presence of arterial disease.[3]

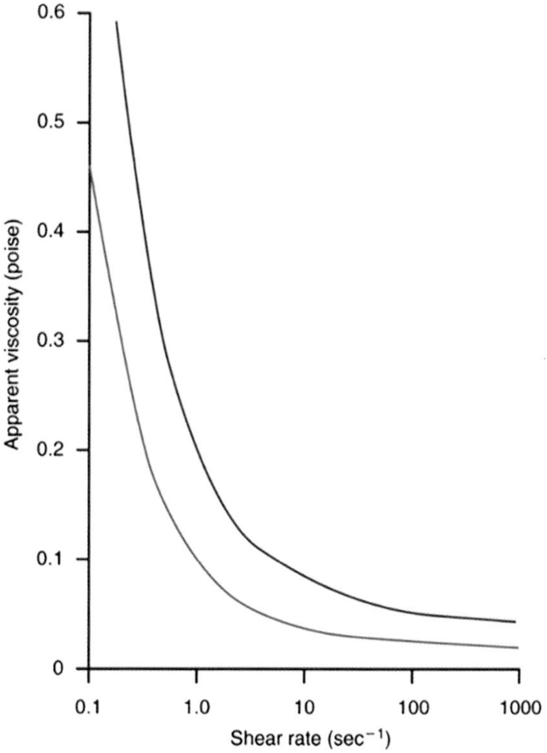

FIGURE 9-2 Relationship between blood viscosity and shear rate. (Modified with permission Whitmore RL. *Rheology of the Circulation*. New York, NY: Pergamon Press; 1968.)

NORMAL PRESSURE AND FLOW

The systolic pressure rises as the arterial pressure pulse moves distally, whereas the diastolic pressure falls and the pulse pressure widens. The decrease in mean arterial pressure (MAP) between the heart and ankle is normally less than 10 mmHg. The ratio of ankle systolic pressure to brachial systolic pressure (ankle-brachial index, ABI) normally has a mean value of 1.11 ± 0.10 in resting states.[4]

Cardiac systole results in the initial large forward flow phase; this is followed by a brief second phase of reversed flow in early diastole and a third smaller phase of forward flow in late diastole. The reversed flow phase is caused by the reflected waves produced when the initial surge of forward-flowing blood encounters the high resistance imposed by the arterioles. The triphasic flow pattern is modified by numerous factors, including proximal arterial disease and changes in vascular resistance. For example, warm exposure causes vasodilation and decreased resistance which tends to eliminate the reversed flow phase. Opposite effects are seen with cold exposure as resistance increases.

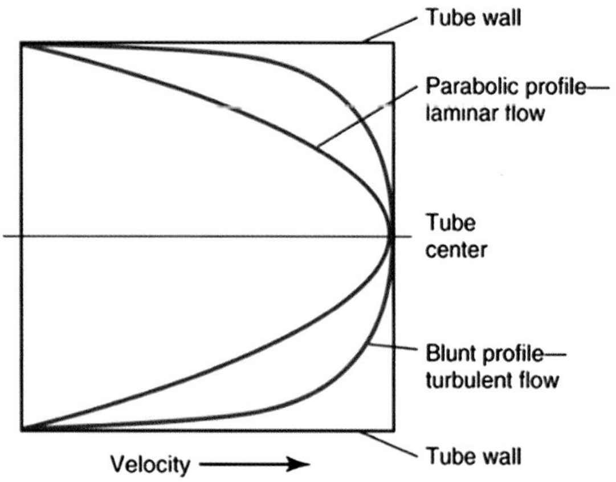

FIGURE 9-4 Parabolic velocity profile. (Reproduced with permission from Rutherford RB. *Vascular Surgery.* Philadelphia, PA: WB Saunders; 1977.)

BLOOD FLOW PATTERNS

LAMINAR FLOW

In the idealized conditions specified by Poiseuille's law, all flow streamlines move parallel to the walls of the tube and the fluid is arranged in a series of concentric layers or laminae, exemplified in the laminar flow pattern (Figure 9-3). The velocity is lowest adjacent to the tube wall and increases toward the center of the tube; however, the velocity within each lamina remains constant. This results in a parabolic velocity profile (Figure 9-4).

TURBULENT FLOW

In contrast to the linear streamlines of laminar flow, turbulence is an irregular flow state in which velocity varies rapidly with respect to space and time. These irregular changes in velocity cause fluid energy to dissipate as heat, resulting in greater energy losses compared to a laminar flow state. Under conditions of turbulent flow, the velocity profile changes from the parabolic shape of laminar flow to a rather rectangular or blunt shape (Figure 9-4).

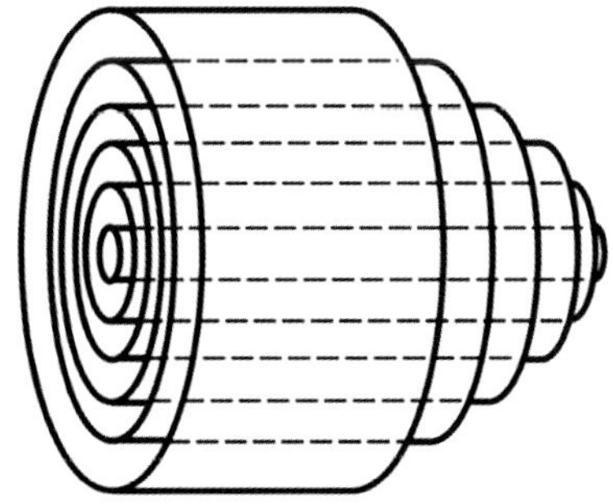

FIGURE 9-3 Laminar flow pattern. (Reproduced with permission from Strandness DE, Sumner DS. *Hemodynamics for Surgeons.* New York, NY: Grune and Stratton; 1975.)

Although turbulent flow is uncommon in normal arteries, the arterial flow pattern is often disturbed. This condition of disturbed flow is an intermediate state between stable laminar flow and frank turbulence. It is a transient disruption in the laminar streamlines that disappear as downstream flow proceeds. This is commonly seen at points of branching and curvature. Turbulence resulting from a stenotic arterial lesion generally occurs immediately downstream from the stenosis and may be present only during cardiac systole when velocities peak.

BOUNDARY LAYER SEPARATION

When fluid flows through a tube, the portion of fluid adjacent to the tube wall is referred to as the boundary layer. This layer is subject to both frictional interactions with the tube wall and viscous forces generated by the more rapidly moving fluid toward the center of the tube. When the tube geometry changes, such as at points of curvature, branching, or alteration in lumen diameter, small pressure gradients are created that cause the boundary layer to stop or reverse direction. This results in a complex, localized flow pattern known as an *area of boundary layer separation or flow separation*.[6,7] Areas of flow separation have been observed in models of arterial anastomoses and bifurcations (Figure 9-5). In a carotid artery bifurcation, the rapid central flow stream of the common carotid artery is compressed along the inner wall of the carotid bulb, producing a region of high shear stress, with an area of flow separation along the outer wall of the carotid bulb that includes helical flow patterns and flow reversal. The region of the carotid bulb adjacent to the separation zone is subject to relatively low shear stresses. Distal to the bulb, in the internal carotid artery, flow reattachment occurs, and a more laminar flow pattern is present.[21]

The flow patterns described in the carotid bifurcation models have also been documented in human subjects by pulsed Doppler studies.[8,9] The Doppler spectral waveform obtained near the inner wall of the carotid bulb is typical of the forward flow pattern found in the internal carotid artery. However, sampling of flow along the outer wall of the bulb demonstrates lower velocities with periods of both forward and reverse flows that are consistent with flow separation (Figure 9-6). Flow separation in the carotid bulb can also be seen with color-flow imaging (Figure 9-7). These findings are considered to be normal and are particularly common in young individuals. As increasing age causes alterations in arterial distensibility and wall-thickening in the carotid bulb, flow separation becomes less prominent.[10]

The clinical importance of boundary layer separation is that these localized flow disturbances may contribute to the formation of atherosclerotic plaques.[11] Intimal thickening and atherosclerosis tend to occur along the outer wall of the carotid bulb, whereas the inner wall is relatively spared during examinations of human carotid bifurcations, both at autopsy and during surgery. These findings suggest that atherosclerotic lesions form near areas of flow separation and low shear stress.

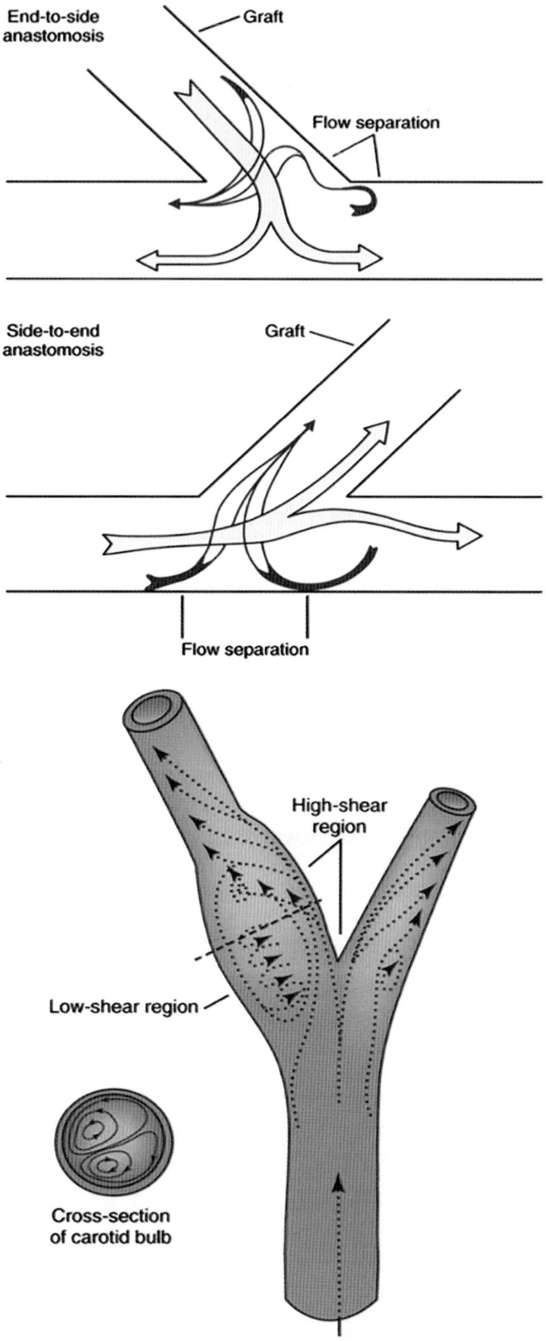

FIGURE 9-5 Areas of flow separation, in anastomosis and carotid artery bulb. (For bottom art: Reproduced with permission from Bergan JJ, Yao JST. Cerebrovascular Insufficiency. New York, NY: Grune and Stratton; 1983.)

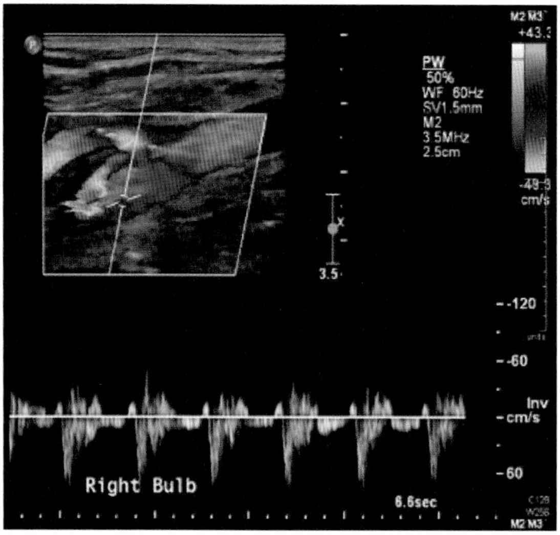

FIGURE 9-6 Flow separation with areas of foreword and reversal of flow. (Reproduced with permission from Moore WS. *Moore's Vascular and Endovascular Surgery: A Comprehensive Review*. Philadelphia, PA: Elsevier; 2018.)

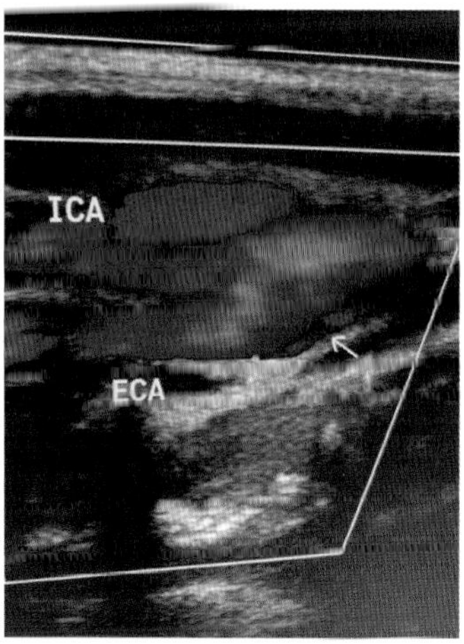

FIGURE 9-7 Flow separation in carotid artery bulb in a young 24-year-old male patient. (Reproduced with permission from Munier Nazzal MD, MBA, FRCS, FACS.)

PULSATILE FLOW

Pressure and flow vary continuously with time in a pulsatile system. The prior hemodynamic principles discussed are all based on a steady flow system, and they cannot be applied to the pulsatile flow system. However, they can be used to determine the minimum energy losses occurring in a specific flow system. The resistance or opposition offered by a peripheral vascular bed to pulsatile blood flow describes vascular impedance.[5] Pulsatile flow seems to be critical for optimal organ function, and studies have shown, for example, that kidneys perfused by a steady flow instead of pulsatile flow had reductions in urine volume and sodium excretion. High-resistance pulsatile flow is expected to exert pressure on the wall and thus allows either permeation of fluids or nutrients through the wall and allows the exchange of substances across the wall such as in the intestine and kidneys. However, low-resistance flow improves flow and oxygenation to an end organ such as the lower extremity.

BIFURCATIONS AND BRANCHES

Sudden changes in the flow pattern that occurs with the branching of the arterial system are potential sources of energy loss. Branching flow patterns are determined by the area ratio and the branch angle. The area ratio is defined as the combined area of secondary branches divided by the area of the primary artery.[12] A decline in the area ratio is associated with an increase in both the velocity of flow and the amount of reflected pulsatile energy. The branch angle also plays a role in flow disturbance and energy loss. As the angle between branches widens, the tendency to develop turbulent or disturbed flow increases. This is of significance in constructing anastomosis between different vessels or grafts and vessels.

HEMODYNAMICS OF ARTERIAL STENOSIS

ENERGY LOSSES

According to Poiseuille's law, which describes the viscous energy losses, the radius of a stenosis has a much greater effect on viscous energy losses than its length. The energy losses that occur at the entrance (contraction effects) and exit (expansion effect) of a stenotic segment are known as inertial energy losses. These are proportional to the square of blood velocity. The geometry of a stenotic segment also has an effect on energy losses. A vessel with an abrupt change in lumen size results in more energy loss than a gradually tapering vessel. This is why energy lost at the exit of the stenotic segment can be quite significant because of the sudden expansion of flow and dissipation of kinetic energy in a zone of turbulence.

CRITICAL STENOSIS

Arterial narrowing that produces a significant reduction in blood pressure or flow is called critical stenosis. As previously noted, energy losses associated with a stenosis are inversely proportional to the fourth power of the radius. This creates an exponential relationship between energy loss (pressure drop) and reduction in the lumen size (Figure 9-8).[13,14] Pressure drop across a stenosis varies with flow rate. Since flow velocity is dependent on distal hemodynamic resistance, the critical stenosis value will also vary with the resistance of the runoff vessel. The autoregulation mechanism observed in many vascular beds allows it to maintain a constant level of blood flow over a wide range of perfusion pressures. This is demonstrated by the constriction of resistance vessels in response to an increase in blood pressure and the dilation of resistance vessels when blood pressure decreases. In peripheral arteries with physiologic flow rates, the critical stenosis value is reached at approximately a 50% reduction in lumen diameter or a 75% reduction in cross-sectional lumen area. However, a stenosis may not be significant at resting flow rates but becomes critical when flow rates are increased by reactive hyperemia or exercise. For example, a stenotic lesion that does not appear severe by arteriography may be associated with significant pressure gradients during exercise. Therefore, it is

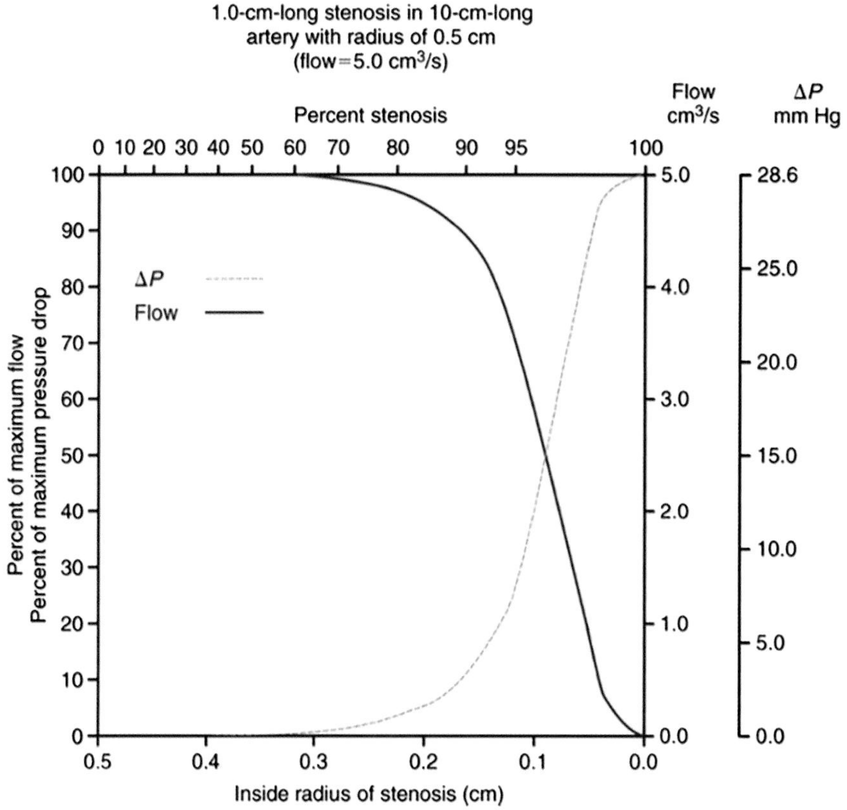

FIGURE 9-8 Relationship between energy loss and flow. (Reproduced with permission from Strandness DE, Sumner DS. *Hemodynamics for Surgeons*. New York, NY: Grune and Stratton; 1975.)

difficult to predict the hemodynamic significance of a lesion based on the apparent reduction in lumen size and physiologic testing by blood pressure measurement must be used to document the clinical severity of arterial lesions.

STENOSIS LENGTH AND MULTIPLE STENOSES

The radius of a stenosis has a much greater effect on viscous energy losses than its length. Doubling the length of stenosis results in doubling the viscous energy losses, however reducing the radius by half increases energy losses by a factor of 16. Since inertial energy losses are mainly due to the entrance and exit effects, they are independent of stenosis length. Therefore, separate short stenoses are usually more significant than a single longer stenosis. It has been shown that when stenoses that are not significant individually are arranged in series, large reductions in pressure and flow can occur.[15] Thus, multiple subcritical stenoses may have the same effect as a single critical stenosis.

BRUITS AND POSTSTENOTIC DILATATION

An audible sound or bruit over an artery is usually regarded as a clinical sign of arterial disease. Narrowing or irregularity of the vessel lumen produces turbulent flow patterns that cause vibrations in the arterial wall. These vibrations generate displacement waves that radiate through surrounding tissue and can be detected as audible sounds. A bruit may be absent when an artery is nearly occluded or when flow rates are extremely low.

Poststenotic dilation is a common clinical finding and has been seen in the thoracic aorta below coarctations and distal to atherosclerotic lesions. This is most likely explained by the arterial wall vibrations resulting in structural weakness of elastin fibers.

ABNORMAL PRESSURE AND FLOW

When an arterial lesion is hemodynamically significant at resting flow rates, there will be a measurable reduction in distal blood pressure. In general, limbs with a lesion at one anatomic level have ankle-brachial indices between 0.90 and 0.50, whereas limbs with lesions at multiple levels have ankle-brachial indices less than 0.50. The ankle-brachial index can also correlate with the clinical severity of disease; in limbs with intermittent claudication, the index has a mean value of 0.59 ± 0.15; in limbs with ischemic rest pain, 0.26 ± 0.13.[4] Patients with intermittent claudication have limited capacity to increase limb blood flow during exercise, and pain occurs in the muscles that have been rendered ischemic. As the occlusive disease progresses and becomes more severe, a decrease in peripheral vascular resistance can no longer compensate and resting flow drops causing signs and symptoms of ischemia at rest.[16]

COLLATERAL CIRCULATION

Collateral circulation is a mechanism that compensates for the hemodynamic effects of a stenosis or obstruction. These are preexisting pathways that enlarge when flow through the parallel major artery is reduced. The abnormal pressure gradient across the collateral system and increased velocity of flow through the midzone vessels are the main stimuli for collateral development. Collateral vessels are smaller, longer, more numerous, and have higher resistance compared to the native artery. In addition, the acute changes in collateral resistance during exercise are minimal.[16] Collateral systems have three components: (1) stem arteries (distributing branches), (2) a midzone of smaller intramuscular channels, and (3) reentry vessels that join the major artery distal to the point of obstruction, Figure 9-9.[5,22]

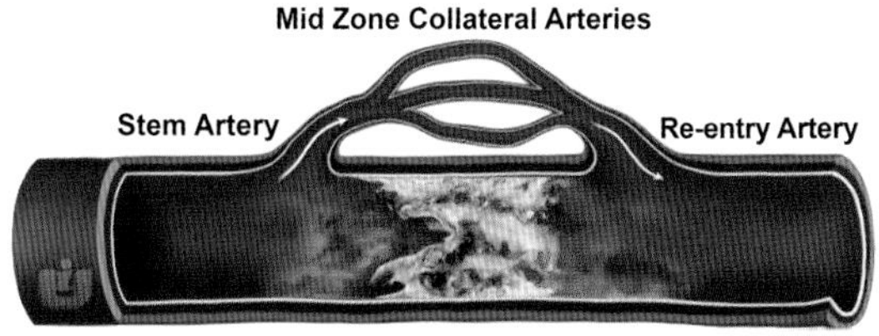

FIGURE 9-9 Collateral circulation. (Reproduced with permission from Size GP. Vascular physiology and hemodynamics. In: *Inside Ultrasound Vascular Reference Guide*. Inside Ultrasound; Vail, 2013.)

DISTRIBUTION OF VASCULAR RESISTANCE AND BLOOD FLOW

As opposed to collateral resistance, the resistance of a peripheral runoff bed is highly variable. Peripheral resistance is regulated by the muscular arterioles, which is mainly determined by the sympathetic nervous system. Vascular resistance in the lower limb is divided into segmental and peripheral components. Segmental resistance consists of the relatively fixed parallel resistances of the major normal or diseased artery and the bypassing collateral vessels. Peripheral resistance includes the highly variable resistances of the distal calf muscle arterioles and cutaneous circulation. Normally, resting segmental resistance is low and peripheral resistance is high. With exercise, the peripheral resistance drops and flow through the segmental arteries increases by up to a factor of 10, with little or no pressure drop.

With moderate arterial disease, the segmental resistance is increased due to collateral flow and abnormal pressure drop is present across the thigh. However, due to a compensatory decrease in peripheral resistance, the total resistance of the limb and resting blood flow often remain in the normal range. During exercise, the segmental resistance remains high and fixed, whereas peripheral resistance decreases but the capacity of peripheral circulation to compensate is limited resulting in calf muscle ischemia and claudication. When arterial disease becomes severe, the compensatory decrease in peripheral resistance may be unable to provide normal blood flow at rest, causing an even larger pressure drop across the involved segments and with little or no increase in blood flow with exercise. This causes severe claudication or even ischemic rest pain or ulceration.

VASCULAR STEAL

Vascular steal occurs when two runoff beds with different resistances are supplied by a limited source of arterial inflow. One example of the steal phenomenon is the subclavian steal syndrome. During which reversal of flow in the vertebral artery is associated with subclavian artery occlusion and symptoms of brainstem ischemia. When occlusion is present in the left proximal subclavian artery or the innominate artery on the right, the pressure at the origin of the ipsilateral vertebral artery is reduced. This may result in a reversal of flow in the vertebral artery, which then becomes the source of collateral flow to the arm. During arm exercise, the reversed flow is augmented due to increased demand, and the patient may then experience ischemia of the brainstem. Similar principles can be applied in extra-anatomic bypass grafts in which a single donor artery supplies several vascular beds. For example, in the case of a femoral-femoral graft, one iliac artery is the donor artery, the ipsilateral leg is the donor limb, and the contralateral leg is the recipient limb. This results in a doubling of blood flow in the donor artery.[17] The ankle-brachial index improves on the recipient side even if there is significant occlusive disease. On the other hand, there may be a decrease in the ankle-brachial index on the donor side; however, a symptomatic steal is uncommon unless there is stenosis of the donor iliac artery.

HEMODYNAMIC PRINCIPLES IN THE TREATMENT OF ARTERIAL DISEASE

The high fixed segmental resistance of disease arteries and collaterals is responsible for decreased blood flow. Therefore, therapy must be directed toward lowering this high segmental resistance in order to improve blood flow since peripheral resistance has already been lowered to compensate for the increased segmental resistance.[18] Walking exercise therapy has been shown to improve collateral flow, but the degree of clinical improvement is not sufficient enough to improve moderate-to-severe arterial disease.[19]

The best method for reducing the fixed segmental resistance is a direct intervention by open surgical or catheter-based techniques. Arterial grafts are frequently used, and the same hemodynamic principles are applied. Since vessel diameter is the main determinant of hemodynamic resistance, the diameter of a graft is considerably more important than its length. However, graft diameter is often limited by arterial size. The diameter of a graft should be somewhat similar to the adjacent artery to minimize energy losses associated with entrance and exit effects. Similarly, end-to-end anastomoses are theoretically preferable to end-to-side anastomoses due to the elimination of energy losses resulting from curvature and angulation. However, these losses appear to be minimal and not clinically significant under physiologic conditions.

ANEURYSMS AND ARTERIAL WALL STRESS

Aneurysms form when the structural components of the arterial wall are weakened. Rupture occurs when the tangential stress within the arterial wall becomes greater than its tensile strength. Tangential stress is directly proportional to pressure and radius but inversely proportional to wall thickness. Stress has the dimensions of force per unit area of the tube wall (dynes per square centimeter).[20] For example, when the diameter of a tube increases by three-fold and assuming the pressure remains constant, the wall stress would increase by a factor of 12 (Figure 9-10).

Clinical applications of Physics principles in vascular disease:

- Blood flows in arteries propelled by left ventricle.
- The volume in an artery or its branches is constant.
- The diameter of an artery affects blood flow. If the diameter is reduced by 50%, the velocity of flow increases by four times.

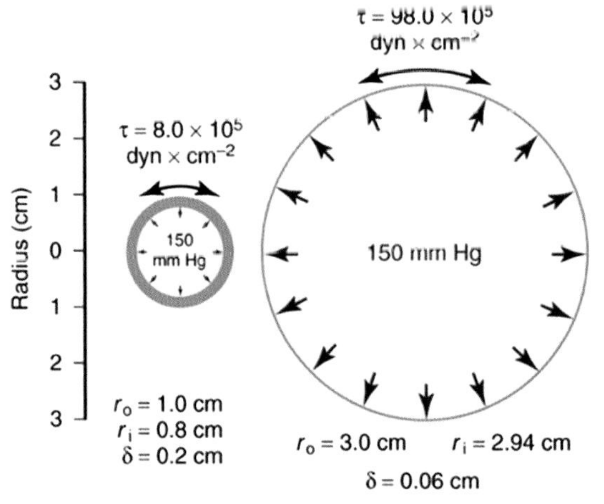

FIGURE 9-10 Relationship between diameter and wall stress. (Reproduced with permission from Rutherford RB. *Vascular Surgery*, 2nd ed. Philadelphia, PA: WB Saunders; 1984.)

- Pressure fall is much greater in small vessels like those in the microcirculation. Viscosity's effect on flow in large arteries is minimal.
- Flow in blood vessels differs; based on arterial dilatation, blood closest to the wall of the artery is slowest. This can result in the deposition of materials on the wall of blood vessels that can lead to pathological diseases such as atherosclerosis.
- Change in flow such as in anastomosis areas can lead to a change in velocity of flow such as stagnant flow which might cause restenosis.
- Normal blood flow is laminar.
- Flow can become turbulent in areas of dilatation, stenosis, curved segments, angulation, bifurcation, and branching. Examples of such areas: the aortic bifurcation, common femoral bifurcation, and carotid bulb.
- Turbulent flow can result in reversal of flow and stagnation which can contribute to the deposition of blood materials that can cause plaque formation and neointimal hyperplasia such as in the graft artery or graft veins anastomosis.
- Areas of turbulence in blood flow beyond areas of stenosis or in the graft-vein anastomosis can lead to chaotic flow. This can result in areas of dilatation or stenosis in the arterial areas distal to the stenosis.
- Loss of energy at areas of stenosis is exaggerated with exercise due to reduced resistance to flow and results in reducing pressure.
- 50% reduction in diameter is equivalent to a 75% area reduction.
- In areas of stenosis, blood flow decreases and peak systolic velocity increases which becomes significant at 50% diameter stenosis. Once stenosis reaches a certain point (90%–95%), a sharp fall in peak systolic velocity occurs.
- Resistance to flow is higher in smaller vessels. As resistance increases, flow decreases. Therefore, blood flow is lowest in smaller vessels "microcirculation" than in larger vessels "macrocirculation."

- Certain circulation beds are high resistance such as the small intestine, external carotid, and limbs leading to low flow in diastole. Other vascular beds such as the brain and kidneys have low resistance and thus have forward flow in diastole.
- Resistance in vascular bed can change during exercise (limbs), postprandial (small intestine), and sympathetic blockade (skin). Autoregulation changes resistance as needed.
- Collateral flow in occluded vessels has higher total resistance than native arteries. In response to exercise, collateral resistance becomes greater leading to a less hyperemic response.
- Exercise causes vasodilatation in the high-resistance circulation in the lower extremities. In normal conditions, blood flow increases 10–20 times. In areas of stenosis and occlusion, the collateral circulation is high resistance and does not allow such an increase which delays the removal of pain-producing metabolites from the circulation and thus causes pain in the lower extremities. Normally, pain-producing metabolites are removed in less than 60 seconds. In cases of arterial stenosis and occlusion, metabolites accumulate in the circulation causing pain.
- A bruit results from vibrant flow in vessels causing transmitted vibration heard via stethoscope.
- In aneurysmal disease, as the diameter of an aneurysm increases the tension in the wall increases and the thickness of the wall decreases resulting in rupture of the wall.
- Vasoconstriction causes a decrease in venous flow, while vasodilatation causes an increase in venous flow.
- Blood flow in veins mostly from the contraction of muscles such as calf muscles.
- Respiratory variations in venous flow are noticed in proximal veins but not apparent in distal veins.
- During inspiration, venous flow increases in the upper extremities and decreases in the lower extremities due to changes in the intrathoracic pressures.
- Valsalva, coughing, and straining cause a decrease in venous flow in all extremities.
- Larger veins have more blood flow. Smaller veins have slower blood flow resulting in more potential for thrombosis.

REFERENCES

1. Gauer OH, Thron HL. Postural changes in the circulation. In: Hamilton WF, Dow P, eds. *Handbook of Physiology. Sect 2: Circulation*. Vol. III. Washington, DC: American Physiological Society; 1965:2409.
2. Guyton AC. Venous return. In: Hamilton WF, et al. eds. *Handbook of Physiology. Sect 2: Circulation*. Vol. II. Washington, DC: American Physiological Society; 1963:1099.
3. Burton AC. *Physiology and Biophysics of the Circulation*. 2nd ed. St Louis, MO: Mosby–Year Book; 1972.
4. Yao JST. Hemodynamic studies in peripheral arterial disease. *Br J Surg*. 1970;57:761-766.
5. Strandness DE Jr, Sumner DS. *Hemodynamics for Surgeons*. New York: Grune & Stratton; 1975.
6. Gutstein WH, Schneck DJ, Marks JO. In vitro studies of local blood flow disturbance in a region of separation. *J Atheroscler Res*. 1968;8:381-388.
7. Logerfo FW, Soncrant T, Teel T, Dewey F. Boundary layer separation in models of side-to-end arterial anastomoses. *Arch Surg*. 1979;114:1364-1373.
8. Ku DN, Giddens DP, Phillips DJ, et al. Hemodynamics of the normal human carotid bifurcation—In vitro and in vivo studies. *Ultrasound Med Biol*. 1985;1:13-26.
9. Phillips DJ, Greene FM Jr, Langlois Y, et al. Flow velocity patterns in the carotid bifurcations of young, presumed normal subjects. *Ultrasound Med Biol*. 1983;1:39-49.
10. Reneman RS, van Merode V, Hick P, et al. Flow velocity patterns in and distensibility of the carotid artery bulb in subjects of various ages. *Circulation*. 1985;71:500-509.
11. Fox JA, Hugh AE. Localization of atheroma: a theory based on boundary layer separation. *Br Heart J*. 1966;28:388-394.
12. McDonald DA. Steady flow of a liquid in cylindrical tubes. *Blood Flow in Arteries*. 2nd ed. London: Edward Arnold; 1974:17-54.
13. Berguer R, Hwang NHC. Critical arterial stenosis—a theoretical and experimental solution. *Ann Surg*. 1974;180:39-50.

14. May AG, Van de Berg L, DeWeese JA, Rob CG. Critical arterial stenosis. *Surgery*. 1963;54:250-259.
15. Flanigan DP, Tullis JP, Streeter VL, et al. Multiple subcritical arterial stenosis: effect on poststenotic pressure and flow. *Ann Surg*. 1977;186:663-668.
16. Sumner DS, Strandness DE Jr. The relationship between calf blood flow and ankle blood pressure in patients with intermittent claudication. *Surgery*. 1969; 65:763-771.
17. Ludbrook J. Collateral artery resistance in the human lower limb. *J Surg Res*. 1966;6:423-434.
18. Shin CS, Chaudhry AG. The hemodynamics of extra-anatomic bypass grafts. *Surg Gynecol Obstet*. 1979; 148:567-570.
19. Gardner AW, Poehlman ET. Exercise rehabilitation programs for the treatment of claudication pain: a meta-analysis. *JAMA*. 1995;274:975-980.
20. Sidawy AN, Perler BA. Arterial hemodynamics. In: *Rutherford's Vascular Surgery and Endovascular Therapy, E-book*. Elsevier Health Sciences; 2018:87-96.
21. Philadelphia, PA, Moore WS. Hemodynamics for the vascular surgeon. In: *Moore's Vascular and Endovascular Surgery E-book: A Comprehensive Review*. Elsevier Health Sciences; 2018:64-84.
22. Pearce, AZ, Size GP. Vascular physiology and hemodynamics. In: *Inside Ultrasound Vascular Reference Guide*. Davies Publishing; 2013:25-43.

SELF-ASSESSMENT STUDY QUESTIONS AND ANSWERS

Questions

1. Poiseuille's law states that the pressure gradient between two points along a tube is inversely proportional to which of the following?
   A. Mean flow velocity
   B. Blood viscosity
   C. Tube radius
   D. Volume flow rate
   E. Tube length

2. The value of critical stenosis of a particular artery depends on which of the following?
   A. Compliance of the arterial wall
   B. Blood viscosity
   C. Length of the arterial segment
   D. Flow rate and peripheral resistance of the vessel
   E. Tangential stress

3. In flowing blood, inertial energy losses are related to which of the following?
   A. Changes in velocity and direction of flow
   B. Mean blood pressure
   C. Blood viscosity
   D. Specific gravity of blood
   E. Friction between adjacent layers of moving blood

4. Tangential stress is inversely proportional to which of the following?
   A. Mean blood pressure
   B. Radius of the vessel
   C. Flow rate
   D. Vessel wall thickness
   E. Blood viscosity

5. Vascular steal from the donor limb is most likely to occur in which of the following circumstances?
   A. There is an occlusive lesion in the donor artery.
   B. There is an occlusive lesion in the recipient artery.
   C. The donor limb is hemodynamically normal.
   D. The recipient limb has a mild occlusive disease.
   E. There is an occlusive disease in both the donor and recipient limbs.

6. Which of the following statements about collateral circulation is true?
   A. Collateral artery resistance is usually less than that of the original unobstructed parallel artery.
   B. The midzone of the collateral bed consists of small intramuscular vessels.
   C. Collateral vessels are new pathways that run perpendicular to the major artery that is occluded.
   D. The vascular resistance of the collateral bed is variable.
   E. Normal pressure gradient across the collateral system stimulates the development of collateral pathways.

7. The Bernoulli principle states that:
   A. Increased pressure increases velocity.
   B. Increased velocity decreases pressure.
   C. Decreased pressure decreases velocity.
   D. Decreased velocity decreases pressure.

8. Which of the following is a function of the calf muscle pump?
   A. It improves arterial blood flow to the exercising muscle.
   B. It decreases venous return to the right heart.
   C. It minimizes the accumulation of interstitial fluid in the distal limb.
   D. It increases venous pressure in the dependent limb.
   E. It increases venous volume in the exercising limb.

9. Which of the following statements about venous return is true?
   A. During inspiration, venous return is increased.
   B. During inspiration, venous return is decreased.
   C. During inspiration, venous flow is decreased in the upper extremities.
   D. During inspiration, venous flow is increased in the lower extremities.
   E. During inspiration, the intrathoracic pressure is increased.

SELF-ASSESSMENT STUDY QUESTIONS AND ANSWERS

10. Venous flow is influenced by all of the following except

A. Respirations
B. Filling pressure of the right heart
C. Body position
D. The activity of the calf muscle pump
E. All of the above

SELF-ASSESSMENT STUDY QUESTIONS AND ANSWERS

Answers

1. C.
2. D.
3. A.
4. D.
5. A.
6. B.
7. B.
8. C.
9. A.
10. E.

CHAPTER

10 Vascular Surgical Techniques: Open Surgical Exposure of Arteries, Veins, and Other Open Techniques for Occlusive Disease and Anterior Spine Exposure

Rebecca Kelso

OUTLINE

VESSEL EXPOSURE AND CONTROL
- Anatomy
- Incision
- Retractors
- Dissection
- Redo Dissection
- Vessel Control
- Vascular Clamping
- Balloon Occlusion
- Tourniquet

ARTERIOTOMY AND ENDARTERECTOMY
- Endarterectomy
- Vessel Reconstruction

ANTERIOR SPINE EXPOSURE

Vascular surgeons are unique from other specialty surgeons as their focus is on a broad spectrum of blood vessels which is only exclusive of the heart and intracerebral vessels. With this anatomic scope are a variety of surgical approaches and treatment options that can be adapted to all situations. Each vascular open operation has the goal of identifying the inflow and outflow vessels that will then be locally reconstructed or bypassed to improve perfusion. Hybrid vascular surgery is a label that has been developed in the last two decades to refer to cases with an open and endovascular component, as endovascular surgery has taken root in the management of vascular disease especially for occlusive and aneurysmal disease. Its innovation has been led by vascular surgeons and knowledge of both open and endovascular techniques and is a necessity in the current treatment of vascular patients.

Regardless of innovation, skillful management of the blood vessels is important as even minor errors can be relentless and unforgiving. As such, the basics of vessel dissection and anastomosis remain constant. This chapter will focus on the basic techniques of exposure, vessel control, endarterectomy, and vessel reconstruction. Specifics regarding conduits will be covered in Chapter 14. As the iliac vessels are often exposed with a retroperitoneal approach, vascular surgeons often have the unique opportunity to participate in spine surgery and thus the techniques of anterior spinal exposure are also presented.

VESSEL EXPOSURE AND CONTROL

ANATOMY

Anatomic awareness is essential to all exposures. A majority of exposures have been developed by pioneers in vascular surgery using muscle-sparing paths in naturally occurring planes. Given the multitude of possible management options, there are a plethora of approaches with some locations having different options based on the situation. One example is the approach to the popliteal artery which is most commonly accessed from a medial exposure for a bypass or thrombectomy. However, when performing popliteal aneurysm repair, a posterior approach can be very effective. A specific incision may also be selected based upon the surrounding tissue structures or previous surgery. This is often a consideration when choosing the lateral or medial approach to the profunda femoris artery. In general, the extremity vessels are often in close proximity to other structures particularly peripheral nerves and associated veins. Central abdominal incisions, by contrast, have fewer options for locations. Truncal exposure requires a deeper knowledge of associated organs and tubular structures (bowel, ureter, lymphatics, etc.) in addition to variations in the abdominal wall. Arterial anomalies are more common with the trunk vessels. Redo surgery carries additional risk and complexity as the natural planes are often fused with scar tissue, rotational flaps, or synthetic material. Similar situations like radiation and infection can also affect the natural tissue causing radiation fibrosis, inflammation, and edematous phlegmons. Situational awareness and proper caution can minimize local injury and enhance outcomes. Despite these differences, some constant techniques remain.

INCISION

Incisions are primarily longitudinal along the direction of the vessels to allow more exposure of the underlying vessel. In the extremity, they tend to extend a few centimeters past the expected length needed. The longitudinal nature allows easy extension as the surgery progresses. One of the most frequent incisions is the groin incision for exposure of the femoral artery. A longitudinal incision here often crosses the groin crease and can be a difficult area for patients to manage, but an extension for additional dissection of the superficial femoral artery or profunda can be quite simple. Oblique incisions are used for smaller cases, such as thrombectomy and delivery of aortic devices, as minimal femoral artery exposure is usually acceptable and the need for an extension is rare.[1] In this area, oblique incisions have been associated with decreased wound complications including infection, lymphatic leak, and seroma.[1,2] This difference is related to the decrease in soft tissue dissection and lymphatic interruption.

RETRACTORS

Self-retaining retractors are an important assist during the dissection as they provide visualization by holding the subcutaneous and muscle tissues out of the way. An assortment of sizes in addition to table-held retractors are available to accommodate various depths and amounts of tissue. While invaluable, they can also cause local soft tissue trauma including the avulsion of small veins and lymphatics. Improper pressure or retraction can cause a nerve injury (i.e., marginal mandibular neuropraxia during carotid endarterectomy). During the dissection, the position of the retractor is usually sequentially adjusted as the dissection continues to the level of the vessel.

DISSECTION

Dissection can often be guided by the palpable pulse of the artery through soft tissue. In cases of occlusion, when the pulse is not present, a calcific tubular structure can still be appreciated. In other situations, a sterile Doppler can be used to not only identify the location of a vessel but also confirm patency. Assessing patency is of greater importance in distal vessels as confirmation of the preoperative imaging target for a successful bypass. Unfortunately, a Doppler can also pick up the monophasic flow of a paired vein and thus the probe requires careful positioning directly on the surface of small arteries for correct identification.

Direct dissection of the artery and veins includes a couple of basic concepts. The first is sharp dissection with scissors directly around the vessel. The

Metzenbaum or Potts-Smith dissecting scissors are the most commonly used scissors. They are preferred due to their blunt tips and cutting blades which leads to precise dissection with decreased injury from sharper tips. Manipulation of the vessel and surrounding soft tissue is best done using the atraumatic Debakey forceps. "Traction and counter traction" is a mantra of dissection. This technique of retracting the surrounding tissue is critical to expose the correct planes. It allows identification of the peri-areolar tissue surrounding the vasa vasorum of the vessel and thus parallel dissection in this plane. By dissecting directly on the vessel, there is a decreased incidence of injury to the surrounding tissue while providing easier identification of smaller vessel branches or crossing vessels. Specific crossing vessels can identify major arterial branches, such as the lateral circumflex vein at the level of the profunda artery. Other veins, like the venae comitantes in the tibial region, can not only identify the tibial artery origins but their variable communications can also be numerous. Close dissection to the artery can identify the necessary branches that need to be ligated to properly expose the artery.

REDO DISSECTION

In the re-operative field, direct sharp dissection can be relatively tedious. Scar tissue is often too dense for regular scissors to cut. Two techniques often employed in this are the use of a No. 15 blade scalpel and a Freer elevator. These two instruments are used in more of a stroking/scraping manner parallel to the vessel. The scalpel can be used to cut through the thicker tissue, while the Freer can be used to recreate and extend the peri-advential space when identified. Luckily, even when vessels have a heavy anterior plane of scar tissue, as seen over a patch from an endarterectomy, the sides and posterior aspect usually maintain a semblance of peri-aerolar tissue.

VESSEL CONTROL

The order of dissection usually identifies first the proximal and then the distal vessel. This allows for inflow control as needed during the remaining dissection. Silicon vessel loops can be used to help mobilize the vessel and provide additional traction. This is especially useful in the more fragile veins in lieu of forceps, whereas veins do not tolerate the same tissue handling as the muscular arteries. Crush or avulsion injuries can occur. In saphenous vein harvest, crush injuries can lead to future conduit compromise and bypass failure. In vessels with at-risk plaque such as the carotid artery, a classic teaching is the concept of dissecting the tissue away from the vessel to minimize plaque disruption. This technique can also help dissect smaller branches rather than cutting them during direct artery dissection. Double looping the vessel loop in the areas of control is termed "to Potts" or the "Potts loop" and allows atraumatic occlusion of the vessel, traction for intermittent control as desired during a thrombectomy, and facilitates clamp placement (Figure 10-1).

VASCULAR CLAMPING

Vascular clamps are preferred for more secure control. Like other instruments, they come in a variety of sizes, lengths, and curvatures for maneuverability and positioning out of one's working visual *field of view* while providing occlusion of flow. If used inappropriately, they can cause vessel trauma and stenosis or stricture despite their atraumatic design. Clamps are usually placed distal first to protect the outflow and prevent any distal embolization of plaque. Prior to any prolonged vascular occlusion, patients are anticoagulated with heparin. Initial dosing is

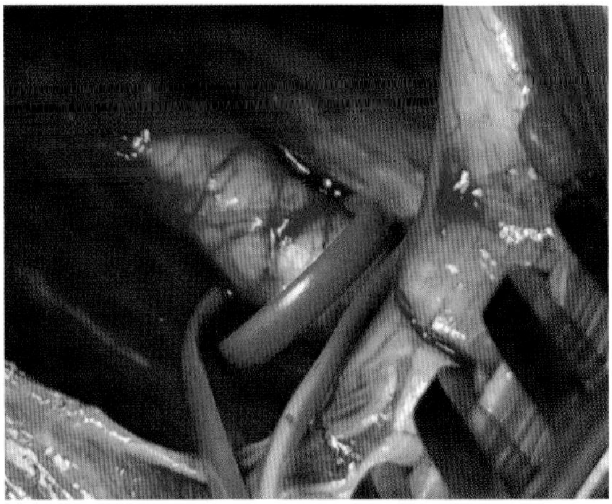

FIGURE 10-1 Vessel control is obtained by using the Pott's technique of a double loop around a vessel.

75–100 U/kg to elevate the activated clotting time (ACT) to twice the baseline, and intermittent boluses to maintain anticoagulation as necessary during the case. Heparin and other blood thinners should be avoided at the beginning of a case to maintain a clean and dry dissection field. Bleeding not only impairs visualization but also distorts tissue color and the natural identifying features of arteries, veins, and nerves.

Heavily calcified lesions may not respond to vessel occlusion through any of the above techniques. While it is ideal to clamp soft nondiseased vessels, most patients requiring vascular surgery have atherosclerotic plaques throughout. Proper caution and technique can minimize complications such as plaque rupture with embolization, dissection, or puncture of the vessel wall. Most common are vessels with a soft anterior wall and a posterior plaque (Figure 10-2). Clamps applied transversely in an anterior-posterior direction are able to minimize the risk of injury to the plaque while obtaining the best occlusion. Soft jaw clamps (i.e., Fogarty Hydragrip) have rubber inserts that help conform the soft portion of the artery to the irregularity of the plaque surface, also improving occlusion.

BALLOON OCCLUSION

In some situations, occlusion using a balloon catheter can be considered. The appropriately sized conformable balloon is inserted into the vessel lumen and slowly inflated until occlusion is complete. Inflation is maintained using a 3-way stopcock. A dual lumen catheter with an irrigation port can also be considered in vessels where access for distal infusion is beneficial with heparin, saline, or cold perfusate. This option is especially useful in the vessels that may be difficult to dissect due to scar tissue. For various reasons, dissection along the posterior portion of the artery may not be possible or unsafe. For example, in a common femoral pseudoaneurysm, the posterior lying profunda femoral artery is often difficult to identify. Opening the pseudoaneurysm sac to directly visualize the origin and placing an intraluminal occlusion balloon for control is often more efficient than circumferential dissection. In another example, right iliac control during a retroperitoneal aneurysm repair can be more difficult given the lateral positioning and depth of the vessel. Iliac occlusion in this situation of difficult access, or in arteries with heavy circumferential calcification, can often be also assisted by balloon occlusion with less risk to the patient. Finally, aortic balloon occlusion can be performed during situations of rupture to allow control of bleeding and hemodynamic stability while other steps of dissection or repair are completed.

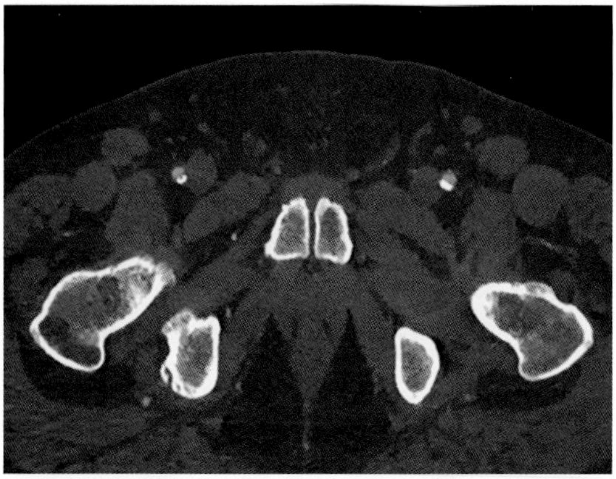

FIGURE 10-2 CT scan of femoral vessels demonstrating posterior plaque. Clamping of this vessel is best performed using an anterior to posterior clamp orientation rather than side to side.

TOURNIQUET

Tourniquets were not readily used until published by Scheinin and Lindfors in 1979 during treatment of a popliteal aneurysm[3] and Bernhard et al. in 1980[4] during use in lower leg revascularization. Sterile tourniquets have become more common for performing small vessel anastomosis of the popliteal and tibials, graft revision, and upper extremity arteriovenous fistulas for dialysis. The use of a tourniquet minimizes intimal injury from clamps and also decreases the amount of dissection involved to control the vessel. The use of a tourniquet decreases the extent of exposure and the need for circumferential control. By only dissecting the anterior surface of the vessel, disruption of the vaso vasorum is decreased with less risk of ischemic injury to the adventitia.

The technique includes the use of an Esmarch bandage to exsanguinate the leg prior to inflation to 250 mmHg. Vessels with heavier calcification, as seen in end-stage renal failure, may be more noncompressible requiring an increase of the tourniquet to 300 mmHg or additional inflow occlusion to eliminate ongoing bleeding. The paired tibial veins are also decompressed during this period of time, further improving the view of the artery. In addition, not only can clamps and vessels loop obstruct the visual field and make work in the wound cumbersome, they can distort or rotate these smaller vessels. Removing them allows the artery to lay open and facilitates a more precise anastomosis. However, heavily calcified vessels may prevent effective occlusion of the arteries by use of a tourniquet and increase bleeding because of venous outflow obstruction.

ARTERIOTOMY AND ENDARTERECTOMY

Arteriotomies are either longitudinal or transverse. Longitudinal arteriotomies are usually performed for endarterectomy or bypass anastomosis as they can be extended and provide a good look at the lumen and any intimal disease. A transverse arteriotomy is used for access to the vessel for remote work such as thrombectomy or delivery of an endovascular device. They are both performed by using a No. 11 scalpel. The scalpel is used with the blade pointed up in a stabbing motion while held at 45° to the surface of the artery. The angle Potts scissors can then be used to extend the incision as far as necessary. Extension is often carried into a major branch when the origin is diseased or an endarterectomy is intended. A transverse incision can be closed without narrowing the lumen, with either continuous or interrupted sutures. However, in smaller lumens, interrupted sutures are preferred to prevent constriction. Longitudinal incisions are best closed with patch angioplasty to minimize the risk of narrowing the lumen, especially if it extends into a smaller branch like the profunda femoris or internal carotid arteries.

ENDARTERECTOMY

Endarterectomy, while used in more vessels prior to the arrival of endovascular techniques, remains the dominant method of management of carotid and femoral occlusive disease. It is also used for the management of atherosclerotic disease at the beginning and/or end of a bypass and at orifices such as the renal artery. Atherosclerosis forms primarily within the intima and adjacentlayer of the media. Endarterectomy removes the internal disease by creating a plane in this layer which leaves the outer media and adventitia behind to re-endothelialize the vessel. In many instances, the plaque can be divided in the middle to allow dissection in each direction individually for better control. Proximally the plaque is usually transected within the normal artery leaving the cut end flush in the direction of flow. The distal endpoint is more carefully created as the direction of flow can evert any residual flap and obstruct flow. The distal plaque is tapered to a more normal or "feathered" endpoint and often tacked in place using interrupted sutures. The remaining wall can be cleared of all residual loose fibers.

In addition to direct endarterectomy, there are two other types: eversion and remote. Eversion endarterectomy was first described by DeBakey in 1959 for the management of the internal carotid artery and was originally described with transection of the common carotid (Figure 10-3).[5] Most carotid eversion today involves transection of the internal carotid artery origin. Eversion is performed by placing traction on the specimen and turning the distal vessel inside out (Figure 10-3C). Endarterectomy is performed under direct visualization until the endpoint is created with the use of a Freer. Once the endpoint is complete, the vessel is reverted to its normal configuration. Remote endarterectomy is a term for endarterectomy performed without direct visualization of the plane. Originally described using Cannon or Mollring cutters, remote endarterectomy is most frequently performed by extending the Freer into the vessel circumferentially past the endpoint of the arteriotomy. The remaining plaque is then pulled out sharply. This technique may lead to a tapered endpoint versus breaking in a sharp endpoint. If the distal end needs to be managed, a counter arteriotomy can be made at the distal endpoint to suture tack the flap followed by an arterial patch. Hybrid surgery uses remote endarterectomy to manage the distal iliac artery and "tack" the distal endpoint with a stent as seen in the iliofemoral or popliteal sections.

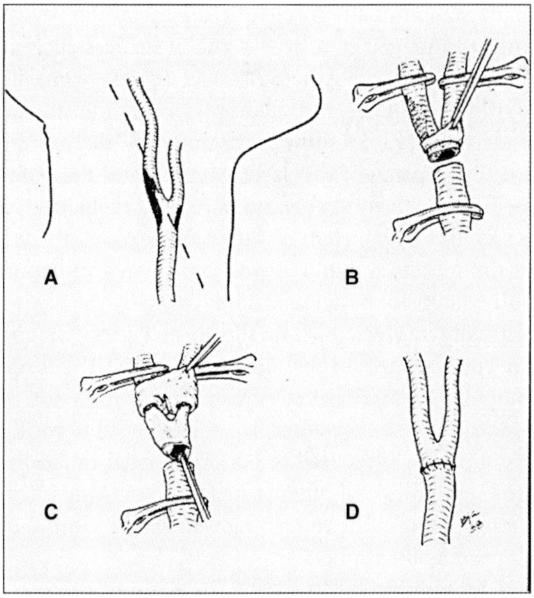

FIGURE 10-3 Original images of DeBakey's eversion endarterectomy with transection of the common carotid artery (A), eversion (B), removal of plaque (C) and end-to-end reconstruction (D). (Reproduced with permission from Debakey ME, Crawford ES, Cooley DA, et al. Surgical considerations of occlusive disease of innominate, carotid, subclavian, and vertebral arteries. *Ann Surg.* 1959;149(5):690-710.)

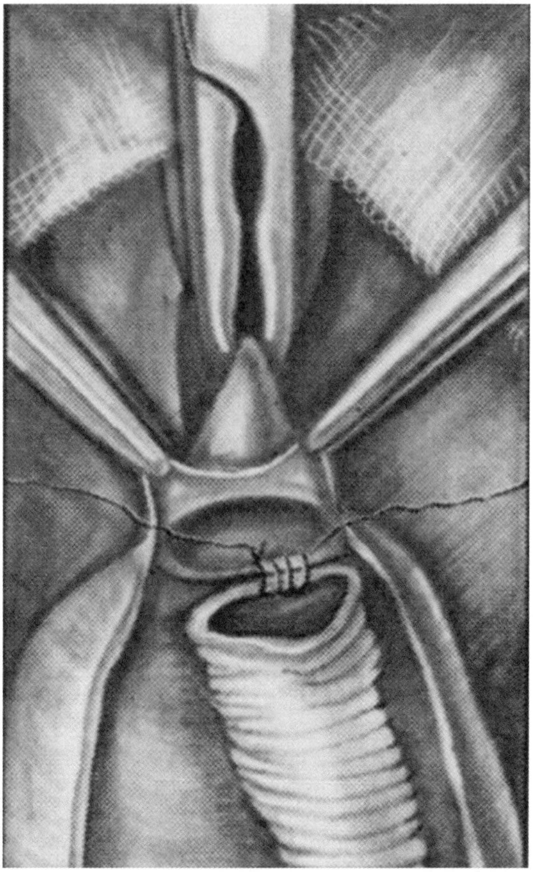

FIGURE 10-4 Creech technique as originally described for the proximal aortic anastomosis incorporating both the top and bottom portions of the artery for a double thickness wall. (Reproduced with permission from Creech, O Jr. Endo-aneurysmorrhapy and treatment of aortic aneurysm. *Ann Surg.* 1966; 164 (6):935-946.)

VESSEL RECONSTRUCTION

Vessel reconstruction is probably the most exciting portion of vascular surgery to beginning trainees and becomes routine with practice. The saying "in to out on the artery and out to in on the vein (graft)" is repeated throughout this early phase of training. It refers to suturing from within the arterial intima to out of the adventitia to ensure the intima does not separate or in-fold from the remaining vessel and occlude the lumen. Sutures are usually placed in a continuous fashion to close the arteriotomy with primary closure, patch angioplasty, or bypass anastomosis. A second saying of "1-mm apart and 1-mm deep perpendicular sutures" is also chanted to minimize leakage and promote the eversion of the vessels. Eversion also allows for better tacking of the intima. Two techniques of bypass anastomosis bear mention: parachute and Creech. The parachute technique is used when direct visualization of each stitch is important like in the corner or heel/toe of the arteriotomy. Continuous stitches are placed while the bypass is held above like a parachute suspended on its strings. Once several sutures have been placed around the corner, the bypass is brought down to its final position. Creech refers to Dr Oscar Creech's description of his management of the proximal aorta in aneurysm repair. His 1966 paper described suturing the posterior wall of the aorta by using a double thickness suture from the top to the bottom wall of the aorta than transecting the aorta (Figure 10-4).[6] It is often used as a verb as "to Creech".

Patch angioplasty can be performed with autogenous or nonautogenous patches, and today is most commonly performed with a bovine pericardial patch due to ease of availability, pliability, and decreased infection risk compared to their synthetic counterparts. The native greater saphenous vein and endarterectomized superficial femoral artery are common autogenous tissues used mostly in an infected field or when encountered during the exposure (i.e., anterior accessory saphenous vein during femoral artery exposure). They can be used as a patch or bypass. Harvesting a vein, while often needing a second incision, rarely increases the morbidity of a procedure. Due to the risk of degeneration, the saphenous vein at the ankle is no longer used. The patch is often tapered at the ends and trimmed as needed to approximate the arterial defect.

Bypass anastomoses are most commonly described as "end-to-side" and "end-to-end," although "side-to-side" is occasionally encountered. End-to-side is the most commonly created anastomosis. There is less dissection to the vessel and surrounding branches compared to its end-to-end counterparts. In addition, maintaining access to the native artery circulation has its benefits. It allows both retrograde and antegrade flow into the remaining vessels and collaterals. A classic example is the retrograde flow into the native external and internal iliac arteries from an aorto-bi-femoral bypass. Maintaining antegrade access can also be beneficial for future procedures. Recanalization of native arteries can be performed in these cases when the graft has failed or needs to be resected such as in infection. This technique is only possible in occlusive disease as in aneurysmal situations, when all direct flow into the aneurysm sac needs to be excluded. Side-to-side anastomoses are no longer common as they were primarily used to create portocaval shunts. These have largely been replaced by medical management and transjugular intrahepatic portosystemic shunts (TIPS).

End-to-side anastomoses are usually created with a beveled angle of about 30°; however, a more perpendicular degree is often seen in anastomoses such as carotid-subclavian bypass or radio-cephalic fistula. In a beveled anastomosis (Figure 10-5), the ends of the vessel are referred to as the heel and toe of the bypass. The orientation is similar to the foot in that the heel side is the closest corner to the remaining bypass and the toe is the farthest away. The anastomosis is then started at the heel of the bypass and sewn around to the toe. This method has been adopted as it provides the best visualization of the heel corner while allowing adjustments to the length of the toe depending on the desired length of the anastomosis. Some surgeons also prefer to parachute the toe of an anastomosis. Spacing at the heel and toe is important as incorrect suturing can lead to narrowing of the anastomosis and/or bleeding. A perpendicular anastomosis (Figure 10-6), by contrast, starts the suture in the middle of the back wall and sews around the edges to the front. With all anastomosis, it is important to gauge the size of each vessel and trim them appropriately to ensure they match.

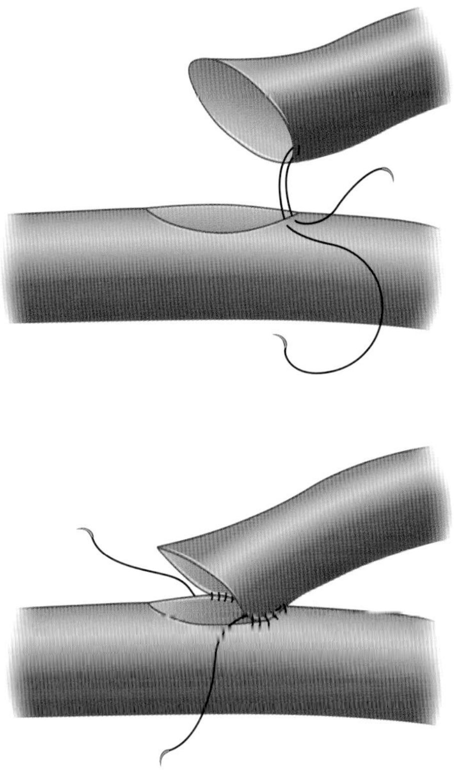

FIGURE 10-5 **Beveled end-to-side anastomosis.** (**A**) The bypass conduit is cut at a 45° angle and sewn starting at the heel. (**B**) Sutures are placed along both sides to midway (**B**) prior to completing around the toe to the front.

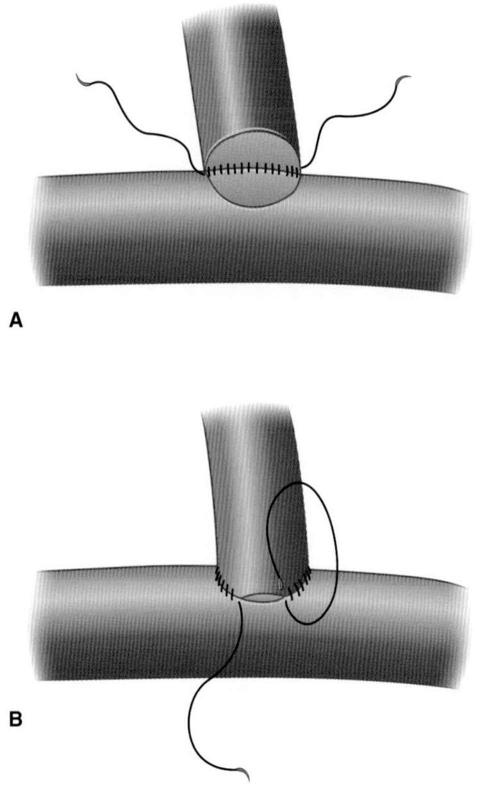

FIGURE 10-6 Perpendicular end-to-side anastomosis. (**A**) The straight end of the bypass is sewn first along the back wall. (**B**) It is sewn around both directions to complete in the front.

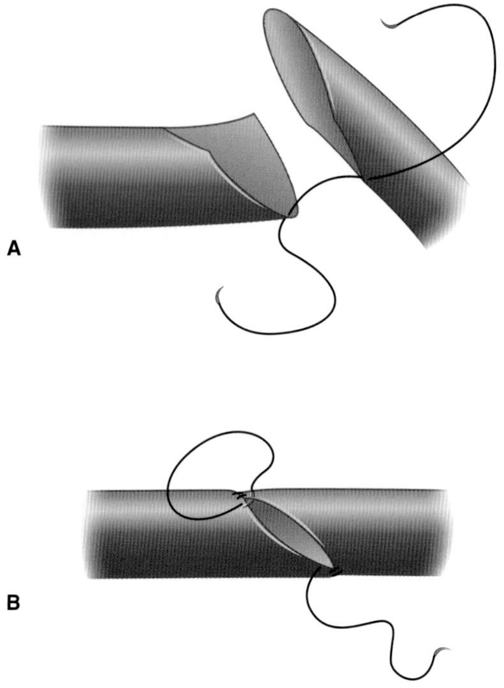

FIGURE 10-7 End-to-end anastomosis. (**A**) Each end is spatulated to create an oblique opening. Sutures are then started along the bottom corner. (**B**) Each suture is sewn around the opening to complete on the top.

End-to-end anastomoses (Figure 10-7) are performed primarily to reconnect native vessels together if there is enough mobility to provide a tension-free connection. It can also be used to describe a direct anastomosis of an end vessel to graft or vein bypass. Corner sutures are frequently applied to orient the vessels while creating the anastomosis. Pulling this suture too tightly can cause an anastomotic stricture and can be minimized by allowing flow in the vessel prior to tying, or creating a beveled rather than perpendicular anastomosis. A beveled connection, also termed spatulated, is created by slitting the posterior aspect of the inflow vessel and the anterior aspect of the receiving side. The two ends can then be sewn together creating an oblique longer anastomosis.

ANTERIOR SPINE EXPOSURE

Anterior interbody lumbar fusion (AILF) has become a standard part of a spine surgeon's armamentarium to treat predominantly degenerative disc disease, spondylothisthesis, and scoliosis. As part of the exposure, an access surgeon is often used to access the retroperitoneum and specifically the iliac vessels. While there are similarities to other lower abdominal operations, there are specific nuances to the technique. The majority of exposure surgery currently uses a version of the mini retroperitoneal dissection popularized in a technical paper by Salvador Brau in 2002 rather than the transabdominal approach in order to eliminate the need to manipulate the intestines.[7] With today's spine technology, operations are often performed in a lateral position lending to exposures using a lateral ALIF or oblique/anterior to the psoas technique. This chapter will focus predominantly on the supine ALIF technique as a foundation to which other exposures are related.

Like other preoperative preparation for surgery, proper awareness of previous abdominal operations is important to consider candidacy and risk for additional surgery. A history of abdominal wall surgery is of lower risk compared to previous retroperitoneal dissections, such as iliac lymph node dissection, kidney transplant, and aorto-bi-iliac bypass. The contents of abdominal wall include only the musculature and the epigastric vessels. That being said, surgeries with extensive dissection within the peritoneal space (i.e., TRAM or component of parts separation) have significant scar tissue or synthetic mesh that obliterates the usual anterior peritoneal plane used to gain entrance to the retroperitoneum. These operations are often considered a contraindication to retroperitoneal surgery. The retroperitoneum, by comparison, contains important structures including the ureter, spermatic cord, and iliac vessels. The less visible structures include small lymph nodes and sympathetic pelvic nerves. Previous surgery in the retroperitoneal space or radiation can produce a variable amount of scar tissue but is often less than the amount of scarring secondary to infection or abscess from discitis or diverticulitis. Surgical judgment is essential in considering risk in a re-operative or previously operated space as this may be a relative contraindication.

Incision placement in the lower abdomen can be accomplished through a mini incision centered over the desired spinal level(s). Horizontal versus vertical placement is often related to surgeon preference and the number of levels planned in the fusion. Often a vertical incision can use an existing lower midline incision; it also allows for ease of extension and increased versatility in patients with a high pelvic incidence (PI). With more levels, an oblique or paramedian longer incision is usually used. Incisions can often be centered by palpating the sacral promontory and iliac crest as landmarks to the L5/S1 and L4/5 discs, respectively. In certain cases, preoperative radiographic visualization with a skin marking for localization can be beneficial. The rectus sheath is opened usually in a paramedian fashion to allow lateral retraction and entrance to the retroperitoneum caudal to the arcuate line.

Dissection of the retroperitoneum uses the landmarks of the psoas and the iliac artery. The peritoneum in the midline can be very thin and careful dissection should be performed to minimize peritoneal defects. This is especially true in patients with previous midline surgery or hernia repairs. Once the psoas and genitofemoral nerve are identified, the entire peritoneal contents contained in the retroperitoneal fat, including the ureter, should be mobilized medially en bloc medial to the iliac vessels (Figure 10-8). Given the symmetry of the iliac vessels in the pelvis, the dissection to L5/S1 can be performed from the left or right flank. Since dissection for L4/5 and higher requires lateral to medial mobilization under the iliac vein, this should be performed using a left-sided approach. This avoids manipulation of the right-sided IVC which is fraught with vascular complications (Figure 10-8). The author prefers a right-sided approach for all L5/S1 to preserve the left plane for future proximal surgeries, reduced manipulation of the left iliac vein, and

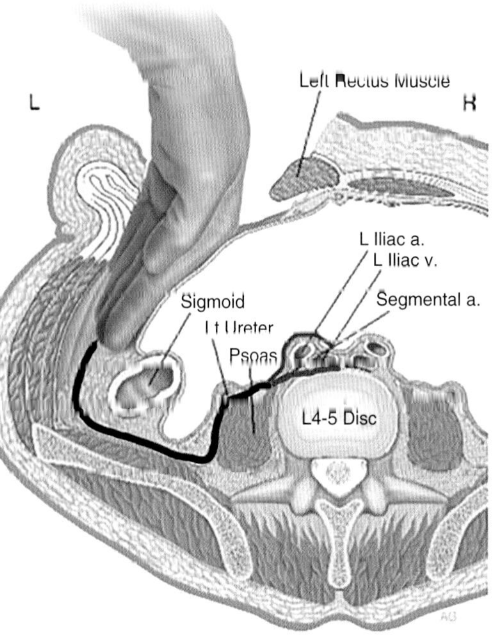

FIGURE 10-8 Retroperitoneal dissection for L4/5 and L5/S1. The dissection is completed in the retroperitoneal space for both dissections (black line). The L4/5 dissection then continues lateral to the left iliac vein to identify the iliolumbar vein for ligation (blue line). L5/S1 dissection continues anterior to the left iliac artery and medial to the vein to the presacral space between the vessels (red line). (Reproduced with permission from Brau SA. Mini-open approach to the spine for anterior lumbar interbody fusion: description of the procedure, results and complications. *Spine J.* 2002;2(3):216-223.)

decreased dissection around the hypogastric plexus fibers. These fibers are more prevalent on the left and aggressive manipulation is theorized to increase the risk of retrograde ejaculation. In patients without previous surgical exposure, this plane can often be manipulated with blunt dissection and the planes of the vascular structures are easily identified. Frequently used instruments in this dissection include Wiley retractors (SpinalTech), sponge sticks, Kittners, and retractor-based lighting or a headlight. These allow a deep dissection through a small incision with maximal exposure and eliminate the need for manual dissection. More obese patients may even require instruments associated with laparoscopic surgery, including laparoscopic Kittners, knot pushers, and clip appliers.

Several vessels may need to be ligated to achieve visualization of the target disc level. After exposure of the anterior spinal column between the vessels, the median sacral vessels need to be ligated for exposure of L5/S1. During exposure of L4/5, the iliolumbar vein along the lateral aspect of the iliac vein must be identified and ligated prior to mobilization to the right side of the vertebral body to prevent an avulsion injury.[8] This vessel can have several anatomic variants including an ascending lumbar[9]; thus, the entire lateral spine must be bluntly dissected free to expose the lateral aspect of the iliac vein and associated branches. Occasionally, the iliolumbar vein will be absent or very distal such that ligation is not necessary. The more cranial exposures will also require ligation of the segmental lumbar arteries and veins.

Once mobilization of the proper vessels has been achieved, exposure of the disc space can be accomplished by additional blunt dissection to visualize the anterior spine ligament and the lateral aspects of the vertebral body. Additional manual retraction will be required to expose the edge of the vertebral body on the opposite side. Use caution in this mobilization, as there can be small veins directly from the anterior spine which need to be controlled with bi- or monopolar cautery.

In patients with previous retroperitoneal surgery or even previous posterior spine surgery or osteophytes, inflammation and scar tissue can be present to varying degrees obscuring the anterior ligament and vessels. In these cases, dissection needs to be intentional and careful to prevent vessel injury. Vein injuries are more common than arterial injuries given their thinner wall. Injuries need to be carefully manipulated as attempts to gain hemostasis can lead to further injury. Depending on the size of the injury, bleeding can be controlled with hemostatic agents, hemoclips, or sutures. Catastrophic injuries may need to be controlled with ligation or endovascular covered stents.

Once dissection is complete, a self-retaining table-held retractor can be positioned. There are many versions of the anterior lumbar retractor. However, they all have similarities including multiple 1 in radiolucent blades of varying depth. Many systems have blades from 60 cm to 220 cm and some even have various widths and directions of the blade tips to accommodate additional situations. Newer designs have incorporated attachments for lights directly onto the blade. Blades are held in place with one of the two options: articulations at the handle that allow adjustable angles at the tip of the blade ("toe-in") or reverse tip blades which are positioned on the lateral wall of the vertebral body. Retractors need to be positioned to allow a direct anterior-posterior access to the target disc (Figure 10-9). Additional retractors may be needed inferiorly or superiorly to assist in the

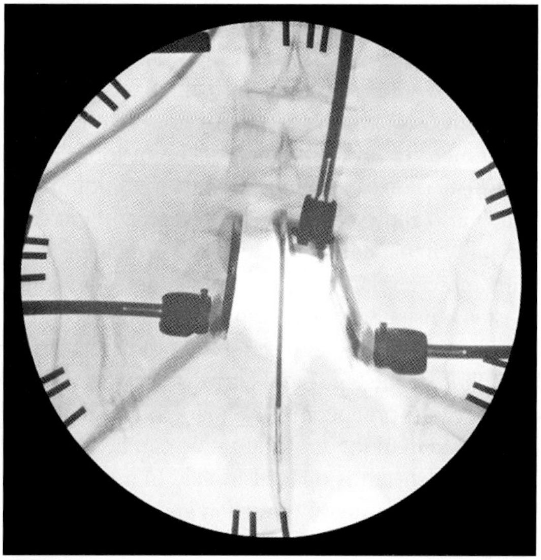

FIGURE 10-9 Retractor blades are positioned along the lateral aspect of the vertebral body to provide visualization of the entire anterior disc space. A needle marks the middle of the space.

exposure. Adjustments to the exposure may need to be made to adapt to anatomic variations of the spine and vessels. A preoperative review of the MRI or CT scan can be useful in helping to identify variations including transitional spinal levels, iliac vein anomalies, and both high and low iliac vein bifurcations. Preoperative identification of these variations allows for advance planning as poor preparation can lead to limited exposure or injury to unexpected structures.

REFERENCES

1. Caiati JM, Kaplan D, Gitlitz D, Hollier LH, Marin ML. The value of the oblique groin incision for femoral artery access during endovascular procedures. *Ann Vasc Surg*. 2000;14 (3):248-253.
2. Swinnen J, Chao A, Tiwari A, Crozier J, Vicaretti M, Fletcher J. Vertical or transverse incisions for access to the femoral artery: a randomized control study. *Ann Vasc Surg*. 2010;24(3):335-341.
3. Scheinin TM, Lidfors O. Simplified repair of popliteal aneurysms. *J Cardiovasc Surg*. 1979;20:189-192.
4. Berhnard VM, Boren CH, Towne JB. Pneumatic tourniquet as a substitute for vascular clamps in distal bypass surgery. *Surgery*. 1980;87:709-713.
5. DeBakey ME, Crawford ES, Cooley DA, Morris GC Jr. Surgical considerations of occlusive disease of innominate, carotid, subclavian and vertebral arteries. *Ann Surg*. 1959;149:690-710.
6. Creech O. Endo-aneurysmorrhapy and treatment of aortic aneurysm. *Ann Surg*. 1966;164(6):935-946.
7. Brau S. Mini-open approach to the spine for anterior lumbar interbody fusion: description of the procedure, results and complications. *Spine J*. 2002;2:216-223.
8. Sivakumar G, Paluzzi A, Freeman B. Avulsion of ascending lumbar and iliolumbar veins in anterior spinal surgery: an anatomical study. *Clin Anat*. 2007; 20:553-555.
9. Jasani V, Jaffray D. The anatomy of the iliolumbar vein; a cadaver study. *J Bone Joint Surg [Br]*. 2002; 84-B:1046-1049.

CHAPTER

11 Techniques of Amputation in Vascular Disease

Jeff M. Cross and Nabil A. Ebraheim

OUTLINE

GENERAL CONSIDERATIONS AND HISTORY
- Brief History
- Anatomic Variants
- Epidemiology

CLINICAL FINDINGS

DIAGNOSIS AND PREOPERATIVE CONSIDERATIONS
- Tissue Evaluation Methods
  - Toe pressures (TBP)
  - Ankle-Brachial Index (ABI)
  - Transcutaneous Oximetry ($TcPO_2$)
  - Skin Perfusion Pressure (SPP)
  - Fluorescence Imaging
  - Angiography
- Preoperative Planning
- Staged Amputation
- Ambulation Rate
- Ambulation Energy

MANAGEMENT AND SURGICAL TECHNIQUE
  - Anesthesia
  - Antibiotics
  - Blood Vessels
  - Nerves
  - Muscles
  - Bone
- Digit/Ray Resection
- Transmetatarsal (TMA)
- Technique
- Lisfranc
- Technique
- Hindfoot (Chopart, Boyd, and Pirigoff)
- Technique
- Syme (Ankle Disarticulation)
- Technique
- Transtibial (TTA)
- Technique
- Knee Disarticulation (KD)
- Technique
- Gritti-Strokes Amputation (GSA)
- Technique (Modifications From KD)
- Transfemoral (TFA)
- Technique
- Cryoamputation (Physiologic Amputation)
- Technique

POSTOPERATIVE MANAGEMENT
- Routine Care
- Complications
  - Mortality
  - Thromboembolic Events
  - Infection
  - Pain
  - Contracture

GENERAL CONSIDERATIONS AND HISTORY

BRIEF HISTORY

Amputation has been described in Roman and Greek literature 2000 years old, with techniques of preoperative planning, vascular control, bone preparation, and soft tissue flap coverage similar to those of modern times.[1,2] Because of the high mortality and minimal anesthesia, emphasis was placed on speed, with most surgeons using large "amputation knives" to complete the soft tissue cleavage in a single, circular cut, some of which can still be found in many surgical trays even today (Figure 11-1).[3] Lending to this, the word "amputation" takes its roots from the Latin *ambi* (around) and *putare* (to prune). Much like the rest of western medicine, the practices of amputation suffered a dramatic setback during the next millennium, and little is known about the evolution of the procedure during this time. Arabic surgeon Albucasis made many great innovations during the medieval period, including publishing an illustrated surgical text, but his work was slow to spread to other countries.[1] With the advent of high-powered weapons came a higher demand for battlefield amputations during the fifteenth century, which was subsequently delegated to barbers in order to offload overworked physicians. These dirt to doctor individuals were referred to as "barber surgeons," whose ranks gave rise to many of the innovators of modern amputation techniques over the following century.[4]

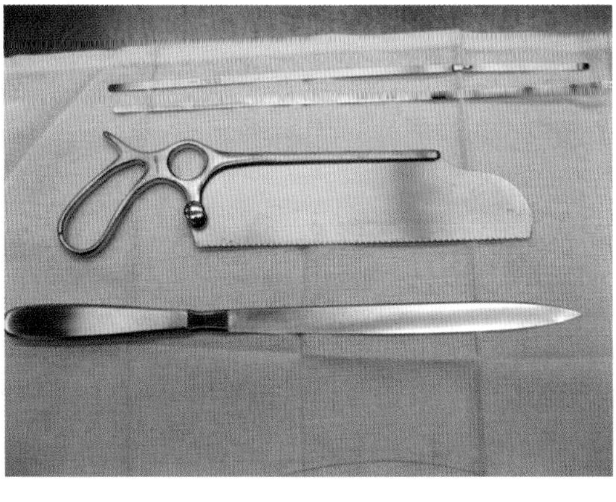

FIGURE 11-1 Traditionally styled amputation knife and bone saw still found in modern surgical trays.

Still, the practices used at the time were far from technical or precise. After swiftly cutting down to bone, vessels were then found in the proximal mass and quickly controlled with clamps, thermocautery, and hemostatic materials. It wasn't until the sixteenth century that the development and popularization of vessel ligatures by French surgeon Ambroise Pare, and subsequently the tourniquet by Petit, made the procedure exceedingly safer for patients. Although others had previously described the importance of planning soft-tissue coverage, seventeenth-century English surgeon C. Lowdham is credited with the innovation of flap coverage in order to allow for a lower tension closure.[1,3] The nineteenth century saw further advancement with Lister's introduction of antiseptic technique, as well as the widespread use of general anesthetics, which allowed not only for fewer complications, but increased surgical time to achieve better hemostasis, better bone preparation, and a more meticulous closure.[1,5]

With these and further advancements, amputation has become a routine life-saving procedure used for an increasing number of indications. The sentiment that these procedures should not be considered a salvage operation, but rather a comprehensive treatment option to improve patient outcomes is echoed throughout the modern history of amputation and the vascular community in general. In this chapter, we will primarily focus on lower extremity amputations in the setting of vascular disease, and provide a framework for providers in evaluating, planning, performing, and postoperatively managing these procedures.

ANATOMIC VARIANTS

Variations in lower extremity vascular anatomy are relatively uncommon, with the majority of anomalies happening at the level of the foot and ankle terminal branches and anastomoses. While these structures will be covered in other chapters, it is important for the surgeon to consider how these variants might affect surgical approach and dissection type. Examining any preoperative angiographic imaging is especially helpful, as a majority of patients undergoing a vascular amputation have had this performed prior to this stage but should not be routinely performed for surgical planning purposes.[6] The branching patterns of the popliteal artery are also an area of significant interest in vascular surgery; however, the clinical significance of this in amputations is only relevant to knee disarticulations, and the anatomic variant rate is estimated to be less than 8% of the population. Nervous anatomy at the knee is less predictable, as the origin points of the tibial, common fibular, and sural cutaneous can vary widely from patient to patient. Even though rates of natural anatomic anomalies in lower extremity vasculature are low, a patient with a dysvascular limb may have had previous bypass interventions, stents, or vein harvests. A thorough history and physical, as well as previous operative reports, should be obtained prior to intervention to avoid iatrogenic injury to aberrant structures.

EPIDEMIOLOGY

Though total amputation rates are decreasing worldwide, the incidence of amputations due to peripheral arterial disease (PAD) has been steadily climbing for several decades. Heavily contributing to this is a global surge in diabetes mellitus (DM), which places patients at a nearly 10-fold risk of amputation compared to healthy individuals. In fact, over two-thirds of all-cause amputees are diabetics, although the rate of amputation in the diabetic population seems to be falling recently. While this is hopefully a sign of improved treatment, this phenomenon is also likely confounded by lead-time bias thanks to improved screening.[7] It is undeniable that populations with higher rates of DM and decreased access to healthcare, especially vascular surgeons, have the highest rates of amputation. In the United States, this has historically been rural, African American, and Native American patients.[8] Socioeconomic disparity, rather than biology, is largely to blame for uncontrolled diabetes, failed revascularization, and advanced wounds at presentation.[9,10] Still, advances in revascularization procedures and surgeon training have decreased the percentage of patients with PAD ending with major amputation, and hope remains that endovascular interventions on the horizon may further push back this threshold.

CLINICAL FINDINGS

Amputations in patients with PAD should be considered only after exhausting revascularization options, and likewise, after antibiotic and wound care options have failed in patients with gangrenous wounds. Recent reviews comparing open and endovascular limb salvage procedures for patients with critical limb ischemia indicate equivalent future amputation rates, corroborating the findings of the randomized BASIL trial. However, the same studies noted an odds ratio for amputation of 1.05 at 2 to 3 years, suggesting that revascularization may only temporarily delay the inevitable for this population.[11,12] These techniques will be described elsewhere in the text but should only be attempted if there exists a good likelihood of success, and primary amputation should not be discounted as a first-line treatment if the patient is unlikely to benefit. The Rutherford classification is widely used as a functional scale to describe patients with PAD, offering surgeons criteria for intervention, whether that be revascularization or amputation.[13] Still, the decision to pursue amputation is often multifactorial, as patients may present with overlapping acute and chronic wounds or infections. To aid the clinician, the Society for Vascular Surgery combined this and several other validated classification systems to incorporate wound, ischemia, and foot infections (WIfI) into a single score, grouped into clinical stages 1–4. Two-thirds of the patients classified as Stage 4 are likely to have amputation performed within the next year, with a 30% to 40% mortality rate among those who do not. This is in stark contrast with Stage 3 patients (<10% amputation and mortality rates).[14–16] Further refining is needed, but this system may eventually provide surgeons with evidence-based criteria for amputation.

Given the scope of this book, this chapter will not discuss amputation indications and techniques for traumatic, oncologic, or complex deformity cases, and surgeons should beware that each of these carries with it their own considerations and nuances.

DIAGNOSIS AND PREOPERATIVE CONSIDERATIONS

TISSUE EVALUATION METHODS

In determining the likelihood of a patient healing a wound in the setting of diabetes or PAD, the

TABLE 11-1 Commonly Cited Values for Reliable Wound Healing

Test	Normal	Healing Threshold
$TcPO_2$	50-70 mmHg	>40 mmHg
SPP	50-80 mmHg	>30-40 mmHg
TBP	70-110 mmHg	>30 mmHg
ABI	0.9-1.4	>0.9

surgeon has a variety of noninvasive tests that may guide further management. While no individual test is superior in terms of accuracy or precision, some consensus exists regarding which are most reliable for predicting both wound healing and future amputation rates. Table 11-1 highlights these commonly cited values, and below is a further discussion on each based on available meta-analyses.

Toe pressures (TBP)

Toe pressures are taken using a specialized toe cuff, and photoplethysmography is employed to determine flow distal to the cuff. This can be done manually but is typically performed using a dedicated automatic sphygmomanometer. Below 30 mmHg, the risk of incomplete wound healing doubles for diabetic foot wounds, as well as the risk of nonhealing surgical wounds for foot and ankle amputations. Toe-brachial index has not been extensively studied and does not offer the surgeon much confidence in its predictive ability.[17–20]

Ankle-Brachial Index (ABI)

Despite being a popular test in evaluating PAD, its use in predicting wound healing has poor sensitivity and specificity when compared to other methods. Some studies have shown that an ABI > 0.9 is strongly predictive of wound healing in partial foot amputations and diabetic wounds; however, values within the normal range are uncommon in most vascular patients, and measurements are unreliable in diabetics.[18,20] Both ABI and TBP also are limited to distal amputations and cannot guide transtibial or transfemoral level selection.

Transcutaneous Oximetry ($TcPO_2$)

In this method, electrodes are placed on the skin in the area of interest, as well as a control area, such as the chest. The electrodes induce local hyperemia by imparting heat, and subsequently measure the oxygen tension of the tissue below. Normal tension is between 50 and 70 mmHg with a variation of around 10%, and the test should be done in conjunction with pulse oximetry to ensure systemic or environmental causes of hypoxia are not skewing the results.[21] This does not require expensive equipment, rare isotopes, or advanced training, and can be performed quickly for same day evaluation. Little consensus exists on threshold values, but >40 mmHg is associated with near 100% wound healing, and less than 20 mmHg with near 100% failure, with some studies suggesting that >30 mmHg may also be an appropriate cutoff.[22–24] Additionally, an oxygen challenge test may be performed, by comparing the $PtcO_2$ value when the patient is switched to breathing 100% normobaric oxygen, which has been proposed as a marker for severe ischemia.[25] An increase of less than 10 mmHg is associated with failure of wound healing, but this has not been extensively studied.[26]

Skin Perfusion Pressure (SPP)

Much like a traditional arterial blood pressure measurement, this value corresponds to the external pressure needed to overcome capillary blood flow in the underlying skin. This was initially determined using injectable radiotracers, measuring the speed at which they washed out from the tissue in question. Because this test required access and patient exposure to rare isotopes, it was quickly replaced with photoplethysmography, which instead measures blood flow using a laser doppler probe. By directly measuring tissue perfusion like $TcPO_2$, this test is not confounded by arterial calcifications or other large vessel disease, can be performed in spite of prior great toe amputations, and is much quicker and easier than transcutaneous oximetry. This comes at the expense of poor precision, and several authors advocate for confirming results with TcPO2 regardless. Using a thermostatic heating probe has been recently proposed to improve detectability and precision, but the clinical significance of this remains unclear.[27] Meta-analyses suggest that 30 to 40 mmHg may be an appropriate cutoff, with sensitivity and specificity similar to $TcPO_2$ at 75% to 85%.[28–30]

Fluorescence Imaging

This emerging test works similarly to radioisotope imaging in SPP, but with the benefit of administering safer and more accessible fluorescent dyes such as indocyanine green instead. While it has a variety of proposed applications, including determining tissue viability intraoperatively, there is not enough evidence to guide its use in determining tissue viability for amputation.[20,31–33]

Angiography

Though around half of lower extremity amputation candidates will have had prior angiographic studies performed, it is a less reliable method and does not correlate well with wound healing. It is therefore not recommended to obtain routine angiographic studies for surgical planning, but if available, the surgeon may use as an adjunct to assist in level selection.[6,34]

PREOPERATIVE PLANNING

The level of amputation should first and foremost be dictated by the proximity of the patient's disease process. As previously discussed, the extent of the patient's pathology should be investigated prior to surgery, and the surgeon should choose a level at which the patient has the capacity to heal their surgical wound. Soft tissue and skin coverage may also impact the surgeon's level and timing, as patients with active wounds or an insufficient soft tissue envelope may preclude amputation at the desired level. Finally, the patient's functional status and goals should guide the surgeon in choosing from the viable amputation options remaining. A thorough history and physical should include the following:

- Recent ambulation status and lifestyle demand
- Social support and living situation
- Ankle, knee, and hip strength and range of motion, noting any contractures or arthropathies
- Presence or lack of skin sensation at planned level
- Evaluation of presence or likelihood of contralateral amputation
- Evaluation of functional upper extremities in aiding ambulation

Positive patient factors associated with achieving both basic and advanced mobility after amputation include younger age, married, and higher education, while negative patient factors include diabetes, COPD, dialysis, and anxiety/depression. Interestingly, basic mobility has been found to peak in patients with a BMI of 30 kg/m^2, while advanced mobility is more likely in lower BMI patients. In aggregate, these factors may help set expectations for the surgeon and patient for postoperative recovery and function. Several validated tools exist to assist the surgeon in making these calculations and are readily available online, such as AMPREDICT.[35,36] In baseline ambulatory patients, preserving function and planning for prosthetic fitting is of utmost importance. In nonambulatory patients, on the other hand, consideration should be given to facilitating transfers and upright positioning.

Several studies have advocated for the use of a multidisciplinary care team to aid preoperative risk reduction and postoperative rehabilitation, which has been found to drastically improve healing rates, hospital stays, and time to ambulation.[37] Such a team is typically consistent of the surgeon, physical and occupational therapist, dietitian/diabetic consultant, social worker, prosthetist, and in appropriate cases, a counselor or psychiatrist. Early multidisciplinary action has even been shown to significantly reduce the rate of amputation by nearly half in some patients and should therefore be implemented promptly in the patient's care.[38,39] Preoperative laboratory studies should be obtained to screen for malnutrition, glycemic control, and cytopenia, then optimized prior to surgery if at all possible. Typically, a serum albumin >2.5 g/dL and lymphocyte count >1500 e recommended for better wound healing outcomes. Lifestyle modifications such as diet improvement and smoking cessation are also important, and any significant comorbidity should be evaluated by the appropriate specialist. Cardiopulmonary comorbidities, especially, are not just important for preoperative clearance, but even more so for postoperative monitoring, as the procedure will significantly change the patient's physiology and may require more frequent checks by their other providers. A bariatric referral can be warranted in patients with significant obesity, as an overweight habitus will limit prosthetic options, exponentially increase energy expenditure with ambulation, lead to excessive wear on the stump, etc. Preoperative physical therapy to address any flexion contractures or weakness also can improve postop return to function, and failure to overcome contractures that would preclude prosthetic ambulation should make the surgeon consider amputation at or above that joint. Any anticipated durable medical equipment needed postoperatively should ideally be delivered to the home in advance.

Delayed presentation of patients with critical limb ischemia or gangrenous infection may not allow for these preoperative considerations, but at a minimum, preoperative inpatient physical therapy and social work consults may help both the patient and surgeon set reasonable expectations for postoperative plans and outcomes.

STAGED AMPUTATION

When treating a septic patient, amputation may be necessary to improve the overall clinical condition, but nonviable tissue may not yet be fully demarcated, or the patient may not be medically optimized for a successful operation. A staged amputation may be indicated in these situations, with an initial procedure performed quickly to minimize perioperative complications, followed by a formal revision to a higher level in the near future. Staged amputation patients have superior 30-day mortality, readmission, and reoperation rates when compared to primary amputation patients, which is surprising as these patients typically have a greater and more acute burden of illness.[40–44] This first stage is often referred to as a "guillotine" amputation, named (despite his adamant objection) for the French physician Joseph-Ignace Guillotine, who proposed the use of the device during the French Revolution as a quicker, more painless form of execution. As implied, this stage should be swift with emphasis on hemostasis, and soft tissue closure is usually not necessary.

However, critically ill patients may not even tolerate anesthesia or blood loss for a guillotine procedure, and a bedside cryoamputation should be considered. The technique will be described later in this chapter, but despite selection for more unstable patients, studies have reported excellent, if not superior, healing and mortality outcomes.[45–48] Once the patient has clinically improved, the surgeon can assess and plan for a formal revision. In both of these staged procedures, it is essential that the surgeon treat the patient's gangrenous ischemia with maximal therapeutic intent, while simultaneously taking into consideration the likely level of amputation in the second stage. "Best some healthy tissue be removed rather than leave any disease tissue" — Celsus.[4]

AMBULATION RATE

The likelihood of patients to achieve ambulation after different levels of amputation is widely studied, but results are fraught with confounding variables. For example, a recent meta-analysis of knee disarticulations revealed ambulation rates ranging from 13% to 75%, citing poor outcome measures, lack of follow-up, and failure to control for comorbidities or preoperative ambulation status.[49] Nevertheless, the literature is largely in agreeance on several things:

- Amputations placed more distal and with better likelihood of prosthetic fit result in a higher chance of the patient regaining ambulatory status by 6 months
- Return to ambulation is multifactorial, and more likely dependent on individual patient factors such as age, physical fitness, and presence of comorbidities.
- Level of amputation should not dictate a patient's candidacy for a prosthetic, as even hip disarticulation patients are able to achieve ambulation.[50,51]

AMBULATION ENERGY

Although less variable than ambulation rate, the increase in metabolic cost of ambulation also tends to be difficult to quantify but trends with residual limb length.[52,53] Interestingly, amputation at the level of the ankle seems to be favorable to midfoot amputation.[52] Many studies have used oxygen consumption and heart rate as a measure of energy requirement, but it is also known that patients with amputations have a compensatory decrease in their self-selected walking speed (SSWS). This decrease is multifactorial (limitations from stump pain or prosthetic design, age, etc.) and does not always align with the most metabolically efficient speed.[54] It should also be noted that patients with vascular amputations reportedly have a significantly higher energy expenditure with ambulation than traumatic amputations.[54] Much of this research is dated, and more recent meta-analyses and reviews have confirmed these trends but suggest that selection bias and poor design may overestimate the commonly cited values. Hindfoot and ankle amputations increase ambulation energy as little as 15%, while transfemoral amputees may see an increase up to 50%.

In terms of stump length, early reports indicated that transtibial amputation proximity was proportional to the increase in oxygen consumption, but more recent studies have not reproduced this, and also found no evidence for the effect in transfemoral amputations.[55–57] Successful myodesis is also thought to decrease metabolic costs by improving motor efficiency and stabilization, taking the burden off of less efficient proximal muscle groups. Bilateral amputees are rarely examined, with the most commonly cited studies using only a handful of patients to calculate their findings and are likely not reliable numbers. The use of a short nonarticulating pylon prosthesis (SNAPP, or "stubby") in bilateral transfemoral amputees is associated with better return to ambulation and confidence, despite significant decreases in walking speeds, efficiency, ability to perform activities of daily living (ADLs), and cosmesis.[58,59] Still, there exists a role for low demand patients or occasional use in home ambulation. Regardless of these specifics, the takeaway to the surgeon remains the same: a lower level of amputation leads to lower energy expenditure, making them preferrable for patient outcomes, especially in a population plagued by compromised cardiovascular health.

MANAGEMENT AND SURGICAL TECHNIQUE

There are many technical aspects to consider for each amputation procedure, but in general, surgeons should approach every case with the same core principles in mind:

- Soft tissue flaps should be oversized and trimmed to ensure tension-free coverage and layered closure.
- Good hemostasis should be achieved within visibly viable soft tissues, and treated delicately.
- End bone should be flattened, and edges chamfered, to prepare it for weight-bearing.
- Joint forces should be balanced to prevent contractures via tenodesis, myodesis, tendon transfer, and/or tenotomy.

Anesthesia

The ACS-NSQIP reviewed a large series of patients to determine if regional or general anesthesia is preferrable for major amputation. While general offers the surgeon the option of paralysis and a faster time to surgery, it is considered to be a greater physiologic burden on a likely already sick patient. There was no difference in operative times, postoperative morbidity and mortality, or length of stay. This decision should therefore be made on a case-by-case basis in collaboration with the anesthesia team.[60]

Antibiotics

Literature to support preoperative antibiotic prophylaxis specifically in amputations is scarce, but recent SCIP guidelines and the nightmare-inducing thought of a postoperative stump infection should convince any surgeon.[61] IDSA guidelines from 2012 and several recent studies have advocated for the use of a five-day postoperative antibiotic course in patients receiving amputation for diabetic foot infections, which appears to significantly lower infection rate as well as reduce hospital stay. In this population, oral agents have been shown to be a safe alternative to intravenous to facilitate earlier discharge. It is important to note that these guidelines apply to amputations that have removed all infected tissue, and an extended course of organism-specific antibiotics is warranted otherwise.[62–65] Open wounds may present a problem for surgical field sterility and should be washed thoroughly prior to prepping the limb, and sealed off using an adherent dressing or stockinette.

Blood Vessels

To ensure a good night's sleep after performing an amputation, the surgeon must be certain that the vasculature is ligated in a safe and secure fashion. The most common suture is silk as it is both braided and nonabsorbable to provide excellent knot integrity for an extended period. There is a concern that circumferential ties may roll off the end of the vessel with movement since they rely only on friction. Stick ties, which involve piercing the vessel to anchor the suture in place, maximize security but are traumatic to the vessel. Bleeding can still occur through the holes created, which may chronically lead to pseudoaneurysm or fistula formation. Since standard practice is to double ligate, a good technique is to use a stick tie first, which serves as a backstop for a more proximal hand tie. This method creates a more secure hand tie while minimizing possible complications from the more distal stick tie.

Tourniquet use is hotly debated, with orthopedic surgeons anecdotally much more likely to use them than their vascular surgery counterparts. Several high-quality studies have found that tourniquets reduce operative blood loss, postoperative transfusions, and duration of surgery owing to better visualization in a bloodless field.[66–68] Evidence-based guidelines recommend their use based on these benefits, but the tourniquet does not come without downsides.[69] Raising and lowering the tourniquet increases and decreases the systemic vascular resistance and central venous pressure, creating unnecessary cardiac stress during an already physiologically jarring procedure. The release of the tourniquet results in reactive hyperemia at the surgical site, which some posit may compromise tissue closure and result in greater postoperative bleeding.[5,66,70] Reports of arterial wall damage are rare, but neuropraxia and postoperative local pain are not as infrequent. Tourniquet use should therefore be strongly considered during amputation, but not without caution and proper technique.

Nerves

There are numerous intraoperative nerve-handling methods proposed, with the most common being transecting the nerve while under tension. This way, it retracts into tissue far from the operative site, thereby protected from scarring and pressure from the weight-bearing area. Many surgeons inject the nerve with local anesthetic prior to cutting as well. While bleeding vessels are easily visualized, nerves, especially those in the subcutaneous tissues, are often difficult to locate. Failure to do so can result in a painful stump that discourages ambulation and may require revision. The surgeon should be well versed in the nervous anatomy of the lower limb and take care to identify and isolate them (Figure 11-2).

A technique called targeted muscle reinnervation (TMR), originally developed as a method of repositioning nerves for use in a myoelectric prosthesis, has recently also been noted to significantly decrease the postoperative neuropathic pain complications of amputation. The surgeon locates a motor nerve branch that is no longer necessary after amputation and removes a short segment. The distal end of the larger sensory or mixed nerve being divided is anastomosed to this free graft, then placed within the motor nerve's original muscle target. Rather than form a neuroma, TMR creates a channel for fascicles to grow down, allowing them to find physiologic targets within the muscle such as motor end plates and proprioceptors. "TMR gives the regenerating fascicles 'somewhere to go and something to do,'" preventing the formation of pathways that may cause postoperative phantom and residual limb pain (RLP).[71] Although currently very rarely performed and technically difficult for surgeons untrained in nerve grafting, studies have shown clear benefit to performing this primarily in amputations and should be considered in patients with a high likelihood of postoperative pain complications.[71–75]

Muscles

Muscle represents the largest component of soft tissue in the amputated extremity and provides both

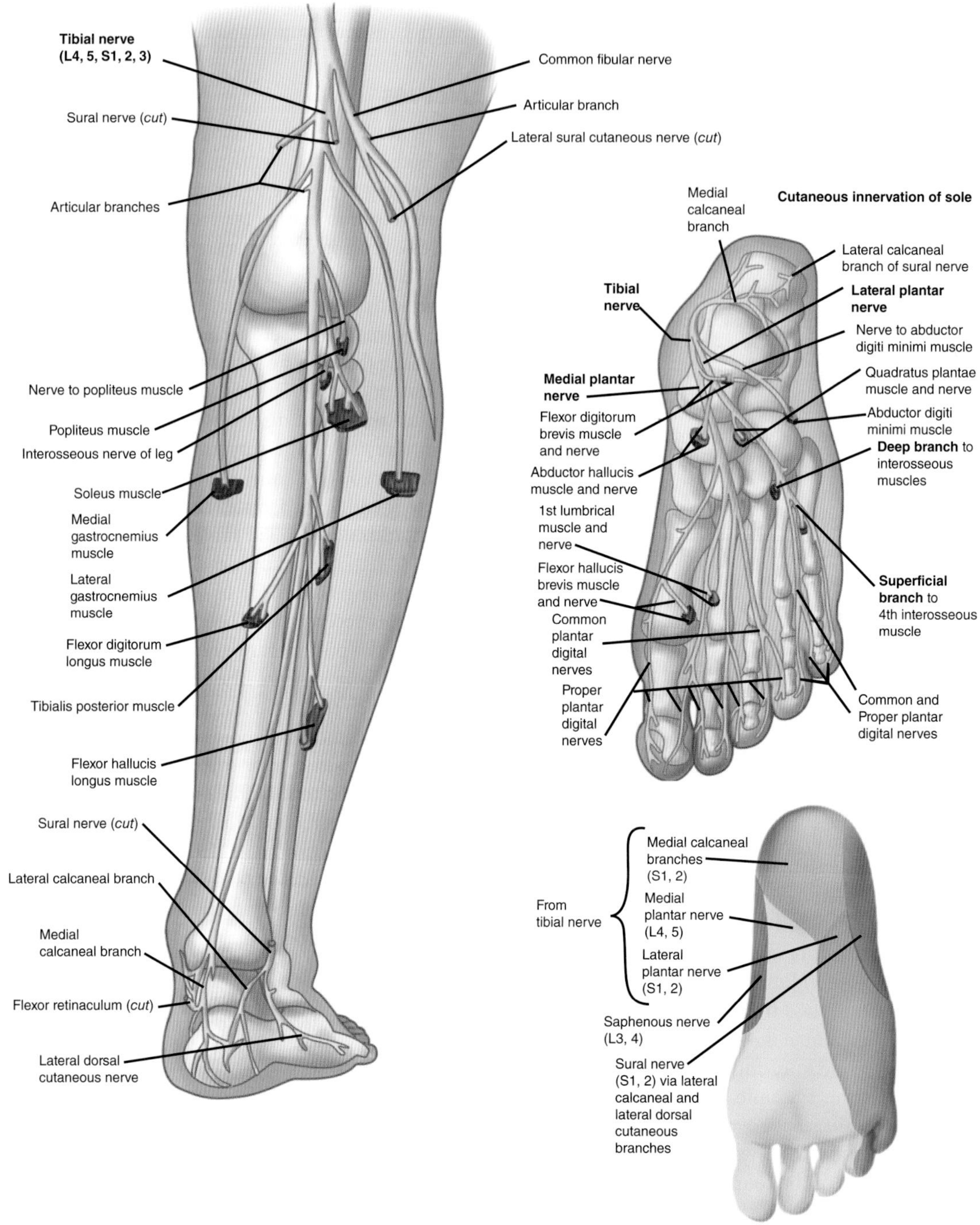

FIGURE 11-2 Nervous anatomy of the lower extremity illustrated with muscular and dermatomal innervations. Reproduced with permission from Amato AA, Russell JA. *Neuromuscular Disorders*, 2nd ed. New York, NY: McGraw Hill; 2016.

bone coverage and padding as well as motor function and proprioception. Poorly managed muscle tissue will lead to wound complications, stump pain, unbalanced contractures, and lack of residual function. Below are the most common methods of securing muscle tissue following amputation:

- Myodesis (or tenodesis) involves securing the muscle (or tendon) directly to the bone, typically through drill holes in the cortex using nonabsorbable suture. This is desirable as it directly restores muscle function, increasing the likelihood of successful ambulation and prevention of contractures. Care should be taken to avoid iatrogenic fracture, and soft tissues should be shielded from bone debris during drilling.
- Myoplasty is an anastomosis of two opposing muscle groups by their fascia over the distal bone. While technically simpler to perform, it solves the problem of balancing forces without any guarantee of good motor function. If it does not scar down to the underlying bone, this muscular belt glides back and forth over the stump, causing irritation. However, for patients unlikely to achieve ambulation, performing myoplasty decreases surgical time and provides potentially superior coverage due to decreased tissue loss during mobilization.[76]
- Myofascial closure, also known as creating a "tobacco-pouch" is the final type, whereby the fascia of a single muscle is closed and not attached to any other structure. This is not recommended but can be an alternative if myodesis or myoplasty is not possible.

Bone

Though the bone cut is one of the simplest parts of the procedure, "prep and polish" cannot be overlooked for optimal results. Periosteum should be sharply excised 1- to 2-cm proximal to the planned cut, and all soft tissues should be retracted and completely shielded with sponges. These actions prevent the growth of aberrant bone spikes and development of soft tissue calcifications in the stump. While some advocate for a sleeve of elevated periosteum

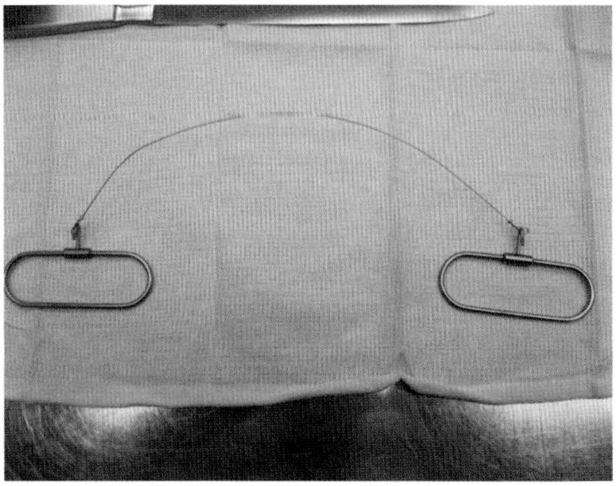

FIGURE 11-3 Flexible Gigli saw blade attached to hook-handles.

to cap the distal bone, there is no literature to suggest improved healing, and doing so introduces the possibility of revision for bony overgrowth. Excessive proximal periosteal stripping will devitalize the bone and should be avoided. The cut should be made perpendicular to the diaphysis to evenly distribute pressure, and the edges lightly beveled and smoothed with rasps or the saw, creating an atraumatic weight-bearing surface. Oscillating saws are ideal for this task, using a blade that is just large enough to perform the cut in one pass to ensure smoothness. An assistant should continuously cool the blade with saline to avoid thermal injury to the bone.[77] In guillotine transmetatarsal amputations and rare instances of retained intramedullary hardware, a Gigli (jee-lyee) saw can be used instead (Figure 11-3).

This latter half of this chapter will discuss indications, techniques, and pitfalls of the most common lower extremity vascular amputations. An overview of the different levels, as well as a review of the relevant axial anatomy, can be found in Figure 11-4. While we will not discuss pediatric amputations in this chapter, the surgeon should be aware that skeletally immature patients will not only continue to grow through all open physes but are subject to appositional bone growth from the end of any cut bone. Measures to cap the end of the bone, such as grafting the calcaneus to the tibia, performing an Ertl bone bridge, or securing a synthetic bone cap are all

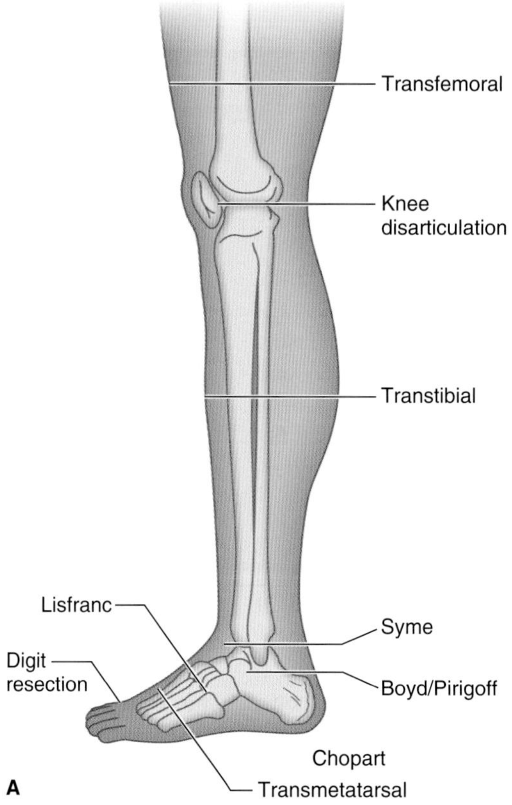

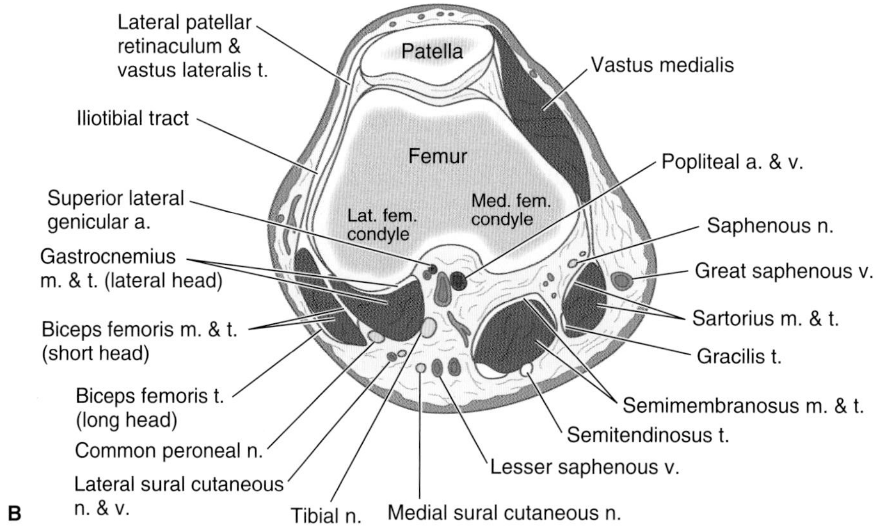

FIGURE 11-4 **(A) Common levels for lower extremity vascular amputations and associated axial anatomy at the (B) transfemoral**

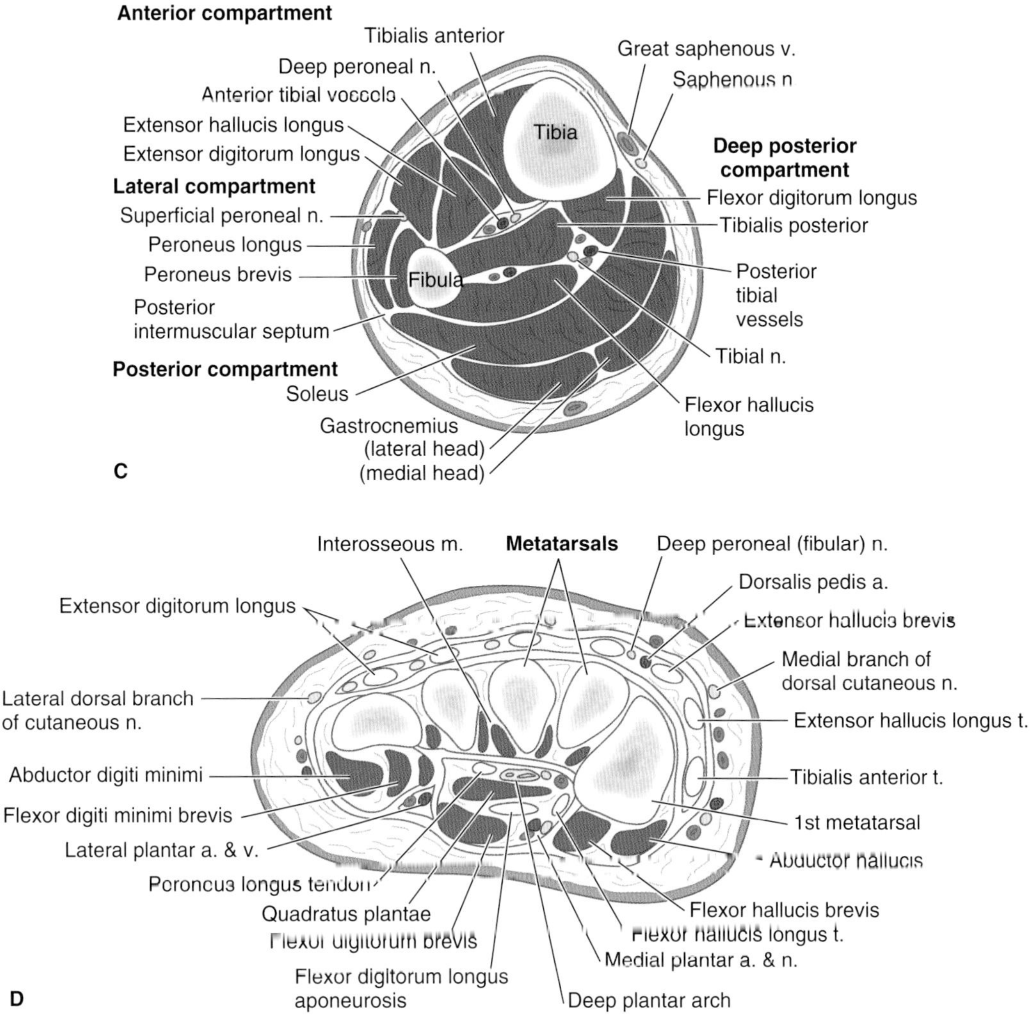

FIGURE 11-4 Continued (C) transtibial, and (D) transmetatarsal levels.

potential options to prevent or slow this from requiring a stump revision.

DIGIT/RAY RESECTION

Amputation of a single digit for a nonhealing wound is simple, straightforward, and may be done at any level distal to the metatarsal head. Flexor and extensor tendons can be cut and allowed to retract, and the digital neurovascular bundles should be easy to identify and divide. The "tennis-racquet" flap for the hallux and 5th digit is a popular technique, and longitudinal fish mouth flaps can be used for the remainder, although some advocate for these wounds to be left open to heal by secondary intention. Partial resection of the metatarsal head may be necessary for closure, but not in excess, which would preclude weight-bearing, especially the hallux. That said, it is estimated that at least 20% of hallux amputations are later revised to a more proximal level.[78–80] Still, given the ease of performing these procedures and minimal risk of failure, this should be considered a perfectly acceptable success rate.

Wounds directly over the metatarsal head plantarly are not amenable to a simple digit resection but may benefit from a single ray resection if they are isolated. Resection of the 2nd digit often results in a hallux valgus deformity and offers another indication for performing a ray resection. The incisions for the digit amputation are extended to excise the wound plantarly and combined into a longitudinal incision over the metatarsal shaft dorsally, excising the diaphysis but leaving the base intact. This is critical to preserve the attachments of the peroneals (1st and 5th) as well as the ligamentous stability of the Lisfranc joint between the 1st and 2nd. In this case, care should be taken to avoid the deep plantar structures, including the vasculature, aponeurosis, and fat pad. Ray resection of the 1st digit should be avoided in ambulatory patients due to the significant role of the hallux and first metatarsal in normal stride, and primary transmetatarsal amputation should be considered. Despite narrowing the forefoot, patients are typically still able to ambulate with normal footwear, sometimes assisted by custom inserts.

TRANSMETATARSAL (TMA)

At its origin, TMA was used to treat trench foot during WWII, and continues to be an excellent partial foot amputation widely used today. It allows the surgeon to aggressively treat forefoot gangrene while still preserving the TMT joints for ambulation. Despite its popularity, it is still prone to high rates of wound complications, with around 25% requiring reoperation, and 1 in 3 is later revised to a major amputation.[81] Healing predictors are also unreliable at this level, and studies have had a difficult time discerning prognostic risk factors, if any exists.[82] Additionally, losing extensor hallucis and digitorum function tends to result in an equinus contracture, which can be solved through either a split tibialis anterior transfer to the medial cuneiform, gastrocnemius recession, and/or tendoachilles lengthening.[83]

TECHNIQUE

- The exact proximity of the amputation should be dictated by the location of the patient's pathology, but skin and bone cuts should follow the natural parabola of the metatarsals and create a viable plantar flap that closes dorsally.
- Extensor hallucis and digitorum tendons are cut and allowed to retract. If performing a proximal TMA, take care to preserve the dorsalis pedis as it passes between the first and second metatarsals.
- The metatarsals are dissected subperiosteally, taking care to preserve interosseous soft tissue.
- Starting with the second, the metatarsals are then cut starting using an oscillating saw angled slightly proximal plantarly, taking great care to avoid the soft tissues essential for successful wound healing.
- The metatarsals are gently dissected off the plantar flap, and the amputated forefoot removed. The sesamoids should also be removed, allowing the flexor hallucis tendons to retract.
- If the digital nerves are identifiable, they may be cut under tension.
- Smoothing of the cut surfaces of the metatarsals can be done with a rasp or a rongeur.
- At this point, the wound may be left open if soft tissues are not yet amenable to closure.
- After good hemostasis is achieved and the wound copiously irrigated, the plantar fascia is brought up and secured to the dorsal metatarsal periosteum, or attached using drill holes, then closed in a layered fashion.
- If desired, a split anterior tibial tendon transfer, gastrocnemius recession, and/or tendoachilles lengthening can be performed to prevent equinus.

LISFRANC

Despite the majority of Jacques Lisfranc's career being focused on his gynecologic work, his special interest in midfoot amputations for diabetic gangrene led to numerous anatomic eponyms in this anatomic area.[84] His amputation technique is notable for speed since it is primarily a disarticulation, while still preserving the midfoot as in a TMA. Like other disarticulations discussed in this chapter, high failure rates owed to poor soft tissue balancing have caused this procedure to be much more rarely performed. While surgeon preference may continue to lean toward TMA, Lisfranc amputations may be a viable option if the degree of gangrene does not allow for the former.

TECHNIQUE

- The medial TMT joint is marked, and the medial side of the plantar flap is extended distally along the entire length of the metatarsal shaft. The lateral incision is made similarly along the metatarsal shaft extending from the articulation with the cuboid. They are connected dorsally and plantarly.
- An attempt to find and appropriately transect distal sensory branches of the peroneal and medial/lateral plantar nerves should be made. The dorsalis pedis is found diving into the first dorsal space and ligated.
- Extensor tendons should be sharply transected but tagged for later tenodesis, with care taken not to release the tibialis anterior from the cuboid. The flexor tendons are cut under tension and allowed to retract.
- The metatarsal bones are disarticulated at the TMT joints. Optionally, the base of the 5th metatarsal may be cut in order to preserve the attachment of the peroneus brevis.
- If the peroneus brevis is released, the peroneus longus should be passed through a drill hole in the cuboid, and tenodesis performed between the two tendons and the plantar cuboid periosteum. This should be performed with the ankle in neutral.
- A gastrocnemius recession or Achilles lengthening/transection may be performed at the surgeon's discretion, but it is recommended to prevent eventual equinus.
- The extensor hallucis is secured to the lateral cuneiform in a similar fashion.
- Plantar fascia is then secured dorsally to the periosteum, and the remainder of the plantar flap is closed in layers.[85]

HINDFOOT (CHOPART, BOYD, AND PIRIGOFF)

Hindfoot amputations have traditionally been favored for trauma or deformity cases, but a few studies have looked at their efficacy in treating vascular disease. When forefoot pathology becomes too overwhelming for a TMA or a Lisfranc to adequately treat, these operations may be the last possibility of maintaining the patient's limb length. A recent review has found that patients are often very satisfied with an amputation at this level, and most retain the ability to walk short distances without a prosthesis.[86] Despite the preservation of the anatomic weight-bearing surfaces, including the specialized fibrofatty heel pad, patients have suboptimal outcomes attributed to poor wound healing and high rates of revision. In select patients with good wound healing capabilities, hindfoot amputations still may be beneficial, but are often so technically challenging that the risks outweigh any minimal benefit over a transtibial amputation. Patients must also have a patent posterior tibial artery to supply the posterior heel pad, which must be disease-free, otherwise the procedure should be abandoned and a transtibial amputation performed. Lastly, some authors feel that securing the tibialis anterior to the talus, sometimes augmenting with a transferred posterior tibial tendon, can balance the now unopposed Achilles tendon to prevent a contracture. However, given that ankle motion is now redundant, consider a simple percutaneous Achilles tendon release instead.[86–89]

TECHNIQUE

- The talonavicular joint is palpated and marked, a small needle may be useful here to confirm positioning. Amputation will occur at this level and should ideally be covered with a posterior flap or fish mouth. Skin coverage should be planned according to the availability of viable tissue.
- Begin by performing an Achilles tenotomy, which can be done percutaneously using a #11 blade. It is imperative to avoid the posterior tibial artery during this step.

- Dorsally, the neurovascular structures are appropriately divided, and all tendinous structures may be transected under tension and allowed to retract.

Chopart:

- The talonavicular joint is identified and incised, releasing the capsular attachments circumferentially. The same is done with the calcaneocuboid joint, and the midfoot is removed.

Pirigoff / Boyd:

- After incising the anterior capsule to expose the tibiotalar joint, release the ligamentous attachments of the talus to the tibia and fibula, taking care to protect the posterior tibial artery medially. This should allow the talus to be dislocated. If difficulty is encountered here, the talus can be removed piecewise with an osteotome, or a smooth wire can be used to skewer it for better control.
- An osteotomy is made transversely through the distal tibia and fibula just proximal to the joint line.
- Another osteotomy is made in the calcaneus. In the Pirigoff technique, it is made starting just proximal to the posterior facet and aimed slightly distal to remove all three facets, while in the Boyd technique, the posterior and middle facets are taken off with an anteriorly directed osteotomy, and the anterior facet removed with a more vertical osteotomy.
- The two subchondral bone surfaces are then fixed to each other using crossed retrograde cannulated screws, with the calcaneus placed in 15 degrees of external rotation and slightly posterior.[87,89]
- With the tourniquet released, good hemostasis is ensured, and a thorough irrigation and debridement is performed.
- Using nonabsorbable suture, the heel pad can be secured to holes drilled into the anterior cortex of the talus (Chopart) or calcaneus/tibia (Pirigoff/Boyd). Skin flaps can now be trimmed and closed.

SYME (ANKLE DISARTICULATION)

Initially described nearly 200 years ago in thorough detail, James Syme's amputation for severe infection and trauma remains largely unpopular when compared to transtibial amputation.[90] The key benefits of amputation at this level are largely based on retention of true weight-bearing surfaces, namely, the distal tibial articular surface and heel pad tissue. Other benefits include a longer remaining limb length, as well as better gait dynamics with lower metabolic cost of ambulation, even when compared to a more distal TMA. Reportedly over 40% of ankle disarticulation patients are even able to walk short distances without using a prosthesis, which is a testament to its supporters. However, these virtues have been overshadowed by a history of wound complications, heel pad migration, and poor cosmesis. Wagner initially described a method for performing this as a staged procedure and, with proper preoperative optimization, was able to achieve very high rates of ambulation and wound healing.[91] Pinzur concluded in an RCT that performing a single surgery was just as efficacious, and later proved that diabetic patients, when proper candidates, outperformed similar patients that received a more proximal transtibial amputation.[92,93] Such criteria include a preoperative serum albumin > 2.5 g/dL, ABI > 0.5 or $PtcO_2 > 20$ mmHg, and a patent posterior tibial artery, which supplies the heel pad. Today, a large fraction of Syme's amputations are performed on children for fibular hemimelia and are a niche in the vascular surgery world. Still, in patients with good wound-healing capacity and high preoperative functional status, an ankle disarticulation should be strongly considered for improved return to function.[49,94]

TECHNIQUE

- Ensure proper integrity of the heel pad preoperatively. Identify and mark the medial and lateral malleoli. Create a fish mouth incision using the malleoli as apices, extending directly plantar and across the ankle joint dorsally (Figure 11-5).
- Dorsally, the neurovascular structures are appropriately divided, and all tendinous structures may be transected under tension and

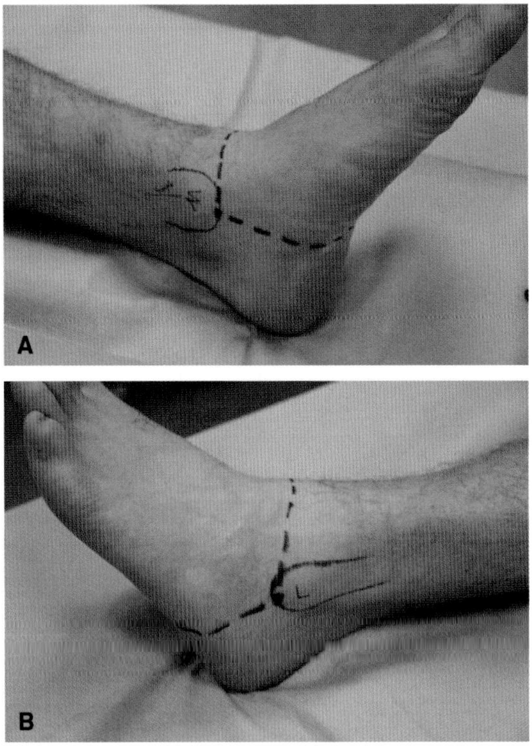

FIGURE 11-5 **(A) Medial and (B) lateral aspects of the Syme incision.**

allowed to retract. Incise the anterior capsule to visualize the tibiotalar joint.

- Release the ligamentous attachments of the talus to the tibia and fibula, taking care to protect the posterior tibial artery medially. This should allow the talus to be dislocated. If difficulty is encountered here, the talus can be removed piecewise with an osteotome, or a smooth wire can be used to skewer it for better control.
- Working laterally and plantar, elevate the heel pad from the calcaneus subperiosteally, taking care not to disrupt its intrinsic structure. The plantar skin is extremely thin near the Achilles tendon insertion, and careful release is crucial.
- Once the foot has been removed, the remaining tendinous and neurovascular structures should be dealt with as they were anteriorly.
- The distal fibula, medial malleolus, and, if necessary, posterior malleolus can now be cut with an oscillating saw to be flush with the tibial plafond. An additional vertical cut can be made to remove the medial malleolar flare.
- With the tourniquet released, good hemostasis is ensured, and a thorough irrigation and debridement is performed.
- Using nonabsorbable suture, the heel pad can be secured to holes drilled into the anterior cortex of the tibia. A pin may be placed through the heel pad into the distal tibia if there is concern for migration, but trauma to this valuable tissue should be minimized if possible. Skin flaps can now be trimmed and closed.

TRANSTIBIAL (TTA)

Transtibial, or "below-knee" amputations are the most commonly performed major amputation, boasting good functional outcomes despite the significant amount of limb loss it entails. While every attempt should be made to preserve the knee joint, surgeons should be aware that the rate of eventual TTA revision to a more proximal level is significant, ranging between 9% and 24%. However, many authors believe this can be minimized using preoperative evaluation tools such as $TcPO_2$, as a majority of these conversions happen early due to nonhealing wounds or perioperative infections.[95–99] Preoperative nonambulatory status and end-stage renal disease are thought to be risk factors for early failure, and the surgeon should consider primary amputation at a higher level for reasons discussed earlier in the chapter.[100] Flap formation is a hotly debated topic in TTA, as there are multiple considerations in terms of scar placement and preserving soft tissue perfusion. The two most common are the Skew and Burgess flaps (described in detail below), and a Cochrane review by Tisi concluded there was no difference between the two aside from minimally earlier time to mobility with the skew flap due to earlier prosthetic fitting.[44] Again, consideration should be given to preexisting wounds, scars, soft tissue imbalances, and surgeon preference when choosing between flap types. Optimal stump length is also controversial, with most surgeons believing the tibia should be cut 8- to 15-cm distal to the tubercle. Since length is favorable for biomechanics and the stump may be shortened in the event of a revision, we recommend at least 12 cm.

TECHNIQUE

- Depending on soft tissues and surgeon preference, skin incisions are made in one of several ways:
  - Skew (sagittal flap): A mark is made anteriorly and posteriorly approximately 12-cm distal to the tubercle. The diameter of the leg at this level is measured, and moving distally the same distance as this measurement, a mark is then made medially and laterally. The elliptical flaps created by connecting these four marks (Figure 11-6a).
  - Burgess (posterior flap): The transverse anterior incision is marked at the level of the planned tibial cut, approximately 12 cm from the tubercle, and the diameter of the limb at this level is measured. The posterior incision is marked distally by half the diameter, then connected to the anterior incision medially and laterally (Figure 11-6b).
- Using blunt dissection, the tibial crest should be easily reached, and an elevator used to clear the periosteum circumferentially.
- Medially the greater saphenous vein should be identified and ligated, and the saphenous nerve should also be isolated and divided under tension.
- The incision is then carried laterally, incising the fascia of the lateral compartment. The superficial peroneal nerve pierces the crural fascia between the peroneus brevis and the extensor digitorum to become superficial approximately one-third of the way down the lower leg. It should be identified and later properly divided.
- Next, the anterior tibial neurovascular bundle should be dissected and appropriately divided, and the remainder of the anterior and lateral compartments incised down to bone.

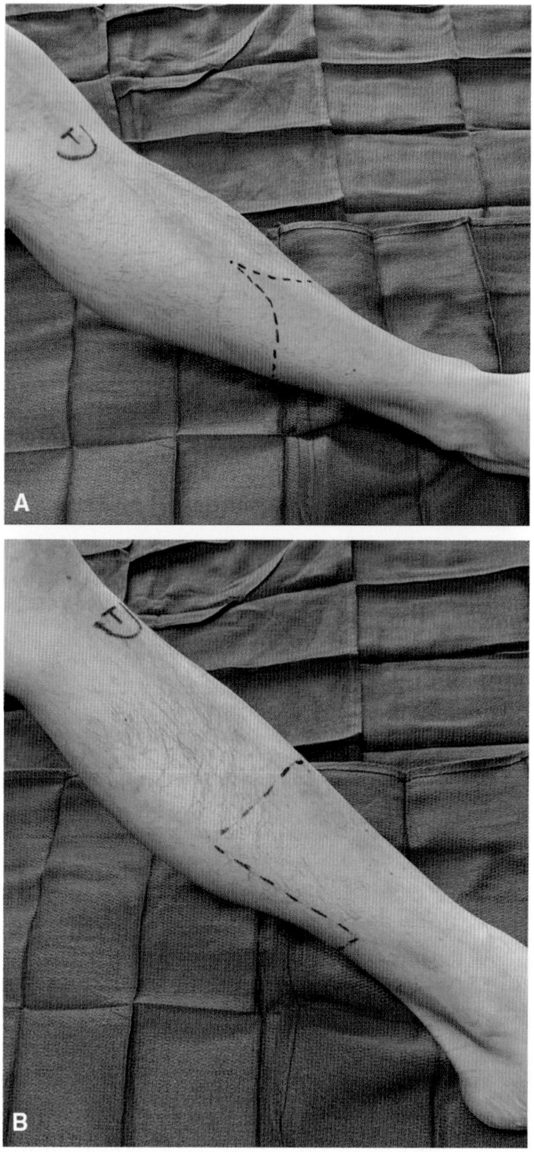

FIGURE 11-6 (A) Depiction of the skew or sagittal flap and (B) Burgess or posterior flap incisions for transtibial amputations.

- With the tibia exposed and soft tissues protected, a cut is made ideally 12- to 15-cm distal to the tubercle. The fibula is similarly cut about 1- to 2-cm proximal to this.
- The posterior compartments are then dissected off the tibia and fibula. It can be helpful

to place the knee in flexion and draw the bones anteriorly for this step. The amputated limb can be removed.

- The tibial and peroneal neurovascular bundles can now be dissected in the deep posterior compartment and appropriately managed. The sural nerve should be present just superficial to the gastrocnemius at this level adjacent to the small saphenous vein, and if possible, identified and divided under tension.
- Many surgeons prefer to bevel the tibia anteriorly with a second 45 degree cut. All bony edges should be smoothed, hemostasis achieved, and the wound copiously irrigated.
- A tenodesis can be performed between the Achilles and the anterior tibial periosteum or through drill holes, and a fascial closure completed between the anterior and posterior compartments.
- The remainder of the wound can be closed in a layered fashion, taking care to the corners of the flaps to avoid redundant skin and dog-ears.

KNEE DISARTICULATION (KD)

Knee disarticulation, or through-knee amputation, is a much less common form of lower limb amputation, accounting for around 1% to 2% of vascular amputations annually.[49,101] Previously, this level was thought to be associated with higher rates of wound complications and difficulty with prosthetic fit, but subsequent higher-quality studies have disproved this, with similar outcomes compared to transfemoral amputation (TFA).[102–104] Benefits include increased stability and proprioception due to intact adductor and quadricep insertion, a longer lever arm for decreased ambulatory metabolic cost and improved sitting posture, and minimal contracture risk.[49] What's more, KD preserves the distal femoral cartilage cap, which creates a true end-weight-bearing stump, decreases the risk of osteomyelitis, and maintains the epiphysis in pediatric patients. Lastly, while return to the OR for revision to a higher level is not ideal, revising a KD to a TFA allows for more preservation of length than a failed TFA requiring revision to an even higher level.

Despite these advantages, many surgeons feel uncomfortable performing this procedure due to a lack of training, citing difficulty forming myocutaneous flaps over the femoral condyles and managing intra-articular structures involved in this method. The Mazet technique proposes a partial solution to this by trimming the condyles, decreasing the size of the needed flap and allowing for suction socket prosthetics. However, some surgeons feel the bulky femoral condyles allow for inherent rotational stability of a future prosthetic and should be left intact. Evidence is not sufficient to support one method over the other in regard to wound healing, ambulation, or reoperation rates, and technique should therefore be selected based on surgeon training.[105,106]

TECHNIQUE

- Identify and mark the patella, tibial tubercle, patellar tendon, and the diameter of the limb at the level of the femoral condyles (X). The anterior incision is marked at the level of the patellar tendon, while the posterior incision should be distal to that by X cm to create a posterior flap (Figure 11-7).
- Incision is made anteriorly, carefully exposing and subperiosteally elevating the patellar tendon from the tibial tubercle.

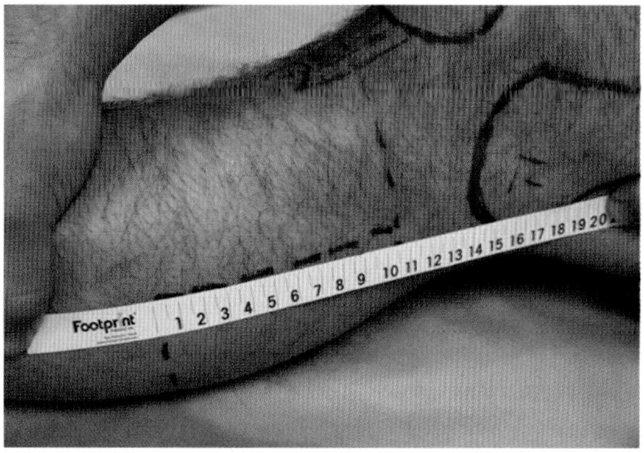

FIGURE 11-7 Planned incision for a knee disarticulation (dotted), located at the level of the patellar tendon anteriorly, then a posterior flap is created the same length as the diameter of the knee.

- As the incision is carried medially, the greater saphenous vein and nerve are encountered and divided. Posteriorly, lesser saphenous vein is encountered and divided, and the incision carried down through the fascia. The medial and lateral sural cutaneous nerves may be ignored as they will be divided more proximally later.
- The capsule is incised anteriorly at the level of the tibial plateau, submeniscally, both medially and laterally. The ACL and PCL are released from their tibial insertions as well. This can be done with the knee in flexion to improve visualization.
- Hoffa's fat pad should be completely removed from the undersurface of the patellar tendon.
- The posterior capsule is incised at the same level, and dissection is carried closely down the posterior tibia to create a musculocutaneous flap by meeting the previous incision.
- Posterior neurovascular structures are isolated and divided (popliteal artery/vein and tibial/common peroneal nerves).
- Checking the posterior flap size, the surgeon should mobilize the posterior muscular structures between the subcutaneous tissue and the fascia and may elect to carefully resect the medial or lateral head of the gastrocnemius if it is too bulky.
- If performing the Mazet technique, the distal femur is trimmed to form a box, ideally using an oscillating saw, avoiding the adductor insertion. The undersurface of the patella is similarly removed to expose subchondral bone.
- At this time, the tourniquet should be deflated to check for adequate vascular control, anticipating that several geniculate artery branches may have been inadvertently cut without ligation. Once hemostasis is achieved with ligation and electrocautery, the tourniquet is re-inflated, and a thorough irrigation is performed.
- Heavy, nonabsorbable sutures are used to create a tenodesis between the patellar tendon and the cruciate ligaments. This tightened with the hip in flexion in order to advance the patella to the level of the condyles, making sure it does not sit inferior to them. If performing the Mazet technique, the tenodesis is instead performed using the quadriceps tendon, advancing the patella to cover the inferior surface of the femur.
- Myoplasty is performed between the gastrocnemius and the preserved anterior capsule/patellar tendon to securely cover the condyles circumferentially. The cutaneous flap can now be trimmed and closed.[107]

GRITTI-STROKES AMPUTATION (GSA)

The Gritti-Stokes amputation is very similar to a KD, somewhat closer in relation to a TFA. Benefits include excellent wound healing rates and a technically simpler procedure; however, it has not been popular among surgeons due to very poor cosmetic satisfaction, ambulation rates, and patellar nonunion. In the nonambulatory patient, GSA could be a viable alternative to KD for preserving length if the surgeon does not feel comfortable handling the intra-articular structures.[49,108–110]

TECHNIQUE (MODIFICATIONS FROM KD)

- The incision creates and anterior flap that is positioned distal to the tibial tubercle and meets the posterior flap at the level of the femoral condyles.
- Dissection is carried out similar to KD, and like the Mazet technique, the undersurface of the patella is cut to expose subchondral bone.
- A transcondylar cut is made in the femur using an oscillating saw, angled to create a 15 degree bevel that is distal anteriorly and proximal posteriorly.
- The undersurface of the patella is secured to this cut either with drill holes and heavy suture, crossed pins, or other type of stout fixation.

TRANSFEMORAL (TFA)

When TTA or KD is not an option or has failed, TFA becomes the patient's last chance at a salvageable limb. Ambulation rates, energy consumption, and rates of prosthetic usage are discussed earlier in this chapter, with TFA having inferior outcomes compared to more distal amputations. Due to the very proximal insertion sites of hip flexors and abductions, and the more distal insertions of the extensors and adductors, patients are prone to unbalanced contractures postoperatively.[107,111,112] With a long working length, there is much debate over the optimal level for the level at which the femur should be transected. Enough room should be left above the knee joint for a prosthesis to attach and articulate; however, amputating proximal to Hunter's canal risks the insertion site of the adductor magnus, leading to worsened abduction contractures and control of the residual limb. Expert opinion and several studies agree this level, if possible, should be 12 to 15 cm above the knee joint.[113] The same group also advocates for a sagittal fish mouth with a medial flap that allows for myodesis of the adductor magnus insertion that is detached from the medial condyle. This is in contrast to the popular technique of creating a posterior or fish mouth flaps in the coronal plane, though neither has been proved superior, and the surgeon should take into account individual patient factors when deciding.

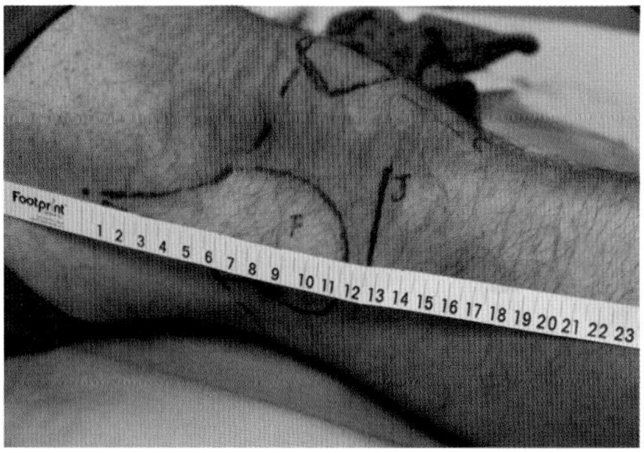

FIGURE 11-8 Fishmouth flap incision (dotted) for a transfemoral amputation, which converge 12-cm proximal to the joint line (J) in line with the femoral condyles (F).

TECHNIQUE

- Prior to scrubbing, the surgeon may check if there will be enough room on the thigh for a nonsterile tourniquet, which often cannot be placed proximally enough to still allow for adequate exposure after draping. Consider using a sterile tourniquet in these cases.
- Identify and mark the knee joint medially and laterally, as well as the medial and lateral femoral condyles to ensure the leg is positioned in neutral rotation.
- Marks are made 12- to 15-cm proximal to the knee joint both medially and laterally. The anterior and posterior fish mouth flaps are then drawn, extending distally from these marks to a point equal to half the diameter of the leg at the amputation level (Figure 11-8).
- Incision is made circumferentially down through fascia, identifying and ligating the saphenous vessels medially, then carried down to bone anteriorly and laterally. Any suprapatellar synovial tissue should be completely removed.
- Elevating soft tissues and periosteum off the femur, the amputation site is exposed, cut, and chamfered using an oscillating saw and rasps.
- The medial and posterior neurovascular structure can now more easily be dissected and divided: superficial and deep femoral vessels, the saphenous nerve, and the tibial and common peroneal nerves. It should not be assumed, at this level, that the tibial and common peroneal nerves will still be concomitant, keeping an eye out for early sural nerve branching.
- The adductor tubercle should be identified, and the adductor magnus insertion subperiosteally elevated off and tagged.
- The amputation is completed through the remaining soft tissues, tagging the hamstring tendons to prevent retraction. The tourniquet should be deflated to check for adequate

hemostasis, and once obtained, it can be reinflated, and the site thoroughly irrigated.

- Drill holes are made in the anterior, lateral, and posterior cortices through the distal end of bone. Using heavy, nonabsorbable suture, myodesis can be performed with the previously tagged adductor magnus to cover the distal femur by anchoring it first laterally, then secured anteriorly and posteriorly. This should be done with the thigh in maximal adduction.
- The quadriceps and hamstring tendons may also undergo tenodesis through the same holes, keeping the hip in flexion and extension, respectively, for adequate tension.
- The remaining vastus and tensor fascia lata can now undergo myoplasty with absorbable suture to the previous myodesis. Cutaneous flaps may not be trimmed and closed.
- With short residual limbs, it may be necessary to secure the dressings by wrapping the elastic bandage around the hip several times.

CRYOAMPUTATION (PHYSIOLOGIC AMPUTATION)

As previously discussed, cryoamputation is an excellent option in patients too unstable for formal amputation but still requiring urgent amputation to decrease their burden of infection or rhabdomyolysis. The term "physiologic" refers to the notion that the limb remains physically attached but does not have any appreciable physiologic impact due to lack of blood flow and metabolic activity. However, it is very rarely utilized, owing to lack of materials or knowledge. Complications of the cryoamputation are related to improper technique, including accidental damage to more proximal tissues, the contralateral limb, or surrounding medical equipment such as IV lines. Below is a very safe and effective method modified from Chen et al. using simple equipment readily available at nearly any hospital (or nearby grocery store).[114] It not only allows for simple maintenance by floor staff, but easily protects the contralateral limb while still allowing for easy inspection.

TECHNIQUE

- Begin by determining and marking the desired level of amputation, and measure both the largest diameter (D) and distal length (L) of the extremity from here. Cut a hole several centimeters larger than D in the side of a Styrofoam cooler that has a length of at least L (Figure 11-9a and b). It may be necessary to "anastomose" two coolers together with foam tape if the amputation is very proximal.
- 6-in cotton roll is then wrapped around the limb several times, centered over the previous mark. Optionally, a skin temperature probe may be applied under the proximal edge of the padding for easier monitoring later.
- Using foam tape, secure a piece of foam cushion to the bottom edge of the hole for the limb to rest on, as well as the inside of the cooler where the heel will rest. If the hole is cut too high, a blanket at the bottom of the cooler may be necessary.
- If the foot is unable to pass through the hole, a V-shaped wedge can be cut above this. The limb can then be lowered into the hole, and the wedge secured back to the cooler with more tape. If the hole is very oversized, securing more foam around the edges will safely decreases the diameter.
- Once inside, the amputation line should be flushed with the outer edge of the cooler. A heat source will need to be applied to the limb from the edge of the cooler extending proximally. Chen uses a water-circulated thermal wrap at ~36°C, which is ideal for temperature control and tissue protection, but if this is unavailable, an air-circulated warmer or frequently changed warmed blankets may be used.
- The hole can now be sealed using 2-in cotton padding around the limb inside and outside the cooler and secured with more foam tape. This also secures the cooler in place around the limb and prevents movement that would result in a different level of amputation (Figure 11-9c).

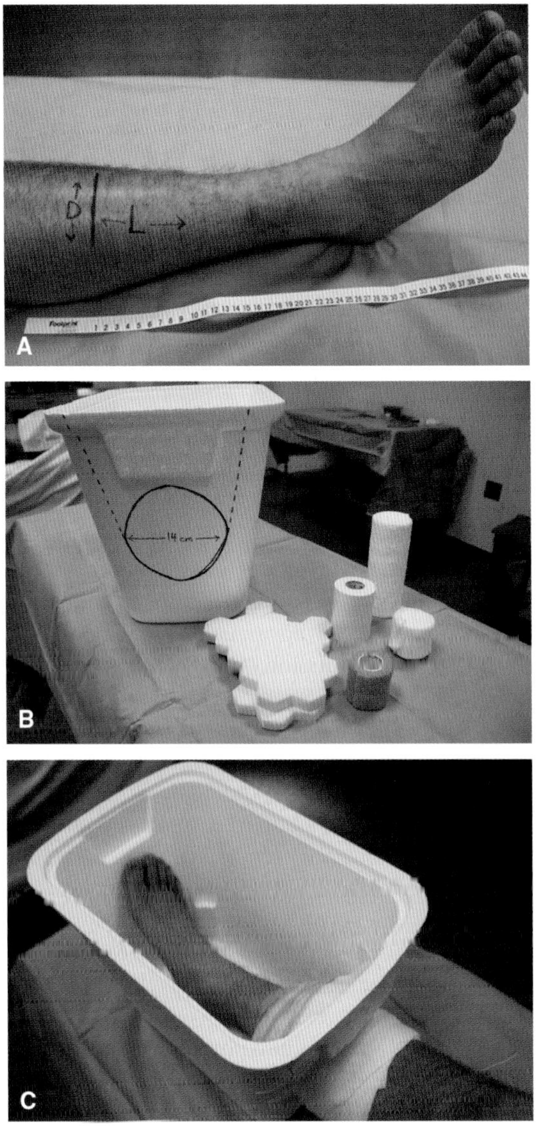

FIGURE 11-9 Demonstration of proposed technique for cryoamputation. (**A**) The planned level of amputation is marked, and the diameter D is measured as well as the distal length L. (**B**) Materials used for the adapted cryoamputation method, including a styrofoam cooler marked 2-cm larger than D, cotton roll, elastic bandage, foam tape, and foam padding. (**C**) The limb is placed into the cooler and secured.

- Some authors advocate for applying a venous tourniquet to prevent ascending cooling. If desired, this can be placed using an elastic bandage or Penrose drain just distal to the cotton wrap.
- Prior to icing, the patient may get IV pain control or sedation if needed and should only be required for the first few minutes at most. Some patients will tolerate this just fine with a circumferential application of local anesthetic near the amputation line.
- After filling the cooler with dry ice above the level of the leg, loosely secure the lid. Heavy gloves should be used when handling the ice, and it can be broken into small pieces to ensure even contact with the limb. Keep the contralateral leg covered with a blanket in case an errant piece falls onto the bed unnoticed.
- Frequent monitoring of the proximal skin temperature and dry ice levels should be performed initially and can be performed twice per shift after this. This is continued until the patient is safe to proceed with formal amputation.

POSTOPERATIVE MANAGEMENT

ROUTINE CARE

The surgeon's choice of postoperative wound care consists of traditional soft dressings or rigid dressings made of plaster, plastic, or fiberglass. Supporters of rigid dressing argue that it offers greater protection from trauma, greater compression, and early joint contracture prevention, which would allow for earlier wound healing and prosthetic fitting.[115] More advanced rigid orthoses called immediate postoperative prosthetics (IPOP) are becoming popular in current literature as they tout the benefits of a rigid dressing but are removable and also can be fabricated preoperatively. These typically increase cost substantially and require adequate preparation and resources that may not be available to all surgeons. On the other hand, rigid dressings carry a higher risk of skin breakdown, and most don't allow the surgeon to examine the surgical site postoperatively. Additionally, there are no contracture-prevention benefits for above knee procedures, which are more likely amenable to soft dressings. However, there exists no sufficient evidence to support any supposed risks or benefits of either type and this decision should be made on a case-by-case basis.[116–118] Elastic bandages such as stump shrinkers should also be avoided until the wound is healed to avoid incisional tension; however, some practices will allow graduated use within a week after surgery.

Negative pressure incisional wound therapy is also widely researched for diabetic wounds, but there is minimal evidence to support its use in routine amputation.[119] Surgeons may still consider negative pressure dressings for guillotine amputations or patients on anticoagulation with a high risk of bleeding. While postoperative fluid collections have not been associated with higher infection rates, most surgeons elect to place a drain that is pulled within 24 to 72 hours to avoid large hematomas that may cause wound complications or early return to the operating room.[120] The drain should not be sutured to allow for easy removal without disturbing the surgical dressings.

Perineural catheters that slowly administer local anesthetic to large nerves in the immediate postoperative period are a commonly used strategy in multimodal pain management. These can be easily placed by the surgeon during the procedure, and removed without difficulty, even by the patient. Although there is minimal evidence regarding their use in lower extremity amputation, it is likely that they reduce opioid consumption and, to a lesser degree, pain scores. Several randomized trials are ongoing to confirm this, but there is no indication that they decrease the likelihood of residual and phantom leg pain.[121]

Early weight-bearing is an advantage of IPOPs as previously mentioned, which can be advantageous for rehabilitation in traumatic amputations. However, vascular amputations carry a much higher concern for wound healing, and patients are often much frailer and more susceptible to falls. Literature is scarce and inconclusive about postoperative weight-bearing, but surgeons are cautioned to allow for complete wound healing and adequate physiotherapy prior to allowing the patient to ambulate.[122]

Postoperatively, partial foot amputations should be placed in neutral with an external splint, and the knee and hip should be allowed to rest in full extension using either an external cast, brace, or by simply placing pillows under the ankle and avoiding them under the knee/thigh. If possible, patients should be encouraged to lay prone for a period of time during the day and begin work with physical therapy as soon as possible.

COMPLICATIONS

Mortality

Despite advances in surgical techniques, mortality rates following amputation remain extremely high, owing largely to patients' pre-existing disease burden and postoperative loss of mobility. Major amputations (above the ankle) performed for dysvascular limbs have 30-day mortality rates around 8%, increase to roughly 35%, 65%, and 80% at 1, 5, and 10 years, and are higher in TFAs at all time points when compared to transtibial.[99,123–126] Minor amputations have expectedly better survival, reportedly near 10% and 45% for 1- and 5-year mortality.[127] Other commonly cited risk factors for mortality include age >74, cardiovascular and renal comorbidities, prior amputation, and dementia. Diabetes is also a risk factor for increased mortality, but to a much smaller extent.[123–125,127,128] Recent literature in multiple specialties has focused on assimilating these factors in order to create frailty indices. These scores would give more patient-specific mortality and complication rates, but it is still unclear if they have any role in surgical decision-making for amputation.[129–131] Patients who are successfully fitted with a prosthesis and who are discharged to an inpatient rehabilitation facility are noted to have markedly lower mortality rates, seemingly even when controlling for confounding comorbidities and physical frailty.[132,133]

Thromboembolic Events

Minimal and low-quality evidence exists regarding VTE following amputation, but the reported rate of postoperative VTE is consistently between 10% and 20%. It is important to note that some studies have noted a significant percentage of patients who present with DVT preoperatively, owing to immobility from their disease process. Surgeons should be cautious about aggressive anticoagulation due to the potentially catastrophic effects of a stump hematoma and the patient's high fall-risk. Although chemoprophylaxis is typically avoided because of this, some evidence suggests low-molecular-weight and unfractionated heparin are viable and equivalent prophylactic options.[134–137]

Infection

Infection rates reported in the literature vary widely, owing to different definitions of infection, as well as underdiagnosing and underreporting. Still, the rate of revision for wound complications is not insignificant, between 4% and 30%, and this continues to be the largest cause for readmission.[138] Factors associated with higher rates of infection include diabetes, smoking within 1 year, use of a drain and skin staples, and TTA (fourfold when compared to TFA), while the use of a nerve catheter, operating room time, and type of suture are not significant.[139–142] Prompt workup with CT imaging should be performed, and if possible, any stump fluid aspirated for culture prior to broad-spectrum antibiotic administration. Abscesses should be surgically drained, and if the infection appears to communicate with the bone, it should be aggressively debrided and sent for culture as well. In cases of more significant osteomyelitis, revision to a higher level should be considered, but is not always necessary if the bone can be safely resected to leave a functional limb.[143] While it is often tempting to attempt to salvage a previously successful amputation with more conservative treatment of the infection, it is wise to remember that the patient's already high mortality risk increases dramatically the longer they are non-weight-bearing, and a proximal amputation for definitive treatment may improve recovery time and quality of life.

Pain

Phantom limb pain (PLP) is experienced both acutely and chronically by an increasingly reported number of patients due to normalization of symptoms, as high as 85%.[144–146] While there is still much debate over the mechanism and risk factors, surgeons should be diligent to use multimodal pain control in the postoperative period and have a low threshold for early pain management referral. Opioids, NMDA antagonists, antidepressants, anticonvulsants such as gabapentin, and local injectable analgesics are all appropriate pharmacologic options, but should be paired with behavioral therapies such as mental imagery and mirror/virtual reality therapy, both of which highly effective in reducing PLP symptoms.[147]

RLP, on the other hand, is typically caused by painful stump neuromas, which are infrequent and occur in less than 5% of lower extremity amputations.[147] While all transected nerves heal by neuroma formation, those that become symptomatic can be difficult to treat, with options ranging from radiofrequency ablation to open excision, none of which are particularly successful. A proper physical exam is all that is necessary for diagnosis, with the most common finding being a positive Tinel's sign, elicited by reproducing symptoms by manually tapping on the tissue over the neuroma. Earlier, TMR was discussed as a method for preventing both PLP and RLP, and recent studies have also demonstrated excellent success with treating both postoperatively with TMR as well.

Contracture

Flexion contracture can be devastating to the chances of successful prosthetic fit, ambulation, and hinder positioning while seated. If a significant contracture develops, physical therapy, adaptive prosthetics, and serial casting are first line, but if the patient is making slow or minimal improvement, early surgical intervention should be discussed to get the patient back to normal ambulation. Equinus contractures may develop in unbalanced midfoot amputations, and can be rectified with a gastrocnemius recession, percutaneous Achilles lengthening, or Achilles tenotomy. Knee flexion contractures in hindfoot or transtibial amputations can be managed with a manipulation under anesthesia with postoperative casting, followed by hamstring release if unsuccessful. Hip flexion/abduction contractures in TFAs are mitigated by performing an adequate adductor myodesis, and the need for a psoas tenotomy is rare. A myodesis repair or tendon transfer may be considered but may cause more wound and immobility complications than it solves. If these strategies are unsuccessful and the contracture significantly hinders the patient's function, revision to or above the level of the affected joint should be considered.

REFERENCES

1. Markatos K, Karamanou M, Saranteas T, Mavrogenis AF. Hallmarks of amputation surgery. *Int Orthop.* 2019;43(2):493-499.
2. Celsus AC. Ad optimas editiones collati praemittitur notitia literaria studiis Societatis Bipontinae. Editio ac- curata. In: *De Medicina Libri Octo Ad Optimas Editiones Collati Praemitittur Notitia Literaria Studiis Societatis Bipontinae.* Biponti: Ex typographia Societatis; 1786:495-496.
3. Sachs M, Bojunga J, Encke A. Historical evolution of limb amputation. *World J Surg.* 1999;23(10):1088-1093.
4. Ham R, Cotton L. The history of amputation surgery and prosthetics. Chapman & Hall London In: *Limb Amputation: From Aetiology to Rehabilitation.* Springer, New York, NY, 1991.
5. Saied A, Mousavi AA, Arabnejad F, Heshmati AA. Tourniquet in surgery of the limbs: a review of history, types and complications. *Iran Red Crescent Med J.* 2015;17(2):e9588.
6. Hardy DM, Lyden SP. The majority of patients have diagnostic evaluation prior to major lower extremity amputation. *Ann Vasc Surg.* 2019;58:78-82.
7. Li Y, Burrows NR, Gregg EW, Albright A, Geiss LS. Declining rates of hospitalization for nontraumatic lower-extremity amputation in the diabetic population aged 40 years or older: U.S., 1988-2008. *Diabetes Care.* 2012;35(2):273-277.
8. Unwin N. Epidemiology of lower extremity amputation in centres in Europe, North America and East Asia. *BJS.* 2000;87(3):328-337.
9. Eslami MH, Zayaruzny M, Fitzgerald GA. The adverse effects of race, insurance status, and low income on the rate of amputation in patients presenting with lower extremity ischemia. *J Vasc Surg.* 2007;45(1):55-59.
10. Newhall K, Spangler E, Dzebisashvili N, Goodman DC, Goodney P. Amputation rates for patients with diabetes and peripheral arterial disease: the effects of race and region. *Ann Vasc Surg.* 2016;30:292-298.e1.
11. Jones WS, Dolor RJ, Hasselblad V, et al. Comparative effectiveness of endovascular and surgical revascularization for patients with peripheral artery disease and critical limb ischemia: systematic review of revascularization in critical limb ischemia. *Am Heart J.* 2014;167(4):489-498.e7.
12. Bradbury AW, Adam DJ, Bell J, et al. Bypass versus angioplasty in severe ischaemia of the leg (BASIL) trial: a survival prediction model to facilitate clinical decision making. *J Vasc Surg.* 2010;51(Suppl 5):52S-68S.
13. Rutherford RB, Baker JD, Ernst C, et al. Recommended standards for reports dealing with lower extremity ischemia: Revised version. *J Vasc Surg.* 1997;26(3):517-538.
14. Darling JD, McCallum JC, Soden PA, et al. Predictive ability of the society for vascular surgery wound, ischemia, and foot infection (WIfI) classification system after first-time lower extremity revascularizations. *J Vasc Surg.* 2017;65(3):695-704.
15. Mills JL, Conte MS, Armstrong DG, et al. The society for vascular surgery lower extremity threatened limb classification system: risk stratification based on wound, ischemia, and foot Infection (WIfI). *J Vasc Surg.* 2014; 59(1):220-234.e1-2.
16. Zhan LX, Branco BC, Armstrong DG, Mills JL. The society for vascular surgery lower extremity threatened limb classification system based on wound, ischemia, and foot infection (WIfI) correlates with risk of major amputation and time to wound healing. *J Vasc Surg.* 2015;61(4):939-944.
17. Linton C, Searle A, Hawke F, Tehan PE, Sebastian M, Chuter V. Do toe blood pressures predict healing after minor lower limb amputation in people with diabetes? A systematic review and meta-analysis. *Diab Vasc Dis Res.* 2020;17(3):1479164120928868.
18. Wang Z, Hasan R, Firwana B, et al. A systematic review and meta-analysis of tests to predict wound healing in diabetic foot. *J Vasc Surg.* 2016;63(2 suppl):29S-36S.e1-2.
19. Tay WL, Lo ZJ, Hong Q, Yong E, Chandrasekar S, Tan GWL. Toe pressure in predicting diabetic foot ulcer healing: a systematic review and meta-analysis. *Ann Vasc Surg.* 2019;60:371-378.
20. Forsythe RO, Apelqvist J, Boyko EJ, et al. Performance of prognostic markers in the prediction of wound healing or amputation among patients with foot ulcers in diabetes: a systematic review. *Diabetes Metab Res Rev.* 2020; 36(Suppl 1):e3278.
21. Coleman LS, Dowd GSE, Bentley G. Reproducibility of tcPO2 measurements in normal volunteers. *Clin phys physiol meas.* 1986;7(3):259-263.
22. Nishio H, Minakata K, Kawaguchi A, et al. Transcutaneous oxygen pressure as a surrogate index of lower limb amputation. *Int Angiol.* 2016;35(6):565-572.
23. Arsenault KA, Al-Otaibi A, Devereaux PJ, Thorlund K, Tittley JG, Whitlock RP. The use of transcutaneous oximetry to predict healing complications of lower limb amputations: A systematic review and meta-analysis. *Eur J Vasc Endovasc Surg.* 2012;43(3):329-336.
24. Christensen KS, Klarke M. Transcutaneous oxygen measurement in peripheral occlusive disease. an indicator of wound healing in leg amputation. *J Bone Joint Surg Br.* 1986;68(3):423-426.

25. Bongard O, Krahenbuhl B. Predicting amputation in severe ischaemia. The value of transcutaneous PO2 measurement. *J Bone Joint Surg Br*. 1988;70(3):465-467.
26. Harward TR, Volny J, Golbranson F, Bernstein EF, Fronek A. Oxygen inhalation-induced transcutaneous PO2 changes as a predictor of amputation level. *J Vasc Surg*. 1985;2(1):220-227.
27. Watanabe Y, Masaki H, Kojima K, et al. Assessment of the characteristics and detectability of skin perfusion pressure measured using a thermostatic heating probe. *Ann Vasc Dis*. 2013;6(4):718-724.
28. Pan X, You C, Chen G, Shao H, Han C, Zhi L. Skin perfusion pressure for the prediction of wound healing in critical limb ischemia: a meta-analysis. *Arch Med Sci*. 2018;14(3):481-487.
29. Yamada T, Ohta T, Ishibashi H, et al. Clinical reliability and utility of skin perfusion pressure measurement in ischemic limbs-Comparison with other noninvasive diagnostic methods. *J Vasc Surg*. 2008;47(2):318-323.
30. Pan X, Chen G, Wu P, Han C, Ho JK. Skin perfusion pressure as a predictor of ischemic wound healing potential (Review). *Biomed Rep*. 2018;8(4):330-334.
31. de Silva GS, Saffaf K, Sanchez LA, Zayed MA. Amputation stump perfusion is predictive of post-operative necrotic eschar formation. *Am J Surg*. 2018;216(3):540-546.
32. Hutchison D, Cuff R, Liao T, et al. Pilot study to assess the use of a fluorescence imaging system for assessment of amputation healing. *J Wound Care*. 2019;28(Suppl 2):S24-S29.
33. van den Hoven P, Ooms S, van Manen L, et al. A systematic review of the use of near-infrared fluorescence imaging in patients with peripheral artery disease. *J Vasc Surg*. 2019;70(1):286-297.e1.
34. Dwars BJ, van den Broek TAA, Rauwerda JA, Bakker FC. Criteria for reliable selection of the lowest level of amputation in peripheral vascular disease. *J Vasc Surg*. 1992;15(3):536-542.
35. Czerniecki JM, Turner AP, Williams RM, et al. The development and validation of the AMPREDICT model for predicting mobility outcome after dysvascular lower extremity amputation. *J Vasc Surg*. 2017;65(1):162-171.e3.
36. Gailey RS, Roach KE, Applegate EB, et al. The amputee mobility predictor: an instrument to assess determinants of the lower-limb amputee's ability to ambulate. *Arch Phys Med Rehabil*. 2002;83(5):613-627.
37. Malone JM, Moore W, Leal JM, Childers SJ. Rehabilitation for lower extremity amputation. *Arch Surg*. 1981;116(1):93-98.
38. Musuuza J, Sutherland BL, Kurter S, Balasubramanian P, Bartels CM, Brennan MB. A systematic review of multidisciplinary teams to reduce major amputations for patients with diabetic foot ulcers. *J Vasc Surg*. 2020;71(4):1433-1446.e3.
39. Albright RH, Manohar NB, Murillo JF, et al. Effectiveness of multidisciplinary care teams in reducing major amputation rate in adults with diabetes: a systematic review & meta-analysis. *Diabetes Res Clin Pract*. 2020;161:107996.
40. Cheun TJ, Jayakumar L, Sideman MJ, et al. Short-term contemporary outcomes for staged versus primary lower limb amputation in diabetic foot disease. *J Vasc Surg*. 2020;72(2):658-666.e2.
41. Silva LR, Fernandes GM, Morales NU, et al. Results of one-stage or staged amputations of lower limbs consequent to critical limb ischemia and infection. *Ann Vasc Surg*. 2018;46:218-225.
42. Fisher DF, Clagett GP, Fry RE, Humble TH, Fry WJ. One-stage versus two-stage amputation for wet gangrene of the lower extremity: a randomized study. *J Vasc Surg*. 1988;8(4):428-433.
43. Desai Y, Robbs JV, Keenan JP. Staged below-knee amputations for septic peripheral lesions due to ischaemia. *BJS*. 1986;73(5):392-394.
44. Tisi PV, Than MM. Type of incision for below knee amputation. *Cochrane Database Syst Rev*. 2014;2014(4):CD003749.
45. Hunsaker RH, Schwartz JA, Keagy BA, Kotb M, Burnham SJ, Johnson G. Dry ice cryoamputation: a twelve-year experience. *J Vasc Surg*. 1985;2(6):812-816.
46. Still JM, Wray CH, Moretz WH. Selective physiologic amputation: a valuable adjunct in preparation for surgical operation. *Ann Surg*. 1970;171(1):143-151.
47. Bunt TJ. Physiologic amputation. Preliminary cryoamputation of the gangrenous extremity. *AORN J*. 1991;54(6):1220-1224.
48. Winburn GB, Wood MC, Hawkins ML, et al. Current role of cryoamputation. *Am J Surg*. 1991;162(6):647-650; discussion 650-1.
49. Murakami T, Murray K. Outcomes of knee disarticulation and the influence of surgical techniques in dysvascular patients: a systematic review. *Prosthet Orthot Int*. 2016;40(4):423-435.
50. Fortington LV, Rommers GM, Geertzen JHB, Postema K, Dijkstra PU. Mobility in elderly people with a lower limb amputation: a systematic review. *J Am Med Dir Assoc*. 2012;13(4):319-325.
51. Kahle JT, Highsmith MJ, Schaepper H, Johannesson A, Orendurff MS, Kaufman K. Predicting walking ability

following lower limb amputation: an updated systematic literature review. *Technol Innov*. 2016;18(2-3):125-137.
52. Pinzur MS. Gait analysis in peripheral vascular insufficiency through-knee amputation. *J Rehabil Res Dev*. 1993;30(4):388-392.
53. Waters RL, Perry J, Antonelli D, Hislop H. Energy cost of walking of amputees: the influence of level of amputation. *J Bone Joint Surg Am*. 1976;58(1):42-46.
54. Wezenberg D, van der Woude LH, Faber WX, de Haan A, Houdijk H. Relation between aerobic capacity and walking ability in older adults with a lower-limb amputation. *Arch Phys Med Rehabil*. 2013;94(9):1714-1720.
55. Gonzalez EG, Corcoran PJ, Reyes RL. Energy expenditure in below knee amputees: correlation with stump length. *Arch Phys Med Rehabil*. 1974;55(3):111-119.
56. Waters RL, Mulroy S. The energy expenditure of normal and pathologic gait. *Gait Posture*. 1999;9(3):207-231.
57. Bell JC, Wolf EJ, Schnall BL, Tis JE, Potter BK. Transfemoral amputations: is there an effect of residual limb length and orientation on energy expenditure? *Clin Orthop Relat Res*. 2014;472(10):3055-3061.
58. Wright DA, Marks L, Payne RC. A comparative study of the physiological costs of walking in ten bilateral amputees. *Prosthet Orthot Int*. 2008;32(1):57-67.
59. Huang CT, Jackson JR, Moore NB, et al. Amputation: energy cost of ambulation. *Arch Phys Med Rehabil*. 1979;60(1):18-24.
60. Moreira CC, Farber A, Kalish JA, et al. The effect of anesthesia type on major lower extremity amputation in functionally impaired elderly patients. *J Vasc Surg*. 2016;63(3):696-701.
61. McIntosh J, Earnshaw JJ. Antibiotic prophylaxis for the prevention of infection after major limb amputation. *Eur J Vasc Endovasc Surg*. 2009;37(6):696-703.
62. Sadat U, Chaudhuri A, Hayes PD, Gaunt ME, Boyle JR, Varty K. Five day antibiotic prophylaxis for major lower limb amputation reduces wound infection rates and the length of in-hospital stay. *Eur J Vasc Endovasc Surg*. 2008;35(1):75-78.
63. Shah SP, Negrete A, Self T, Bergeron J, Twilla JD. Comparison of three antimicrobial strategies in diabetic foot infections post-amputation. *Ther Adv Infect Dis*. 2019;6:2049936119864542.
64. Johnson SW, Drew RH, May DB. How long to treat with antibiotics following amputation in patients with diabetic foot infections? Are the 2012 IDSA DFI guidelines reasonable? *J Clin Pharm Ther*. 2013;38(2):85-88.
65. Lipsky BA, Berendt AR, Cornia PB, et al. 2012 infectious diseases society of America clinical practice guideline for the diagnosis and treatment of diabetic foot infections. *Clin Infect Dis*. 2012;54(12):e132-e173.
66. Wied C, Tengberg PT, Holm G, et al. Tourniquets do not increase the total blood loss or reamputation risk in transtibial amputations. *World J Orthop*. 2017; 8(1):62-67.
67. Wolthuis AM, Whitehead E, Ridler BMF, Cowan AR, Campbell WB, Thompson JF. Use of a pneumatic tourniquet improves outcome following trans-tibial amputation. *Eur J Vasc Endovasc Surg*. 2006;31(6):642-645.
68. Choksy SA, Lee Chong P, Smith C, Ireland M, Beard J. A randomised controlled trial of the use of a tourniquet to reduce blood loss during transtibial amputation for peripheral arterial disease. *Eur J Vasc Endovasc Surg*. 2006; 31(6):646-650.
69. Geertzen J, van der Linde H, Rosenbrand K, et al. Dutch evidence-based guidelines for amputation and prosthetics of the lower extremity: amputation surgery and postoperative management. Part 1. *Prosthet Orthot Int*. 2015; 39(5):351-360.
70. Silver R, de la Garza J, Rang M, Koreska J. Limb swelling after release of a tourniquet. *Clin Orthop Relat Res*. 1986;(206):86-89.
71. Valerio IL, Dumanian GA, Jordan SW, et al. Preemptive treatment of phantom and residual limb pain with targeted muscle reinnervation at the time of major limb amputation. *J Am Coll Surg*. 2019;228(3):217-226.
72. Souza JM, Cheesborough JE, Ko JH, Cho MS, Kuiken TA, Dumanian GA. Targeted muscle reinnervation: a novel approach to postamputation neuroma pain. *Clin Orthop Relat Res*. 2014;472(10):2984-2990.
73. Mioton LM, Dumanian GA, Cheesborough J, Valerio I. 117 Targeted muscle reinnervation successfully treats neuroma pain and phantoms in major limb amputees: a randomized clinical trial. *Neurosurgery*. 2018;65: 86.
74. Bowen JB, Ruter D, Wee C, West J, Valerio IL. Targeted muscle reinnervation technique in below-knee amputation. *Plast Reconstr Surg*. 2019;143(1):309-312.
75. Dumanian GA, Potter BK, Mioton LM, et al. Targeted muscle reinnervation treats neuroma and phantom pain in major limb amputees: a randomized clinical trial. *Ann Surg*. 2019;270(2):238-246.
76. Geertzen JHB, van der Schans SM, Jutte PC, Kraeima J, Otten E, Dekker R. Myodesis or myoplasty in transfemoral amputations. What is the best option? An explorative study. *Med Hypotheses*. 2019;124:7-12.
77. Krause WR, Bradbury DW, Kelly JE, Lunceford EM. Temperature elevations in orthopaedic cutting operations. *J Biomech*. 1982;15(4):267-275.
78. Borkosky SL, Roukis TS. Incidence of re-amputation following partial first ray amputation associated with diabetes mellitus and peripheral sensory neuropathy: a systematic review. *Diabet Foot Ankle*. 2012;3.

79. Kadukammakal J, Yau S, Urbas W. Assessment of partial first-ray resections and their tendency to progress to transmetatarsal amputations: a retrospective study. *J Am Podiatr Med Assoc*. 2012;102(5):412-416.
80. Häller TV, Kaiser P, Kaiser D, Berli MC, Uçkay I, Waibel FWA. Outcome of ray resection as definitive treatment in forefoot infection or ischemia: a cohort study. *J Foot Ankle Surg*. 2020;59(1):27-30.
81. Thorud JC, Jupiter DC, Lorenzana J, Nguyen TT, Shibuya N. Reoperation and reamputation after transmetatarsal amputation: a systematic review and meta-analysis. *J Foot Ankle Surg*. 2016;55(5):1007-1012.
82. Landry GJ, Silverman DA, Liem TK, Mitchell EL, Moneta GL. Predictors of healing and functional outcome following transmetatarsal amputations. *Arch Surg*. 2011;146(9):1005-1009.
83. McCallum R, Tagoe M. Transmetatarsal amputation: a case series and review of the literature. *J Aging Res*. 2012;2012:797218.
84. DeCotiis MA. Lisfranc and chopart amputations. *Clin Podiatr Med Surg*. 2005;22(3):385-393.
85. Greene CJ, Bibbo C. The lisfranc amputation: a more reliable level of amputation with proper intraoperative tendon balancing. *J Foot Ankle Surg*. 2017;56(4):824-826.
86. Andronic O, Boeni T, Burkhard MD, Kaiser D, Berli MC, Waibel FWA. Modifications of the pirogoff amputation technique in adults: a retrospective analysis of 123 cases. *J Orthop*. 2019;18:5-12.
87. Langeveld ARJ, Meuffels DE, Oostenbroek RJ, Hoedt MTC. The Pirogoff amputation for necrosis of the forefoot: Surgical technique. *J Bone Joint Surg Am*. 2011;93(Suppl 1):21-29.
88. Nather A, Wong KL. Distal amputations for the diabetic foot. *Diabet Foot Ankle*. 2013;4. doi: 10.3402/dfa.v4i0.21288.
89. Tosun B, Buluc L, Gok U, Unal C. Boyd amputation in adults. *Foot Ankle Int*. 2011;32(11):1063-1068.
90. Malcolm-Smith NA. Syme and his amputation. *Surgeon*. 2004;2(2):91-98.
91. Wagner FW. Amputations of the foot and ankle. Current status. *Clin Orthop Relat Res*. 1977;(122):62-69.
92. Pinzur MS, Stuck RM, Sage R, Hunt N, Rabinovich Z. Syme ankle disarticulation in patients with diabetes. *J Bone Joint Surg Am*. 2003;85(9):1667-1672.
93. Pinzur MS, Osterman H, Smith D. Syme ankle disarticulation in peripheral vascular disease and diabetic foot infection: the one-stage versus two-stage procedure. *Foot Ankle Int*. 1995;16(3):124-127.
94. Dillingham TR, Pezzin LE, MacKenzie EJ. Limb amputation and limb deficiency: epidemiology and recent trends in the United States. *South Med J*. 2002;95(8):875-883.
95. Yip VSK, Teo NB, Johnstone R, et al. An analysis of risk factors associated with failure of below knee amputations. *World J Surg*. 2006;30(6):1081-1087.
96. Keagy BA, Schwartz JA, Kotb M, Burnham SJ, Johnson G. Lower extremity amputation: the control series. *J Vasc Surg*. 1986;4(4):321-326.
97. Columbo JA, Nolan BW, Stucke RS, et al. Below-knee amputation failure and poor functional outcomes are higher than predicted in contemporary practice. *Vasc Endovascular Surg*. 2016;50(8):554-558.
98. Taylor SM, Kalbaugh CA, Cass AL, et al. "Successful outcome" after below-knee amputation: an objective definition and influence of clinical variables. *Am Surg*. 2008;74(7):607-612; discussion 612-3.
99. Aulivola B, Hile CN, Hamdan AD, et al. Major lower extremity amputation: outcome of a modern series. *Arch Surg*. 2004;139(4):395-399; discussion 399.
100. Wu JT, Wong M, Lo ZJ, et al. A series of 210 peripheral arterial disease below-knee amputations and predictors for subsequent above-knee amputations. *Ann Vasc Dis*. 2017;10(3):217-222.
101. Lim S, Javorski MJ, Halandras PM, Aulivola B, Crisostomo PR. Through-knee amputation is a feasible alternative to above-knee amputation. *J Vasc Surg*. 2018;68(1):197-203.
102. Hagberg E, Berlin K, Renström P. Function after through-knee compared with below-knee and above-knee amputation. *Prosthet Orthot Int*. 1992;16(3):168-173.
103. Hughes J. Biomechanics of the through-knee prosthesis. *Prosthet Orthot Int*. 1983;7(2):96-99.
104. Pinzur MS, Gold J, Schwartz D, Gross N. Energy demands for walking in dysvascular amputees as related to the level of amputation. *Orthopedics*. 1992;15(9):1033-1036; discussion 1036-7.
105. Jansen K, Jensen JS. Operative technique in knee disarticulation. *Prosthet Orthot Int*. 1983;7(2):72-74.
106. Albino FP, Seidel R, Brown BJ, Crone CG, Attinger CE. Through knee amputation: technique modifications and surgical outcomes. *Arch Plast Surg*. 2014;41(5):562-570.
107. Jaegers SM, Arendzen JH, de Jongh HJ. Changes in hip muscles after above-knee amputation. *Clin Orthop Relat Res*. 1995;(319):276-284.
108. Theriot J, Bhattarai P, Finlay DJ. A Reevaluation of the Gritti-Stokes (Above-Knee) amputation for the nonambulatory patient. *Ann Vasc Surg*. 2019;60:468-473.
109. Yusuf SW, Baker DM, Wenham PW, Makin GS, Hopkinson BR. Role of Gritti-Stokes amputation in

peripheral vascular disease. *Ann R Coll Surg Engl.* 1997;79(2):102-104.
110. Taylor BC, Poka A, Mehta S, French BG. Gritti-Stokes amputation in the trauma patient: tips and techniques. *JBJS Essent Surg Tech.* 2012;2(2):e7.
111. Geertzen JHB, de Beus MC, Jutte PC, Otten E, Dekker R. What is the optimal femur length in a trans-femoral amputation? A mixed method study: scoping review, expert opinions and biomechanical analysis. *Med Hypotheses.* 2019;129:109238.
112. Gottschalk F. Transfemoral amputation: biomechanics and surgery. *Clin Orthop Relat Res.* 1999;(361):15-22.
113. Chen SL, Kuo IJ, Kabutey NK, Fujitani RM. Physiologic cryoamputation in managing critically ill patients with septic, advanced acute limb ischemia. *Ann Vasc Surg.* 2017;42:50-55.
114. Schon LC, Short KW, Soupiou O, Noll K, Rheinstein J. Benefits of early prosthetic management of transtibial amputees: a prospective clinical study of a prefabricated prosthesis. *Foot Ankle Int.* 2002;23(6):509-514.
115. Kwah LK, Webb MT, Goh L, Harvey LA. Rigid dressings versus soft dressings for transtibial amputations. *Cochrane Database Syst Rev.* 2019;6(6):CD012427.
116. Zayan NE, West JM, Schulz SA, Jordan SW, Valerio IL. Incisional negative pressure wound therapy: an effective tool for major limb amputation and amputation revision site closure. *Adv Wound Care.* 2019;8(8):368-373.
117. Kotha V, Walters E, Stimac G, Kim P. Incisional application of negative pressure for nontraumatic lower extremity amputations: a review. *Surg Technol Int.* 2019;34:49-55.
118. Stenqvist CP, Nielsen CT, Napolitano GM, et al. Does closed incision negative wound pressure therapy in nontraumatic major lower-extremity amputations improve survival rates? *Int Wound J.* 2019;16(5):1171-1177.
119. Polfer EM, Hoyt BW, Senchak LT, Murphey MD, Forsberg JA, Potter BK. Fluid collections in amputations are not indicative or predictive of infection. *Clin Orthop Relat Res.* 2014;472(10):2978-2983.
120. Ehde DM, Czerniecki JM, Smith DG, et al. Chronic phantom sensations, phantom pain, residual limb pain, and other regional pain after lower limb amputation. *Arch Phys Med Rehabil.* 2000;81(8):1039-1044.
121. Bosanquet DC, Glasbey JCD, Stimpson A, Williams IM, Twine CP. Systematic review and meta-analysis of the efficacy of perineural local anaesthetic catheters after major lower limb amputation. *Eur J Vasc Endovasc Surg.* 2015;50(2):241-249.
122. Ülger Ö, Yıldırım Şahan T, Çelik SE. A systematic literature review of physiotherapy and rehabilitation approaches to lower-limb amputation. *Physiother Theory Pract.* 2018;34(11):821-834
123. Meshkin DH, Zolper EG, Chang K, et al. Long-term mortality after nontraumatic major lower extremity amputation: a systematic review and meta-analysis. *J Foot Ankle Surg.* 2021;60(3):567-576.
124. Thorud JC, Plemmons B, Buckley CJ, Shibuya N, Jupiter DC. Mortality after nontraumatic major amputation among patients with diabetes and peripheral vascular disease: a systematic review. *J Foot Ankle Surg.* 2016;55(3):591-599.
125. Belmont PJ, Davey S, Orr JD, Ochoa LM, Bader JO, Schoenfeld AJ. Risk factors for 30-day postoperative complications and mortality after below-knee amputation: a study of 2,911 patients from the national surgical quality improvement program. *J Am Coll Surg.* 2011;213(3):370-378.
126. van Netten JJ, Fortington LV, Hinchliffe RJ, Hijmans JM. Early post-operative mortality after major lower limb amputation: a systematic review of population and regional based studies. *Eur J Vasc Endovasc Surg.* 2016;51(2):248-257.
127. López-Valverde ME, Aragón-Sánchez J, López-de-Andrés A, et al. Perioperative and long-term all-cause mortality in patients with diabetes who underwent a lower extremity amputation. *Diabetes Res Clin Pract.* 2018;141:175-180.
128. Stern JR, Wong CK, Yerovinkina M, et al. A Meta-analysis of long-term mortality and associated risk factors following lower extremity amputation. *Ann Vasc Surg.* 2017;42:322-327.
129. Kraiss LW, Beckstrom JL, Brooke BS. Frailty assessment in vascular surgery and its utility in preoperative decision making. *Semin Vasc Surg.* 2015;28(2):141-147.
130. Wang J, Zou Y, Zhao J, et al. The impact of frailty on outcomes of elderly patients after major vascular surgery: a systematic review and meta-analysis. *Eur J Vasc Endovasc Surg.* 2018;56(4):591-602.
131. Andersen JC, Gabel JA, Mannoia KA, et al. 5-Item modified frailty index predicts outcomes after below-knee amputation in the vascular quality initiative amputation registry. *Am Surg.* 2020;86(10):1225-1229.
132. Dillingham TR, Pezzin LE. Rehabilitation setting and associated mortality and medical stability among persons with amputations. *Arch Phys Med Rehabil.* 2008;89(6):1038-1045.
133. Singh RK, Prasad G. Long-term mortality after lower-limb amputation. *Prosthet Orthot Int.* 2016;40(5):545-551.
134. Herlihy DR, Thomas M, Tran QH, Puttaswamy V. Primary prophylaxis for venous thromboembolism in people undergoing major amputation of the lower extremity. *Cochrane Database Syst Rev.* 2020;7(7):CD010525.

135. Huang ME, Johns JS, White J, Sanford K. Venous thromboembolism in a rehabilitation setting after major lower-extremity amputation. *Arch Phys Med Rehabil.* 2005;86(1):73-78.
136. Bani-Hani M, Titi M, Al-khaffaf H. Deep Venous thrombosis after arterial surgery a literature review. *Eur J Vasc Endovasc Surg.* 2008;36(5):565-573.
137. Toth S, Flohr TR, Schubart J, Knehans A, Castello MC, Aziz F. A meta-analysis and systematic review of venous thromboembolism prophylaxis in patients undergoing vascular surgery procedures. *J Vasc Surg Venous Lymphat Disord.* 2020;8(5):869-881.e2.
138. Dormandy J, Heeck L, Vig S. Major amputations: clinical patterns and predictors. *Semin Vasc Surg.* 1999;12(2):154-161.
139. Coulston JE, Tuff V, Twine CP, Chester JF, Eyers PS, Stewart AHR. Surgical factors in the prevention of infection following major lower limb amputation. *Eur J Vasc Endovasc Surg.* 2012;43(5):556-560.
140. Hasanadka R, McLafferty RB, Moore CJ, Hood DB, Ramsey DE, Hodgson KJ. Predictors of wound complications following major amputation for critical limb ischemia. *J Vasc Surg.* 2011;54(5):1374-1382.
141. Phair J, DeCarlo C, Scher L, et al. Risk factors for unplanned readmission and stump complications after major lower extremity amputation. *J Vasc Surg.* 2018;67(3):848-856.
142. Stone PA, Flaherty SK, AbuRahma AF, et al. Factors affecting perioperative mortality and wound-related complications following major lower extremity amputations. *Ann Vasc Surg.* 2006;20(2):209-216.
143. Dutronc H, Gobet A, Dauchy FA, et al. Stump infections after major lower-limb amputation: a 10-year retrospective study. *Med Mal Infect.* 2013;43(11-12):456-460.
144. Alviar MJM, Hale T, Dungca M. Pharmacologic interventions for treating phantom limb pain. *Cochrane Database Syst Rev.* 2016;10(10):CD006380.
145. Chan BL, Witt R, Charrow AP, et al. Mirror therapy for phantom limb pain. *N Engl J Med.* 2007;357(21):2206-2207.
146. Mercier C, Sirigu A. Training with virtual visual feedback to alleviate phantom limb pain. *Neurorehabil Neural Repair.* 2009;23(6):587-594.
147. Penna A, Konstantatos AH, Cranwell W, Paul E, Bruscino-Raiola FR. Incidence and associations of painful neuroma in a contemporary cohort of lower limb amputees. *ANZ J Surg.* 2018;88(5):491-496.

SELF-ASSESSMENT STUDY QUESTIONS AND ANSWERS

Questions

1. Which of the following epidemiologic factors is associated with higher rates of amputation?
   A. Native American
   B. Diabetes Mellitus
   C. Rural residence
   D. All of the above

2. Which preoperative evaluation indicates reliable wound healing for a transtibial amputation?
   A. Toe blood pressure of 30 mmHg
   B. $TcPO_2$ of 45 mmHg
   C. Skin perfusion pressure of 25 mmHg
   D. Angiographic study showing patency of the popliteal artery and proximal branches

3. Staged amputations, when compared to single-stage primary amputations, have been shown to have higher
   A. 30-day mortality.
   B. Unplanned reoperation.
   C. Readmission.
   D. None of the above are correct.

4. Which of the following is false regarding tourniquet use for lower extremity amputations?
   A. Operative blood loss is reduced
   B. Duration of surgery is reduced
   C. Postoperative bleeding is reduced
   D. Transfusion risk is reduced

5. An example of myodesis would be
   A. Securing the fascia of the adductor magnus to the femur via sutures passed through drill holes.
   B. Closure of the quadriceps fascia to itself, creating a blind pouch.
   C. Anastomosis of the anterior and posterior compartment fascias in a transtibias amputation.
   D. Securing the quadriceps to the femur by suturing the patellar tendon to the cruciates in a knee disarticulation.

6. Which of the following amputations is not a disarticulation?
   A. Lisfranc
   B. Syme
   C. Boyd
   D. Chopart

7. Which of the following has been shown to significantly prevent or treat residual limb pain?
   A. Injection of the nerves with local anesthetic prior to cutting
   B. Targeted muscle reinnervation
   C. Postoperative gabapentin
   D. Perineural catheter placement

8. Which incisional flap layout is superior for wound healing in transtibial amputations?
   A. Burgess
   B. Skew
   C. Sagittal
   D. They each have equivalent wound healing rates

9. What is the primary purpose of performing an adductor myodesis in transfemoral amputations?
   A. Preserving adductor function for improved ambulation
   B. Preventing abduction contractures
   C. Improving bone coverage
   D. None of the above

10. Which of the following is not associated with a significantly higher mortality rate following lower extremity amputation?
    A. Diabetes mellitus
    B. Transfemoral amputation level
    C. Renal disease
    D. Prior amputation

SELF-ASSESSMENT STUDY QUESTIONS AND ANSWERS

Answers

1. D.
2. B.
3. D.
4. C.
5. A.
6. C.
7. B.
8. D.
9. B.
10. A.

CHAPTER

12 Basics on Endovascular Diagnosis and Treatment

J. Ignacio Torrealba and Mohamed F. Osman

OUTLINE

ACCESS
- **Femoral Artery**
- **Superficial Femoral Artery**
- **Popliteal Artery**
- **Tibial Access**
- **Axillary Artery**
- **Brachial Artery**
- **Radial Artery**

SPECIAL SITUATION
- **Scarred Groins**
- **Hemostasis**
  - Manual pressure
  - Closure devices
    - *Extravascular plugs*
    - *Suture mediated*
    - *Mechanical closure*
  - Compression devices
- **Equipment**
  - Needles
  - Guidewires
    - *0.035-in guidewires*
    - *0.018 and 0.014-in guidewires*
  - Sheaths
  - Guiding catheters
  - Catheters
- **Treatment Devices**
  - Balloon angioplasty
  - Stents
  - Embolization tools

MECHANICAL

PARTICLES

LIQUID AGENTS

Endovascular therapy has evolved steadily throughout the past two decades. Devised as a form of minimally invasive therapy, it has often replaced or complemented open surgical therapy. From the initial descriptions of balloon angioplasty to treat peripheral vessel disease, endovascular therapy has expanded into more complex procedures involving practically every vessel in our body. To understand and confidently manage endovascular therapy, we have to start from the basic principles and learn the different access options and devices that can be used to treat a wide array of diseases.

ACCESS

The very first step of any endovascular procedure is to choose the best-suited access for the intervention. Depending on the site of intervention, type of disease, and diameter of devices, there can be numerous different access possibilities.

FEMORAL ARTERY

The common femoral access is the most versatile arterial access.

Through this artery, we can perform upper extremity, cerebrovascular, thoracic, abdominal, and lower extremity interventions. Most of the ancillary elements for endovascular therapy have been designed with the femoral access as the entry point.

Given its usual big diameter (8–9 mm),[1] it can accommodate most devices, even large bore diameter sheaths (up to 26 Fr).

Access can be either percutaneous or open. Based on previous images or intraoperative ultrasound (US), the exact point of entry is chosen to avoid calcified plaques.

US-guided puncture is highly recommended, gaining access to the anterior aspect of the artery, below the inguinal ligament and above the femoral bifurcation (which can be easily recognized under US). In this position, the artery lies in front of the femoral head, so manual pressure can be applied for hemostasis after sheath removal. Other less-useful guiding techniques involve radiographic guidance based on the femoral head or the presence of calcium in the artery.

When the puncture is too low, there is a risk of puncturing the superficial femoral artery (SFA) or the profunda femoral artery, which can be troublesome for hemostasis given the lack of a bone prominence to hold the artery against. Such a low entry might also occlude the origin of the vessel with some closure devices (Figure 12-1).

After gaining needle access, it is important to carefully advance the guidewire under fluoroscopy and observe its smooth advancement. If any resistance is met, there should be liberal use of contrast angiography to assess the plaque burden in the iliac arteries to avoid dissections and false lumen passages. Microsheaths come with smaller and softer wires and are a good option when iliac disease is suspected.

When treating lower extremity disease, the common femoral artery is usually punctured in a retrograde fashion, towards the Aorta, and after inserting the sheath, the wire is advanced to the aortic bifurcation and contralateral access is gained. It can also be punctured under the US guidance in an antegrade fashion, pointing towards the distal vasculature.[2]

With obese patients, the skin fold is usually much lower than the femoral bifurcation and relying only on superficial anatomical features can lead to lower punctures, with the aforementioned complications.

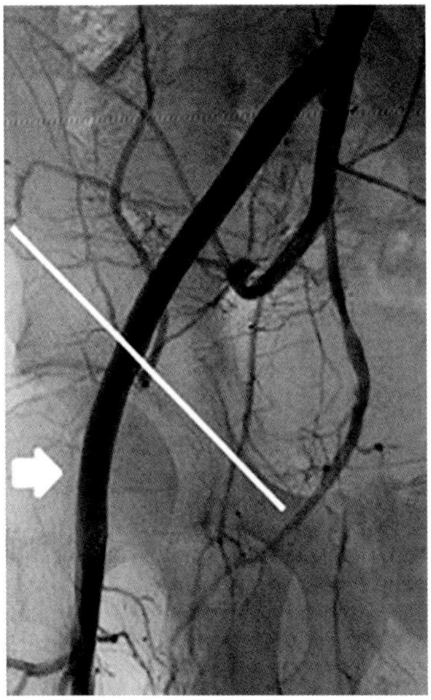

FIGURE 12-1 White arrow showing the adequate position for arterial puncture in the common femoral artery. Puncture cannot be above the inguinal ligament (white line) where potential hemorrhagic complications can occur due to the lack of bony structures to hold pressure after sheath removal.

Antegrade access affords better pushability for ipsilateral intervention but can increase the radiation exposure to the operator standing closer to the image intensifier.

SUPERFICIAL FEMORAL ARTERY[3]

The SFA can be used in an antegrade fashion for angioplasty or endovascular treatment of popliteal aneurysms, or it can also be used in a retrograde manner when extensive scarring in the groin has to be avoided. Hemostasis has to be obtained with a closure device since manual pressure often results in hematoma or pseudoaneurysm formation in this location. For the safe use of a closure device, the inner SFA arterial diameter must be at least 4 to 5 mm.

POPLITEAL ARTERY[4]

Described for lower extremity interventions, the popliteal artery can be accessed under US and used to cross femoropopliteal lesions in a retrograde fashion, especially those involving SFA flush occlusions. This access might be somehow uncomfortable since the posteriorly placed popliteal artery has to be punctured, in a prone position.

It also requires completion hemostasis by a closure device.

TIBIAL ACCESS[5]

Described for lower extremity interventions, distal access can be gained in the anterior or posterior tibial artery, the pedal artery, and even in the peroneal artery. Extensive calcification might make this access very hard to puncture and navigate with guidewires.

To avoid vessel damage, it is recommended to initially use a 4-Fr sheath inner dilator and introduce a 0.014 wire up through the dilator. Subsequently, a 0.014 catheter or balloon can be directly advanced through the artery, without the need for a transition sheath. Once the lesion is crossed, wire access has to be gained through the lesion from above (either by snaring or by balloon-assisted flap rupture and distal wire reentry) and beyond the tibial access. Wire and catheter from the tibial access are withdrawn and hemostasis is achieved with balloon inflation (Figure 12-2).

AXILLARY ARTERY[6]

The axillary artery is a readily available access through either open or percutaneous approach. This is especially useful if there is a need for multiple or large bore diameter sheaths for fenestrated endovascular aneurysm repair (FEVAR), branched endovascular aneurysm repair (BEVAR), or chimney endovascular aneurysm repair (chEVAR).

BRACHIAL ARTERY[7]

More commonly accessed on the left side, the brachial artery can also be used on the right side if preoperative images show no atherosclerotic disease in the aortic arch.

It can be accessed percutaneously or through an open approach.

The 3- to 5-mm brachial artery can accept profiles up to 6 Fr for manual hemostasis, while anything larger should undergo an open repair of the artery. Closure devices are not recommended in this location, given the small diameter of the artery.

When accessing percutaneously under the US guidance, the vessel puncture should be at the level of the elbow at the humeral condyle to obtain hemostasis after sheath withdrawal (Figure 12-3).

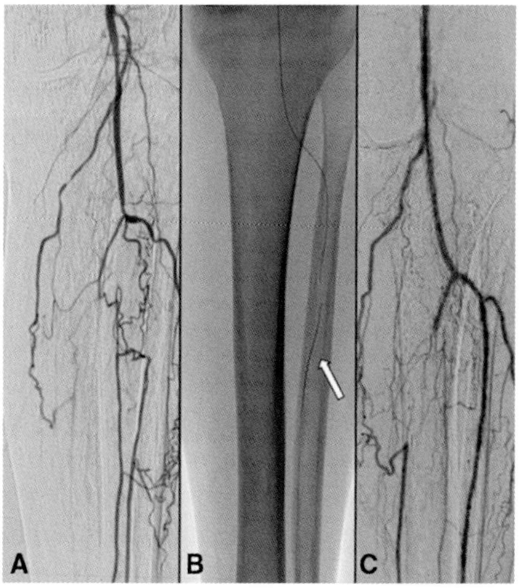

FIGURE 12-2 **(A) Left anterior tibial artery occlusion before PTA, (B) during antegrade and retrograde tibial access wire crossing (white arrow), and (C) after PTA achieved with retrograde tibial access.**

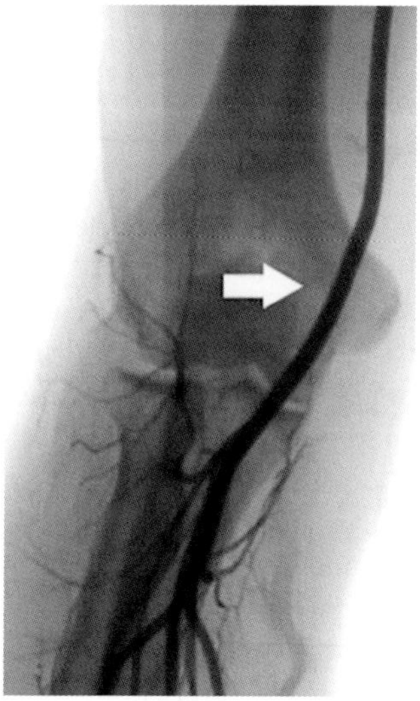

FIGURE 12-3 **White arrow pointing at the correct puncture site, over the humeral condyle.**

Immediately after arterial access, an heparin bolus is recommended if aortic arch manipulation is intended.

In case of visceral or lower extremity percutaneous interventions, it is advised to introduce a long-braided sheath into the descending or abdominal aorta. The braided configuration helps to avoid kinking in the subclavian–aorta interphase.

In case of brachial to femoral "through-and-through access", a long-braided sheath advanced into the descending aorta should always be secured to protect the subclavian origin from the alternating wire friction that could potentially "saw" the subclavian artery takeoff.

RADIAL ARTERY[8]

Classically used for coronary interventions, radial access is a straightforward access. It can accommodate profiles up to 6 fr. The radial artery is prone to spasms; therefore, it is usually flushed with vasodilators (e.g., Nitroglycerin) after sheath access.

Fistulograms and upper extremity angioplasty can be straightforwardly performed. Visceral and iliac interventions can also be performed through this access. As technology advances, longer devices are being introduced for lower extremity interventions through this access. The same principles for protecting the subclavian origin apply to this access.

SPECIAL SITUATION

SCARRED GROINS

Access through scarred tissue can prove to be very difficult. In the case of a scarred groin, some special measures have to be employed.

When using a micropuncture set, after gaining needle and wire access, the microsheath has to be introduced. There are stiff micropuncture sheaths for this purpose, but sometimes, it is preferable to access with an 18-gauge needle, so a stiffer 0.035 guide can be advanced from the beginning.

After sheath access, a stiff guidewire with a soft tip has to be advanced as high as possible in the abdominal aorta. Sequential dilation starting with a 4-5-6 Fr sheath inner dilator is done to be able to introduce the associated sheath. In case the sheath still does not track through the scar, an even stiffer wire has to be placed. Another option is to advance a low-profile crossing catheter over the wire (OTW) without a sheath, up to the aorta and then exchange for a Lunderquist or Amplatz stiff guidewire. After this, sequential dilation can be performed and access gained.

HEMOSTASIS

Manual pressure

Once the procedure is completed, the sheath has to be withdrawn. Manual compression is the gold standard to achieve hemostasis. It is advisable to check an activated clotting time (ACT) and to ensure that there is no uncontrolled elevated systolic blood pressure. Manual pressure has to be focused on the entry site, with enough pressure to stop any bleeding but without occluding the vessel. At all times, the pulse should be felt. Pressure times vary depending on the profile of the sheath, but a good algorithm is to hold 10 minutes for a 5 Fr sheath and 5 minutes extra for every 1 Fr increase. It is advisable to check the puncture site with US to ensure flow distally and to rule out any pseudoaneurysm development, especially in groins with a hematoma.

Closure devices

Several different closure devices permit obtaining hemostasis after percutaneous access with similar efficacy.[9] They are suture mediated, intra or extravascular plugs, and compression devices, among others.

Extravascular plugs *Angioseal* (Terumo Interventional Systems) is an extravascular collagen plug that 'sandwiches' the arterial wall against an absorbable anchor left inside the vessel wall. It is available in 6 and 8 Fr. The minimum recommended vessel diameter is 5 mm. The vessel cannot be re-punctured within 90 days of the procedure due to the risk of embolization.

Exoseal (Cordis): Extravascular re-absorbable plug that expands inside the femoral fascia and maintains hemostasis. It is available in 5, 6, and 7 Fr.

Mynx Grip (Cordis): Extravascular polyethylene glycol (PEG) plug that expands inside the femoral fascia (Figure 12-4). While the plug is expanding, a

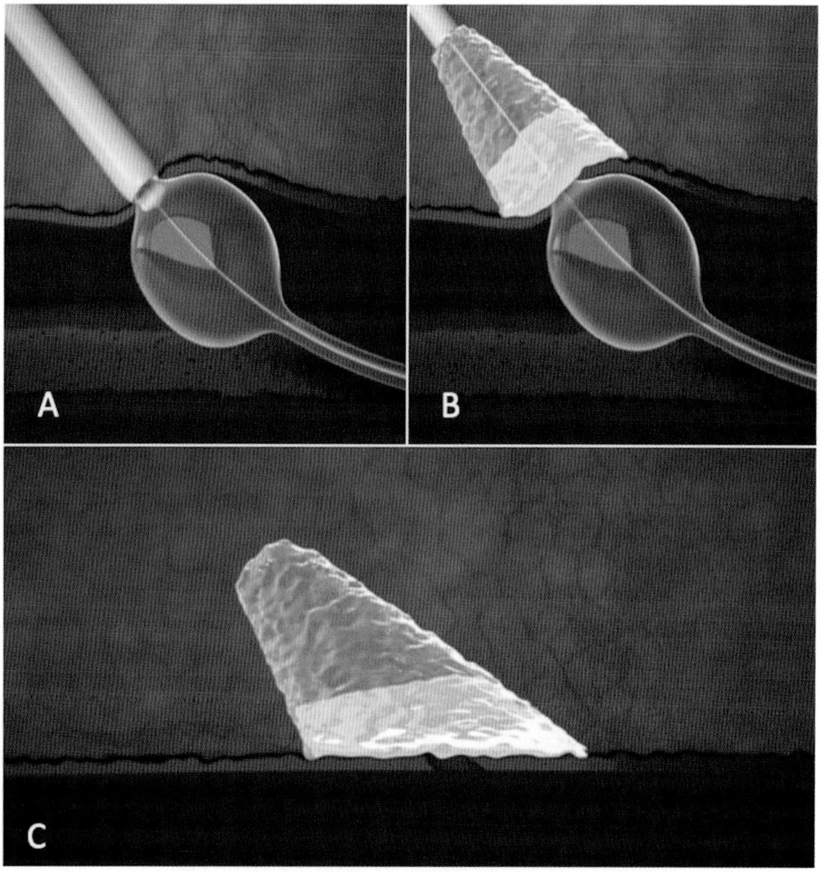

FIGURE 12-4 **Mynx device.** Once the balloon is inflated within the arterial lumen and pulled against arterial wall ensuring proper positioning (**A**), the sealant is placed in the extravascular tissue track (**B**). The sealant expands to maintain hemostasis after the device is withdrawn (**C**).

balloon is kept inflated inside the vessel to achieve hemostasis. This is available in 5 and 6 Fr.

Vascaid (Cardiva Medical): Extravascular collagen patch that expands inside the femoral fascia. While the plug is expanding, hemostasis is achieved with expansion of an intra-luminal nitinol cage on its tip that is then retracted and removed. This is available in 5, 6, and 7 Fr.

Manta (Essential Medical): Similar to the Angioseal, it relies on an intra-vessel re-absorbable toggle that helps to "sandwich" the wall with an extravascular bovine collagen pad to achieve hemostasis. The device is intended for large bore diameters, available in 14 and 18 Fr, achieving hemostasis for arteriotomies up to 22 Fr. It takes 6 months for the components to be reabsorbed.

Suture mediated *Proglide* (Abbott Vascular): A 6-Fr device, it delivers a polypropylene stitch with a premade knot that is tightened after sheath removal. In a preclosed fashion, two sutures can be deployed to close arteriotomies up to 26 Fr.

Prostar (Abbott Vascular): A 10-Fr device, it delivers two-braided sutures that have to be manually knotted. It can also be used as a preclosed system for larger bore sheaths.

Mechanical closure *Starclose* (Abbott Vascular): A 6-Fr device, it delivers a nitinol extravascular clip that "grabs" the adventitia and closes the arteriotomy. It can be punctured for subsequent endovascular procedures.

Compression devices

Femostop (Abbott Vascular): An external compression device, it consists of a strap with an inflation device that can be controlled through a bulb with a manometer. It creates compression against the femoral head to achieve hemostasis. Pressure has to be controlled and kept well under systemic blood pressure, due to the risk of femoral artery thrombosis.

Catalyst III (Cardiva Medical): A manual compression assist device, it consists of a nitinol disk deployed inside the artery through the existing sheath. It contains protamine sulfate to aid in hemostasis. The device is pulled against the arterial wall and pressure is held for 15 min. Finally, the device is withdrawn, and extra manual pressure is maintained for an additional 5 min.

EQUIPMENT

Needles

Interventions are mostly performed with 18 gauge access needles that accept 0.035 wires or 21-gauge needles for 0.014 or 0.018 wires (also called micropuncture). It is advised to use micropuncture access whenever possible and especially in diseased and small vessels.

Guidewires

There are several different guidewires. Interventionalists usually use 0.035, 0.018, and 0.014-in guidewires.

The 0.035 wires are usually constructed with an outer spring coil welded to an inner wire that can vary its diameter depending on the desired stiffness. It also can be coated with hydrophilic materials (Teflon preferentially) to decrease friction and increase navigability.

The 0.018 and 0.014 wires have only the inner wire, and the tip can have different configurations depending on the type of lesion encountered.

0.035-in guidewires There are several different lengths, 180- or 260-cm lengths are most commonly used.

Starter wires: These are soft tip wires usually used to introduce sheaths. They provide enough support with low damaging risk. They are not usually steerable enough to cannulate branch vessels (e.g., Starter, Bentson wire; Cook Medical).

Navigating guidewires: These have soft tips (either J-form or straight) and commonly have a hydrophilic coating (e.g., Glidewire; Terumo Interventional Systems) to navigate and select different vessels.

They can be floppy or stiffer. Stiff guidewires add support but with a higher risk of vessel damage. It is advised to use floppy wires for cannulation.

Support wires: These are used to obtain support to deliver different devices like catheters, balloons, and stents to the target vessel. Once catheter access to the selected site is obtained, navigating wires are exchanged for these stiffer wires. There are several different degrees of stiffness for different interventions (e.g., Rosen wire; Amplatz wire; Lunderquist wire in order of increasing stiffness; Cook Medical).

Exchange wires: These long wires, usually >300 cm, are used to get "through and through access" (e.g., Metro wire; Cook Medical).

0.018 and 0.014-in guidewires Classically used for small vessel interventions such as tibial vessels, they are also used for carotid and visceral interventions. Lengths may vary, with at least 260 cm necessary for most peripheral interventions.

Depending on the tip weight and coating, they can be navigating wires (with hydrophilic low-weight tips), support wires (usually with a floppy tip and stiffer body), and crossing wires (heavy 12 gr weigh tip, useful for crossing occlusions).

Sheaths

After arterial access is secured, a sheath with a hemostatic valve (plastic or inflatable) is introduced to act as an interphase with the blood vessel.

It has an inner dilator that helps the smooth transition inside the artery without damaging its wall. Sheaths are available in different diameters, lengths, and forms, ranging from short 4- to 26-Fr sheaths.

Sheath profile is measured from the inside diameter; therefore, the outer diameter is always slightly larger.

There are also preformed sheaths for specific uses such as the Ansel sheath for visceral or Balkin sheath (Figure 12-5) for hypogastric access.

Sheaths can be in a braided or nonbraided configuration with the first being kink-resistant but bulkier. It is important to note that any time an angulated vessel or bifurcation has to be crossed with a sheath (e.g., aortic bifurcation, visceral artery, arch vessel cannulation), nonbraided sheaths have to be avoided given their tendency to kink.

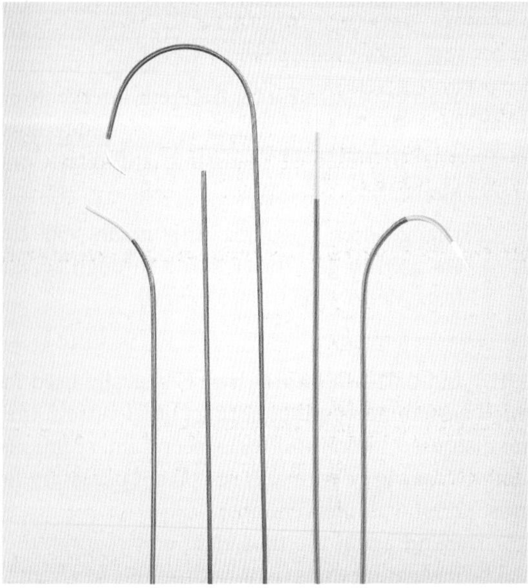

FIGURE 12-5 Different straight and preformed sheaths for vessel access. (Courtesy Cook Medical)

Steering sheaths have recently appeared on the market, allowing rotation of the tip of the sheath depending on the angulation of the vessel to cannulate, facilitating the selection and device delivery with very good support.

Guiding catheters

These catheters were created to engage distal arteries with their preformed tips and thus deliver interventional devices directly to the target vessels. Mostly used in coronary interventions, they do not have valves, so they often have to be used inside a sheath. Their profile is measured by their outer diameter.

Catheters

Catheters can also vary in profile, length, and forms depending on the intended vessel to image or treat.

Diagnostic catheters: Intended for contrast injection and imaging in big vessels. They have multiple lateral openings, usually in the last 15 mm from their tip, to allow for a homogeneous flush of contrast. They are normally radiopaque on their tip and can be marked with 1-cm distance platinum marks for precise measurements (Omniflush, Straight, Pigtail; see Figure 12-6).

Selective catheters: They come in a different array of forms, with single curves being the simplest and usually used to select vessels lying straight ahead (Glidecatheter; Terumo; Kumpe; Cook Medical; see Figure 12-7). They are also often used to exchange wires after selecting or crossing lesions.

Double curve catheters are used to engage vessels with more acute angles that are not easily entered with the single curve catheters (Cobra, Headhunter).

Reverse curve catheters are completely curved catheters that need to be formed in the aorta to select desired vessels. Most often

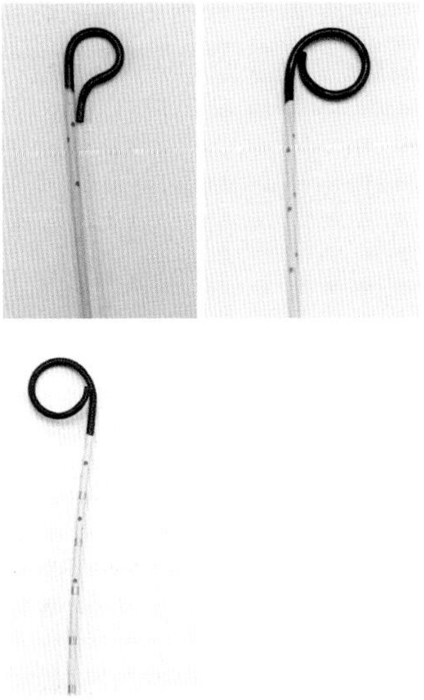

FIGURE 12-6 Diagnostic catheters. Although the tips have different shapes, multiple holes at the tip provides rapid and high-volume contrast injection. (Image courtesy of AngioDynamics, Inc. and its affiliates)

used to select caudally oriented vessels in the abdominal aorta (VS1, SOS) or aortic arch vessels (Simmons 2, VTek).

Crossing catheters: Specially designed to cross stenotic or occluded lesions, they are also useful to access angulated vessels when no extra support is achieved (e.g., difficult angle for visceral cannulation without enough wire support). There are different types and brands and they can be braided, tapered, or marked.

TREATMENT DEVICES

Balloon angioplasty

Plain old balloon angioplasty (POBA): Angioplasty was first performed by Dotter and Judkins in 1964[10] by dilation of an iliac artery. After some failed attempts of balloon angioplasty with fully compliant balloon catheters, it was in 1974 that Gruntzig performed the first POBA with a semi-compliant balloon catheter in an SFA.[11]

It involves the inflation of the balloon within a stenosis or occlusion to generate a controlled rupture of the vessel plaque, with focal dissection and "ironing" of the stenosis, allowing to increase the luminal diameter. It is important to dilate only the diseased segment, avoiding damage to the nondiseased areas of the artery.

Balloons can be found in different brands, with different profiles, lengths, diameters, and shaft lengths (Figure 12-8).

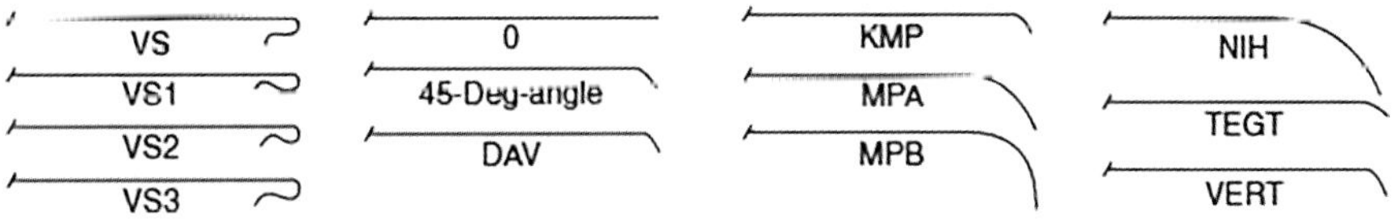

FIGURE 12-7 Catheters. Some common single and reverse curve catheters. (Courtesy of Cook Medical)

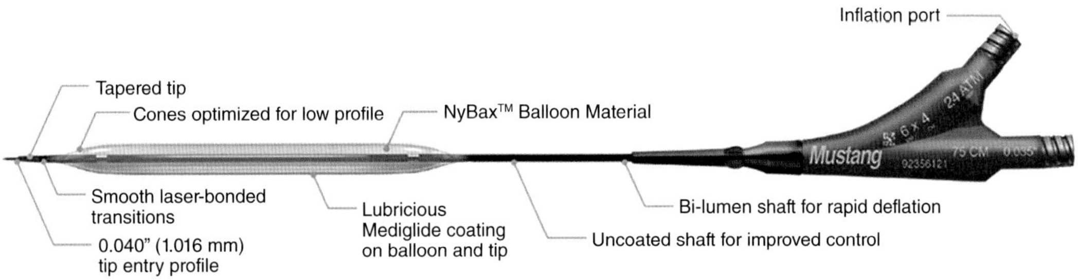

FIGURE 12-8 POBA. Illustration of balloon dilation with controlled rupture and "ironing" of the plaque. (Image provided courtesy of Boston Scientific. © 2023 Boston Scientific Corporati on or its affiliates. All rights reserved.)

0.035 Balloons: These are made of plastic polymers, available in compliant, semi-compliant, or noncomplaint configurations. Vessel angioplasty usually utilizes the latter two.

There are several different diameters from 3 to 15 mm and with different lengths.

They come in monorail or OTW configurations that gives more pushability to the system.

0.014–0.018 Balloons: These are also made of polymers, usually in semi-compliant configurations. There are nontapered and tapered balloons with different diameters usually ranging from 1.5 to 4 mm in the 0.014 profile and 2 to 10 mm in diameter for the 0.018 balloons. They can come in an OTW or single-operator exchange (SOE, or rapid exchange). SOE allows one to use shorter wires and gives easier handling, but with less pushability.

Cutting balloon (Boston scientific): These balloons have longitudinal micro-blades attached, allowing for plaque cutting and rupture in a controlled fashion. They need to be inflated very slowly to allow homogeneous inflation of the balloon avoiding the risk of vessel perforation or pseudoaneurysm formation. They come in 0.014 profiles from 2 to 4 mm of diameter and in 0.035 profile from 5 to 8 mm of diameter and 20 mm in length, requiring introducers up to 7 Fr.

Scoring balloon (AngioSculpt XL; Spectranectics): It consists of a semi-compliant balloon mounted inside a nitinol "cage" formed by the scoring components. The objective of the cage is to score the plaque, generating a more controlled plaque rupture, thus lowering the chance for vessel dissection.

Drug coated balloons (DCB): Semi-compliant balloon with a cytotoxic drug coating (typically Paclitaxel) embedded in different solvents. The objective is to deliver the drug to the lesion, inflating it typically for 3 min to achieve drug transference to the plaque. In order to avoid loss of drug during lesion crossing, the vessel has to be "prepared" with POBA prior to DCB delivery. Paclitaxel aims to decrease smooth-cell proliferation and decrease neointimal hyperplasia formation.[12]

Used mostly in the SFA treatment, it has sparked recent controversy for reports attributing higher overall mortality in patients treated with this technique.[13]

Stents

During mid-1980s, stents were first introduced to improve angioplasty results of POBA. The first were self-expanding coronary stents[14] followed in 1987 by the introduction of balloon-expandable stents (BES) by Palmaz et al.,[15] allowing treatment of recoil, residual stenosis, and dissection.

There are several different types of stents. A useful distinction can be made based on whether they are covered or uncovered and whether they are self-expanding or BES.

Uncovered stent: Also known as bare metal stent, they come in different designs, typically with struts between the metal scaffold allowing blood flow to pass through. There are two types of uncovered stents, self-expanding stents (SES), and BES:

Self-expanding stents: Most SES are composed of Nitinol (Nickel/Titanium alloy) which gives them unique characteristics such as flexibility, ability to accommodate changes in diameter, and high radial force. Usually laser-cut from a single metal piece, they re-form to their pre-configured shape and size when exposed to 37°C inside the artery. They come in different lengths and diameters up to 14 mm.

SES are crimped inside a delivery catheter. When the outer cover is retrieved, the stent self-expands. They are used in several different locations in the body, including carotid (where stents can be open or closed-cells configurations), supra-aortic vessels, visceral arteries, iliac, and SFA (Figure 12-9).

When placed in areas of bending, they might have the potential risk for fracture and occlusion (as it occurs in the SFA). New

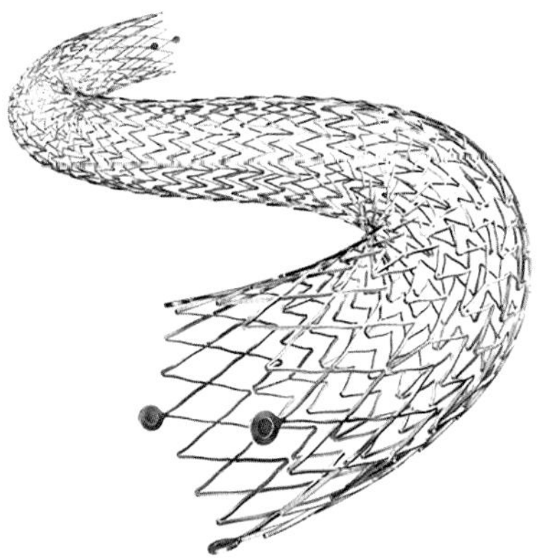

FIGURE 12-9 Self-expanding stent, specifically designed for SFA intervention. (Image provided courtesy of Boston Scientific. © 2022 Boston Scientific Corporation or its affiliates. All rights reserved.)

braided Nitinol stents have been designed to better adapt to bending areas, promising better long term results in these areas (Supera stent).[16]

Some stents have added Paclitaxel on their surface (Zilver PTX; Cook) in an effort to obtain better long-term patency.[17]

Wallstent (Boston Scientific) is one of the oldest and a different type of SES. It is made of braided Eligloy (cobalt-alloy stainless steel) wires, with less radial force than other SES but is available in bigger diameters (up to 24 mm). For years, it was the only venous stent available.

Recently, larger Nitinol SES have appeared, with diameters of 20 mm and up, dedicated to the treatment of venous occlusive diseases (Figure 12-10).

Balloon expandable stents (BES): Composed of stainless steel or chromium/cobalt alloy, they are mounted on a balloon and deployed by balloon inflation. They have high hoop strength (ability to push plaque or calcium aside) but accommodate poorly to bends or kinks. The diameter BES reach is determined by the size of the balloon used to deploy them and can be postdilated with bigger balloons to reach bigger diameters.

BES can be found in 0.014, 0.018, and 0.035 profiles. Since they do not have a protecting sheath, it is advisable to advance a sheath through the lesion, then insert and position the stent in the desired location and then withdraw the sheath before deployment.

BES are commonly used in ostial disease such as common iliac, visceral, or supra-aortic disease (Figure 12-11).

The Palmaz stent (Cordis) is a BES that needs to be manually loaded onto a big-diameter balloon. It can reach large diameters depending on the balloon size. Usually, it is used within the aorta for stenosis or type Ia endoleaks after EVAR.

Covered stents: Also known as stent-grafts, they are constructed with one or more layers of fabric (usually PTFE) coating onto a metal scaffold, making them impermeable. Usually used in the endovascular treatment of aneurysms, pseudoaneurysms, or arterial perforation, they are also useful for "bridging" target vessels to the main aortic graft in fenestrated/branched EVAR.

Self-expanding stent grafts: Composed of a nitinol scaffold with PTFE coating, they can accommodate bends and curves, with the Viabahn (Gore & Associates) stent graft especially devised for this.

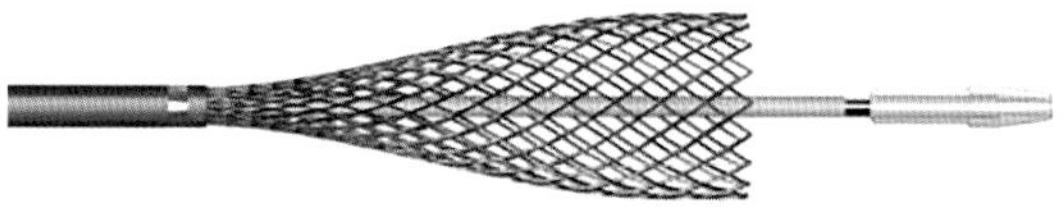

FIGURE 12-10 Wallstent being deployed. Composed of braided Eligloy. (Image provided courtesy of Boston Scientific. © 2022 Boston Scientific Corporation or its affiliates. All rights reserved.)

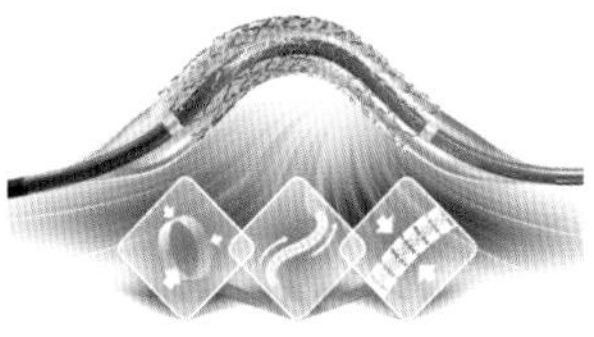

FIGURE 12-11 Visipro—an example of a balloon expandable stent. (Image provided courtesy of Boston Scientific. © 2023 Boston Scientific Corporati on or its affiliates. All rights reserved.)

One of the drawbacks of the SES stent grafts is the need for high profiles (up to 12 Fr) that can be partially overcome with 0.018 devices.

Self-expanding covered stents have been used for the treatment of arteriovenous fistulas, visceral and popliteal aneurysms, arterial pseudoaneurysms, vessel rupture, bridging stents for branched EVAR, chimney EVAR, or iliac or femoropopliteal occlusive disease.

Balloon expandable covered stent: Composed of a stainless-steel scaffold, they are mounted on a balloon and have lower profiles than SES stent grafts.

Classically stiffer than SES, new stents have emerged with better conformability and ability to reach diameters up to 16 mm (VBX; Gore & Associates).

They have been used for ostial disease (SMA restenosis, supra-aortic vessels), and for bridging target vessels to aortic grafts in FEVAR (Figure 12-12).

Atherectomy devices: There are several different atherectomy devices available. Their objective is to debulk the plaque burden in a diseased vessel. There are directional devices, with blades cutting through plaque (Hawkone, Turbohawk, and Silverhawk; Medtronic), and orbital devices that can pulverize calcific plaque (Diamondback 360; Cardiovascular Systems) or drill through the plaque while aspirating the debris (Jetstream; Boston Scientific). Laser atherectomy devices are based on high-energy beam of light debulking the plaque.

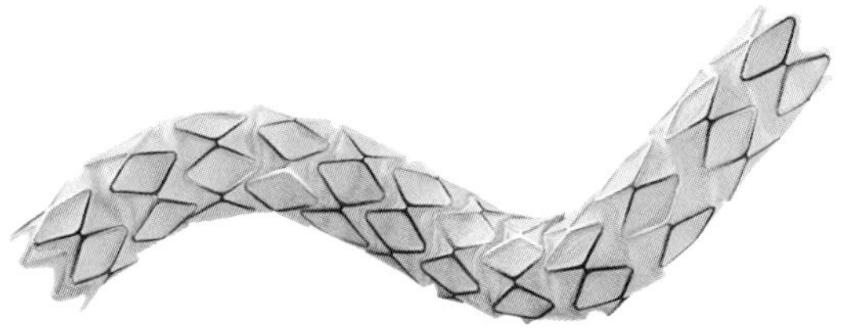
GORE® VIABAHN® VBX Balloon Expandable Endoprosthesis

FIGURE 12-12 VIABAHN—covered stent. (Reproduced with permission from W. L. Gore & Associates, Inc., Flagstaff, AZ.)

They normally require at least 6- to 7-Fr sheaths and 0.018 profiles.

Despite the theoretical advantages of atherectomy, they show similar results as "sole modality for treatment" as other techniques[18] (Figure 12-13).

Embolization tools

Embolization techniques have also evolved over time.

Several situations might need vessel embolization, such as acute bleeding in deep vessels, arteriovenous malformation treatment, endoleaks after EVAR, aneurysm or pseudoaneurysm treatment, tumor or cancer treatment, and venous interventions.

The different options for embolization can be classified as mechanical, particle, or liquid agents.

MECHANICAL

These rely on the delivery of a device that mechanically induces thrombosis and long-term inflammation leading to fibrosis of the embolized vessel. It depends on the ability of the patient to create thrombus.

Coils: Coils are embolization devices that are delivered to different vascular beds to promote their thrombosis. The original Gianturco coil was composed of a coiled segment of 0.038 steel guidewire. Coils have undergone enormous progress with current coils made of stainless steel or platinum onto which are added Dacron, nylon fibers, polyester, wool, silk, or hydrogel to increase its thrombogenicity.

There are a wide range of lengths (2–60 cm) and sizes (2–20 mm diameter when totally deployed), with a wide variety of forms (helical, conical, tornado shape, 3D configurations) helpful to embolize from small (e.g., intracranial) to bigger vessels such as the subclavian or hypogastric arteries.

Depending on the coil size, they can be delivered through either a 0.035 (catheter) or 0.018 profile (microcatheter). There are pushable coils that can be pushed with a wire or a saline flush and detachable coils, which are released once the intended position is

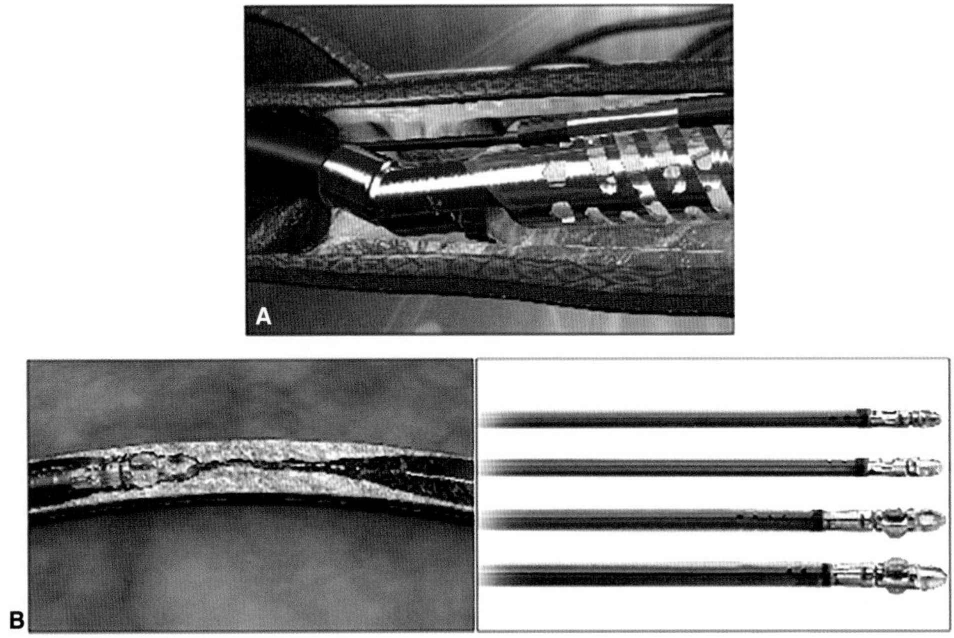

FIGURE 12-13 **Atherectomy.** (**A**) The TurboHawk plaque excision system (Covidien). (**B**) Jetstream atherectomy catheters (Bayer Healthcare) feature expandable blades down/blades up technology, enabling treatment of multiple vessel sizes with a single device. (**A:** Reproduced with permission from Medtronic, Boulder, CO. **B:** Image provided courtesy of Boston Scientific. ©2022 Boston Scientific Corporation or its affiliates. All rights reserved.)

reached, allowing them to be retrieved and repositioned if needed.

Coils have to be oversized 20% of the vessel to be effective, and on occasion, multiple coils are needed (Figure 12-14).

Plugs: Several different plugs are available to generate thrombosis by halting blood flow at their delivery site.

The most popular peripheral plugs are the Amplatzer plugs (Abbott Vascular). They are composed of a Nitinol mesh that creates a cylinder. They come in four configurations, with the Amplatzer II plug most often used for subclavian or hypogastric artery embolization before coverage with a stent graft in order to avoid retrograde flow and endoleaks.

Amplatzer plugs come in different sizes from 3 to 22 mm in diameter and lengths from 6 to 18 mm. The smaller diameter plugs are placed through a 4- to 5-Fr sheath; plugs with a diameter of 14 mm or more require a 6 or 7 Fr. The plug is delivered through a sheath into the target vessel and once in position is detached from the delivery system. It can also be repositioned, if needed, before detachment. They should be oversized by 40%. Despite being more expensive than coils, they may reduce the need for multiple coils to achieve vessel occlusion.

There are new plugs that come with a fabric lining achieving thrombosis of the vessel by stopping blood flow distally. They come in different sizes (2–11 mm) and can be delivered in 0.018 or 0.035 profiles.

PARTICLES

The first embolic agents developed were designed to be delivered in the distal arterial bed and generate stagnation of blood flow and thrombosis of small vessels. As with the mechanical agents, they rely on the patient's ability for thrombus creation.

PVA particles: Made of a polyvinyl alcohol foam sheet that is dried and rasped into small

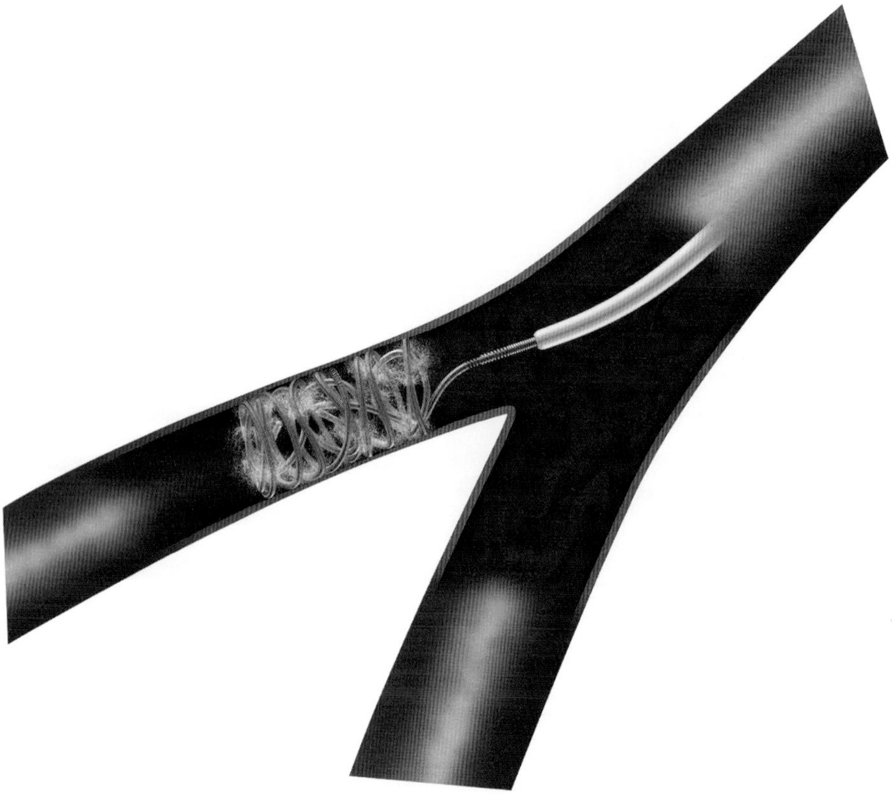

FIGURE 12-14 Coil embolization. (Courtesy of Cook Medical)

particles. They are irregular in form, with sizes from 100 to 1100 um. Given their shape irregularity, they might aggregate causing occlusion to more proximal vessels rather than just the distal target.

Gelfoam has also been used as embolic agent, in form of particles, also irregular and with tendency to aggregate.

Microspheres: Like the other particles, they were also designed to be delivered in the distal arterial bed. They have proven very useful in the treatment of AVMs, prostate, uterine fibroids, and other tumor embolizations. Unlike particles, they do not tend to aggregate and, therefore, are more accurate.

The first microspheres were made of a polymer matrix impregnated and embedded with gelatin. There are also PVA microspheres, and even drug-eluting beads (delivering doxorubicin or irinotecan to localized tumors). They are well calibrated and regular in shape, available in different seizes from 40 to 1200 um. They are packaged in prefilled 20-mL syringes with 2 mL of microspheres (Figure 12-15).

LIQUID AGENTS

As opposed to mechanical or particle agents, liquid agents do not depend on the ability for thrombus creation, since the aim is to reach the vessel, precipitate, and polymerize, thus occupying the vessel and stopping blood flow.

Ethanol: Used as a sclerosing agent in AVMs, it denaturalizes protein, leading to endothelial damage and vessel occlusion.

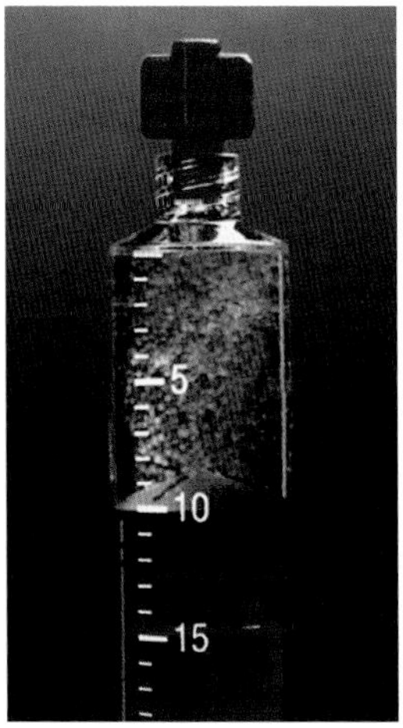

FIGURE 12-15 **A 20-mL syringe with 2 cc of microspheres.** (© Merit Medical, Reprinted by Permission.)

n-Butyl cyanoacrylate (NBCA): Initially designed for cerebral AVMs treatment, it is used in several other locations such as peripheral AVMs and type II endoleaks among others. It reacts in the presence of anionic environment, like blood or water, therefore delivery catheters have to be flushed only with D5W. It can be added to tantalum powder to allow for radioscopic visualization. NBCA tends to polymerase rapidly, so rates can be altered by varying NBCA concentrations. The faster the flow it will be injected into, the faster it has to polymerize to avoid distal embolization.

Ethylene Vinyl Alcohol Copolymer (EVOH): Onyx (Medtronic) was also designed for the treatment of cerebral AVMs. EVOH is added to dimethyl sulfoxide (DMSO) as a solvent. In contact with blood, DMSO diffuses away, allowing EVOH to precipitate and polymerize. For its delivery, Onyx requires DMSO compatible catheters. As opposed to NBCA, Onyx is nonadhesive, thus allowing longer injection times without occluding the catheter. Onyx is toxic and therefore injection rates have to be slow, with < 0.3 cc injected over 40 seconds.

REFERENCES

1. Sandgren T, Sonesson B, Ahlgren AR, Länne T. The diameter of the common femoralartery in healthy human: Influence of sex, age, and body size. *J Vasc Surg.* 1999;29:503-510.
2. Biondi-Zoccai G, Agostoni P, Sangiorgi G, et al. Mastering the antegrade femoral artery access in patients with symptomatic lower limb ischemia: learning curve, complications, and technical tips and tricks. *Catheter Cardiovas Inter.* 2006;68(6):835-842.
3. Blumberg S, Sadek M, Maldonado T, et al. Safety and effectiveness of antegrade superficialfemoral artery access in an office-based ambulatory setting. *J Vasc Surg.* 2017; 65(6S):117S.
4. Komshian S, Cheng T, Farber A, et al. Retrograde popliteal access to treat femoropopliteal artery occlusive. *J Vasc Surg.* 2018;68:161-167.
5. Montero-Baker M, Schmidt A, Braunlich S, et al. Retrograde approach for complex popliteal and tibioperoneal occlusions. *J Endovasc Ther.* 2008;15:594-604.
6. Harris E, Warner C, Hnath J, Sternbach Y, Darling RC III. Percutaneous axillary artery access for endovascular interventions. *J Vasc Surg.* 2018;68(2):555-559.
7. Alvarez-Tostado JA, Moise M, Bena J, et al. The brachial artery: a critical access for endovascular procedures. *J Vasc Surg.* 49:378-385.
8. Kumar A, Jones L, Kollmeyer K, Chen J, Richmond J, Ahn S. Radial artery access for peripheral endovascular procedures. *J Vasc Surg.* 2017;66(3):820-825.
9. Noori V, Eldrup-Jorgensen J. A systematic review of vascular closure devices for femoral artery puncture sites. *J Vasc Surg.* 2018;68(3):887-899.
10. Dotter CT, Judkins M. Transluminal treatment of arteriosclerotic obstruction, description of a new technique and a preliminary report of its application. *Circulation.* 1964;30:654-670.
11. Barton M, Gruntzig J, Husmann M, Rosch J. Balloon angioplasty – the legacy of Andreas Grüntzig, M.D. (1939–1985). *Front Cardiovasc Med.* 2014;1:15.
12. Laird J, Schneider P, Jaff M, et al. Long-term clinical effectiveness of a drug-coated balloon for the treatment of femoropopliteal lesions. Five-year outcomes from the IN.PACT. *Circ Cardiovasc Interv.* 2019;12(6):e007702.
13. Katsanos K, Spiliopoulos S, Kitrou P, Krokidis M, Karnabatidis D. Risk of death following application of paclitaxel-coated balloons and stents in the femoropopliteal artery of the leg: a systematic review and meta-analysis of randomized controlled trials. *J Am Heart Assoc.* 2018;7(24):e011245.

14. Sigwart U, Puel J, Mirkovitch V, Joffre F, Kappenberger L. Intravascular stents to prevent occlusion and restenosis after transluminal angioplasty. *N Engl J Med.* 1987;316(12):701-706.
15. Palmaz JC, Kopp DT, Hayashi H, et al. Normal and stenotic renal arteries: experimental balloon-expandable intraluminal stenting. *Radiology*. 1987;164(3):705-708.
16. Garcia L, Rosenfield K, Metzger C, et al. SUPERB final 3-year outcomes using interwoven nitinol biomimetic supera stent. *Catheter Cardiovasc Interv.* 2017;89(7):1259-1267.
17. Dake M, Ansel G, Jaff M, et al. Durable clinical effectiveness with paclitaxel-eluting stents in the femoropopliteal artery. 5-Year Results of the Zilver PTX randomized trial. *Circulation*. 2016;133:1472-1483.
18. Diamantopoulos A, Katsanos K. Atherectomy of the femoropopliteal artery: a systematic review and meta-analysis of randomized controlled trials. *J Cardiovasc Surg (Torino)*. 2014;55(5):655-665.

CHAPTER

13 Vascular Graft Conduits: Types and Patency

Heitham Albeshri and Daniel Katz

OUTLINE

INTRODUCTION
AUTOGENOUS VEIN GRAFTS
- Lower Extremity Veins
- Upper Extremity Veins
- Vein Graft Preparation
- Vein Graft Configuration

PROSTHETIC GRAFT
GRAFT PATENCY
GRAFT SURVEILLANCE

INTRODUCTION

Atherosclerosis is a leading cause of peripheral artery disease (PAD) which can be silent or present with a variety of symptoms and signs of ischemia. Ideal treatment includes a multidisciplinary approach involving the vascular surgeon, primary care provider, podiatrist, and plastic surgeon. The goal of the treatment is to prevent further progression of the disease using lifestyle modification and to reestablish blood flow to the affected end organ. Traditionally, the open surgical bypass was the only option to reestablish perfusion. Currently, percutaneous endovascular therapy adds a very reliable and attractive option with lower morbidity and mortality. Yet, both approaches to revascularization are important and necessary as part of an aggressive limb salvage program and are core skills for any vascular surgeon. In this chapter, we will discuss the different available bypass conduits, their characteristics, patency, and factors affecting their patency.

AUTOGENOUS VEIN GRAFTS

In general, autogenous conduits are the preferred option for vascular bypass, with great saphenous vein proving to be the most durable, but their use may be limited by the availability of suitable veins of appropriate diameter, length, and quality. In this section, we describe both upper and lower extremity venous options which can be used for arterial bypass.

LOWER EXTREMITY VEINS

In the lower extremity, there are three veins group: The deep veins (within the muscular compartments), the superficial veins (between the dermis and superficial to the muscular fascia), and the perforators which connect the other two groups. The superficial veins include the great saphenous vein (GSV, the greater or long saphenous vein) and the small saphenous vein (SSV, the lesser or short saphenous vein). The GSV runs between the superficial and aponeurotic deep fascia (Figure 13-1).[1] It begins just anterior to the medial malleolus, crosses the tibia, traverses medial to the knee, ascends in the medial-posterior aspect of the thigh to the groin, and then enters the fossa ovalis (approximately 4-cm inferior and lateral to the pubic tubercle) to drain into the anterior surface of the common femoral vein. The SSV begins lateral to the Achilles tendon in the calf. It runs posteriorly in the calf, pierces the muscular fascia, and courses between the medial and lateral heads of the

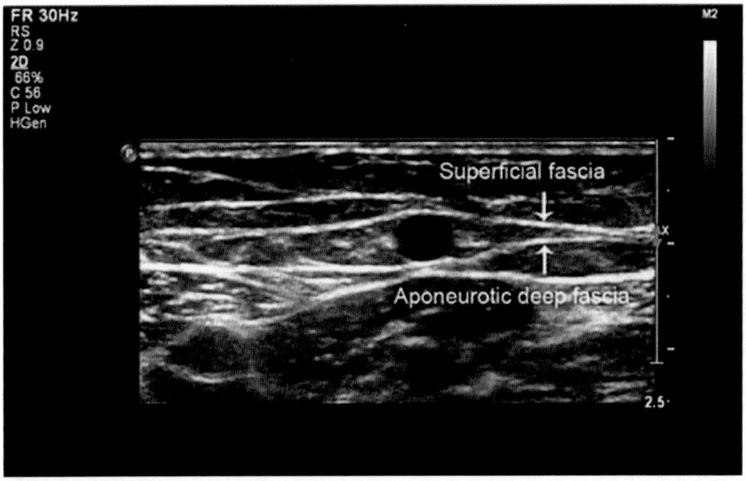

FIGURE 13-1 In a transverse view, the saphenous eye or "Egyptian" eye is featured with the LSV located between the superficial and aponeurotic deep fasciae. (Reproduced with permission from Chen SS, Prasad SK. Long saphenous vein and its anatomical variations. *Australas J Ultrasound Med.* 2009;12(1):28-31.)

gastrocnemius and joins the popliteal vein in the popliteal fossa about 5-cm proximal to the knee crease.

UPPER EXTREMITY VEINS

Two groups have been described in the upper extremity: the superficial (cephalic vein, basilic vein, and the median cubital vein) and deep groups (brachial and axillary vein). The cephalic vein starts at the posterolateral aspect of the wrist, runs across the lateral portion of the forearm, ascends lateral to the biceps muscle into the deltopectoral groove, and passes through the clavipectoral fascia to join the axillary vein. The basilic vein begins at the posteromedial side of the forearm, runs lateral to the antecubital fossa, and ascends medially in the upper arm, where it passes through the deep fascia and joins the brachial veins to become the axillary vein. The median cubital vein starts at the apex of the antecubital fossa as a branch of the cephalic vein and ascends medially to enter the basilic vein.

VEIN GRAFT PREPARATION

Preparing a vein graft for the bypass starts with appropriate preoperative planning with venous duplex mapping and critical perioperative handling and preparation considerations.

Preoperative venous conduit mapping allows for identification using a high-resolution B-mode ultrasound to determine available venous size and quality. Duplex mapping minimizes the need for dissection during vein harvest. In the lower extremity, the GSV vein is examined along its entire course from the groin to the ankle with the patient in a modified reversed Trendelenburg position to assess the diameter, the degree of compressibility, and thickness of the vein wall in each of six locations (Figure 13-2). Ideally, the vein conduit should measure greater than 3 mm in diameter.[2] Alternatively, the small saphenous vein, contralateral GSV, or upper extremity superficial veins can be used. Hence, complete preoperative venous mapping of both upper and lower extremities may be advisable if the ipsilateral GSV is deemed inadequate.

Endothelial injury during venous harvesting can induce platelet deposition and growth factors and subsequently stimulate smooth muscle proliferation and matrix deposition, which lead to early development of intimal hyperplasia.[3] Therefore, maintenance of an intact endothelial layer and practicing a harvest technique that help to reduce endothelial injury is crucial to achieve optimal patency. This should be considered during dissecting the vein by practicing "no-touch" technique as much as possible by using a vessel loop and limiting handling of the vein.[4]

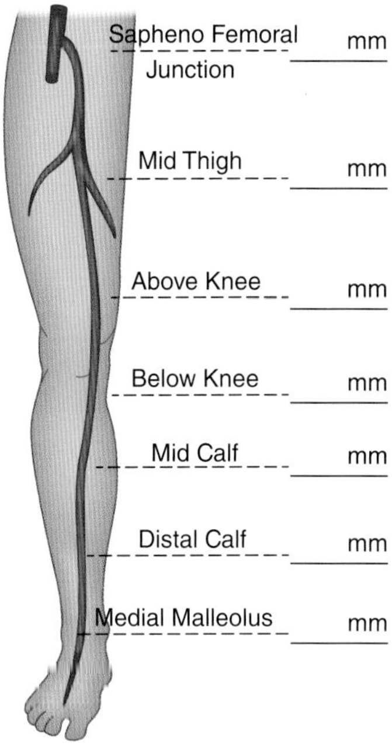

FIGURE 13-2 Location of the six standard measurements of lower extremity venous mapping. (Reproduced with permission from Seeger JM, Schmidt JH, Flynn TC. Preoperative saphenous and cephalic vein mapping as an adjunct to reconstructive arterial surgery. *Ann Surg.* 1987;205(6):733-739.)

Another technical aspect of vein harvest is to ligate branches away from the wall (about 0.5 cm) with 3-0 silk ties to minimize the risk of inducing vein graft stenosis.[5] Once the vein is harvested, minimal manual pressure distention with a heparinized buffered, balanced salt solution at neutral pH (e.g., Plasmalyte A), Heparin (5–10 units/mL), and a vasodilator (e.g., papaverine 12 mg/dL) are commonly used.[6]

VEIN GRAFT CONFIGURATION

There are three basic configurations of lower limb bypass vein grafts: *in-situ*, reversed, and nonreversed. Choosing the right configuration depends on several factors such as vein graft proximal and distal diameter with a desire to avoid size mismatch between the artery and the vein graft. Furthermore, patient factors such as obesity and high risk of wound complications can also determine the surgeon's preference of avoiding too much dissection and choose *in-situ* instead of another configuration.

In-situ vein graft technique was introduced during the late 1950s by Rob and Hall.[7] It requires only proximal and distal dissection of the saphenous vein while leaving the vein in its normal anatomical location and preserving the vasa vasorum. In addition, ligation of vein branches using skip incisions (that minimize skin complications) prevents arteriovenous fistula formation.[7] The larger caliber greater saphenous vein in the proximal thigh can be anastomosed with the larger common femoral artery; similarly, the smaller sized greater saphenous vein in the calf can be anastomosed with the smaller caliber popliteal or tibial artery. This more appropriate approximation of vein conduit to artery size minimizes size mismatch. Disruption of the venous valves by a valvulotome is mandatory in *in-situ* grafts and allows antegrade perfusion of the vein bypass.

The other two configurations (reverse and non-reverse) require complete harvesting of the vein from its anatomical bed and tunneling as preferred by the surgeon. In reversed vein grafts, the vein is harvested from its anatomical bed and reversed so that the venous valves are positioned to afford antegrade flow. In the reversed configuration, the smaller caliber calf vein is anastomosed to the larger caliber inflow artery while the larger thigh saphenous vein is anastomosed to the smaller recipient outflow artery. The nonreversed translocated technique combines a complete vein harvest from the normal vein anatomical bed with valvulotomy and is usually used with tunneling of the vein bypass in a subcutaneous nonanatomical location. Different valvulotome instruments are available such as *Modified Mills*, *LeMaitre*, or *Uresil* valvulotome (Figure 13-3).[8]

Finally, when a single segment GSV is not long enough, multiple venous segments (either small saphenous vein or arm vein) can be sewn together to create a bypass conduit of an appropriate length. It has a comparable patency with other autogenous vein grafts and is still a preferred option over a synthetic graft.[9]

PROSTHETIC GRAFT

In patients who do not have adequate autogenous vein, prosthetic grafts may become a viable option. Unlike

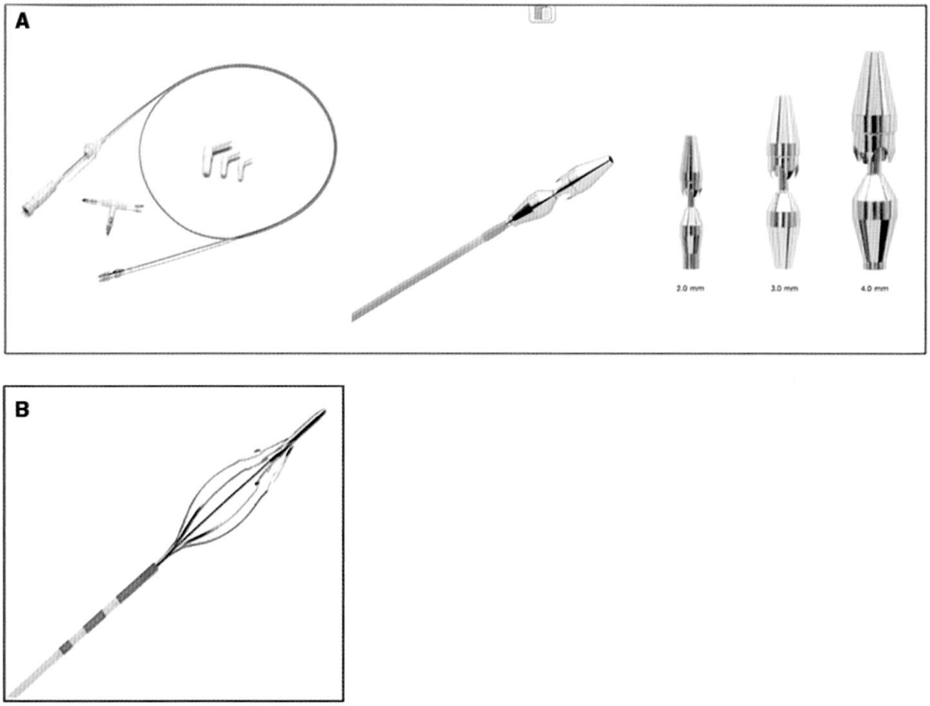

FIGURE 13-3 (**A**) *Uresil* valvotome. (**B**) *LeMaitre* valvotome. (Reproduced with permission from LeMaitre Vascular, Inc. Burlington, MA.)

vein grafts, prosthetic grafts lack an endothelial cell lining which is thought to be protective against clotting. It was first introduced by Voorhees in 1952 using Porous Vinyon "N" cloth tubes.[10] Throughout the last decades, prosthetic material engineering has advanced and a large variety of prosthetic grafts are currently available. The most commonly used prosthetic materials are polyester Dacron (knitted or woven) and expanded polytetrafluoroethylene (ePTFE) (Figures 13-4 and 13-5).[11,12] The Dacron graft has good compliance compared to the PTFE and may make it a better option for the large artery bypass like the aorta. Because of its increased porosity and higher risk of leak, the modern Dacron graft is coated with collagen to minimize graft porosity. In the lower extremity, ePTFE is most commonly the preferred option for the lower extremity bypass over Dacron.[13] External ring addition to the ePTFE provides increased resistance against external compression and using a heparin bonding to the inner layer of the graft can improve the patency of these grafts.[14] Other prosthetic options such as polypropylene and polyurethane are less likely used due to poor biostability and loss of compliance after implantation.[15]

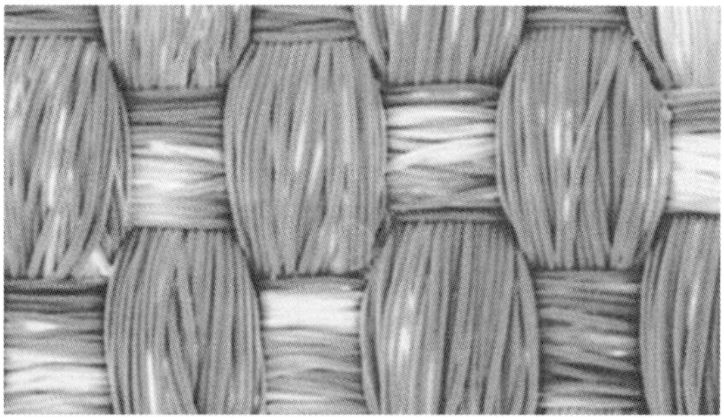

FIGURE 13-4 **Woven Dacron graft (×50).** (Reproduced with permission from Salzmann DL, Kleinert LB, Berman SS, et al: Inflammation and neovascularization associated with clinically used vascular prosthetic materials. *Cardiovasc Pathol.* 1999;8(2):63-71.)

Composite sequential grafting is another configuration option that can be used when sufficient vein length for a completely autogenous distal bypass is not available. This will use a combination of both vein graft

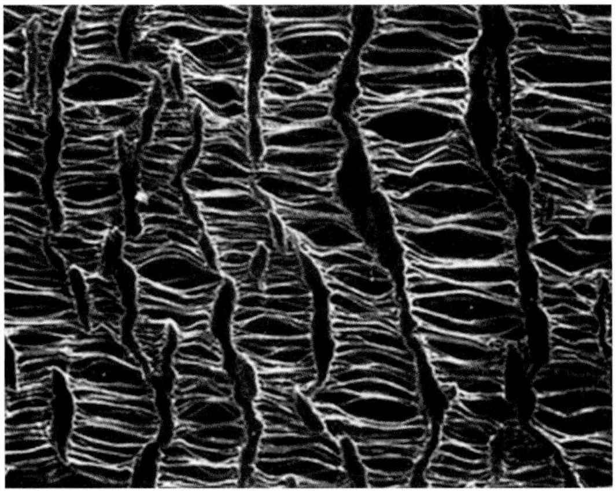

FIGURE 13-5 Scanning electron microscopy of node-fibril structure in expanded polytetrafluoroethylene grafts (original magnification ×500). (Reproduced with permission from Lumsden AB, Chen C, Coyle KA, et al: Nonporous silicone polymer coating of expanded polytetrafluoroethylene grafts reduces graft neointimal hyperplasia in dog and baboon models. *J Vasc Surg*. 1996;24(5):825-833.)

and polytetrafluoroethylene (PTFE) graft. It consisted of PTFE femoropopliteal segment (above or below the knee) and a harvested great saphenous vein graft with its proximal anastomosis placed directly over the distal PTFE hood in end-to-side anastomosis fashion and distal anastomosis to the target vessel (Figure 13-6). This will benefit from having additional outflow at the native artery and using an autogenous graft below the knee.[16,17] Finally, although cryopreserved allografts are expensive, they can be a very viable option in an infected field.

GRAFT PATENCY

In randomized and observational studies, prosthetic grafts were found to be comparable to autogenous graft when used for the femoropopliteal above knee bypass. Overall primary patency rates with saphenous vein grafts were 86%, 72%, and 51% at 1, 5, and 10+ years, respectively, and secondary patency rates were 92%, 83%, and 63%. For ePTFE, primary rates at 1, 5, and 10+ years were 77%, 51%, and 32%, respectively, and secondary patency rates were 79%, 62%, and 24%. However, for the femoropopliteal below knee bypass, the autogenous vein grafts were found to have a significantly better primary and secondary patency in short and long terms. These results were

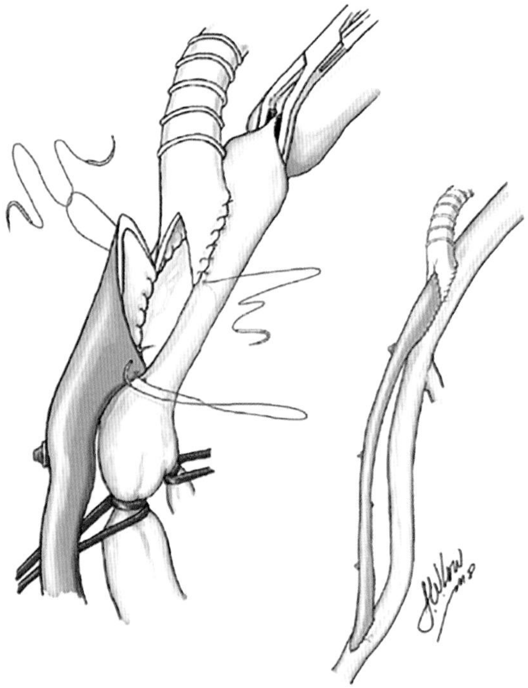

FIGURE 13-6 Drawing shows the diamond anastomosis, with an expanded polytetrafluoroethylene (ePTFE) graft proximally and an autologous vein graft anastomosed to the proximal and distal portions of the popliteal arteriotomy, respectively. (Reproduced with permission from David Low, MD, Perelman School of Medicine, University of Pennsylvania.)

also constant for the femoral to distal (tibial) bypass, where primary patency rates of the vein graft were 82%, 69%, and 48% at 1, 5, and 10+ years, respectively, and secondary patency rates were: 88%, 79%, and 60%, compared to ePTFE which has primary patency of 60% and 24%, and secondary patency of 65% and 28% at 1 and 5 years, respectively.[18,19] To overcome this inferior patency of the prosthetic grafts, some distal anastomosis adjunct configurations have been suggested like a vein patch or Miller vein cuff (Figure 13-7). Miller vein cuff was shown to improve the long-term patency up to 70% of the prosthetic graft.[20] This is due to the lower intimal hyperplasia seen with Miller cuff compared to PTFE alone. This improved patency can be explained by the reduction in compliance mismatch in Miller cuff anastomosis as it acts as a mechanical adapter enhancing wall shear stress and the elastic matching

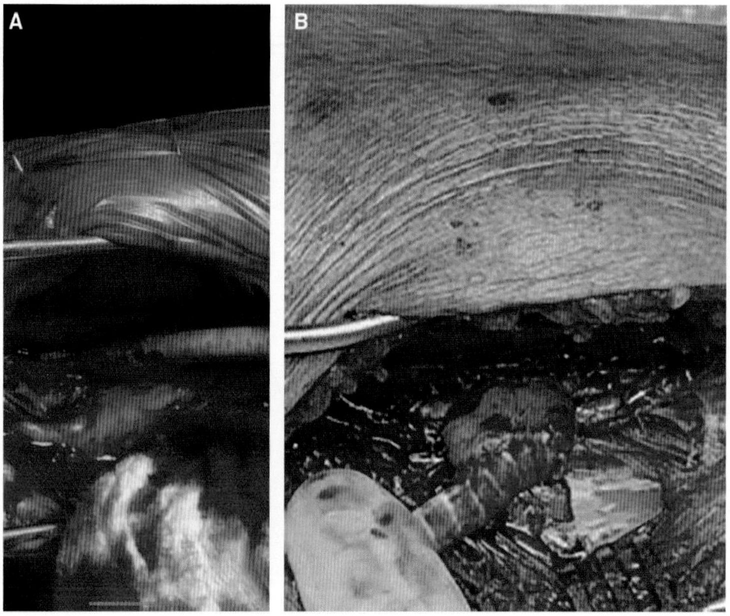

FIGURE 13-7 **Distal anastomosis prosthetic graft configuration using:** (**A**) Vein patch. (**B**) Miller vein cuff.

between ePTFE and the native artery, resulting in an early decrease of intimal hyperplasia.[21] The Miller cuff acts as a mechanical adapter enhancing wall shear stress and the elastic matching between ePTFE and the native artery, resulting in an early decrease of intimal hyperplasia.

Most vascular patients will continue on antiplatelets medication to help maintain patency of the bypass. The Clopidogrel and Acetylsalicylic Acid in Bypass Surgery for Peripheral Arterial Disease (CASPAR) trial showed similar overall incidence of graft occlusion, amputation, or death between the groups compared to single antiplatelet agent.[22] Recently, in a double-blind trial (VOYAGER-PAD trial), patients with PAD who had undergone revascularization were randomly assigned to receive rivaroxaban (2.5 mg twice daily) plus aspirin or placebo plus aspirin and showed significantly lower incidence of the composite outcome of acute limb ischemia, major amputation for vascular causes, myocardial infarction, ischemic stroke, or death from cardiovascular causes with the patient who received rivaroxaban plus aspirin compared to aspirin alone.[23]

GRAFT SURVEILLANCE

It is very critical to follow patients after revascularization. Serial arterial duplex is performed every 3 months for 1 year, every 6 months for 2 additional years, and annually thereafter. Significant proximal or distal anastomosis stenosis or stenosis in the body of the vein graft are noted to be present in up to 25% of patients. A peak systolic velocity greater than 300 cm/s or a velocity ratio greater than 3.5 to 4.0 indicates 70% stenosis of the graft and needs to be treated.[24]

REFERENCES

1. Chen SS, Prasad SK. Long saphenous vein and its anatomical variations. *Australas J Ultrasound Med.* 2009;12:28-31.
2. Seeger JM, Schmidt JH, Flynn TC. Preoperative saphenous and cephalic vein mapping as an adjunct to reconstructive arterial surgery. *Ann Surg.* 1987;205:733-739.
3. Conte MS, Mann MJ, Simosa HF, Rhynhart KK, Mulligan RC. Genetic interventions for vein bypass graft disease: a review. *J Vasc Surg.* 2002;36:1040-1052.

4. Gottlob R. The preservation of the venous endothelium by "dissection without touchin" and by an atraumatic technique of vascular anastomosis. The importance for arterial and venous surgery. *Minerva Chir.* 1977;32:693-700.
5. Souza DS, Dashwood MR, Tsui JC, et al. Improved patency in vein grafts harvested with surrounding tissue: results of a randomized study using three harvesting techniques. *Ann Thorac Surg.* 2002;73:1189-1195.
6. Zhao J, Andreasen JJ, Yang J, Rasmussen BS, Liao D, Gregersen H. Manual pressure distension of the human saphenous vein changes its biomechanical properties-implication for coronary artery bypass grafting. *J Biomech.* 2007;40:2268-2276.
7. Connolly JE. In situ saphenous vein bypass—forty years later. *World J Surg.* 2005;29(Suppl 1):S35-S38.
8. https://www.lemaitre.com/products/eze-sit-valvulotome
9. McGinigle KL, Pascarella L, Shortell CK, Cox MW, McCann RL, Mureebe L. Spliced arm vein grafts are a durable conduit for lower extremity bypass. *Ann Vasc Surg.* 2015;29:716-721.
10. Voorhees AB Jr., Jaretzki A 3rd, Blakemore AH. The use of tubes constructed from vinyon "N" cloth in bridging arterial defects. *Ann Surg.* 1952,135:332-336.
11. Salzmann DL, Kleinert LB, Berman SS, Williams SK. Inflammation and neovascularization associated with clinically used vascular prosthetic materials. *Cardiovasc Pathol.* 1999;8:63-71.
12. Lumsden AB, Chen C, Coyle KA, et al. Nonporous silicone polymer coating of expanded polytetrafluoroethylene grafts reduces graft neointimal hyperplasia in dog and baboon models. *J Vasc Surg.* 1996;24:825-833.
13. Branchereau A, Rudondy P, Gournier JP, Espinoza H. The albumin-coated knitted Dacron aortic prosthesis: a clinical study. *Ann Vasc Surg.* 1990;4:138-142.
14. Uhl C, Grosch C, Hock C, Topel I, Steinbauer M. Comparison of long-term outcomes of heparin bonded polytetrafluoroethylene and autologous vein below knee femoropopliteal bypasses in patients with critical limb ischaemia. *Eur J Vasc Endovasc Surg.* 2017;54:203-211.
15. Kapadia MR, Popowich DA, Kibbe MR. Modified prosthetic vascular conduits. *Circulation.* 2008;117:1873-1882.
16. McCarthy WJ, Pearce WH, Flinn WR, McGee GS, Wang R, Yao JS. Long-term evaluation of composite sequential bypass for limb-threatening ischemia. *J Vasc Surg.* 1992;15:761-769; discussion 9-70.
17. Rogers AC, Reddy PW, Cross KS, McMonagle MP. Using the diamond intermediate anastomosis in composite sequential bypass grafting for critical limb ischemia. *J Vasc Surg.* 2016;63:1116-1120.
18. Ziegler KR, Muto A, Eghbalieh SD, Dardik A. Basic data related to surgical infrainguinal revascularization procedures: a twenty year update. *Ann Vasc Surg.* 2011;25:413-422.
19. Dalman RL, Taylor LM Jr. Basic data related to infrainguinal revascularization procedures. *Ann Vasc Surg.* 1990;4:309-312.
20. Miller JH, Foreman RK, Ferguson L, Faris I. Interposition vein cuff for anastomosis of prosthesis to small artery. *Aust N Z J Surg.* 1984;54:283-285.
21. Cabrera Fischer EI, Bia Santana D, Cassanello GL, et al. Reduced elastic mismatch achieved by interposing vein cuff in expanded polytetrafluoroethylene femoral bypass decreases intimal hyperplasia. *Artif Organs.* 2005;29:122-130.
22. Thomson L. Review of an article: Results of the randomized, placebo-controlled clopidogrel and acetylsalicylic acid in bypass surgery for peripheral arterial disease (CASPAR) trial. Jill J.F. Belch, MD, FRCP, John Dormandy, MD, FRCS, and the CASPAR Writing Committee, Dundee and London, United Kingdom (*J Vasc Surg.* 2010,52:825-33). *J Vasc Nurs.* 2012;30:29-30.
23. Bonaca MP, Bauersachs RM, Anand SS, et al. Rivaroxaban in peripheral artery disease after revascularization. *N Engl J Med.* 2020;382:1994-2004.
24. Olojugba DH, McCarthy MJ, Naylor AR, Bell PR, London NJ. At what peak velocity ratio value should duplex-detected infrainguinal vein graft stenoses be revised? *Eur J Vasc Endovasc Surg.* 1998;15:258-260.

SELF-ASSESSMENT STUDY QUESTIONS AND ANSWERS

Questions

1. Which of the following is an example of lower extremity superficial vein?
A. Popliteal vein
B. Deep femoral vein
C. Basilic vein
D. Great saphenous vein
E. Brachial vein

2. A 63-year-old male with nonhealing lower leg wound. In preparation of femoral to below knee popliteal bypass using saphenous vein, which of the following is a critical step to perform this procedure?
A. Arterial duplex of the lower leg to assist size of the artery.
B. Upper and lower extremity vein mapping.
C. ESR and CRP to rule out vasculitis.
D. Lower leg venous duplex to rule out reflux disease.
E. Carotid duplex scan.

3. Which of the following is true about small saphenous vein?
A. It begins behind the knee and runs distally to the ankle.
B. It runs at the medial aspect of the thigh.
C. It courses between the medial and lateral heads of the gastrocnemius
D. It cannot be used as a conduit for arterial bypass.
E. It is part of the lower leg deep vein system.

4. Which of the following is found to induce endothelial injury during venous harvesting?
A. Practicing "no-touch" technique as much as possible.
B. Using minimal manual pressure distention with a heparinized balanced salt solution.
C. Ligate the vein branches as close as possible from the wall.
D. Placing the harvested vein in a well-balanced solution at neutral PH
E. Using heparin (5–10 units/mL) and a vasodilator (e.g., papaverine 12 mg/dL) in the harvesting solution.

5. One-year primary patency of femoral below the knee bypass of autogenous vein vs PTFE prosthetic graft?
A. 60% vs 79%
B. 90% vs 50%
C. 80% vs 60%
D. 55% vs 68%
E. No studies show patency rates

SELF-ASSESSMENT STUDY QUESTIONS AND ANSWERS

Answers

1. D.

2. B.

3. C.

4. C.

5. C.

CHAPTER

14 Complex Regional Pain Syndrome

Ahmed Bosaily and Munier Nazzal

OUTLINE

OVERVIEW AND HISTORY
PATHOPHYSIOLOGY
CLINICAL FINDINGS
DIFFERENTIAL DIAGNOSIS
DIAGNOSIS
MANAGEMENT OF THE CRPS
SUMMARY

OVERVIEW AND HISTORY

Complex regional pain syndrome (CRPS), in the past known as reflex sympathetic dystrophy (RSD), is characterized by severe pain, swelling, skin color change, limited range of motion, vasomotor instability, and bone demineralization usually that affects the limbs.

First was described in the sixteenth century by a French surgeon and barber; he described severe and persistent pain syndrome in the limbs after phlebotomy.[1] In 1864, Silas Weir Mitchell reported a specific type of pain that resulted from penetrating wounds during the civil war, which was the first description of the syndrome in North America.[1] In 1872, Mitchell named this finding with the term causalgia. Sudeck's atrophy was described in 1900. He described posttraumatic bone atrophy. RSD was described by Evans in 1946.[2]

After that, multiple articles were published with different names for the same presentation until 1993, when the International Association for the Study of Pain (IASP) reviewed the nomenclature and developed criteria. In 1994, a new nomenclature was developed, CRPS, noting that it is a complex disorder, which tends to begin in a region of the body, usually the distal aspect of an extremity, where the pain is a necessary component with a presentation of a variety of clinical symptoms.

The etiology of CRPS is unknown, but it can be precipitated by trauma, including fractures, crush injuries, sprain, or surgery. In a retrospective study of 74 cases of CRPS, the most frequent reported etiologies were fractures (46%) and sprain (12%).[3]

PATHOPHYSIOLOGY

The pathophysiology of CRPS is not well known and seems to be multifactorial. Some proposed mechanisms include inflammation of deep tissue, neurogenic, and/or changes in pain perception in the Central Nervous System.[4] A significant increase in proinflammatory cytokines IL-beta, IL-2, IL-6, and TNF-alfa occurs in the affected tissue, plasma, and CSF.[5–8]

Marinus J et al. found that IL-8 elevated in the blood during the acute phase of CRPS. During the chronic phase, several proinflammatory mediators, including TNFα, interferon-γ (IFNγ), IL-2, monocyte chemoattractant protein-1 (MCP-1), and bradykinin increased. Also, IL-6, MCP-1, and macrophage inflammatory protein 1β (MIP-1β) were found in the affected limb.[8]

With neurogenic inflammation, neuropeptides may be released, including substance P, neuropeptide Y, and calcitonin gene-related peptide. Pain can be explained on the basis of central sensitization, where the activity of nociceptive afferent signals increases.[4] In a study by Birklein et al. of 145 patients with CRPS found that 97% of patients manifested motor dysfunction such as tremors, exaggerated reflexes, dystonia, and myoclonic jerks.[9] However, a systematic review revealed that there was no notable change in the motor cortex of the affected limb.[10] The sympathetic nervous system dysfunction plays a role in many chronic CRPS patients.[11] Autonomic dysfunction can cause local or systematic manifestations like hyper or hypohidrosis, skin color changes, or differences in extremity temperature.[12] Systematically, it can cause increased heart rate, reduced heart rate variability, and impaired orthostatic response in the acute warm phase of CRPS, norepinephrine release decreases from the sympathetic fiber. This causes an increase in cutaneous blood flow. However, in the cold, chronic phase, blood flow decreases because of increased α-adrenoceptors sensitivity to circulating catecholamines.[13]

Psychological and genetic factors might play a role in pathogenesis, especially HLA-DQ1.[14] A multicentric study and a systemic review concluded that there was no association with a specific personality or the presence of psychological predictors of the CRPS.[15,16] However, patients with certain psychological conditions with coping problems may overreact to pain. In general, the underlying mechanism for developing CRPS involves abnormal neuronal transmission, central sensitization, and autonomic dysregulation.

CLINICAL FINDINGS

Symptoms of CRPS include pain, sensitivity loss, motor symptoms, autonomic symptoms, and trophic changes in the affected extremities. The pain is regional to specific areas and not related to nerve dermatomes, usually having a distal predominance of abnormal sensory, motor, pseudo motor, vasomotor, and/or trophic findings.[17] The syndrome is divided into two types. CRPS type 1, formerly known as reflex sympathetic dystrophy (RSD), and CRPS type 2, formerly known as causalgia.[18] While both types occur typically after trauma, the key distinguishing feature is the presence of a definite nerve injury, which is absent in type 1, but present in type 2 CRPS.

There are two phases of CRPS based on symptoms: First, acute inflammation or "warm" phase, during which the affected limb shows classical signs of inflammation.[19] Symptoms usually appear distally to the area of trauma like a glove or stocking.[20] Patients usually describe a constant, deep pain that exacerbates with movement or temperature changes.[21] The second, chronic, or "cold" phase starts 6 months after the inflammation phase. The quality of pain is different, more persistent while resting, and challenging to treat. Muscular spasms may be experienced by some patients.[20]

DIFFERENTIAL DIAGNOSIS

CRPS is difficult to diagnose with certainty. It is a clinical diagnosis whose symptoms can be part of other clinical conditions. The risk of both overdiagnosis and under-diagnosis is present due to the nonspecificity of symptoms. It is a diagnosis of exclusion. The differential diagnosis includes a number of clinical conditions such as neuropathy of the small or large fiber sensorimotor type, cellulitis, Reynaud's disease, vascular insufficiency, vasculitis, and erythromyalgia. Other conditions that should be ruled out include central nerve system stroke, neoplasm, encephalitis, and spinal cord disease such as trauma, myelitis, syringomyelia. Additionally, multiple sclerosis and poliomyelitis can present with similar symptoms. Generally, the differential diagnosis can be divided into central nerve lesions such as spinal tumors, peripheral nervous system lesions, connective tissue disorders, inflammatory disorders, vascular disease, or malignancy. Peripheral nervous system lesions, including nerve compression in cervicobrachial or lumbosacral plexus, acute sensory polyneuropathy, neuritis, autoimmune (e.g., posttraumatic vasculitis), and infectious (e.g., borreliosis). Inflammatory conditions include cellulitis, myositis, vasculitis, arthritis, osteomyelitis, and fasciitis. Vascular conditions include traumatic vasospasm, vasculitis, arterial insufficiency, thrombosis, Raynaud's syndrome, thromboangiitis obliterans (Buerger's syndrome), lymphedema, and secondary erythromelalgia. While malignant conditions include conditions such as Pancoast tumor/paraneoplastic syndrome.

The multiplicity of conditions explains the difficulty in reaching a diagnosis and the fact that CRPS is a diagnosis of exclusion.

DIAGNOSIS

The diagnosis of CRPS is difficult, mostly clinical, and is based on excluding other potential causes of the symptoms. There is no definitive diagnostic test (Figure 14-1).[22] Certain tests have been described to be useful in confirming a diagnosis of CRPS, most importantly, three-phase bone scintigraphy. Others include side-by-side radiographs and skin temperature measurements.[23]

The Budapest consensus panel proposed a set of clinical criteria that help in the diagnosis of CRPS. The sensitivity of those criteria is 85%, and the specificity is 70% (Table 14-1). The basic symptom includes continuing pain which is out of proportion to a causative event with a number of symptoms and signs. As shown in the finger patients should report at least one symptom and display 1 sign at the time of evaluation in two or more categories in Table 14-1.

MANAGEMENT OF THE CRPS

A multidisciplinary approach is suggested for the management of CRPS.[23] The earlier the treatment is administered, the better the result is, that is, before radiological changes are seen.[24] All treatment options aim to decrease symptoms and restore the functionality of the affected limb as no definitive treatment exists.

Treatment options (Table 14-2) include psychosocial and behavioral management, physical and

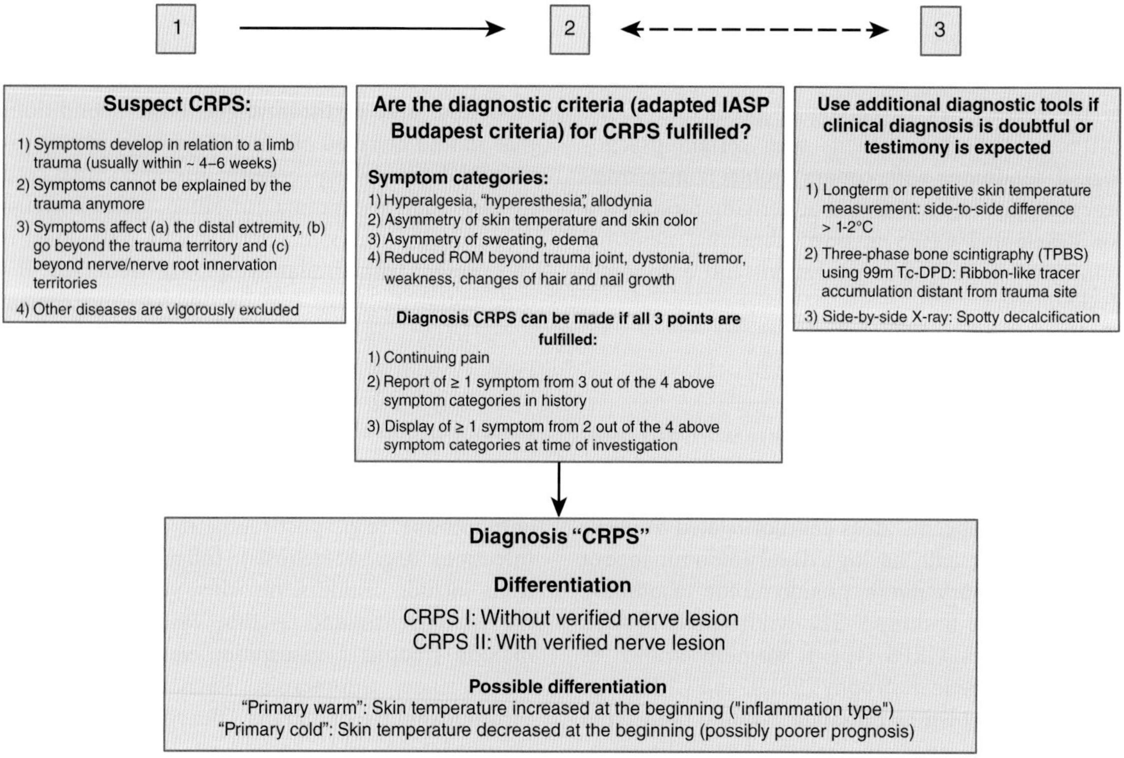

FIGURE 14-1 Rational diagnostic approach to complex regional pain syndrome. (Reproduced with permission from Birklein F, O'Neill D, Schlereth T. Complex regional pain syndrome: an optimistic perspective. *Neurology*. 2015;84(1):89-96.)

TABLE 14-1 The Budapest Criteria for Complex Regional Pain Syndrome (CRPS)

Patient should have continuous pain disproportional to the inciting event and:
1. At least one symptom in ≥3 of the following categories: • **Sensory** (hyperesthesia, allodynia) • **Vasomotor** (temperature asymmetry, skin colour changes, skin color asymmetry) • **Sudomotor/Edema** (edema, sweating changes, sweating asymmetry) • **Motor/Trophic** (decreased range of motion, weakness, tremor, dystonia, trophic changes affecting the skin, nails, hair)
2. At least one sign present upon evaluationin ≥2 of the following categories : • **Sensory** (Evidence of hyperalgesia and/or allodynia) • **Vasomotor** (Evidence of temperature asymmetry and/or skin color changes/asymmetry • **Sudomotor/Edema** (Evidence of edema and/or sweating changes/asymmetry) • **Motor/Trophic** (Evidence of decreased range of motion and/or weakness, tremor, dystonia and/or trophic changes affecting the skin, nails, hair)
Absence of another diagnosis that would better explain the symptoms and signs
A patient is diagnosed with CRPS, if all four criteria are met. For research classification, at least one symptom from all four categories and at least one sign from all categories should be attested.

TABLE 14-2 Summary for Treatment Options for CRPS

Pharmacological treatments:	• A nonsteroidal anti-inflammatory drugs (NSAIDs) • An anticonvulsant, such as gabapentin or pregabalin • A tricyclic or other antidepressant drug that is effective for neuropathic pain • Bisphosphonates • Topical lidocaine cream
Psychosocial and behavioral management.	
Physical Therapy (PT)and occupational therapy (OT).	
Interventional procedures:	• Trigger/tender point injections • Regional sympathetic nerve block • Spinal cord stimulation • Epidural clonidine • Chemical or mechanical sympathectomy

occupational therapy, pharmacologic approaches (nonsteroidal anti-inflammatory drugs (NSAIDs), anticonvulsants such as gabapentin or pregabalin, tricyclic or other antidepressant drugs that are effective for neuropathies pain, bisphosphonates, topical lidocaine cream, and interventional procedures (trigger/tender point injections, regional sympathetic nerve blocks, spinal cord stimulation, epidural clonidine, and chemical or mechanical sympathectomy). Therapy options differ from case to case. In general, physical therapy (PT) and occupational therapy (OT) are considered first-line treatments for CRPS.[23]

The intravenous regional block involves the injection of therapeutic agents directly into the venous circulation of the affected limb after sparing the circulation with a tourniquet. Only one study reported an increased analgesic duration using local analgesia with bretylium.[25]

Sympathetic block (stellate ganglion, thoracic, and lumbar sympathetic chains) was targeted in multiple studies as a treatment option for CRPS. Multiple randomized controlled trials reported a beneficial effect of the sympathetic block. In children lumbar sympathetic block with lower limb CRPS for a short duration (<12 hours) while a longer duration of action in adults with upper limb CRPS (12 months) with thoracic sympathetic block. Continuous infraclavicular brachial plexus blocks may offer an exciting alternative to stellate ganglion blocks. Compared to the conventional landmark-based technique, ultrasound guidance can increase the analgesic duration of stellate ganglion blocks.[26]

TABLE 14-3 Summary of Randomized Hyperbaric Oxygen Therapy in CRPS

Name of Study	Type of Study	Number of Patients	Type of Intervention
Tuter et al.: The treatment of a complex regional pain syndrome[28]	Prospective	35	20 patients treated with HBOT 15 patients treated with caffetin
Kiralp et al.: Effectiveness of hyperbaric oxygen therapy in the treatment of complex regional pain syndrome[25]	Double-blinded, randomized control study	71	37 patients treated with HBOT 34 patients treated with normal air

The 2013 Cochrane Review of Interventions for CRPS concluded that although a broad range of therapeutic approaches have been proposed for the treatment of CRPS pain and disability, there is a critical lack of high-quality evidence evaluating the effectiveness of most of these therapies.[27]

Hyperbaric oxygen therapy (HBOT) was suggested as a potential treatment for CRPS in a number of randomized studies (Table 14-3). The results showed HBOT decreased pain and wrist edema while increasing wrist flexion. There was no effect on wrist extension.[29] HBOT is an intermittent inhalation of 100% oxygen in a hyperbaric chamber at a pressure higher than one absolute atmosphere (1 ATA = 760 mmHg, the normal atmospheric pressure at sea level). Multiple treatment pressures suggested ranging from 1 to 3 ATA. The duration of an HBOT treatment session varies from 30 to 120 minutes. CRPS is not an accepted indication for HBOT. With HBOT, the dissolved oxygen increases to 6 mL/dL. Both tissue hypoxia and acidosis are considered as contributing mechanisms for CRPS symptoms. In addition, hypoxia contributes to atrophy and ulceration in chronic CRPS, while acidosis increases the pain perception in affected limbs. Using HBOT improves both hypoxia and acidosis, and this may contribute to its effectiveness. Another suggested mechanism is related to hyperoxia-induced vasoconstriction locally, which leads to a decrease in vasogenic edema.

SUMMARY

CRPS presented itself with multiple symptoms with a wide range of differential diagnoses including central nervous system conditions, peripheral conditions, inflammatory conditions, vasculitis, and vascular disease. The constellation of symptoms and signs are on the basic principles behind the diagnosis of CRPS. The treatment of this condition is multifactorial with variable responses to treatment. It is a diagnosis of exclusion with no diagnostic test that can be used to prove or disprove the diagnosis. Management is multidisciplinary and might include different modalities from chemical therapy, nerve block, psychological therapy, surgical intervention in the form of sympathectomy, and hyperbaric oxygen therapy.

REFERENCES

1. Feliu MH, Edwards CL. Psychologic factors in the development of complex regional pain syndrome: history, myth, and evidence. *Clin J Pain*. 2010;26(3):258-263.
2. Gellman H. Reflex sympathetic dystrophy: alternative modalities for pain management. *AAOS Instr Course Lect*. 2000;49:549-557.
3. Sandroni P, Benrud-Larson LM, McClelland RL, Low PA. Complex regional pain syndrome type I: incidence and prevalence in Olmsted county, a population-based study. *Pain*. 2003;103(1-2):199-207.

Result	Strength	Weakness
HBOT decreased pain intensity and edema with an increase in ROM. Increase quality of life from 56% to 63%.	Prospective	Not enough data about randomization, patient age, and health condition Small population
HBOT decreased the wrist pain and edema with an increase in wrist flexion.	Randomized Double blinded Prospective	Small population Young and healthy sample Short time between injury and receiving treatment (1.5 months)

4. Bussa M, Guttilla D, Lucia M, Mascaro A, Rinaldi S. Complex regional pain syndrome type I: a comprehensive review. *Acta Anaesthesiol Scand.* 2015;59(6):685-697.
5. Munnikes RJ, Muis C, Boersma M, Heijmans-Antonissen C, Zijlstra FJ, Huygen FJ. Intermediate stage complex regional pain syndrome type 1 is unrelated to proinflammatory cytokines. *Mediators Inflamm.* 2005;2005(6):366-372.
6. Alexander GM, van Rijn MA, van Hilten JJ, Perreault MJ, Schwartzman RJ. Changes in cerebrospinal fluid levels of pro-inflammatory cytokines in CRPS. *Pain.* 2005;116(3):213-219.
7. Uçeyler N, Eberle T, Rolke R, Birklein F, Sommer C. Differential expression patterns of cytokines in complex regional pain syndrome. *Pain.* 2007;132(1-2):195-205.
8. Parkitny L, McAuley JH, Di Pietro F, et al. Inflammation in complex regional pain syndrome: a systematic review and meta-analysis. *Neurology.* 2013;80(1):106-117.
9. Maihofner C, Baron R, DeCol R, et al. The motor system shows adaptive changes in complex regional pain syndrome. *Brain.* 2007;130:2671-2687.
10. Di Pietro F, McAuley J, Parkitny L, et al. Primary motor cortex function in complex regional pain syndrome: A systematic review and meta-analysis. *J Pain.* 2013;14:1270-1288.
11. Vogel T, Gradl G, Ockert B, et al. Sympathetic dysfunction in long-term complex regional pain syndrome. *Clin J Pain.* 2010;26:128-131.
12. Urits I, Shen A, Jones M, Viswanath O, Kaye A. Complex regional pain syndrome, current concepts and treatment options. *Curr Pain Headache Rep.* 2018;22:10.
13. Terkelsen A, Mølgaard H, Hansen J, Finnerup N, Krøner K, Jensen T. Heart rate variability in complex regional pain syndrome during rest and mental and orthostatic stress. *Anesthesiology.* 2012;116:133-146.
14. Kemler MA, van de Vusse AC, van den Berg-Loonen EM, Barendse GA, van Kleef M, Weber WE. HLA-DQ1 associated with reflex sympathetic dystrophy. *Neurology.* 1999;53(6):1350-1351.
15. Beerthuizen A, Stronks D, Huygen F, Passchier J, Klein J, Spijker A. The association between psychological factors and the development of complex regional pain syndrome type 1 (CRPS1): a prospective multicenter study. *Eur J Pain.* 2011;15:971-975.
16. Beerthuizen A, van 't Spijker A, Huygen FJ, Klein J, de Wit R. Is there an association between psychological factors and the complex regional pain syndrome type 1 (CRPS1) in adults? A systematic review. *Pain.* 2009;145:52-59.
17. Harden RN, Bruehl S, Stanton-Hicks M, Wilson PR. Proposed new diagnostic criteria for complex regional pain syndrome. *Pain Med.* 2007;8(4):326-331.
18. Merskey H, Addison RG, Beric A, et al. Detailed descriptions of pain syndromes. In: Merskey H, Bogduk N, eds. *Classification of chronic pain: descriptions of chronic pain syndromes and definitions of pain terms.* 2nd ed. Seattle, WA: IASP Press; 1994:40-43.
19. Bussa M, Mascaro A, Cuffaro L, Rinaldi S. Adult complex regional pain syndrome type I: a narrative review. *PMR.* 2017;9:707-719.
20. Veldman P, Reynen H, Arntz I, Goris R. Signs and symptoms of reflex sympathetic dystrophy: Prospective study of 829 patients. *Lancet.* 1993;342:1012-1016.

21. GalveVilla M, Rittig-Rasmussen B, Moeller Schear Mikkelsen L, Groendahl Poulsen A. Complex regional pain syndrome. *Man Ther*. 2016;26:223-230.
22. Fife CE, Eckert KA, Workman WT. Ethical issues, standards and quality control in practice of hyperbaric medicine. In: Jain KK, ed. *Textbook of Hyperbaric Medicine*. 6th ed. New York, NY: Springer; 2016.
23. Harden RN, Oaklander AL, Burton AW, et al. Reflex Sympathetic Dystrophy Syndrome Association; complex regional pain syndrome: practical diagnostic and treatment guidelines, 4th ed. *Pain Med*. 2013;14(2):180-229.
24. Harden RN, Swan M, King A, et al. Treatment of complex regional pain syndrome: functional restoration. *Clin J Pain*. 2006;22: 420-424.
25. Hord AH, Rooks MD, Stephens BO, Rogers HG, Fleming LL. Intravenous regional bretylium and lidocaine for treatment of reflex sympathetic dystrophy: a randomized, double-blind study. *Anesth Analg*. 1992;74: 818-821.
26. Duong S, Bravo D, Todd KJ, et al. Treatment of complex regional pain syndrome: an updated systematic review and narrative synthesis. *Can J Anesth*. 2018;65: 658-684.
27. O'Connell NE, Wand BM, McAuley J, Marston L, Moseley GL. Interventions for treating pain and disability in adults with complex regional pain syndrome. *Cochrane Database Syst Rev*. 2013(4):CD009416.
28. Tuter NV, Danilov AB, Poliakova LV. The treatment of a complex regional pain syndrome. *Zh Nevrol Psikhiatr Im S S Korsakova*. 1997;97:33-35.
29. Kiralp MZ, Yildiz S, Vural D, et al. Effectiveness of hyperbaric oxygen therapy in the treatment of complex regional pain syndrome. *J Int Med Res*. 2004;32:258-262.

SELF-ASSESSMENT STUDY QUESTIONS AND ANSWERS

Questions

1. What is the difference between complex regional pain syndrome (CRPS) Type 1 and Type 2?
   A. Absence of pain
   B. Nerve injury
   C. Joint stiffness
   D. Excess sweating

2. A 40-year-old female presents with burning pain, allodynia, swelling, and intermittent blue discoloration in her right hand and most of the forearm to the elbow. This occurred 5 months ago when he suffered a skateboarding accident and fell onto her right arm. Workup is negative for infection, nonunion fracture, and vasculitis. She reports that instead of improving, the pain has worsened and spread proximally. A procedural intervention is considered for pain control to help the patient tolerate physical therapy. Which of the following would be most appropriate?
   A. Right regional ganglion block
   B. Right median nerve block
   C. Spinal cord stimulation
   D. Right ulnar nerve block

3. Which of the following is a characteristic of complex regional pain syndrome (CRPS) II?
   A. Focal neurological deficit
   B. Muscle weakness
   C. Sweating
   D. Osteoporosis

4. What is the most common psychological disorder associated with complex regional pain syndrome?
   A. Anorexia
   B. Bipolar
   C. Psychosis
   D. Anxiety

5. Which is the first line of management for Complex Regional Pain Syndrome?
   A. Psychotherapy
   B. Physical therapy
   C. Sympathetic block
   D. Steroids

6. A 35-year-old male presented with severe pain in the left foot after sustaining a crush injury. He described the pain as fluctuating and burning. The pain is worse at night. The foot is inflamed and discolored. What is the most likely diagnosis?
   A. Morton neuroma
   B. Acute limb ischemia
   C. Complex regional pain syndrome
   D. Compartment syndrome

7. A patient presented to your office after he was diagnosed with a left shoulder complex regional pain syndrome of his right shoulder to discuss the management options. Based on current evidence, which of the following treatments has been shown to help patients with this disorder?
   A. Arthroscopic surgery
   B. Physical therapy
   C. Steroidal therapy
   D. Regional ganglion block

SELF-ASSESSMENT STUDY QUESTIONS AND ANSWERS

8. A 52-year-old male presents with the inability to move his left ankle joint. The patient's ankle was hit during a soccer game 3 weeks ago, which caused him mild discomfort, but he was able to ambulate comfortably. There was no swelling or deformity at that time. The following week, the ankle joint became swollen and painful. He took over-the-counter acetaminophen, but it did not give him much relief. Today, the patient woke up from his sleep due to severe pain in his ankle that he never felt before. He says that the sensation of his jeans rubbing over his ankle causes him discomfort. He had to come to the hospital in a wheelchair, as he cannot walk on his left leg. He denies numbness, paresthesia, headache, and back pain. On examination, vitals are within normal limits. The left ankle joint is swollen, sweaty, and warm compared to the right ankle. There is a blueish discoloration over the skin around the ankle. There is excruciating pain when the ankle joint is moved in any direction. The dorsalis pedis and popliteal pulses are palpable in both legs. X-ray of the ankle reveals bone demineralization. Which of the following is the best treatment for this patient?

A. Bisphosphonates
B. Patient-controlled analgesia pump
C. Regional sympathetic nerve block
D. Ankle cast for 6 weeks

9. A 25-year-old female steps off a curb and sustains a grade three inversion injury to her left ankle. The physical examination reveals a markedly swollen ankle, the neurovascular exam is intact, and radiographs are negative for a fracture. She is placed in a short leg cast and returns 3 weeks later complaining of cold intolerance, a swollen foot, with diffuse numbness, tingling, and pain with weight-bearing. What is the most likely diagnosis?

A. Neuropraxia sural nerve
B. Injury to the posterior tibial artery
C. Early chronic regional pain syndrome
D. Tarsal tunnel

10. A 45-year-old male presented with pain to his left hand after traumatic injury, which of the following is NOT one of Budapest symptoms to diagnose complex regional pain syndrome?

A. Asymmetry of skin temperature and color
B. Reduced ROM beyond trauma joint
C. Symmetrical sweating and edema
D. Allodynia

SELF-ASSESSMENT STUDY QUESTIONS AND ANSWERS

Answers

1. B.
2. A.
3. A.
4. D.
5. B.
6. C.
7. B.
8. C.
9. C.
10. C.

SECTION II Venous Disease

CHAPTER

15 Venous Anatomy and Physiology

Eric Goldschmidt and John Blebea

OUTLINE

INTRODUCTION
EMBRYOLOGY OF THE VENOUS SYSTEM
General Considerations
Vitelline System
Umbilical System
Cardinal System
HISTOLOGY OF THE VENOUS SYSTEM
ANATOMY OF THE MATURE VENOUS SYSTEM
Lower Extremity
Upper Extremity
Thorax/Neck
Abdomen/Pelvis
ANOMALIES OF THE MATURE VENOUS SYSTEM
Superior Vena Cava Anomalies
Inferior Vena Cava Anomalies
Renal Vein Anomalies
PHYSIOLOGY OF THE VENOUS SYSTEM
Introduction
Venous Volume
Venous Return
Venous Resistance
Muscle Pump
Venous Valve Cycle
Hemodynamic Role of Perforating Veins
ACKNOWLEDGMENT

INTRODUCTION

A conceptual understanding of the events during venous embryology and development will be of great help in understanding the anatomy of the mature venous system as well as its common anatomic variations. Similarly, knowledge of the histologic structure of veins and their valves will facilitate an understanding of venous physiology. This chapter aims to present the development and structure of the venous system in an organized fashion so that its physiology is easily correlated.

EMBRYOLOGY OF THE VENOUS SYSTEM

GENERAL CONSIDERATIONS

The embryo has three major venous systems that have distinct functional roles during development and which ultimately differentiate into the adult venous system. The formation of these segments begins early in week 3 of development through a process called vasculogenesis, and by week 4, these three systems have formed (Figure 15-1). The *vitelline* system drains the yolk sac, developing gastrointestinal tract and foregut derivatives. The *umbilical* system carries oxygenated blood from the maternal placental vessels to the embryo, while the *cardinal* system drains blood from the developing body wall, head, neck, and limbs into the sinus horns of the embryonic heart. These three systems are bilaterally symmetric initially but undergo substantial remodeling and lose their symmetry during development. Far greater variation is present in the mature venous system compared to the arterial, which is a reflection of the highly variable organization in the networks of primitive venous channels as well as the extensive remodeling. Small and large disturbances in the remodeling process

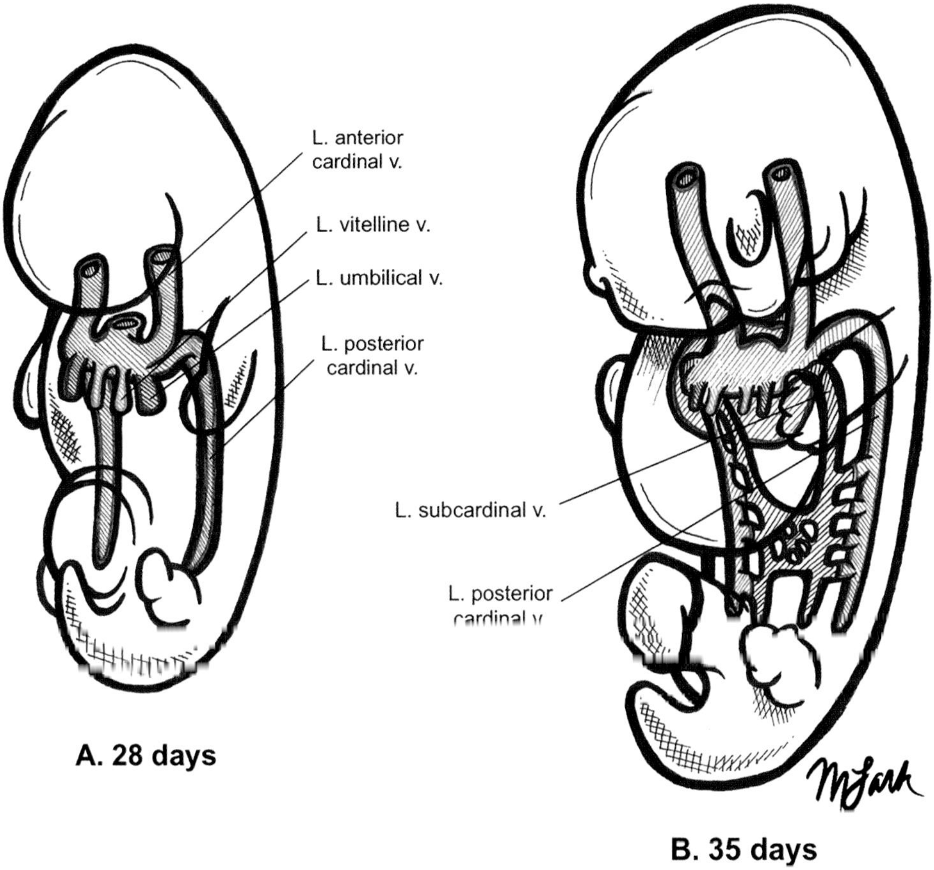

FIGURE 15-1 Venous embryologic development at 4 and 5 weeks. (Reproduced with permission from Meghan Lark.)

lead to variations in the mature venous system as well as commonly recognized anomalies.

VITELLINE SYSTEM

The developing vitelline system originates in the capillary plexuses of the yolk sac and includes part of the vessels that drain the embryonic gastrointestinal tract and gut derivates. This system empties into the sinus horns of the developing heart through the paired vitelline veins. These veins are also connected to symmetric right and left vitelline plexuses that project into the developing liver parenchyma, which form the hepatic sinusoids. The left vitelline vein begins to diminish as the left sinus horn regresses to form the coronary sinus. These events preferentially shunt blood from the developing gastrointestinal tract and yolk sac through the right vitelline vein and liver via several transverse anastomoses. One of these transverse anastomoses within the liver becomes dominant and forms the ductus venosus, which serves to shunt oxygenated blood into the right atrium. By the end of the third month, the left vitelline vein adjacent to the sinus venosus has completely disappeared, and all blood from the vitelline system is directed through the liver and into the future right atrium via the right vitelline vein (Figure 15-2). The cranial-most portion of the right vitelline vein between the liver and right heart becomes the suprahepatic inferior vena cava. The portion of the right

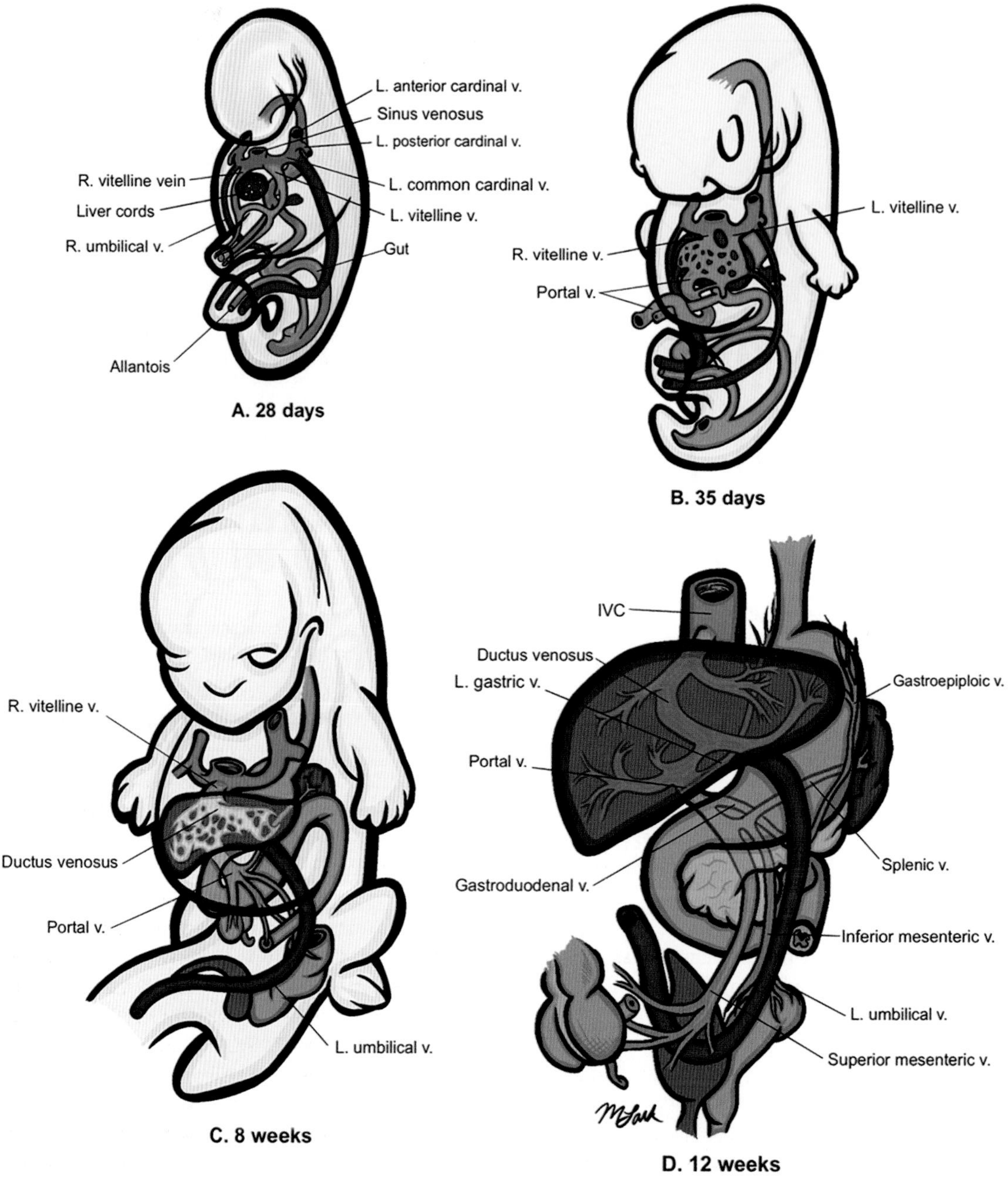

FIGURE 15-2 Embryologic development of the venous system through 12 weeks. (Reproduced with permission from Meghan Lark.)

vitelline vein caudal to the liver becomes the portal vein and superior mesenteric vein, while several of the most cranial transverse anastomoses between the left and right vitelline veins develop into the splenic and inferior mesenteric veins. Therefore, the mature vitelline system serves to drain portions of the foregut, hindgut, and entire midgut into the right atrium through the liver.

UMBILICAL SYSTEM

The umbilical venous system returns oxygenated blood from the placenta to the developing heart. Initially, the umbilical veins are paired, but as the vitelline system undergoes extensive remodeling during development the right umbilical vein is obliterated while the left umbilical vein persists. This is in contrast to the developing vitelline and cardinal venous systems in which the left portion of the respective system regresses. As occurs during the development of the vitelline system, the left umbilical vein loses connectivity to the left sinus horn but establishes a new anastomosis to the ductus venosus enabling oxygenated blood from the placenta to reach the inferior vena cava and right heart while bypassing the developing hepatic sinusoids. After birth both the ductus venosus and the left umbilical vein atrophy to become the ligamentum venosum and ligamentum teres hepatis contained within the falciform ligament.

CARDINAL SYSTEM

The cardinal venous system is the primitive blueprint for the future somatic venous drainage and drains the developing head, neck, limbs, and body wall. The major named vessels include the paired anterior and posterior (cranial and caudal to the heart, respectively) cardinal veins, the paired subcardinal veins, and the paired supracardinal veins. The anterior and posterior cardinal veins converge to form the paired common cardinal veins before emptying into the sinus horns of the embryonic heart. The left and right posterior cardinal veins run adjacent to paired subcardinal and supracardinal veins that run in the body wall medial to the posterior cardinal veins. Ultimately, the posterior cardinal veins are largely replaced by these separate, paired vessels which, similar to the other embryonic venous systems, undergo extensive remodeling during the process of development between weeks 4 and 12.

The paired left and right subcardinal veins each sprout anterior and medially from their respective left and right posterior cardinal veins and develop caudally along the body wall. As these paired veins mature a series of anastomoses develop between them allowing for the shunting of blood between the left and right subcardinal veins. The most cranial portion of these connections occurs at the level of the future kidney. Ultimately, the left subcardinal vein experiences regression of multiple longitudinal segments such that the segmental tributaries drain into the right subcardinal vein. Simultaneously, the right subcardinal vein loses its original connection to the right posterior cardinal vein and gains communication to the right vitelline vein inferior to the heart. This portion of the right subcardinal vein ultimately forms the segment of the inferior vena cava between the kidneys and liver, and the cranial-most transverse anastomosis between the left and right subcardinal veins forms the future left renal vein. There are both anterior and posterior vessels surrounding the aorta that make up this anastomosis, but ultimately in normal development, the posterior portion regresses allowing the mature left renal vein to lie anteriorly to the aorta. This does not always occur and persistence of the posterior vessel into adulthood leads to paired renal veins in front of and behind the aorta. This is clinically relevant during the repair of abdominal aortic aneurysms when clamping the aorta can tear the posterior vein leading to life-threatening hemorrhage.

While the subcardinal veins are undergoing development and remodeling a second pair of veins sprout from the base of the right and left posterior cardinal veins named the supracardinal veins. Like the others, these veins are symmetric and run parallel to the subcardinal veins, draining the dorsal body wall via a series of laterally branching collateral vessels that mature into the intercostal veins. As the new supracardinal veins develop, they take over the function of the embryonic posterior cardinal veins which are obliterated except for the most caudal portion. These caudal remnants form islands, which sprout anastomoses to the caudal supracardinal veins and form the primitive common iliac veins and caudal-most segment of the inferior vena cava.

The abdominal portion of the left supracardinal vein is obliterated during subsequent remodeling, while the right supracardinal vein joins with the right subcardinal vein to form the infrarenal inferior vena cava.

The thoracic portions of the supracardinal veins also undergo significant remodeling. As already mentioned, the cranial-most portions of the supracardinal veins join with the posterior cardinal veins. In this region, a transverse median anastomosis exists between the left and right supracardinal veins, with the dorsal body wall being drained via a series of transverse veins that extend laterally called the intercostal veins. The cranial-most segment of the left supracardinal vein loses its connection to the left posterior cardinal vein and drains across midline into the right supracardinal vein. The right supracardinal vein similarly loses its connection to the right posterior cardinal vein and forms a new anastomosis with the anterior cardinal vein. The end result is drainage of blood from the left supracardinal vein into the right supracardinal vein and ultimately the right anterior cardinal and common cardinal veins. This relationship corresponds to the recognized anatomic arrangement between the hemiazygos vein, azygous vein, and superior vena cava.

The mature interior vena cava thus has its origins in multiple embryonic venous systems including the vitelline and cardinal systems. The superior-most portion of the inferior vena cava, extending from the liver to the right atrium, is derived from the right vitelline vein. The right subcardinal vein gives rise to the portion of the inferior vena cava extending from the renal veins to the liver, while the infrarenal inferior vena cava and confluence arise from the right supracardinal vein and left and right posterior cardinal veins, respectively.

The left and right anterior cardinal veins lie superior to the heart and drain blood from the head and neck into the paired left and right common cardinal veins which in turn empty into the left and right sinus horns. The most cranial portion of both the left and right anterior cardinal veins develops into the internal jugular vein which develops a connection to the corresponding external jugular vein that drains the face. Between weeks 7 and 10, a medial connection develops between the left and right anterior cardinal veins while the continuity between the left sinus horn and the left anterior cardinal vein is lost. This new connection allows the shunting of blood from the left upper limb, head, and neck into the right anterior cardinal vein, and this ultimately develops into the left brachiocephalic (innominate) vein. The venous plexuses within the developing limbs coalesce proximally into the left and right subclavian veins which anastomose with the corresponding anterior cardinal vein. The short segment of the right anterior cardinal vein that lies between this junction and the previously formed intercardinal anastomosis corresponds to the right brachiocephalic (innominate) vein, and the right common cardinal vein caudal to this becomes the superior vena cava. The caudal most portion of the left anterior cardinal vein below the left brachiocephalic vein regresses and the left common cardinal vein and left sinus horn to develop into the future coronary sinus.[1]

HISTOLOGY OF THE VENOUS SYSTEM

The venous wall is composed of three layers, often referred to as tunics. From the lumen outward, these layers are the tunica intima, tunica media, and tunica adventitia. The tunica intima consists of three components: a single layer of epithelium lining the vessel lumen called the endothelium, the basal lamina consisting of collagen fibers and glycoproteins, and the subendothelial layer made up of loose connective tissues. The tunica media is composed primarily of smooth muscle fibers arranged circumferentially around the tunica intima that are surrounded by sheets of elastic fibers called the internal and external elastic membranes. The external elastic membrane separates the tunica media from the more peripheral tunica adventitia. This adventitial layer is composed primarily of longitudinally oriented collagen and elastic fibers that merge with the loose connective tissue surrounding the vessel. Also, present in the adventitial layer of large veins are the vasa vasorum which supplies blood to the vessel wall itself. Compared to the arterial equivalents the tunics of veins are not as well-defined or distinct, and the elastic and muscular components are far less prominent. These histological differences underlie venous morphology and enable them to serve as capacitance vessels rather than conductance vessels like their arterial counterparts.

Veins can be divided into four subtypes based on diameter: large veins (>10 mm), medium veins (1–10 mm), small veins (0.1–1 mm in diameter), and venules (<0.1 mm). In large veins, the tunica media is relatively thin while the adventitial layer is prominent. This reflects the large amount of longitudinally organized smooth muscle fibers in the adventitia while the media contains only a few layers of circumferentially organized smooth muscle fibers. Examples of large veins include the superior and inferior vena cava, iliacs, and the portal vein.

The three tunics of medium veins are the most distinct of all veins. Similar to large veins, the tunica media contains far fewer layers of circular smooth muscle fibers than the equivalent artery and the thick adventitial layer is the most developed layer. Examples of medium veins include the femoral, popliteal, tibial, and brachial veins. Medium veins are usually found running in parallel to their equivalently named artery.[2]

Finally, the small veins and venules which represent the smallest elements of the venous system exhibit a progressively thicker smooth muscle component. The postcapillary venules that drain the capillary beds lack smooth muscle layers entirely. As the postcapillary venules coalesce, they increase in diameter and begin to acquire concentric layers of smooth muscle. As they increase in size, the postcapillary venules become muscular venules.

Venous valves are a unique feature of the venous system without an arterial equivalent. Valves are fibroelastic projections of the tunica intima and consist of two semilunar leaflets lined by endothelium with the free edge oriented in the direction of blood flow. These structures serve to prevent the reflux of blood in a retrograde fashion and are typically found in veins >2 mm in diameter. They are critically important in maintaining blood flow cephalad, from the foot to the heart, against the pull of gravity. Valvular dysfunction is an important contributor to the signs and symptoms of chronic venous insufficiency in adults.

ANATOMY OF THE MATURE VENOUS SYSTEM

LOWER EXTREMITY

The venous drainage of the lower limb can be separated into superficial, deep, and perforating systems (Figure 15-3). The superficial system of veins lies within the subcutaneous tissue of the leg and above the deep fascial layer. The deep system lies beneath the deep fascia, and its veins are paired with accompanying named arteries. The numerous veins of the perforating system allow the deep and superficial systems to freely communicate with each other with preferential flow from the superficial into the larger capacitance deep system.

The two major named veins of the superficial system are the great and small saphenous veins. The great saphenous vein originates in the dorsal venous arch and medial foot, passes anterior to the medial malleolus, and then ascends the leg along the posterior border of the medial tibia. As it reaches the knee, the vein passes posterior to the medial condyle of the femur and ascends in the medial portion of the thigh to the groin in the saphenous opening (fossa ovalis) of the fascia lata where it joins the common femoral vein of the deep system. Just prior to this junction, the great saphenous vein is joined by the accessory saphenous, superficial external pudendal, superficial epigastric, and superficial circumflex iliac veins. Importantly, the great saphenous vein contains between 8 and 12 valves along its length which function to prevent the retrograde reflux of blood down the leg.

The small saphenous vein arises on the lateral aspect of the foot and the dorsal venous arch. It passes posterior to the lateral malleolus and ascends along the lateral edge of the calcaneal tendon toward the posterior midline of the leg. As it approaches the popliteal fossa, the small saphenous vein penetrates the deep fascia and runs between the medial and lateral heads of the gastrocnemius muscle where it empties into the popliteal vein of the deep system behind the knee.

Along the course of the great and small saphenous veins, there are numerous perforating veins that penetrate the deep fascia and allow blood from the superficial system to drain into the deep system. This keeps the diameter of the saphenous veins relatively uniform despite receiving numerous tributaries along their length.

The deep system, usually in pairs, accompanies all the major named arteries of the lower extremity. In the distal lower leg, the anterior tibial veins drain a

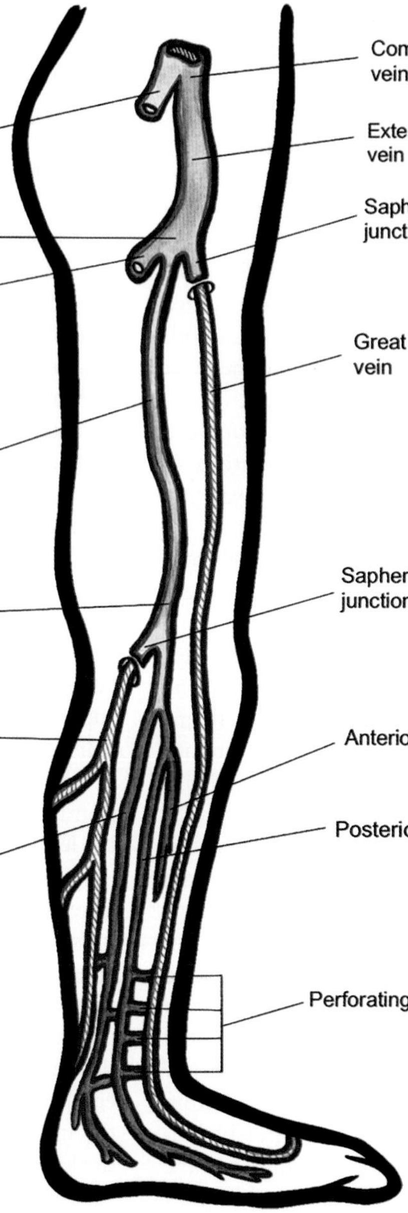

FIGURE 15-3 **Superficial and deep venous system of the leg.**

minority of the dorsal venous arch. The posterior tibial and peroneal veins receive blood from the plantar surface of foot. These three deep veins from the lower extremity merge below the knee to form the popliteal vein which traverses the popliteal space before transitioning into the femoral vein at the upper border of the popliteal fossa. The femoral vein ascends adjacent to the superficial femoral artery, beginning laterally then posteriorly and medially before it reaches the groin. The profunda femoris vein drains the muscle bellies of the deep thigh and merges with the femoral vein to form the common femoral vein just inferior to the inguinal ligament. The common femoral vein passes deep to the inguinal ligament and becomes the external iliac vein which runs through the pelvis.

UPPER EXTREMITY

Similar to the pattern of the venous drainage in the lower limb, the veins of the upper limb can be divided into superficial, deep, and perforating systems (Figure 15-4). The cephalic vein originates on the lateral edge of the dorsum of the hand and ascends along the anterolateral edge of the forearm towards the elbow. At the level of the cubital fossa, the cephalic vein communicates with the median cubital which provides a connection with the basilic vein. It is a common site for venipuncture. The main cephalic vein continues superiorly on the lateral margin of the arm, passes in the deltopectoral groove at the shoulder, and then pierces the clavipectoral fascial to join the axillary vein.

In a parallel fashion to the cephalic vein, the basilic vein originates from tributaries on the medial aspect of the dorsal venous network of the hand and ascends along the medial edge of the forearm. As the basilic vein traverses the cubital fossa, it also communicates with the median cubital vein before entering the arm. Approximately one-third of the distance to the shoulder, the basilic vein penetrates the brachial fascia and enters the deep compartment where it runs parallel to the brachial artery. Ultimately, the basilic vein merges with the paired brachial veins and transitions into the axillary vein which crosses the axilla.

There is a third highly variable superficial vein of the forearm called the median antebrachial vein, which originates at the ventral surface of the base of the thumb. This vein ascends between the cephalic and basilic veins and may communicate through collaterals with either the cephalic or the basilic vein in the forearm before the main trunk joins the median cubital and basilic junction.

The deep venous system of the arm parallels the arterial supply as in the leg. Beginning in the hand, the deep and superficial venous arches coalesce along the medial and lateral margins of the anterior wrist to form the paired radial veins laterally and the paired ulnar veins medially. These paired veins traverse the elbow before converging to form the paired brachial veins that run immediately adjacent to the brachial artery. These vessels ultimately merge with the basilic vein distal to the axilla to form the axillary vein.

THORAX/NECK

The major relevant veins of the neck and thorax drain the head, neck, and limbs and serve to return blood to the right atrium (Figures 15-5 and 15-6). As described previously, the venous outflow of the upper extremities to the thorax is via the axillary and cephalic veins. As the axillary vein traverses medially, the cephalic vein drains into its superior aspect proximal to the clavicle. When the axillary vein reaches the margin of the first rib, it transitions into the subclavian vein which courses medially until it merges with the internal jugular vein. This merger marks the transition of the subclavian vein into the right brachiocephalic (innominate) vein, which merges with the left brachiocephalic vein to form the superior vena cava and finally drain into the right atrium.

The venous drainage of the head and neck (Figure 15-6) is primarily through the internal jugular veins which lie in the deep neck adjacent to the internal carotid and common carotid arteries within the carotid sheath. The most common location is for the internal jugular vein to lie anterior and lateral to the carotid arteries within the carotid sheath. The internal jugular vein begins at the jugular foramen of the skull and drains blood from the brain, face, deep cervical structures, and superficial neck. As it courses inferiorly, it exists the neck posterior to the sternocleidomastoid muscle and sternoclavicular joint where it drains into the subclavian vein to form the brachiocephalic (innominate) vein.

ABDOMEN/PELVIS

The veins of the abdominal and pelvic regions (Figure 15-7) can be separated into two systems that communicate through the hepatic veins: the caval system and the portal venous system. The caval system drains the lower extremities, pelvis, posterior

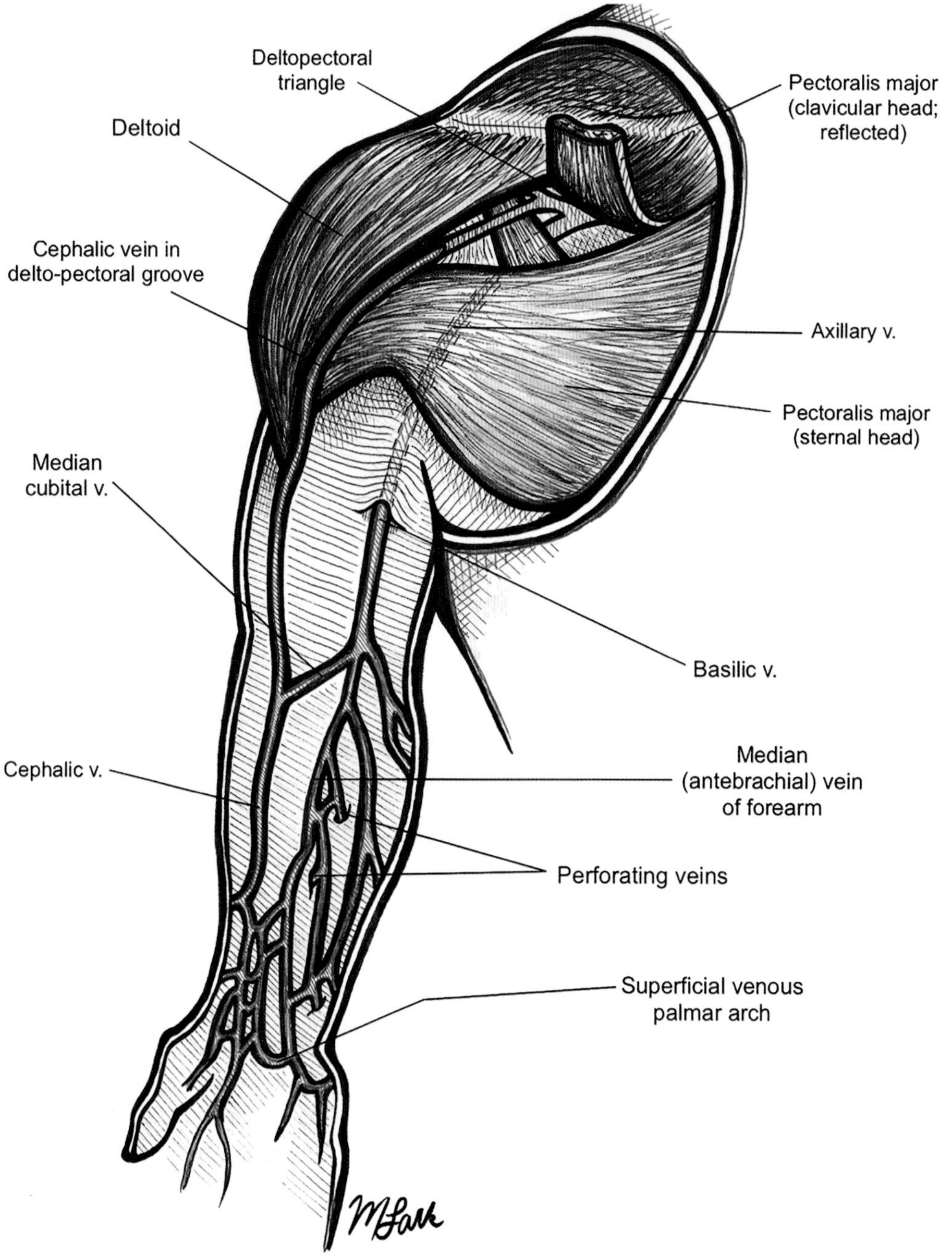

FIGURE 15-4 Superficial veins of the upper extremity. (Reproduced with permission from Meghan Lark.)

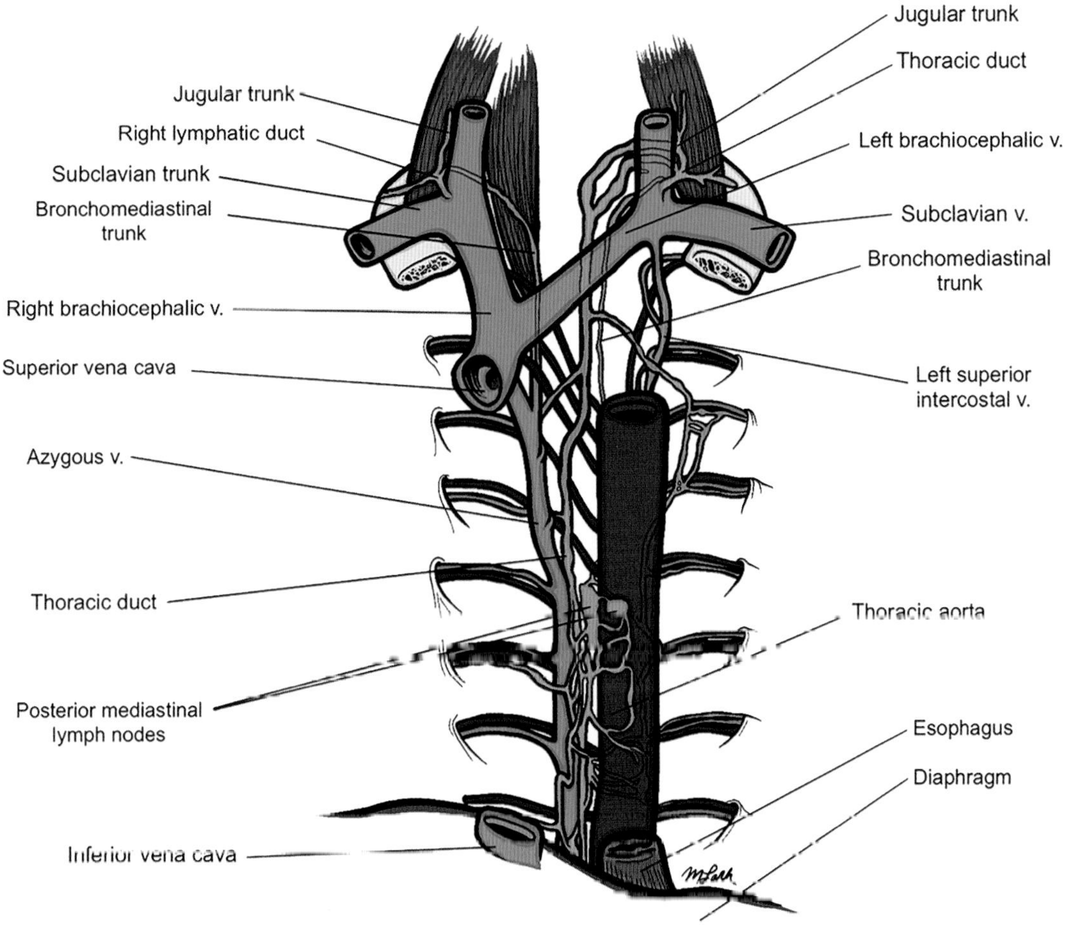

FIGURE 15-5 **Venous system of the thoracic cavity.** (Reproduced with permission from Meghan Lark.)

body wall, kidneys, and adrenal glands, while the portal system serves to deliver blood to the liver from the small and large intestines, stomach, and spleen.

The inferior vena cava is the largest vein found in the body lying to the right of the midline and anterior to the lumbar spine. It originates at the confluence of the left and right common iliac veins at the level of the L5 vertebra and extends to the right atrium. As it passes superiorly, it receives blood from the paired lumbar veins, renal veins, right gonadal vein, right adrenal vein, phrenic veins, and hepatic veins before traversing the diaphragm at the level of T8. The left adrenal and gonadal veins empty into the left renal vein. A collateral pathway for venous drainage exists between the inferior and superior vena cava through the ascending lumbar veins and the azygous vein.

The portal vein forms posterior to the duodenum from the merger of the superior mesenteric and splenic veins. The inferior mesenteric vein joins the splenic vein typically posterior to the pancreas. The main portal vein lies anterior to the inferior vena cava and extends superiorly to the liver within the porta hepatis ultimately dividing into the left and right portal veins which supply the left and right lobes of the liver. The liver then drains blood into the inferior vena cava via the left, right, and middle hepatic veins posterior to the liver.[3]

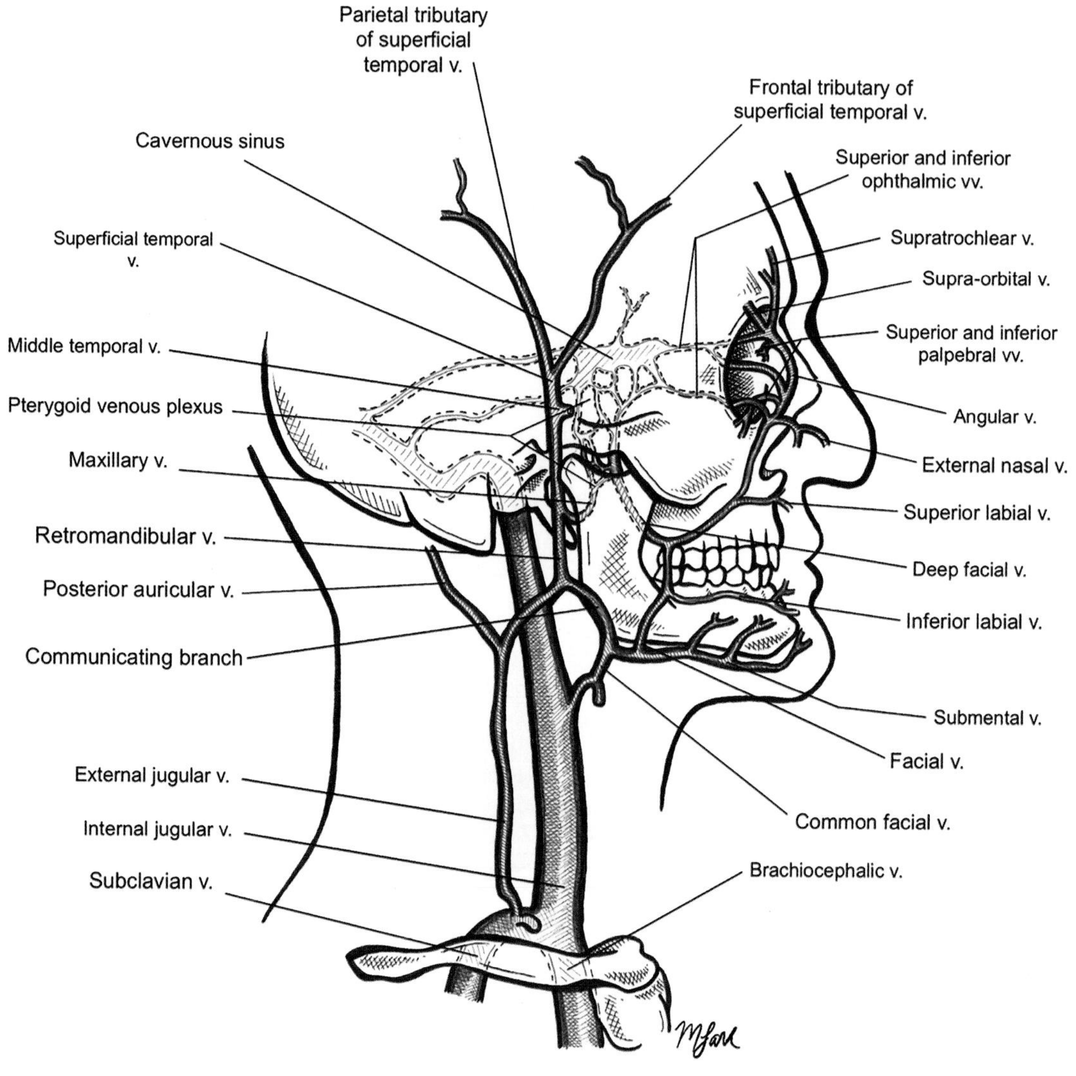

FIGURE 15-6 Major veins of the neck. (Reproduced with permission from Meghan Lark.)

ANOMALIES OF THE MATURE VENOUS SYSTEM

SUPERIOR VENA CAVA ANOMALIES

Two described, although infrequent, anomalies exist involving the superior vena cava and include a double (persistent left) superior vena cava and a left-sided superior vena cava. A double superior vena cava arises when the caudal segment of the left anterior cardinal vein fails to obliterate. There is variable formation of the intercardinal anastomosis during development in these patients so that the left brachiocephalic vein may be diminutive or completely absent. Likewise, a left-sided superior vena cava occurs when the caudal portion of the right anterior cardinal vein is obliterated with persistence of the left anterior cardinal vein. In either case, the left upper extremity, face, and neck will drain into the coronary sinus through the

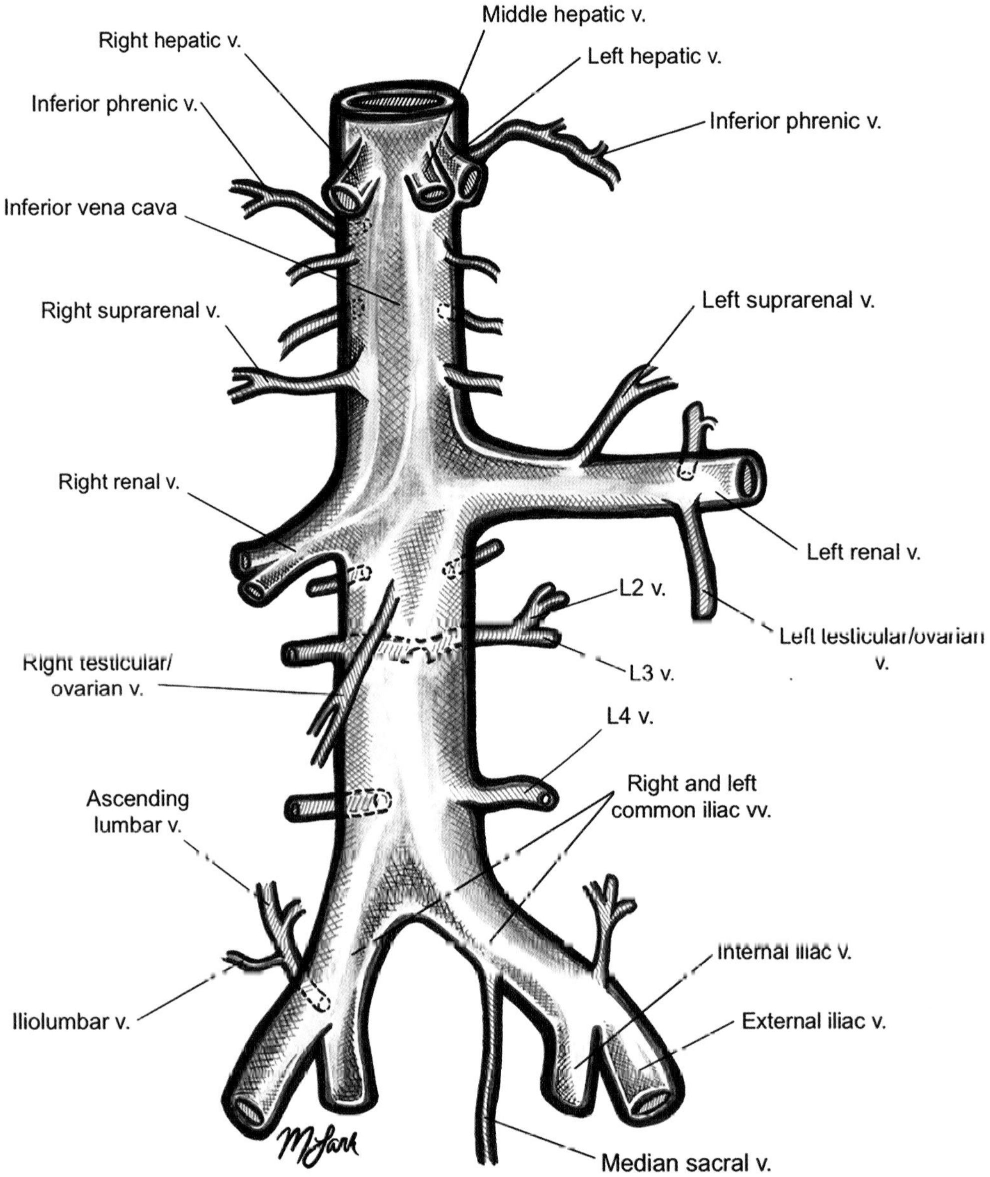

FIGURE 15-7 Caval venous anatomy of the abdomen and pelvis. (Reproduced with permission from Meghan Lark.)

abnormal super vena cava on the left side. In the single left-sided super vena cava, the azygous system is also drained into the right atrium via the coronary sinus. In a very small subset of patients with either a double superior vena cava or left-sided superior vena cava, the abnormal venous drainage occurs directly into the left atrium. Physiologically, superior vena cava anomalies are not important but may present incidentally as abnormal findings on radiographic studies of the chest or found during interventional procedures.[4]

INFERIOR VENA CAVA ANOMALIES

A rare clinical entity termed duplicated inferior vena cava arises with failed regression of the caudal left supracardinal vein. In this instance, there are two infrarenal inferior vena cavas with communication at the level of the renal veins. Cephalad drainage from the left-sided cava can also occur through the left renal vein or via the hemiazygos vein. Finally, a single left-sided inferior vena cava can develop when the right supracardinal vein obliterates with persistence of the left supracardinal vein. In this case, the inferior vena cava lies to the left of midline below the renal arteries but crosses to the right at this level. With a left-sided inferior vena cava, the right adrenal and gonadal veins adopt the drainage pattern of the left adrenal and gonadal veins observed in a normal inferior vena cava configuration and drain into the right renal vein. Similarly, the left adrenal and gonadal veins drain into the abnormal inferior vena cava.[5]

RENAL VEIN ANOMALIES

The most common clinically relevant renal vein anomaly is the retro-aortic left renal vein. This entity occurs when the posterior vessels traversing between the left and right subcardinal veins persist while the anterior vessels regress allowing for the mature left renal vein to pass posterior to the aorta. A closely related left renal vein anomaly also exists when both the anterior and posterior segments of the traversing branches persist between the left and right subcardinal vein which allows the aorta to be completely encircled by the left renal veins. This entity is termed a circum-aortic left renal vein. In both situations, awareness of the abnormal configuration is important during dissection of the abdominal aorta and renal arteries in this region.[6]

PHYSIOLOGY OF THE VENOUS SYSTEM

INTRODUCTION

Venous function is an integral part of blood circulation. In addition to serving as conductors between the microcirculation and the heart, veins are capacitance vessels that provide the ability to sequester significant volumes of blood and recruit necessary volume back into the circulation as needed.

Anatomically, the venous system differs significantly from the arterial side of the circulation. The venous wall is structurally different, which underlies the unique mechanical properties such as collapsibility and compliance. Additionally, the organization of the veins of the extremities into deep and superficial networks connected by perforating vessels has no arterial equivalent. Furthermore, intramuscular sinusoids and valves are also unique to the venous system. These key differences reflect the distinct functions of the venous system. In describing venous physiology, this section will concentrate on the unique functions of venous capacitance and volume and the mechanisms involved in venous return.

VENOUS VOLUME

At any given time, up to 80% of the intravascular blood volume resides in veins, underscoring the physiological importance of venous capacitance. The reservoir function of veins enables them to adjust blood return to the heart and thus affect cardiac preload and output to match the immediate physiologic needs of the body. Changes in body position, exercise, or digesting a meal trigger a redistribution of the blood volume within the vascular system such that cardiac function would be reduced if preload was not increased. This compensatory change is mediated by increasing venous blood return to the right heart.[7] Likewise, a reduction in blood volume due to dehydration or bleeding can be compensated for through the recruitment of blood from the veins.

Changes in venous volume are mainly determined by the mechanical properties of the venous wall and the activity of smooth muscle cells (venous tone). The measure of the responsiveness of the venous wall to pressure changes is called compliance. Compliance is defined as the ratio of the change in volume to the change in transmural pressure. When transmural pressure is low, the compliance of the venous wall is high, and small changes in pressure cause large volume changes. At high levels of transmural pressure, venous compliance is very low, and large changes in pressure cause very small volume changes. When pressure outside the vein exceeds intramural pressure, the vein can collapse, and the compliance is low.

In the normal physiologic range of venous pressures (3–10 mmHg), high venous compliance exists which allows for significant shifts in blood volume with changes in body position. For example, the transition from a supine to a standing position changes the hydrostatic pressure, leading to a rapid increase in leg vein volume by approximately 400 mL, with an additional increase of 100 mL after 1 minute.[8] Such volume shifts trigger a range of vasoactive responses to maintain constant cardiac output while blood flow through the liver, kidney, and mesenteric vessels significantly decrease.[9] Failure or delay in the action of these mechanisms may result in syncope from the reduced cardiac output.

Venous volume and blood flow are regulated through venous tone. Changes in smooth muscle activity in the tunica media are mediated through multiple bioactive substances released by nerves, endothelium, or circulating blood and are controlled largely by sympathetic alpha-adrenergic activity. When veins contract to augment cardiac preload and output, their resistance increases, but this increase is usually offset by arteriolar dilation and the activity of the muscle pump. Intramuscular sinusoids lack adrenergic innervation and do not constrict, maintaining the ability of the muscle pump to accumulate the necessary volume of blood.[10]

Veins also play a role in the body's thermoregulation, which is a product of their ability to change volume and resistance. These changes can be mediated by sympathetic activity but also directly by temperature changes in the environment. Dilated superficial veins serve as heat exchangers while constricted veins conserve energy in a cold environment.

VENOUS RETURN

In general, blood moves because of and in the direction of an energy gradient. Two components of total blood energy are kinetic and potential energy. Kinetic energy is related to the energy of a moving mass and is directly proportional to the velocity and specific gravity of the blood. Potential energy is associated with a set of forces that act on a body in a way that depends on the body's position in space. It is frequently associated with gravitational energy, which is possessed by virtue of height above the surface of the earth. It is important to mention that other components of potential energy are actively involved in the dynamic of the venous flow. An example is the potential energy of the blood in the intramuscular sinusoid during muscle relaxation. The kinetic energy of muscle contraction converts this energy of the blood into kinetic energy of the flow.

Venous return refers to the volume of blood that returns to the right atrium and is typically in the range of 5 L/min in a healthy individual. This volume is determined primarily by the pressure differential between the blood in the peripheral veins and the blood in the central veins. In an individual at rest, the pressure differential between the peripheral veins and the right atrium is small as the venous system is at low pressure. Pressure within the large named peripheral veins is roughly between 8 and 10 mmHg while the central venous pressure, which is a surrogate of right atrial pressure, usually ranges from 0 to 6 mmHg.[11] Venous return is facilitated by multiple factors including venous tone, venous valves, the skeletal muscle pump, cardiac suction effect, and negative intrathoracic pressure during inspiration. These factors act to increase the pressure gradient between the venous blood in the periphery and the right atrium, which promotes venous return and increased cardiac preload.

Blood flow in the veins of the lower extremities is largely influenced by conditions in the more proximal veins. Changes in volume and pressure of the veins traversing the abdominal and thoracic compartments affect the venous return from more distal veins. Changes in hydrostatic pressure in the abdominal veins are impacted by changes in intraabdominal pressure with breathing and diaphragmatic movement. Subatmospheric pressure in the thorax maintains positive transmural pressure in the intrathoracic veins despite intravascular pressure drops caused by the heart. The influence of respiration on the pattern of blood flow in the veins of the lower extremities is the result of movements by the diaphragm. The diaphragm descends during inspiration, which increases intraabdominal pressure and decreases blood flow through the femoral veins.

During expiration, the diaphragm rises and intraabdominal pressure decreases, allowing increased blood flow in the femoral and iliac veins. As the relative role of the diaphragm in the respiratory cycle changes with the position of the body, so does the pattern of venous flow. In a slightly head-down position, venous flow in the femoral veins depends solely on the cardiac cycle, whereas in a standing position, it depends more upon the respiratory cycle.[12]

Blood flow in individual veins and regions may change dramatically over time without affecting the total venous return to the heart or venous return from the region or organ. Bending the knee or elbow, for example, can temporarily stop venous flow in some of the extremity's veins, but the resulting venous outflow from this extremity over time remains equal to arterial inflow. During acute venous thrombosis (except in rare cases of phlegmasia), increased collateral flow develops over a very short time, balancing the venous outflow with arterial inflow. The term "venous stasis" describes a chronic phenomenon in the lower extremities with valvular dysfunction and less efficient venous return.

VENOUS RESISTANCE

Venous resistance (R) is the ratio of the total energy gradient across the segment (ΔE) over the flow rate through this segment (Q): $R = \Delta E/Q$. For practical purposes, the dynamic pressure gradient (ΔPd) is substituted for the total energy gradient. Resistance of a venous segment is not constant, but changes with the velocity of blood flow, variations of transmural pressure, and blood viscosity. Around venous valves, the constantly changing position of the cusps and the dimensions of the sinus cause continuous changes in resistance. The collapsibility of veins also contributes to the changing resistance, leading to very complex flow dynamic phenomena.

The high compliance of the venous wall plays an important role in adjusting venous resistance to the needs of the venous return. The veins easily extend, decreasing resistance when a larger conductance or capacitance is needed. In the postthrombotic disease, this function is significantly impaired. Inflammation in and around the venous wall during the acute episode of thrombosis results in fibrosis of the wall and loss of compliance. In many cases, thrombus resolution is not complete, and fibrotic structures (synechia) remain in the vein lumen for many years. Synechia restricts venous distention, elevating resistance when blood flow increases. Preexisting collateral veins attempt to compensate by increasing their caliber and conductance over time. The main vein size and flow volume can be increased mechanically with the insertion of a stent in the affected region.

Muscle Pump

The concept of the muscle pump is similar to a "bellows" where the intramuscular veins and sinusoids fill with blood during muscle relaxation and empty by muscle contraction. This produces increased venous flow, reduced venous volume, and a drop in venous pressure. Retrograde blood flow does not occur due to the presence of unidirectional venous valves in the veins cephalad to the muscle combined with high resistance of the microvasculature. The net result is the flow of venous blood from the periphery to the right heart.

The effectiveness of the muscle pump is dependent on the functional competency of venous valves to create an appropriate pathway for blood displaced from intramuscular veins. Competent valves in perforating veins secure unidirectional flow from the superficial to the deep veins. Competent valves in the superficial veins are necessary for further flow into more proximal deep veins. Incompetent valves allow blood to return inappropriately to the intramuscular veins and sinusoids and decrease the effectiveness of the muscle pump.

Venous Valve Cycle

The venous valve cycle describes the time period between two consecutive closures of the valve, which has been described in four phases.[13] During the *opening phase,* the valve cusps move from the closed position toward the sinus wall to open. After reaching a certain point, the cusps cease opening and enter the *equilibrium phase.* During this phase, the leading edges remain suspended in the flowing stream and undergo oscillations. The valve is maximally open during this phase yet the cusps maintain their position some distance from the wall, creating a partial narrowing of the flow lumen. The cross-sectional area between the leaflets is approximately two-thirds of the cross-sectional area of the vein distal to the valve. The flow accelerates in this narrowed area, forming a proximally directed jet. The impact of the jet against the layer of slower-moving blood proximal to the valve results in a reversal of flow in the parts of the stream closer to the wall. While the larger stream located in the center of the vessel is directed cephalad along the vein axis, the smaller part of the flow turns retrograde into the sinus pocket behind the valve cusp, forming a vortex along the sinus wall and mural side of the valve cusp before reemerging in the mainstream in the vein, creating vortical flow.

As vortical flow persists, it applies pressure upon the mural surface of the valve cusps. When the pressures on the mural and luminal sides of the cusp are in equilibrium, the valve remains open and the cusps float in the stream. When the venous flow rate increases, as occurs during foot movements or muscle contraction, the velocity of the flow between the valve cusps rapidly increases and keeps the valves open. As flow and intraluminal pressure decreases, the valve cusps start moving toward the center of the vessel. With rising pressures on the mural side and falling pressures on the luminal side of the cusps, valve closure is favored, and the *closing phase* ensues. The valve cusps move synchronously toward the center until they reach a symmetrical position. The last phase is the *closed phase*, during which the cusps close together to prevent retrograde and backward flow of blood.

HEMODYNAMIC ROLE OF PERFORATING VEINS

The venous system contains numerous interconnections between its individual vessels, which establish collateral circulatory routes. These connections prevent disruption of blood flow during changes in body and extremity position and compression of the veins by contracting muscles during locomotion or by external pressure. Perforating veins are unique structures that cross the deep fascia of the extremity and connect the superficial and the deep venous systems of extremities. Although some anatomical studies have demonstrated that all perforating veins have valves, others have shown some are avalvular.[14,15] Under normal physiologic conditions perforating veins enable blood to flow from the superficial to the deep system. However, during pathological states of incompetence or occlusion of the proximal deep veins, blood is inappropriately directed from the deep system and into the superficial system, which can contribute to lower extremity swelling and chronic venous changes.

ACKNOWLEDGMENT

Special thanks to Meghan Lark, MS for the illustrations.

REFERENCES

1. Schoenwolf GC, Bleyl SB, Brauer PR, Francis-West PH. Development of the vasculature. In: *Larsen's Human Embryology*. 4th ed. Philadelphia, PA: Elsevier; 2009:385-433.
2. Ross MH, Pawlina W. Cardiovascular system. In: *Histology: Text and Atlas*. 6th ed. Baltimore, MA: Wolters Kluwer; 2011:400-440.
3. Agur AMR, Dalley AF, Moore KL. *Clinically Oriented Anatomy*. United Kingdom: Wolters Kluwer Health/Lippincott Williams & Wilkins; 2010.
4. Verma M, Pandey NN, Ojha V, Kumar S, Ramakrishnan S. Developmental anomalies of the superior vena cava and its tributaries. what the radiologist needs to know? *Br J Radiol*. 2021;94(1118):20200856.
5. Jacobowitz G, Sadek M. Congenital occlusion/absence of the inferior vena cava. In: *Rutherford's Vascular Surgery and Endovascular Therapy*. 2-Volume Set. 9th ed. Cambridge, MA: Elsevier; 2019:2145-2153.
6. Sonawane GB, Moorthy KH, Pillai BS. Newer variants of retroaortic left renal vein. *Indian J Urol*. 2020;36(2):142-143.
7. Koeppen BM, Stanton BA. Properties of the vasculature. In: *Berne and Levy Physiology*. 6th ed. Cambridge, MA: Elsevier; 2010:342-343.
8. Rushmer RF. *Cardiovascular Dynamics*. 4th ed. Philadelphia, PA: Saunders; 1976.
9. Culbertson JW, Wilkins RW, Ingelfinger FJ, Bradley SE. The effect of the upright posture upon hepatic blood flow in normotensive and hypertensive subjects. *J Clin Invest*. 1951; 30:305-311.
10. Shepherd JT. Role of the veins in the circulation. *Circulation*. 1966;33:484-491.

11. Tansey EA, Montgomery LEA, Quinn JG, Roe SM, Johnson CD. Understanding basic vein physiology and venous blood pressure through simple physical assessments. *Adv Physiol Educ*. 2019;43(3):423-429.
12. Moneta GL, Bedford G, Beach K, Strandness DE. Duplex ultrasound assessment of venous diameters, peak velocities, and flow patterns. *J Vasc Surg*. 1988;8:286-291.
13. Lurie F, Kistner RL, Eklof B, Kessler D. Mechanism of venous valve closure and role of the valve in circulation: a new concept. *J Vasc Surg*. 2003;38:955-961.
14. Cotton LT. Varicose veins. Gross anatomy and development. *Br J Surg*. 1961;48:589-598.
15. Thomson H. The surgical anatomy of the superficial and perforating veins of the lower limb. *Ann R Coll Surg Engl*. 1979;61:198-205.

SELF-ASSESSMENT STUDY QUESTIONS AND ANSWERS

Questions

1. All of the following are major venous systems found in developing embryo except for what?
   A. Vitelline
   B. Cardinal
   C. Umbilical
   D. Azygous

2. The mature inferior vena cava originates from what embryologic venous system(s)?
   A. Vitelline system
   B. Cardinal system
   C. Vitelline and cardinal system
   D. Umbilical and vitelline system
   E. Vitelline, cardinal, and umbilical system

3. In normal veins, most of the smooth muscle cells are located in what layer?
   A. Tunica intima
   B. Tunica media
   C. Tunica adventitia
   D. None of the above—veins lack smooth muscle

4. Which of the following regarding anomalies found in the mature venous system is true?
   A. Double SVC occurs when the caudal segment of the right anterior cardinal vein fails to obliterate.
   B. Double SVC occurs when the caudal portion of the right anterior cardinal vein is obliterated with persistence of the left anterior cardinal vein.
   C. Duplicated IVC occurs when the caudal right supracardinal vein fails to regress.
   D. Retroaortic left renal vein occurs when the anterior vessels traversing between the left and right subcardinal veins persists while anterior vessels regress.

5. All of the following regarding the physiology of the venous system are true, except:
   A. About 50% of the intravascular blood volume resides in veins.
   B. Normal pressure in peripheral veins ranges from 8 to 10 mmHg.
   C. Normal pressure in central veins ranges from 0 to 6 mmHg.
   D. The ratio of the change in venous volume to transmural pressure is known as compliance.

6. All of the following facilitate venous blood return to the heart except for:
   A. Skeletal muscle contraction
   B. Venous valves
   C. Increased intraabdominal pressure
   D. Diaphragmatic movement

7. Which of the following regarding the venous valve cycle is true?
   A. Venous valves are maximally open during the equilibrium phase
   B. Opening phase follows equilibrium phase
   C. Movement of the valve cusps toward the sinus wall occurs during the opening phase
   D. The closing phase precedes equilibrium

8. All of the following regarding perforating veins is true, except.
   A. Perforating veins extend between the deep and superficial venous system.
   B. Perforating veins do not cross the deep fascia.
   C. The majority of perforating veins contain valves.
   D. Under normal physiologic conditions blood flows from the superficial to the deep system.

SELF-ASSESSMENT STUDY QUESTIONS AND ANSWERS

9. Which of the following statements regarding venous resistance is true?

A. Venous resistance is the ratio of flow over the dynamic pressure gradient.
B. Venous resistance is inversely proportional to the blood flow through a particular segment.
C. Resistance to blood flow during postthrombotic disease is due to increased compliance.
D. Resistance of a venous segment is constant.

10. All of the following regarding the veins of the lower extremity are true, except:

A. Veins of the lower extremity can be divided into deep, superficial and perforating veins.
B. The GSV originates on the dorsal surface of the foot and passes posterior to the medial malleolus.
C. The site in the proximal thigh where the GSV passes across the fascia before joining with the femoral vein is called the fossa ovalis.
D. The SSV originates on the lateral aspect of the foot and passes posterior to the lateral malleolus to the posterior midline of the leg.
E. The anterior tibial vein drains blood from the dorsal surface of the foot while the posterior tibial and peroneal veins drain blood from the plantar surface.

SELF-ASSESSMENT STUDY QUESTIONS AND ANSWERS

Answers

1. D.
2. C.
3. B.
4. D.
5. A.
6. C.
7. A.
8. B.
9. B.
10. B.

CHAPTER

16 Deep Venous Thromboembolism

Sriganesh B. Sharma and Andrea Obi

OUTLINE

GENERAL CONSIDERATIONS
- Epidemiology and Risk Factors for DVT
- Pathophysiology

CLINICAL FINDINGS

DIFFERENTIAL DIAGNOSIS

DIAGNOSIS
- Rationale
- Imaging

MANAGEMENT OF CLINICAL PROBLEM
- Modalities of Treatment
  - Pharmacologic—Anticoagulation
  - Interventional
- Treatment of DVT Based on Anatomic Location
  - Upper Extremity DVT (UE DVT)
  - Lower Extremity DVT (LE DVT)
    - *Severe Obstructive Proximal (Iliofemoral) DVT*
    - *Acute LE DVT with Large Central Vein Thrombosis*
    - *Distal (Calf) DVT*

CASE PRESENTATION

ACKNOWLEDGMENT

GENERAL CONSIDERATIONS

Venous thromboembolism (VTE), which includes both deep venous thrombosis (DVT) and pulmonary embolism (PE), represents one of the most common preventable causes of hospital death and is associated with substantial long-term morbidity and mortality. The incidence of DVT exceeds 250,000 patients a year while more than 200,000 patients a year develop PE.[1,2] The total incidence of VTE is estimated between 300,000 and 600,000 individuals in the United States per year.[3] The widespread impact of VTE on healthcare spending ranges in the order of billions of dollars.[4] Therefore, the incidence, prevalence, cost, morbidity, and mortality from VTE represent a significant public health burden. As such, understanding the underlying risk factors, diagnostic approaches, and factors that affect prophylaxis and treatment of DVTs and PEs is paramount.

EPIDEMIOLOGY AND RISK FACTORS FOR DVT

The annual incidence of DVT in the United States has remained constant since the 1980s at approximately 50 per 100,000 person-years, However, the incidence varies with the comorbidities of each population studied, and this fact highlights the influence of genetic, environmental, and socioeconomic factors in predisposing to DVT formation. There are racial differences with African Americans having the highest incidence of VTE, Whites having an intermediate incidence, and Hispanics and Asian/Pacific Islanders having the lowest incidence.[1,5] Patient factors that predispose to the increased risk of DVT formation include trauma and malignancy. Pregnancy results in uterine compression of venous outflow, contributing to an increased VTE risk. Hospitalization is a particularly potent risk factor for DVT formation with hospitalized patients displaying an increased risk of DVT as compared to matched outpatients. Events occurring during hospitalization, such as surgery and immobilization, increase the risk for DVT, with patients undergoing elective neurologic and orthopedic surgeries demonstrating the greatest risk. When considering hospitalized patients and outpatients alike, risk factors such as increasing age, obesity, certain disease states (e.g., inflammatory bowel disease, systemic lupus erythematosus, malignancies), inherited thrombophilias and hypercoagulability syndromes, the presence of varicose veins, and estrogen hormone therapies (oral contraceptives or hormone replacement therapy) further independently predispose patients to DVT formation.[6] Analysis of these factors has enabled the development of risk assessment models, such as the Padua (for medial patients) or Caprini (for surgical patients) scores, which employ these factors to risk-stratify patients and guide their thromboprophylaxis during hospitalization.

PATHOPHYSIOLOGY

The pathophysiologic underpinnings of DVT formation were first proposed by Virchow approximately 150 years ago as a triad of venous stasis, hypercoagulability, and endothelial injury. The specific mechanisms of each component and how they interact with one another is not completely understood and remains the subject of ongoing studies. As such, it is not surprising that disease processes that serve to impede venous outflow (e.g., immobility), favor blood clot formation (e.g., inherited thrombophilias), and alter endothelial integrity (e.g., sepsis and infection) greatly increase DVT formation risk. Furthermore, certain disease states such as malignancy alter the balance of mediators of hemostasis, such as tissue factor (TF) and platelet adhesion molecules such as glycoprotein Ib and IIb/IIIa, thereby resulting in the activation of coagulation mechanisms. At the same time, clot resolution may also be perturbed in certain patients such as those in the postsurgical state, where levels of plasminogen activator inhibitor-1 (PAI-1) are upregulated, thereby yielding an overall antifibrinolytic milieu that favors thrombus stabilization and amplification. Our current understanding of thrombus and vein wall biology, the inflammatory response to venous thrombus formation, and the physiology of thrombus resolution and vein recanalization represents a refinement of these primary principles and enables us to better formulate prophylaxis and future treatment strategies for DVT.[7]

CLINICAL FINDINGS

The clinical manifestations of DVT span a wide spectrum ranging from asymptomatic to limb-threatening venous gangrene. They commonly include the acute onset of extremity pain, edema, cyanosis, and rarely fever. This range of symptomatology results from many factors related to thrombus formation. The anatomic distribution of the thrombosed veins, including the extent of occlusion, the presence of preexisting venous insufficiency, local and systemic inflammation, and acuteness of thrombosis are all factors that affect the severity of the presenting clinical symptoms of a DVT. Symptoms are much more severe when the proximal venous segments are involved (i.e., iliofemoral DVT) when compared to distal leg segments (e.g., tibial calf DVT). Although the majority of DVT occurs in the legs, approximately 5% to 15% is present in the upper extremities and involves the subclavian and axillary venous segments. Not uncommonly, a silent asymptomatic leg DVT can be discovered during the investigation of a PE.

DIFFERENTIAL DIAGNOSIS

Unfortunately, the clinical signs and symptoms of a DVT lack sufficient specificity for the diagnosis of DVT by clinical examination alone because they can be associated with many other disease processes. For example, studies have found that calf pain alone, though demonstrating a 75% to 91% sensitivity for DVT, only has a specificity of 3% to 5%. Alternate diagnoses must therefore be considered when evaluating a patient for DVT because so many other diagnoses share similar symptoms. Such differential diagnoses include local trauma, cellulitis, arthritis, musculoskeletal pathologies, lymphedema, and complex regional pain syndrome. Systemic diseases that can lead to extremity swelling commonly include congestive heart failure, renal insufficiency, or liver

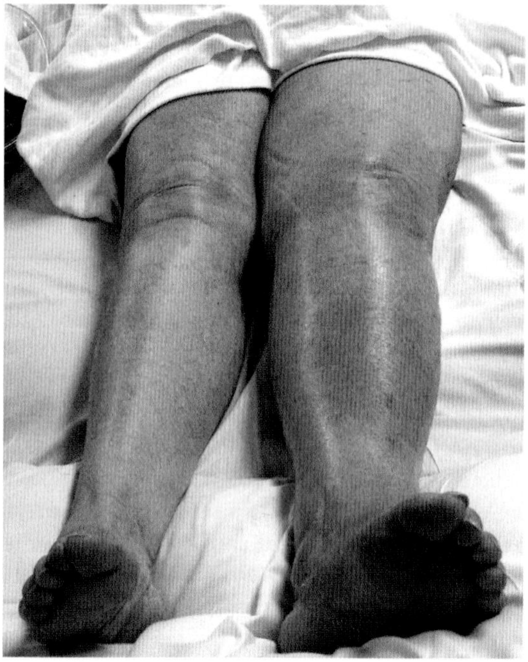

FIGURE 16-1 Pronounced left leg swelling in the presence of extensive ilio-femoral deep venous thrombosis. Erythematous discoloration is also evident in the lower leg as compared to the contralateral right side. (Reproduced with permission from John Blebea, MD)

failure. One should also be cognizant that each of these pathologies may also coexist with a DVT. In order to assist in the clinical diagnosis of DVT, prediction tools such as the Wells criteria have been developed which consider a combination of patient risk factors (e.g., active malignancy, paralysis, immobilization) and presenting symptoms (e.g., calf edema with affected extremity >3 cm larger than uninvolved extremity) to assist in the clinical diagnosis of DVT Figure 16-1). Such tools can be helpful in the initial evaluation of a patient with possible DVT.

DIAGNOSIS

RATIONALE

In the absence of reliable and specific clinical findings, the Wells criteria are a useful tool that can help stratify patients in regard to their probable diagnosis of DVT.[8] Patients identified as intermediate or high risk for DVT have a 16.6% to 74.6% prevalence of DVT, whereas those stratified as low risk have a very low 3% probability. This risk stratification is very useful in determining which patients would benefit from additional diagnostic testing. Those at high risk should get additional studies, usually a duplex ultrasound. Wells low-risk patients, in association with a normal D-dimer level (a product of fibrinolysis), have a negative predictive value approaching 100%. In such a circumstance, this combination effectively excludes the diagnosis of DVT without the need for further studies. Similar results have been observed for intermediate-risk patients with a normal D-dimer who were found to have only a 0.6% incidence of DVT at 3 months. A negative D-dimer level is less useful in high-probability patients per the Wells criteria, and thus, high-risk patients must undergo additional diagnostic testing. The D-dimer level has also been suggested as a predictor for recurrent DVT after treatment has been completed.[9]

IMAGING

Duplex ultrasonography is the current first-line imaging test for diagnosing lower extremity DVTs (Figures 16-2 and 16-3). Duplex imaging combines both B-mode anatomic imaging of venous clots and Doppler flow analysis. It has a sensitivity and specificity of greater than 95% in proximal DVT diagnosis in patients with appropriate Wells pretest probability. Duplex ultrasonography involves visualizing the entire length of a venous segment and is advantageous over other imaging modalities such as computed tomography [CT] or magnetic resonance imaging [MRI]) because it is painless, does not expose the patient to contrast or radiation, is safe in pregnancy, and is relatively inexpensive. However, compared to the other modalities, duplex ultrasonography is operator dependent and is not as accurate for calf veins or the common iliac and subclavian veins that are relatively inaccessible, and visualization may be hindered by patient factors such as obesity. The primary diagnostic criteria for acute DVT by duplex ultrasonography are the inability to collapse the affected venous segment on compression and the absence of flow augmentation with compression.

Venography is an additional modality for establishing a diagnosis of DVT (Figure 16-4). Venography

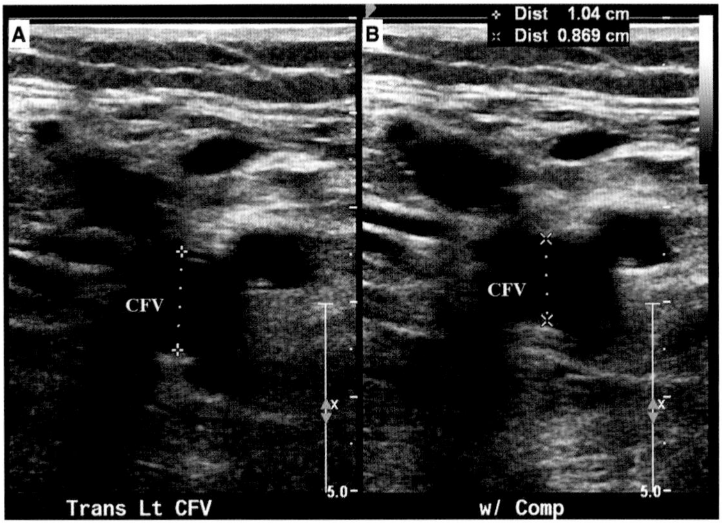

FIGURE 16-2 Transverse Duplex ultrasound image of the left common femoral vein (CFV) for the diagnosis of DVT. In the acute setting, the DVT is iso-echoic on ultrasound and is not directly visible (**A**). However, external compression with the ultrasound probe (**B**) is not able to compress the wall of the CFV. By direct measurement, the anterior-posterior dimension of 1.04 cm is only decreased to 0.07 cm with compression. (Reproduced with permission from John Blebea, MD)

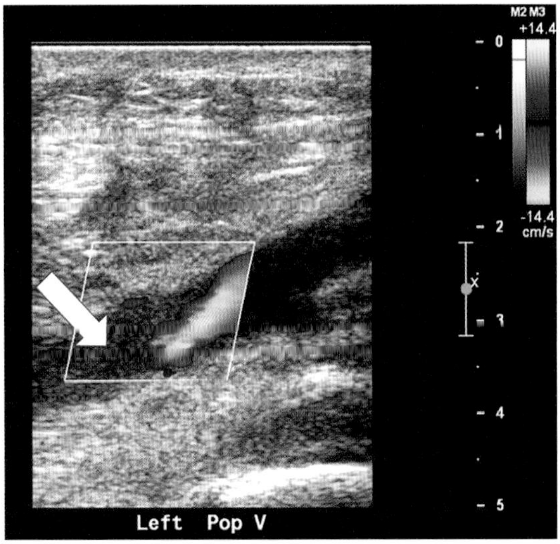

FIGURE 16-3 Longitudinal Duplex ultrasound image of a less-acute popliteal vein DVT. In this case, the thrombus is echogenic and visible on ultrasound (arrow) and obstructs cephalad blood blow, shown in blue. (Reproduced with permission from John Blebea, MD)

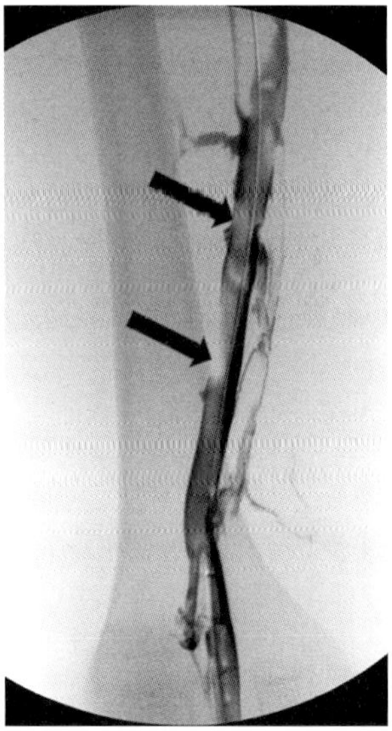

FIGURE 16-4 Venography performed through a catheter in the popliteal vein in preparation for thrombolysis. Thrombus (arrows) is represented by the areas of nonfilling by the injected black contrast. (Reproduced with permission from John Blebea, MD)

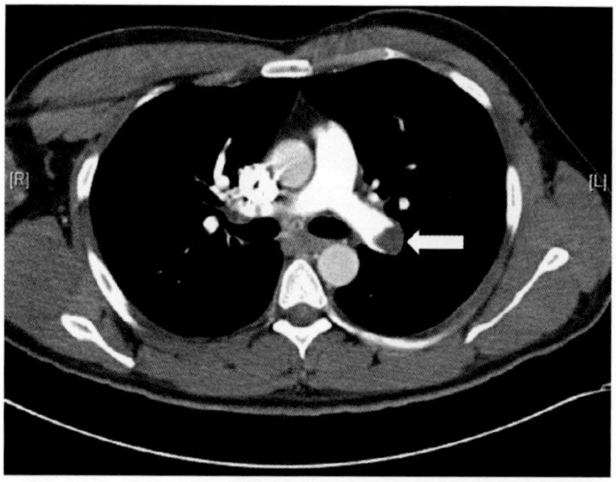

FIGURE 16-5 Cross-sectional computed tomography image demonstrating a pulmonary embolus (arrow) in the left main pulmonary artery. (Reproduced with permission from John Blebea, MD)

may be performed through direct percutaneous contrast injection or utilizing high-resolution CT or MR. Although providing a more detailed and extensive visualization of the veins, each of these modalities has its own disadvantages when compared with duplex ultrasonography. They are invasive and include the administration intravenous of contrast, which can expose the patient to the risk of an allergic reaction and nephrotoxicity. There is an exposure to radiation in the case of both contrast venography and CT, and all are more expensive than ultrasound. CT and MR are considered advantageous for diagnosing PEs (Figure 16-5) and for assessing pelvic vein thrombosis, respectively.

MANAGEMENT OF CLINICAL PROBLEM

Treatment of DVT involves stabilization of the developed thrombus, prevention of thrombus extension and embolization from deep veins, and the facilitation of the innate fibrinolytic systems to encourage clot resolution (Figure 16-6). Therapy may vary depending on acuity and severity of presentation, as well as the anatomic location of affected venous segments. To this end, pharmacologic (anticoagulation) and interventional therapies may be undertaken. In addition to these therapies, the elevation of the affected extremity and compression therapy should be employed for symptomatic relief for DVT.[10,11]

MODALITIES OF TREATMENT

Pharmacologic—Anticoagulation

Anticoagulation represents the mainstay therapy for patients diagnosed with DVT (Figure 16-7).[12] In patients without contraindications, anticoagulation should be initiated when there is a high level of suspicion for DVT and should not be delayed if imaging is not readily available. Current first-line therapy for the treatment of acute VTE in patients without contraindications as recommended by the ACCP is direct oral anticoagulants (DOACs) (Figures 16-1 and 16-2).[13,14] Most patients can be treated as outpatients with only those with acute iliofemoral DVT and severe symptoms requiring hospitalization (Figure 16-1). Oral anticoagulation can also be achieved with vitamin K antagonists such as warfarin. Vitamin K antagonists, although inexpensive, require frequent monitoring of anticoagulant activity (i.e., prothrombin time or INR). Unlike these agents, DOACs do not require monitoring and dose adjustments but may need dose reduction depending on the patient's hepatic and renal function. In general, the bleeding potential for the DOACs is less compared to vitamin K antagonists, especially the incidence of intracranial hemorrhage, although bleeding may still occur in 5% to 10% of cases, commonly from the GI tract.

Anticoagulation also can be achieved through the administration of intravenous unfractionated heparin or subcutaneous low molecular weight heparins (LMWH). LMWHs are preferred in patients with DVT in the setting of a GI malignancy and in pregnancy. Some evidence indicates that LMWH may decrease the severity of the postthrombotic syndrome.[15] Unfortunately, these heparins predispose a small fraction of patients to develop an immune reaction and hypercoagulability in the form of heparin-induced thrombocytopenia (HIT). In patients with HIT or suspected HIT requiring parenteral anticoagulation, direct thrombin inhibitors, such as bivalirudin, lepirudin, and argatroban, can be used via the parenteral route in the patients who require anticoagulation. The length of anticoagulation depends on a number of factors, the most important being the thrombotic risk at the time of the initial DVT. In terms

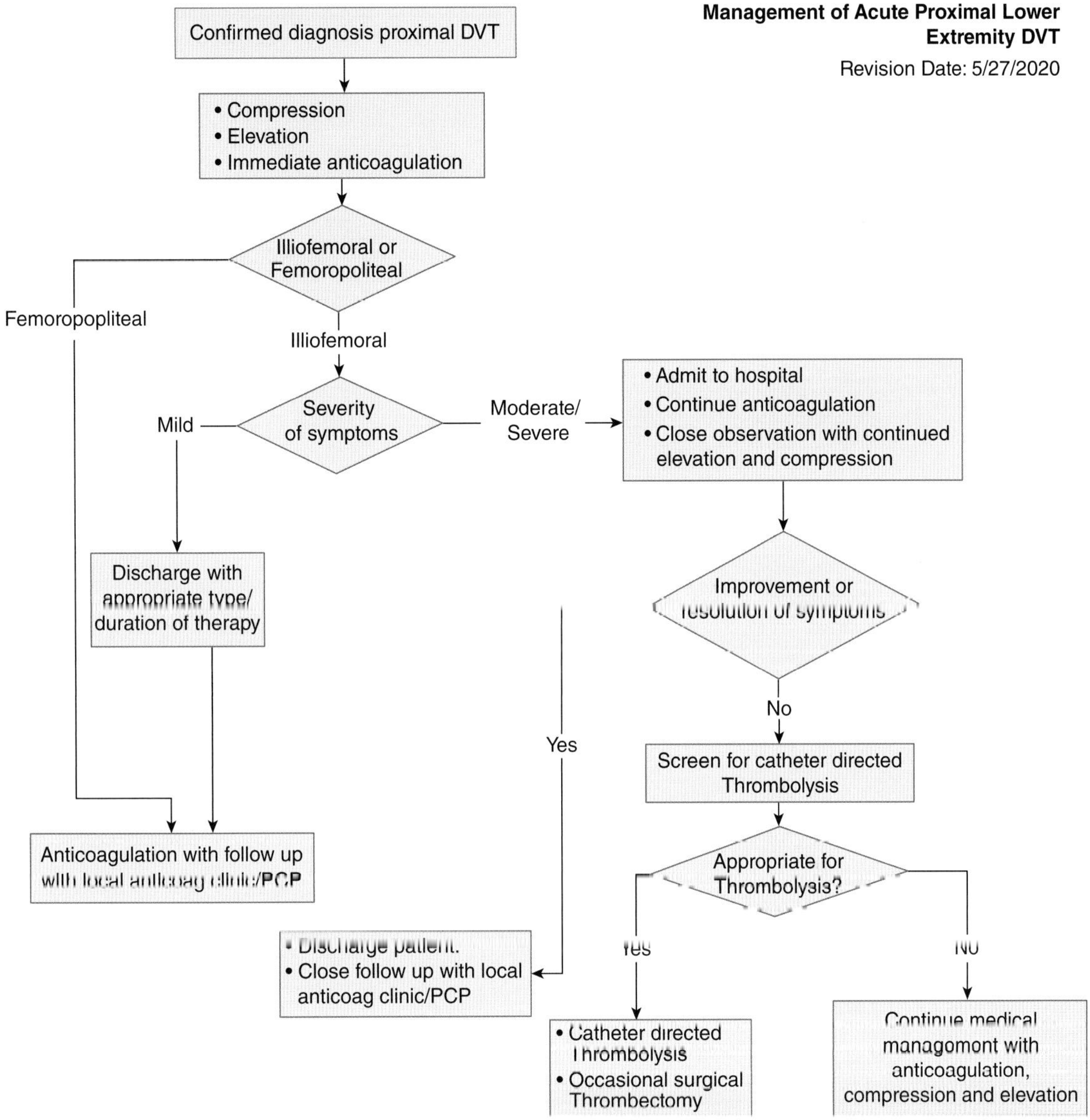

FIGURE 16-6 Management of acute proximal lower extremity DVT. (Reproduced with permission from Grant PJ, Courey AJ, Hanigan S, et al. *Guidelines of Clinical Care Inpatient, Special Topics in Venous Thromboembolism [Internet]*. Ann Arbor, MI: Michigan Medicine University of Michigan; 2019 Feb.)

of a DVT without evident or transient reversible risk factors (such as surgery under general anesthesia > 30 minutes, major trauma, acute illness with immobilization), anticoagulation is usually indicated for a period of time longer than 3 months.[16] In the presence of reversible risk factors, 3 months for a first-time DVT is recommended. Following completion of full-dose anticoagulation, reduced-dose rivaroxaban or apixaban may be prescribed to mitigate the risk of recurrent VTE.[17] Alternatively, aspirin 100 mg reduces the risk of recurrent VTE, although to a lesser degree (Figure 16-2).[18]

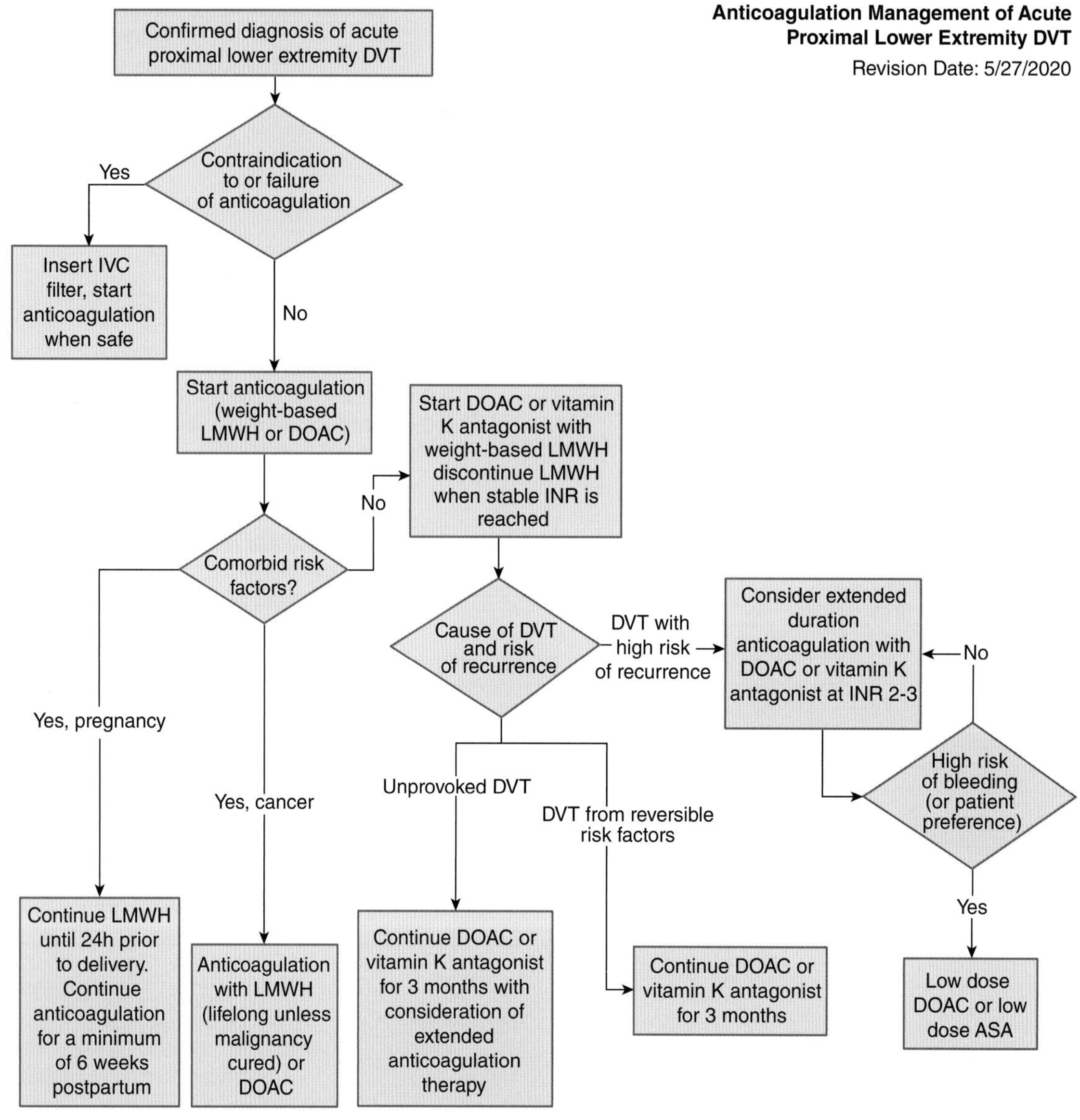

FIGURE 16-7 Anticoagulant considerations for management of lower extremity DVT. (Reproduced with permission from Grant PJ, Courey AJ, Hanigan S, et al. *Guidelines of Clinical Care Inpatient, Special Topics in Venous Thromboembolism [Internet]*. Ann Arbor, MI: Michigan Medicine University of Michigan; 2019 Feb.)

Interventional

A select group of patients with iliofemoral DVT and more severe symptoms are candidates for interventional treatment for acute DVT such as catheter-directed thrombolysis, thrombectomy, and venous stenting.[19] Rarely, this therapy is employed for limb salvage in the setting of venous gangrene, and phlegmasia cerulean dolens. More commonly, it is employed to decrease limb morbidity from the development of postthrombotic syndrome in patients with severe obstructive iliofemoral DVT.[20] Patients mostly likely to benefit from invasive therapies are those with good functional status with >2-year life expectancy with extensive acute iliofemoral DVTs.[21] Contraindications to catheter-directed thrombolysis include DVTs that do not involve the iliac system, DVTs with symptoms lasting > 28 days, active bleeding, recent surgery, active malignancy, severe hypertension, and those with poor functional status. Importantly, catheter-directed thrombolysis does not decrease the risk of PE or mortality and comes with the risk of increased bleeding, points that must be discussed with the patient.

TREATMENT OF DVT BASED ON ANATOMIC LOCATION

Upper Extremity DVT (UE DVT)

Upper extremity DVT may involve the brachiocephalic, axillary, and subclavian veins. These DVTs may be primary (spontaneous) or secondary (provoked). Primary UE DVT risk increases with thoracic outlet syndrome, where the subclavian vein is compressed by the first rib, a cervical rib, the clavicle, subclavius muscle, or anterior scalene muscle. A manifestation of thoracic outlet syndrome (TOS) anatomy is the Paget–Schroetter syndrome which is effort thrombosis of the subclavian vein associated with repetitive motion, such as baseball pitching. Secondary UE DVTs account for the majority of UE DVTs, and the most common causes of these DVTs include indwelling catheters, malignancy, or surgery/trauma to the affected upper extremity.[22]

The choice of anticoagulant and duration of anticoagulation is determined by patient comorbidities and the presence of reversible risk factors, similar to lower extremity DVT. For catheter-associated DVTs, the catheter should be removed as soon as possible and anticoagulation continued for 3 months after the catheter is removed if there is no contradiction. If the catheter is still needed, then it can remain in place with the patient continuing on anticoagulation.[23] Thrombolysis may be considered in patients with an acute UE DVT with TOS, those with severe symptoms, or those dependent on dialysis access in the affected arm. For patients with TOS, surgical release of the vein via cervical or first rib resection should be performed expeditiously to prevent rethrombosis following thrombolysis.

Lower Extremity DVT (LE DVT)

Severe Obstructive Proximal (Iliofemoral) DVT

Anticoagulation is indicated for all the patients with proximal LE DVT, involving the popliteal vein and higher. Thrombus removal may be considered in patients with iliofemoral DVTs for relief of acute symptoms and prevention of severe PTS if they meet specific criteria: phlegmasia alba dolens progressing to phlegmasia cerulea dolens, characterized by massive painful limb swelling with or without cyanosis, skin blisters and/or necrosis, and loss of or diminished arterial pulses (Figure 16-1). Aggressive therapies for phlegmasia include both thrombolysis and occasionally venous thrombectomy should the patient not respond to initial extremity elevation, fluid resuscitation, and aggressive systemic anticoagulation. Surgical thrombectomy is reserved for those who have contraindications to thrombolysis.

Acute LE DVT with Large Central Vein Thrombosis

Extensive acute LE DVT may occur in the setting of chronic thrombosis of the central veins such as the inferior vena cava or the iliac veins. The acute thrombus may be treated with a similar approach to proximal LE DVTs described in the previous section.

Distal (Calf) DVT

There are two recommended options for the management of distal (calf) DVTs: anticoagulation of the same duration as for proximal DVT or serial duplex monitoring and anticoagulation if there is thrombus extension. Patients who are high risk, including those with elevated D dimer, severe symptoms, cancer, VTE history, no identifiable reversible risk factor, hospitalized, thrombus > 5 cm long, involving multiple veins, >7 mm diameter, or in close proximity to the popliteal vein should be treated with anticoagulation. For low-risk patients, serial duplex ultrasonography may be performed over a 2-week interval to assess for clot propagation, and anticoagulation therapy for 3 months duration prescribed, if the extension of the thrombus is identified. A review of the literature shows that the rate of clot extension into the popliteal vein ranges from 0.9% to 5.7% in untreated patients. It should be noted that calf DVTs involving the gastrocnemius and soleus vein in isolation do not generally require anticoagulation therapy. The most recent randomized controlled trial on this subject found no advantage for LMWH anticoagulation in reducing the risk of proximal extension or VTE events in low-risk patients with symptomatic calf DVT; however, anticoagulation did predispose patients to an increased bleeding risk.[24]

CASE PRESENTATION

A 56-year-old woman presents with a 2-day history of a painful, swollen left lower extremity. She was recently prescribed hormone replacement therapy for menopause but otherwise denies any significant medical history. On examination, her left lower extremity is swollen from her ankle to her thigh and is tender to palpation. Her motor and sensory faculties are intact with preserved palpable pedal pulses.

This patient underwent compression with a single layer stretch bandage in the emergency department and was fitted for compression stockings 20 to 30 mmHg several days later. She was initially treated as an inpatient with heparin infusion and leg elevation. Her symptoms improved with medical therapy and she did not undergo interventional therapy. She was discharged after 3 months with apixaban and estrogen-containing hormone replacement therapy was discontinued. After 3 months, she began a maintenance program of low-dose apixaban.

ACKNOWLEDGMENT

Special thanks to Thomas Wakefield, MD for his assistance and support.

REFERENCES

1. Heit JA, Ashrani A, Crusan DJ, McBane RD, Petterson TM, Bailey KR. Reasons for the persistent incidence of venous thromboembolism. *Thromb Haemost.* 2017;117:390-400.
2. Heit JA, Spencer FA, White RH. The epidemiology of venous thromboembolism. *J Thromb Thrombolysis.* 2016;41:3-14.
3. Beckman MG, Hooper WC, Critchley SE, Ortel TL. Venous thromboembolism: a public health concern. *Am J Prev Med.* 2010;38:S495-501.
4. Grosse SD, Nelson RE, Nyarko KA, Richardson LC, Raskob GE. The economic burden of incident venous thromboembolism in the United States: a review of estimated attributable healthcare costs. *Thromb Res.* 2016;137:3-10.
5. White RH, Keenan CR. Effects of race and ethnicity on the incidence of venous thromboembolism. *Thromb Res.* 2009;123(Suppl 4):S11-S17.
6. Caprini JA, Arcelus JI, Reyna JJ. Effective risk stratification of surgical and nonsurgical patients for venous thromboembolic disease. *Semin Hematol.* 2001;38:12-19.
7. Wakefield TW, Myers DD, Henke PK. Mechanisms of venous thrombosis and resolution. *Arterioscler Thromb Vasc Biol.* 2008;28:387-91.
8. Wells PS, Anderson DR, Rodger M, et al. Evaluation of D-dimer in the diagnosis of suspected deep-vein thrombosis. *N Engl J Med.* 2003;349:1227-1235.
9. Bruinstroop E, Klok FA, Van De Ree MA, Oosterwijk FL, Huisman MV. Elevated D-dimer levels predict recurrence in patients with idiopathic venous thromboembolism: a meta-analysis. *J Thromb Haemost.* 2009;7:611-618.
10. Amin EE, Bistervels IM, Meijer K, et al. Reduced incidence of vein occlusion and postthrombotic syndrome after immediate compression for deep vein thrombosis. *Blood.* 2018;132:2298-2304.
11. Kahn SR, Shapiro S, Wells PS, et al. Compression stockings to prevent post-thrombotic syndrome: a randomised placebo-controlled trial. *Lancet.* 2014; 383:880-888.
12. Weitz JI, Jaffer IH, Fredenburgh JC. Recent advances in the treatment of venous thromboembolism in the era of the direct oral anticoagulants. *F1000Res.* 2017;6:985.
13. Ahmed Z, Hassan S, Salzman GA. Novel oral anticoagulants for venous thromboembolism with special emphasis on risk of hemorrhagic complications and reversal agents. *Curr Drug Ther.* 2016;11:3-20.

14. Gross PL, Weitz JI. New anticoagulants for treatment of venous thromboembolism. *Arterioscler Thromb Vasc Biol*. 2008;28:380-386.
15. Hull RD, Pineo GF, Brant R, et al. Home therapy of venous thrombosis with long-term LMWH versus usual care: patient satisfaction and post-thrombotic syndrome. *Am J Med*. 2009;122:762-769, e3.
16. Kearon C, Akl EA. Duration of anticoagulant therapy for deep vein thrombosis and pulmonary embolism. *Blood*. 2014;123:1794-801.
17. Vasanthamohan L, Boonyawat K, Chai-Adisaksopha C, Crowther M. Reduced-dose direct oral anticoagulants in the extended treatment of venous thromboembolism: a systematic review and meta-analysis. *J Thromb Haemost*. 2018;16:1288-1295.
18. Simes J, Becattini C, Agnelli G, et al. Aspirin for the prevention of recurrent venous thromboembolism: the INSPIRE collaboration. *Circulation*. 2014;130: 1062-1071.
19. Elsharawy M, Elzayat E. Early results of thrombolysis vs anticoagulation in iliofemoral venous thrombosis. A randomised clinical trial. *Eur J Vasc Endovasc Surg*. 2002;24:209-214.
20. Kahn SR, Julian JA, Kearon C, et al. Quality of life after pharmacomechanical catheter-directed thrombolysis for proximal deep venous thrombosis. *J Vasc Surg Venous Lymphat Disord*. 2020;8:8-23, e18.
21. Vedantham S, Goldhaber SZ, Julian JA, et al. Pharmacomechanical catheter-directed thrombolysis for deep-vein thrombosis. *N Engl J Med*. 2017;377: 2240-2252.
22. Kucher N. Clinical practice. Deep-vein thrombosis of the upper extremities. *N Engl J Med*. 2011;364:861-869.
23. Crawford JD, Liem TK, Moneta GL. Management of catheter-associated upper extremity deep venous thrombosis. *J Vasc Surg Venous Lymphat Disord*. 2016;4:375-379.
24. Righini M, Galanaud JP, Guenneguez H, et al. Anticoagulant therapy for symptomatic calf deep vein thrombosis (CACTUS): a randomised, double-blind, placebo-controlled trial. *Lancet Haematol*. 2016;3:e556-e562.

SELF-ASSESSMENT STUDY QUESTIONS AND ANSWERS

Questions

1. Initial treatment of acute femoropopliteal DVT involves all of the following except:
   A. Full systemic anticoagulation
   B. Leg compression
   C. Leg elevation
   D. Immediate thrombolysis
   E. Ambulation once anticoagulation is therapeutic

2. What is the diagnostic test that is the gold standard for the diagnosis of DVT?
   A. Contrast venography
   B. CT scanning
   C. Duplex ultrasonography
   D. Contrast arteriography
   E. MRI

3. Match each DOAC with its mechanism (only one is correct):
   A. Dabigatran and inhibition of Factor Xa
   B. Rivaroxaban and inhibition of Factor Xa
   C. Apixaban and inhibition of Factor IIa
   D. Rivaroxaban and inhibition of Factor IIa
   E. Edoxaban and inhibition of Factor IIa

4. What is the correct way to reverse the following anticoagulants?
   A. Fresh frozen plasma and warfarin
   B. Protamine and warfarin
   C. Vitamin K and LMWH
   D. Vitamin K and heparin
   E. Andexanet alfa and dabigatran

5. When is pharmacomechanical thrombolysis (PMCT) indicated to be used (choose one)?
   A. Asymptomatic acute femoropopliteal DVT
   B. Asymptomatic acute iliofemoral DVT
   C. Symptomatic acute femoropopliteal DVT
   D. Symptomatic acute infrapopliteal DVT
   E. Symptomatic acute iliofemoral DVT

6. An example of a reversible risk factor for DVT is
   A. Cigarette smoking
   B. Hyperlipidemia
   C. Major surgery
   D. Metastatic pancreatic cancer
   E. Protein C deficiency

7. Axillary subclavian thrombosis in a young athlete should prompt evaluation for what underlying condition?
   A. Malignancy
   B. Thoracic outlet syndrome
   C. Hemophilia
   D. Prothrombin gene mutation
   E. SVC syndrome

8. Prior to obtaining imaging, clinical risk stratification in a patient with symptoms concerning for DVT should be calculated via what scoring system?
   A. Caprini risk assessment tool
   B. Padua score
   C. Eagle's criteria
   D. Revised cardiac risk index
   E. Wells score

9. Patient with calf DVT and which findings may be followed with serial ultrasound rather than treated with anticoagulation?
   A. Outpatient, very swollen painful calf
   B. Inpatient, minimal ankle edema
   C. Inpatient, no symptoms, elevated D dimer
   D. Outpatient, >5 cm long, prior DVT
   E. Outpatient, <5 cm long, recent major surgery

10. Which of the following combination therapies reduces the risk of DVT recurrence?
    A. Full dose anticoagulation, low-dose DOAC therapies, aspirin
    B. Aspirin, clopidogrel, ACE inhibitors
    C. Low dose DOAC, aspirin, compression stockings
    D. Full dose anticoagulation, low-dose DOAC, alteplase
    E. Aspirin, cilostazol, statin therapy

SELF-ASSESSMENT STUDY QUESTIONS AND ANSWERS

Answers

1. D.
2. C.
3. B.
4. A.
5. E.
6. C.
7. B.
8. E.
9. E.
10. A.

CHAPTER

17 Pulmonary Embolism

Emily A. Malgor and Rafael D. Malgor

OUTLINE

GENERAL CONSIDERATION AND HISTORY
DIFFERENTIAL DIAGNOSIS
DIAGNOSIS
MANAGEMENT OF THE CLINICAL PROBLEM

GENERAL CONSIDERATION AND HISTORY

Pulmonary emboli (PE), along with deep vein thrombi (DVT), comprise the spectrum of diagnoses referred to as venous thromboembolism (VTE). PE are associated with significant morbidity and mortality: their prevention and treatment are important as they are one of the principal causes of sudden cardiovascular death, third in line after strokes and heart attacks.[1] This high rate of mortality makes PE the most important short-term complication of a DVT. Thus, prevention of a PE is critical, and DVT treatment guidelines are aimed at achieving this goal.[2]

Patients with PE may not display any signs or symptoms that would suggest a PE; this can happen in up to 75% of the patients.[3] One of the explanations for this high incidence of asymptomatic PE is based on the dual blood supply of the lung through the bronchial and pulmonary arteries along with the small size of the majority of PE. However, the higher the thrombus load and greater the number of affected locations, the greater the clinical severity of the PE. The Prospective Investigation of Pulmonary Embolism Diagnosis II (PIOPED II) study documented that most patients with symptomatic PE will present with sudden onset dyspnea, pleuritic chest pain, cough, orthopnea, calf/thigh pain with associated swelling suggestive of DVT, or signs compatible with thrombophlebitis (redness and tenderness to palpation of erythematous superficial veins in the legs).[4]

The American Heart Association (AHA) has proposed three categories to stratify patients with PE: nonmassive, submassive, and massive.[5] The reason for stratifying patients into these categories is to aid in mortality risk assessment and to assist in determining the best treatment strategies. A *nonmassive PE*, also referred to as a low-risk PE, includes those patients who have experienced a PE yet have normal blood pressure, normal levels of cardiac biomarkers, and normal right heart (specifically, right ventricle) function on imaging. Normal blood pressure includes a systolic blood pressure ranging from 90 mmHg to 120 mmHg and a diastolic blood pressure ranging from 60 to 80 mmHg. Cardiac biomarkers used to assess PE stress include troponins and natriuretic peptides. Imaging modalities used to assess the right ventricle include an echocardiogram ("echo") and CT scan. Additionally, an electrocardiogram ("EKG") is used to identify patients at risk of adverse outcomes in acute PE.

A *submassive PE* is defined as an acute PE with a normal systolic blood pressure ($\geq$90 mmHg) but with right ventricular (RV) dysfunction or the presence of ischemic heart muscle (myocardial necrosis). RV dysfunction is determined by dilation of the RV on imaging, abnormal findings on an EKG, or elevation of cardiac biomarkers (described above). Myocardial necrosis is defined by the elevation of troponins (a type of cardiac biomarker). A *massive PE* refers to those patients in whom an acute PE has occurred with a resulting systolic blood pressure of <90 mmHg for more than 15 minutes or requiring intravenous medications to normalize it, with no other identifiable cause. Patients experiencing a massive PE have a significantly increased risk of death, both during their initial hospital stay and 90 days beyond the event.

DIFFERENTIAL DIAGNOSIS

Determining the probability that a PE has occurred is the first step a physician will take in evaluating PE. Other possible diagnoses to be considered include, but are not limited to, musculoskeletal pain, inflammation involving the lungs (pleuritis), inflammation involving the heart (pericarditis), hyperventilation, lung trauma, or inflammation of the central part of the chest (mediastinitis).

An efficient and cost effective way of determining the likelihood of a PE and the need for more rigorous and costly diagnostic tests is to calculate a clinic probability score. More than one tool exist to determine this, with the Wells Short Clinical Score commonly used. Briefly, a score of ≤2 is considered low, a score between 2 and 6 is moderate, and a score ≥7 is high. Table 17-1 shows the Wells Short Clinical Score.[6] The low- and moderate-scoring patients can have a diagnosis of PE ruled out with a D-dimer test and an additional imaging study.

TABLE 17-1 Wells Short Clinical Score for Predicting PE[6]

Criteria	Score
Clinical signs and symptoms of deep venous thrombosis: minimal swelling of the leg and pain on palpation of the deep leg veins	3.0
Pulmonary embolism more likely than an alternative diagnosis	3.0
Heartbeat frequency >100 beats per minute	1.5
Recent immobilization or surgery within <4 weeks	1.5
Documented history of deep venous thrombosis and/or pulmonary embolism	1.5
Hemoptysis	1.0
Recent history of malignancy <6 months (treatment or palliative treatment)	1.0

DIAGNOSIS

The clinical findings listed above, whether witnessed or described by the patient, make the diagnosis of PE a possibility, particularly if a DVT is suspected or confirmed (see Chapter 16 for symptoms and signs of DVT). Once a patient who has been evaluated is suspected of having a PE as a result of their history and physical examination, additional tests should follow. Those patients in whom there is a low or moderate probability of PE (based upon the Wells Short Clinical Score, Table 17-1) will undergo a blood draw to obtain a D-dimer level. This protein fragment develops when a blood clot dissolves. It is a highly sensitive test, so it can effectively rule *out* the presence of a PE. In other words, if its result is negative (normal), no treatment is indicated for a PE. On the other hand, it has only moderate specificity, so it is limited in its ability to rule *in* PE. This is why a positive D-dimer warrants imaging capable of accurately visualizing the pulmonary arteries, typically CT angiography (Figure 17-1). Figure 17-2 illustrates

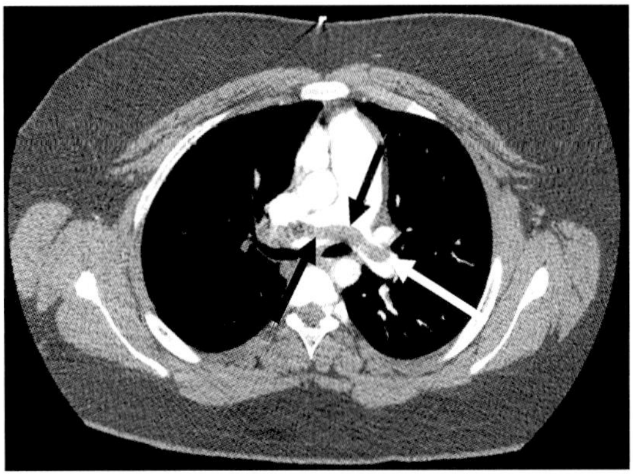

FIGURE 17-1 Cross-sectional CT angiogram demonstrating saddle embolus obstructing both the right and left pulmonary arteries. (Reproduced with permission from John Blebea, MD.)

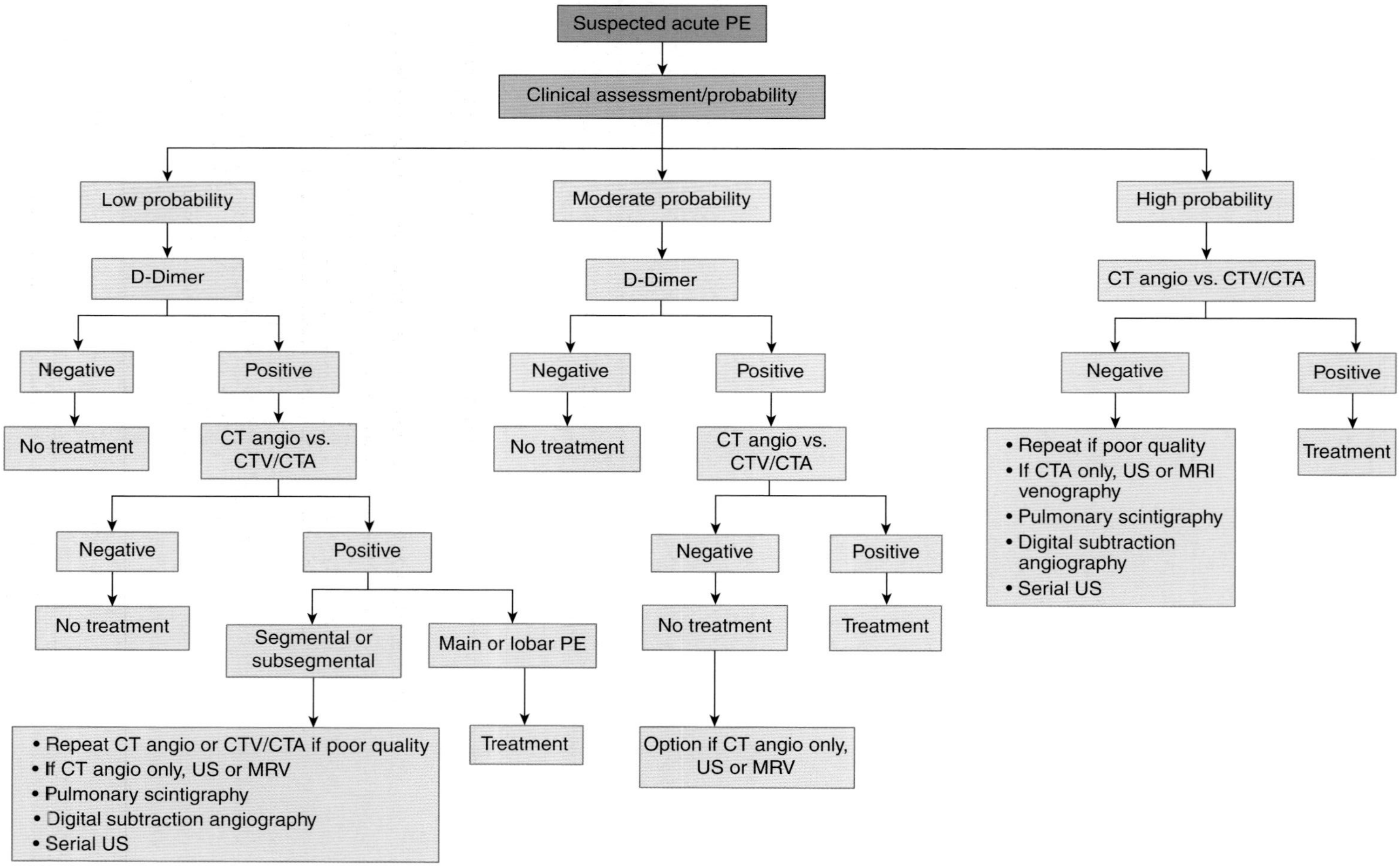

FIGURE 17-2 Algorithm for the diagnosis of PE. CT, computed tomography; CTA, computed tomographic angiography; CTV, computed tomographic venography; MRI, magnetic resonance imaging; MRV, magnetic resonance venography; US, ultrasound. (Reproduced with permission from Gloviczki P, Forum AV. *Handbook of Venous and Lymphatic Disorders: Guidelines of the American Venous Forum*. 4th ed. Boca Raton, FL: CRC Press; 2017.)

a diagnostic algorithm applied to patients with suspicion of PE.[7]

MANAGEMENT OF THE CLINICAL PROBLEM

Different approaches to treat a confirmed acute PE exist. The selected treatment varies greatly based on the levels of severity of the PE and its clinical effect on the patient. However, all patients with a confirmed PE will be systemically anticoagulated, will have biomarkers obtained via a blood draw, and will undergo an EKG.

Low-risk patients have normal systolic blood pressure (>90 mmHg), normal cardiac biomarkers, normal EKG, and low PE severity as determined by different types of clinical scores (such as the AHA classification and the Pulmonary Embolism Severity Index, or PESI).[5,7,8] The simplified version of the PESI (sPESI) contains a more limited number of parameters and is commonly used in clinical practice (Table 17-2). *Nonmassive PE* falls into this category.[5] These patients can be monitored as an outpatient, and admission to a hospital is optional. Anticoagulation is always initiated if there are no contra-indications.

Patients considered to be at *moderate risk* have a normal systolic blood pressure, but they demonstrate any one of the following: persistently lowered blood oxygen saturation levels below 94%, an EKG showing signs of increased pressure in the pulmonary arteries (pulmonary hypertension), elevated cardiac biomarkers, an echo demonstrating decreased movement (hypokinesis) of the right ventricle of the heart, and an elevated PE severity score, among other things. Thus, in addition to initiating an anticoagulant, it is recommended that these patients can be admitted to the hospital for ongoing monitoring.[7]

TABLE 17-2 Simplified Pulmonary Embolism Severity Index[7,8]

Parameters Assessed	Points*
Age >80 years	1
History of cancer	1
Chronic cardiopulmonary disease	1
Pulse ≥110/min	1
Systolic blood pressure <100 mmHg	1
Arterial oxygen saturation <90%	1

*Low risk=0, high risk ≥1.

Should a patient develop new or worsening signs, a repeat set of cardiac biomarkers, echo, and risk assessment are indicated. Importantly, when patients exhibit moderate distress, they represent a more severe presentation of moderate risk. These patients demonstrate severe right ventricular hypokinesis on echo or a worsening EKG. In addition to anticoagulation, most of these patients will be admitted to an intensive care unit (ICU) and will receive fibrinolytics. *Submassive PE* falls into the more severe moderate-risk category.[5] The *high-risk* category specifically describes patients with low systolic blood pressure and who are in distress, as you would see in the setting of a *massive PE*. These patients will all be admitted to the ICU and initiated on fibrinolytic agents unless contraindicated.[5,7]

When a patient with PE presents to the emergency department or via the transfer center, the pulmonary embolism response team (PERT) is contacted if such a regional team has been established.[9] This is a multidisciplinary team that includes cardiothoracic surgeons, interventional radiologists or cardiologists, vascular surgeons, pulmonologists, and intensivists. This team of cardiopulmonary and vascular specialists will discuss the patient's risk category and decide on the best therapeutic approach among the treatment modalities that are available to treat patients with PE. The primary initial treatment remains the so-called conservative treatment with intravenous systemic heparin anticoagulation. However, the treatment should be tailored to each patient's clinical status and risk of bleeding with anticoagulation (Figure 17-3). The utilization of a prophylactic inferior vena cava filter in patients with PE has attracted much attention in the past with some controversy remaining. There is, however, no beneficial long-term data and a lack of level 1 evidence to recommend its empirical and routine use.[2,10]

Conservative (medical) therapy. The mainstay treatment of PE remains anticoagulation for the vast majority of patients with PE. Anticoagulation is ideally complemented with cardiorespiratory support in an intensive care setting. The primary goal of anticoagulation is to prevent thrombus propagation and new thrombus formation, and to a lesser extent, to trigger the patient's fibrinolytic system to achieve thrombus resolution over time.

Anticoagulation protocols may vary from institution to institution based on different societal guidelines. A protocol must be tailored to each patient's specific risk of bleeding (low or standard heparinization dose protocols). Most of the heparinization protocols recommend 80 to 100 units/kg bolus and then a drip rate of 18 units/kg/h of intravenous unfractionated heparin.[2] Patients who are not candidates for anticoagulation but who have a proximal deep vein thrombosis should be offered an inferior vena cava filter to reduce the risk of a fatal PE in a patient with existing cardiorespiratory compromise. At least 3 to 6 months of anticoagulation is recommended for patients with acute PE without identified underlying thrombophilia or ongoing risk factors. Many patients have these associated conditions and will be maintained on life-long anticoagulation.

Systemic thrombolysis is also part of the algorithm for medical treatment of PE in patients who present with hypotension (e.g., systolic BP <90 mmHg) and who do not have a high bleeding risk (Grade 2B evidence).[2] Some patients presenting with hypotension and who have a higher risk of bleeding are better served with catheter-direct thrombectomy or pharmacomechanical thrombectomy, although this does not entirely eliminate the bleeding risk. Potential limitations include a lack of resources or operator familiarity necessary to do such procedures.

Contraindications to systematic thrombolysis can be found in Table 17-3. However, most of the patients with PE will not necessitate *systematic* thrombolysis; a stronger level of recommendations argues against using systemic thrombolysis in these patients (Grade 1B).[2] Those not presenting with hypotension alone but with severe symptoms of significant cardiopulmonary impairment are at higher risk of deterioration and, therefore, must be monitored closely in an ICU setting. Care in these patients includes continuous hemodynamic monitoring (including blood pressure, heart rate, tissue perfusion, and gas exchange via invasive or noninvasive capnography/oximetry) and trending cardiac biomarkers (troponins, BNP).

TABLE 17-3 Contraindications to Thrombolytics in Patients with PE[2]

Absolute Contraindications	Relative Contraindications
Any prior ICH	Oral anticoagulant therapy
Known structural cerebral vascular lesion (e.g., arteriovenous malformation)	Significant hypertension on presentation (SBP >180 mmHg or DBP >110 mmHg)
Known malignant intracranial neoplasm (primary or metastatic)	History of chronic, severe, poorly controlled hypertension
Ischemic stroke within 3 months[†]	Known intracranial pathology not covered in absolute contraindications
Suspected aortic dissection	Pregnancy, active peptic ulcer
Active bleeding or bleeding diathesis (excluding menses)	History of prior ischemic stroke >3 months
Significant closed-head or facial trauma within 3 months	Traumatic or prolonged (>10 min) CPR
Intracranial or intraspinal surgery within 2 months	Major surgery (<3 weeks)
Severe uncontrolled hypertension[*]	Recent (within 2–4 weeks) internal bleeding

[*]Unresponsive to emergency therapy.

[†]except acute ischemic stroke within 4.5 hours.

CPR, cardiopulmonary resuscitation; DBP; diastolic blood pressure; ICH, intracranial hemorrhage; SBP, systolic blood pressure; and STEMI, ST-elevation myocardial infarction.

Endovascular therapy. As endovascular therapy for PE becomes more widely utilized within the US, more data have been generated for different clinical scenarios. The most common indication for catheter-based therapy remains submassive PE or intermediate-risk PE. The main goal for endovascular therapy in these circumstances is a faster reduction in thrombus burden through a minimally invasive approach. Three modalities are currently available: catheter-directed thrombolysis (CDT), suction thrombectomy without associated thrombolytic agents, and pharmaco-mechanical thrombectomy (PMT). These techniques have essentially rendered rotational fragmentation of the thrombus with a pigtail catheter a secondary and outdated strategy in the endovascular treatment of PE.

Catheter-directed thrombolysis. Over the past decade, CDT has become an attractive treatment modality because of its availability and ease of use compared to other endovascular techniques.[11,12] The primary goals of CDT are to reduce right ventricular afterload and to improve gas exchange. With this in mind, the ideal location of the catheter with its multiple side holes is inside the thrombus.

Two of the most common infusion catheters available and used in the United States are the Uni-Fuse® (Angiodynamics, Latham, NY) and Cragg-McNamara™ Micro Therapeutics Infusion Catheter® (eV3 Inc, Plymouth, MN) catheters. Both are approved by the Food and Drug Administration (FDA) for thrombolysis in the peripheral vasculature, without specific indications to treat PE. The Uni-Fuse® catheter is a multihole catheter with an inner wire that occludes its distal tip, distributing the thrombolytic agent out the side holes to percolate directly into the thrombus. The Cragg-McNamara® catheter can be utilized with or without a tip-occluding guidewire in place, allowing thrombolytic infusion from the Prostream™ Infusion Wire.

Technical steps. Access from either the femoral or the jugular vein is obtained and a 5 F or larger sheath is advanced through the right ventricle into the main pulmonary artery. Caution must be exercised when performing venography as it can inadvertently push thrombus further into the right and left pulmonary arteries resulting in rapid hemodynamic deterioration, shock, and cardiopulmonary arrest. Once specific access to the right and left pulmonary arteries is obtained, venography is performed to delineate the anatomy and to determine the location of the most severe thrombus burden. A guidewire is then advanced into the appropriate segmental pulmonary artery, followed by the placement of a multiside hole catheter for infusion.

A tissue plasminogen activator (t-PA) infusion dose of 0.5 to 1.0 mg/h through both the right and left pulmonary artery catheters is initiated. Some interventionalists prefer to place a Swan-Ganz catheter within the main pulmonary artery to monitor hemodynamic changes in the PA and guide the duration of therapy. Additional preferences include following up with a transthoracic echocardiogram within 24 hours of lysis initiation. Once pulmonary artery pressure is significantly reduced or normalized, the catheters and sheaths can be discontinued at the bedside without the use of fluoroscopy.

Lately, ultrasound-assisted infusion of thrombolytic agents (USAT) has been advocated as an alternative to CDT with a multiside hole catheter.[13–16] The Ekos System® (Ekos Corp., Bothell, WA) utilizes an ultrasonic core to generate an acoustic field, dispersing the fibrinolytic agent into the clot. This is felt to disaggregate thrombus through the separation of fibrin crosslinks, accelerating clot thrombolysis. The system consists of a 5.4 French infusion catheter with markers delineating the active ultrasound core. Figure 17-4 depicts a typical setup for PE CDT.

Outcomes. A recent systematic review and meta analysis of CDT to treat intermediate- and high-risk PE was conducted.[17] Fourteen retrospective studies, six prospective studies, one registry, and one randomized controlled trial were analyzed. The authors concluded that CDT achieved a high clinical success rate in patients with intermediate- and high-risk PE; however, these findings were based on sparse high-quality, level 1 evidence.

Complications. The most daunting complication of PE lytic treatment is major bleeding. Major bleeding is defined by the International Society of Thrombosis and Hemostasis (ISTH) as "fatal bleeding or symptomatic bleeding in a critical area or organ, such as intracranial, intraspinal, intraocular resulting in vision changes, retroperitoneal, intraarticular, pericardial, or intramuscular causing compartment syndrome. Along with fatal and symptomatic bleeding in a critical location, a drop in hemoglobin ≥2 g/dL or bleeding requiring transfusion of ≥2 units of whole blood or pack of red cells are considered major bleeding."[18] It is possible to have nonmajor bleeding episodes while on lysis. This is defined as any bleeding that does not fit the ISTH major bleeding definition but requires medical intervention by a healthcare professional, leads to hospitalization

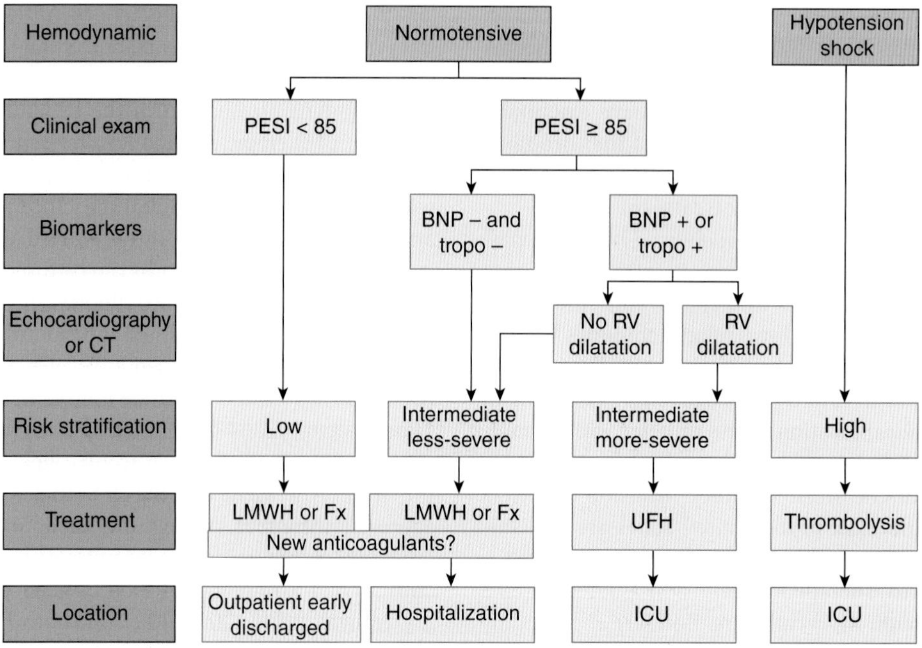

FIGURE 17-3 Algorithm for the treatment of acute PE. BNP, brain natriuretic peptide (cardiac biomarker); Fx, fondaparinux; ICU, intensive care unit; LMWH, low molecular weight heparin (a medication class that includes enoxaparin); PESI, Pulmonary Embolism Severity Index; RV, right ventricle; tropo, troponin (cardiac biomarker); UFH, unfractionated heparin. (Reproduced with permission from Penaloza A, Roy PM, Kline J. Risk stratification and treatment strategy of pulmonary embolism. *Curr Opin Crit Care.* 2012;18(4):318-325)

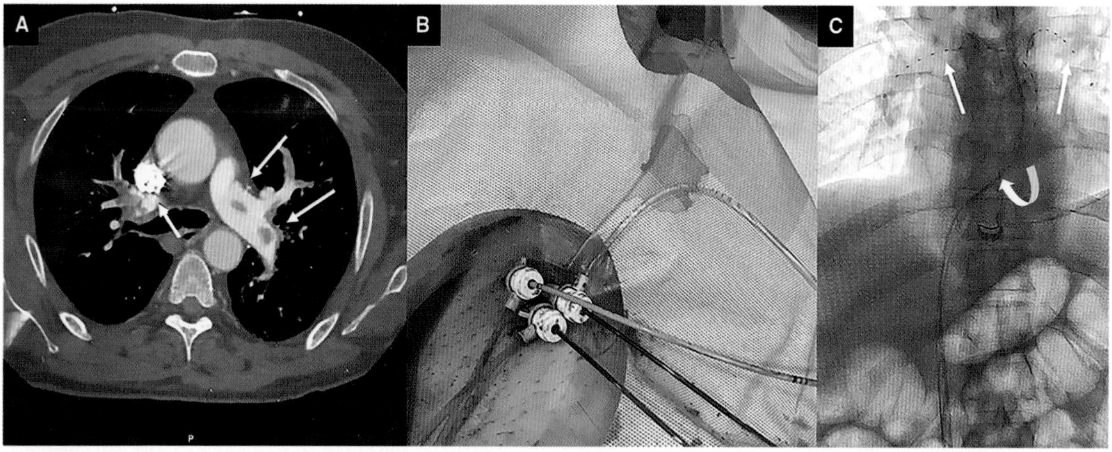

FIGURE 17-4 Ultrasound-assisted infusion of thrombolytic agents in a patient presenting with lower extremity acute DVT and PE following a motor vehicle accident. (**A**) Computed tomography angiography of the chest showing bilateral segmental and subsegmental pulmonary embolism (white arrows). (**B**) Right femoral vein access with two EKOS® infusion catheters and a Swam-Ganz catheter to monitor pulmonary artery pressure (blue catheter). (**C**) Fluoroscopic image showing bilateral pulmonary artery lysis catheter placements (straight arrows) while a Swan-Ganz catheter is placed within the main pulmonary artery (curved arrow).

or increased level of care, or prompts a face-to-face evaluation.[19] The importance of close monitoring of fibrinogen, platelets, hemoglobin, and hematocrit levels cannot be overemphasized. Thrombolysis must be avoided or discontinued in patients presenting with any major or minor active bleeding, and interventions must be taken to address any bleeding at risk of causing permanent organ or limb dysfunction.

Suction thrombectomy and pharmacomechanical thrombectomy. Three catheter-based techniques exist to physically debulk PE: suction/aspiration of the PE, mechanical fragmentation of the PE, and saline-jet fragmentation of the PE combined with aspiration (rheolysis).

The AngioVac System® (Angiodynamics, Latham, NY) is a veno-venous bypass system designed for en bloc suction thrombectomy through a funnel-shaped inflow tip. It is composed of the AngioVac® Cannula and the AngioVac® Circuit. A filter is positioned between the inflow and outflow cannulae to trap thrombotic debris. This system requires a perfusion team to manage the veno-venous bypass circuit and entails large-bore access (26 French inflow and 16–20 French outflow access). The use of AngioVac® for PE thrombectomy is not widely reported, likely due to the difficulty in safely steering such a large-bore catheter into the right ventricular outflow tract and pulmonary arteries.[20] Design improvements in the last few years have been made in order to overcome challenges with navigating the cannula. Figure 17-5 exemplifies the use of the AngioVac® device.

The Penumbra Indigo® System (Penumbra, Inc., Alameda, CA) uses mechanical thrombus engagement with a mechanized continuous aspiration to remove the thrombus. The system was originally designed to remove thrombus from peripheral

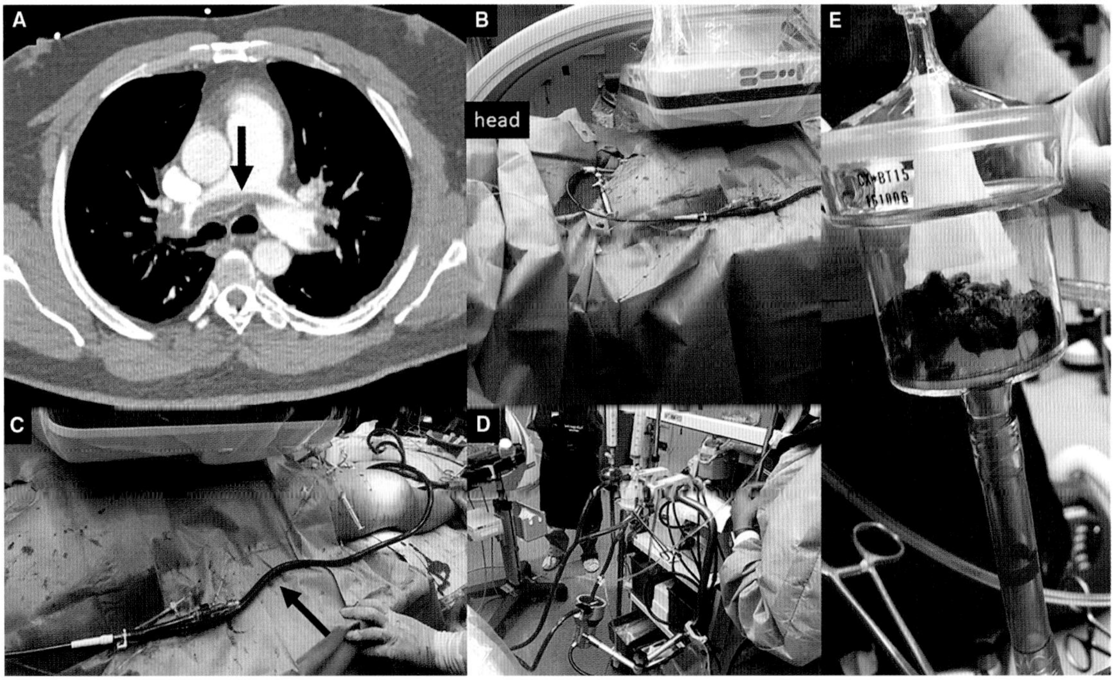

FIGURE 17-5 The AngioVac thrombectomy system in a patient with acute shortness of breath and altered mental status. (**A**) Computed tomography angiography shows a saddle pulmonary embolus (arrows). (**B**) Jugular thrombectomy cannula inserted for thrombus extraction. (**C**) The cannula is connected via tubing (arrow) for blood return through the common femoral vein. (**D**) A centrifugal blood pump maintains suction and flows in the cannula circuit. (**E**) Large clot burden removed from the pulmonary arteries.

arteries and veins, utilizing catheters as large as 12 French. A system designed specifically for the pulmonary arteries (Penumbra Indigo® Aspiration System) is in its trial phase, currently available only to those institutions with an investigative device exemption (IDE). The EXTRACT-PE Trial recently met primary safety and efficacy endpoints in November 2019. However, there is still a paucity of data on PE treatment.[21] The advantages of this system over other endovascular PE treatments are the portability and flexibility of the catheters without the need for thrombolytic agents (Figure 17-6A).

The FlowTriever® Retrieval/Aspiration System (Inari Medical, Irvine, CA) is the first mechanical suction thrombectomy catheter specifically approved to treat PE (Figure 17-6B). A retractable aspirator creates a vacuum to extract large thrombi, which is one of the most appealing uses of this system. Other advantages are the lack of need for an ICU admission, the lack of need for use of thrombolytics, and possible treatment in a single session. Despite all these advantages, caution must be exercised while navigating the pulmonary artery and its branches to prevent heart and pulmonary arterial injuries due to the large catheter size and associated inflexibility of the system. A prospective trial analyzing the safety and efficacy of FlowTriever® enrolled 106 patients with intermediate-risk PE. This showed significant improvement in the RV/LV ratio (reduction of 0.38; 25.1%, $P < 0.001$) and minimal major bleeding events (1%).[22]

The AngioJet™ System (Boston Scientific, Minneapolis, MN) is a pharmaco-mechanical thrombectomy system utilizing the Venturi-Bernoulli effect via high-velocity, high-pressure saline jets (mechanical effect) following impregnation of the thrombus with a thrombolytic agent (pharmacological effect). The catheter comes in multiple sizes up to the 8 French ZelanteDVT™ Catheter, which can provide better impregnation of thrombus with thrombolytic agents. Advantages related to PMT with Angiojet™ are seen in the reduction of contrast and thrombolytic agents needed and the possibility of treating submassive and massive PE in a single session.[23] The major adverse events related to this PMT system are the release of thrombus byproducts that can cause severe bradycardia and asystole and pigments that can cause acute renal failure.

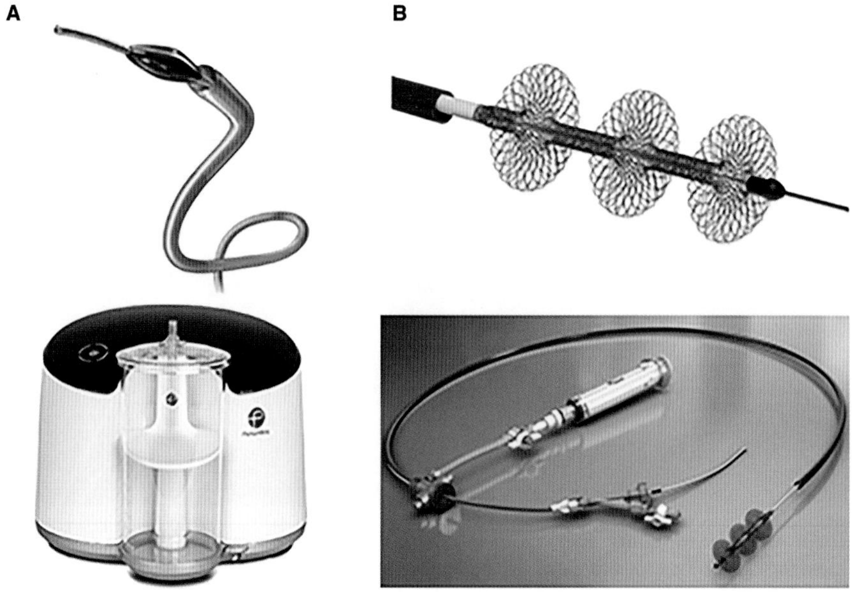

FIGURE 17-6 Suction thrombectomy systems to treat PE. (**A**) The Penumbra Indigo™ with its catheter (top) and automated suction pump (bottom). (**B**) The FlowTriever system™ with its catheter and syringe suction system.

Open surgery. In patients with massive PE, emergency surgical pulmonary embolectomy (SPE) via a median sternotomy may be necessary. Open surgery is indicated in massive PE or in patients with a submassive PE with contraindications to thrombolysis. Candidates for open surgery have a surgically accessible, centrally located thrombus rather than multiple peripheral emboli. Other indications for open surgery are active bleeding, rapid deterioration despite systemic thrombolysis or CDT, thrombus-in-transit, the presence of a large patent foramen ovale and/or severe right ventricular dysfunction.

Operative steps. Access to the pulmonary artery is gained via a median sternotomy. The patient is then placed on full cardiopulmonary bypass by cannulating the ascending aorta and the superior vena cava; anticoagulation with an activated clotting time target of at least ≥350 to 400 seconds is necessary. Cardioplegia is initiated, and a 2-cm longitudinal main pulmonary arteriotomy is made and extended to the proximal left pulmonary artery, distal to the pulmonic valve, and short of the pulmonary artery bifurcation. A combination of forceps and suction catheters is employed to remove a saddle PE. If a thrombus is found in the right pulmonary artery, an arteriotomy on the right pulmonary artery between the aorta and the superior vena cava is made. In certain circumstances, the pleural cavity can be entered and the lungs compressed to direct smaller, more peripheral thrombi to the larger proximal vessels to be aspirated. In cases where a thrombus is located in the right atrium or ventricle, a right atriotomy or ventriculotomy can be performed. The use of hypothermia can be avoided when cardiopulmonary bypass time is anticipated to be short. Patients treated via open surgery are ideally cared for postoperatively in cardiothoracic intensive care units where vital signs, oxygenation, and heart function parameters are closely monitored.

Outcomes. In a systematic review and meta-analysis on 1579 patients with pooled data regarding PE outcomes, all-cause mortality was 26.3% and surgical site complications 7%. Gastrointestinal and pulmonary bleeding amounted to 3% and 4%, respectively. A major issue with this study was the large dispersion of data pooled from 56 studies with different inclusion criteria, but it provided valuable information nonetheless.[24]

Complications. Major complications can ensue during or after emergency pulmonary embolectomy. Some of the intraoperative or immediate postoperative complications include the inability to wean the patient from cardiopulmonary bypass, persistent RV dysfunction, and cardiac tamponade. Other postoperative complications include poststernal wound infection and postoperative bleeding. The most important factor in avoiding these complications is a meticulous operative technique followed by attempts to minimize cardiopulmonary bypass time. Additionally, timely and early intervention for open surgery in patients with worsening hemodynamics and respiratory parameters increases the success of operative treatment.

Extracorporeal life support (ECLS). ECLS uses extracorporeal membrane oxygenation (ECMO) to bypass the lungs and heart. It provides hemodynamic and respiratory support in patients with high-risk PE. ECLS is an available alternative when the patient cannot withstand immediate surgery or when a surgical team is not immediately available. The role of ECLS is to counteract hypoxia and to provide cardiopulmonary support until the thrombus burden is reduced and pulmonary blood flow is adequately reestablished.

A common limitation of ECLS is the lack of a dedicated team to perform the procedure. ECLS can be started within 30 minutes in centers with adequate resources and trained personnel. It is often used as a bridge for more definitive open or endovascular treatment. Typically, the femoral vein and artery are accessed with cannulas to create a circuit with a membrane oxygenator and blood pump. Alternative access includes the axillary artery and the jugular vein. Upon placement of cannulas, the patient is fully heparinized for a target ACT between 160 and 220 seconds. Patients with respiratory failure due to PE recover within 48 to 72 hours, compared to other respiratory-failure-generating entities, such as ARDS, that require an average of 12 days of ECLS. Decannulation should be performed in the operating room with the repair of the access vessels at that time.

REFERENCES

1. Beyth RJ, Cohen AM, Landefeld CS. Long-term outcomes of deep-vein thrombosis. *Arch Intern Med.* 1995;155(10):1031-1037.
2. Kearon C, Akl EA, Ornelas J, et al. Antithrombotic therapy for VTE disease: CHEST guideline and expert panel report. *Chest.* 2016;149(2):315-352.
3. Kistner RL, Ball JJ, Nordyke RA, Freeman GC. Incidence of pulmonary embolism in the course of thrombophlebitis of the lower extremities. *Am J Surg.* 1972;124(2):169-176.
4. Beckman MG, Hooper WC, Critchley SE, Ortel TL. Venous thromboembolism: a public health concern. *Am J Prev Med.* 2010;38(Suppl 4):S495-S501.
5. Jaff MR, McMurtry MS, Archer SL, et al. Management of massive and submassive pulmonary embolism, iliofemoral deep vein thrombosis, and chronic thromboembolic pulmonary hypertension: a scientific statement from the American Heart Association. *Circulation.* 2011;123(16):1788-1830.
6. Prandoni P, Lensing AWA, Prins MH, Barbar S. On the true prevalence of pulmonary embolism in patients hospitalized for a first syncopal event. *J Am Coll Cardiol.* 2019;74(23):2950-2951.
7. Gloviczki P, Forum AV. *Handbook of Venous and Lymphatic Disorders: Guidelines of the American Venous Forum.* 4th ed. CRC Press; 2017.
8. Aujesky D, Obrosky DS, Stone RA, et al. Derivation and validation of a prognostic model for pulmonary embolism. *Am J Respir Crit Care Med.* 2005;172(8):1041-1046.
9. Rosovsky R, Chang Y, Rosenfield K, et al. Changes in treatment and outcomes after creation of a pulmonary embolism response team (PERT), a 10-year analysis. *J Thromb Thrombolysis.* 2019;47(1):31-40.
10. Mismetti P, Laporte S, Pellerin O, et al. Effect of a retrievable inferior vena cava filter plus anticoagulation vs anticoagulation alone on risk of recurrent pulmonary embolism: a randomized clinical trial. *JAMA.* 2015;313(16):1627-1635.
11. Bloomer TL, El-Hayek GE, McDaniel MC, et al. Safety of catheter-directed thrombolysis for massive and submassive pulmonary embolism: results of a multicenter registry and meta-analysis. *Catheter Cardiovasc Interv.* 2017;89(4):754-760.
12. Chen H, Ren C, Chen H. Thrombolysis versus anticoagulation for the initial treatment of moderate pulmonary embolism: a meta-analysis of randomized controlled trials. *Respir Care.* 2014;59(12):1880-1887.
13. Kuo WT, Banerjee A, Kim PS, et al. Pulmonary embolism response to fragmentation, embolectomy, and catheter thrombolysis (PERFECT): initial results from a prospective multicenter registry. *Chest.* 2015;148(3):667-673.
14. Tapson VF, Sterling K, Jones N, et al. A Randomized trial of the optimum duration of acoustic pulse thrombolysis procedure in acute intermediate-risk pulmonary embolism: the OPTALYSE PE trial. *JACC Cardiovasc Interv.* 2018;11(14):1401-1410.
15. Piazza G, Hohlfelder B, Jaff MR, et al. A prospective, single-arm, multicenter trial of ultrasound-facilitated, catheter-directed, low-dose fibrinolysis for acute massive and submassive pulmonary embolism: the SEATTLE II study. *JACC Cardiovasc Interv.* 2015;8(10):1382-1392.
16. Kucher N, Boekstegers P, Muller OJ, et al. Randomized, controlled trial of ultrasound-assisted catheter-directed thrombolysis for acute intermediate-risk pulmonary embolism. *Circulation.* 2014;129(4):479-486.
17. Avgerinos ED, Saadeddin Z, Abou Ali AN, et al. A meta-analysis of outcomes of catheter-directed thrombolysis for high- and intermediate-risk pulmonary embolism. *J Vasc Surg Venous Lymphat Disord.* 2018;6(4):530-540.
18. Schulman S, Kearon C; Subcommittee on Control of Anticoagulation of the Scientific and Standardization Committee of the International Society on Thrombosis and Haemostasis. Definition of major bleeding in clinical investigations of antihemostatic medicinal products in non-surgical patients. *J Thromb Haemost.* 2005;3(4):692-694.
19. Kaatz S, Ahmad D, Spyropoulos AC, Schulman S; Subcommittee on Control of Anticoagulation. Definition of clinically relevant non-major bleeding in studies of anticoagulants in atrial fibrillation and venous thromboembolic disease in non-surgical patients: communication from the SSC of the ISTH. *J Thromb Haemost.* 2015;13(11):2119-2126.
20. Al-Hakim R, Park J, Bansal A, Genshaft S, Moriarty JM. Early experience with angiovac aspiration in the pulmonary arteries. *J Vasc Interv Radiol.* 2016;27(5):730-734.
21. Al-Hakim R, Bhatt A, Benenati JF. Continuous aspiration mechanical thrombectomy for the management of submassive pulmonary embolism: a single-center experience. *J Vasc Interv Radiol.* 2017;28(10):1348-1352.
22. Tu T, Toma C, Tapson VF, et al. A prospective, single-arm, multicenter trial of catheter-directed mechanical thrombectomy for intermediate-risk acute pulmonary embolism: the FLARE study. *JACC Cardiovasc Interv.* 2019;12(9):859-869.

23. Villalba L, Nguyen T, Feitosa RL Jr, Gunanayagam P, Anning N, Dwight K. Single-session catheter-directed lysis using adjunctive power-pulse spray with AngioJet for the treatment of acute massive and submassive pulmonary embolism. *J Vasc Surg*. 2019;70(6):1920-1926.

24. Kalra R, Bajaj NS, Arora P, et al. Surgical embolectomy for acute pulmonary embolism: systematic review and comprehensive meta-analyses. *Ann Thorac Surg*. 2017;103(3):982-990.

SELF-ASSESSMENT STUDY QUESTIONS AND ANSWERS

Questions

1. A 38-year-old otherwise healthy man presents to the emergency department complaining of shortness of breath and fatigue. He has no family history or previous history of venous thromboembolism. A moderate probability of pulmonary embolism is suspected. What is the recommended next step in this patient's workup?
A. Computer tomography angiography (CTA) of the chest
B. Duplex venous scan of bilateral lower extremities
C. Ventilation perfusion scan
D. Catheter-based pulmonary venography
E. D-dimer blood test

2. Which of the following best defines submassive PE?
A. A 60-year-old patient presenting with acute chronic, recurrent PE, a systolic blood pressure of 100 mmHg, and troponins and brain natriuretic peptide within normal limits.
B. A 45-year-old patient presenting with acute PE, deep vein thrombosis, and an oxygen saturation of 92% on room air.
C. An 80-year-old patient with acute PE, normal troponins, and a blood pressure of 80 mmHg.
D. A 32-year-old patient with acute PE, a right-to-left ventricular ratio of 1, and a systolic blood pressure of 80 mmHg.
E. A 52-year-old patient with acute PE, a systolic blood pressure of 90 mmHg, a right-to-left ventricular ratio of 1, and elevated troponins.

3. A 63-year-old female experiences sudden shortness of breath and chest pain 2 hours after eating a typical dinner. She has a history of Factor V Leiden and has been on warfarin for years for recurrent episodes of deep vein thrombosis. On admission to the local emergency department, her international normalized ratio is 1.6 and her troponins are 4.5. Which imaging modality provides the emergency department physician with a quick and accurate assessment of right ventricular (RV) dysfunction?
A. Computed tomography pulmonary angiography (CTA)
B. Magnetic resonance venography (MRV) of the chest
C. Ventilation-perfusion scan (VQ scan)
D. Catheter-based angiography with pulmonary artery pressure measurement
E. Transesophageal echocardiogram (TEE)

4. Which one of the findings below are not compatible with right ventricular dysfunction demonstrated on computed tomography pulmonary angiography?
A. An elevated right-to-left ventricular ratio
B. Interventricular septal bowing
C. Reflux of contrast into the hepatic veins
D. Inferior vena cava contrast reflux
E. Pulmonary artery dilation

5. A 51-year-old patient is brought by ambulance to the hospital after endotracheal intubation was performed in the field following brief cardiopulmonary resuscitation. He remains hypotensive (systolic blood pressure 80 mmHg) and tachycardic (heart rate 125 beats per minute). A computed tomography angiography confirms a saddle pulmonary embolism. Your local hospital does not have cardiopulmonary bypass capabilities. The patient is expeditiously placed on extracorporeal life support (ECLS). What is the role of ECLS in patients with pulmonary embolism?
A. Normalizes hemodynamics while improving systemic perfusion
B. Provides cardiopulmonary support while thrombus burden is reduced
C. Offloads the right ventricle and provides extracorporeal oxygenation
D. Decreases inflammatory response and improves hemodynamic parameters
E. Provides extracorporeal oxygenation and blood pressure support

SELF-ASSESSMENT STUDY QUESTIONS AND ANSWERS

6. Which of the following is not an indication for open pulmonary artery thrombectomy in patients with acute pulmonary embolism?

A. Active bleeding
B. Rapid deterioration despite thrombolysis systemically or via catheter
C. Thrombus-in-transit
D. Moderate right ventricular dysfunction
E. Large patent foramen ovale

7. Which of the following is an absolute contraindication to systemic thrombolysis in patients with massive pulmonary embolism?

A. Prior intracranial hemorrhage
B. Pregnancy, first trimester
C. History of prior ischemic stroke >3 months
D. Traumatic or prolonged (>10 min) CPR
E. History of chronic, severe, poorly controlled hypertension

8. The concept behind a pulmonary embolism response team (PERT) is to assist in caring for or transferring patients to centers with a multidisciplinary team. Which one of the following medical specialties is unlikely to be part of a PERT?

A. Interventional radiologists or cardiologists
B. Cardiothoracic surgeons
C. Pulmonologists
D. Hematologists
E. Vascular surgeons

9. A 75-year-old otherwise healthy gentleman on postoperative day 2 after a prostatectomy for benign prostatic hyperplasia has some chest discomfort and calls for his nurse. On primary assessment, his arterial oxygen saturation is 81%, systolic blood pressure is 90 mmHg, and heart rate is 125 bpm. Advanced cardiac life support measures are initiated. He is later diagnosed with a pulmonary embolism and his cardiopulmonary status improves with anticoagulation. Considering this patient has a high-risk PE based on the simplified PE severity index (sPESI), which of the following parameters is not part of the sPESI?

A. History of cancer
B. History of chronic cardiopulmonary disease
C. Congestive heart failure with ejection fraction <25%
D. Systolic blood pressure <100 mmHg
E. Arterial oxygen saturation <90%

10. The advent of endovascular therapy has changed the landscape of pulmonary embolism treatment. Several devices are approved to treat PE in the US. Which of the devices below can be utilized for the mechanical and pharmacological treatment of PE?

A. EkoSonic™ Endovascular System
B. AngioJet™ System
C. AngioVac® System
D. Penumbra™ System
E. Cragg-McNamara™ Infusion Catheters

SELF-ASSESSMENT STUDY QUESTIONS AND ANSWERS

Answers

1. E.
2. E.
3. A.
4. E.
5. B.
6. D.
7. A.
8. D.
9. C.
10. B.

CHAPTER

18 Chronic Venous Disease

Pamela S. Kim and Antonios P. Gasparis

OUTLINE

GENERAL
PATHOPHYSIOLOGY
CLINICAL FINDINGS
DIAGNOSIS/DIFFERENTIAL DIAGNOSIS
TESTING
MANAGEMENT
CONCLUSIONS

GENERAL

Chronic venous disease (CVD) is a common and often underappreciated problem with significant socioeconomic impact.[1-3] Encompassing any abnormality of the venous system of long duration, it can manifest with symptoms and/or signs ranging from telangiectasias to mild leg discomfort to venous claudication or ulcers. At its advanced stages, it is known as chronic venous insufficiency (CVI), when abnormalities of the venous system produce edema, skin changes, or ulcers.[2,3]

CVD is most prevalent in western populations (50%-85%) and is a disease with a considerable rate of progression. The Bonn Vein study found that over 6 years, the incidence of varicose veins and CVD reached 14%. About 13 years of follow-up in the Edinburgh Vein Study demonstrated that 58% of 334 patients with CVD progressed to a more advanced stage. In the Framingham study of 3822 patients, the annual incidence of varicose veins was 2.6% in women and 1.9% in men. Risk factors for the development of CVD and its progression include increasing age, pregnancy, excess body weight, low physical activity, sedentary living habits or occupations, and genetics. With an aging population and increasingly sedentary habits, the already 2% to 3% of national health care budget expenditure on CVD is anticipated to increase considerably.[1,4-9]

PATHOPHYSIOLOGY

The lower extremity venous system includes deep veins, superficial veins, and connecting perforating veins. The deep veins lie beneath the muscle facia and drain the leg muscles. The superficial veins are above the fascia and drain the cutaneous tissues. Perforating veins penetrate the fascia, connecting the superficial and deep veins, while communicating veins connect veins within the same compartment. Bicuspid valves are found in the deep, superficial, and most perforating veins.[9,10]

The main function of the venous system is to return blood to the heart. Success depends on the interaction of a central pump, a pressure gradient, a peripheral venous pump, and competent venous valves. Hydrostatic gravitational pressures in the lower limbs reflect the vertical distance below the atrium. Thus, pressure is highest in the upright and motionless positions. Actual pressures, however, also reflect several other extrinsic factors. Contraction of the diaphragm during inspiration increases intraabdominal and lower extremity venous pressures, as does obesity and the presence of ascites. Normally in the standing position, blood is pumped against gravity via the muscle pumps of the leg and venous valves ensure the blood flows only in the cephalad direction. Relaxation of the muscle pump allows blood to flow back in from the surrounding tissue. This contraction and relaxation of the muscle pump, intact valves, and healthy vein walls all work to return peripheral blood to the heart. A dysfunction in any of these components will lead to increased venous pressure.[1,7,10,11]

Venous pathology may result from valvular incompetence (reflux), venous obstruction, or a combination of these mechanisms. It can occur in the superficial veins, deep veins, perforator veins, or a combination of the above. This is exacerbated by multiple other factors such as dysfunction of the muscle pump system and obesity. Valvular incompetence may be due to preexisting weakness in the vessel wall or valve leaflets, or as a result of direct injury or excess distention due to hormonal effects or persistent high pressure. Deep venous valves are most commonly damaged by previous deep vein thrombosis (DVT). The incompetence of the valves results in venous reflux. Reflux describes the retrograde flow of blood of abnormal duration in a venous segment, which leads to increased hydrostatic pressures during walking. Obstruction of the deep veins may limit the flow of blood, also leading to increased venous pressures. This can be due to chronic postthrombotic changes, venous stenosis, or extrinsic compression. Postthrombotic etiologies of venous pathology are frequent, even with the use of adequate anticoagulation. This process unfortunately has a more rapid progression of the disease, particularly in advanced stages of CVI. Extrinsic compression is mostly seen in the iliac venous system with anatomic iliac vein compression by the overlying artery or malignancy. An ineffective calf muscle pump leads to ineffective emptying of blood from the distal lower limbs. This can be secondary to leg immobility from prolonged sitting or standing, obesity, arthritis, or inactivity. Musculo-fascial weakness, loss of joint motion, and various foot static disorders can also contribute to the failure of the muscle pump. All of these mechanisms lead to increased venous pressures and venous hypertension.[2,7–9,12,13]

The signs and symptoms of CVD and its progression are due to persistent venous hypertension and inflammation. Ultimately, ambulatory venous hypertension, or a failure to reduce venous pressures with exercise, becomes the final pathway to the more severe manifestations of CVI. Ambulatory venous pressures are determined by venous reflux, venous obstruction, as well as the calf muscle pump function. With the progressive deterioration of each of these factors as CVD advances, the prolonged blood pooling leads to distension of the vein wall and disturbances in the endothelium. This precipitates adherence and activation of leukocytes that initiate an inflammatory cascade. This in turn leads to increased capillary permeability, interstitial fluid accumulation and edema, and impaired lymphatic flow which all contribute to progressive venous disease and its manifestations.[1,8,10,11,14]

CLINICAL FINDINGS

It has been shown that hemodynamic venous deterioration parallels the clinical severity of disease, as does QOL.[15] Typical symptoms include lower limb tingling, pain or discomfort, heaviness, aching, fatigue, and itchiness. These symptoms may be exacerbated by heat or prolonged dependency and relieved with leg elevation. Visible manifestations of dilated veins from telangiectasias to varicose veins will develop (Figure 18-1). Episodes of superficial thrombophlebitis may develop in the varicosities, typically with painful and indurated areas along the vein. Varicosities of any size may bleed. Additionally, worsening leg edema can progress to skin changes with hemosiderin staining, lipodermatosclerotic changes, and ultimately ulcers in the most advanced stages (Figure 18-2). Edema begins in the perimalleolar region and ascends the leg as it develops. In advanced CVI, this progresses to phlebolymphedema as the lymphatic system cannot compensate to remove the increased interstitial fluid. Additionally, obstruction of the deep venous system, particularly in the iliac veins, may also contribute to venous hypertension. Ultimately, progressive symptoms can limit the ability to take part in occupational, social, and other physical activities with significant attendant socioeconomic detriment.[2,6,9,11]

Based on the presence of these clinical signs, the clinical presentation of venous disease is described by the Clinical Etiological Anatomical Pathophysiological (CEAP) classification system. Developed originally by an international consensus conference in 1993 and recently updated in 2020, it provides a

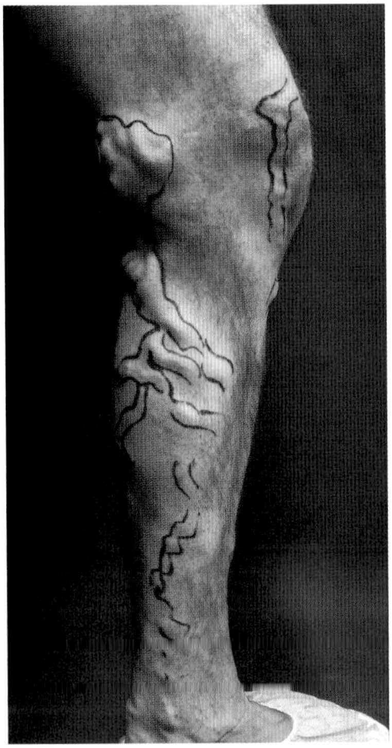

FIGURE 18-1 Prominent large varicosities (outlined with ink) reflected of severe underlying venous insufficiency.

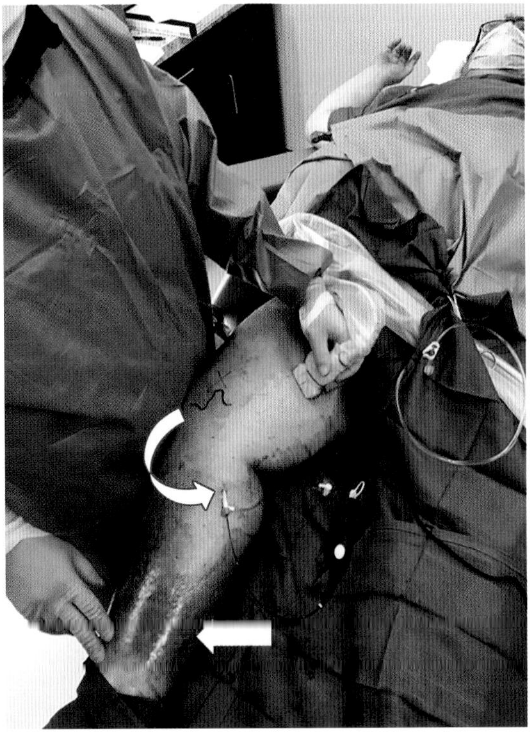

FIGURE 18-2 Leg demonstrating brownish discoloration above the ankle with lipodermatosclerosis reflecting CEAP class C4 disease (straight arrow) undergoing radiofrequency ablation with the entry of the catheter into the great saphenous vein (curved arrow) under ultrasound guidance.

reproducible description and classification of the many manifestations of CVD. The clinical classification has seven categories (C0-C6) modified by the presence or absence of symptoms. An etiologic category defines congenital, primary, and secondary causes of venous dysfunction. The anatomic classification describes superficial, deep, and perforating venous systems that may be involved, while the pathophysiologic classification illustrates the underlying mechanism of the dysfunction (reflux or obstruction).[10,16]

To complement CEAP and further define the severity of the venous disease, the Venous Severity Score (VSS) was developed. This includes a Venous Clinical Severity Score (VCSS), a Venous Segmental Disease Score (VSDS), and a Venous Disability Score (VDS). Furthermore, the use of disease-specific quality of life (QOL) questionnaires such as the Chronic Venous Disease Quality of Life Questionnaire (CIVIQ), the Aberdeen questionnaire, and the VEINES-QOL are used to evaluate patients perceived severity of disease and treatment success outcomes.[3,9–11]

DIAGNOSIS/DIFFERENTIAL DIAGNOSIS

A thorough history and physical examination are essential in the initial evaluation of CVD. In particular, a history of varicose veins, prior DVT, or events that could have provoked a DVT, personal or family history of clotting issues, and prior venous interventions should be obtained. Additionally, a history of abdominal or pelvic surgery, malignancy, or radiation is important. The most common presenting symptoms of CVD which include swelling and discomfort of the lower limb are seen in a variety of etiologies. As such, it is important to determine the duration of the symptoms. A complete medication list and recent changes in that regimen should also be obtained.[9,17–20]

The physical examination should not focus solely on the lower limbs. An evaluation of the heart, lungs, and abdomen is also needed to assess for systemic etiologies or contributing factors. The abdominal examination should include an evaluation for any stigmata of vena cava obstruction such as the presence of abdominal wall collaterals. Additionally, both lower limbs and feet need to be assessed, even if the complaint is only in one. This is preferably done with the legs dependent or in a standing position for optimal assessment of swelling and visualization of varicosities. If swelling is present, its distribution and the presence of pitting should be noted. The skin needs a thorough examination with attention to the presence of varicose veins, areas of hemosiderin staining, eczematous dermatitis or atrophy blanche, lipodermatosclerotic changes, and active or healed ulcers. Range of motion, pain/tenderness, and the presence of neurologic abnormalities also should be explored. A peripheral pulse examination is also important to evaluate for combined venous and arterial dysfunction.[9,17–20]

Many of the symptoms and clinical manifestations of CVD are seen in other etiologies, so it is important to have a broad differential diagnosis in mind. Acute symptoms (<72 hours) can be due to acute DVT, infection, trauma, and exacerbation of a medical condition or medication changes. Chronic issues can include along with CVD, lymphatic dysfunction, longstanding medical etiologies, and static foot disorders. The aching, heaviness, and fatigue of the legs due to CVD, however, typically worsens with dependency throughout the day and improves with elevation. Lower limb swelling is one of the most common complaints encountered and can be due to several etiologies. Assessment for systemic disease is essential, particularly in older patients who have multiple comorbid conditions. Swelling can result from new onset or exacerbations of cardiac, pulmonary, renal, hepatic, or endocrine issues. Obesity contributes to central venous obstruction and leads to venous hypertension causing or contributing to the signs and symptoms of CVD. Numerous medications, particularly calcium channel blockers, have been identified as causing lower limb edema. Also, a history of unexplained weight loss or adenopathy may suggest a malignant process causing venous compression. The distribution of swelling is also important. In lipedema, there is disproportionate swelling of the lower limbs from the ankles to the waist when compared with the torso. The feet are generally spared, and there is no pitting of the swelling. A similar distribution of swelling may also be seen in the upper limbs. In contrast to CVD, lymphedema typically affects the dorsum of the foot. It is also associated with squaring of the toes and foot, toenail deformities, skin thickening with the inability to pinch a skin fold on the dorsum of the base of the second toe (Kaposi–Stemmer sign), and hyperkeratotic skin in its advanced stages. The above classic findings of lymphedema are not always present, however, especially in the early stages of the disease. It should also be noted that patients with advanced CVI usually have combined venous and lymphatic disease. Persistent venous hypertension can overload the lymphatic fluid transport, leading to phlebolymphedema and its associated hyperkeratotic skin changes.[9,17–20]

TESTING

Duplex ultrasound imaging (DUS) is the recommended method of assessing the lower extremity venous system. It provides a noninvasive, reproducible method of viewing anatomy, identifying obstruction, and measuring valvular incompetence, with sensitivity and specificity rates of >80% and a positive predictive value nearing 100%. DUS can also be used to evaluate the iliac venous system and the IVC. Because of this, DUS has become frequently the only diagnostic tool used for the identification of venous disease. With any test, however, accurate and reliable results depend on the expertise of the technologist performing the study and the physician interpreting the images. Nonetheless, established protocols attempt to standardize the results. It is recommended to evaluate both lower limbs at the initial investigation with the patient upright and with augmentation of flow through distal limb compression or during a

Valsalva maneuver. Pathologic venous reflux is present with retrograde flow ≥0.5 second in the superficial saphenous veins and ≥1.0 second in the femoral and popliteal veins. Each evaluation examines the sapheno-femoral junction for incompetence, lower saphenous vein reflux, vein diameters and potential sources for filling of superficial varices. Variations in venous anatomy are noted such as veins that are hypoplastic, atretic, or duplicated. The state of the deep venous system, including valvular competence and evidence of previous thrombosis, is documented, and abnormal perforating veins are reported. The information gained from DUS is often sufficient to guide appropriate therapy. However, if a further understanding of global hemodynamics is required, plethysmographic techniques can be employed.[10,21-26]

Photoplethysmography (PPG) and air plethysmography (APG) use measurements of venous volume to quantify limb reflux. They can evaluate the impact of reflux and obstruction on overall venous function with a noninvasive approach. The gold standard of assessing hemodynamics, however, is ambulatory venous pressure monitoring. This is an invasive technique involving the insertion of a needle into a dorsal foot vein connected to a pressure transducer. It is now rarely used in practice because of the availability of noninvasive options. All of these techniques typically need to be combined with DUS for anatomic localization because plethysmographic studies only provide hemodynamic information.[9,10]

If additional anatomic imaging, particularly of the abdomen and pelvis, needs to be obtained after DUS, contrast-enhanced venous phase computed tomography (CT) or magnetic resonance (MR) imaging are excellent options. Deep venous anatomy, the presence of thrombus, mass effect by tumor or enlarged lymph nodes, and iliocaval compression/obstruction can be easily visualized.[9,10,27]

Contrast venography is another modality used to directly visualize the venous system. This can be performed by an ascending approach with contrast injection in the dorsum of the foot, or a descending approach to evaluate reflux with proximal contrast injection in a semivertical position on a tilt table. Venography, however, has almost completely been replaced by DUS except when performed during therapeutic interventional procedures. For visualization of the iliocaval system, contrast venography with intravascular ultrasound (IVUS) is a modality available for both assessment and treatment of abdominal/pelvic etiologies of CVD. Although it is an invasive approach, venous lesions, stenoses, and compression can be assessed with sensitivity >85%. It is considered the gold standard method of diagnosing iliocaval obstruction. Treatment with venoplasty and stenting can be performed in the same setting if needed.[9,10,28]

MANAGEMENT

The goal of initial management of CVD involves conservative interventions that reduce venous hypertension and inhibit the inflammatory cascade to alleviate symptoms and subsequently QOL. Weight control and regular exercise to rehabilitate the muscle pump will help with symptoms, as well as the use of compression therapy. Various choices for compression include elastic, inelastic, and pneumatic options to oppose the hydrostatic forces of venous hypertension. The use of graded elastic compression stockings is a mainstay in the management of CVD to control swelling and its positive effect on the microcirculation of the skin. Multilayered medicated compression is the treatment of choice for the treatment of venous stasis ulcers. However, compression therapy is hampered by low patient compliance, failure to treat the underlying pathology, and no definitive data that prevents the progression of disease.[1,8,9,29] Pharmacologic therapies utilize venoactive drugs to improve venous tone and capillary permeability. Micronized purified flavonoid fraction (MPFF) is a venoactive drug that reduces leukocyte activation and in turn decreases the release of inflammatory molecules in CVD. Studies have found that in CVD patients, the use of MPFF significantly reduced leg pain over 8 weeks and overall improved leg discomfort and heaviness as well as the QOL.[1,7,11]

Indications for intervention in CVD are variable and depend on symptom severity, the options for intervention, and the functional and medical status of the patient. This is approached after a trial of conservative therapy, with many insurance providers first requiring a trial of compression therapy. Specific treatment options take into consideration

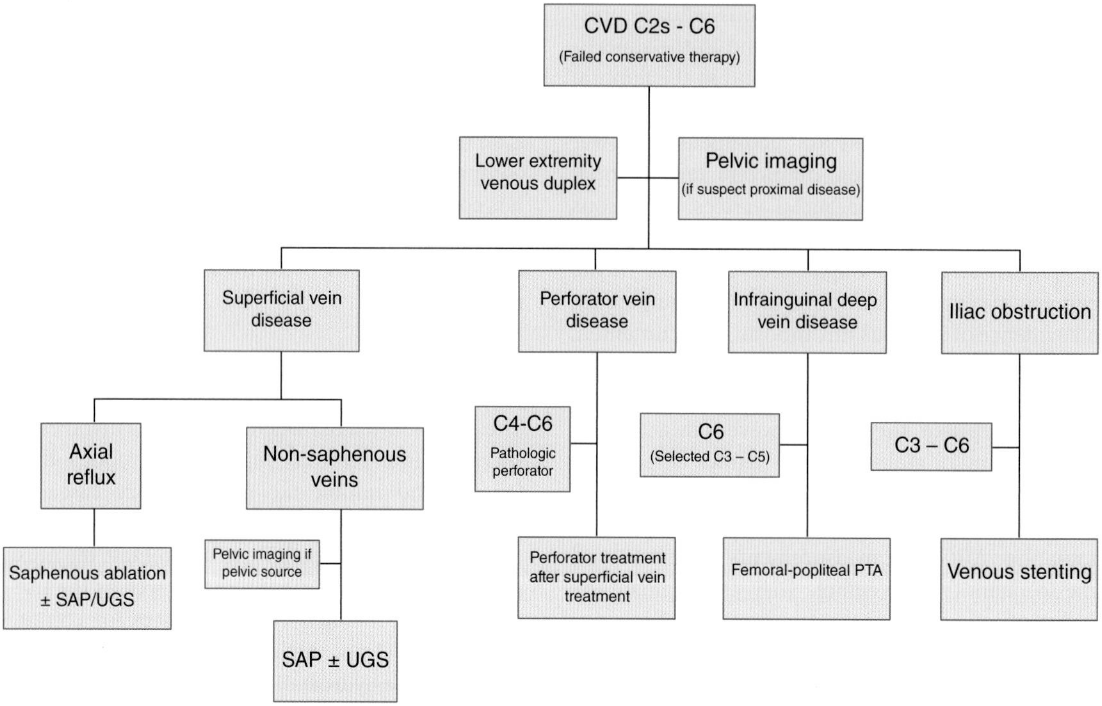

FIGURE 18-3 Diagnostic and treatment algorithm for patients with chronic venous insufficiency. PTA, percutaneous transluminal angioplasty; SAP, surgical ambulatory phlebectomy; UGS, ultrasound-guided sclerotherapy.

the etiology, anatomy, and pathophysiology of each patient (Figure 18-3).[26] Most CVD is due to superficial venous insufficiency with nonthrombotic etiologies as discussed previously. Insufficiency can occur in the great saphenous vein (GSV), the small saphenous vein (SSV), or the anterior accessory GSV (AAGSV) and their associated tributaries. Reflux in perforators is often seen but is not relevant unless there is advanced CVI (pathologic perforator), especially in the presence of ulcers. In the deep venous system, most disease is postthrombotic. Postthrombotic syndrome (PTS) develops in approximately 50% of patients with DVT, with the incidence and severity of symptoms affected by the location and extent of obstruction. Obstruction at the level of the femoropopliteal vein leads to PTS in about 40% of patients, while approximately 60% of patients will develop PTS after DVT in the iliac vein. Nonthrombotic compression of the iliac veins, while a common finding in the adult population, may not necessarily lead to symptoms.[26,30] As a result, a thorough history, physical examination, and appropriate diagnostic testing are essential in formulating an appropriate treatment plan.

CVD is a progressive condition. Rates of disease progression, even in those patients with C2 disease, are estimated to be 4.3% per year. In 13 years of follow-up, nearly one-third of patients with varicose veins progressed to more advanced stages with skin changes.[4,5] As such, treatment for axial superficial reflux of the GSV (uninterrupted reflux from the groin to the calf) is recommended for symptomatic C2 disease and higher. For GSV reflux below the knee, treatment for advanced C4-C6 disease may be appropriate. However, the evidence for recommendations on segmental reflux is lacking. The above recommendations are similar to SSV reflux. The AAGSV, although not commonly an initial location for CVD, is a frequent cause of recurrence after the treatment of the GSV and patients will benefit from treatment of AAGSV for symptomatic reflux.[26] The traditional treatment for saphenous vein insufficiency was high ligation with or without stripping of the GSV and ligation of the sapheno-popliteal junction for SSV insufficiency. This approach however requires either general or epidural anesthesia with complications of nerve damage, scarring, postoperative pain, and high incidence of recurrent reflux (30% GSV and 50% SSV). Minimally invasive techniques were then developed with the aim of reducing surgical trauma and improving long-term success. Thermal tumescent (TT) methods include endovenous laser (EVLA) and radiofrequency ablation (RFA) (Figure 18-2). These procedures utilize heat to cause thermal injury to the vein wall, causing thrombosis and fibrosis. Tumescence anesthesia is used to minimize thermal injury on the surrounding tissue as well as induce vasospasm to maximize the effect of heat on the vein wall. Unlike traditional ligation and stripping, these techniques only require local anesthesia and have fewer complications with minimal scarring, less postprocedural pain and faster recovery times. In particular, EVLA and RFA have been the most studied minimally invasive techniques with excellent proven efficacy and durability at long term, equivalent to ligation and stripping with improved QOL.[24–33]

A new generation of ablative technology for the treatment of saphenous vein insufficiency has been developed in the form of nonthermal nontumescent (NTNT) methods. These require only a local anesthetic and can be more safely utilized for the below knee saphenous vein segment with a lower risk of nerve injury. The first NTNT technology was mechanochemical ablation (MOCA). This procedure utilizes a rotating wire that abrades the venous endothelium, along with a liquid sclerosant that is injected at the same time. Only local anesthetic at the catheter entry site is needed. A systematic review of the use of MOCA in saphenous vein ablation revealed anatomical success rates of 92% for the GSV and 87% for the SSV at more than 2 years.[34,35] Another recent method is cyanoacrylate closure (CAC). Cyanoacrylate glue is delivered through a specifically designed catheter into the saphenous vein. When the glue mixes with blood or plasma, it polymerizes causing an acute inflammatory reaction that ultimately leads to lumen occlusion. Twenty-four-month results from a randomized, multicenter clinical trial comparing CAC to RFA revealed equivalent (>94%) closure rates with similar improvement in symptoms and QOL.[34,36] Five-year follow-up of the same study found freedom from recanalization in 91% in the CAC group and 85% in the RFA group.[37] Finally, foam sclerosant can also be used to close the saphenous veins. Polidocanol endovenous microfoam (PEM) utilizes a proprietary device to produce low nitrogen (0.8%), oxygen/carbon dioxide (65:35) ratio foam. It is delivered percutaneously into the vein without the need for an anesthetic and can be used to treat not only saphenous vein insufficiency but its varicosities and tributaries in the same setting. It is useful in the treatment of tortuous axial veins because it does not require the insertion of a catheter into the length of the vein to be treated. Additionally, it can be used in veins with scarring, vascular beds beneath ulcerations, groin neovascularization and venous malformations. Compared with physician compounded foams, PEM has shown to have better stability and cohesive properties. A recent prospective study described closure rates of 93% at 6 months, comparable to other NTNT technologies as well as TT modalities.[38]

For patients with identified perforator pathology, treatment is recommended only in class C5-C6 disease where patients have an associated ulcer nearby. It should be noted however that compression is still the treatment of choice for ulcer healing. Perforator ablation is to prevent the recurrence of ulcers and is usually performed after axial insufficiency, and associated tributary disease has been treated. For those who may benefit from treatment, ablation with TT methods or ultrasound guided sclerotherapy is recommended over open techniques.[26]

Treatment of symptomatic tributary disease and varicose veins is appropriate in association with class C2 disease and higher. For patients with diseased tributaries in association with saphenous reflux, the tributaries can be managed concomitantly with the saphenous ablation or as a staged procedure. Several studies show that saphenous ablation is associated with regression of remaining tributaries in 30% to 60% of cases, so treatment of previously identified diseased tributaries and varicose veins is no longer needed. Nontruncal varicose veins are common manifestations of CVD and have a high association with saphenous disease. However, nontruncal tributaries may also require primary treatment in cases such as bleeding and superficial thrombophlebitis without needing to treat the truncal vein.[26] Treatment options for tributaries and varicosities include sclerotherapy and ambulatory microphlebectomy. Sclerotherapy utilizes chemical agents (detergents) to disrupt the venous wall and achieve endoluminal fibrosis. It is injected as liquid or foam directly into the vein without the need for an anesthetic. In contrast to the proprietary PEM, physician compounded foams are not as effective in the treatment of axial veins (anatomic success of 34% at 5 years). However, it is widely utilized for the obliteration of varicose veins and tributaries as well as reticular veins and telangiectasias. Liquid sclerotherapy can be used for smaller veins, while liquid sclerotherapy in higher concentrations or foam sclerotherapy is more effective with larger veins. The sclerosant as a foam allows for enhanced interaction with the vein wall. Ultrasound guidance is utilized for the deeper veins, while visual sclerotherapy may be done for the more superficial, visible veins. Multiple treatments may be required to successfully ablate the target veins.[9,26,39] Ambulatory microphlebectomy is used for the removal of symptomatic varicose veins. This can be performed with local tumescent anesthesia which augments dissection as well as provides pain management and hemostasis. Again, concomitant or staged phlebectomies of varicose veins during treatment of saphenous insufficiency (ablation) are typically performed.[26,40]

Patients with deep venous disease and PTS commonly have more advanced diseases than patients with isolated superficial venous insufficiency. Most patients are initially managed conservatively with leg elevation and compression to help alleviate venous hypertension. However, many patients do not have sufficient relief of symptoms due to poor compliance with compression, inability to tolerate adequate high levels of compression, and severe disease. Among the available interventions for the treatment of postthrombotic or nonthrombotic iliac vein lesions, the endovascular approach has surpassed surgical bypass as a safer and more effective treatment option. Angioplasty and stenting have been shown to establish and maintain venous outflow with high technical success rates, excellent long-term patency, and a lower incidence of perioperative complications (Figure 18-4). The majority of such patients have significant clinical improvement regardless of the presence of remaining reflux, adjunct saphenous procedures, or etiology of obstruction.[12,26,41–44] Stenting may be a reasonable first-line approach for the treatment of iliac or IVC

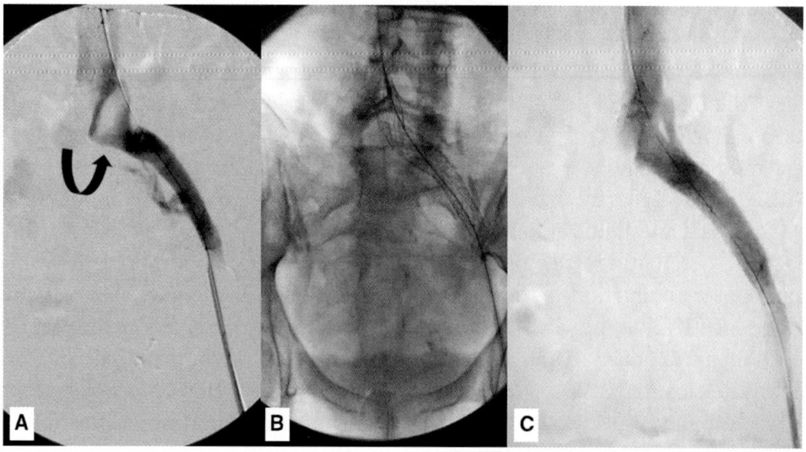

FIGURE 18-4 Intraoperative venogram of the left iliac system demonstrating (A) stenosis at the junction of the common iliac vein to the inferior vena cava (arrow) reflected by diminished contrast flow; (B) successful placement of stent extending from the length of the common iliac vein into the IVC; (C) even density of contrast flow following stenting demonstrating alleviation of the stenosis.

obstruction in patients with symptomatic C4-C6 disease. For patients with both superficial axial reflux and iliocaval obstruction, either initial treatment of the superficial system or initial treatment of the deep system is possible. With the associated complication rates of iliac interventions, a strategy of treating the superficial system first is preferred due to fewer procedural risks.[26] In contrast to the iliocaval segment, treatment options for infrainguinal deep vein disease are more limited and often ineffective. Compared with the iliac system, the femoropopliteal veins are more challenging due to their particular hemodynamics, anatomy, and technical aspects in addressing deep venous reflux. What works in the iliocaval segment does not necessarily work in the femoropopliteal segment. Angioplasty and stenting are also options in the lower limb, but published studies have small sample sizes and include both suprainguinal as well as infrainguinal vein results. Generally, thrombolysis is combined with venoplasty and stenting for optimal results. However, the lack of dedicated venous stents for use in the infrainguinal segment, along with persistent concern for increased risk of acute thrombosis, stent fracture, and restenosis, have precluded widespread utilization of this technique. Open procedures such as valvuloplasty, vein transposition, vein transplantation, and synthetic valves are all considerations, but many of these procedures are technically challenging and have low efficacy, with variable success in a few centers around the world. There has been a long history of attempts to construct a biological or artificial valve, some with endovascular deployment. A number are in various stages of development, but nothing is currently available that has success rates equivalent to what can be accomplished in the suprainguinal system. Accordingly, intervention for infrainguinal deep vein insufficiency is performed only selectively in patients with advanced CVI with disabling symptoms.[30]

CONCLUSIONS

CVD is a common problem with significant socioeconomic impact. It is a progressive disease stemming from persistent venous hypertension and inflammation. Careful diagnosis is needed, and decisions on its management should be guided by the severity of the disease and its anatomic and pathologic considerations (Figure 18-3).

REFERENCES

1. Nicolaides AN, Labropoulos N. Burden and suffering in chronic venous disease. *Adv Ther*. 2019;36:S1-S4.
2. Eklof B, Perrin M, Delis KT, Rutherford RB, Gloviczki P. Updated terminology of chronic venous diorders: the VEIN-TERM transatlantic interdisciplinary consensus document. *J Vasc Surg*. 2009;49:498-501.
3. Onida S, Davies AH. Predicted burden of venous disease. *Phlebology*. 2016;31:74-79.
4. Robertson L, Lee AJ, Evans CJ, et al. Incidence of chronic venous disease in the Edinburgh Vein Study. *J Vasc Surg Venous Lymphat Disord*. 2013;1:59-67.
5. Lee AJ, Robertson LA, Boghossian SM, et al. Progression of varicose veins and chronic venous insufficiency in the general population in the Edinburgh Vein Study. *J Vasc Surg Venous Lymphat Disord*. 2015:3:18-26.
6. Davies, A. The seriousness of chronic venous disease: a review of real-world evidence. *Adv Ther*. 2019;36:S5-S12.
7. Bush R, Comerota A, Meissner M, Raffetto JD, Hahn SR, Freeman K. Recommendations for the medical management of chronic venous disease: the role of micronized purified flavonoid fraction (MPFF). *Phlebology*. 2017;32:3-19.
8. Labropoulos N. How does chronic venous disease progress from the first symptoms to the advanced stages? A review. *Adv Ther*. 2019;36:S13-S19.
9. Eberhardt RT, Raffetto JD. Chronic venous insufficiency. *Circulation*. 2014;130:333-346.
10. Meissner MH, Moneta G, Burnand K, et al. The hemodynamics and diagnosis of venous disease. *J Vasc Surg*. 2007;46:4S-24S.
11. Mansilha A, Sousa J. Pathophysiological mechanisms of chronic venous disease and implications for venoactive drug therapy. *Int J Mol Sci*. 2018;19:1669.
12. Seager MJ, Busuttil A, Dharmarajah B, Davies AH. A systematic review of endovenous stenting in chronic venous disease secondary to iliac vein obstruction. *Eur J Vasc Endovasc Surg*. 2016;51:100-120.
13. Labropoulos N, Gasparis AP, Pefanis D, Leon LR Jr, Tassiopoulos AK. Secondary chronic venous disease progresses faster than primary. *J Vasc Surg*. 2009;49:704-710.
14. Ligi D, Croce L, Mannello F. Chronic venous disorders: the dangerous, the good, and the diverse. *Int J Mol Sci*. 2018;19:2544.

15. Labropoulos N, Delis K, Nicolaides AN, Leon M, Ramaswami G, Volteas N. The role of the distribution and anatomic extent of reflux in the development of signs and symptoms in chronic venous insufficiency. *J Vasc Surg*. 1996;23:504-510.
16. Lurie F, Passman M, Meisner M, et al. The 2020 update of the CEAP classification system and reporting standards. *J Vasc Surg Venous Lymphat Disord*. 2020;8:342-352.
17. Evans NS, Ratchford EV. The swollen leg. *Vascular Medicine*. 2016;21:562-564.
18. Ely JW, Osheroff JA, Chambliss ML, et al. Approach to leg edema of unclear etiology. *J Am Board Fam Med*. 2006;19:148-160.
19. Trayes KP, Studdiford JS, Pickle S, et al. Edema: diagnosis and management. *Am Fam Physician*. 2013;88:102-110.
20. Rockson SG. Current concepts and future directions in the diagnosis and management of lymphatic vascular disease. *Vasc Med*. 2010;15:223-231.
21. Lurie F, Comerota A, Eklof B, et al. Multicenter assessment of venous reflux by duplex ultrasound. *J Vasc Surg*. 2012;55:437-445.
22. Coleridge-Smith P, Labropoulos N, Partsch H, Myers K, Nicolaides A, Cavezzi A. Duplex ultrasound investigation of the veins in chronic venous disease of the lower limbs – UIP consensus document. *Eur J Vasc Endovasc Surg*. 2006;31:83-92.
23. Garcia R, Labropoulos N. Duplex ultrasound for the diagnosis of acute and chronic venous diseases. *Surg Clin N Am*. 2018;98:201-218.
24. Labropoulos N, Tiongson J, Pryor L, et al. Definition of venous reflux in lower-extremity veins. *J Vasc Surg*. 2003;38:793-798.
25. Lim KH, Hill G, Tarr G, van Rij A. Deep venous reflux definitions and associated clinical and physiological significance. *J Vasc Surg Venous Lymphat Disord*. 2013;1:325-332.
26. Masuda E, Ozsvath K, Vossler J, et al. The 2020 appropriate use criteria for chronic lower extremity venous disease of the American Venous Forum, the Society for Vascular Surgery, the American Vein and Lymphatic Society, and the Society of Interventional Radiology. *J Vasc Surg Venous Lymphat Disord*. 2020;8:505-525.e4.
27. Sermsathanasawadi N, Pruekprasert K, Pitaksantayothin W, et al. Prevalence, risk factors, and evaluation of iliocaval obstruction in advanced chronic venous insufficiency. *J Vasc Surg Venous Lymphat Disord*. 2019;7:441-447.
28. Saleem T, Knight A, Raju S. Diagnostic yield of intravascular ultrasound in patients with clinical signs and symptoms of lower extremity venous disease. *J Vasc Surg Venous Lymphat Disord*. 2020;8(4):634-639.
29. Paranhos T, Paiva CSB, Cardoso FCI, et al. Assessment of the use of Unna boot in the treatment of chronic venous leg ulcers in adults: systematic review protocol. *BMJ Open*. 2019;9:e032091.
30. Garcia, R, Labropoulos N, Gasparis AP, Elias S. Present and future options for treatment of infrainguinal deep vein disease. *J Vas Surg: Venous and Lym Dis*. 2018;6: 664-671.
31. Rasmussen LH, Lawaetz M, Bjoern L, Vennits B, Blemings A, Eklof B. Randomized clinical trial comparing endovenous laser ablation, radiofrequency ablation, foam sclerotherapy and surgical stripping for great saphenous varicose veins. *Br J Surg*. 2011;98: 1079-1087.
32. vanEekeren RRJP, Boersma D, DeVries JPPM, Zeebregts CJ, Reijnen MMPJ. Update of endovenous treatment modalities for insufficient saphenous veins: a review of literature. *Semin Vasc Surg*. 2014;27:118-136.
33. van den Bos R, Arends L, Kockaert M, Neumann M, Nijsten T. Endovenous therapies of lower extremity varicosities: a meta-analysis. *J Vasc Surg*. 2009;49: 230-239.
34. Whiteley MS. Glue, steam and Clarivein: best practice techniques and evidence. *Phlebology*. 2015;30:24-28.
35. Witte, ME, Zeebregts CJ, Jan de Borst G, Reijnen MMPJ, Boersma D. Mechanochemical endovenous ablation of saphenous veins using the ClariVein: a systematic review. *Phlebology*. 2017;32:649-657.
36. Gibson K, Morrison N, Kolluri R, et al. Twenty-four month results from a randomized trial of cyanoacrylate closure versus radiofrequency ablation for the treatment of incompetent great saphenous veins. *J Vasc Surg Venous Lymphat Disord*. 2018;6:606-613.
37. Morrison N, Gibson K, Vasquez M, Weiss R, Jones A. Five-year extension study of patients from a randomized clinical trial (VeClose) comparing cyanoacrylate closure versus radiofrequency ablation for the treatment of incompetent great saphenous veins. *J Vasc Surg Venous Lymphat*. 2020;8(6):978-989.
38. Kim PS, Elias S, Gasparis A, Labropoulos N. Results of polidocanol endovenous microfoam in clinical practice. *J Vasc Surg Venous Lymphat Disord*. 2021;9(1):122-127.
39. Paravastu SC, Horne M, Dodd PD. Endovenous ablation therapy (laser or radiofrequency) or foam sclerotherapy versus conventional surgical repair for short saphenous varicose veins. *Cochrane Database Syst Rev*. 2016;11:CD010878.
40. Geersen DF, Shortell CEK. Phlebectomy techniques for varicose veins. *Surg Clin North Am*. 2018;98:401-414.

41. Neglen P, Hollis K, Olivier J, Raju S. Stenting of the venous outflow in chronic venous disease: long-term stent-related outcome, clinical, and hemodynamic result. *J Vasc Surg*. 2007;46:979-990.
42. Wen-da W, Yu Z, Yue-zin C. Stenting for chronic obstructive venous disease: a current comprehensive meta-analysis and systematic review. *Phlebology*. 2016;31:376-389.
43. Razavi MK, Jaff MR, Miller LE. Safety and effectiveness of stent placement for iliofemoral venous outflow obstruction. *Circ Cardiovas Interv*. 2015;8:e002772.
44. Gagne PJ, Gagne N, Kucher T, Thompson M, Bently D. Long-term clinical outcomes and technical factors with the wallstent for treatment of chronic iliofemoral venous obstruction. *J Vasc Surg: Venous and Lym Dis*. 2019;7:45-55.

SELF-ASSESSMENT STUDY QUESTIONS AND ANSWERS

Questions

1. The estimated incidence of varicose veins and chronic venous disease is
   A. 14%
   B. 27%.
   C. 53%.
   D. 81%.

2. A patient with chronic venous insufficiency has
   A. Venous claudication.
   B. Painful varicose veins.
   C. A healed venous ulcer.

3. Symptoms associated with chronic venous disease include
   A. Pain, pulselessness, paresthesia, paralysis, and poikilothermia.
   B. Heaviness, aching, swelling, throbbing, and itching.
   C. Nonpitting edema, inability to pinch a skin fold on the dorsum of the toe, hyperkeratosis, lymphangectasia, and papillomatosis.
   D. Enlarged joints, swelling, tenderness at joints.

4. The signs and symptoms of CVD develop from
   A. Venous hypertension.
   B. Inflammation.
   C. Impaired lymphatic flow.
   D. All of the above.

5. The CEAP classification is
   A. Venous severity scale used to show improvement with treatment.
   B. Venous classification used to guide evaluation and management.
   C. Better than VCSS and VEINSES-QOL in describing severity.
   D. Outdated classification system no longer used.

6. A patient presents with worsening bilateral lower extremity edema. They report a recent change in their heart medication by the cardiologist they see for congestive heart failure. Which of the following are appropriate differential diagnoses?
   A. DVT
   B. Medication reaction
   C. Cardiogenic edema
   D. All of the above

7. A 58-year-old male patient presents for evaluation of left lower extremity swelling of several months' duration. The previous week he developed a bleeding varicose vein and went to the emergency room where a compressive dressing was applied. Removal of his dressing shows a varicose vein with an overlying scab. His left leg calf diameter is 4 cm greater than the right and with a dark color just above the ankle. In addition to a detailed history and physical examination, the next appropriate step would be
   A. Duplex ultrasound.
   B. CTV/MRV.
   C. Thermal ablation of bilateral GSV.
   D. Ambulatory micro-phlebectomy of offending vein.

8. Treatment is warranted for symptomatic C2 disease to
   A. Improve aesthetics.
   B. Reduce pain or discomfort.
   C. Prevent progression to skin changes.
   D. Prevent later DVT.

9. A patient with deep venous disease and symptomatic postthrombotic syndrome warrants:
   A. CTV or MRV
   B. Ablation of axial veins
   C. Low pressure 10 to 20 mmHg knee-high compression
   D. Venography and endovascular treatment

SELF-ASSESSMENT STUDY QUESTIONS AND ANSWERS

Answers

1. A.
2. C.
3. B.
4. D.
5. B.
6. D.
7. A.
8. B.
9. A.

CHAPTER

19 Superficial Venous Insufficiency and Varicose Veins

Anastasiya Shchatsko and John Blebea

OUTLINE

DEFINITIONS
EPIDEMIOLOGY
HISTORY
ANATOMY AND PHYSIOLOGY
TYPES OF VEINS
RISK FACTORS
ETIOLOGY AND PATHOPHYSIOLOGY
DIAGNOSIS
Symptoms
Differential Diagnosis
DUPLEX ULTRASOUND
MANAGEMENT
Indications for Treatment
Treatment
Thermal Tumescent Methods
Comparison of Interventional Methods
FUTURE DIRECTIONS
ACKNOWLEDGMENT

DEFINITIONS

Chronic venous disease (CVD), varicose vein disease, venous reflux disease, and superficial venous insufficiency are many times used interchangeably and reflect both the presence of visible varicose veins and the underlying cause of valvular reflux and venous insufficiency. Varicose veins are defined as bulging dilated or tortuous veins that are located superficially under the skin of the lower extremities and correspond to CEAP class C1 and C2 (classification to be explained later). Chronic venous insufficiency (CVI), on the other hand, involves symptoms and skin changes that are more extensive than just the presence of varicose veins and includes venous disease starting from CEAP class C3 and higher. They also reflect the presence of valvular reflux and insufficiency but of a more severe and chronic nature. Chronic venous insufficiency is discussed more specifically in Chapter 8, while this chapter will focus on superficial venous insufficiency and varicose veins.

EPIDEMIOLOGY

The prevalence of venous disease is greatly underestimated in the USA and worldwide. Twice more frequent than coronary heart disease, and as prevalent as diabetes, venous disease affects approximately 25 million Americans, with almost one million people in the United States having venous ulcers. The overall cost is estimated at $21 to $46 billion annually.[1,2]

HISTORY

It has been proposed that humankind has been suffering from varicose veins ever since we started walking on two legs. Venous disease has similarly been recognized for a long time. The first documented case of varicose veins was recorded around 1550 BC in the papyrus of Ebers. Hippocrates noticed a connection between varicose veins and ulcers and started to treat varicose veins with compression and cautery. The first phlebectomy by mini-incisions was performed by Celsus (26 BC – 50 AD), but it was so painful that the patient reportedly refused further treatment. Vesalius described the anatomy of veins in 1543, Harvey then discovered the direction of venous flow to the heart, and Valsalva in 1710 described the pumping effect of muscles on venous flow. Risk factors for developing varicose veins, such as pregnancy and long travel, were identified by Paré in 1545. Fabricius first attributed varicose veins to valvular incompetence (1603) and a century later Dionis and Petit additionally attributed varices to proximal compression and obstruction. Rudolf Virchow in 1846 was the first to point out the hereditary tendency of varicose veins. In the 1880s, Briquet elucidated the role of abnormal flow from deep veins via the perforators in varicose vein pathogenesis. In terms of treatment, the first attempt at sclerotherapy was performed by Pravaz in the nineteenth century after the invention of the syringe and hypodermic needle but it was associated with numerous complications and was not further pursued. In 1884, Madelung proposed longitudinal incisions to perform phlebectomy but a less traumatic stripping technique was described by Charles Mayo in 1904. The hook phlebectomy, still in frequent use today, was introduced by Muller in 1956. Modern sclerotherapy developed only more recently in the 1960s with the development of safer sclerosants for injection. Endovascular techniques (radiofrequency ablation and laser ablation) began to be implemented in the 1990s and revolutionized superficial venous treatment as an alternative to stripping with less pain and a much quicker recovery. Evolution has continued with even less invasive methods and treatments now available.

ANATOMY AND PHYSIOLOGY

The anatomical nomenclature of the venous system was updated in 2002.[3,4] The lower extremity venous system consists of three major parts: superficial veins, deep veins, and perforator veins. The deep venous system, accompanying the major arteries of the leg, carries approximately 80% to 90% of the lower limb venous blood (Figure 19-1). The superficial system is associated with the visible varicose veins and is the most frequent target of therapeutic interventions. It is divided into two networks. The first network includes the great saphenous vein (GSV) and small saphenous vein (SSV) located subcutaneously in the superficial fascial compartments (Figures 19-2 and 19-3). The second network consists of tributaries of GSV and SSV which are also known as the communicating veins, which are different entities than perforators, and are located above the superficial fascia (Figure 19-3). The GSV drains into the common femoral vein and its terminal segment is called the sapheno-femoral junction (SFJ). Duplicated GSVs occur in 8% of people in the thigh and up to 25% in the calf.[5] There are also important accessory saphenous veins (ASVs) in the thigh, which travel anterior and posterior to the GSV, which can be important routes for venous reflux, particularly after ablation of the GSV.[6–9] The SSV drains into the popliteal vein and creates the sapheno-poplitial junction. In addition to these two junctions, the superficial veins connect to the deep venous system (in the deep compartment) by means of perforators (Figure 19-4). The most well-described and the most clinically important perforators are the medial calf perforators involving the posterior tibial veins, but there are more than 150 perforators in the leg that could be of clinical importance in specific patients.[10]

Healthy lower extremity veins have axial, unidirectional venous blood flow to the heart. This flow is maintained by the combined effects of the venous valves, lower extremity muscular pump compressive action, and negative intra-abdominal and intrathoracic pressure. It is crucial to have normal valvular function in all three venous systems to support antegrade venous flow. The calf muscle pump is a crucial component as it compresses the largest venous volume in the lower extremity (soleal and gastrocnemius sinusoids) and creates the highest pressure.[11]

An appreciation of the relevant nerves that are close to the saphenous veins is important for physicians to be able to prevent injury and potentially

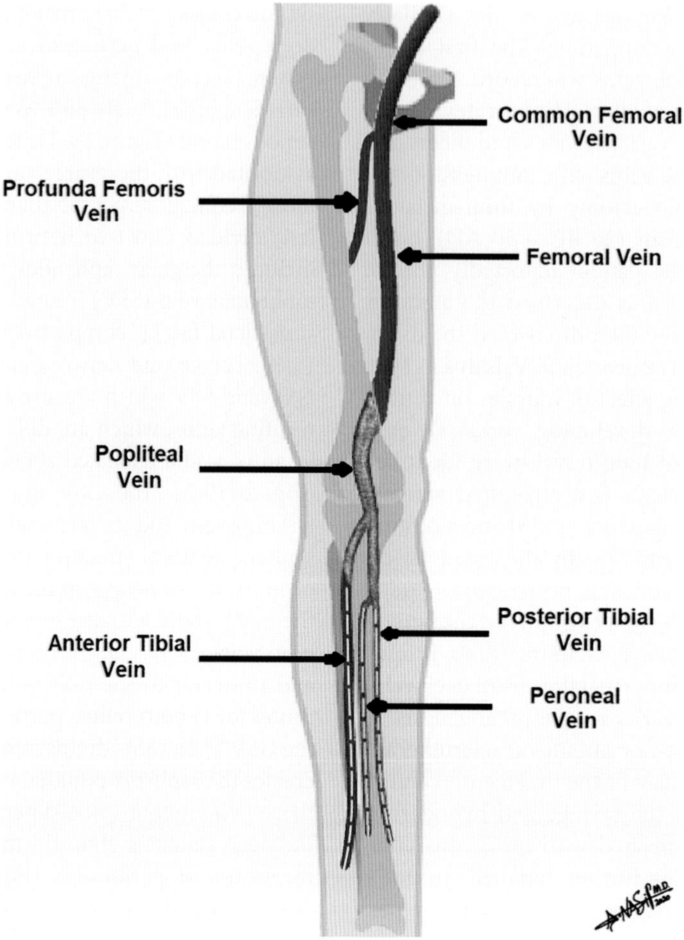

FIGURE 19-1 Deep venous system illustrating the paired tibial veins joining to form the popliteal which subsequently ascends to become the femoral vein. After its junction with the profunda (deep) femoral vein, it becomes the common femoral vein. (Reproduced with permission from Abdullah Nasif, MD.)

identify them with ultrasound. The *saphenous nerve* emerges from deep to superficial just above the knee and then runs closely to GSV in the distal two-thirds of the calf. It is a sensory nerve, but injury to it can cause neuropathic pain or loss of sensation on the medial portions of the lower leg. Because of its location and to prevent nerve injury, thermal ablation techniques of the GSV are most commonly not performed below the knee. The *sural nerve* originates from the tibial nerve below the knee and runs along the lateral aspect of the SSV. It is also a sensory nerve. Nonthermal ablation of the SSV will diminish the risk of injury to the sural nerve. The *common peroneal nerve* is relatively superficial and located laterally close to the fibular head, below the knee, and could potentially be damaged during open phlebectomies. Since it is both a motor and sensory nerve, injury can cause both loss of sensation and a foot drop.

TYPES OF VEINS

The CEAP classification recognizes four types of lower extremity veins associated with venous disease: telangiectasias, reticular veins, varicose veins, and corona phlebectatica (Figure 19-5). *Telangiectasias*, commonly referred to as "spider veins," are visibly

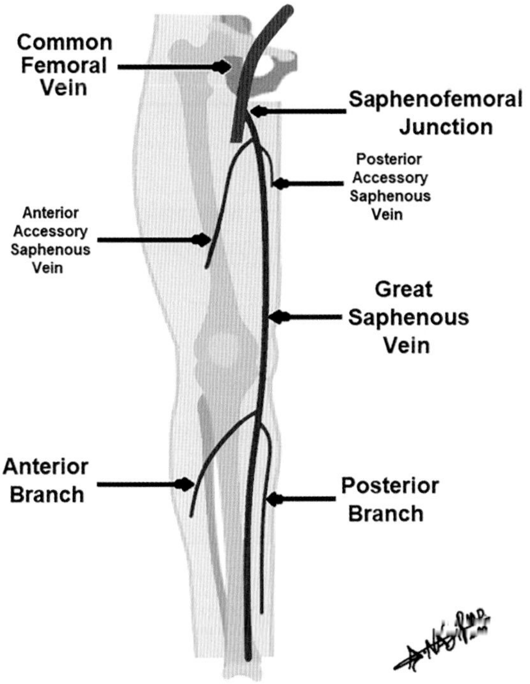

FIGURE 19-2 The great saphenous vein is located on the medial aspect of the leg, ascending from the medial malleolus at the ankle to the groin where it joins the common femoral vein at the saphenofemoral junction. (Reproduced with permission from Abdullah Nasif, MD.)

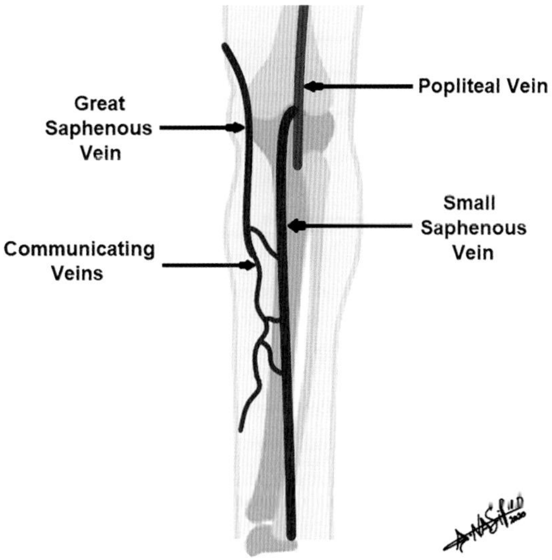

FIGURE 19-3 The small saphenous vein starts on the lateral aspect of the ankle, runs in the midline of the posterior calf for most of its path, and joins the deep venous system behind the knee at the popliteal vein. Communicating veins are collateral branches linking the great and small saphenous veins. (Reproduced with permission from Abdullah Nasif, MD.)

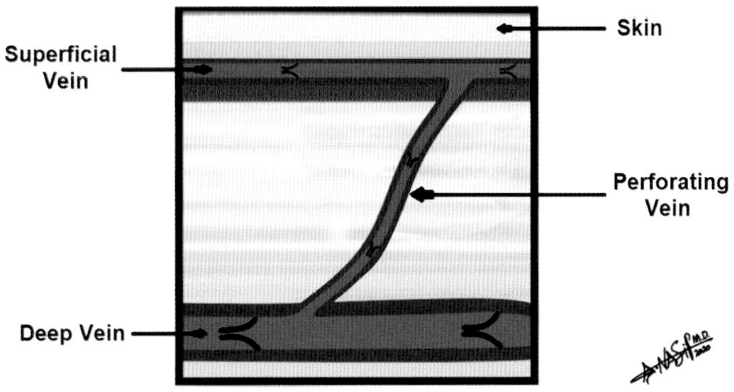

FIGURE 19-4 The perforating veins normally direct blood flow from the superficial to the larger capacitance deep veins through means of unidirectional valves. (Reproduced with permission from Abdullah Nasif, MD.)

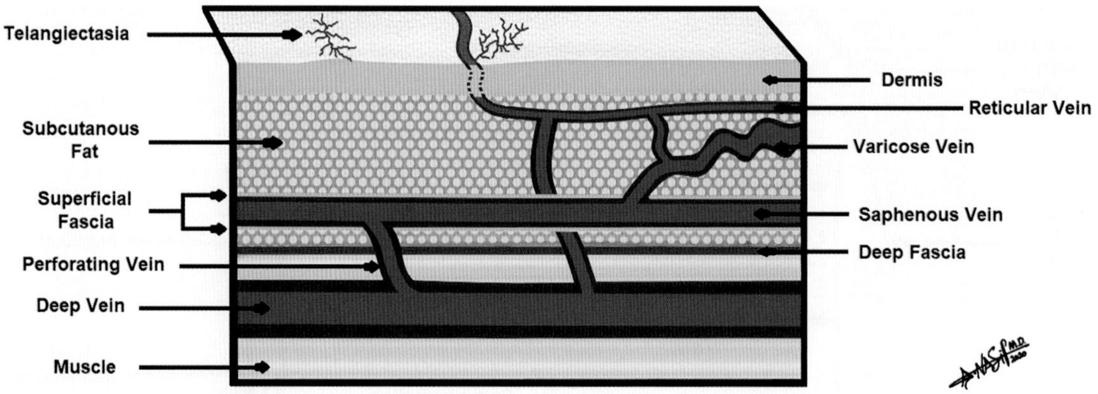

FIGURE 19-5 Sagittal anatomic illustration representing the relative locations and connections of the different types of veins of the legs. (Reproduced with permission from Abdullah Nasif, MD.)

dilated venules less than 1 mm in diameter. *Reticular veins*, sometimes called "blue veins" or "subdermal varices," are bluish subdermal veins 1 to 3 mm in diameter. They usually are tortuous and should not be confused with normally visible veins in thin people with transparent skin. True *varicose veins* are deeper subcutaneous dilated veins measuring greater than 3 mm in diameter when measured in the upright position. They typically involve tributaries of the saphenous veins, are usually tortuous, and are secondary to reflux from the axial saphenous system or perforating veins. *Corona phlebectatica*, "malleolar flare," or "ankle flare" is a fan-shaped pattern of multiple small intradermal veins on the medial or lateral aspects of the ankle. Essentially a group of blue telangiectasias, it has been recently recognized as an early sign of a more advanced disease in the 2020 CEAP revision.

RISK FACTORS

Risk factors for venous disease include family history,[12] female gender, pregnancy,[13] increasing age, obesity,[7] increased height,[14] standing occupations, and a history of deep venous thrombosis.[7,9] Elevated estradiol levels seen after menopause have been cited as a risk factor.[15] However, the effect of hormone replacement therapy is unclear, and oral contraceptives do not appear to increase the risk.[8]

There are several known genetic disorders associated with varicose veins. Klippel–Trenaunay syndrome is characterized by a triad of asymmetric limb hypertrophy, localized capillary malformation ("port-wine stain"), and congenital lower extremity varicosities. Parkes–Weber syndrome is similar to Klippel–Trenaunay syndrome but with the addition of arteriovenous fistulas. Ehlers–Danlos syndrome is characterized by connective tissue weakness and early-onset varicose veins. Mutations in the FOXC2 gene have been found to be associated with primary venous valve failure in the superficial and deep veins of the lower limb.[16–19] Significant progress has been made in gaining a better understanding of the molecular basis of CVD: structural changes of the vessel wall, extracellular matrix abnormalities, impaired balance between growth factors or cytokines, genetic alterations, etc.[20]

ETIOLOGY AND PATHOPHYSIOLOGY

Venous disease etiology is defined as being primary, secondary, or congenital with the associated pathophysiological mechanisms being associated with either reflux or obstruction. The most common pathophysiological mechanism is reflux due to valve malfunction leading to retrograde flow of blood and producing clinical symptoms and dilated varicose veins (Figure 19-6). Primary valvular incompetence of the superficial venous system is the most common. The "primary" designation points toward a primary

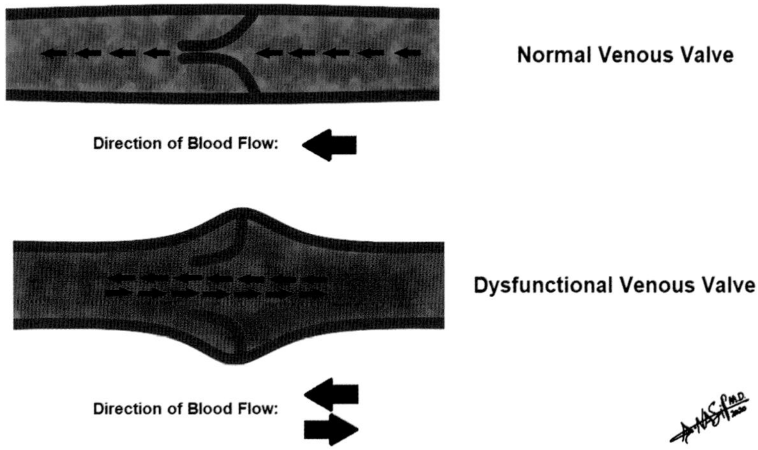

FIGURE 19-6 Normal bicuspid venous valves are meant to maintain unidirectional cephalad flow back to the heart. When dysfunctional, there is delayed closure of the valve leaflets allowing retrograde blood flow in a caudal direction and resulting venous hypertension in the lower extremities. (Reproduced with permission from Abdullah Nasif, MD.)

weakness in the vein wall[21,22] which leads to dilation of the vein and separation of the cusps of the valves resulting in valvular dysfunction. Secondary valvular incompetence, seen more frequently in the deep venous system, develops after deep venous thrombosis or superficial thrombophlebitis. Although therapeutic or intrinsic thrombolysis may dissolve the clot and restore blood flow through the vein, scarring at the base of the valve cusps limits their subsequent movement and ability to close effectively ("frozen valve").[11] Congenital valve absence is rare. Obstruction, caused by lack or incomplete recanalization of DVT in the deep system, leads to necessary venous return through collateral channels, often requiring retrograde flow through perforators, overload of the superficial veins, and their secondary dilatation and reflux.

Venous reflux and insufficiency most commonly affects more than one venous system. Isolated deep vein reflux is the least common while the superficial system is most frequently affected.[23] Incompetence of one venous system is usually associated with minimal signs of chronic venous insufficiency. However, incompetence in all three is much more frequently associated with ulcer development.[23] Gravitational effects when standing worsen any valvular insufficiency.

DIAGNOSIS

SYMPTOMS

Among the typical complaints of patients with CVD are leg heaviness, achiness, swelling, throbbing, and itching (HASTI) and the visible presence of varicose veins with associated concerns about their appearance (Figure 19-7). The symptoms of pain and achiness are most likely related to local inflammation due to venous stasis. Diffuse pain is often related to axial venous reflux, whereas dysfunctional venous flow in bulging varicosities may produce more focal discomfort. Patients may also complain about unpleasant sensations that are difficult to describe (heaviness, cramps, tension, pruritus, throbbing, burning) which can negatively impact their quality of life.[24] Symptoms are generally worse at the end of the day and exacerbated by leg dependency. They may be ameliorated by leg elevation or the use of compression stockings. Infrequently, acute superficial vein thrombosis (thrombophlebitis) may develop, manifested by local pain, erythema, and tenderness. Even more rarely, focal trauma or erosion of the skin overlying varicosity may lead to bleeding.

The effect of varicose disease on quality of life has been well described. Although there are several scales to measure and report the severity of symptoms, assessment using the Revised Venous

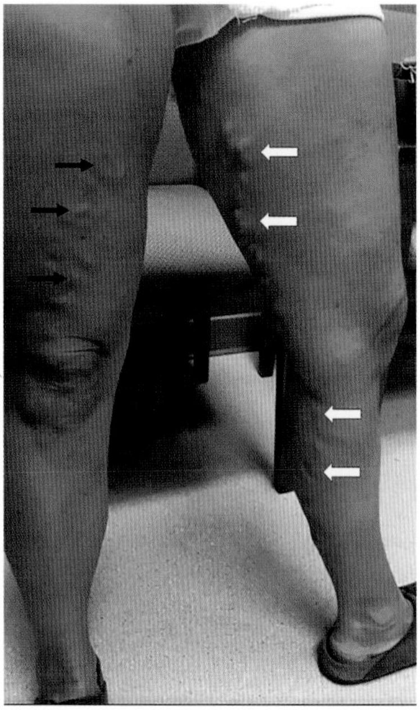

FIGURE 19-7 Varicose veins involving the great saphenous vein on the left leg (white arrows) extending from above to below the knee. On the right leg, the varicosities reflect insufficiency of the anterior accessory saphenous vein (black arrows).

Clinical Severity Score (VCSS) is clinically useful and has been validated (Table 19-1).[25] This assessment is patient-reported and quantifies the severity of chronic venous disease, progression, and response to treatment.[26–28]

Medical history is helpful in establishing the etiology of primary, secondary, or congenital varicosities and to differentiate chronic venous disease from other medical conditions causing similar symptoms. Although the patients may only complain about the visible varicose veins, their medical history will identify the presence of causative risk factors,[29,30] associated congenital abnormalities, and possible contraindications for treatment (pregnancy, allergy, severe coagulopathy, recent DVT, and limited life span).

A *physical examination* should be performed with the patient standing in a well-lit, warm room and the legs fully exposed. The presence of telangiectasia, reticular veins (C1), varices (C2), as well as their size, location, and distribution should be noted. The location of varicose veins is important as deviations from the classic distribution along the saphenous veins could suggest other conditions. Varices in the groin, perineum, and vulva could be related to iliac vein obstruction or pelvic reflux. Varices on the lateral thigh could be a sign of a congenital pathology (Klippel–Trenaunay syndrome). Aneurismal dilation of the great saphenous vein near SFJ could be misdiagnosed as a femoral hernia. Areas of clustered varicosities should be examined for the presence of a thrill or bruit which would suggest the presence of an arterio-venous malformation or fistula. Attention should be also paid to signs of more severe disease (edema, skin changes, and ulcers), and signs suggestive of thrombophlebitis (focal redness, tenderness, and palpable cords). The presence of a soft tissue mass, abdominal mass, or groin lymphadenopathy may be an indicator of external venous compression and obstruction to outflow via the iliac veins causing secondary leg swelling and pain.

An evaluation of the arterial pulses is important to differentiate co-existent peripheral arterial disease which may confound the patients' symptoms or require attention before venous interventions. Evaluating sensory and motor nerve function helps to diagnose diabetic neuropathy and also provides a baseline for nerve function before venous interventions.

DIFFERENTIAL DIAGNOSIS

The clinical diagnosis of venous disease is usually straightforward, although the symptoms are not specific and should be differentiated from other possible conditions. Leg pain could be due to degenerative joint disease, sciatica, arthritis, fibromyalgia, and peripheral arterial disease. The physical presence of telangiectasias, reticular veins, and varicosities is helpful but shared with some rare conditions. In Klippel–Trenaunay syndrome, varicosities are usually on the lateral aspect of the thigh as it represents a persistent embryonic vein, and capillary malformations are also more common.[31] Parkes Weber syndrome is a rare condition that has characteristic limb overgrowth along with the presence of arteriovenous malformations and fistulas. Rare cases of pulsatile varicose veins have been described due to tricuspid valve regurgitation.[32] All patients with venous disease should be classified objectively using the CEAP classification (Table 19-2).

TABLE 19-1 Revised Venous Clinical Severity Score (VCSS)

Attribute	Absent (0)	Mild (1)	Moderate (2)	Severe (3)
Pain or discomfort	None	Occasional	Daily, not preventing daily activity	Daily, limits daily activity
Varicose Veins	None	Few	Continued to calf/thigh	Involves calf/thigh
Venous Edema	None	Limited to foot and ankle	Above ankle but below the knee	Extends to knee and above
Skin Pigmentation Presumes venous origin Does not include focal pigmentation or pigmentation due to other chronic diseases	None or focal	Limited to peri malleolar area	Diffuse over the lower third of the calf	Wider distribution above lower third of calf
Inflammation (erythema, cellulitis, dermatitis, venous eczema)	None	Limited to peri malleolar area	Diffuse over the lower third of the calf	Wider distribution above lower third of calf
Induration Presumes venous origin Includes white atrophy	None	Limited to peri malleolar area	Diffuse over the lower third of the calf	Wider distribution above lower third of calf
No. Active Ulcers	None	1	2	>3
Active Ulcer Size (diameter)	None	<2 cm	2–6 cm	>6 cm
Ulcer Duration	None	<3 months	3–12 months	>1 year
Compression Therapy	None	Intermittent	Most days	Fully compliant

Adapted with permission from Vasquez MA, Rabe E, McLafferty RB, et al. Revision of the venous clinical severity score: venous outcomes consensus statement: special communication of the American Venous Forum Ad Hoc Outcomes Working Group. *J Vasc Surg*. 2010;52(5):1387-1396.

TABLE 19-2 CEAP Classification[33]

C – Clinical Class		E – Etiologic	A – Anatomic	P – Pathophysiologic
C0 No visible or palpable signs of venous disease	**C4a** – Pigmentation or eczema	**Ep** – Primary	**As** – Superficial	**Pr** – Reflux
C1 – Telangiectasias or reticular veins	**C4b** – Lipodermatosclerosis or atrophie blanche	**Es** – Secondary	**Ad** – Deep	**xPo** – Obstruction
C2 – Varicose veins	**C4c** – Corona phlebectatica	**Esi** – Secondary intravenous	**Ap** – Perforator	**Pr,o** – Reflux and obstruction
C2r – Recurrent varicose veins	**C5** – Healed ulcer	**Ese** – Secondary extravenous	**An** – No venous anatomic location identified	**Pn** – No pathophysiology identified
C3 – Edema	**C6** – Active venous ulcer			
C4 – Changes in skin and subcutaneous tissue secondary to CVD	**C6r** – Recurrent active venous ulcer			

A, asymptomatic; r, recurrent; s, symptomatic.

Adapted with permission from Lurie F, Passman M, Meisner M, et al. The 2020 update of the CEAP classification system and reporting standards. *J Vasc Surg Venous Lymphat Disord*. 2020;8(3):342-352.

DUPLEX ULTRASOUND

Duplex ultrasound is an essential component in the evaluation of patients with chronic venous disease. It is a safe, noninvasive, cost-effective, and reliable diagnostic method to complement the clinical examination.[30] For most patients, it is used to (1) exclude the presence of acute or chronic DVT; (2) document and quantify the presence of reflux in all three venous systems (superficial, deep, perforators); and (3) define the extent of superficial system reflux for potential therapeutic intervention.[30] The deep venous system is examined in the supine position to rule out DVT, as this may be a contraindication for superficial venous system ablation. The major goal of the superficial system evaluation is to assess both anatomy and hemodynamics. It should be performed in an upright position if technically possible and safe for the patient.[34] It can reveal anatomic anomalies such as duplication, areas of obstruction, or stenosis from prior episodes of phlebitis, and irregular entry points into the deep venous system. The presence and duration of reflux are examined following distal leg compression and release (Figure 19-8). A Valsalva maneuver can also be used in evaluating the common femoral vein or sapheno-femoral junction. For the superficial system, abnormal reflux is retrograde flow longer than 0.5 seconds, but clinically significant if more than 1 second regardless of the vein diameter.[30,35,36] To be appropriate for catheter cannulation to perform an ablation, an abnormal vein should generally be 4 mm or larger in diameter. Duplex ultrasound has high sensitivity and specificity with an overall 94% accuracy for detecting reflux. It is also recommended for follow-up of patients after venous interventions and for patients with recurrence varicose veins.

Other diagnostic modalities such as computed tomography venography, magnetic resonance venography, ascending and descending contrast venography,

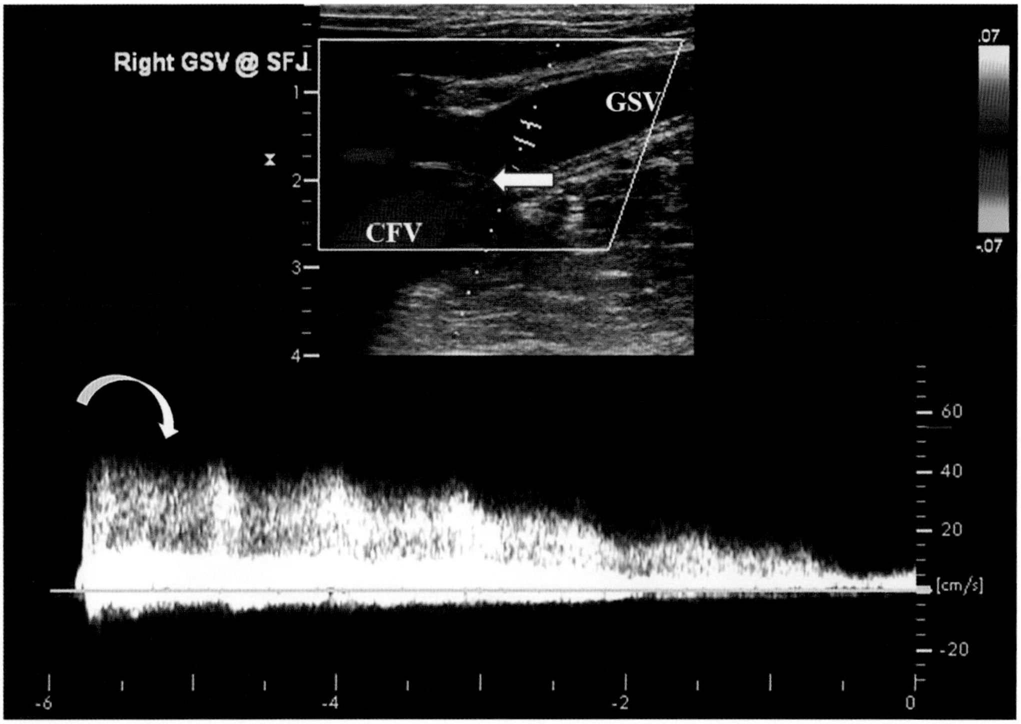

FIGURE 19-8 Longitudinal color Duplex ultrasound of the great saphenous vein (GSV) as it drains cephalad into the common femoral vein (CFV). The terminal valve at the saphenofemoral junction (straight arrow) is incompetent with resultant retrograde flow of 6 seconds (bottom *x*-axis) as documented by Doppler velocity scale (curved arrow).

and intravascular ultrasonography are occasionally helpful but rarely required for C0-C2 disease.[37]

MANAGEMENT

INDICATIONS FOR TREATMENT

For CEAP class C0-C2 patients, the indications for intervention are lifestyle-limiting symptoms and complications such as bleeding from varices and thrombophlebitis. Cosmesis is also an appropriate indication for treatment but is generally not covered by insurance companies. The latter often also has a policy requiring a trial of compression therapy for up to 3 months, but there is no scientific support to require a compression therapy trial prior to intervention in symptomatic patients. According to the REACTIVE trial, surgery for symptomatic saphenous reflux was proven to be more successful and cost-effective than compression therapy alone.[38,39] The appropriate use criteria for chronic lower extremity venous disease, developed by several professional societies in 2020, are a helpful reference for treatment guidelines (Table 19-3).[34]

It is important to differentiate axial from segmental reflux. Axial reflux is sequential reflux in the GSV, AASV, or SSV that extends from its junction with the deep system distally in continuity to the knee or ankle level. Segmental reflux is localized retrograde flow in the thigh or calf but is not in the continuity from the junction to the deep system in the groin or popliteal fossa. It can involve any part of a venous system including the superficial, deep, or perforators. Segmental reflux is associated with less clinically severe disease.[40–42] However, segmental below-knee GSV reflux is more commonly associated with symptomatic and more advanced disease than above-knee reflux.[40,43]

TREATMENT

Endovenous ablation describes treatment methods of venous closure as opposed to the historical

TABLE 19-3 Treatment Guidelines

Ablation	**Appropriate for**	GSV has axial reflux with or without SFJ reflux
	CEAP C2 symptomatic disease with ultrasound-proven reflux when	AAGSV with an axial reflux
		SSV with a symptomatic reflux
		Below knee GSV reflux
	Rarely appropriate for	AAGSV is without reflux but GSV has reflux
		Asymptomatic disease and visible veins, CEAP class C1-2 with no reflux in GSV
		Perforator veins in symptomatic C1-2 patient
Sclerotherapy, ambulatory phlebectomy, or powered phlebectomy	**Appropriate for**	Nontruncal varicose veins
	Symptomatic varicose veins with ultrasound-proven reflux, C2	Tributaries of an ablated saphenous vein, either simultaneous or staged procedure
It is never appropriate to		Ablate a saphenous vein without reflux
		Treat a perforator vein in asymptomatic C1-2 patients (excludes cosmetic indications)
		Perform stenting of iliac vein or IVC in asymptomatic C1 patients with obstructive disease as incidental findings

Data from Masuda E, Ozsvath K, Vossler J, et al. The 2020 appropriate use criteria for chronic lower extremity venous disease of the American Venous Forum, the Society for Vascular Surgery, the American Vein and Lymphatic Society, and the Society of Interventional Radiology. *J Vasc Surg Venous Lymphat Disord*. 2020;8(4):505-525.e4.

method of venous stripping and removal. Ablation can utilize thermal energy (using radiofrequency, laser, or high-intensity ultrasound), chemicals sclerosants (sclerotherapy), or a combination of mechanical and chemical ablation (mechanical occlusion chemically assisted [MOCA]). All of these procedures are performed in an outpatient setting without general anesthesia, typically done in the office, and under ultrasound guidance for percutaneous catheter placement. They can be divided into two major categories. Thermal tumescent (TT) procedures include radiofrequency ablation (RFA) and endovenous laser ablation (EVLA) which require perivenous injection of anesthetic agents because of the painful high heat produced within the vein by these methods. Nonthermal, nontumescent (NTNT) techniques do not require tumescent anesthesia and include mechanochemical, foam sclerotherapy, and medical glue injection to occlude the saphenous veins.

Thermal Tumescent Methods

Thermal ablation methods utilize heat from either alternating electrical current (RFA) or a laser (EVLA) to induce direct thermal injury to the wall of the vein leading to fibrosis and permanent lumen closure (Figure 19-9). Because of the high heat induced, up to 120°C, they require perivenular tumescent anesthesia, up to a volume of 500 mL of normal saline along with a lidocaine anesthetic, bicarbonate, and epinephrine. This injection separates the vein from adjacent skin and soft tissues to prevent injury, induces vasospasm to improve thermal ablation efficacy, and alleviates pain both during and after the procedure. RFA and EVLA have been proven to be safe and effective and are recommended for the treatment of saphenous incompetence in C2 patients with symptomatic varicose veins.

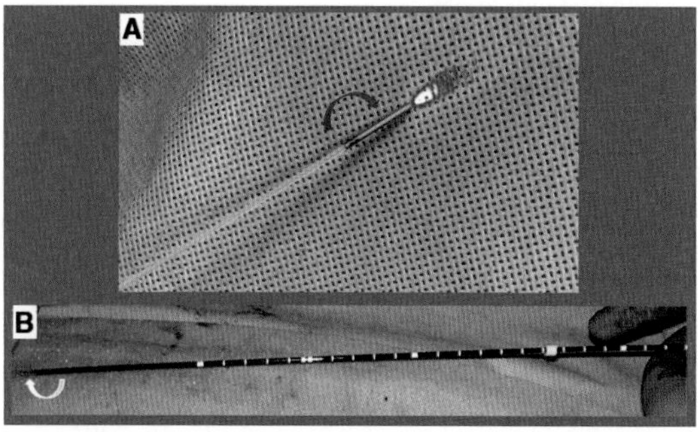

FIGURE 19-9 Thermal ablation techniques utilize either a laser (A) or radiofrequency (B) catheter as a source of heat arising from the tip (arrows) which collapses and closes the vein as it it withdrawn along its length.

Patient selection criteria take into account vein diameter and vein tortuosity. Generally, it is not recommended to attempt ablation of veins much smaller than 4 mm as they could be difficult to cannulate while those with a diameter greater than 2.5 cm may not close. Aneurysmal dilations at the saphenofemoral junctions may be better treated with surgical excision and stripping. Prior thrombophlebitis with a partially obstructed saphenous vein can make catheter advancement difficult. Patients with extensive occlusive deep vein thrombosis should only selectively undergo superficial ablation as the saphenous system plays an essential role for venous outflow in those cases.[44] Other relative contraindications to thermal ablation (EVLA or RFA) are uncorrectable coagulopathy, liver dysfunction that limits local anesthetic use, pregnancy, breastfeeding,[30] congenital venous abnormalities (e.g., Klippel–Trenaunay syndrome), and severe peripheral arterial disease.

Preprocedural considerations—Antiplatelet agents, nonsteroidal anti-inflammatory, and anticoagulation medications can be continued but may increase postoperative bruising and ecchymosis.[45,46] DVT prophylaxis is used only in high-risk patients (as determined by Caprini score) as a single dose of low-molecular-weight heparin before the procedure.[47]

RFA and EVLA Procedure Description—Ultrasound is utilized during the procedure to provide visualization of the vein to be treated (GSV, SSV, accessory vein), mark its path, and give guidance for cannulation. The percutaneous entry point is either above or below the knee for the GSV depending on the easiest accessibility, size of the vein, and its proximity to the surface, as well as the extent of the reflux. Ablation itself is usually limited to the above-the-knee segment of the vein, to avoid injury to the saphenous nerve, which lies in close proximity to the GSV in the calf. The Seldinger technique is used to insert a vascular sheath and the ablation catheter is advanced under ultrasound guidance. In order to prevent the development of thrombus within the common femoral vein (endovenous heat-induced thrombosis, EHIT), the tip of the catheter should be positioned distal to the entry of the superficial epigastric vein and 2.5 cm or more from the SFJ.[30,48] Once the ablation catheter is fixed in the proper location, tumescent anesthesia under ultrasound guidance is infiltrated circumferentially around the vein.[37] At the completion of the procedure, an ultrasound is used to confirm successful GSV obliteration and the absence of a thrombus in the common femoral vein. If obliteration is not achieved due to a technical failure, repeat ablation is not recommended as re-advancing the catheter might perforate the vessel. Instead, follow the patient clinically and use sclerotherapy or surgical intervention if later needed.[23]

Postprocedural care (common for all ablations) includes compression therapy, early ambulation, and follow-up with Duplex ultrasound. The most recent clinical practice guidelines[49] suggest using compression therapy after thermal ablation and stripping when possible. Compression pressures >20 mmHg in combination with eccentric pads, placed directly over the treated vein, provides the greatest reduction in postoperative pain (GRADE – 2; LEVEL OF EVIDENCE – B). There is no convincing evidence about the duration of compression which is why societal guidelines recommend using the best clinical judgment. In our clinical practice, we keep circumferential Ace wrappings on for 48 hours followed by stockings thereafter. There is no benefit in wearing compression stockings for more than 1 week, according to extrapolated data from a UK study about the duration of elastic compression after stripping.[50] Prior guidelines recommended postprocedural duplex scanning at 48 to 72 hours. However, in view of the low incidence of DVT and PE, many clinicians now perform a follow-up ultrasound within a week of the procedure in order to document successful venous closures and examine for possible development of endovenous heat-induced thrombosis (EHIT).[23]

Outcomes for RFA reported in the literature reflect as a mix of different types of RFA technology used over time. However, anatomical occlusion rates usually range between 89% and 95%[36,51–54] with 94% being the most recently reported randomized controlled study with 5-year follow-up.[55] Symptomatic improvement is reported by almost all patients. Similar results have been seen with EVLA with an occlusion rate of 88% at 5 years[56] (Table 19-4). A Cochrane review[57] indicates no difference in clinical or symptomatic recurrences between ablation and surgical ligation and stripping. Current guidelines, therefore, recommend endovenous thermal ablation of the incompetent saphenous vein over open surgery because they are associated with much less pain, less morbidity, faster recovery, higher quality of life scores, faster return to normal activities, and lower total cost.[30] Recurrences can develop due to recanalization or neovascularization in up to 22% of cases with long-term follow-up, a percentage similar to that after surgery.[58] Recanalization, however, is usually asymptomatic in 70% to 80% of patients. Recurrent varicose veins may be treated with another intervention, usually phlebectomy or sclerotherapy.

Complications of thermoablation methods are fewer when compared with surgical stripping. Possible complications include technical failures and later recanalization, superficial vein phlebitis (6.5%–8.8%), deep venous thrombosis or endovenous heat-induced thrombosis or EHIT (1.4%), hyperpigmentation (5%), paresthesia due to nerve injury (2.4%), ecchymosis, hematoma (1.2%–3.6%), pain and skin burn (0.5%–1.2%), infection at the vein access site (0.2%), and very rarely AV fistula.[30,57,59–66] The most bothersome complication is nerve injury causing hypoesthesia that may occur from thermal damage due to the close proximity of the saphenous nerve to the vein below the knee. That is why it is recommended to limit RFA to the proximal third of the GSV below the knee. Injury to the proximal common peroneal, tibial, and distal sciatic nerves after treatment of the small saphenous vein and the common peroneal nerve is associated with ablation of the vein of Giacomini. Knowledge of the relevant anatomy and sufficient tumescent anesthesia infiltration helps to prevent these complications. Skin burns are prevented by sufficient tumescent infiltration to protect the skin. EHIT is a heat-induced localized DVT and an extension of thrombus from the superficial-ablated vein (GSV, SSV) into the deep

TABLE 19-4 Comparison of Venous Treatment Methods

Procedure	Occlusion Rate	Pros	Cons
EVLA	85%–93% (5 years)	• known long-term outcomes • approved for truncal veins	• risk of thermal nerve injury • earlier lasers had greater bruising and discomfort compared to RFA • skin burns • phlebitis • EHIT
RFA	94% (5 years)	• known long-term outcomes • approved for truncal veins	• risk of thermal nerve injury • skin burns • phlebitis • EHIT
MOCA	85% (6–12 months)	• good for saphenous veins below the knee • no tumescent anesthesia • almost painless • minimal risk for nerve injury • no skin burns	• hyperpigmentation • not approved for tributary veins • limited follow-up data
Glue	82% (3 years)	• good saphenous veins below the knee • no tumescent anesthesia • almost painless • minimal risk for nerve injury • no skin burns	• not approved for tributary veins • max vein diameter: 12 mm • phlebitis • permanent foreign body • limited follow-up data
Sclerotherapy (liquid and foam)	23%–82% (5 years)	• truncal veins and tributaries, tortuous veins • tributary vein treatment combined with thermal methods for truncal veins gives excellent result • cost-effective • no tumescent anesthesia • almost painless • minimal risk for nerve injury • no skin burns	• inferior GSV occlusion compared to thermal methods but with similar clinical improvement in symptoms • hyperpigmentation • rare embolic complications (cerebral symptoms) • phlebitis • rare skin necrosis
Phlebectomy		• good for tortuous veins • nontruncal varicose veins • tributaries of an ablated saphenous vein, either simultaneous or staged procedure	• ecchymoses/hematomas • paresthesia • wound infections • possible nerve injury

TABLE 19-4 Comparison of Venous Treatment Methods—Continued

Procedure	Occlusion Rate	Pros	Cons
Ligation and Stripping	77%–94% (5 years)	• good for multiple recurrences • good for tortuous veins and aneurysmal dilation of SFJ	• pain • ecchymoses/hematomas • longer return to normal activities and work • Hematomas • Wound complications • Saphenous nerve injury

vein (femoral or popliteal vein).[67] EHIT is a form of DVT characterized by a more benign clinical picture than an unprovoked DVT. It is believed that EHIT is most likely to occur when the ablation catheter is placed too close to the SFJ, and therefore, a distance of greater than 2.5 cm from SFJ is now recommended. Unified American Venous Forum EHIT classification system described four types of EHIT, differentiated by the degree of thrombus extension into the deep vein.[68] Type I EHIT is a thrombus "flush" to the junction between a superficial and a deep vein. In Type II EHIT, the thrombus extends <50% into the deep vein, Type III has a thrombus extending >50%, while type IV EHIT is characterized by complete occlusion of the deep vein (occlusive DVT).

According to the guidelines, there is usually no need for treatment of EHIT types I and II. Type II should undergo weekly surveillance with duplex ultrasound until the resolution of the thrombus. On the other hand, for high-risk patients with EHIT II, additional antiplatelet or anticoagulation along with surveillance may be considered. After thrombus retraction to the SFJ or SPJ, such treatment should be stopped. Treatment for EHIT III consists of oral therapeutic anticoagulation (usually with a Factor Xa inhibitor) and ultrasound surveillance. Similarly, anticoagulation treatment should be stopped after the thrombus retracts to the SFJ or SPJ. Treatment for EHIT IV should be individualized, taking into the account the risks and benefits to the patient and treated in accordance with CHEST guidelines for the treatment of DVT.[68]

Tips for RFA and ELVA Treatment

- **Preoperative complete duplex ultrasound**
- **May continue antiplatelets, anticoagulants, and NSAIDs**
- **Ultrasound during procedure to mark vein, location of SFJ, choose an entry point**
- **Do not advance ablation catheter into the common femoral vein**
- **Start ablation 2.5-cm distally to SFJ, distal to superficial epigastric vein**
- **Tumescent anesthesia around the whole length of the vein**
- **ACE wrap/compression to decrease bruising and pain**
- **Postprocedural ultrasound**

Nontumescent nonthermal (NTNT) methods employ chemical and mechanochemical agents to provoke luminal fibrosis and obliteration. No thermal energy is applied, so these methods do not require tumescent anesthesia and the risk for nerve injury is minimal, and there is no risk for skin burns.

Mechanochemical ablation, also known as MOCA, is a relatively new type of ablation that combines mechanical abrasion to the venous wall and chemical ablation. *Technique.* The catheter contains a wire with an angled tip that rotates 3500 times a minute to cause mechanical damage to the endothelium of the venous wall. Concomitantly, a sclerosant is infused inside the injured vein as the guidewire rotates.[69] *Efficacy.* According to randomized controlled trials, MOCA has the same short-term technical, quality of life, and safety results as RFA.[70] Its rate of nerve injury, DVT, and skin burns is lower than thermal ablation; however, it has lesser anatomical success with 82% GSV occlusion at 1 year's follow-up.[71] There is less long-term experience compared to RFA and EVLA.[72] *Complications* include induration (12%–18%), thrombophlebitis (2%–13%), ecchymosis (8%–10%),[73] hyperpigmentation (5%), and deep venous thrombosis (0%–1%).

Cyanoacrylate adhesive (glue) vein ablation is the most recently approved nonthermal nontumescent technique and is only registered for truncal vein ablation. *Technique.* It is a catheter-based endovenous occlusion technique, so the endovenous procedure is similar to RFA and EVLA except that the catheter should be placed 5 cm distal to the SFJ to decrease thrombus formation in SFJ and DVT development. The glue is injected at 3 cm intervals, and external pressure is applied to the treated segments. The cyanoacrylate polymer begins rapid polymerization after contact with blood and the vein wall. Occlusion is initially caused by the glue itself followed by an inflammatory reaction and fibrotic occlusion of the vein. It should not be used in the superficial epifascial vein segments as it is more likely to cause visible phlebitis. The glue remains as a permanent foreign body in the vein lumen. *Efficacy:* in a randomized clinical trial, glue ablation was shown to be noninferior to RFA in the treatment of truncal veins. Occlusion rates previously varied from 76%[74,75] to 97%[76,77] at 1 year. The most recent 2018 randomized study showed that the 2-year complete closure rate was 95%, while symptoms, quality of life improvement, and safety were all similar to the RFA group.[78] Longer-term follow-up is not yet available. *Contraindications* include patients with a history of hypersensitivity to cyanoacrylate, DVT, or sepsis. The vein diameter should not be larger than 12 mm as safety and effectiveness have not been proven for larger veins. *Complications* are most commonly manifested by a phlebitic reaction to the glue (up to 4%–20%), glue extension through the SFJ, and hyperpigmentation (2.4%).[75,77]

Sclerotherapy involves the method of injection of a sclerosing agent (most commonly polidocanol or sodium tetradecyl sulfate) into the vein to obtain ablation. It can be used in the both truncal saphenous vein and individual varicosities or tributaries. It is particularly useful after recurrence following tumescent or nontumescent ablation techniques when the main saphenous vein is no longer patent for endovascular access. Foam sclerotherapy prepared by mixing the sclerosant and physiologic gas (CO_2, O_2, or room air), displaces the intraluminal blood and allows for greater contact of the sclerosant with the venous endothelium. It is particularly useful in the truncal veins and large branches and in tortuous veins. It is not used for telengiectasias. Severe *complications* after sclerotherapy are extremely rare ($<0.01\%$). Inadvertent arterial injection and skin necrosis are rare. More frequent complications are phlebitis (10%), matting, and hyperpigmentation (4.5%) particularly when higher concentrations are used. With foam sclerotherapy, transient neurologic adverse events (visual disturbances, migraine, confusion), chest tightness, and dry cough are rare but concerning and are more frequent in patients with patent foramen ovale when the foam bubbles can transit from the right side of the heart into the arterial and cerebral circulation. *Efficacy.* Truncal foam sclerotherapy occlusion rates are lower than RFA and ELVA. However, when used for tributary veins together with endothermal ablation of the truncal veins, foam sclerotherapy has high rates of success.[79]

Additionally, patient-reported quality of life scores were not as good at 5 years as compared to EVLA (Van der Velden 2015).[80] However, the technique is useful for nontruncal branches and individual varicosities when there is no truncal reflux.[30]

Surgery, exemplified by ligation of the great saphenous vein and stripping/removal in its entirety, used to be the gold standard in treatment but has now been supplanted in developed countries by the described less-invasive ablation techniques. Indications for stripping have been restricted to tortuous GSV superficially located and aneurysmal dilation of SFJ. Ambulatory phlebectomy (also known as a stab or hook phlebectomy, miniphlebectomy), however, continues to be a frequently used modality for the treatment of nontruncal varicosities. The technique includes stab incisions and removal of the veins using a hook or hemostat (Figure 19-10). Varicose veins

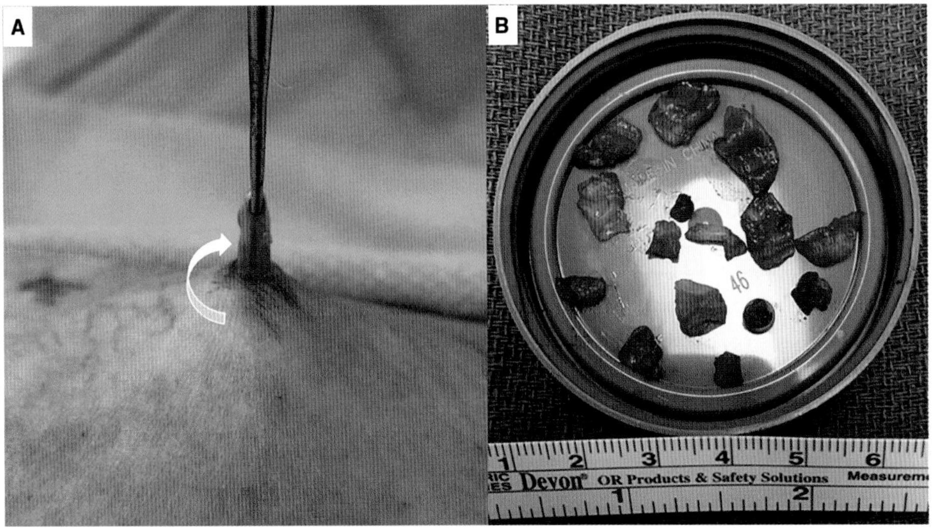

FIGURE 19-10 **Phlebectomy is performed by making a small stab incision on the skin through which a hook is inserted and the vein (vein) is pulled out (A). The vein is ligated at each end and the resulting specimens are resected and removed (B).**

are marked preoperatively with tumescent or local anesthesia applied. *Complications* vary significantly, ecchymosis and hematoma are reported in about 5% cases, paresthesias and nerve injury in 9%, superficial phlebitis in 2%, edema in 5%, hyperpigmentation in 1%, residual or recurrent varicose veins in 9%, and DVT in less than 1%. *Efficacy:* there is no recurrence of the excised veins but other varicosities may develop over time. Powered phlebectomy used to have a similar complication profile. Selected centers have less complications, hematoma (6%), ecchymosis (33%), cellulitis (1%), skin pigmentation (2%), saphenous neuropathy (0.3%), and no DVT. The limiting factor and its relatively infrequent use is post-procedural pain.[59]

Comparison of Interventional Methods

Major decision points about treatment modality choice are outlined in Figure 19-11 and Table 19-4. They are mainly based on the size of a vein, its location, and surrounding structures. Large saphenous veins are typically treated with RFA, ELVA, MOCA, medical glue, or with ultrasound-guided foam sclerotherapy. Saphenous veins above the knee are treated with either TT or NTNT methods. Below knee saphenous veins are adjacent to sensor nerves, and thus nonthermal methods are preferred. Branch vessels and individual varicosities are treated with either sclerotherapy or stab phlebectomy.

Noninterventional therapy includes changes in lifestyle (exercise, weight loss, elevating the legs when resting) and wearing compression stockings or garments. *Compression therapy*, exemplified by Class II (20–30 mmHg) and class III (30–40 mmHg) stockings, decreases ambulatory venous hypertension and thereby helps control reflux and venous hypertension in the leg.[23] Compression helps to decrease leg swelling and pain. Compression therapy is also indicated after thermal ablation, stripping, and sclerotherapy to decrease postoperative pain. However, there is no evidence that it decreases the progression of disease or prevents recurrence after an intervention. In terms of *efficacy*, the REACTIV randomized clinical trial proved that venous ablation provides better symptomatic relief and improvements in QOL than management with compression therapy and lifestyle modifications in patients with uncomplicated varicose veins.[38] Although a trial of compression

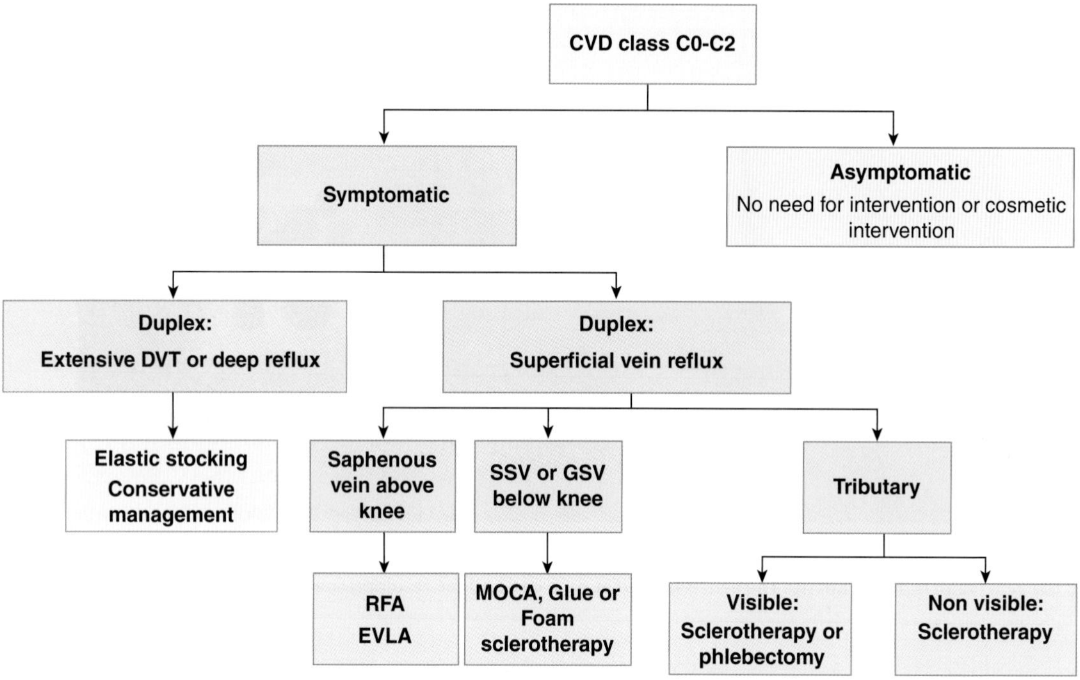

FIGURE 19-11 Flowchart for the treatment of venous disease. DVT, deep venous thrombosis; EVLA, endovenous laser ablation; GSV, great saphenous vein; MOCA, mechanical occlusion chemically assisted; RFA, radiofrequency ablation; SSV, small saphenous vein.

stockings is sometimes required by insurance companies before approval for ablation interventions, it is not medically recommended to use compression therapy as a primary treatment of symptomatic varicose veins (class C2) in patients who are candidates for saphenous vein ablation.[30] Possible *complications* are skin excoriations or ulcerations from inappropriate fitting. More often, obese and elderly patients may have difficulties in using elastic stockings and therefore compliance is low.

Medical therapy is not used often in the United States but is more frequently prescribed in Europe and South American countries. Diosmin, hesperidin, and micronized purified flavonoid fraction have shown the most efficacy among venoactive medications. The most recent Cochrane review[81] evaluated these medications and found that moderate-quality evidence confirms their beneficial effects on edema, cramps, restless legs, swelling, and paresthesia. The most frequent adverse effects mentioned were gastrointestinal disorders.

FUTURE DIRECTIONS

Devices and therapeutic approaches will continue to evolve in the future. One such promising modality is *High Intensity Focused Ultrasound* (HIFU)[82]—a completely noninvasive intervention based on the heat produced by percutaneous ultrasound energy. HIFU does not require venous cannulation nor tumescence anesthesia and could be potentially safer for patients on therapeutic anticoagulation. The transducer is placed on the skin above the vein and a focused ultrasound is directed on the vein to be treated. Although only a limited number of patients have so far been treated with HIFU, the technology is promising and potentially could be applicable to a wide number of patients.

ACKNOWLEDGMENT

Special thanks to Abdullah Nasif, MD, for the illustrations in this chapter.

REFERENCES

1. Chronic venous disease (CVD), epidemiology, costs and consequences. The Sage Group. https://www.thesagegroup.us/reports/chronic-venous-disease-cvd-epidemiology-costs-and-consequences/. Accessed April 19, 2021.
2. Davies AH. The seriousness of chronic venous disease: a review of real-world evidence. *Adv Ther.* 2019;36(S1):5-12.
3. Caggiati A, Bergan JJ, Gloviczki P, et al. Nomenclature of the veins of the lower limbs: an international interdisciplinary consensus statement. *J Vasc Surg.* 2002;36(2):416-422.
4. Kachlik D, Pechacek V, Hnatkova G, et al. The venous perforators of the lower limb: a new terminology. *Phlebology.* 2019;34(10):650-668.
5. Thomson H. The surgical anatomy of the superficial and perforating veins of the lower limb. *Ann R Coll Surg Engl.* 1979;61(3):198-205.
6. García-Gimeno M, Rodríguez-Camarero S, Tagarro-Villalba S, et al. Duplex mapping of 2036 primary varicose veins. *J Vasc Surg.* 2009;49(3):681-689.
7. Bush RG, Bush P, Flanagan J, et al. Factors associated with recurrence of varicose veins after thermal ablation: results of the recurrent veins after thermal ablation study. *Sci World J.* 2014;2014:505843.
8. Proebstle TM, Möhler T. A longitudinal single-center cohort study on the prevalence and risk of accessory saphenous vein reflux after radiofrequency segmental thermal ablation of great saphenous veins. *J Vasc Surg Venous Lymphat Disord.* 2015;3(3):265-269.
9. Winokur RS, Khilnani NM, Min RJ. Recurrence patterns after endovenous laser treatment of saphenous vein reflux. *Phlebology.* 2016;31(7):496-500.
10. Van Limborgh J. L'Anatomie du systeme veineux de l'extremite inferieure relation avec la pathologie variqueuse. *Folia Angiol.* 1961;8:240-257.
11. Kamel MK, Blebea J. Pathophysiology of edema in patients with chronic venous insufficiency. *Phlebolymphology.* 2020;27(1):3-10.
12. Cornu-Thenard A, Boivin P, Baud JM, et al. Importance of the familial factor in varicose disease. Clinical study of 134 families. *J Dermatol Surg Oncol.* 1994;20(5):318-326.
13. Jukkola TM, Mäkivaara LA, Luukkaala T, et al. The effects of parity, oral contraceptive use and hormone replacement therapy on the incidence of varicose veins. *J Obstet Gynaecol.* 2006;26(5):448-451.
14. Fukaya E, Flores AM, Lindholm D, et al. Clinical and genetic determinants of varicose veins: prospective, community-based study of ≈500 000 individuals. *Circulation.* 2018;138(25):2869-2880.
15. Ciardullo AV, Panico S, Bellati C, et al. High endogenous estradiol is associated with increased venous distensibility and clinical evidence of varicose veins in menopausal women. *J Vasc Surg.* 2000;32(3):544-549.
16. Jacob AG, Driscoll DJ, Shaughnessy WJ, et al. Klippel-trénaunay syndrome: spectrum and management. *Mayo Clinic Proceedings.* 1998;73(1):28-36.
17. Gordeuk VR, Sergueeva AI, Miasnikova GY, et al. Congenital disorder of oxygen sensing: association of the homozygous Chuvash polycythemia VHL mutation with thrombosis and vascular abnormalities but not tumors. *Blood.* 2004;103(10):3924-3932.
18. Saiki S, Sakai K, Saiki M, et al. Varicose veins associated with CADASIL result from a novel mutation in the Notch3 gene. *Neurology.* 2006;67(2):337-339.
19. Mellor RH, Brice G, Stanton AWB, et al. Mutations in FOXC2 are strongly associated with primary valve failure in veins of the lower limb. *Circulation.* 2007;115(14):1912-1920.
20. Segiet OA, Brzozowa-Zasada M, Piecuch A, et al. Biomolecular mechanisms in varicose veins development. *Annals of Vascular Surgery.* 2015;29(2):377-384.
21. Wali MA, Eid RA. Changes of elastic and collagen fibers in varicose veins. *Int Angiol.* 2002;21(4):337-343.
22. Pocock ES, Alsaigh T, Mazor R, et al. Cellular and molecular basis of venous insufficiency. *Vasc Cell.* 2014;6(1):24.
23. Blebea J. The pathophysiology and hemodynamics of chronic venous insufficiency of the lower limb. In: *Handbook of Venous and Lymphatic Disorders.* Boca Raton, FL: CRC Press; 2017.
24. Perrin M. From venous pain to surgery. https://vein-academy.servier.com/book/from-venous-pain-to-surgery/. Accessed April 19, 2021.
25. Vasquez MA, Rabe E, McLafferty RB, et al. Revision of the venous clinical severity score: venous outcomes consensus statement: special communication of the American Venous Forum Ad Hoc Outcomes Working Group. *J Vasc Surg.* 2010;52(5):1387-1396.
26. Kaplan RM, Criqui MH, Denenberg JO, et al. Quality of life in patients with chronic venous disease: San Diego population study. *J Vasc Surg.* 2003;37(5):1047-1053.
27. Smith JJ, Guest MG, Greenhalgh RM, et al. Measuring the quality of life in patients with venous ulcers. *J Vasc Surg.* 2000;31(4):642-649.
28. Smith JJ, Garratt AM, Guest M, et al. Evaluating and improving health-related quality of life in patients with varicose veins. *J Vasc Surg.* 1999;30(4):710-719.
29. Bermudez KM, Knudson MM, Nelken NA, et al. Long-term results of lower-extremity venous injuries. *Arch Surg.* 1997;132(9):963-967; Discussion 967-968.

30. Gloviczki P, Comerota AJ, Dalsing MC, et al. The care of patients with varicose veins and associated chronic venous diseases: clinical practice guidelines of the Society for Vascular Surgery and the American Venous Forum. *J Vasc Surg*. 2011;53(5):2S-48S.
31. Wang SK, Drucker NA, Gupta AK, et al. Diagnosis and management of the venous malformations of Klippel-Trénaunay syndrome. *J Vasc Surg Venous Lymphat Disord*. 2017;5(4):587-595.
32. Li X, Feng Y, Liu Y, Zhang F. Varicose veins of the lower extremity secondary to tricuspid regurgitation. *Ann Vasc Surg*. 2019;60:477.e1-477.e6.
33. Lurie F, Passman M, Meisner M, et al. The 2020 update of the CEAP classification system and reporting standards. *J Vasc Surg Venous Lymphat Disord*. 2020;8(3):342-352.
34. Masuda E, Ozsvath K, Vossler J, et al. The 2020 appropriate use criteria for chronic lower extremity venous disease of the American Venous Forum, the Society for Vascular Surgery, the American Vein and Lymphatic Society, and the Society of Interventional Radiology. *J Vasc Surg Venous Lymphat Disord*. 2020;8(4):505-525.e4.
35. Practice Guidelines for Superficial Venous Disease. American Vein & Lymphatic Society. https://www.myavls.org/member-resources/clinical-guidelines.html. Accessed April 19, 2021.
36. Labropoulos N, Tiongson J, Pryor L, et al. Definition of venous reflux in lower-extremity veins. *J Vasc Surg*. 2003;38(4):793-798.
37. Vuylsteke ME, Klitfod L, Mansilha A. Endovenous ablation. *Int Angiol*. 2019;38(1):22-38.
38. Michaels JA, Campbell WB, Brazier JE, et al. Randomised clinical trial, observational study and assessment of cost-effectiveness of the treatment of varicose veins (REACTIV trial). *Health Technol Assess*. 2006;10(13):1-196,
39. Michaels JA, Brazier JE, Campbell WB, et al. Randomized clinical trial comparing surgery with conservative treatment for uncomplicated varicose veins. *Br J Surg*. 2006;93(2):175-181.
40. Labropoulos N, Leon M, Nicolaides AN, et al. Superficial venous insufficiency: correlation of anatomic extent of reflux with clinical symptoms and signs. *J Vasc Surg*. 1994;20(6):953-958.
41. Danielsson G, Arfvidsson B, Eklof B, et al. Reflux from thigh to calf, the major pathology in chronic venous ulcer disease: surgery indicated in the majority of patients. *Vasc Endovascular Surg*. 2004;38(3):209-219.
42. Lim KH, Hill G, Tarr G, et al. Deep venous reflux definitions and associated clinical and physiological significance. *J Vasc Surg Venous Lymphat Disord*. 2013;1(4):325-332
43. Labropoulos N, Delis K, Nicolaides AN, et al. The role of the distribution and anatomic extent of reflux in the development of signs and symptoms in chronic venous insufficiency. *J Vasc Surg*. 1996;23(3):504-510.
44. Hong K, Georgiades C. Radiofrequency ablation: mechanism of action and devices. *J Vasc Interv Radiol*. 2010;21(Suppl 8):S179-S186.
45. Sharifi M, Mehdipour M, Bay C, et al. Effect of anticoagulation on endothermal ablation of the great saphenous vein. *J Vasc Surg*. 2011;53(1):147-149.
46. Enzler MA, Russell D, Schimmelpfennig J. Thermal ablation in the management of superficial thrombophlebitis. *Eur J Vasc Endovasc Surg*. 2012;43(6):726-728.
47. Gould MK, Garcia DA, Wren SM, et al. Prevention of VTE in nonorthopedic surgical patients: antithrombotic therapy and prevention of thrombosis, 9th ed: american college of chest physicians evidence-based clinical practice guidelines. *Chest*. 2012;141(Suppl 2):e227S-e277S.
48. Sadek M, Kabnick LS, Rockman CB, et al. Increasing ablation distance peripheral to the saphenofemoral junction may result in a diminished rate of endothermal heat-induced thrombosis. *J Vasc Surg Venous Lymphat Disord*. 2013;1(3):257-262.
49. Lurie F, Lal BK, Antignani PL, et al. Compression therapy after invasive treatment of superficial veins of the lower extremities: clinical practice guidelines of the American Venous Forum, Society for Vascular Surgery, American College of Phlebology, Society for Vascular Medicine, and International Union of Phlebology. *J Vasc Surg Venous Lymphat Disord*. 2019;7(1):17-28.
50. Biswas S, Clark A, Shields DA. Randomised clinical trial of the duration of compression therapy after varicose vein surgery. *Eur J Vasc Endovasc Surg*. 2007;33(5):631-637.
51. Goode SD, Chowdhury A, Crockett M, et al. Laser and radiofrequency ablation study (LARA study): a randomised study comparing radiofrequency ablation and endovenous laser ablation (810 nm). *Eur J Vasc Endovasc Surg*. 2010;40(2):246-253.
52. Lurie F, Creton D, Eklof B, et al. Prospective randomized study of endovenous radiofrequency obliteration (Closure procedure) versus ligation and stripping in a selected patient population (EVOLVeS study). *J Vasc Surg*. 2003;38(2):207-214.
53. Nordon IM, Hinchliffe RJ, Brar R, et al. A prospective double-blind randomized controlled trial of radiofrequency versus laser treatment of the great saphenous vein in patients with varicose veins. *Ann Surg*. 2011;254(6):876-881.

54. Balint R, Farics A, Parti K, et al. Which endovenous ablation method does offer a better long-term technical success in the treatment of the incompetent great saphenous vein? Review. *Vascular*. 2016;24(6):649-657.
55. Lawaetz M, Serup J, Lawaetz B, et al. Comparison of endovenous ablation techniques, foam sclerotherapy and surgical stripping for great saphenous varicose veins. Extended 5-year follow-up of a RCT. *Int Angiol*. 2017;36(3):281-288.
56. Hamann SAS, Giang J, De Maeseneer MGR, et al. Editor's choice: five year results of great saphenous vein treatment: a meta-analysis. *Eur J Vasc Endovas Surg*. 2017;54(6):760-770.
57. Nesbitt C, Bedenis R, Bhattacharya V, et al. Endovenous ablation (radiofrequency and laser) and foam sclerotherapy versus open surgery for great saphenous vein varices. *Cochrane Database Syst Rev*. 2014;(7):CD005624 .doi:10.1002/14651858.CD005624.pub3
58. O'Donnell TF, Balk EM, Dermody M, et al. Recurrence of varicose veins after endovenous ablation of the great saphenous vein in randomized trials. *J Vasc Surg Venous Lymphat Disord*. 2016;4(1):97-105.
59. Lin PH, Matos JM, Chen A, et al. Treatment outcomes and lessons learned from transilluminated powered phlebectomy for varicose veins in 1034 patients. *Vasc Endovascular Surg*. 2016;50(4):277-282.
60. Anwar MA, Lane TRA, Davies AH, et al. Complications of radiofrequency ablation of varicose veins. *Phlebology*. 2012;27(Suppl 1):34-39.
61. Dexter D, Kabnick L, Berland T, et al. Complications of endovenous lasers. *Phlebology*. 2012;27(Suppl 1):40-45.
62. Wittens C, Davies AH, Bækgaard N, et al. Editor's choice: management of chronic venous disease: clinical practice guidelines of the European society for vascular surgery (ESVS). *Eur J Vasc Endovasc Surg*. 2015;49(6):678-737.
63. Merchant RF, Pichot O, Closure Study Group. Long-term outcomes of endovenous radiofrequency obliteration of saphenous reflux as a treatment for superficial venous insufficiency. *J Vasc Surg*. 2005;42(3):502-509; Discussion 509.
64. Ahmad A, Sajjanshetty M, Mandal A, et al. Early arteriovenous fistula after radiofrequency ablation of long saphenous vein. *Phlebology*. 2013;28(8):438-440.
65. Rudarakanchana N, Berland TL, Chasin C, et al. Arteriovenous fistula after endovenous ablation for varicose veins. *J Vasc Surg*. 2012;55(5):1492-1494.
66. Ziporin SJ, Ifune CK, MacConmara MP, et al. A case of external iliac arteriovenous fistula and high-output cardiac failure after endovenous laser treatment of great saphenous vein. *J Vasc Surg*. 2010;51(3):715-719.
67. Healy DA, Kimura S, Power D, et al. A systematic review and meta-analysis of thrombotic events following endovenous thermal ablation of the great saphenous vein. *Eur J Vasc Endovasc Surg*. 2018;56(3):410-424.
68. Kabnick LS, Sadek M, Bjarnason H, et al. Classification and treatment of endothermal heat-induced thrombosis: recommendations from the american venous forum and the society for vascular surgery. *J Vasc Surg Venous Lymphat Disord*. 2021;9(1):6-22.
69. Van Eekeren RRJP, Boersma D, Elias S, et al. Endovenous mechanochemical ablation of great saphenous vein incompetence using the ClariVein device: a safety study. *J Endovasc Ther*. 2011;18(3):328-334.
70. Lane T, Bootun R, Dharmarajah B, et al. A multi-centre randomised controlled trial comparing radiofrequency and mechanical occlusion chemically assisted ablation of varicose veins: final results of the Venefit versus Clarivein for varicose veins trial. *Phlebology*. 2017;32(2):89-98.
71. Vähäaho S, Mahmoud O, Halmesmäki K, et al. Randomized clinical trial of mechanochemical and endovenous thermal ablation of great saphenous varicose veins. *Br J Surg*. 2019;106(5):548-554.
72. Holewijn S, van Eekeren RRJP, Vahl A, et al. Two year results of a multicenter randomized controlled trial comparing mechanochemical endovenous ablation to radiofrequency ablation in the treatment of primary great saphenous vein incompetence (MARADONA trial). *J Vasc Surg Venous Lymphat Disord*. 2019;7(3):364-374.
73. Boersma D, van Eekeren RRJP, Werson DAB, et al. Mechanochemical endovenous ablation of small saphenous vein insufficiency using the Clarivein® device: one-year results of a prospective series. *Eur J Vasc Endovasc Surg*. 2013;45(3):299-303.
74. Chan YC, Law Y, Cheung GC, et al. Cyanoacrylate glue used to treat great saphenous reflux: measures of outcome. *Phlebology*. 2017;32(2):99-106.
75. Gibson K, Ferris B. Cyanoacrylate closure of incompetent great, small and accessory saphenous veins without the use of post-procedure compression: initial outcomes of a post-market evaluation of the VenaSeal System (The WAVES study). *Vascular*. 2017;25(2):149-156.
76. Proebstle TM, Alm J, Dimitri S, et al. Twelve-month follow-up of the european multicenter study on cyanoacrylate embolization of incompetent great saphenous veins. *J Vasc Surg Venous Lymphat Disord*. 2014;2(1):105-106.
77. Chan YC, Law Y, Cheung GC, et al. Predictors of recanalization for incompetent great saphenous veins treated with cyanoacrylate glue. *J Vasc Interv Radiol*. 2017;28(5):665-671.

78. Gibson K, Morrison N, Kolluri R, et al. Twenty-four month results from a randomized trial of cyanoacrylate closure versus radiofrequency ablation for the treatment of incompetent great saphenous veins. *J Vasc Surg Venous Lymphat Disord.* 2018;6(5):606-613.
79. Cartee T, Wirth P, Blebea J, et al. Ultrasound guided foam sclerotherapy is safe and effective in the management of superficial venous insufficiency of the lower extremity. *J Vasc Surg Venous Lymphat Disord.* 2021; In Press.
80. Van der Velden SK, Biemans AAM, De Maeseneer MGR, et al. Five-year results of a randomized clinical trial of conventional surgery, endovenous laser ablation and ultrasound-guided foam sclerotherapy in patients with great saphenous varicose veins. *Br J Surg.* 2015;102(10):1184-1194. doi:10.1002/bjs.9867
81. Martinez-Zapata MJ, Vernooij RW, Uriona Tuma SM, et al. *Phlebotonics for venous insufficiency*. Cochrane Vascular Group, ed. Cochrane Database of Systematic Reviews. Vol. 4, 2016. https://www.cochranelibrary.com/cdsr/doi/10.1002/14651858.CD003229
82. Whiteley MS. High intensity focused ultrasound (HIFU) for the treatment of varicose veins and venous leg ulcers – a new non-invasive procedure and a potentially disruptive technology. *Curr Med Res Opin.* 2020;36(3):509-512.

SELF-ASSESSMENT STUDY QUESTIONS AND ANSWERS

Questions

1. What is C2 disease according to the CEAP classification?
A. Varicose veins
B. No visible or palpable signs of venous disease
C. Telangiectasias or reticular veins
D. Ulcer
E. Edema

2. What are the indications for treatment of saphenous veins in C2 class varicose veins?
A. Insurance approval
B. Symptoms or bleeding
C. Noncompliance with compression stockings
D. Presence of AV fistulas
E. Deep venous thrombosis

3. What is the primary goal of Duplex ultrasound evaluation prior to intervention for varicose veins?
A. Rule out external venous compression
B. Examine for presence of AV fistulas
C. Confirm vein dilatation
D. Confirm the presence of axial reflux
E. Identify location of phlebitis

4. What is the current standard for C2 varicose veins treatment?
A. HIFU
B. Surgical ligation/stripping
C. Compression therapy
D. Vasoactive medications
E. Endovenous ablation

5. Is hose compression therapy trial required before treatment of symptomatic reflux disease?
A. Absolutely necessary
B. Necessary in most circumstances
C. Not required
D. Has no role in varicose vein treatment
E. Does not improve postprocedural pain

6. What are the major advantages of thermal ablation techniques over surgical ligation/stripping?
A. Faster recovery, less morbidity
B. Has no advantage, it is comparable
C. Not complicated by DVT
D. Does not cause nerve injuries
E. Not complicated by EHIT

7. Where should the tip of an RFA or laser catheter be located before starting endovenous ablation?
A. In the common femoral vein
B. In the femoral vein
C. At the saphenofemoral junction
D. 2.5 cm from inferior epigastric vein (Correct)
E. 5 cm from inferior epigastric vein

8. What treatment methods are preferred for the saphenous veins below the knee?
A. Thermal ablation methods
B. Compression therapy
C. Nonthermal ablation methods (MOCA or glue)
D. Phlebectomy
E. Radiofrequency ablation

9. What method is the best for treatment of tributary veins?
A. Thermal ablation
B. Nonthermal ablation
C. Compression therapy
D. Ligation/stripping
E. Sclerotherapy/phlebectomy

10. Choose the most appropriate treatment option for EHIT with thrombus extension into common femoral vein, more than 50% of its diameter?
A. Duplex ultrasound surveillance
B. Therapeutic anticoagulation with apixaban
C. Aspirin
D. Aspirin and plavix
E. Therapeutic anticoagulation with warfarin

SELF-ASSESSMENT STUDY QUESTIONS AND ANSWERS

Answers

1. A.
2. B.
3. D.
4. E.
5. C.
6. A.
7. D.
8. C.
9. E.
10. B.

CHAPTER

20 Chronic Venous Disease of the Upper Extremities and Central Veins

Leah Gober and Karl A. Illig

OUTLINE

INTRODUCTION

ANATOMY

- **Overview**
- **Notable Upper Arm Relationships**
  - Deltopectoral Groove/Triangle and the Cephalic Vein
  - The Costoclavicular Junction (CCJ) and the Subclavian Vein
  - Intrathoracic Venous Problems

CLINICAL PRESENTATION

SPECIFIC PROBLEMS

- **Venous Thoracic Outlet Syndrome**
  - Intermittent Positional Stenosis (McCleery's Syndrome)
  - Postphlebitic Obstruction (Chronic Paget–Schroetter Syndrome)
- **Arteriovenous Access-Related VTOS**
  - Peripheral Stenoses
  - Cephalic Arch Stenosis
  - Costoclavicular Junction Stenosis
  - Intrathoracic Venous Stenosis
  - The HeRO Graft
- **Pacemaker and Catheter-Induced Obstruction**
- **Obstruction Secondary To Malignancy**

ALGORITHM FOR CARE

CONCLUSIONS

INTRODUCTION

The venous system, with its complex network of one-way valves, communicating branches, and peripheral pumping mechanisms, connects in a progressive fashion that culminates in an effective system to return blood to the heart even when working against gravity. Venous embryologic development is understood as passing through three main stages: first, as an undifferentiated capillary network composed of primitive mesenchymal tissues; second, differentiation into large plexiform structures; and third, maturation into isolated macroscopic channels, the vein.[1,2] The upper extremity, in particular, is unique in that it needs to return blood while being located intermittently both above and below the right atrium to which it flows.[3]

Veins also act as both conduit and capacitance vessels. The volume of blood contained within a vein can change drastically with only minor changes in pressure, allowing for dynamic adaptations to optimize cardiovascular stability. With less gravity to work against, the valves of the upper extremity are not as numerous as that of the lower extremity, and gravity does not have the same chronic effects on the upper extremity veins as it does that of the lower limbs.

Chronic venous disease in the upper extremities is much less common than in the lower extremities largely because of less gravitational stress. Venous disease does occur, however, in several well-defined situations, which will be the subject of this chapter. In general, problems arise due to increased pressure in the veins, which is caused by central obstruction (with or without iatrogenically increased pressure in the setting of arteriovenous [AV] access). This intraluminal pressure, in turn, creates varying degrees of fluid extravasation which leads to swelling and pain. Skin changes are uncommon and true varicose veins and ulceration, in contrast to lower extremities, are vanishingly rare.

Upper extremity venous disease can conveniently be divided into four broad categories, several of which overlap: chronic venous thoracic outlet syndrome (VTOS), caused by chronic compression and/or injury to the subclavian vein at the costoclavicular junction (CCJ); AV access-associated swelling and dysfunction, caused by stenosis or occlusion at the CCJ or more central veins and exacerbated by the delivery of high pressure to the system; iatrogenic injury from intraluminal devices; and malignancies that affect the central vessels.

ANATOMY

OVERVIEW

Similar to the lower extremities, the upper limbs have both a superficial and deep venous system, the latter of which is generally paired and follows the corresponding artery. The twin radial and ulnar veins run deep to the fascia and join to form the brachial vein at the antecubital fossa. The brachial veins are also generally paired and tend to coalesce at the axilla where they become the single axillary vein and transition into the subclavian vein at the lateral border of the first rib. The superficial veins arise from the dorsum of the hand to drain into the cephalic vein laterally and the basilic medially (Figure 20-1). The cephalic vein, anatomically analogous to the great saphenous vein, and the basilic vein, analogous to the small saphenous vein, coalesce in varying patterns at the antecubital fossa, most commonly producing a dominant antecubital vein. From there, the cephalic vein consistently runs fairly superficially up the lateral border of the arm, diving deeply as the cephalic arch to join the axillary vein, while the basilic vein enters

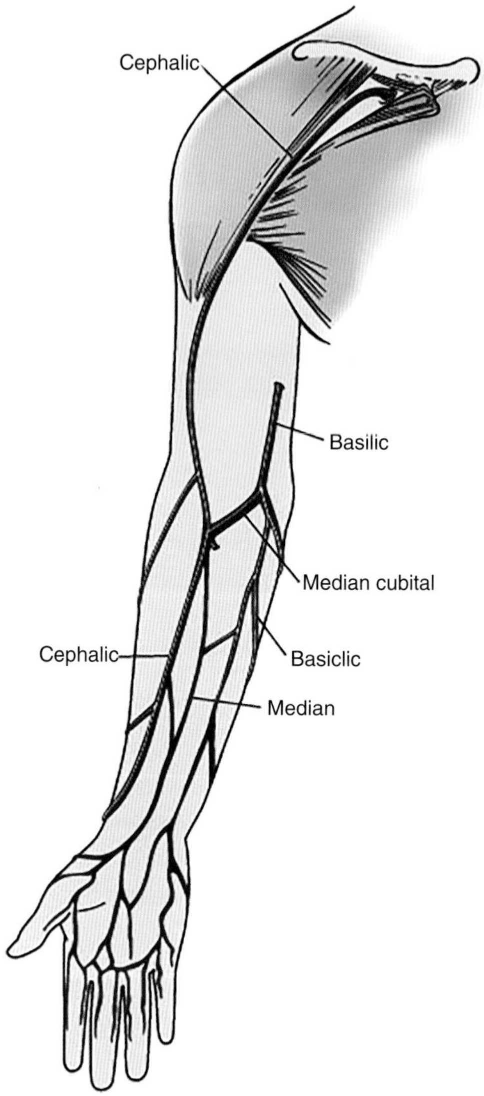

FIGURE 20-1 Superficial venous anatomy of the right arm. Note that the basilic vein penetrates the superficial fascia to join the brachial veins at a variable point in the upper arm. (Reproduced with permission from Gloviczki P, Forum AV. *Handbook of Venous and Lymphatic Disorders: Guidelines of the American Venous Forum*, 4th ed. Boca Raton, FL: CRC Press; 2017.)

the deep brachial vein variably between the mid-upper arm and axilla. Notably, the basilic vein is deep to the superficial fascia, a fact of importance when considering its use for AV access. The median cubital vein of the superficial system is commonly used for phlebotomy and intravenous cannulation. The

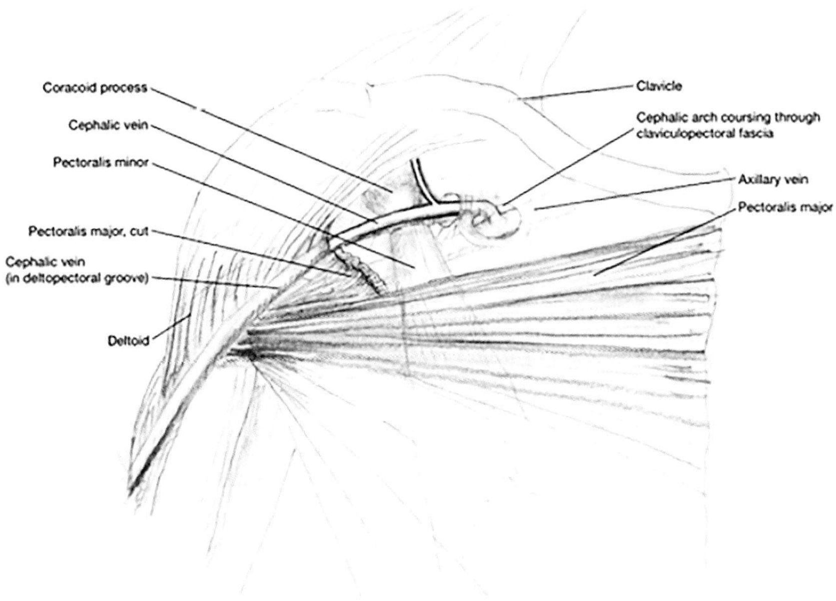

FIGURE 20-2 A drawing of the cephalic arch, showing its course superficial to the muscles before diving deep to the clavipectoral fascia. (Reproduced with permission from Sivananthan G, Menashe L, Halin NJ. Cephalic arch stenosis in dialysis patients: review of clinical relevance, anatomy, current theories on etiology and management. *J Vasc Access*. 2014;15(3):157-162.)

perforating veins run the length of the upper limb, bridging flow from the superficial to deep systems.[2]

Centrally, the right subclavian receives the internal jugular vein to form the relatively short right brachiocephalic vein. The left-sided anatomy is topologically similar although the left brachiocephalic vein is longer and runs across the midline. Both brachiocephalic veins coalesce to form the superior vena cava (SVC) initially outside the pericardial sac and then enter the right atrium at the sternal angle.[4,5] As with most vasculature of the human body, a fair amount of variation exists in the source and drainage of the upper extremity venous system.[6]

NOTABLE UPPER ARM RELATIONSHIPS

Deltopectoral Groove/Triangle and the Cephalic Vein

While the CCJ is critical in the pathophysiology of subclavian vein obstruction, the contributions of the deltopectoral groove and cephalic arch are less well understood. As the cephalic vein ascends the arm, it passes between the medial deltoid and lateral pectoralis muscles to enter the deltopectoral triangle, bounded by the previously mentioned muscles in addition to the inferior border of the clavicle (Figure 20-2). It is at this location that the vein is protected by a fat pad and can be accessed for pacemaker wire insertion by exploiting the separation between the deltoid and pectoralis muscles. The cephalic arch is a very common site of stenosis and failure in cephalic vein-based AV access procedures. Although the exact reasons are poorly understood, it may be due to external compression by the adjacent muscles and shear forces due to the curvature of the vessel at this location.[6–8]

The Costoclavicular Junction (CCJ) and the Subclavian Vein

The scalene triangle, composed of the anterior scalene muscle, middle scalene muscle, and first rib, surrounds the brachial plexus and subclavian artery as they communicate with the arm.[6] The subclavian

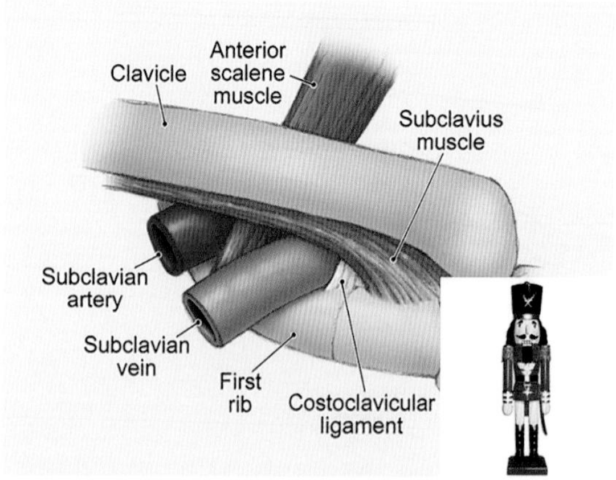

FIGURE 20-3 The venous thoracic outlet is a second-degree lever, like a nutcracker—the fulcrum, anteriorly, is the connection of the clavicle and first rib at the sternum, held together by the costoclavicular ligament. The subclavius muscle and tendon also compress the vein superiorly.

vein is located *anterior* to the anterior scalene muscle. Although not technically fully bounded by fixed structures, the relationship of the vein to the clavicle and anterior portion of the first rib at the CCJ is critical (Figure 20-3). The clavicle and first rib are attached anteriorly by the ligamentous structures that hold the two bones (the costoclavicular ligament) and the tendinous insertion of the subclavius muscle. Both of these structures also directly compress the vein as well as creating a fulcrum at the CCJ. Finally, although the clavicle and first rib do not normally have much movement, when they do they act as a second-class degree lever—akin to a nutcracker—and compress whatever is between them with significant force (Figures 20-3 and 20-4).[9,10] As more fully discussed below, this pinching action produces two problems: symptoms induced by the extrinsic compression itself and chronic injury to the vein leading to later scarring and thrombotic occlusion.

Intrathoracic Venous Problems

While CCJ stenosis is likely exacerbated by subclavian vein dialysis catheters (and thus for this reason are almost never used today), dialysis catheters are also associated with brachiocephalic vein and SVC stenosis, and catheter duration seems to correlate with the risk of stenosis (Illig, Ross, unpublished data). Outside of iatrogenically induced pathology, however, intrathoracic venous problems can arise as a sequela of congenital malformations or aberrant arterial anomalies. Symptomatic compression of the left brachiocephalic vein between the arterial

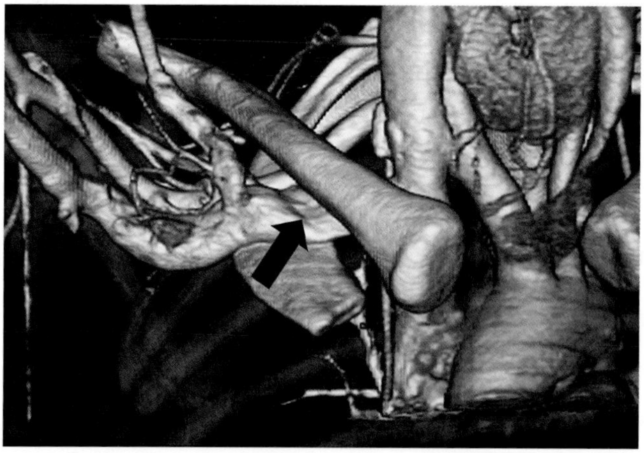

FIGURE 20-4 CT reconstruction of a patient with right-sided venous thoracic outlet syndrome clearly showing the point of compression at the anterior thoracic outlet. The void directly below the clavicle (arrow) is the digitally subtracted subclavius muscle, illustrating the importance of this structure. The arm is in a raised position. (Reproduced with permission from Illig KA, Thompson RW, Freischlag JA, et al. *Thoracic Outlet Syndrome*, 2nd ed. Switzerland, AG: Springer; 2021.)

structures and sternum exists but is probably rare, with the first case presented by Wurtz in 1989.[11] This "aortosternal venous compression" may be associated with an aberrant right subclavian artery or a leftward origin of the innominate artery.[12] Injury and resultant ligation can also occur during CABG; however, this is seemingly rare.

CLINICAL PRESENTATION

In general, three groups of symptoms are seen, depending on the clinical scenario. All have in common the fact that the venous outflow from the limb is obstructed. Simple physics demonstrates that the amount of blood flowing out of the limb must equal the amount of blood flowing into the limb or else the arm will swell. This is exactly what happens, although specifics vary by circumstances.

In the simplest case, the vein is obstructed (fully or partially) at the thoracic outlet (Figures 20-3 and 20-4). In an otherwise healthy person (VTOS, discussed below). In the acute setting, the limb will become swollen, with a blue discoloration, and will feel heavy and painful. Rarely, an acute total occlusion will be associated with the phlegmasia cerulea, limb-threatening ischemia due to lack of arterial inflow because there is no venous outflow. In the more chronic setting due to partial obstruction, arm swelling will persist but will be mitigated by increased flow through collateral vessels seen in the upper arm, shoulder, and chest (Figure 20-5). Because of these collaterals, and less of a gravity effect compared to the legs, skin changes are relatively uncommon and venous ulceration almost unheard of.

The second pattern seen is when blockage is more centrally located, involving the brachiocephalic veins and SVC. In addition to the limb symptoms above, SVC syndrome can develop, with concomitant obstruction to jugular venous return of blood flow from the face and head. These patients can have facial and neck swelling and discomfort, and dyspnea occasionally requiring airway control or even tracheostomy. Such symptoms are pathognomonic for significant central venous obstruction.

Lastly, a patient with an AV access will have the most extreme such symptoms because their arterial inflow is so much higher requiring greater volumes of venous outflow. Dialysis patients with brachiocephalic occlusion can develop SVC syndrome as their access outflow is usually in part via the jugular veins, which become overloaded. In addition, they will have the sequelae seen during dialysis – high pressure, increased recirculation and impaired clearance, prolonged postcannulation bleeding, and pulsatility, for example. They often present with significant arm swelling and visible, dilated collateral veins (Figure 20-5).

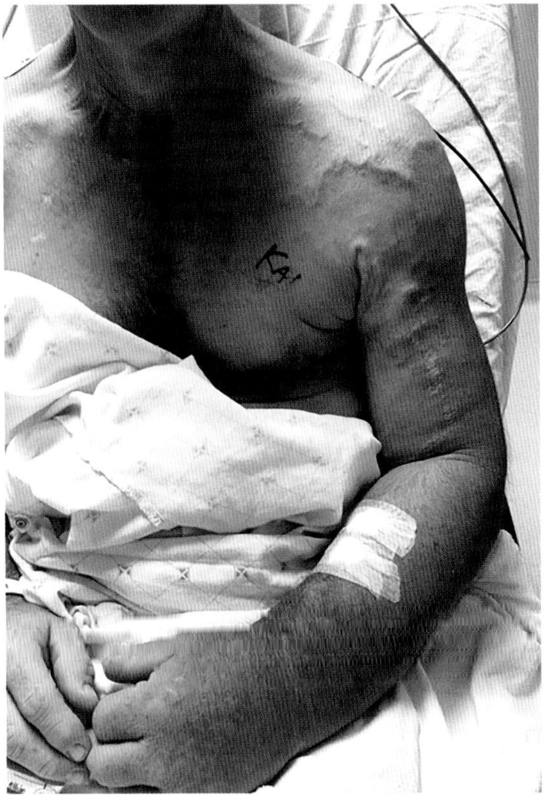

FIGURE 20-5 A patient with an AV fistula and occlusion at the costoclavicular junction. Note the swollen arm, dilated shoulder collaterals, and readiness for surgery (surgeon's initials at the operative site).

In general, while the muscular arteries have evolved to constrain high pressure, the veins have not. Any obstruction to venous outflow will increase the pressures within the veins, which in turn will lead to fluid extravasation and tissue swelling.

SPECIFIC PROBLEMS

VENOUS THORACIC OUTLET SYNDROME

Venous thoracic outlet syndrome (VTOS) is the condition whereby the subclavian vein is adversely affected by the rib and clavicle at the CCJ as described above (Figure 20-4). This can be simply extrinsic compression with arms in a "stress" position (almost always overhead), temporary thrombosis, or chronic occlusion.

Intermittent Positional Stenosis (McCleery's Syndrome)

Swelling of the upper extremity without thrombosis is indicative of McCleery's syndrome, defined by intermittent extrinsic compression with no clear occlusion.[13,14] Symptoms arise solely when the arms are elevated or with exertion, affecting a patient population of otherwise, healthy, young, active patients that resolve with arm descent and adduction. These patients present similarly to those with Paget–Schroetter syndrome, with intermittent exercise-related arm swelling causing a purplish discoloration and over time resulting in notable collaterals.

Since upper extremity venous drainage system is anatomically normal at rest and without elevation, diagnosis can be challenging. An experienced ultrasound technician is needed to assess vein patency, requiring abduction and elevation of the arm to induce compression and hindrance of flow. McCleery's syndrome and VTOS, in general, are associated with a high rate (21%) of false negatives elicited on ultrasound in patients with confirmed disease.[15] Venography thus remains the gold standard for diagnosis. Even with a positive duplex examination, the potential for obstruction of the central veins and SVC needs to be evaluated and is best done with an imaging study. On venogram, venous flow is normal with the arm adducted in a dependent position but, with abduction and elevation, a smooth, tapered cut-off with numerous collaterals is seen proximal to the shoulder indicating compression of the subclavian vein as it passes under the clavicle. Another potential cause in such circumstances is pectoralis minor syndrome where compression is caused by the muscle and tethering of the brachial plexus at the pectoralis minor space. Recognition of this condition is important, as the treatment differs (first rib resection for classic McCleery's syndrome, pectoralis minor tenotomy for venous pectoralis minor syndrome).

Data regarding the natural history of McCleery's syndrome are sparse. In one study from Johns Hopkins, three of the 19 patients were found to have some degree of nonobstructive chronic thrombus.[14] Because these are usually young, active patients with low surgical risk and generally a long lifespan, the general recommendation for treatment is surgical decompression by means of a first rib resection. Transaxillary first rib resection is largely successful in alleviating symptoms and is well-tolerated long term in young patients, as well as providing a cosmetically pleasing result.

Postphlebitic Obstruction (Chronic Paget–Schroetter Syndrome)

In addition to discovering a rare bone disease and a breast cancer that later bore his name, James Paget also described the formation of a thrombus in the subclavian vein "in an otherwise perfectly healthy individual".[16] A decade later, the etiology of this thrombus was uncovered as repeated trauma by Leopold von Schroetter; however, it was not until the next century that E. S. Hughes gave "effort thrombosis" a formal name, honoring its' original discoverers.[17] In most cases, the cause is long-term, repetitive compression usually associated with arms overhead activity eventually leading to intimal damage of the vein, secondary inflammation and scarring, and stenosis with decreased venous outflow or thrombus formation.

While some patients present with McCleery's syndrome before thrombosis occurs, most are asymptomatic until the vein occludes and present with arm discoloration and swelling. Unfortunately, most patients, and a surprising number of physicians, are not aware of the available treatment algorithms and success for acute Paget–Schroetter syndrome. Two classes of patients are at risk for chronic symptoms: those who do not receive proper treatment and those in whom treatment fails.

When a patient presents with arm swelling in the absence of an intraluminal device of more than a few months duration, chronic un- or mis-treated subclavian vein stenosis should be suspected. Patients who are treated with anticoagulation alone, for example, have some degree of long-term symptomatology in up to 75% of cases.[16] Treatment depends on three factors: the symptom status of the patient, the risks of intervention, and the anatomic status of the vein. Obviously, the greater the symptoms and lower the surgical risk, the more aggressive one can be with treatment. By contrast, patients with minimal symptoms, especially if only a few months out, can be observed as many will improve as sufficient collaterals develop.

Two general categories of anatomic blockage can be present: stenosis or occlusion. If the vein is patent but stenotic and symptoms are significant, it is tempting to treat the lesion endovascularly with either balloon angioplasty or stenting. Unfortunately, these patients essentially all end up with a stent, as vessel recoil or lack of initial efficacy after initial angioplasty is almost inevitable. Placing a stent across the *nondecompressed* thoracic outlet is associated with negative outcomes, increasing the risk of recurrence and contributing to stent fragmentation, vessel damage, and complicating future repair.[18–20] The reason for angioplasty failure and stent fracture is the continued crushing effects of the clavicle and first rib (Figure 20-4). It is for this reason that first rib resection is the best option.[21] Removal of the first rib alone may allow recanalization of the vein in those with total occlusion and alleviation of the extrinsic compression in symptomatic patients with vein stenosis. An additional theoretical benefit of decompression is to provide more room for periclavicular collaterals to dilate, although this has not been proven. Finally, once the extrinsic bony compression has been removed, stenting can be considered, although results are still not as good as in other areas of the body.[22]

Finally, if the vein is chronically occluded and of long duration, symptom status and surgical risk are important considerations as surgical repair or bypass can be challenging. The subclavian and brachiocephalic vein can be repaired directly or bypassed, although exposure and reconstructive options are complex. Reconstruction, for example, can be performed by means of patch angioplasty, interposition grafting," endovascular bypass" by means of a covered stent after decompression and wire passage, or subclavian to atrial bypass.[23,24] Decompression and surgical bypass in patients without other endovascular options are associated with symptomatic relief in >90% of cases in carefully selected patients.

ARTERIOVENOUS ACCESS-RELATED VTOS

By definition, AV access involves connecting a high pressure, low capacitance arterial system to a low pressure, high capacitance venous system. The resulting increases in blood volume, turbulence, and alterations in venous blood flow along with endothelial damage due to repeated intraluminal line introduction can result in stenoses that create high venous pressures. These high pressures result in hemodynamic sequelae during dialysis and clinical arm swelling problems that all can be described as chronic venous insufficiency in the arm.

Peripheral Stenoses

The most common location for hemodialysis AV graft stenosis occurs at the outflow anastomosis with 80% of stenoses/occlusions being found at the junction of the prosthetic graft and the vein.[25] Under the influence of high pressures, venous endothelium undergoes neointimal hyperplasia.[26] Increased levels of fibroblast and platelet-derived growth factors stimulate aggressive proliferation of the smooth muscle layer.[27] In a physiologically successful graft with unobstructed venous outflow, the luminal pressures are low. If stenosis or obstruction develops, however, pressure increases and the resultant increased capillary pressure increases endothelial permeability and leads to fluid extravasation. These factors contribute to the clinical presentation seen on examination of patients with venous thrombosis: generalized upper extremity heaviness, persistent swelling, and erythematous skin changes.

Treatment of such venous stenoses (the venous anastomosis of an AV graft) is straightforward. Historically, balloon angioplasty alone has been the initial treatment of choice, but while effective in the short-term, recurrence rates are high. Recently, several prospective randomized trials have shown a clear benefit to covered stents in this situation.[28,29] Unfortunately, such stents are much more expensive than balloons alone, so the overall role (and institutional cost:benefit analysis) is not completely clear.

Cephalic Arch Stenosis

Before it joins the axillary vein, the cephalic arch runs perpendicularly from the deltopectoral groove into the deep vein. This naturally tortuous segment of the vein is particularly prone to stenosis in patients with cephalic vein outflow.[30] This area is uniquely affected in brachiocephalic fistulas because of its proximity to the anastomosis and high valvular density, leading to a 39% stenosis rate, compared to a 2% rate for radiocephalic fistulas.

Treatment options include endovascular interventions, including stenting and angioplasty, along with open surgical solutions. Unfortunately, this lesion is technically difficult to treat due to the high pressures required during angioplasty, not uncommonly resulting in technical failure or rupture, and, even when successful, associated with low primary patency rates (29%–45% at 12 months).[31,32] Covered stents may be associated with better results compared to balloon angioplasty alone with one series showing primary patency rates of 74% and 60% at 6- and 12-month follow-up, respectively.[33] Finally, in healthier and younger patients, surgical intervention with transposition or bypass remains the superior option for long-term patency and lower rates of reintervention compared to both angioplasty and stenting.[34,35]

Costoclavicular Junction Stenosis

Patients with an AV access have the same anatomy at the CCJ as do those with venous TOS. External compression of the vein occurs by both tissue and bone due to its intimate relationship with the subclavius muscle and first rib superiorly.[16,36] The problem seems to be more aggressive in these patients, however, for several possible reasons. First, the high flow initially and elevated pressures later thicken the wall of the vein, rendering it less compliant. Secondly, the high flow means that a minor stenosis, or even periodic narrowing due to arm positioning, is more likely to induce turbulence, which acts as a stimulus for further intimal hyperplasia. This produces a positive feedback loop where a relatively stenosis induces turbulence, which then induces intimal hyperplasia, which worsens the stenosis, leading to more turbulence, and so on. Finally, although the era of subclavian dialysis catheters is in the past, far too many of these patients have iatrogenic intimal damage at multiple sites along their journey to dialysis.

Historically, these lesions were treated endovascularly, since these interventions are chiefly performed in a patient population less suitable for general anesthesia and open surgery, and AV access interventionalists, be they surgeons or radiologists, have not been familiar with the principles of venous TOS. Primary angioplasty has variable outcomes, with patency rates at 1-year follow averaging around 30%.[32] Again, stent placement has acceptable short-term efficacy, but dismal long-term patency, ranging from 17% to19% at 1 year[37,38] due to the unaltered bony compression (Figure 20-4). In the early 2000s, it was recognized that this was a form of venous TOS and that the lesion would be unlikely to improve without removal of the extrinsic compression. At that time, our group began an aggressive practice of thoracic outlet decompression in appropriate patients.[36] In our first series, patients with threatened and dysfunctional AV access who underwent decompression achieved fistula salvage in 80% of cases.[39,40] Another option is medial claviculectomy, which involves the removal of the clavicle at its junction with the sternum and allows extensive exposure of the vein. In a recent series, while primary patency was only 28%, secondary patency at 18 months was 84%.[41] Full analysis of our experience (now approximately 110 patients) is in progress.

Intrathoracic Venous Stenosis

Stenosis of the intrathoracic veins, thought to affect up to 40% of patients on dialysis, is complicated and poorly understood with optimal treatment still evolving.[32] Stenoses are caused by a combination of factors with chronic indwelling dialysis catheters most strongly implicated.[42] The left side is more commonly affected, probably due to the more tortuous course of the left brachiocephalic vein. Catheter insertion via the subclavian vein carries a 49% higher rate of complications when compared to the internal jugular.[43,44] Patients have the same peripheral swelling and high pressure within the fistula, but typically also have more centrally focused and dramatic manifestations, including face, chest, and arm swelling or even dyspnea (SVC syndrome). Truly durable outcomes are difficult to achieve and most institutions have settled on repeated angioplasty as the best-practice. Long-term patency rates at 1 year approach 30% for primary angioplasty and 21% for primary stenting.[32] Of particular risk are tight stenoses at the junction of the right atrium and SVC. Fatal rupture can occur with angioplasty, and there are no landing zones for insertion of covered stents in this location (personal communication, John Ross, MD).

The HeRO Graft

In patients who have exhausted other options for hemodialysis access due to recurrent and irreparable outflow vein stenosis from the CCJ to the SVC, the Hemodialysis Reliable Outflow (HeRO) graft (Merit Medical, Salt Lake City UT) allows for outflow into the atrium, bypassing the venous problem. The reported 12-month primary (26%–58%) and secondary patency (56%–90%) rates are very good.[45–47] A technique that has recently emerged for patients with SCV and/or brachiocephalic occlusion is an "inside out" wire recanalization to the skin, followed by catheter placement and subsequent conversion to a HeRO graft, often staged to reduce the risk of infection.[18] Using this technique, we have documented a mean procedure time of less than 60 minutes, access for hemodialysis within 36 hours in 89% of patients, and a 30 day infection rate of 2% for the HeRO component.[19]

PACEMAKER AND CATHETER-INDUCED OBSTRUCTION

A common sequela of catheter insertion in the large upper extremity veins is secondary deep vein thrombosis. The pathophysiology itself is secondary to vessel wall damage induced during insertion, medication infusion, an ongoing trauma to the venous wall along the body of the catheter. The presence of a catheter induces a local inflammatory response through IL-6, while altering the wall shear stress and increasing stasis.[50,51] During infusion, shear stress in the vicinity of the catheter tip can increase up to 3,000 times the physiological normal, inflicting significant damage to the surrounding endothelium. Additionally, both lead infections and temporary wire insertions prior to more permanent solutions are associated with increased risks of venous stenosis and catheter complications.[52]

Catheter-induced thrombosis is often asymptomatic and infrequently reported, with embolic and significant thrombotic complications occurring in 0.6% to 3.5% of patients.[53,54] Despite a low rate of major complications, up to 50% of patients will present with partial thrombosis.[55] In addition to SVC syndrome if occlusion is central, patients may present with recurrent pulmonary emboli. Once identified, the best option is pacemaker wire removal. When removal is impossible (as with pacemaker or AICD wires), the best treatment is anticoagulation and prevention of thrombus propagation. Catheter-directed thrombolysis and pharmacomechanical techniques are interventional options for removal of fresh significant thrombus. Pharmacomechanical lysis is associated with a shorter hospital stay and lower overall costs.[56] A common theme among upper extremity thrombosis treatment algorithms is time to intervention. If intervened within a few days, the success rate is almost 100%. If delayed within 6 weeks, the success rate drops to 50%.[16] In addition, even after successful salvage, the patient should be closely monitored for signs of chronic thrombosis arising from fibrous stenosis.

A final but common issue arises when a stenosis with significant recoil is found along the track of pacemaker or defibrillator wires. It is tempting to place a stent in this situation, but the worry is that the wires will be "jailed" by the stent. A counterargument is that the wires will never be removed – if they could have been, they already would have been removed per the algorithm in the paragraph above. A small study from Toronto suggested that no short-term problems are created by stenting across wires in this scenario although follow-up was limited.[57]

OBSTRUCTION SECONDARY TO MALIGNANCY

Cancer-associated thrombosis resulting in venous thromboembolism is a direct cause of mortality in patients with systemic malignancies and is their second leading eventual cause of death.[58] A diagnosis of upper extremity DVT, in the axillary, subclavian, brachial, or more proximal veins (assuming conventional VTOS is not present) is a strong clinical marker of occult cancer, with up to 49% of patients so identified having tumor eventually found. The subclavian vein is the most common site of upper extremity thrombotic presentation (62%), just ahead of the internal jugular (45%) and axillary vein (45%), with many patients presenting with multiple and concurrent thrombi.[59]

A combination of factors contributes to the formation of DVT in malignancy, including immobilization, indwelling catheters, a malignancy-induced prothrombotic state, and chemotherapeutic side effects. Both tissue factor and phosphatidylserine are produced by tumor cells, and their presence triggers the coagulation cascade and provides a negatively charged surface for catalyzation, respectively. Additionally, cancer cells induce local activation through fibrin deposition and platelet aggregation.[60]

What was once a manifestation of infection, SVC syndrome is now (in a patient not on dialysis) almost always caused by malignancy.[61] Presenting as dyspnea, neck engorgement, facial swelling, and cough, it can be caused by primary lung cancers, especially Pancoast tumors of the pulmonary apex, non-Hodgkin lymphoma, and thymomas. Nonmalignancy provoked SVC syndrome, in addition to being caused by AV access-related problems, can be a result of infection, most often from tuberculosis, fibrosing mediastinitis, and thoracic abdominal aneurysms.

Radiation therapy is the first step for nonthrombotic SVC syndrome associated with malignancy, and although the tumor is rarely cured, it often regresses relatively quickly allowing relief of obstruction and symptomatic improvement.[61,62] If the vessels are patent but acutely thrombosed, the same algorithm as with any thrombus should be followed. The American College of Chest Physicians suggest anticoagulation alone is preferable to thrombolysis in patients with "proximal upper extremity DVTs".[63] Because upper extremity DVTs tend to be asymptomatic until devastating complications ensue, demonstrated by a 9% incidence of concurrent PE and a 6% 1-month mortality rate, great care should be taken to identify those at risk and properly anticoagulate if indicated.[60] In selected cases, reconstruction can be safely performed with secondary patency rates of 74% at 5 years.[64]

ALGORITHM FOR CARE

An overall algorithm for care in these patients is presented in Figure 20-6. When a patient presents with signs and symptoms suggestive of chronic upper extremity venous disease, the first step is to determine what the major underlying cause is: chronic VTOS, AV access-associated swelling, pacemaker or other device or catheter-associated obstruction, or malignancy. Based on the discussion above, this initial triage should be straightforward in almost all cases.

If chronic VTOS (acute onset of swelling months ago in a healthy patient, occlusion or stenosis at the CCJ by venography), four options exist: conservative care (as clot is chronic and organized, anticoagulation is not usually needed), thoracic outlet decompression alone, thoracic outlet decompression with endovascular intervention, or thoracic outlet decompression with surgical reconstruction. How aggressive to be and how much risk to assume will depend on the symptom severity and the health of the patient. In most cases, however, the asymptomatic patient does not need any intervention.

If swelling is present in a patient with an AV access, the first step is to determine the location of the outflow problem, best done with a fistulogram. If outflow or cephalic arch stenosis is found, treatment options include angioplasty, covered stent placement, and/or surgical repair. If stenosis is present at the CCJ, the general health and life expectancy of the patient should be assessed, as well as the state of the existing access. If favorable, consideration should be given to CCJ decompression with angioplasty or stenting. If unfavorable, replacement with a HeRO graft or moving the dialysis access to the other limb are good options. If the latter option is chosen, the original access should be ligated to treat the arm swelling. Finally, if the problem is intra-thoracic, recanalization as a conduit for HeRO graft placement can be considered, or access can be moved to the lower extremity.

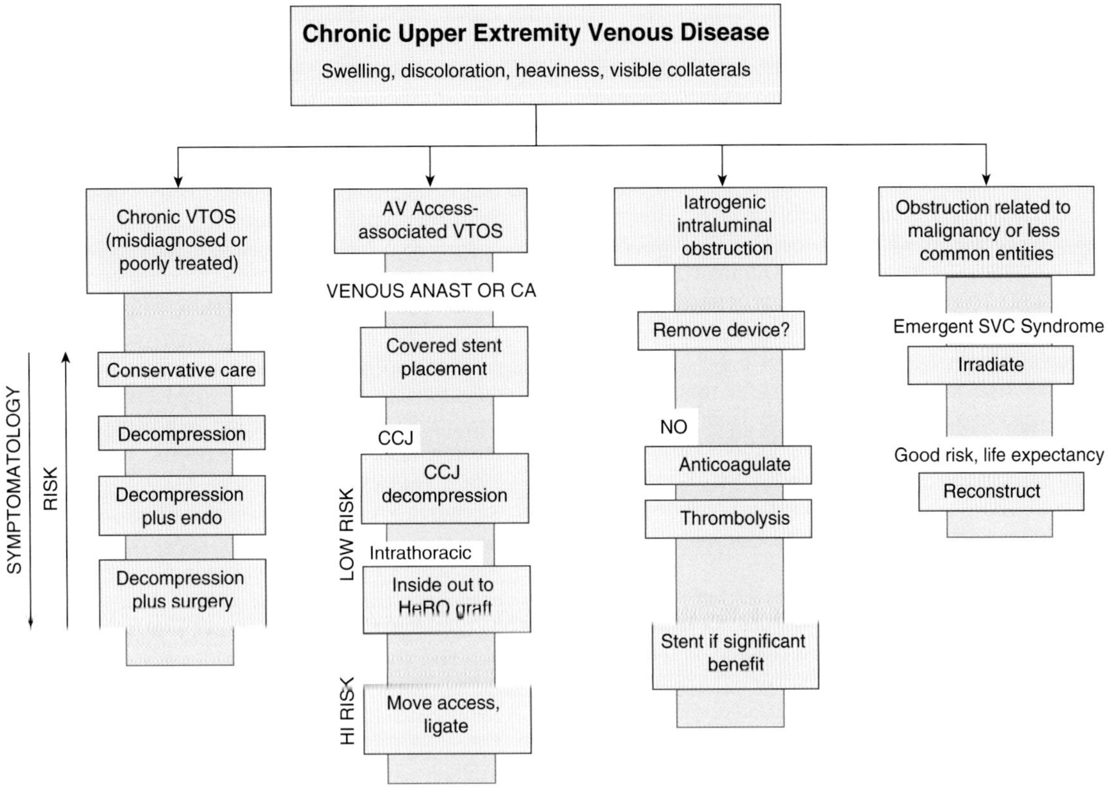

FIGURE 20-6 Algorithm for the treatment of patients with chronic upper extremity venous disease, as described in the text. AV, arteriovenous; CA, cephalic arch; CCJ, costoclavicular junction; SVC, superior vena cava syndrome; VTOS, venous thoracic outlet syndrome.

If a pacemaker or other conduit is present, the first step is to inquire whether the device can be removed, particularly, if it is a dialysis catheter. In many cases, transvenous pacemakers and defibrillators can be replaced with epicardial devices, but if not, thrombolysis can be used for acute symptomatic thrombosis while anticoagulation may be of value in the long term. Most feel that stenting across a pacemaker lead is not recommended but what little data exist suggests that it is well tolerated.

Finally, in a patient with SVC syndrome and no obvious cause being evident, malignancy should be suspected. If found by imaging, radiation therapy is the first step for short-term palliation, while long-term care is individualized according to cause and anatomy. Reconstruction can be considered if life expectancy permits, but this is complex, high-risk surgery.

CONCLUSIONS

Venous disease of the upper extremity differs from that of the lower extremity in that gravity is a minor causative factor. However, venous outflow in the arm passes through the CCJ, a "pinch point" that has no analog in the leg. This area is implicated in the vast majority of cases, whether causing classic VTOS, acting as an obstruction to venous outflow in patients with AV access, or becoming the narrowest point in the outflow tract in patients with pacemakers, defibrillators, or the like. Such obstruction will cause arm swelling and increased pressure within an AV access, and, if sufficiently central, SVC syndrome. Treatment depends on the health and life expectancy of the patient, and on the specific anatomic problem present.

REFERENCES

1. Woollard HH. The development of the principal arterial stems in the forelimb of the pig. *Contrib Embryol.* 1922;14, 139-154.
2. Gloviczki P, Mozes G. Development and anatomy of the venous system. In: Gloviczki P, ed. *Handbook of Venous and Lymphatic Disorders: Guidelines of the American Venous Forum.* 3rd ed. Boca Raton, FL: CRC Press; 2008.
3. Tansey EA, Montgomery LEA, Quinn JG, Roe SM, Johnson CD. Understanding basic vein physiology and venous blood pressure through simple physical assessments. *Adv Physiol Educ.* 2019;43: 423-429.
4. Claasz AA, Chorley DP. A study of the relationship of the superior vena cava to the bony landmarks of the sternum in the supine adult: implications for magnetic guidance systems. *J Assoc Vasc Access.* 2007;12: 138-139.
5. Chukwuemeka A, Currie L, Ellis H. CT anatomy of the mediastinal structures at the level of the manubriosternal angle. *Clin Anat.* 1997;10:405-408.
6. Kusztal M, Weyde W, Letachowicz K, Golebiowski T, Letachowicz W. Anatomical vascular variations and practical implications for access creation on the upper limb. *J Vasc Access.* 2014;15(Suppl 7):S70-S75.
7. Deslauriers J. Anatomy of the neck and cervicothoracic junction. *Thorac Surg Clin.* 2007;17:529-547.
8. Fructuoso M, Ferreira J, Sousa P. Surgical treatment of cephalic arch problems in arteriovenous fistulas: a center experience. *Ann Vasc Surg.* 2018;48:253.e11-253.e16.
9. Loukas M, Myers CS, Wartmann Ch T, et al. The clinical anatomy of the cephalic vein in the deltopectoral triangle. *Folia Morphol (Warsz).* 2008;67(1):72-77.
10. Urschel HC Jr, Pool JM, Patel AN Anatomy and pathophysiology of VTOS. In: Illig KA, Thompson RW, Freischlag JA, Donahue DM, Jordan SE, Edgelow PI, eds. *Thoracic Outlet Syndrome.* London: Springer; 2013:339.
11. Hernandez JA, Walser EM, Swischuk LE. Aortosternal venous compression in patients with aberrant right subclavian arteries. *AJR Am J Roentgenol.* 2005;184: 1434-1436.
12. Lee S, Lee JG, Cho SH. Aortosternal venous compression: innominate vein compression by the innominate artery. *Ann Thorac Surg.* 2011;92:361.
13. McCleery CR, Kesterson JE, Kirtley JA, Love RB. Subclavius and anterior scalene muscle compression as a cause of intermittent obstruction of the subclavian vein. *Ann Surg.* 1951;133:588-602.
14. Likes K, Rochlin DH, Call D, Freischlag JA. McCleery syndrome: etiology and outcome. *Vasc Endovascular Surg.* 2014;48:106-110.
15. Brownie ER, Abuirqeba AA, Ohman JW, Rubin BG, Thompson RW. False-negative upper extremity ultrasound in the initial evaluation of patients with suspected subclavian vein thrombosis due to thoracic outlet syndrome (Paget-Schroetter syndrome). *J Vasc Surg Venous Lymphat Disord.* 2020;8:118-126.
16. Illig KA, Doyle AJ. A comprehensive review of Paget-Schroetter syndrome. *J Vasc Surg.* 2010;51:1538-1547.
17. Hughes ES. Venous obstruction in the upper extremity. *Br J Surg.* 1948;36:155-163.
18. Meier GH, Pollak JS, Rosenblatt M, Dickey KW, Gusberg RJ. Initial experience with venous stents in exertional axillary-subclavian vein thrombosis. *J Vasc Surg.* 1996;24(6):974-981; discussion 981-973.
19. Urschel HC, Patel AN. Paget Schroetter syndrome therapy: failure of intravenous stents. *Ann Thor Surg.* 2003;75(6):1693-1696.
20. Rajendran S, Cai TY, Loa J, et al. Early outcomes using dedicated venous stents in the upper limb of patients with venous thoracic outlet syndrome: a single centre experience. *CVIR Endovasc.* 2019;2(1):22.
21. de Leon RA, Chang CC, Busse C, et al. First rib resection and scalenectomy for chronically occluded subclavian veins: what does it really do? *Ann Vasc Surg.* 2008;22:395-401.
22. Kreienberg PB, Chang BB, Darling RC III, et al. Long-term results in patients treated with thrombolysis, thoracic inlet decompression, and subclavian vein stenting for Paget-Schroetter syndrome. *J Vasc Surg.* 1998;27(3):576-81.
23. Wooster M, Fernandez B, Summers KL, Illig KA. Surgical and endovascular central venous reconstruction combined with thoracic outlet decompression in highly symptomatic patients. *J Vasc Surg Venous Lymphat Disord.* 2019;7:106-112.e103.
24. Edwards JB, Brooks JD, Wooster MD, Fernandez B, Summers K, Illig KA. Outcomes of venous bypass combined with thoracic outlet decompression for treatment of upper extremity central venous occlusion. *J Vasc Surg Venous Lymphat Disord.* 2019;7:660-664.
25. Maya ID, Oser R, Saddekni S, Barker J, Allon M. Vascular access stenosis: comparison of arteriovenous grafts and fistulas. *Am J Kidney Dis.* 2004;44:859-865.
26. Roy-Chaudhury P, Kelly BS, Zhang J, et al. Hemodialysis vascular access dysfunction: from pathophysiology to novel therapies. *Blood Purif.* 2003;21:99-110.
27. Scholz SS, Vukadinović D, Lauder L, et al. Effects of arteriovenous fistula on blood pressure in patients with end-stage renal disease: a systematic meta-analysis. *J Am Heart Assoc.* 2019;8: e011183.
28. Haskel ZJ, Trerotola S, Dolmatch B, Schuman E, Altman S, Mietling S. Stent graft versus balloon

angioplasty for failing dialysis-access grafts. *N Engl J Med*. 2010;362:494-503.
29. Mohr BA, Sheen AL, Roy-Chaudhury P, Schultz SR, Aunry J. Clinical and economic benefits of stent grafts in dysfunctional and thrombosed hemodialysis access graft circuits in the REVISE randomized trial. *J Vasc Interv Radiol*. 2019;30:203-211.
30. Hammes M, Funaki B, Coe FL. Cephalic arch stenosis in patients with fistula access for hemodialysis: relationship to diabetes and thrombosis. *Hemodial Int*. 2008;12:85-89.
31. Rajan DK, Clark TW, Patel NK, Stavropoulos SW, Simons ME. Prevalence and treatment of cephalic arch stenosis in dysfunctional autogenous hemodialysis fistulas. *J Vasc Interv Radiol*. 2003;14,567-573.
32. Bakken AM, Protack CD, Saad WE, Lee DE, Waldman DL, Davies MG. Long-term outcomes of primary angioplasty and primary stenting of central venous stenosis in hemodialysis patients. *J Vasc Surg*. 2007;45:776-783.
33. Miller GA, Preddie DC, Savransky Y, Spergel LM. Use of the Viabahn stent graft for the treatment of recurrent cephalic arch stenosis in hemodialysis accesses. *J Vasc Surg*. 2018;67:522-528.
34. Davies MG, Hicks TD, Haidar GM, El-Sayed HF. Outcomes of intervention for cephalic arch stenosis in brachiocephalic arteriovenous fistulas. *J Vasc Surg*. 2017;66:1504-1510.
35. Sigala F, Saßen R, Kontis E, Kiefhaber LD, Förster R, Mickley V. Surgical treatment of cephalic arch stenosis by central transposition of the cephalic vein. *J Vasc Access*. 2014;15: 272-277.
36. Illig KA. Management of central vein stenoses and occlusions: the critical importance of the costoclavicular junction. *Semin Vasc Surg*. 2011;24:113-118.
37. Maya ID, Saddekni S, Allon M. Treatment of refractory central vein stenosis in hemodialysis patients with stents. *Semin Dial*. 2007;20:78-82.
38. Oderich GS, Treiman GS, Schneider P, Bhirangi K. Stent placement for treatment of central and peripheral venous obstruction: a long-term multi-institutional experience. *J Vasc Surg*. 2000;32:760-769.
39. Glass C, Dugan M, Gillespie D, Doyle A, Illig K. Costoclavicular venous decompression in patients with threatened arteriovenous hemodialysis access. *Ann Vasc Surg*. 2011;25:640-645.
40. Illig KA, Gabbard W, Calero A, et al. Aggressive costoclavicular junction decompression in patients with threatened AV access. *Ann Vasc Surg*. 2015;29:698-703.
41. Auyang PL, Chauhan Y, Loh TM, Bennett ME, Peden EK. Medial claviculectomy for the treatment of recalcitrant central venous stenosis of hemodialysis patients. *J Vasc Surg Venous Lymphat Disord*. 2019;7:420-427.
42. Oguzkurt L, Tercan F, Yildirim S, Torun D. Central venous stenosis in haemodialysis patients without a previous history of catheter placement. *Eur J Radiol*. 2005;55: 237-242.
43. Bambauer R, Inniger R, Pirrung KJ, Schiel R, Dahlem R. Complications and side effects associated with large-bore catheters in the subclavian and internal jugular veins. *Artif Organs*. 1994;18:318-321.
44. Salgado OJ, Urdaneta B, Colmenares B, Garcia R, Flores C. Right versus left internal jugular vein catheterization for hemodialysis: complications and impact on ipsilateral access creation. *Artif Organs*. 2004;28:728-733.
45. Al Shakarchi J, Houston JG, Jones RG, Inston N. A review on the hemodialysis reliable outflow (HeRO) graft for haemodialysis vascular access. *Eur J Vasc Endovasc Surg*. 2015;50:108-113.
46. Gage SM, Katzman HE, Ross JR, et al. Multi-center experience of 164 consecutive Hemodialysis Reliable Outflow [HeRO] graft implants for hemodialysis treatment. *Eur J Vasc Endovasc Surg*. 2012;44:93-99.
47. Cline BC, Gage SM, Ronald J, et al. Treatment of arm swelling in hemodialysis patients with ipsilateral arteriovenous access and central vein stenosis: conversion to the hemodialysis reliable outflow graft versus stent deployment. *J Vasc Interv Radiol*. 2020;31:243-250.
48. Hentschel DM, Minarsch L, Vega F, Ebner A: The surfacer inside-out access system for right-side catheter placement in dialysis patients with thoracic venous obstruction. *J Vasc Access*. 2020;21(4):411-418.
49. Illig KA, Louden MJ, Aruny J, Ross JR. Safe and effective HeRO graft placement: technique and results. *J Vascular Access*. 2022. In press.
50. Chabot K, Lavoie ME, Bastard JP, Rabasa-Lhoret R. Intravenous catheters induce a local inflammatory response. *Cytokine*. 2018;111:470-474.
51. Piper R, Carr PJ, Kelsey LJ, Bulmer AC, Keogh S, Doyle BJ. The mechanistic causes of peripheral intravenous catheter failure based on a parametric computational study. *Sci Rep*. 2018;8:3441.
52. Da Costa SS, Scalabrini Neto A, Costa R, Caldas JG, Martinelli Filho M. Incidence and risk factors of upper extremity deep vein lesions after permanent transvenous pacemaker implant: a 6-month follow-up prospective study. *Pacing Clin Electrophysiol*. 2002;25:1301-1306.
53. Phibbs B, Marriott HJ. Complications of permanent transvenous pacing. *N Engl J Med*. 1985;312:1428-1432.
54. Bernstein V, Rotem CE, Peretz DI. Permanent pacemakers: 8-year follow-up study. Incidence and management of congestive cardiac failure and perforations. *Ann Intern Med*. 1971;74:361-369.

55. Stoney WS, Addlestone RB, Alford WC Jr, Burrus GR, Frist RA, Thomas CS Jr. The incidence of venous thrombosis following long-term transvenous pacing. *Ann Thorac Surg*. 1976;22:166-170.
56. Mahmoud O, Vikatmaa P, Räsänen J, et al. Catheter-directed thrombolysis versus pharmacomechanical thrombectomy for upper extremity deep venous thrombosis: a cost-effectiveness analysis. *Ann Vasc Surg*. 2018;51: 246-253.
57. Borsato GW, Rajan DK, Simons ME, Sniderman KW, Tan KT. Central venous stenosis associated with pacemaker leads: short-term results of endovascular interventions. *J Vasc Intervent Radiol*. 2012;23(3):363-367.
58. Khorana AA. Venous thromboembolism and prognosis in cancer. *Thromb Res*. 2010;125:490-493.
59. Lee JA, Zierler BK, Zierler RE. The risk factors and clinical outcomes of upper extremity deep vein thrombosis. *Vasc Endovascular Surg*. 2012;46:139-144.
60. Lima LG, Monteiro RQ. Activation of blood coagulation in cancer: implications for tumour progression. *Biosci Rep*. 2013;33(5):e00064.
61. Markman M. Diagnosis and management of superior vena cava syndrome. *Cleve Clin J Med*. 1999;66: 59-61.
62. Cheng S. Superior vena cava syndrome: a contemporary review of a historic disease. *Cardiol Rev*. 2009;17:16-23.
63. Kearon C, Akl EA, Ornelas J, et al. Antithrombotic therapy for VTE disease: chest guideline and expert panel report. *Chest*. 2016;149:315-352.
64. Alimi YS, Gloviczki P, Vrtiska TJ, et al. Reconstruction of the superior vena cava: benefits of postoperative surveillance and secondary endovascular interventions. *J Vasc Surg*. 1998;27:287-301.

SELF-ASSESSMENT STUDY QUESTIONS AND ANSWERS

Questions

1. As compared to the lower extremities, gravity plays what role in the arms in terms of venous outflow?
A. It is LESS IMPORTANT.
B. It is MORE IMPORTANT.
C. It is EQUALLY IMPORTANT.
D. It plays NO ROLE in either.

2. The basilic vein is considered:
A. A collateral vein
B. A deep vein
C. A central vein
D. A superficial vein

3. The cephalic arch is unusual in that it:
A. Loops around the humeral head.
B. Curves sharply and penetrates fascia.
C. Merges with the basilic vein.
D. Inserts upon the jugular vein.

4. In the thoracic outlet, the subclavian vein passes:
A. Posterior to the middle scalene muscle
B. Through the scalene triangle
C. Anteriorly between the first rib and clavicle
D. Below the first rib

5. A swollen head and chest with visible chest wall collaterals can be a sign of:
A. Superior vena cava syndrome
B. Stenosis at the venous anastomosis of a forearm loop AVG
C. Unilateral jugular vein occlusion with otherwise normal anatomy
D. Leriche syndrome

6. A person with McCleery's syndrome will have swelling of the arm:
A. With the arm dependent
B. With the arm overhead
C. In the arm at all times
D. In the face at all times

7. A young athlete with sudden swelling of one arm is most likely to have:
A. Acute arterial insufficiency
B. A lymphoid or hematogenous malignancy
C. A hypercoagulable syndrome and no other abnormality
D. Acute venous thoracic outlet syndrome (Paget–Schroetter syndrome)

8. The most commonly accepted treatment for acute subclavian vein thrombosis is:
A. Observation with serial ultrasounds only
B. Heparin followed by long term Coumadin
C. Catheter-directed thrombolysis followed by first rib decompression
D. Thoracic outlet decompression only after 3 months

9. In general, the first choice for therapy in a patient with cephalic arch stenosis is:
A. Balloon venoplasty with covered stent placement for recoil
B. Surgical exploration of the arch and subclavian vein insertion
C. Cephalic vein to deep vein transposition
D. Abandonment of the access

10. A HeRO graft is ordinarily used for patient with:
A. Multiple thromboses of AV grafts
B. Poor arterial inflow to the access
C. A scarred axilla with patent veins
D. Poor venous outflow to the atrium

SELF-ASSESSMENT STUDY QUESTIONS AND ANSWERS

Answers

1. A.
2. D.
3. B.
4. C.
5. A.
6. B.
7. D.
8. C.
9. A.
10. D.

CHAPTER

21 Arteriovenous Malformations

Byung-Boong Lee and James Laredo

OUTLINE

DEFINITION
INCIDENCE
ETIOLOGY: GENETIC ASPECT
Pathophysiology
CLASSIFICATION
DIAGNOSTIC EVALUATION
TREATMENT
Surgical/Excisional Therapy
Endovascular/Embolo-Sclerotherapy
FOLLOW-UP
CONCLUSION

DEFINITION

Arteriovenous malformation (AVM) is one of the family of congenital vascular malformations (CVMs) which has an anatomic defect allowing for the inappropriate direct shunting of arterial blood to the venous system in varying degrees.[illegible] AVMs are relatively rare in comparison to other malformation lesions (e.g., venous malformation; lymphatic malformation), but most AVMs are clinically much more serious than other malformation with potentially limb or life-threatening condition.[5-8]

Because of their associated AV shunting of high velocity, low resistance blood flow from the arterial vasculature directly into the venous system,[4-6] AVMs cause profound alterations in cardiovascular hemodynamics. These alterations occur centrally, peripherally, and locally, thus making the AVM the most hemodynamically complex type of CVM.[7-9] In addition, the hemodynamic alterations affect the entire cardiovascular system, including the arterial, venous, and the lymphatic systems. These can produce cardiac failure, peripheral arterial insufficiency (e.g., gangrene), chronic venous insufficiency, and lymphatic overload through venous hypertension. They can also have local effects with direct compression to the surrounding tissues and organs causing significant morbidity and high recurrence rates following treatment[1,4,5] so that the AVM retains its notorious reputation as the most dangerous of all CVMs.[2,10,11]

INCIDENCE

The incidence and prevalence of the CVMs as well as AVM, reported before the ISSVA and Hamburg CVM Classification systems were established, are not accurate with limited reliability of data because they were often misrepresented based on confusing terminology of the prior traditional name-based classification.[3,5,12,13] Nevertheless, among the group of various birth defects involving the vascular system, an overall incidence of CVMs is known to be 1.2% as reported by Tasnadi G et al.,[14] with a male–female ratio of 1:1 and with more than 90% evident at the time of birth.[1,4,13] Peripheral AVMs were reported to be the least common CVM accounting for approximately 10% to 15% among all clinically significant CVM lesions.[4,15] Indeed, the AVM is a much more rare condition among all CVMs as classified by the Hamburg Classification[5,12] (Table 21-1). A majority of CVMs

TABLE 21-1 Hamburg Classification of Congenital Vascular Malformations (CVMs)

Primary classification*
• Arterial malformation (AM)
• Venous malformation (VM)
• Arteriovenous malformation (AVM)
• Lymphatic malformation (LM)
• Capillary/Microvascular malformation (CM)
• Combined vascular malformation: Hemolymphatic malformation (HLM)
Embryological Subclassification†
Extratruncular forms (formerly "angioma")
• Diffuse, infiltrating
• Limited, localized
Truncular forms
• Obstruction and/or Stenosis
– Aplasia; Hypoplasia; Hyperplasia
– Membrane; Congenital spur
• Dilatation
– Localized (aneurysm)
– Diffuse (ectasia)

*Modified based on the consensus on CVM through the international workshop in Hamburg, Germany 1988 and Seoul, Korea 1995.

†Developmental arrest at the different stages of embryonal life: earlier stage—extratruncular form; later stage—truncular form. Both forms may exist together; may be combined with other various malformations (e.g., capillary, arterial, AV shunting, venous, hemolymphatic and/or lymphatic); and/or may exist with hemangioma.

are either the venous malformation (VM)[16,17] or the lymphatic malformation (LM)[18,19] with VMs comprising more than two-thirds of all CVMs.[16,17,20]

A vast majority of AVMs belong to the "extratruncular" (formerly angiomatous) type[4] and exist alone as independent lesions. The "truncular" AVM lesions are extremely rare in the form of genuine fistulous lesions with a direct communication between an artery and a vein, without a nidus interposed (e.g., Patent Ductus Arteriosus (PDA) or pulmonary AV fistula).[1,2,4] AVM lesions, however, infrequently exist with an associated VM and/or LM together as a mixed CVM lesion, classified as being a hemolymphatic malformation (HLM)[5,12] which makes their management both confusing and even more difficult (e.g., Parkes–Weber syndrome).[21,22] To date, no racial, demographic, or environmental risk factors for AVMs have been identified.[4]

ETIOLOGY: GENETIC ASPECT

Several gene mutations have been identified leading to defective development during embryogenesis and resulting in dysplastic vessels which become high-flow AV shunts.[4,6,23–26] These causative genes have been identified for a number of rare inheritable vascular malformations such as Osler-Weber-Rendu syndrome (Hereditary Hemorrhagic Telangiectasia), Blue Rubber Bleb Nevus syndrome (Bean's syndrome), RASA 1 mutations, PTEN mutations.[23–26]

As an example, hemorrhagic telangiectasia (HHT), an inheritable autosomal dominant condition, is caused by loss-of-function mutations in the genes encoding for activin receptor-like kinase-1 (ACVRL1) and endoglin (ENG), part of the transforming growth factor-beta (TGF-β) superfamily of receptors. Most AVM lesions associated with HHT develop progressively over time in the brain, lungs, liver, and intestine so that they are generally diagnosed later in adult life. Visceral HHT AVM lesions, such as Rendu-Osler syndromes, cause bleeding more frequently than the sporadic type of visceral AVM. The sporadic type AVM, therefore, rarely required intestinal resection to control the bleeding.[23]

Another autosomal dominant condition known as combined capillary malformations (CM) and AVM syndrome is caused by a RASA1 mutations affecting the brain, spine, face, and extremities.[24,27]

Such familial/syndrome-based AVM also behaves differently from the sporadic type which account for the majority of AVMs. AVMs caused by the RASA1 mutation generally remain relatively stable with minimal progression. However, the symptomatology varies with different anatomical locations and the AVM lesion at the central nervous system often accompanies significant mass effect and hemorrhage.[4,6,23–26] Parkes Weber syndrome (PWS) can also be associated with the RASA1 mutation to cause AVM with "micro-shunting" lesions. Together with other vascular malformation components (VM and LM), they often result in marked tissue overgrowth of affected muscle, bone, and subcutaneous fat. However, PWS *without* the RASA1 mutation generally are not associated with multiple additional CM lesions.[25] AVMs lesion affecting the lower limb as a part of PWS are slower in progression in comparison to the sporatic AVMs, and they subsequently have less risk of amputation.[4,6,23–26]

PTEN mutations are also responsible for focal tissue overgrowth in hamartomas that frequently contain AVMs as a part of the syndromes of tissue overgrowth (e.g., Cowden and Banyan Riley Ruvalcaba syndromes). Multiple AVM lesions are common, often affecting the muscles of the limbs, paraspinal muscles, and the dura mater of the brain.[4,6,27] Further, this AVM caused by PTEN mutations is known to be the most aggressive type of AVM of all. It recurs not only rapidly following embolization or attempted resection but it is also prone to develop new AVM lesions at different sites.[26]

In terms of the mechanisms involved in the development of AVMs, the endothelial cell turnover rate (ECTR) has been found to be significantly greater, by approximately sevenfold, in AVMs compared to normal blood vessels.[1,6,28] This can be measured through the Ki-67 protein which is present during all active phases of the cell cycle except in resting cells (G (0)). Therefore, nonresting endothelial cells can be identified by use of immunohistochemistry for the Ki-67 antigen. Hence, anti-Ki-67 protein antibodies are an excellent marker to determine the growth fraction of a given cell population.

Increased expression of stromal cell-derived factor-1 (SDF-1) has also been found in AVM suggesting the role of endothelial progenitor cells (EPCs) in maintaining active vascular remodeling within the AVM nidus, which is rarely in normal vessels.[4,6,28,29] Together with mRNA expression of the factors that recruit EPCs [VEGF, SDF-1α, hepatocyte growth factor (HGF) and hypoxia-inducible factor-1 (HIF-1)], increased expression of EPCs among higher-staged AVMs suggests EPCs act as a promoting factor for the evolution of AVM and stimulating their recruitment for neovascularization.[28,29]

PATHOPHYSIOLOGY

AVMs are a unique, complex vascular condition with a direct connection between the arterial and venous-lymphatic systems and bypassing the normal capillary system. Since the pivotal function of the capillary system is to maintain the delicate balance between the two hemodynamically different systems (arterial and venous), homeostasis among these different components of the circulatory system is profoundly disrupted.[1–4,6,30–32] Depending on the location and degree (e.g., size and flow) of the abnormal fistulous connection between the high- and low-pressure systems, the arterial and venous systems give a compensatory hemodynamic response through two distinct phases: the compensation period and the subsequent decompensation period.[4,6]

During the compensation period, increased heart pump function can maintain sufficient arterial flow through the rest of the body and prevent peripheral tissue ischemia even as flow continues into the low-resistance AV fistula. But increased heart pumping subsequently overloads the venous and lymphatic system and eventually the heart itself. Once the compensatory mechanisms reach their maximum capacity, the decompensation period begins. The arterial system is no longer able to maintain adequate arterial blood flow to the peripheral tissues resulting in tissue ischemia distal to the AV fistula. The venous system distal to AVM lesion also fails to hold normal valvular function against retrograde blood flow/pressure. Normal antegrade venous flow/drainage from the peripheral tissues is further impeded by continuous reflux, resulting in severe venous hypertension and subsequently chronic venous insufficiency. There is also increased transudation of fluid into the interstitial space which overcomes the drainage capacity of the lymphatic system.

Hence, the hemodynamics of the AVM affects every vascular component resulting in local, peripheral, and central effects. Proper management of these pathophysiologic effects of the AVM on the entire vascular system warrants precise hemodynamic information on the three pairs of proximal, distal, and collateral arteries and veins at the different stages of the compensatory status.[1–4,6]

CLASSIFICATION

A logical classification system of CVMs was proposed through the consensus workshop held in Hamburg in 1988 to replace the prior traditional nosology-based classification (e.g., Klippel and Trenaunay syndrome), which failed to provide appropriate differentiation of anatomic, pathophysiologic, and clinical differences among various CVMs (Table 21-1).[4,5,12,22,33,34] Based on the morphological differences between the lesions involving the main vessel trunks often with a direct communication ("truncular" form) and the lesions occurring peripherally as separate defects (arteriovenous angiomas), Belov et al. reintroduced an old embryologic term "extratruncular" for the angiomatous-looking AVM lesions to avoid the confusing term of "angioma" (c.f. hemangioma).[4,5,13,30,33,34]

The morphological differences between these two groups were further classified based on their distinctively different embryological characteristics during the different stages of embryogenesis/ angiogenesis. Defective development that occurred in the earlier embryogenic stage would remain primitive amorphous vascular clusters with no direct involvement of the matured vessels. Those defects occurring in the later stage of vascular trunk formation would directly affect mature vascular structures and cause visible deformed conditions.[5,34-36] The Hamburg Classification was further refined with the adoption of an embryological concept for a "modified" Hamburg Classification[4,5,12,34] (Table 21-1).

Mulliken et al. introduced another classification to accommodate hemangiomas as vascular tumors and vascular malformations together under one term of "vascular anomaly." This new classification was later adopted as the ISSVA Classification[4,5,13] (Table 21-2). In addition, two more classifications were adopted for AVM to improve clinical management, the Schobinger and the Arteriographic Classification.[4,6,37,38] The Schobinger Classification[37] defined the level of clinical progression in AVM to provide a more accurate assessment of lesions at different clinical stages and to serve as a practical guideline in the management of AVMs (Table 21-3). The Arteriographic Classification of AVMs[38] exclusively classifies extratruncular AVM lesions based on the radiographic morphology of the nidus.

TABLE 21-2 ISSVA Classification of CVM

Vascular Malformations:
• Fast-Flow Lesions:
– Arterial malformation (AM)
– Arteriovenous malformation (AVM)
– Arteriovenous fistula (AVF)
• Slow-Flow Lesions:
– Capillary malformation CM (port wine stain, telangiectasia, angiokeratoma)
– Venous malformation (VM)
– Lymphatic malformation (LM)
– Combined vascular malformation (CVM, CLM, CLVM, CAVM, CLAVM)
Vascular Tumors:
• Infantile Hemangioma
• Congenital Hemangioma
• Other

This classification is helpful not only for better management of extratruncular lesions with embolosclerotherapy but also for predicting outcome of the therapy (Figure 21-1).

Of note, the term "nidus" is NOT a histological term nor an anatomic or pathologic term but a

TABLE 21-3 Schobinger Classification of AVM

Stage I	Quiescence: Pink-bluish stain, warmth, and arteriovenous shunting are revealed by Doppler scanning. The arteriovenous malformation mimics a capillary malformation or involuting hemangioma.
Stage II	Expansion: Stage I plus enlargement, pulsations, thrill, bruit, and tortuous/tense veins.
Stage III	Destruction: Stage II plus dystrophic skin changes, ulceration, bleeding, tissue necrosis. Bony lytic lesions may occur.
Stage IV	Decompensation: Stage III plus congestive cardiac failure with increased cardiac output and left ventricle hypertrophy.

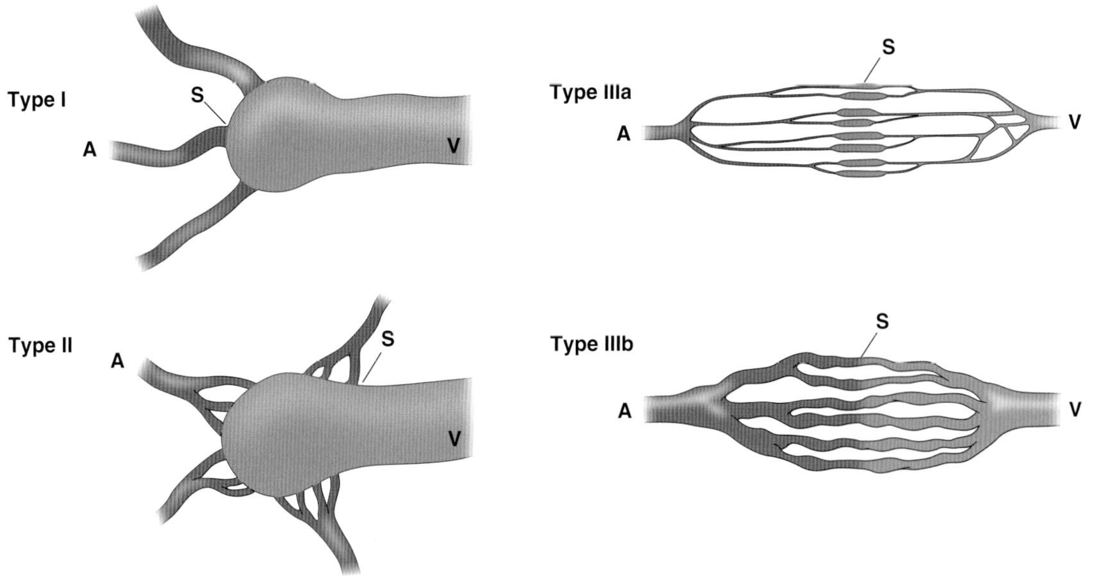

FIGURE 21-1 Arteriographic classification of AVM. Type I (arterio-venous fistulae): at most three separate arteries shunted to a single draining vein. Type II (arteriolo-venous fistulae): multiple arterioles shunted into a single draining vein. Type III a & b (arteriolo-venulous fistulae): multiple shunts between the arterioles and venules.

descriptive radiological/clinical term of a conglomerate of dysplastic minute blood vessels which failed to mature into normal capillary vessels, thus constituting the AVM. They appear as clusters of small-sized AV connections or fistulae, primitive reticular networks filled with contrast on arteriography.[4,6,38]

These nidus lesions are classified into three types: Type I (arterio-venous fistulae), Type II (arteriolo-venous fistulae), and Type III a & b (arteriolo-venulous fistulae). In contrast, truncular AVM lesions will NOT have a nidus on arteriogram but instead will have a large and direct connection between the artery and vein.

DIAGNOSTIC EVALUATION

Clinical manifestation of the AVM depends on the progression of the lesions, invariably producing symptoms (pain, ulceration, and bleeding) and tissue ischemia by the arterial steal and venous hypertension, both of which reduce tissue perfusion.[1-4] Symptoms further depend on anatomical location. Centrally located lesions are more prone to precipitate cardiac failure, while arterial and venous insufficiency more commonly are produced by peripherally located lesions (e.g., ulceration and gangrene).[1-4]

Therefore, a complete systematic evaluation is mandated together with a thorough history and physical examination before proceeding with noninvasive diagnostic imaging to distinguish AVMs from other CVMs.

The evaluation of an AVM should be started first with basic differential diagnoses from among the various CVMs, although it is very helpful to know that most AVMs occur as single lesions. This is followed by a more specific evaluation and confirmation of the AVM. However, since AVMs may also exist in a combined condition with other CVMs like VM and LM (e.g., Parkes–Weber syndrome), the investigations should rule out the copresence of other CVMs as well.[1-4]

Initially, an appropriate combination of noninvasive to more invasive tests should be selected for appropriate differential diagnosis with other CVMs and then more specific diagnostic procedures to confirm the AVM as a whole would follow with further precise and detailed assessment.[4,6] (Table 21-4).

TABLE 21-4 Lists of Diagnostic Tests for AV Malformation

Non- to Minimally Invasive Tests for Initial Studies:
• Duplex ultrasonography (arterial and venous) (DUS)
• Whole body blood pool scintigraphy (WBBPS)
• Transarterial lung perfusion scintigraphy (TLPS)
• Magnetic resonance imaging (MRI) of T1 and T2 images & MR Angiography (MRA)[26]
• Computed tomography (CT) and CT angiography (CTA) with contrast enhancement, and/or three-dimensional CT
Invasive Tests for Confirmation of the Final Diagnosis*:
• Selective and super-selective arteriography
• Percutaneous direct puncture arteriography
• Standard direct puncture phlebography

*Confirmation of the final diagnosis should be made to create a road map for proper treatment.

When the assessment of the primary AVM lesion is completed, the secondary impact of the AVM lesions on the nonvascular organ/systems should be assessed, especially the musculoskeletal system when indicated. Early detection and timely appraisal of vascular–bone syndrome with long-bone length discrepancy, for example, is essential for appropriate management of the AVM lesions affecting the extremities.[39,40]

Duplex ultrasound sonography (DUS) is the first choice modality following the initial clinical assessment of the patient as it is painless, noninvasive, of low cost and allows for subsequent follow-up evaluations. DUS readily differentiates the AVM from VMs and LMs, with its unique findings of pulsatile flow and a high flow lesion. In addition, B mode and Doppler findings of multiple vascular channels with a honeycomb appearance is characteristic of an AVM, which is absent in vascular tumors.[4,6,41] Together with DUS, MRI is frequently an essential diagnostic test for the AVMs since it is able to provide basic information of lesion extent, severity, and anatomic relationship to the surrounding tissues, structures, and organs. Although standard MRI is usually not able to demonstrate the nidus precisely, with limited demonstration of dilated fast flow vascular channels, it remains a very useful assessment tool for the entire group of CVMs.[4,6,41,42] Alternatively, CT angiography can deliver very specific information on the AVM status before proceeding to the contrast arteriographic confirmation and intervention on the lesion.[4,6] Transarterial lung perfusion scintigraphy (TLPS)[4,6,8] is an optional test for the AVMs together with whole body blood pool scintigraphy (WBBPS),[4,6,9] but has a unique role to assess the status of "micro-AV shunting" among Parkes–Weber syndrome in particular, determining the degree of shunting through AVM lesion located in the extremity. It is extremely valuable to detect micro-AVM lesion, often difficult with conventional arteriography alone.[2,6,8] TLPS also is further valuable for the quantitative measurements of the shunting status during therapy to replace the traditional role of arteriography as a follow-up assessment tool for extremity AVMs.[2,6,8]

TREATMENT

In view of the serious nature of the AVMs with the potential for development of a life- and/or limb-threatening conditions, the treatment of AVMs with early aggressive control is generally mandated with priority over all other CVMs.[1,4,31,32] However, due to the high likelihood of recurrence following a conventional treatment, there has also been in the past an overly aggressive tendency for the AVM management which limited subsequent treatment options. In order to minimize the associated morbidity of available treatment modalities (e.g., ethanol sclerotherapy; radical surgical excision), a "controlled" aggressive approach is warranted but only when the benefit exceeds its risk involved.[4,31,32]

The treatment strategy should be made based on a realistic assessment of the long-term goal of the treatment plan by the many different specialists involved: vascular surgeon, orthopedic surgeon, plastic surgeon, head and neck surgeon, interventional radiologist, physiatrist, etc. The final decision on the need for treatment based on various indication criteria (Table 21-5) and the specific treatment modality selected should be made based on a consensus among the multidisciplinary team.[2,4,7,31,32] The indications for treatment are also

TABLE 21-5 Indications for Treatment of AV Malformation

- Hemorrhage
- High-output heart failure
- Secondary arterial ischemic complications
- Secondary complications of chronic venous hypertension
- Lesions located at a life-threatening region (e.g., proximity to the airway) or located in an area threatening vital functions (e.g., seeing, eating, hearing, or breathing)
- Disabling pain
- Functional impairment
- Cosmetically severe deformity
- Vascular–bone syndrome—abnormal long-bone growth with leg length discrepancy[18,19]
- Lesions located in an area with potentially high risk of complication (e.g., hemarthrosis)

determined based on its urgency after assessment of the extent and severity of the AVM. The contemporary approach to the management of AVMs by fully integrated multidisciplinary teams is now able to provide maximum coordination and has brought tremendous improvements in diagnosis and treatment with substantial reductions in morbidity, mortality and also recurrence rates.[7,10,31] It has helped to develop treatment strategies that maximize the risk–benefit ratio while keeping in mind the ultimate goals of treatment balanced with realistic expectations.

SURGICAL/EXCISIONAL THERAPY[2,4,7,10,22,31,43]

Surgical excision has long been the gold standard for the extratruncular type of AVM lesions as the treatment of choice for many decades and still remains the most ideal treatment to the surgically amenable lesions to give a chance of permanent cure. But the majority of the lesions are not sufficiently localized to allow total excision with minimal morbidity, and total surgical removal often carries prohibitively high morbidity and complication rates (e.g., massive operative blood loss, functional loss).[2,4,7] Indeed, complete radical surgical resection to prevent recurrence is often associated with high complication rates, and *incomplete* control of the lesion is many times inevitable. But, over the last decades the development of endovascular therapy has changed the traditional role of surgical resection. Embolo-sclerotherapy has taken over the lead in AVM management either as an independent treatment modality for "surgically inaccessible" lesions or as an adjunct therapy to improve the possibility for complete open surgical therapy.[2,4,7,22,43]

Surgical excision is still most ideal for "surgically accessible" lesions, but the incorporation of preoperative embolo-/sclerotherapy gives a significant improvement in safety and effectiveness of subsequent surgical therapy with reduced morbidity and complications (e.g., intraoperative bleeding). Preoperative *N*-Butyl-cyanoacrylate glue embolotherapy to surgically excisable lesions can make the glue-filled lesions safe to dissect with minimal collateral damage.[2,4,10] Postoperative supplemental embolo / sclerotherapy can further improve overall efficacy of surgical therapy, especially for the treatment of residual lesions after a limited excision. Embolo-/sclerotherapy is now fully integrated with conventional excisional therapy for "surgically accessible" AVM lesions as well, with much improved outcomes especially among "marginally" accessible lesions (Figure 21-2).

ENDOVASCULAR/ EMBOLO SCLEROTHERAPY

Endovascular embolo-/sclerotherapy is now the primary mode of AVM treatment with various embolo- and sclero-agents for the control of "surgically inaccessible" lesions, in addition to a supplemental role to surgical/excisional therapy of a "surgically accessible" lesion (Figures 21-2 through 21-5).[1,22] Endovascular therapy is now the treatment of choice to the majority of "extratrucular" AVM lesions since they are mostly surgically inaccessible as are the "diffuse infiltrating" type with the extension beyond the deep fascia, into muscle, tendon, and bone[1,2,4,7,15,22,43] (Figure 21-3). However, embolo-sclerotherapy is associated with various acute complications (e.g., tissue necrosis, venous thrombosis,

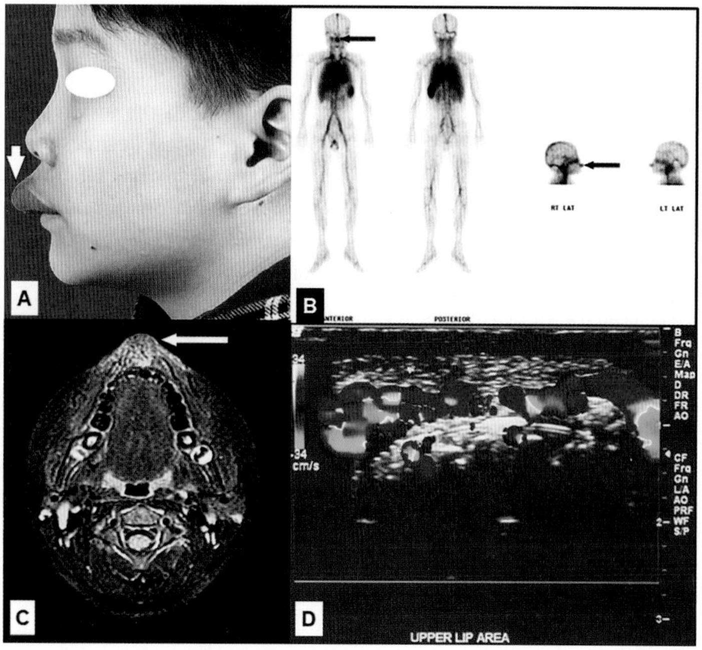

FIGURE 21-2 Surgically "inaccessible" extratruncular AVM lesion treated with multisession embolo-/sclerotherapies as independent therapy. (**A**) Clinical appearance of AVM lesion affecting the upper lip (arrow) with painful swelling. (**B**) Whole body blood pool scintigraphy (WBBPS) findings of AVM lesion localized to upper lip (arrows). Such testing can provide qualitative as well as quantitative measurement for follow-up assessment. (**C**) T2-weighted MRI finding of infiltrating extratruncular AVM lesion (arrow) throughout the entire upper lip. (**D**) Diplex scan findings of hemodynamically very active AVM lesion with turbulent flow (red and blue coloration) affecting the entire upper lip.

pulmonary embolism, nerve damage, and cardiopulmonary arrest) as well as chronic complications (e.g., muscle/tendon contraction) in addition to its related morbidity.[4] Hence, careful assessment of the potential risk of these complications should be considered in the selection of the specific embolo-scleroagent in order to minimize collateral damage to the surrounding tissues—nerve, vessel, cartilage, skin, and soft tissue. The preferred treatment modality should be selected based on a careful risk–benefit analysis of the treatment in which the associated morbidity is justified, such as life- or limb-threatening condition (e.g., hemorrhage, high cardiac output failure).

Embolic agents and liquid agents are two different groups with different chemical properties: absolute ethanol, Onyx, *N*-butyl cyanoacrylate (NBCA), contour particles, and/or coils. These embolo-scleroagents can be utilized in various combinations,[11,42–45] either simultaneously or in multiple separate stages. The liquid agents (e.g., ethanol) are ideal for extratruncular AVM lesions with the critical ability to penetrate to the lesion nidus. Embolic agents (e.g., coils) do NOT have the ability to penetrate the lesion nidus and are limited to function as mechanical occlusion of the vessel lumen.[4,11,46]

Among sclerosing agents, ethanol is the most effective agent and far most commonly used. It, therefore, remains the sclerosing agent of choice for the treatment of extratruncular AVM lesions, especially for the surgically unresectable lesion such as in the diffuse infiltrating type.[4,47,48] The rest of the sclerosing agents (e.g., sodium tetradecyl sulfate, polidocanol and bleomycin) are primarily used in the treatment of low flow venous and lymphatic lesions.[4,22] Absolute ethanol[11,46–50] has curative potential as a powerful sclerosant to denude the endothelial cell layer from the vascular wall and

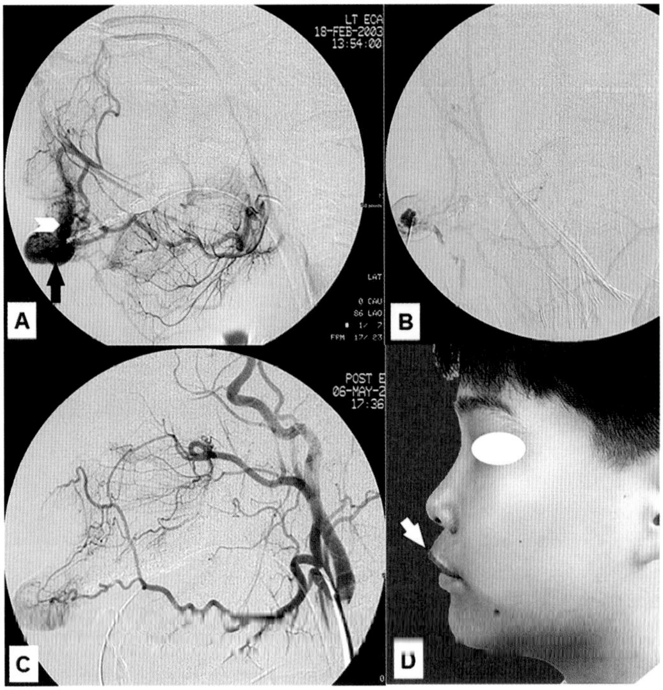

FIGURE 21-3 (**A**) Pretreatment arteriographic findings of upper lip AVM lesion with localized nidus (black arrow) and its extensive collaterals as well as its venous drainage (white arrow). (**B**) Initial ethanol sclerotherapy via direct puncture percutaneous approach with 4.0 mL of 75% of ethanol to control the nidus. (**C**) Arteriographic finding of controlled AVM lesion following two sessions of endovascular treatment. (**D**) Clinical appearance of upper lip with restored normal contour following successful ethanol sclerotherapy. (Reproduced with permission from Gloviczki P, Forum AV. *Handbook of Venous and Lymphatic Disorders: Guidelines of the American Venous Forum*, 4th ed, Boca Raton, FL: CRC Press; 2017.)

permanently eliminate the secretion of chemotactic cellular and angiogenesis factors.[4] However, ethanol sclerotherapy carries a significant risk of cardiopulmonary complications. Pulmonary arterial spasm/hypertension caused by ethanol is a potentially fatal complication that can lead to acute right heart failure and progress to cardiopulmonary arrest. Therefore, close monitoring with a Swan–Ganz catheter is warranted under the general anesthesia.[48,50] Additionally, ethanol sclerotherapy should be performed in multiple sessions, using the most minimal, effective amount of agent during each session in order to minimize the associated risk of complications. A total dose of ethanol of 1 mL/kg of body weight is generally accepted as the maximum volume to be safely administered during a single procedure. Further limiting ethanol administration to 0.14 mL/kg ideal body weight every 10 minutes is recommended when using large volumes of ethanol to treat large lesions.[4,47,50]

NBCA (*N*-butyl-2-cyanoacrylate) or Onyx (ethylene vinyl alcohol copolymer) are the two most commonly used polymerizing agents among liquid agents, but their independent use alone is generally inadequate to provide long-term control of the AVM.[4,10,44,45] Many consider NBCA to be "palliative at best," ideal as a supplemental to enhance the efficacy of surgical dissection, but its long-term effect on the AVM lesions remain controversial when used as single agent therapy. Furthermore, NBCA appears to be resorbed over time resulting in AVM recurrence besides its effects as a foreign body.[4,22,44] Onyx dissolved in dimethyl sulfoxide (DMSO) is a new "less adhesive" liquid polymerizing embolic

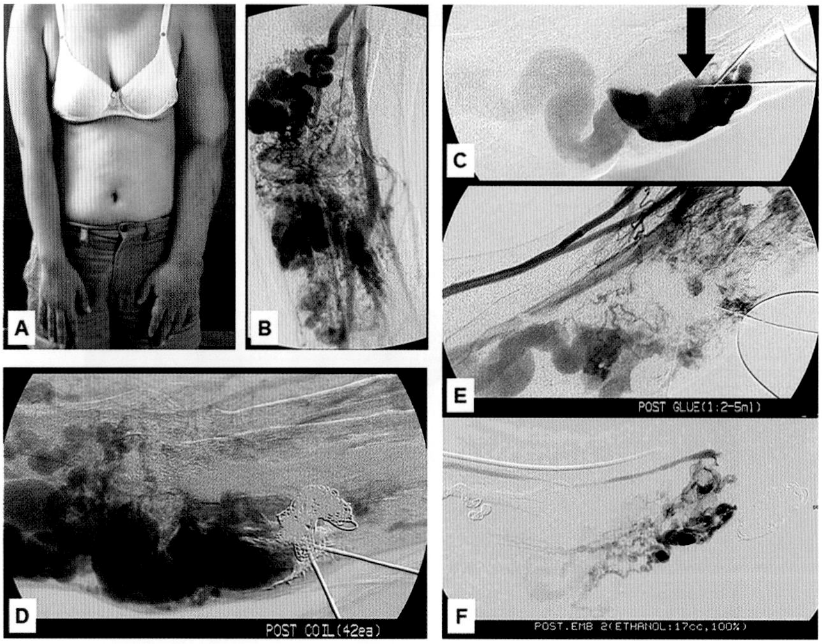

FIGURE 21-4 Multistage embolo-sclerotherapy of multifistulous AVM lesions to control massive high flow. (**A**) Clinical appearance of the left upper extremity affected by AVM lesions along the elbow and forearm region as the cause of massive recurrent bleedings. (**B**) Arteriographic findings of extensive AVM lesions in the multifistulous high flow condition. The feeding arteries are severely dilated and tortuous and its draining veins are also massively dilated. These findings suggest the lesion accompanies extremely high flow to increase the risk of the therapy. (**C**) Massively dilated vein from high flow fistulous connection (arrow). This condition is extremely difficult to manage with a conventional one stage approach. It often requires a multistage-approach with coils and/or glue first before the final treatment with ethanol. (**D**) Angiographic finding of initial coil embolotherapy at the junction of arterio-venous connection to control flow. (**E**) Subsequent nBCA-glue embolotherapy to reduce the flow to lowest possible level before final treatment with ethanol. (**F**) Final stage of endovascular treatment with 17 mL of 100% ethanol. (Reproduced with permission from Gloviczki P, Forum AV. *Handbook of Venous and Lymphatic Disorders: Guidelines of the American Venous Forum*, 4th ed. Boca Raton, FL: CRC Press; 2017.)

agent and has several advantages over NBCA glue including a much lower risk of pulmonary embolism. But onyx is also a palliative agent like NBCA and, many consider, most suitable as preoperative embolic agent for the management of peripheral AVM lesions.[4,45]

Another endovascular alternatives are coils which mechanically occlude the flow and induce thrombosis with no direct effect on the endothelium. This can allow subsequent recanalization of the lesion nidus resulting in recurrence of the lesion.[2,4,49] Coil embolotherapy is therefore not appropriate as sole therapy for extratruncular AVM lesions and additional permanent therapy is required to control the nidus completely, either with absolute ethanol or with surgical excision, if feasible, combined with NBCA.[2,4,7,10,22,49] However, coil embolotherapy is very effective in converting a high-flow lesion to a lower-flow lesion, ideal for a large multifistulous lesion with a prohibitively high risk of complications related to extremely fast shunting blood flow and volume. Initial coil embolization to control the high flow makes the lesion more amenable to ethanol sclerotherapy or NBCA glue embolotherapy and subsequent surgical excision with a reduced risk of complication and morbidity[2,4,49] (Figure 21-4). They can, however, be effective in managing truncular type of fistulous AVM lesions as the primary treatment together with other mechanical occlusive devices (e.g., Amplatz device).

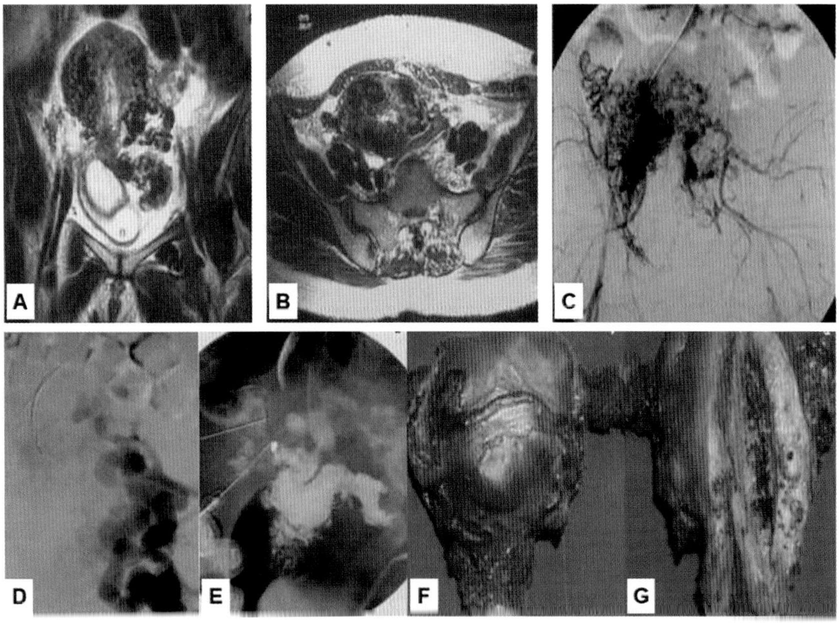

FIGURE 21-5 Surgically "accessible" extratruncular AVM lesion treated with multisession preoperative endovascular treatment and subsequent surgical excision. (**A & B**) T2-weighted MRI findings of pelvic AVM, extensively affecting uterus and para-adnexal soft tissues. This is a life-threatening lesion that can cause massive recurrent uterine bleeding. (**C**) Arteriographic findings of massively infiltrating extratruncular AVM lesions affecting para-adnexal tissue and uterus. (**D**) Massively dilated pelvic veins as venous outflow route for the pelvic AVM. (**E**) *N*-butyl cyanoacrylate injections of the AVM to reduce the risk of intraoperative bleeding during the subsequent surgical excision. (**F**) Surgical specimen of the uterus. (**G**) The inner lumen of the transected uterus shows glue-filled lesion infiltrating all along the endometrium as well as uterine muscle structures, compatible with MRI findings. (Reproduced with permission from Gloviczki P, Forum AV. *Handbook of Venous and Lymphatic Disorders: Guidelines of the American Venous Forum*, 4th ed. Boca Raton, FL: CRC Press; 2017.)

FOLLOW-UP

Careful planning, from diagnosis and treatment to long-term follow-up assessment, is essential for successful AVM management since most of the currently available treatments carry a significant risk of complications, morbidity, and recurrance.[2,4,51] Especially when therapy requires multiple treatment sessions, as is often needed for the majority of AVMs, such careful follow-up evaluation and assessment of treatment results is extremely important. In the majority of cases, the assessment based on duplex scan, whole body blood pool scintigraphy (WBBPS), transarterial lung perfusion scintigraphy (TLPS), CT, and/or MRI are sufficed, although the arteriography remains the gold standard for confirmation of treatment results at its completion.[2,4]

CONCLUSION

A multidisciplinary team approach with fully integrated endovascular and surgical therapy is mandated for effective control of AVM lesions with acceptable complications and morbidity (Figure 21-6). Endovascular therapy is the treatment of choice for the surgically "inaccessible" AVM lesion, whereas surgical therapy, preferably combined with supplemental endovascular therapy, is the best option for the surgically "accessible" lesion. An early aggressive approach is generally required for most AVM lesions to reduce the consequences of AV shunting. However, a careful assessment of the risks and benefits associated with the treatment is warranted for a calculated approach unless the treatment is indicated for a life- or limb-threatening condition (e.g., hemorrhage, high cardiac output failure) (Table 21-6).

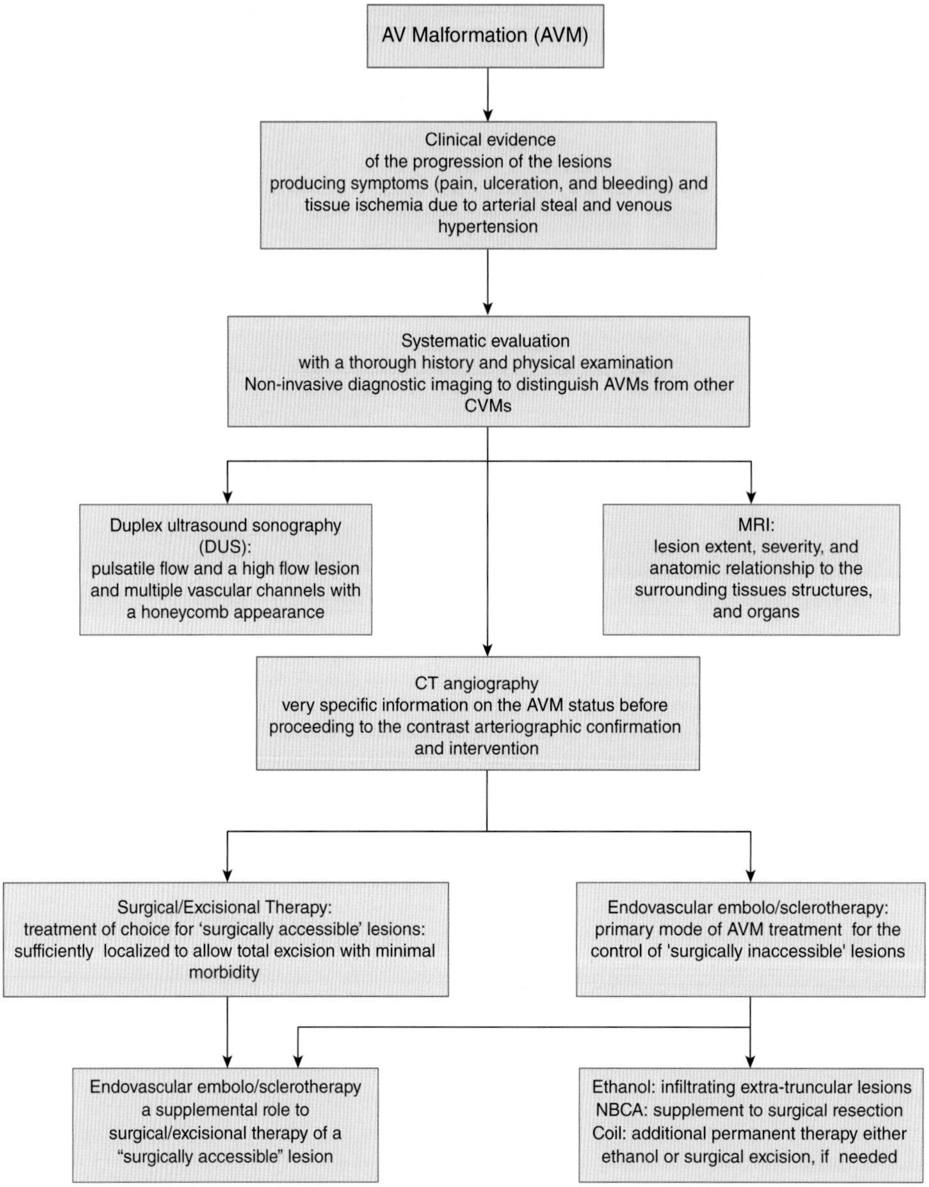

FIGURE 21-6 Evaluation and treatment algorithm for AVMs.

TABLE 21-6 Guidelines 5.4.1 of the American Venous Forum on Arteriovenous Malformations: Evaluation and Treatment

For symptomatic arteriovenous malformations, we recommend endovascular treatment with embolization or sclerotherapy. We recommend it for both definitive treatment of surgically "inaccessible" lesions and for initial therapy of surgically "accessible" lesions (1B)*

*Grade of recommendation (strong/weak): 1. Grade of evidence (A, high quality; B, moderate quality; C, low or very low quality): B.

REFERENCES

1. Gloviczki P, Duncan AA, Kalra M, et al. Vascular malformations: an update. *Perspect Vasc Surg Endovasc Ther.* 2009;21(2):133-148.
2. Lee BB, Lardeo J, Neville R. Arterio-venous malformation: how much do we know? *Phlebology.* 2009;24:193-200.
3. Lee BB. New classification of congenital vascular malformations (CVMs). *Vasc Med Rev.* 2015;3(3):1-5.
4. Lee BB, Baumgartner I, Berlien HP, et al. Consensus document of the international union of angiology (IUA)-2013. Current concept on the management of arterio-venous management. *Int Angiol.* 2013;32(1):9-36.
5. Lee BB, Laredo J. Classification of congenital vascular malformations: the last challenge for congenital vascular malformations. *Phlebology.* 2012;27(6):267-269.
6. Lee BB, Antignani PL, Baraldini V, et al. ISVI-IUA consensus document: diagnostic guidelines on vascular anomalies: vascular malformations and hemangiomas. *Int Angiol.* 2015;34(4):333-374.
7. Lee BB, Do YS, Yakes W, et al. Management of arterial venous shunting malformations (AVM) by surgery and embolosclerotherapy. A multidisciplinary approach. *J Vasc Surg.* 2004;39:590-600.
8. Lee BB, Mattassi R, Kim BT, Park JM. Advanced management of arteriovenous shunting malformation with transarterial lung perfusion scintigraphy (TLPS) for follow up assessment. *Int Angiol.* 2005;24:173-184.
9. Lee BB, Mattassi R, Kim BT, et al. Contemporary diagnosis and management of venous and AV shunting malformation by whole body blood pool scintigraphy (WBBPS). *Int Angiol.* 2004;23:355-367.
10. Lee BB. Statues of new approaches to the treatment of congenital vascular malformations (CVMs): single center experiences. *Eur J Vasc Endovasc Surg.* 2005;30:184-197.
11. Lee BB, Kim DI, Huh S, et al. New experiences with absolute ethanol sclerotherapy in the management of a complex form of congenital venous malformation. *J Vasc Surg.* 2001;33:764-772.
12. Belov S. Classification of congenital vascular defects. *Int Angiol.* 1990;9:141-146.
13. Enjolras O, Wassef M, Chapot R. Introduction: ISSVA classification. In: *Color Atlas of Vascular Tumors and Vascular Malformations.* New York: Cambridge University Press; 2007: 1-11.
14. Tasnadi G. Epidemiology and etiology of congenital vascular malformations. *Semin Vasc Surg.* 1993;6:200-203.
15. Cho SK, Do YS, Shin SW, et al. Arteriovenous malformations of the body and extremities: analysis of therapeutic outcomes and approaches according to a modified angiographic classification. *J Endovasc Ther.* 2006;13(4):527-538.
16. Lee BB, Baumgartner I, Berlien P, et al. Diagnosis and treatment of venous malformations consensus document of the international union of phlebology (IUP): updated 2013. *Int Angiol.* 2015;34(2):97-149.
17. Lee BB. Current concept of venous malformation (VM). *Phlebolymphology.* 2003;43:197-203.
18. Lee B-B, Antignani PL, Baroncelli TA, et al. IUA-ISVI consensus for diagnosis guideline of chronic lymphedema of the limbs. *Int Angiol.* 2015;34(4):311-332.
19. Lee BB, Andrade M, Antignani PL, et al. Diagnosis and treatment of primary lymphedema. Consensus document of the international union of phlebology (IUP)-2013. *Int Angiol.* 2013;32(6):541-574.
20. Lee BB. Hemangioma and venous malformation are as different as an apple and orange! Editorial. *Vasc Invest Ther.* 2019;2(4):85-87.
21. Lee BB, Laredo J, Lee SJ, Huh SH, Joe JH, Neville R. Congenital vascular malformations: general diagnostic principles. *Phlebology.* 2007;22(6):253-257.
22. Lee BB, Laredo J. Hemo-lymphatic malformation: Klippel-Trenaunay Syndrome Review. *Acta Phlebologica.* 2016;17(1):15-22.
23. McDonald J, Bayrak-Toydemir P, Pyeritz RE. Hereditary hemorrhagic telangiectasia: an overview of diagnosis, management, and pathogenesis. *Genet Med.* 2011;13:607-616.
24. Boon LM, Mulliken JB, Vikkula M. RASA1: variable phenotype with capillary and arteriovenous malformations. *Curr Opin Genet Dev.* 2005;15:265-269.
25. Revencu N, Boon LM, Mulliken JB, et al. Parkes Weber syndrome, vein of Galen aneurysmal malformation, and other fast-flow vascular anomalies are caused by RASA1 mutations. *Hum Mutat.* 2008;29:959-965.
26. Tan WH, Baris HN, Burrows PE, et al. The spectrum of vascular anomalies in patients with PTEN mutations: implications for diagnosis and management. *J Med Genet.* 2007;44:594-602.
27. Al-Shahi R, Warlow C. A systematic review of the frequency and prognosis of arteriovenous malformations of the brain in adults. *Brain.* 2001;124(10):1900-1926.
28. Hashimoto T, Mesa-Tejada R, Quick CM, et al Evidence of increased endothelial cell turnover in brain arteriovenous malformations. *Neurosurgery.* 2001;49(1):124-131.
29. Lu L, Mulliken JB, Fishman SJ, Bischoff J, Greene A. Progression of arteriovenous malformation: possible

role of endothelial progenitor cells. Presented at 18th ISSVA Workshop. Brussels, April 2010.
30. Lee BB. All congenital vascular malformations should belong to one of two types: "truncular" or "extratruncular", as different as apples and oranges! Editorial. *Phlebological Review*. 2015;23(1):1-3.
31. Lee BB. Advanced management of congenital vascular malformation (CVM). *Int Angiol*. 2002;21:209-213.
32. Lee BB. Changing concept on vascular malformation: no longer enigma. *Ann Vasc Dis*. 2008;1(1):11-19.
33. Sabin FR. Origin and development of the primitive vessels of the chick and of the pig. *Contrib Embriol Carnegie Inst*. 1917;6-7:61-67.
34. Belov S. Classification, terminology, and nosology of congenital vascular defects. In: Belov S, Loose DA, Weber J, eds. *Vascular Malformations*. Reinbek, Germany: Einhorn-Presse; 1989:25-30.
35. Bastide G, Lefebvre D. Anatomy and organogenesis and vascular malformations. In: Belov St, Loose DA, Weber J, eds. *Vascular Malformations*. Reinbek: Einhorn-Presse Verlag GmbH; 1989: 20-22.
36. Woolard HH. The development of the principal arterial stems in the forelimb of the pig. *Contrib Embryol*. 1922;14:139-154.
37. Shobinger R. In: Proceedings of International Society for the Study of Vascular Anomalies Congress; Rome, Italy, June 23–26, 1996.
38. Kohout MP, Hansen M, Pribaz JJ, Mulliken JB. Arteriovenous malformations of the head and neck: natural history and management. *Plast Reconstr Surg*. 1998;102(3):643-654.
39. Mattassi R. Differential diagnosis in congenital vascular-bone syndromes. *Semin Vasc Surg*. 1993;6:233-244.
40. Kim YW, Do YS, Lee SH, Lee BB: Risk factors for leg length discrepancy in patients with congenital vascular malformation. *J Vasc Surg*. 2006;44:545-553.
41. Lee BB, Mattassi R, Choe YH, et al. Critical role of duplex ultrasonography for the advanced management of a venous malformation (VM). *Phlebology*. 2005;20:28-37.
42. Lee BB, Choe YH, Ahn JM, et al. The new role of MRI (magnetic resonance imaging) in the contemporary diagnosis of venous malformation: can it replace angiography? *J Am Coll Surg*. 2004;198:549-558.
43. Lee BB, Bergan JJ. Advanced management of congenital vascular malformations: a multidisciplinary approach. *Cardiovasc Surg*. 2002;10:523-533.
44. Zanetti PH. Cyanoacrylate/iophenylate mixtures: modification and in vitro evaluation as embolic agents. *J Interv Radiol*. 1987;2:65-68.
45. Numan F, Omeroglu A, Kara B, Cantaşdemir M, Adaletli I, Kantarci F. Embolization of peripheral vascular malformations with ethylene vinyl alcohol copolymer (Onyx). *J Vasc Interv Radiol*. 2004;15(9):939-946.
46. Lee BB, Do YS, Byun HS, et al. Advanced management of venous malformation with ethanol sclerotherapy: midterm results. *J Vasc Surg*. 2003;37:533-538.
47. Jeon YH, Do YS, Shin SW, et al. Ethanol embolization of arteriovenous malformations: results and complications of 33 cases. *J Kor Radiol Soc*. 2003;49:263-270.
48. Yakes WF, Luethke JM, Merland JJ, et al. Ethanol embolization of arteriovenous fistulas: a primary mode of therapy. *J Vasc Intervent Radiol*. 1990;1:89-96.
49. Grady RM, Sharkey AM, Bridges ND. Transcatheter coil embolisation of a pulmonary arteriovenous malformation in a neonate. *Br Heart J*. 1994;71(4):370-371.
50. Shin BS, Do YS, Lee BB, et al. Multistage ethanol sclerotherapy of soft-tissue arteriovenous malformations: effect on pulmonary arterial pressure. *Radiology*. 2005;235:1072-1077.
51. Lee BB. Can "amputation" be justified for arteriovenous-shunting malformations? Editorial. *Phlebology*. 2020; 35(7):445-446.

SELF-ASSESSMENT STUDY QUESTIONS AND ANSWERS

Questions

1. All of the following statements concerning arteriovenous malformations (AVM) are true except for:
   A. They are anatomic defects.
   B. More rare than venous malformations.
   C. More rare than lymphatic malformations.
   D. Less serious clinically than venous/lymphatic malformations.

2. Among congenital vascular malformations (CVM), the most common are
   A. Lymphatic malformations.
   B. Arterial malformations.
   C. Venous malformations.
   D. Arterial-venous malformations.

3. Several gene mutations have been found to cause high-flow AV shunts. These have been associated with all of the following inheritable syndromes except:
   A. Red Rubber Bleb Nevus
   B. Osler-Weber-Rendu
   C. Parkes Weber Syndrome
   D. Banyan Riley Ruvalcaba Syndrome

4. The disruption caused by AVM in the circulatory system is primarily due to the disruption of homeostasis through
   A. Increased heart pumping.
   B. Increased venous return.
   C. Increased lymphatic fluid flow.
   D. Bypassing the capillary system.

5. A more logical and modern classification of CVM, based on morphological and embryological development, was named after the city in which the consensus conference took place:
   A. Paris
   B. Hamburg
   C. London
   D. Washington

6. In the Arteriographic Classification of AVMs, the defining nidus can represent all of the following possible connection between arteries and veins except:
   A. One and one vein
   B. One artery and two veins
   C. Two arteries and one vein
   D. Multiple arterioles and venules

7. Common clinical signs and symptoms of AVMS include all of the following except:
   A. Pain
   B. Ulceration
   C. Bleeding
   D. Hypoesthesia

8. Following a complete history and physical examination, the diagnostic modality that is usually most appropriate is
   A. Duplex ultrasound sonography.
   B. CT angiography.
   C. MR angiography.
   D. Contrast angiography.

9. Surgical excisional therapy for AVMs is
   A. Gold standard of care for AVMs.
   B. Usually resulted in complete removal.
   C. Usually performed in association with embolo-/sclerotherapy.
   D. Associated with minimal morbidity.

10. All of the following concerning endovascular embolo-/sclerotherapy for AVM is true except:
    A. Now the primary mode of AVM treatment.
    B. Liquid agents are used for extratruncular lesions.
    C. Ethanol can cause acute heart failure and arrest.
    D. NBCA (*N*-butyl-2-cyanoacrylate) is better than ethanol.

SELF-ASSESSMENT STUDY QUESTIONS AND ANSWERS

Answers

1. D.
2. C.
3. A.
4. D.
5. B.
6. B.
7. D.
8. A.
9. C.
10. D.

CHAPTER

22 Lymphedema

Stanley G. Rockson

OUTLINE

GENERAL CONSIDERATIONS AND HISTORY
- Lymphatic Anatomy and Physiology
- Lymphedema Causes and Prevalence

CLINICAL FINDINGS

DIFFERENTIAL DIAGNOSIS

DIAGNOSIS
- Lymphoscintigraphy
- Magnetic Resonance Lymphography
- Computed Tomography
- Direct Contrast Lymphangiography

MANAGEMENT OF LYMPHEDEMA
- Medical Management
  - Intermittent Pneumatic Compression
- Surgical Management
  - Suction-Assisted Lipectomy
  - Anastomotic Microsurgical Techniques

GENERAL CONSIDERATIONS AND HISTORY

Lymphedema, characterized by hydrostatic interstitial edema and soft tissue hypertrophy within the affected limb (Figure 22-1), is the disease that develops with end-organ failure of the lymphatic vasculature.

Tissue fluid homeostasis requires the continuous presence of sufficient lymph egress from the limb. When lymph transport capacity is insufficient, interstitial fluid accumulation and regional edema supervene. The presence of lymphedema may reflect either the presence of intrinsic functional defects in lymphatic vascular structure or function, or the advent of lymphatic failure within previously normal vessels as a consequence of sustained circulatory overload. The latter category is predominated by conditions that increase capillary filtration, including right atrial hypertension and chronic venous disease. Intrinsic lymphatic defects can be either primary, on the basis of intrinsic defects, or secondary, caused by disruption of the lymphatic vasculature by surgery, radiation, trauma, or infection. The lymphedema that results from either of these two categories is relatively indistinguishable.

LYMPHATIC ANATOMY AND PHYSIOLOGY

The lymphatic vasculature was first anatomically identified by Gasparo Aselli in the seventeenth century.[1] Appreciation of the more detailed anatomy of this vasculature has grown over the ensuing centuries, through the meticulous work of Pecquet, Bartholinus, Rudbeck, Sappey, von Recklinghausen, and others.[1]

The modern conception of lymphatic anatomy includes a description of the lymphatic capillary as a blind-ended tubular structure comprised of lymphatic endothelial cells. In contrast to the blood vascular capillaries, these structures lack an intact basement membrane, which facilitates the entry of proteins and particulate material that are excluded from blood vascular entry. As the capillaries coalesce into larger, 100- to 200-mm vessels, they acquire a smooth muscle media and an adventitia. The

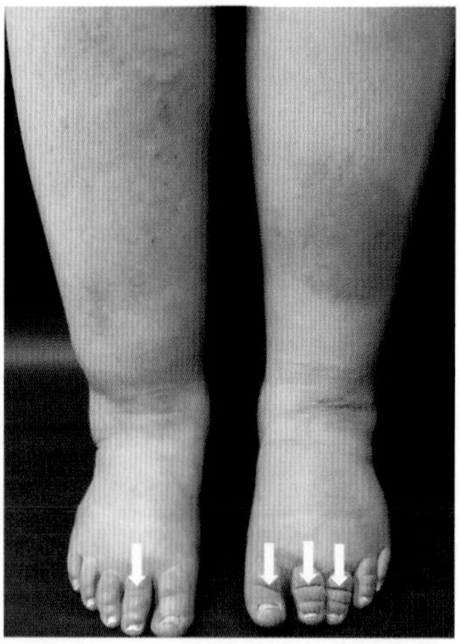

FIGURE 22-1 Primary bilateral lymphedema with swelling of both legs and characteristic exaggerated dorsal toe skin creases (arrows). (Reproduced with permission from Steven Dean, DO.)

lymphatic collectors also have intraluminal valves to ensure unidirectional, central flow.[2,3] In the legs, lymphatic collectors are organized into superficial and deep components. The superficial aspect has medial and lateral channels. The medial channel originates on the dorsum of the foot and follows the course of the saphenous vein. The lateral channel originates on the lateral aspect of the foot and travels to the midleg where, after crossing anteriorly, it follows the course of the medial lymphatics toward the inguinal nodes. The deep lymphatics arise in the subcutaneous compartment and follow the deep blood vasculature as they course toward the inguinal nodes. The deep lymphatics typically communicate with the superficial system only through the popliteal and inguinal lymph nodes. The lymphatic conduits from the lower extremities ultimately gain access to the thoracic duct, the largest of the central lymphatic channels. The thoracic duct transmits the lymph flow from the lower extremities to the central vasculature through its anastomosis with the left brachiocephalic vein.

Lymphatic vascular physiology can best be comprehended through a consideration of the Starling forces that govern fluid flux to and from the interstitial space. Tissue fluid production is governed by the balance between the forces that drive capillary filtration (capillary hydrostatic pressure and tissue oncotic pressure) and those that facilitate reabsorption (interstitial hydrostatic pressure and capillary oncotic pressure). Reabsorption of interstitial fluid at the venous end of the capillary is a relatively trivial phenomenon; in fact, the avoidance of tissue edema relies almost exclusively upon lymph efflux from the limb.[4] The volume and the composition of the interstitial fluid are kept in balance by the lymphatic system. In each 24-hour period, the lymphatics must accommodate 2 to 4 L of interstitial fluid that contains an estimated 100 g of circulatory proteins. In addition to the balance of filtration and reabsorption, the dynamics of lymph production also reflect active transendothelial transport of solutes, lipids, and water.[5]

After interstitial fluid enters the lymphatic endovascular space, its subsequent central transit depends upon both intrinsic and extrinsic pumps,[6] both assisted by the function of the lymphatic valves that ensure unidirectional lymph flow. The behavior of the intrinsic lymphatic pump is determined by the properties of lymphatic smooth muscle and by dynamic changes in lymphatic preload, afterload, spontaneous contractile rate and amplitude, and neural input.[6] The extrinsic pump reflects the augmentation of lymphatic contractility by physical movement, skeletal muscle contraction, arterial pulsations, and extrinsic tissue compression. Upon the entry of lymph into the thorax, the negative intrathoracic pressure generated by diaphragmatic excursion (the "respiratory pump") pulls the fluid into the thoracic duct. These lymphodynamic forces, in aggregate, are critical for normal lymphatic function, and failure of adequate lymph transport, whether from anatomic or functional derangements, will promote the development of lymphedema.

LYMPHEDEMA CAUSES AND PREVALENCE

Lymphedema epidemiology has historically been the subject of some neglect.[7] Estimates of disease prevalence draw heavily upon the observed patterns of disease among cancer survivors.[8] With this in mind, it can be stated that primary lymphedema is a rare disease, affecting an estimated 1:100,000 individuals in the United States[9]; in contrast, secondary, or acquired, lymphedema is common, occurring in 1:1000 Americans.[9]

Cancer diagnosis and treatment, which often entails surgical excision of lymph nodes and radiotherapy, still leads to the development of lymphedema in one of every seven cancer survivors (Figure 22-2).[10] The increasing reliance upon sentinel node techniques has diminished the magnitude of this problem, but has not eliminated the high prevalence of cancer-associated lymphedema. Cancer-associated

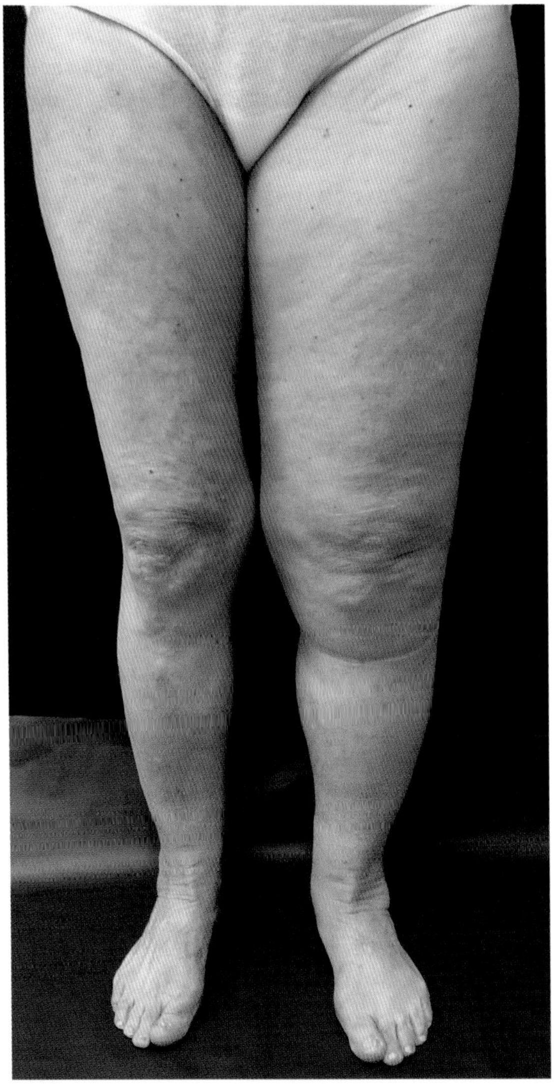

FIGURE 22-2 Secondary lymphedema of the left leg following pelvic lymph node dissection for malignancy illustrating the marked swelling of the entire leg. (Reproduced with permission from Steven Dean, DO.)

secondary lymphoedema can occur as a consequence of cancer treatment or in the setting of advanced neoplastic disease.[10] The common cancers associated with lower extremity lymphedema, with estimates of disease prevalence are: gynecological (37%[11]), melanoma with sentinel node biopsy (35%[12]), melanoma with inguinal lymph node dissection (83%[12]), and genitourinary malignancies (10%[13]). In addition to these treatment-specific causes of lymphedema, chronic edema has been reported in up to 19% of individuals with advanced cancer.[14] This pathogenesis of lymphedema is often multifactorial, relating to factors such as hypoalbuminemia (and its effect on the Starling relationship), metastatic lymphadenopathy, and venous compression (which will increase capillary filtration and, thereby, increase the preload on the lymphatic circulation).

Outside of the cancer setting, the presence of chronic venous disease is a common precursor to the development of lower extremity lymphedema. As previously stated, venous hypertension augments capillary filtration and thereby chronically increases the lymphatic load, ultimately leading to lymphatic fatigue and failure. The epidemiology of phlebolymphedema (the clinical expression of combined venous and lymphatic insufficiency) is similarly difficult to define, but it is estimated that 3% to 11% of the population experience edema and pathological skin changes due to chronic venous insufficiency,[15] many of whom suffer from the aggregate burden of increased lymphatic preload and lymphatic vascular damage from repeated episodes of cellulitis.[16] In addition to intrinsic venous disease, right atrial hypertension can also increase lymphatic preload and thereby lead to lymphedema. Prevalence estimates for lymphedema in congestive heart failure, pulmonary hypertension, and chronic lung disease are not available. Similarly, lymphedema can ensue from surgical and nonsurgical trauma, but the epidemiology of these problems is not well-studied.

CLINICAL FINDINGS

The clinical presentation within the individual patient will depend on the duration and severity of the lymphedema. One or both lower extremities may be involved and, secondarily, the involvement may extend proximally to involve the buttocks or genitalia. The International Society of Lymphology has defined four stages of lymphedema: subclinical disease, early fluid accumulation, edema that persists with leg elevation, and chronic fibrotic disease (elephantiasis).[17,18] In the progression from subclinical disease to early fluid accumulation, the interstitial space becomes distended with an accumulation of protein-enriched fluid. The resulting edema is soft, pitting, and decreases or resolves with limb elevation. In primary lymphedema, and in some cases of acquired disease, squaring of the toes can be seen at this stage. As the patient progresses to the later stages of lymphedema, the pitting quality progressively diminishes and is ultimately lost and, concurrently, limb elevation fails to reduce edema volume.

Ultimately, the affected limb is permanently often grossly, enlarged. The skin may acquire a cobblestone texture. A variety of physical findings reflect these changes: peau d'orange is the result of the cutaneous thickening that stretches the skin pores, and the inelasticity of the skin at the base of the digits (Stemmer's sign; Figure 22-3) is considered to be pathognomic for the presence of lymphedema.[19] Additional cutaneous changes might include acanthosis (thickening caused by hyperplasia), lichenification (leathery thickening that resembles the crusty appearance of slow growing crustose lichens), verrucae (wart like excrescences), and other dystrophic changes.[10] Subdermal and subcutaneous fibrosis is often progressive, and subcutaneous adipose hypertrophy is nearly universal.[20]

DIFFERENTIAL DIAGNOSIS

The differential diagnosis of lymphedema requires a consideration of those entities that can cause hydrostatic edema and those that abnormally thicken the architecture of the skin and subcutis.

Systemic causes of edema (e.g., heart failure, hypoproteinemia, pulmonary hypertension, hypothyroidism, cyclic edema) should certainly be considered in the differential diagnosis, although, as mentioned, lymphedema can supervene in these disorders. Similarly, the various forms of venous incompetence and obstruction should be considered as potentially causes.

Among the disorders that can cause enlargement of the limb with thickening of the tissues, both myxedema and lipedema should be considered. In hypothyroidism, abnormal mucinous deposits create edema and, with chronicity, the skin elasticity is lost and the structural integrity of the dermis is destroyed. In myxedema, there are changes in the glabrous skin of the palms and soles, along with changes at the elbow and knees and xanthous discoloration of the skin, accompanied changes in the hair and nails.

In lipedema, the changes in the limb are caused by a pathological excess of subcutaneous adipose tissues in the leg, with characteristic sparing of the feet. It has been estimated that 10% to 18% of patients referred to a lymphedema clinic have lipedema.[21] Although the pathophysiology of lipedema has not been fully delineated, it appears that the fat disorder arises as a consequence of an underlying disorder in the lymphatic circulation.[22] A characteristic distribution of symmetric adiposity in the lower extremities,

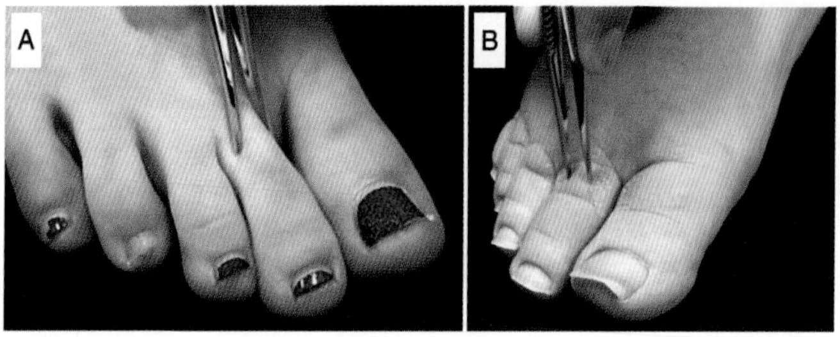

FIGURE 22-3 Stemmer's clinical sign for the diagnosis of lymphedema. (**A**) Normally, the skin fold at the base of the second toe can be easily pinched together with the fingers or a forceps. (**B**) In patients with lymphedema, the thickened skin fold prevents pinching, regardless of the amount of pressure applied. (Reproduced with permission from Steven Dean, DO.)

with sparing of the feet, should suggest consideration of lipedema as a diagnosis. In addition to the history of disproportionately heavy thighs and hips, lipedema patients often complain of pain and easy bruising swelling. The diagnosis of lipedema depends entirely on clinical assessment by physical examination, in the absence of useful diagnostic imaging or biomarker modalities.

DIAGNOSIS

In lymphedema, the diagnosis relies very heavily upon the physical assessment of the patient. In the appropriate risk setting (antecedent cancer therapeutics, surgical trauma, infection, or positive family history), the presence of the characteristic physical findings of edema and tissue changes should lead to the correct diagnosis. The stage of the lymphedema should be appropriately documented[23]; in some cases, this will entail direct measurement of the volume of the affected limb(s). Historically, the diagnosis of lymphedema has relied heavily upon such unidimensional thresholds for excess limb volume[10]; however, a more meaningful set of insights are likely to be gained by a description of symptoms,[24] the presence of pitting,[25] and quantitation of dermal thickness, which can be measured ultrasonographically.[26,27] In addition to these approaches, it is appropriate to look for evidence of clinical or subclinical infection in these patients.[23]

Where the diagnosis remains uncertain, or the differential diagnosis is complex, imaging modalities can assist with the correct identification of a lymphedema diagnosis (Figure 22-4).

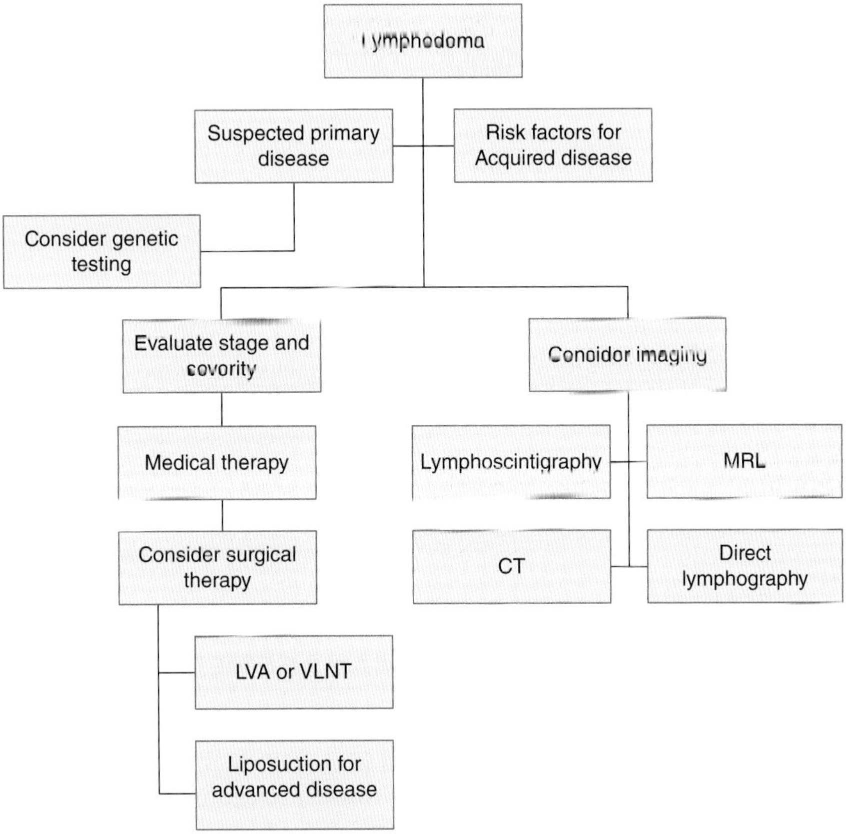

FIGURE 22-4 Diagnostic and treatment algorithm for lymphedema. CT, computed tomography; LVA, lymphaticovenous anastomosis; LVNA, vascularized lymph node transfer; MRL, magnetic resonance lymphography.

LYMPHOSCINTIGRAPHY

Lymphoscintigraphy is performed after the injection of a radiolabeled macromolecule, into the distal subcutaneous tissue of the affected extremity (i.e., the dorsum of the foot). In lymphedema, either primary or secondary, the transit time from injection to the target lymph nodes in the groin is prolonged, and often accompanied by distal accumulation in the dilated channels of the dermis, called "dermal backflow." In cases of primary lymphedema, the lymphatic vasculature is often hypoplastic but, some cases, the vessels are ectatic and incompetent.[28] Quantitative analysis of mean transit times is feasible,[29] and stress lymphoscintigraphy has been proposed as a potentially useful way to predict therapeutic responsiveness.[30]

MAGNETIC RESONANCE LYMPHOGRAPHY

Magnetic resonance can be used to image a honeycomb pattern of subcutaneous thickening that is typical of lymphedema, along with dermal edema and surrounding fibrosis. Dilated lymphatic channels may be seen. In addition, nonenhanced three-dimensional heavily T2-weighted images obtained with two-dimensional prospective acquisition and correction have the capacity to visualize the thoracic duct, cisterna chyli, and lumbar lymphatics.[31] Of late, MR lymphography for the assessment of lymphedema is felt to have a specificity and sensitivity that is superior to that of standard radionuclide lymphoscintigraphy.[32] Magnetic resonance imaging has distinct applicability in the evaluation of lymphedema patients for potential microsurgical interventions.[33]

COMPUTED TOMOGRAPHY

Computed tomography (CT) of a lymphedematous limb can also show a honeycomb pattern in the affected area, but direct imaging of the level of lymphatic obstruction is not feasible with this technique. CT can, however, be used to assess the volume changes within various tissue compartments on the cross-sectional images of the affected limb.[34] The greatest potential impact of CT is provided by the ability to distinguish many of the causes of secondary lymphedema (e.g., lymphedenopathy, lymphoma, pelvic tumor). In addition, CT may shed light on the attributes of other conditions that remain within the differential diagnosis.

DIRECT CONTRAST LYMPHANGIOGRAPHY

Historically, the method of choice for imaging of the lymphatics was the direct introduction of contrast material into the vasculature. The technique required identification of a distal lymphatic through intradermal injection of a vital dye into the metatarsal web spaces. After cannulation, iodinated contrast is injected and serially imaged. More recently, the technique has evolved to entail intranodal injection with dynamic contrast-enhanced magnetic resonance imaging.[35] Direct contrast lymphangiography is not typically warranted in the diagnostic evaluation of isolated lymphedema but is useful in the evaluation and treatment of patients with complex lymphatic vascular disorders.[36]

There are several drawbacks to the procedure, including frequent requirements for surgical exposure in the edematous limb, microsurgical techniques to achieve direct cannulation, and, occasionally, the need for general anesthesia. Of greater importance is the fact that the irritation caused by the contrast agent itself results in lymphangitis in one-third of the studies and potentially can worsen the lymphedema.[37] For these reasons, the use of lymphangiography as a diagnostic modality for the edematous limb has largely been abandoned and is contraindicated in patients with lymphedema; nevertheless, direct lymphangiography is still indicated for the evaluation and interventional treatment of patients with complex lymphatic vascular disorders.[36]

MANAGEMENT OF LYMPHEDEMA

MEDICAL MANAGEMENT

At present, there is no useful pharmacology for the medical management of lymphedema, although there is active investigation that suggests promise for the future.[38,39] Successful therapy of lymphedema relies almost entirely upon physical interventions designed to reduce excess edema volume and to augment residual lymphatic contractility and function.

These interventions are known collectively as complex decongestive physiotherpay (CDP), comprised of an interrelated set of treatment modalities that may include manual lymphatic massage, multilayer bandaging, exercise, and skin care. The guidelines suggest that CDP is pivotal in the management of lymphedema,[18] according to a 1B level of evidence.[23] The required use of graduated compression in the maintenance phase is universally acknowledged.[40] The International Society of Lymphology has endorsed the use of the highest tolerated compression in the range of 20 to 60 mmHg.[17]

Intermittent Pneumatic Compression

Intermittent pneumatic compression (IPC) is an elective component of decongestive physiotherapy that has been historically somewhat controversial. Early observations of complications and lack of efficacy initially reduced enthusiasm for the use of pneumatic compression as standalone therapy. Nevertheless, the incorporation of a multimodal physical approach to the lymphedema patient has long been advocated by some proponents,[41] and more recent formal evaluations of this approach demonstrate that IPC is efficacious, well-tolerated, and remarkably free of complications.[42,43] In addition, it has been shown to provide the benefit of a reduction both in the utilization of medical resources and of health care costs.[44-46] This is particularly true for patients with phlebolymphedema.[16]

A variety of multichamber pneumatic devices are available that intermittently compress the limb; techniques that employ sequential graduated compression (in which the cuffs are inflated sequentially from distal to proximal sites with a pressure gradient from the most distal cuff to the most proximal) are the most efficacious. It is important to ensure that the patient who will undergo IPC has an adequate arterial blood supply to the affected limb; in patients with concomitant peripheral arterial insufficiency, any form of sustained compression can further compromise arterial blood flow.

The guidelines generally support the incorporation of IPC into the treatment regimen for lymphedema while acknowledging that this modality should not be used in a standalone format. The supporting evidence for efficacy is, nevertheless, recognized to be heterogeneous.[18]

SURGICAL MANAGEMENT

The last decade has witnessed a surge of interest in surgical therapies for lymphedema.

Suction-Assisted Lipectomy

In the later stages of lymphedema, the volume excess in the limb is typically predominated by progressive hypertrophy of the subcutaneous adipose compartment. It is now feasible to safely and efficaciously undertake debulking of these limbs in order to facilitate more effective use of external compression and to improve patient mobility and reduce pain.

Suction-assisted lipectomy provides stable, significant reduction of volume excess in lower limb lymphedema. In one recent series, the surgical technique produced a median volume reduction of 79% in primary leg lymphedema and 101% in secondary disease of the lower limb.[47] These favorable outcomes are not influenced by BMI or other patient characteristics, but in suction-assisted lipectomy, volume reduction is unsuccessful without maintenance of chronic compression after surgical intervention.[20] Liposuction combined with long-term decongestive compression therapy is a more effective route to volume reduction than compression therapy alone.

Anastomotic Microsurgical Techniques

Increasingly utilized in the therapeutic approach to lymphedema, anastomotic procedures fall into two broad categories: lymphaticovenous anastomosis (LVA) and autologous, vascularized lymph node transfer (VLNT). A number of these individual strategies have proven to be efficacious,[48] but analyses are based upon small patient numbers, and a lack of long-term follow-up for nonstandardized measurement techniques.[49]

Lymphaticovenous anastomosis is generally recommended for patients with early or mid-stage lymphedema, on the basis of the reported outcome benefits and low complication profile.[50] This recommendation is based upon a systematic review of 12 studies that aggregate the results of 3074 patients. Anatomic considerations also govern the decision to entertain LVA within the treatment approach,[33] inasmuch as lymphatic imaging must demonstrate the presence of patent, functional lymphatic channels for LVA to be feasible, either alone or in combination with VLNT. The latter procedure is associated with a considerably higher risk profile, rendering this technique more appropriate for the advanced stages of lymphedema.[18]

For the surgical management of lymphedema, the American Venous Forum has proposed that all intervention for chronic lymphedema should be preceded by at least 6 months of nonoperative compression treatment (IC recommendation); debulking liposuction should be reserved for patients with late-stage nonpitting lymphedema, who fail conservative measures (2C); and suggests that microsurgical lymphatic reconstructions be performed in centers of excellence, for selected patients with secondary lymphedema, if performed early in the course of the disease.[23]

REFERENCES

1. Kanter MA. The lymphatic system: an historical perspective. *Plast Reconstr Surg*. 1987;79(1):131-139.
2. Baldwin M, Stacker S, Achen M. Molecular control of lymphangiogenesis. *Bioessays*. 2002;24:1030-1040.
3. Gashev A. Physiologic aspects of lymphatic contractile function: current perspectives. *Ann N Y Acad Sci*. 2002;979:178-187.
4. Mortimer PS, Rockson SG. New developments in clinical aspects of lymphatic disease. *J Clin Invest*. 2014;124(3):915-921.
5. Wiig H, Swartz MA. Interstitial fluid and lymph formation and transport: physiological regulation and roles in inflammation and cancer. *Physiol Rev*. 2012;92(3):1005-1060.
6. Scallan JP, Zawieja SD, Castorena-Gonzalez JA, Davis MJ. Lymphatic pumping: mechanics, mechanisms and malfunction. *J Physiol*. 2016;594(20):5749-5768.
7. Rockson SG. LIMPRINT: Elucidating the global problem of lymphedema. *Lymph Res Biol*. 2019;17(2):119-120.
8. Rockson SG, Rivera KK. Estimating the population burden of lymphedema. *Ann N Y Acad Sci*. 2008;1131:147-154.
9. Greene AK. Epidemiology and morbidity of lymphedema. In: Greene AK, Slavin SA, Brorson H, eds. *Lymphedema*. Cham, Switzerland: Springer; 2015:33-44.
10. Rockson SG, Keeley V, Kilbreath S, Szuba A, Towers A. Cancer-associated secondary lymphoedema. *Nat Rev Dis Primers*. 2019;5(1):22.
11. Hayes SC, Janda M, Ward LC, et al. Lymphedema following gynecological cancer: results from a prospective, longitudinal cohort study on prevalence, incidence and risk factors. *Gynecol Oncol*. 2017;146(3):623-629.
12. Gjorup C. *Melanoma Related Limb Lymphoedema and Associated Risk Factors*. Copenhagen, Denmark: University of Copenhagen; 2017.
13. Cormier JN, Askew RL, Mungovan KS, Xing Y, Ross MI, Armer JM. Lymphedema beyond breast cancer: a systematic review and meta-analysis of cancer-related secondary lymphedema. *Cancer*. 2010;116(22):5138-5149.
14. Teunissen SC, Wesker W, Kruitwagen C, de Haes HC, Voest EE, de Graeff A. Symptom prevalence in patients with incurable cancer: a systematic review. *J Pain Symptom Manage*. 2007;34(1):94-104.
15. Nicolaides AN. Investigation of chronic venous insufficiency. *Circulation*. 2000;102(20):e126-e163.
16. Lerman M, Gaebler JA, Hoy S, et al. Health and economic benefits of advanced pneumatic compression devices in patients with phlebolymphedema. *J Vasc Surg*. 2019;69(2):571-580.
17. Executive C. The diagnosis and treatment of peripheral lymphedema: 2016 Consensus document of the international society of lymphology. *Lymphology*. 2016;49(4):170-184.
18. Gianesini S, Obi A, Onida S, et al. Global guidelines trends and controversies in lower limb venous and lymphatic disease. *Phlebology*. 2019;34(Suppl 1):4-66.
19. Stemmer R. A clinical symptom for the early and differential diagnosis of lymphedema. *Vasa*. 1976;5(3):261-262.
20. Brorson H, Ohlin K, Olsson G, Karlsson M. Breast cancer-related chronic arm lymphedema is associated with excess adipose and muscle tissue. *Lymphat Res Biol*. 2009;7(1):3-10.
21. Szolnoky G. Differential diagnosis: lipedema. In: Lee BB, Rockson SG, Bergan J, eds. *Lymphedema: A Concise Compendium of Theory and Practice*. 2nd ed. London: Springer; 2018:239-249.
22. Ma W, Gil HJ, Escobedo N, et al. Platelet factor 4 is a biomarker for lymphatic-promoted disorders. *JCI Insight*. 2020;5(13): e135109.
23. Lee BB, Antignani PL, Baroncelli TA, et al. IUA-ISVI consensus for diagnosis guideline of chronic lymphedema of the limbs. *Int Angiol*. 2015;34(4):311-332.

24. Ridner SH, Dietrich MS. Development and validation of the lymphedema symptom and intensity survey-arm. *Support Care Cancer*. 2015;23(10):3103-3112.
25. Cariati M, Bains SK, Grootendorst MR, et al. Adjuvant taxanes and the development of breast cancer-related arm lymphoedema. *Br J Surg*. 2015;102(9):1071-1078.
26. Dylke ES, Benincasa Nakagawa H, Lin L, Clarke JL, Kilbreath SL. Reliability and diagnostic thresholds for ultrasound measurements of dermal thickness in breast lymphedema. *Lymph Res Biol*. 2018;16(3):258-262.
27. Yang EJ, Kim SY, Lee WH, Lim JY, Lee J. Diagnostic accuracy of clinical measures considering segmental tissue composition and volume changes of breast cancer-related lymphedema. *Lymph Res Biol*. 2018;16(4):368-376.
28. Szuba A, Shin WS, Strauss HW, Rockson S. The third circulation: radionuclide lymphoscintigraphy in the evaluation of lymphedema. *J Nucl Med*. 2003;44(1):43-57.
29. Hvidsten S, Toyserkani NM, Sorensen JA, Hoilund-Carlsen PF, Simonsen JA. A scintigraphic method for quantitation of lymphatic function in arm lymphedema. *Lymphat Res Biol*. 2018;16(1):[illegible].
30. Tartaglione G, Visconti G, Bartoletti R, et al. Stress lymphoscintigraphy for early detection and management of secondary limb lymphedema. *Clin Nucl Med*. 2018;43(3):155-161.
31. Matsushima S, Ichiba N, Hayashi D, Fukuda K. Nonenhanced magnetic resonance lymphoductography: visualization of lymphatic system of the trunk on 3-dimensional heavily T2-weighted image with 2-dimensional prospective acquisition and correction. *J Comput Assist Tomogr*. 2007;31(2):299-302.
32. Bae JS, Yoo RE, Choi SH, et al. Evaluation of lymphedema in upper extremities by MR lymphangiography: Comparison with lymphoscintigraphy. *Magn Reson Imaging*. 2018;49:63-70.
33. Neligan PC, Kung TA, Maki JH. MR lymphangiography in the treatment of lymphedema. *J Surg Oncol*. 2017;115(1):18-22.
34. Vaughan BF. CT of swollen legs. *Clin Radiol*. 1990;41(1):24-30.
35. Itkin M, Nadolski GJ. Modern techniques of lymphangiography and interventions: current status and future development. *Cardiovasc Intervent Radiol*. 2018;41(3):366-376.
36. Itkin M. Lymphatic intervention is a new frontier of IR. *J Vasc Interv Radiol*. 2014;25(9):1404-1405.
37. O'Brien BM, Das SK, Franklin JD, Morrison WA. Effect of lymphangiography on lymphedema. *Plast Reconstr Surg*. 1981;68(6):922-926.
38. Tian W, Rockson SG, Jiang X, et al. Leukotriene B4 antagonism ameliorates experimental lymphedema. *Sci Transl Med*. 2017;19(389):eaal3920.
39. Rockson SG, Tian W, Jiang X, et al. Pilot studies demonstrate the potential benefits of antiinflammatory therapy in human lymphedema. *JCI Insight*. 2018;3(20).
40. Rabe E, Partsch H, Hafner J, et al. Indications for medical compression stockings in venous and lymphatic disorders: an evidence-based consensus statement. *Phlebology*. 2018;33(3):163-184.
41. Leduc O, Leduc A, Bourgeois P, Belgrado JP. The physical treatment of upper limb edema. *Cancer*. 1998;83(12 Suppl American):2835-2839.
42. Szuba A, Achalu R, Rockson SG. Decongestive lymphatic therapy for patients with breast carcinoma-associated lymphedema. A randomized, prospective study of a role for adjunctive intermittent pneumatic compression. *Cancer*. 2002;95(11):2260-2267.
43. Mayrovitz HN. The standard of care for lymphedema: current concepts and physiological considerations. *Lymphat Res Biol*. 2009;7(2):101-108.
44. Brayton KM, Hirsch AT, O'Brien PJ, Cheville A, Karaca-Mandic P, Rockson SG. Lymphedema prevalence and treatment benefits in cancer: impact of a therapeutic intervention on health outcomes and costs. *PLoS One*. 2014;9(12):e114597.
45. Karaca-Mandic P, Hirsch AT, Rockson SG, Ridner SH. The cutaneous, net clinical, and health economic benefits of advanced pneumatic compression devices in patients with lymphedema. *JAMA Dermatol*. 2015;151(11):1187-1193.
46. Karaca-Mandic P, Hirsch AT, Rockson SG, Ridner SH. A comparison of programmable and non-programmable compression devices for treatment of lymphedema using an administrative health outcomes dataset. *Br J Dermatol*. 2017;177(6):1699-1707.
47. Lamprou DA, Voesten HG, Damstra RJ, Wikkeling OR. Circumferential suction-assisted lipectomy in the treatment of primary and secondary end-stage lymphoedema of the leg. *Br J Surg*. 2017;104(1):84-89.
48. Cormier JN, Rourke L, Crosby M, Chang D, Armer J. The surgical treatment of lymphedema: a systematic review of the contemporary literature (2004-2010). *Ann Surg Oncol*. 2012;19(2):642-651.
49. Hadamitzky C, Pabst R, Gordon K, Vogt PM. Surgical procedures in lymphedema management. *J Vasc Surg Venous Lymphat Disord*. 2014;2(4):461-468.
50. Carl HM, Walia G, Bello R, et al. Systematic review of the surgical treatment of extremity lymphedema. *J Reconstr Microsurg*. 2017;33(6):412-425.

SELF-ASSESSMENT STUDY QUESTIONS AND ANSWERS

Questions

1. Secondary lymphedema due to circulatory overload can be described by all of the following except:
A. Right heart failure
B. Portal hypertension
C. Chronic venous insufficiency
D. Radiation therapy

2. Similar to the venous vasculature, the lymphatic system has all of the following except:
A. Basement membrane
B. Smooth muscle media
C. Adventitia
D. Intraluminal valves

3. The lymphatic system of the lower extremities ultimately drains its contents into the central venous circulation through
A. Common femoral vein.
B. Iliac vein.
C. Thoracic duct.
D. Azygous duct.

4. Flow within the lymphatic system is assisted by all of the following except:
A. Intrinsic pump
B. Extrinsic pump
C. Calf muscle pump
D. Respiratory pump

5. Secondary or acquired lymphedema after cancer treatment is estimated to occur among cancer survivors in approximately:
A. 1 out of 2
B. 1 out of 5
C. 1 out of 7
D. 1 out of 10

6. All of the following are cutaneous changes of lymphedema except:
A. Peau d'orange
B. Acanthosis
C. Lichenification
D. Lipodermatosclerosis

7. Clinical physical characteristics of lipedema of the extremities include all of the following except:
A. Symmetric adiposity of the legs
B. Involvement of the arms
C. Sparing of the feet
D. Sparing of the trunk

8. Among the advanced imaging modalities available for patients with lymphedema, the study least likely to be recommended, due to its potential complications, is
A. Computed tomography.
B. Lymphoscintigraphy.
C. Lymphangiography.
D. Magnetic resonance lymphangiography.

9. Effective treatment for lymphedema includes all of the following except:
A. Medical therapy
B. Pneumatic compression
C. Suction lipectomy
D. Lymphaticovenous anastomosis

10. Physical interventions designed to reduce excess lymphedema volume and to augment residual lymphatic contractility are known as complex decongestive physiotherapy (CDP) and include all of the following except:
A. Manual lymphatic massage
B. Intermittent compression therapy
C. Multilayer bandaging
D. Leg elevation

SELF-ASSESSMENT STUDY QUESTIONS AND ANSWERS

Answers

1. D.
2. A.
3. C.
4. C.
5. C.
6. D.
7. B.
8. C.
9. A.
10. D.

CHAPTER

23 Lower Extremity Swelling and Differential Diagnosis

Thomas F. O'Donnell, Jr.

OUTLINE

INTRODUCTION
PATHOPHYSIOLOGY
Starling Principle and Its Revision
Deleterious Effects of Fluid Stasis
Causes of Increased Capillary Filtration
Causes of Reduced Lymphatic Drainage
EPIDEMIOLOGY
CLINICAL DIAGNOSIS
History
Physical Examination
Treatment and Surveillance
INTRODUCTION
PATHOPHYSIOLOGY
The Starling Principle and Its Revision
Deleterious Effects of Fluid Stasis
Causes of Increased Capillary Filtration
Increased Capillary Hydrostatic Pressure
Increased venous pressure
Lipedema
Other causes of increased capillary pressure
Reduced Plasma Oncotic Pressure
Increased Capillary Permeability
Causes of Reduced Lymphatic Drainage
Lymphedema
Obesity as a Cause of Edema
EPIDEMIOLOGY
CLINICAL DIAGNOSIS
History
Patient Reported Symptoms
Positional or temporal changes
Pain
Physical Examination
Duplex Ultrasound in Clinical Diagnosis
Diagnostic Testing
Treatment and Surveillance

INTRODUCTION

This brief section introduces definitions of acute and chronic edema, emphasizing the importance of understanding the modern view of edema pathophysiology and epidemiology for diagnosis. As an organizational principle, the causes of peripheral edema are categorized at their highest level as increased capillary filtration, decreased lymphatic drainage, or a combination of the two.

PATHOPHYSIOLOGY

STARLING PRINCIPLE AND ITS REVISION

This section begins with a review of the dynamics of fluid exchange at the capillary level and reviews the foundational Starling principle of fluid exchange, which has shaped the medical understanding of edema for more than a century, and how this principle has been revised by modern research.

DELETERIOUS EFFECTS OF FLUID STASIS

The deleterious effects of fluid stasis, drawing upon recent research into the cellular and molecular underpinnings of the vicious circle of inflammation, fibrosis, adipose deposition, and recurrent infections seen in chronic edema are reviewed.

CAUSES OF INCREASED CAPILLARY FILTRATION

Causes of increased filtration are subdivided into increased hydrostatic pressure, decreased osmotic pressure, and increased capillary permeability, with individual causative conditions identified.

CAUSES OF REDUCED LYMPHATIC DRAINAGE

Causes of decreased lymphatic drainage (lymphedema) are subdivided into primary and secondary causes. The author explains the varying definitions of lymphedema found in the literature. This section concludes with a brief review of obesity as a growing cause of edema. A figure representing these classifications and divisions is included.

EPIDEMIOLOGY

A brief review of the challenges involved in estimating the incidence and prevalence of chronic edema. Evidenced-based estimates of the prevalence of primary lymphedema, cancer related lymphedema, phlebolymphedema, and lipedema (a primary cause of chronic swelling) are provided.

CLINICAL DIAGNOSIS

A systematic approach to differential diagnosis is supported by a figure outlining key considerations during the exploration of patient history, physical examination, and diagnostic testing. Differentiating between potential systemic versus localized causes of edema is emphasized as a central goal throughout the diagnostic process.

HISTORY

Essentials of patient history include medications, patient or family comorbidities related to potential systemic or localized causes, prior surgeries or cancer treatments, and patient-reported symptoms of pain or positional or temporal changes to edema.

PHYSICAL EXAMINATION

Essentials of the physical examination include observation of unilateral versus bilateral swelling, size and dimension of lymphedematous limbs, skin changes, signs of systemic (cardiac, hepatic, renal) or venous causes, and duplex ultrasound examination when venous causes are suspected. The section concludes with a brief review of the goals of efficient diagnostic testing to explore systemic causes of edema.

TREATMENT AND SURVEILLANCE

This chapter concludes with an emphasis on the importance of ongoing surveillance after treatment to track edema progression and, if needed, continuing evaluation of systemic or localized causes.

INTRODUCTION

Edema is swelling caused by an increase in interstitial fluid volume. Peripheral edema, which usually occurs in the lower extremities, is a common problem presenting to primary care physicians, who frequently refer these patients to vascular specialists. Edema persisting for ≤72 hours is considered acute. This chapter will focus on the differential diagnosis of chronic peripheral edema, which is defined as fluid accumulation in the extremities that persist for >3 months.

Though chronic peripheral edema is a dire outcome for patients, with frequently devastating consequences for their physical, social, and psychological well-being,[1,2] it remains widely misunderstood and underrecognized in clinical practice.[3,4] Differential diagnosis of this condition requires an understanding of its pathophysiology, beginning with the modern view of capillary fluid exchange. Recent epidemiological data are also useful to the clinician, as it underscores the importance of exploring the potential role of venous disease—the predominant cause of chronic peripheral edema—during diagnosis. This chapter begins with a review of these topics, followed by a systematic approach to differential diagnosis.

PATHOPHYSIOLOGY [FIGURE 23-1]

Edema develops when the rate of capillary and venular filtration into the interstitial spaces in tissue exceeds the rate of lymphatic drainage of this fluid for a sustained period. Edema can result from:

- *increased capillary filtration* due to increased hydrostatic pressure, reduced plasma oncotic pressure, or increased capillary permeability, or
- *reduced fluid drainage* due to lymphatic insufficiency.

These phenomena may occur separately, simultaneously, or sequentially. This simple model of the pathophysiology of chronic edema is based on a major revision of the traditional Starling principle[5] of venous-lymphatic fluid exchange. Causes of edema may be categorized as systemic or localized.

THE STARLING PRINCIPLE AND ITS REVISION

Traditionally, it was thought that venous reabsorption accounted for most interstitial-fluid drainage (the Starling principle). In his seminal research,[5] Ernest Starling infused isotonic saline into the interstitial compartment of a dog's hind limb; the fluid appeared in the venous blood as it became hemodiluted. By contrast, when serum instead of saline was injected the fluid was not absorbed. Starling concluded that the walls of the capillary and postcapillary venules are semipermeable membranes and that fluid exchange across the capillary depends on the balance between the osmotic (pulling in) absorption pressure of the plasma proteins, usually defined as colloid osmotic pressure, and the capillary hydraulic pressure (pushing out) produced by the intraluminal blood pressure. According to this classic model, hydrostatic pressure on the arterial end of the capillary drives the filtration of fluid into the interstitial space, while oncotic pressure on the venular end reabsorbs 90% of the fluid. This classic representation of venous reabsorption is still widely referenced.

However, in 2004, Adamson and associates[6] demonstrated that the effect of capillary oncotic pressure on transvascular fluid exchange was much less than predicted by the original Starling model. Based on this discovery, Levick and Michel[7] provided a revision of the Starling model by establishing that capillaries push fluid into the interstitial space *along their entire length*, not just at the arteriolar-capillary junction. In this model, the intercellular cleft of capillaries fosters high local outward fluid velocity while the semipermeable layer of glycocalyx within the capillary blocks the effect of the osmotic pressure of plasma proteins, decreasing the return of fluid on the venular side of the capillary. Starling's theorized reabsorption of all interstitial fluid via the venules does not appear to take place. Rather, the interstitial fluid is returned to central circulation primarily via the lymphatic system.[8]

DELETERIOUS EFFECTS OF FLUID STASIS

It has long been known that fluid stasis is associated with inflammation, fibrosis, and infection,[3,9] as well as morphologic changes in both venous and lymphatic vessels[10,11]—a vicious circle that promotes increased edema and complications. Interstitial fluid stasis has also been associated with compromised adaptive immunity from impaired lymph flow and immune cell trafficking.[8,12] However, recent research suggests a more active role for dysfunctional lymphatics in the suppression of both adaptive and innate immunity. Research in animal models has demonstrated that accumulation of lymphatic fluid triggers adipogenesis and chronic inflammatory response of CD4+ T cells that in itself is both necessary and sufficient for the development of lymphedema.[13] Expression of Th2 cytokines and transforming growth factor-β1 contribute to increased fibrosis, reduced lymphangiogenesis, reduced lymph vessel pumping, and leaky lymphatics,[13] while increased infiltration of T-regulatory cells (Tregs) in lymphedematous extremities contributes to local immunosuppression.[14] Recurrent cellulitis is common in chronic edema, particularly of the lower extremities, regardless of edema etiology.[15,16] Cellulitis may be precipitated by fungal infections, which

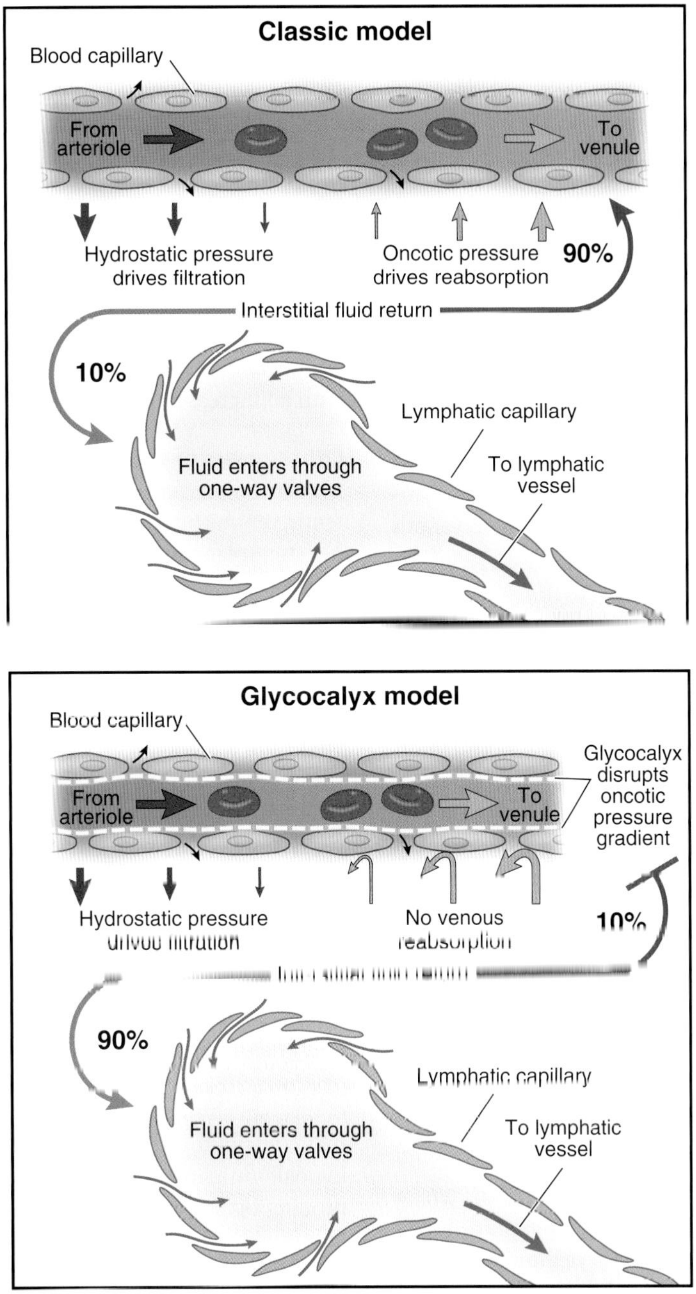

FIGURE 23-1 Revised Starling principle. In the classic model of fluid exchange,[5] osmotic pressure at the venular end of the capillary reabsorbs up to 90% of interstitial fluid for return into circulation. More recent evidence[7] suggests that the glycocalyx layer of capillary walls inhibits osmotic pressure effects from plasma proteins and decreases associated venous reabsorption. Thus, almost all interstitial fluid is returned to circulation via the lymphatic system.

provide an entry point for bacteria and secondary skin infections. Cellulitis damages the lymphatics and can be an independent cause of chronic edema.[17]

CAUSES OF INCREASED CAPILLARY FILTRATION

Increased Capillary Hydrostatic Pressure

Increased venous pressure In chronic venous disease (CVD), elevated pressure from valvular incompetence (reflux) and/or obstruction, often exacerbated by calf-muscle pump dysfunction, increases capillary hydrostatic pressure. Edema forms when the filtration of fluid overwhelms lymphatic drainage capacity. Edema secondary to venous disease (phlebolymphedema) is defined in the clinical classification of chronic venous insufficiency (CEAP) as Clinical Class III and higher.

Lipedema Lipedema, found exclusively in women, is characterized by a symmetric enlargement of the legs secondary to deposits of fat beneath the skin. Unfortunately, lipedema is frequently mischaracterized as obesity; however, the conditions are distinct, and the pathogenesis of lipedema remains unclear. A ready way to distinguish lipedema from obesity is the disproportion between the upper and lower extremities: Lipedema patients may have massive legs and a lean upper body. Differential diagnosis is aided by assessing waist–hip and waist–height ratios.[18] Obesity is distinguished by weight–hip ratios of >85 in women,[19] including for lipedema patients. However, waist–*height* ratios can distinguish patients with obesity and lipedema from patients experiencing obesity alone. Waist–height ratios that demark obesity are >50 for individuals aged under 40 years, between 0.5 and 0.6 for individuals aged 40 to 50 years, and 0.6 for individuals aged 50 years. Lipedema patients have thresholds below these levels.[18] In addition, lipedema usually presents following puberty or around pregnancy or menopause, suggesting a hormonal relationship. In lipedema, there is frequently a history of relatives with enlarged limbs.

Increased interstitial fluid in lipedema (lipolymphedema) is caused by elevated capillary hydrostatic pressure.[20] Indeed, lipedema is commonly mistaken for lymphedema, and while lymphatic dysfunction is found in both conditions they are markedly different. Skin color in unaltered lipedema is unchanged, even as skin loses elasticity. Swelling is bilateral but with symmetrical distribution and—in distinct contrast to lymphedema—there is a lack of swelling in the feet. Typically, lipedema presents with minimal pitting edema but pain and tenderness with easy bruising. While lymphedema starts distally and progresses up the limb, lipedema starts in the buttocks and thighs and moves downward. Unlike lymphedema, unaltered lipedema is not associated with an increased risk of cellulitis.[21]

Other causes of increased capillary pressure Ventricular failure (either one or both sides) causes systemic venous hypertension, that is, congestion of the hepatic, splanchnic, and peripheral circulations. Cirrhosis-related hypertension in the portal venous system can also contribute to lower-extremity edema. Obstructive sleep apnea may cause right-side pulmonary hypertension resulting in peripheral edema. Mild edema is common in pregnancy due to fluid retention, enlargement of the uterus causing vein compression, and/or hormonal changes.

Reduced Plasma Oncotic Pressure

An abnormally low level of plasma proteins (hypoalbuminemia), highly prevalent among critically ill and elderly hospitalized patients, reduces intracapillary osmotic pressure and thereby contributes to increased filtration and edema. Albumin loss in the kidneys (nephrotic syndrome, chronic kidney disease) or gut (protein-losing enteropathy), or a variety of mechanisms in systemic illness and cardiac failure, may contribute to hypoalbuminemia.[22] Uncommonly, hypoalbuminemia may result from decreased protein production secondary to chronic and advanced liver failure. Hypoalbuminemia is also associated with malnutrition, though research has challenged its association with general nutrition status.[23]

Increased Capillary Permeability

Inflammation and trauma increase vascular permeability, facilitating the passage of water and plasma proteins into the extracellular space (edema). A variety of drugs (e.g., calcium channel blocking agents) may also contribute to edema formation through their effects on permeability.[24]

CAUSES OF REDUCED LYMPHATIC DRAINAGE

Lymphedema This cause of edema will be discussed only briefly here because it is well-covered in another. Lymphedema (LED) has traditionally been defined as tissue fluid accumulation that arises from either inherited (primary) or secondary lymphatic drainage impairment.[25] The International Society of Lymphology (ISL) categorizes LED and peripheral venous insufficiency leading to leg swelling separately as conditions of "low-output failure" and "high-output failure," respectively.[26] Others consider any form of chronic edema to be lymphedema, regardless of its primary cause.[24] Indeed, primary LED; LED secondary to cancer treatment (surgery, radiation), trauma, or infection; and venous insufficiency edema present with symptoms and physical findings that are quite similar. The all-encompassing term "edema" is now used for extremity swelling.

OBESITY AS A CAUSE OF EDEMA

Obesity and body mass index (BMI) are known risk factors for developing postsurgical lower extremity edema,[27,28] and severely obese patients (BMI > 59) may develop lower extremity lymphedema spontaneously.[29] As the prevalence of obesity grows, obesity is increasingly recognized in clinical practice as a primary cause of leg edema in the absence of other risk factors.

The mechanisms that regulate leg edema in these patients are not clearly understood. Green and associates[29] have speculated that obesity may reach a threshold at which lymphatic drainage becomes impaired due to compression or inflammation or that elevated capillary pressure in an enlarging limb may overwhelm the lymphatics with the capillary filtrate. Obese cancer patients may have reduced lymphatic reserve prior to surgery or radiation.[30] Obesity also appears to impair the clearance of proinflammatory macromolecules in humans,[31] while preclinical studies have found that adipose tissue in obese mice can promote the abnormal recruitment and inflammatory responses of immune cells.[32] The fatty acids in static lymphatic fluid increase adipose deposition, suggesting a bidirectional relationship between adipose deposition and lymphatic dysfunction.[13]

EPIDEMIOLOGY

Estimating the incidence and prevalence of chronic peripheral edema is complex and is hampered by factors peculiar to this condition. These include frequent under-recognition or misdiagnosis of lymphedema/chronic edema by clinicians,[3,4] widely varying techniques for measurement and diagnosis,[33] and, as noted above, varying definitions of LED itself.

Chronic edema falls under several broad categories, including primary LED, LED secondary to cancer treatment, peripheral edema, and lipedema.[34,35] Primary LED is rare, affecting approximately 1 in 6000 to 10,000 patients.[36] Cancer-related LED, often cited as the most common LED in developed countries, affects approximately 4 million individuals in the United States.[35] In our analysis,[34] breast cancer-related LED was the most common cause of secondary LED, affecting 30% of 17,000 patients with chronic swelling. Pelvic cancers—ovarian, uterine, and cervical—accounted for 9% of cases. Peripheral edema associated with venous insufficiency was next in frequency at 10%, but this is most likely underrepresented because the data analysis based on insurance claims required assigning a specific diagnosis of edema to a patient with chronic venous insufficiency (CVI). Between 3% and 11% of the US population experience symptoms of venous edema, indicating that CVI in its advanced form is the most common cause of chronic peripheral swelling in the United States and developed countries. Lipedema is found in 11% of adult women.[20] Though the exact incidence of lipolymphedema as a primary cause of lower extremity edema is unknown, approximately 15% of women with lymphedema have lipedema as well.[37] Filarial lymphedema, the most common worldwide cause of LED, is not seen in developed countries.

CLINICAL DIAGNOSIS

Most experienced clinicians can diagnose chronic edema by history and characteristic findings on the physical examination. Diagnostic testing to explore potential systemic causes should also be routine during diagnosis. When there is doubt, a lymphoscintigram can be performed to assess lymphatic insufficiency, as recommended in the American Venous Forum guidelines (6.2.1).[38] A systematic approach to differential diagnosis (Figure 23-2) begins with an exploration of potential systemic causes.

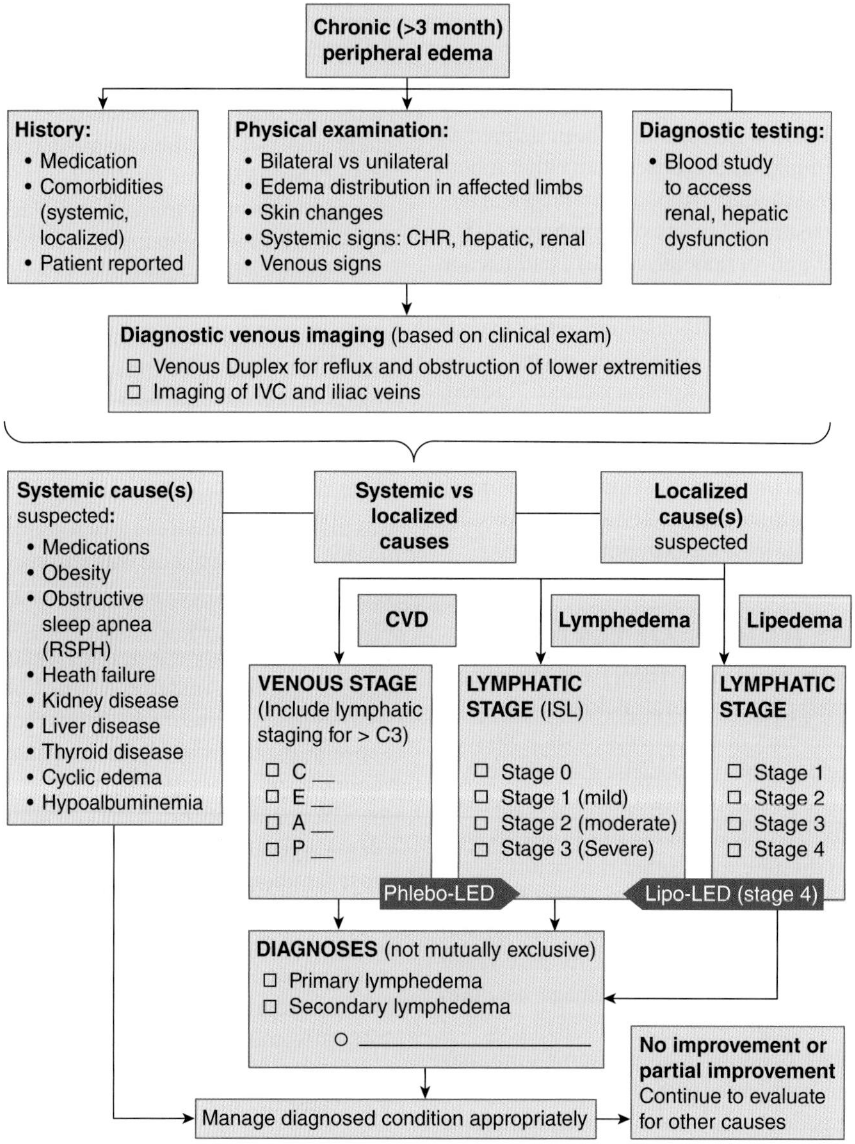

CHF, congestive heart failure; IVC, inferior vena cava; RSPH, right side pulmonary hypertension.

FIGURE 23-2 Differential diagnosis and clinical algorithm for peripheral edema. The diagnostic process begins with the exploration of patient history, physical examination, and diagnostic testing aimed at differentiating between potential systemic or localized causes of edema. The clinician must bear in mind that potential causes of chronic peripheral edema are not mutually exclusive and more than one causative factor may be present.

HISTORY

Systemic and localized conditions associated with edema are found in Table 23-1. Bilateral swelling is more likely to be related to a systemic cause and unilateral swelling to a localized cause (Table 23-2). Well-known systemic causes of edema include heart failure, hepatic disease, and renal disease; more recently, obstructive sleep apnea has also been identified as an edema etiology. Importantly, several commonly used medications are associated with chronic edema, so a review of medication history is essential.

Questions about cardiac disease should be aimed at uncovering symptoms of congestive heart failure, liver disease, or renal disease. Patients with sleep apnea can present with peripheral edema.

Unilateral edema and a history of deep venous thrombosis, outflow obstruction, or chronic venous insufficiency (including varicose veins) point toward a localized venous etiology. The patient should be queried for a family history of venous conditions. By contrast, if a patient has had oncologic surgery and/or radiation therapy, trauma, or recurrent infections, lymphedema secondary to these events may be suspected.

Patient Reported Symptoms

Positional or temporal changes Daily changes in swelling may provide clues to the cause of edema. For example, during the early stages, venous edema worsens over the course of the day due to dependency. Patients typically notice an intensifying tightness of their shoes. Swelling is reduced at night with elevation. By contrast, edema-associated right side pulmonary hypertension in obstructive sleep apnea may be worse in the morning.

Pain Pain is an important historical feature. While heaviness, aching, clumsiness of motion in the edematous limb, and even a bursting sensation are common in venous or lymphatic edema, intense pain is unusual unless there is an underlying episode of cellulitis. Acute pain may also be seen in unilateral swelling due to reflex sympathetic dystrophy, compartment syndrome, or trauma.[39]

PHYSICAL EXAMINATION

The diagnosis of lymphedema relies heavily on the physical examination. Although it is natural to focus on the site of edema, a complete physical examination should be carried out. As mentioned above, this is particularly important to rule out systemic causes. Congestive heart failure characteristically manifests as distended neck veins in a supine position, basilar rales on auscultation of the lungs, and an S-3 gallop on examination of the heart. Signs of liver disease include scleral icterus, a palpable liver, a distended abdomen with ascites, and palmar erythema. A venous etiology is suggested by distended veins in the lower abdomen indicative of potential outflow obstruction, prominent varicose veins in the limb, and pigmentary changes characteristic of advanced chronic venous insufficiency.

The dimension and shape of the edematous limb are characteristic. Swelling secondary to lymphatic deficiency often exhibits a pathognomonic increase in the tissue contour of the dorsum of the forefoot, producing a "buffalo hump." This physical sign is related to the fact that the anterior margin of the ankle joint may be spared out of proportion to the degree of the edema. There is usually a crease across the ankle joint and less edema distally at the metatarsal phalangeal joint line. This distribution of edema contrasts with that of congestive heart failure or venous insufficiency, where the edema is more severe in the dependent or ankle areas.[40]

Lymphedema pits in its early stages. As lymphedema progresses the degree of subcutaneous fibrosis and adipose deposition markedly increases, diminishing tissue compliance and preventing pitting. Lymphedema progression is also marked by skin changes. In the early stages of lymphedema, the skin has a salmon pink color, while lichenification and peau d'orange is observed in later stages. As chronic venous insufficiency progresses to CEAP clinical stage C-4A, eczema as well as cutaneous pigmentary changes are present and lipodermatosclerosis usually occurs. CEAP stages C-5 and C-6 are marked by healed and active ulcers, respectively. Table 23-3 summarizes the typical physical findings in a patient with edema due to CVI. Table 23-4 describes CVI risk factors.

TABLE 23-1 Pathology of Peripheral Edema

Increased Capillary Filtration				Decreased Lymphatic Drainage
Mechanisms	Increased capillary pressure (venous/arterial hypertension and/or increased intravascular volume)	Decreased osmotic pressure (hypoalbuminemia)	Increased capillary permeability	Impaired lymphatics
Systemic and medication-related causes	Venous hypertension: • Obesity • CHF (congestion of hepatic, splanchnic, and peripheral circulations) • Liver disease (portal hypertension) Arterial hypertension: • Obstructive sleep apnea Increased intravascular volume: • Pregnancy • CHF • Renal disease Medications: • Antihypertensives • NSAIDS • Corticosteroids • Hormones • Antidepressants	• Renal (nephrotic syndrome, CKD) • Gut (protein-losing enteropathy) • Cardiac failure • Liver failure • Malnutrition		Primary LED
Localized causes	Venous hypertension: • CVI • Venous outflow obstruction • Lipedema		• Inflammation • Trauma • Reflex sympathetic dystrophy (neurogenic)	• Cancer treatment • Trauma • Infection • Iliac vein compression from venous outflow obstruction or DVT • Malignancy

CHF, congestive heart failure; CVI, chronic venous insufficiency; DVT, deep venous thrombosis; NSAIDS, nonsteroidal anti-inflammatory drugs

TABLE 23-2 Side Predilection of Extremity Swelling

	Unilateral	Bilateral
Acute	• DVT • Cellulitis • Reflex sympathetic dystrophy • Compartment syndrome • Trauma • External venous compression	• Medications • Bilateral DVT
Chronic	• CVI • Postthrombotic syndrome • Secondary LED • Primary LED, esp. precox (female) • AV fistula • Malignancy • Klippel-Trenaunay syndrome	• CHF • Pulmonary hypertension • Lipedema • Renal/hepatic disease • Obesity • Hypoalbuminemia • Lipedema (feet are spared) • Primary LED, esp. precox (male) • Pelvic tumors • Bilateral CVI • Bilateral secondary LED

AV, arteriovenous; CVI, chronic venous insufficiency; DVT, deep venous thrombosis; LED, lymphedema.

(Data from Tretbar LL, Morgan CL, Lee BB, et al. *Lymphedema*. London: Springer-Verlag; 2008.)

TABLE 23-3 Symptoms and Signs of Chronic Venous Insufficiency (CVI)

Ankle edema	Lipodermatosclerosis
Pain and discomfort	Atrophie blanche
Cramps	Ulceration
Pruritus	Superficial thrombophlebitis
Eczema	Varicose vein bleeding
Hyperpigmentation	

TABLE 23-4 Risk Factors for Chronic Venous Insufficiency (CVI)

Risk Factors	Description
CVI with a history of DVT or varicose vein progression	An episode of DVT can damage both vein walls and valves, leading to reflux as well as obstruction by the occlusion of venous segments. Both mechanisms lead to venous hypertension.
Occupational	Occupations that require prolonged standing are associated with venous hypertension and secondary valvular incompetence. A study among Austrian workers—conducted in a compression stocking factory—found that edema in the legs increased between 10.2 mL and 220.3 mL after standing an average of 3.2 hours per day.*
Gender	The vein walls and valves of women are affected by cyclical changes in progesterone concentration. Pregnancy leads to an increase in blood volume and progesterone levels, particularly in the later trimesters.
Age	The incidence of CVI is greater in the older population. Age brings degenerative changes and atrophy of the smooth muscle in the vein wall, with subsequent dilatation.

*Partsch H, Winiger J, Lun B. Compression stockings reduce occupational leg swelling. *Dermatol Surg*. 2004;30(5):737-743.

Duplex Ultrasound in Clinical Diagnosis

As most lower-extremity edema has a venous cause, duplex ultrasound (DUS)—the vascular surgeons' stethoscope—is a critical study in patients with peripheral edema. DUS is utilized specifically to delineate changes in the venous anatomy and can help confirm a venous cause. Studies of valve function and superficial and deep venous systems, as well as studies of morphologic changes, can identify a previous episode of deep venous thrombosis. Changes in the deep venous system may also be marked by recanalization and total obstruction with collateral vessel formation.

As demonstrated by Suehiro and associates, DUS also allows for objective monitoring of edema progression and the progress of treatment.[41] Lower extremity edema typically shows as an epidermal entrance echo that is highly reflective and originates from the outer layers of the epidermis; this is related to alterations in impedance from the coupling medium to the stratum corium. The dermis is portrayed as a display of echoes with various intensities, related to the ultrasound beam reflecting off the interphase between collagen fibers. Finally, with ultrasound, the subcutaneous layer is characterized by either horizontally or obliquely oriented echogenic lines that are related to connected tissue bundles (Figure 23-3). Suehiro was able to correlate ultrasound findings with progressive stages of edema.[42]

DIAGNOSTIC TESTING

After the physical examination, a focused (not shotgun) approach should be taken to additional diagnostic testing. For patients suspected of having a systemic cause of edema, complete blood studies should be obtained to determine whether abnormal values are evident in renal (BUN, creatinine) or hepatic dysfunction (SGOT, SGPT, alkaline phosphatase, and bilirubin).

TREATMENT AND SURVEILLANCE

If a systemic cause of edema is suspected, the primary condition should be managed appropriately. If treatment yields no improvement or only partial improvement of edema, the patient should continue to be evaluated for other causes. It is important to bear in mind that peripheral edema causes are not mutually exclusive and more than one problem may be ongoing.

If chronic venous insufficiency is suspected as the cause of edema, the CEAP stage should be noted. ISL lymphedema staging should also accompany all designations of CEAP ≥ 3, as chronic edema characterizes CVI at this point. Lipedema should also be staged; the presence of lipolymphedema marks stage 4 of the disease.[37]

Again, these potential causes are not mutually exclusive. Differential diagnosis of peripheral edema tests the clinician's acumen in identifying multiple potential causes and how they may combine to produce this chronic condition. Ongoing observation of edema changes is needed to confirm or adjust the initial diagnosis and thereby to guide appropriate treatment.

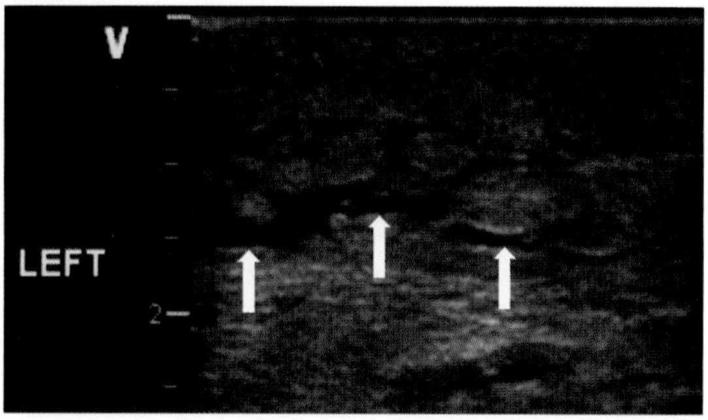

FIGURE 23-3 Longitudinal ultrasound image of the calf illustrating the horizontal anechoic bands (arrows) of subcutaneous edema. (Reproduced with permission from John Blebea, MD.)

REFERENCES

1. Fu MR, Ridner SH, Hu SH, Stewart BR, Cormier JN, Armer JM. Psychosocial impact of lymphedema: a systematic review of literature from 2004 to 2011. *Psycho-oncology*. 2013;22(7):1466-1484.
2. Taghian NR, Miller CL, Jammallo LS, O'Toole J, Skolny MN. Lymphedema following breast cancer treatment and impact on quality of life: a review. *Crit Rev Oncol Hematol*. 2014;92(3):227-234.
3. Farrow W. Phlebolymphedema-a common underdiagnosed and undertreated problem in the wound care clinic. *J Am Col Certif Wound Spec*. 2010;2(1):14-23.
4. Ridner SH, Rhoten BA, Radina ME, Adair M, Bush-Foster S, Sinclair V. Breast cancer survivors' perspectives of critical lymphedema self-care support needs. *Supp Care Cancer*. 2016;24(6):2743-2750.
5. Starling EH. On the absorption of fluids from the connective tissue spaces. *J Physiol*. 1896;19(4):312-326.
6. Adamson R, Lenz J, Zhang X, Adamson G, Weinbaum S, Curry F. Oncotic pressures opposing filtration across non-fenestrated rat microvessels. *J Physiol*. 2004;557(3):889-907.
7. Levick JR, Michel CC. Microvascular fluid exchange and the revised Starling principle. *Cardiovasc Res*. 2010;87(2):198-210.
8. Mortimer PS, Rockson SG. New developments in clinical aspects of lymphatic disease. *J Clin Invest*. 2014;124(3):915-921.

9. Kim D, Huh S, Hwang J, Kim Y, Lee B. Venous dynamics in leg lymphedema. *Lymphology*. 1999;32(1):11-14.
10. Bollinger A, Isenring G, Franzeck UK. Lymphatic microangiopathy: a complication of severe chronic venous incompetence (CVI). *Lymphology*. 1982;15(2):60-65.
11. Scelsi R, Scelsi L, Cortinovis R, Poggi P. Morphological changes of dermal blood and lymphatic vessels in chronic venous insufficiency of the leg. *Int Angiol*. 1994;13(4):308-311.
12. Ruocco E, Brunetti G, Brancaccio G, Lo Schiavo A. Phlebolymphedema: disregarded cause of immunocompromised district. *Clin Dermatol*. 2012;30(5):541-543.
13. Li CY, Kataru RP, Mehrara BJ. Histopathologic features of lymphedema: a molecular review. *Int J Mol Sci*. 2020;21(7):2546.
14. Nores GDG, Ly CL, Savetsky IL, et al. Regulatory T cells mediate local immunosuppression in lymphedema. *J Invest Dermatol*. 2018;138(2):325-335.
15. Ridner SH, Deng J, Fu MR, et al. Symptom burden and infection occurrence among individuals with extremity lymphedema. *Lymphology*. 2012;45(3):113-123.
16. Rodriguez JR, Hsieh F, Huang CT, Tsai TJ, Chen C, Cheng MH. Clinical features, microbiological epidemiology and recommendations for management of cellulitis in extremity lymphedema. *J Surg Oncol*. 2020;121(1):25-36.
17. Morris AD. Cellulitis and erysipelas. *BMJ Clin Evid*. 2008;2008:1708.
18. Reich-Schupke S, Altmeyer P, Stücker M. Thick legs–not always lipedema. *J Dtsch Dermatol Ges*. 2013;11(3):225-233.
19. Obesity: preventing and managing the global epidemic. Report of a WHO consultation. *World Health Organ Tech Rep Ser*. 2000;894:i-xii, 1-253.
20. Buck DW 2nd, Herbst KL. Lipedema: a relatively common disease with extremely common misconceptions. *Plast Reconstr Surg Glob Open*. 2016;4(9):e1043.
21. Fonder MA, Loveless JW, Lazarus GS. Lipedema, a frequently unrecognized problem. *J Am Acad Dermatol*. 2007;57(2):S1-S3.
22. Gounden V, Vashisht R, Jialal I. *Hypoalbuminemia*. Treasure Island, FL: StatPearls; 2020.
23. Soeters PB, Wolfe RR, Shenkin A. Hypoalbuminemia: pathogenesis and clinical significance. *JPEN J Parenter Enteral Nutr*. 2019;43(2):181-193.
24. Partsch H, Lee B. Phlebology and lymphology: a family affair. *Phlebology*. 2014;29(10):645-647.
25. Szuba A, Rockson SG. Lymphedema: classification, diagnosis and therapy. *Vasc Med*. 1998;3(2):145-156.
26. Committee E. The diagnosis and treatment of peripheral lymphedema: 2016 consensus document of the International Society of Lymphology. *Lymphology*. 2016;49(4):170-184.
27. Leray H, Malloizel-Delaunay J, Lusque A, et al. Body mass index as a major risk factor for severe breast cancer-related lymphedema. *Lymphat Res Biol*. 2020;18(6):510-516.
28. Armer JM, Ballman KV, McCall L, et al. Factors associated with lymphedema in women with node-positive breast cancer treated with neoadjuvant chemotherapy and axillary dissection. *JAMA Surg*. 2019;154(9):800-809.
29. Greene AK, Grant FD, Slavin SA. Lower-extremity lymphedema and elevated body-mass index. *N Engl J Med*. 2012;366(22):2136-2137.
30. Savetsky IL, Torrisi JS, Cuzzone DA, et al. Obesity increases inflammation and impairs lymphatic function in a mouse model of lymphedema. *Am J Physiol Heart Circ Physiol*. 2014;307(2):H165-H172.
31. Arngrim N, Simonsen L, Holst JJ, Bülow J. Reduced adipose tissue lymphatic drainage of macromolecules in obese subjects: a possible link between obesity and local tissue inflammation? *Int J Obes*. 2013;37(5):748-750.
32. Zhou C, Su W, Han H, Li N, Ma G, Cui L. Mouse tail models of secondary lymphedema: fibrosis gradually worsens and is irreversible. *Int J Clin Exp Pathol*. 2020;13(1):54-64.
33. Fu MR. Breast cancer-related lymphedema: symptoms, diagnosis, risk reduction, and management. *World J Clin Oncol*. 2014;5(3):241-247.
34. Son A, O'Donnell TF Jr., Izhakoff J, Gaebler JA, Niecko T, Iafrati MA. Lymphedema-associated comorbidities and treatment gap. *J Vasc Surg Venous Lymphat Disord*. 2019;7(5):724-730.
35. Dean SM, Valenti E, Hock K, Leffler J, Compston A, Abraham WT. The clinical characteristics of lower extremity lymphedema in 440 patients. *J Vasc Surg Venous Lymphat Disord*. 2020;8(5):851-859.
36. Lee B-B, Andrade M, Antignani P, et al. Diagnosis and treatment of primary lymphedema. Consensus document of the International Union of Phlebology (IUP)-2013. *Int Angiol*. 2013;32(6):541-574.
37. Földi M, Földi E. Lipedema. In: Földi M, Földi E, eds. *Földi's Textbook of Lymphology*. Munich, Germany: Elsevier Health Sciences; 2006:551.
38. Peller P, Bender C, Gloviczki P. Lymphoscintigrapy and lymphangiography. In: Gloviczki P, ed. *Handbook of Venous Disorders: Guidelines of the American Venous Forum*. 3rd ed. Hachette, UK: Hodder Arnold; 2009:647.

39. Simonian SJ, Morgan CL, Tretbar LL, Blondeau B. Differential diagnosis of lymphedema. In: *Lymphedema*. New York: Springer; 2008:12-20.
40. Trayes KP, Studdiford JS, Pickle S, Tully AS. Edema: diagnosis and management. *Am Fam Physician*. 2013; 88(2):102-110.
41. Suehiro K, Morikage N, Murakami M, et al. Subcutaneous tissue ultrasonography in legs with dependent edema and secondary lymphedema. *Ann Vasc Dis*. 2014;7(1): 21-27.
42. Suehiro K, Morikage N, Murakami M, Yamashita O, Samura M, Hamano K. Significance of ultrasound examination of skin and subcutaneous tissue in secondary lower extremity lymphedema. *Ann Vasc Dis*. 2013; 6(2):180-188.

SELF-ASSESSMENT STUDY QUESTIONS AND ANSWERS

Questions

1. Peripheral edema is swelling in an extremity caused by an increase in interstitial fluid volume. To be considered chronic, peripheral edema has persisted for:
A. More than 24 hours
B. More than 72 hours
C. More than 1 month
D. More than 3 months

2. Edema in the periphery develops in the presence of all of the following except:
A. Increased hydrostatic pressure
B. Increased capillary permeability
C. Increased lymphatic drainage
D. Reduced plasma oncotic pressure

3. Increased capillary pressure can be contributed by all of the following except:
A. Hypoalbuminemia
B. Hypertension
C. Congestive heart failure
D. Nonsteroidal anti-inflammatory drugs

4. The revised Starling principle suggests that most interstitial fluid is:
A. Reabsorbed in the postcapillary venules
B. Reabsorbed by the lymphatic system
C. Fluid is extravasated at the arteriolar-capillary junction
D. Layer of glycocalyx assists in the reabsorption of fluid

5. Lower extremity edema in pregnancy is associated with all of the following except:
A. Fluid retention
B. Hormonal changes
C. Right-sided heart failure
D. Enlarged uterus causing vein compression

6. Clinical history and symptoms are important in the diagnosis of peripheral edema. Early signs and symptoms include all of the following except:
A. Leg swelling worsening through the course of the day
B. Sharp intense pain in the foot
C. Achiness of the entire leg
D. Heaviness of the extremity

7. Signs and symptoms of chronic venous insufficiency (CVI) include all of the following except:
A. Lipodermatosclerosis of the calf
B. Eczema along the leg
C. Ulcerations above the ankle
D. Bluish discoloration of the leg

8. The risk factor associated with the highest risk for the development of chronic venous insufficiency (CVI) is:
A. History of DVT
B. Occupation
C. Gender
D. Age

9. Initial evaluation of the patient with chronic leg edema should include:
A. Cardiac echo to evaluate for heart failure
B. CT of the pelvis for imaging of iliac veins
C. Duplex ultrasound examining vein valve function
D. MRI of the liver for hepatic dysfunction

10. Duplex ultrasound imaging of the legs can also identify subcutaneous edema. The characteristics of edema seen on ultrasound include:
A. Intra-dermal swelling
B. Separation of the superficial and deep fascia
C. Vertical anechoic (black) bands
D. Horizontal anechoic bands

SELF-ASSESSMENT STUDY QUESTIONS AND ANSWERS

Answers

1. D.
2. C.
3. A.
4. B.
5. C.
6. B.
7. D.
8. A.
9. C.
10. D.

SECTION III Arterial Disease

CHAPTER

24 Arterial Anatomy and Pathophysiology

Amy Felsted and Peter Henke

OUTLINE

INTRODUCTION
ARTERIAL ANATOMY
ARTERIAL PATHOPHYSIOLOGY
Atherosclerotic Disease
Aneurysmal Disease
Dissections
Intimal Hyperplasia

INTRODUCTION

The vascular system consists of a complex network of vessels designed to distribute oxygen, fluid, and nutrients to all tissues of the body and remove waste products from the tissue to be excreted from the body. When any component of the vascular system fails, the normal homeostasis is disrupted. Diseases of the arterial system can be particularly catastrophic and constitute the majority of many vascular surgeons' clinical practice. The most common arterial pathologies treated by vascular surgeons include atherosclerotic disease, aneurysmal disease, aortic dissections, and intimal hyperplasia. While distinct entities, each of these pathologies shares similar underlying pathobiological mechanisms, and they often occur synchronously. Optimal preoperative, intraoperative, and postoperative care for arterial disease requires an intimate understanding of arterial wall anatomy and hemodynamics as most arterial diseases progress in generally predictable patterns directly linked to changes in wall anatomy and subsequent alterations in hemodynamics. Knowledge of the basic anatomy and pathophysiology is important for the consideration of therapies (Table 24-1).

ARTERIAL ANATOMY

Each artery wall consists of three tunicae, or layers—the tunica intima, tunica media, and the tunica adventitia. Each layer is structurally distinct and has a unique role in vessel physiology.

On the luminal surface of the tunica intima is the endothelium—a continuous monolayer of endothelial cells. These cells play critical roles in vessel hemostasis, vasomotor tone, vascular thrombosis, and immunity.[1,2] Endothelial cells respond to both physical and chemical stresses at the vessel's luminal surface. They realign parallel to the shear stress on the vessel wall created by constant blood flow.[3] Shear stress also increases production of stress fibers and release of vasodilators by the endothelial cells. In contrast, circumferential stress on the vessel wall due to blood pressure oscillation with each heartbeat induces endothelial cell proliferation. The endothelial cell surface is coated with an antithrombogenic glycocalyx to prevent intraluminal thrombus in intact vessels.[4] The basal lamina of the intima contains significant amounts of collagen, laminin, and fibronectin, providing strength and distributing mechanical stress throughout the artery wall.[5–7] The internal elastic laminal, which separates the tunica

TABLE 24-1 Factors That Contribute to the Development and Progression of Atherosclerotic and Aneurysmal Arterial Disease

Risk Factor	Pro-Atherogenic	Pro-Aneurysmal	Treatment
Age	X	X	None
Male gender		X	None
Family history	X	X	None
Connective tissue disorders		X	Beta blockers and/or losartan
Smoking	X	X	Smoking cessation
Hypertension	X	X	Blood pressure control
Dyslipidemia	X	X	Statin therapy
Atherosclerosis	N/A	X	Treat underlying risk factors
Diabetes	X		Blood glucose control, especially metformin
Obesity	X		Weight loss
Sedentary lifestyle	X	X	Increase physical activity
Chronic inflammation		X	Treat underlying inflammatory disorders

intima from the tunica media is comprised primarily of elastic fibers. The internal elastic lamina serves as a barrier to the movement of macromolecules from in the blood across the vessel wall.[8] Defects in the internal elastic lamina contribute to intimal thickening as macromolecules accumulate in the intima.[9]

The tunica media is bounded luminally by the internal elastic lamina and abluminally by the external elastic laminal. It consists of vascular smooth muscle cells with elastin and collagen filaments surrounded by an extracellular matrix. The medial layer provides structural stability to the arterial wall. The prominence of elastic fibers within the media is greatest in the large proximal arteries, such as the aorta, iliac arteries, and brachiocephalic trunk, and allows them to distend significantly during systole, thereby dampening the oscillations in blood pressure on more distal vessels. More distal arteries have a higher ratio of smooth muscle cells to connective tissue and distend in response to peripheral blood demand via neurohormonal signaling.[10,11]

Beginning at the external elastic lamina and extending to the perivascular connective tissue, the tunica adventitia consists primarily of fibrous connective tissue. Its thickness varies greatly throughout the vascular tree, and it is most prominent in the large muscular arteries. The tunica adventitia contains nerves that contribute to vascular smooth muscle tone, and in vessels greater than 200 μm diameter, it also contains the vasa vasorum which provides nutrition to the adventitia and outer media.

ARTERIAL PATHOPHYSIOLOGY

ATHEROSCLEROTIC DISEASE

Atherosclerosis is a vascular disease in which lipid-rich plaques accumulate intima of arteries throughout the body, and it is the most common underlying pathophysiology treated by the modern vascular surgeon (Figure 24-1). The effects of systemic atherosclerosis manifest throughout the body in a wide range of disease states including myocardial infarction and angina pectoris, ischemic strokes and transient ischemic attacks, intermittent claudication and limb-threatening ischemia, and degenerative arterial

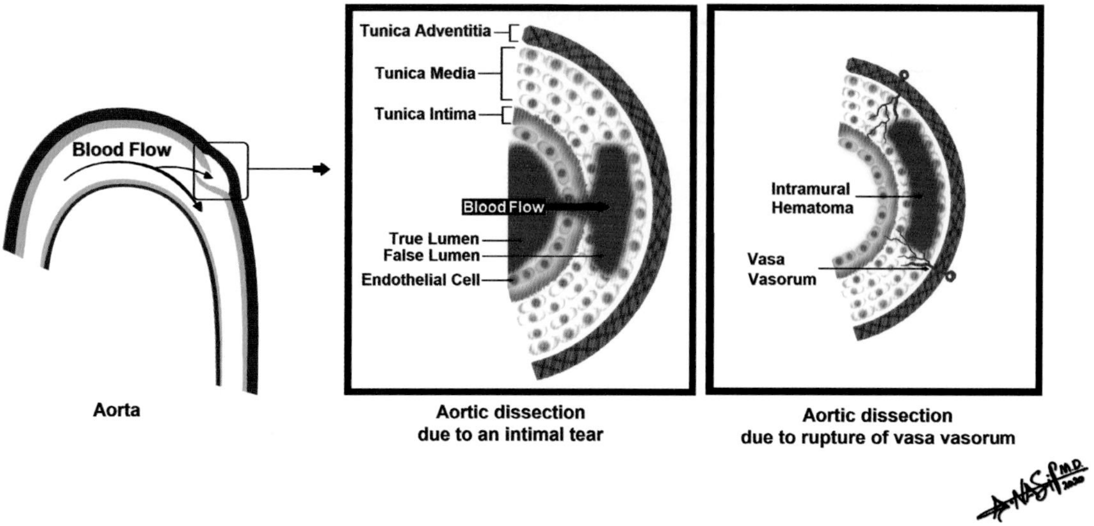

FIGURE 24-1 The pathophysiology of aortic dissection showing both dissection due to intimal tear and dissection sue to rupture of vasa vasorum. (Reproduced with permission from Abdullah Nasif, MD.)

aneurysms. Although the scientific and medical communities' understanding of the complex mechanisms contributing to the development and propagation of atherosclerosis and evolved considerably in recent years, atherosclerotic diseases continue to cause significant morbidity and mortality for our patients.

Excessive low-density lipoprotein (LDL) cholesterol and disorders of lipoprotein metabolism are required for the development of atherosclerosis.[12] Without LDL cholesterol levels beyond that needed for homeostasis, development of arterial fatty streaks by way of LDL cholesterol deposition in the vessel wall could not occur. However, despite the widespread use of statin therapy and popularity of low-fat and low-cholesterol diets, serum cholesterol levels in most of the general population far exceed physiologic needs.[13,14] The arteries of individuals with familial hypercholesterolemia are exposed to excessive levels of LDL cholesterol much earlier in life than the average population. These individuals also develop atherosclerotic lesions and clinically significant diseases much earlier in life.[15–18] In contrast, individuals with loss-of-function mutations of the *PCSK9* gene have increased LDL metabolism and consequently consistently low LDL levels. These individuals have decreased rates of atherosclerotic cardiovascular disease, suggesting that excessive LDL exposure is necessary for the development of atherosclerosis.[19,20]

In the most commonly held schemata of atheroma formation, excess circulating LDL cholesterol particles are deposited in the intima of the arterial wall. Once within the arterial wall, they are shielded from circulating antioxidants. These LDL particles become pro-inflammatory through a series of subsequent modifications, often including oxidation.[21] As the now inflammatory LDL deposits grow, they attract immune cells and additional pro-inflammatory cytokines to the region.[22] Among the cells that infiltrate the vessel's intimal layer in response to the pro-inflammatory cytokine are monocytes (which then can mature into macrophages and ultimately foam cells), T-cells, and smooth muscle cells from the medial layer of the vessel wall. Together with platelets deposited at breaks in the endothelial layer, this conglomerate of cells and deposited cholesterol form the atherosclerotic plaque. Over time, the plaques grow large enough to compromise blood flow through the vessel or may rupture and thrombose the vessel, resulting in clinically significant atherosclerotic disease.

There are likely several other mechanisms that contribute to the formation of atheromatous plaques. LDL cholesterol that has accumulated in the intima may directly enter resident vascular smooth muscle cells via LDL receptor-related proteins, and the lipid-laden cells develop into foam cells inside a plaque.[23,24] Triglyceride-rich lipoproteins and lipoprotein(a) have also been associated with the development of atherosclerotic lesions.[25] Systemic inflammation also likely plays a causal role in the process.[26] Several risk factors for atherosclerosis including tobacco use, hypertension, metabolic syndrome, and diabetes all induce inflammation.[22] Circulating inflammatory cytokines released at distant sites can activate the endothelial lining of vessels increasing their thrombogenic potential and causing immune cells to adhere to immature lipid plaques. Additional evidence supporting the role of inflammation in atherosclerotic disease is the presence of activated T lymphocytes found within atherosclerotic plaques.[27] CRP, a marker of inflammation, has also been found to predict cardiovascular disease and parallel other established risk factors for atherosclerotic disease.[28] The endothelium can also actively contribute to atherogenesis. When healthy, the endothelium is antithrombogenic and secretes vasodilators.[29] However, a high cholesterol diet can activate cellular adhesion molecules on the endothelial surface.[30,31] Aberrations in flow dynamics found at vessel bifurcations or caused by intraluminal thrombus and plaques further interrupt the normal antithrombotic and anti-inflammatory properties of the endothelium.[32] When combined with additional inflammatory risk factors for atherogenesis, the altered endothelium can promote initial plaque formation and propagation.

ANEURYSMAL DISEASE

An arterial aneurysm is defined as a focal dilation of all three layers of the artery wall to more than 150% of the normal vessel diameter.[33] While aneurysms can form anywhere throughout the arterial tree, most occur in the abdominal aorta, and among abdominal aortic aneurysms, the vast majority occur distal to the renal arteries. The primary significance of arterial aneurysms is that as the vessel dilates and the wall weakens, the risk of catastrophic aneurysmal rupture increases. In addition to aneurysmal rupture, the pieces of mural thrombus present in aneurysms can embolize leading to distal arterial occlusion and ischemia.

Most research on aneurysm pathobiology has been performed using tissue samples from ruptured or late-stage aneurysms at the time of surgical intervention. As such, our understanding of the pathophysiology involved is limited, especially in regard to the initiation and early stage progression of the disease. Tissue samples have demonstrated that arterial aneurysms are histologically characterized by oxidative stress and immune cell infiltration of the adventitia, loss of smooth muscle cells in the media, and degradation of elastin and collagen in the extracellular matrix.[34,35] While sharing several risk factors and traditionally thought to arise from atherosclerotic disease, newer data have demonstrated that aneurysmal disease is a separate pathology.[35–38]

Each of the hallmark characteristics of arterial aneurysms evolves through a series of events that positively reinforce each other (Figure 24-[illegible]). Intraluminal thrombus, which often first appears in relation to a fatty plaque or atheroma, also plays an important role in these events. One source of the oxidative stress and immune cell infiltration in the adventitia of the diseased vessel is directly from the intraluminal thrombus. Immune cells, including macrophages and neutrophils trapped within the intraluminal thrombus, are convected into the wall of the vessel where they release oxidases.[39] Additionally, ferrous iron derived from red blood cells sequestered in the intraluminal thrombus catalyzes the released oxidases, thereby accelerating oxidative stress in the vessel wall.[40] As immune cells accumulate in the vessel wall, they trigger the development of tertiary lymphoid organs around the vessel.[41] These structures, similar to traditional lymph nodes, respond to and generate antibodies against neoantigens created during oxidative stress. The neoantigens are then released into circulation and eventually reach their targets resulting in additional adaptive immune cell infiltration at the aneurysmal site.

Intraluminal thrombi also trap circulating bacteria, which recruits immune cells to the area. As neutrophils infiltrate the thrombus to neutralize the bacteria, they release neutrophil extracellular traps (NETs)—complex networks of chromatin and histones capable of sequestering oxidases needed to kill

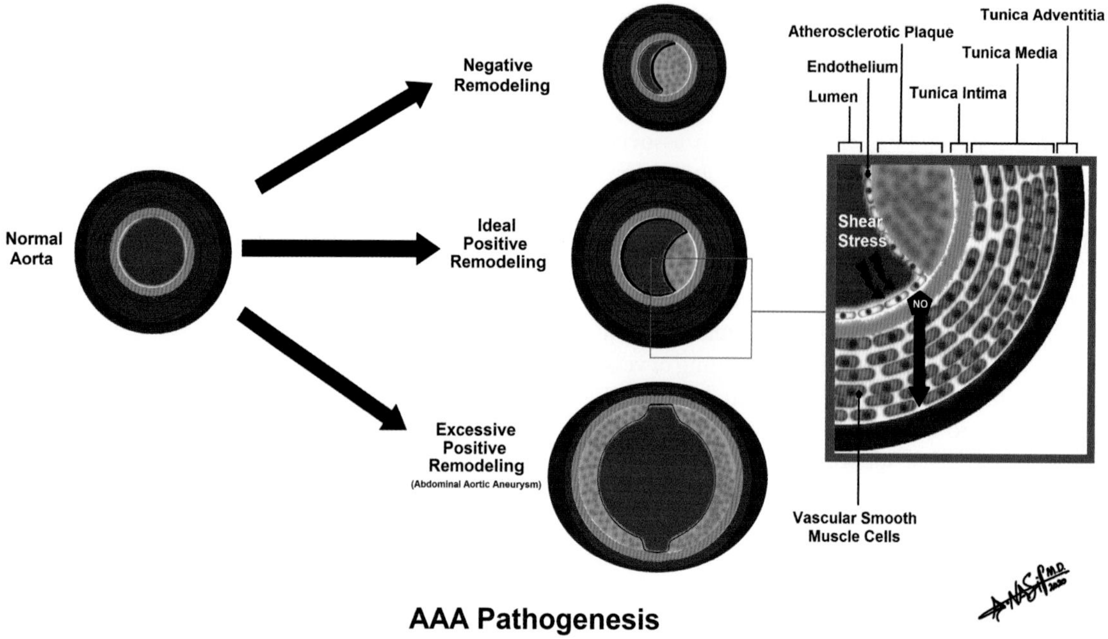

FIGURE 24-2 Figure depicts the pathophysiology of aneurysmal degeneration after aortic dissection. (Reproduced with permission from Abdullah Nasif, MD.)

bacteria. Both the oxidases and the byproducts of bacterial destruction are highly toxic to the vascular smooth muscle cells in the vessel wall. Finally, both circulating proteases and leukocyte-derived proteases are activated on the luminal surface of the intraluminal thrombus before being converted into the aneurysmal vessel wall where they directly degrade the vessel wall's extracellular matrix and induce vascular smooth muscle cell detachment and death.[42,43] These processes work in concert with each other, creating a cycle of inflammation, oxidation, and extracellular matrix degradation that decreases vessel wall strength leading to progressive dilatation and eventual rupture.

DISSECTIONS

Aortic dissections occur when there is loss of aortic wall integrity and bleeding into the medial layer resulting in the elevation of an intimal flap.[44] While the exact mechanisms underlying this pathology are not well understood, both intimal tears and vasa vasorum rupture (with bleeding into the medial layer) may initiate the acute dissection (Figure 24-3). Inflammation and extracellular matrix degeneration are the two most important factors leading to progressive arterial wall compromise and predisposing individuals to dissections.[45,46]

Several connective tissue disorders including Marfan's syndrome, Loeys-Dietz syndrome, and Ehler-Danlos syndrome increase the risk of aortic dissections and aneurysms.[47,48] Marfan's syndrome is caused by a mutation in the *FBN1* or *FBN2* genes, resulting in defects of the glycoprotein fibrillin.[49,50] This in turn leads to weakening of the elastic fibrils in the media and decreased arterial elasticity. Individuals with Marfan's syndrome classically have aortic root dilation and ascending aortic dissections which may become hemodynamically significant or rupture even in childhood. Mutations of the *COL3A1* gene encoding the peptide chains that form type III collagen lead to Ehler-Danlos type IV (vascular type).[51] These individuals have decreased arterial wall tensile strength due to less-stable collagen fibers. They are prone to arterial aneurysms, dissections, and arterial rupture. Unlike Marfan's syndrome and Ehler–Danlos syndrome, Loeys–Dietz syndrome is not caused by a single structural defect in the proteins of the extracellular matrix.

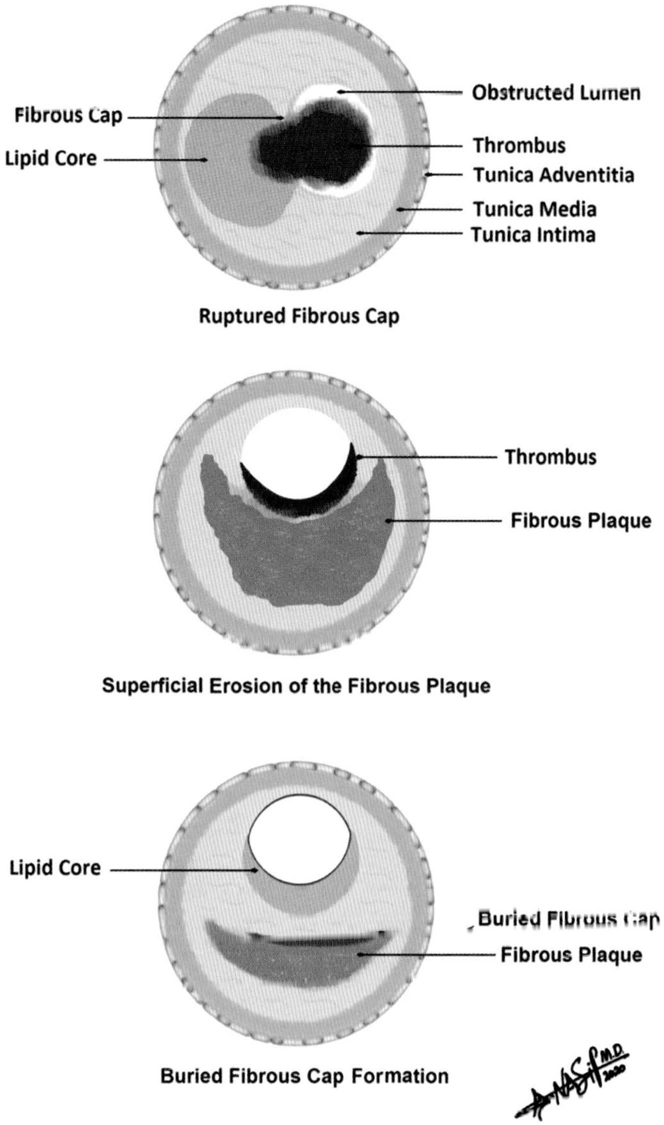

FIGURE 24-3 Figure depicts pathophysiology of aortic dissection. (Reproduced with permission from Abdullah Nasif, MD.)

Rather, it is caused by mutation of one of the several genes involved in TGF-β signaling.[49,52] These mutations lead to increased TGF-β signaling in the vessel wall and ultimately poor collagen formation and a weakened extracellular matrix. Individuals with Loeys–Dietz syndrome develop arterial aneurysms throughout the body and are at high risk of arterial dissections. Mutations of several other genes important to vascular extracellular matrix integrity including SMAD2, ACTA2, and LOX are also associated with arterial dissections, and ongoing research is investigating the roles of these genes in the mechanisms of arterial dissections.[53]

More commonly, aortic dissections occur in individuals without connective tissue disorders. Usually, they occur in the setting of hypertension, aortic aneurysms, and chronic vessel wall inflammation.

Atherosclerosis of the aorta leads to multifactorial aortic wall fragility.[54] Hypertension, and the inflammatory cytokine response it incites, superimposed on the atherosclerotic vessel, causes further degeneration of the vessel wall extracellular matrix and can lead to an intimal tear.[55] Additionally, the repeated trauma of the high-pressure systolic jet on the wall of the proximal aorta may contribute to the predisposition for dissections in the ascending aorta.[44]

INTIMAL HYPERPLASIA

Intimal hyperplasia is the pathologic thickening of the intimal layer of the vessel wall in response to injury.[56] The thickened intima is generally hypercellular and consists of both proliferating endothelial cells and vascular smooth muscle cells, which have migrated from the media and proliferate in the intima. Excessive deposits of extracellular matrix further increase the bulk of the neointima. The mechanisms underlying intimal hyperplasia and normal vessel healing are similar, and it can be difficult to distinguish an injured vessel that is developing intimal hyperplasia from one that will remodel appropriately.[57] Both denuding of the artery's luminal surface and direct injury to vascular smooth muscle cells in the media can result in intimal hyperplasia. When the subendothelial matrix is exposed to the vessel lumen, platelets bind and are activated, and the process of intraluminal thrombus formation begins. This in turn leads to endothelial cell proliferation and ultimately intimal hyperplasia. Similarly, injury to vascular smooth muscle cells leads to their migration into the intima where they can proliferate and lead to intimal hyperplasia.[58-62] Because angioplasty, endovascular stenting, and vascular anastomoses to both prosthetic and native vessels all cause endothelial and smooth muscle cell injury, intimal hyperplasia is a common complication of these interventions. Several therapies have been developed targeting specific components of the mechanism of intimal hyperplasia. While some, such as antiplatelet drugs, can decrease the rate and severity of intimal hyperplasia, there is still no therapy that will completely prevent or reverse pathologic intimal hyperplasia.[63,64]

REFERENCES

1. Sidawy AN, Sumpio B, Clowes AW, Rhodes RS. Basic science curriculum in vascular surgery residency. *J Vasc Surg*. 2001;33(4):854-860.
2. Aird WC. Phenotypic heterogeneity of the endothelium. II. Representative vascular beds. *Circ Res*. 2007; 100(2):174-190.
3. Helmlinger G, Geiger RV, Schreck S, Nerem RM. Effects of pulsatile flow on cultured vascular endothelial cell morphology. *J Biomech Eng*. 1991;113(2):123-131.
4. Levy BI, Tedgui A, eds. *Biology of the Arterial Wall. 1. Basic Science for the Cardiologist*. New York City, New York: Springer, 1999.
5. Wang CX, Shuaib A. Critical role of microvasculature basal lamina in ischemic brain injury. *Prog Neurobiol*. 2007;83(3):140-148.
6. Schnittler HJ, Franke RP, Akbay U, Mrowietz C, Drenckhahn D. Improved in vitro rheological system for studying the effect of fluid shear stress on cultured cells. *Am J Physiol*. 1993;265(1 Pt 1):C289-C298.
7. Laurent S, Boutouyrie P, Lacolley P. Structural and genetic bases of arterial stiffness. *Hypertension (Dallas, Tex.: 1979)*. 2005;45(6):1050-1055.
8. Sims FH. The initiation of intimal thickening in human arteries. *Pathology*. 2000;32(3):171-175.
9. Penn MS, Saidel GM, Chisolm GM. Relative significance of endothelium and internal elastic lamina in regulating the entry of macromolecules into arteries in vivo. *Circ Res*. 1994;74(1):74-82.
10. Wolinsky H, Glagov S. A lamellar unit of aortic medial structure and function in mammals. *Circ Res*. 1967; 20(1):99-111.
11. Hughes AD, Thom SA, Martin GN, et al. Size and site-dependent heterogeneity of human vascular responses in vitro. *J Hypertens Suppl*. 1988;6(4):S173-S175.
12. Goldstein JL, Brown MS. A century of cholesterol and coronaries: from plaques to genes to statins. *Cell*. 2015;161(1):161-72.
13. Hopstock LA, Bønaa KH, Eggen AE, et al. Longitudinal and secular trends in total cholesterol levels and impact of lipid-lowering drug use among Norwegian women and men born in 1905-1977 in the population-based Tromsø study 1979-2016. *BMJ Open*. 2017;7(8):e015001.
14. Schreiner PJ, Jacobs DR, Wong ND, Kiefe CI. Twenty-five year secular trends in lipids and modifiable risk factors in a population-based biracial cohort: the coronary artery risk development in young adults (CARDIA) study, 1985-2011. *J Am Heart Assoc*. 2016; 5(7):e003384.

15. Abifadel M, Varret M, Rabès J-P, et al. Mutations in PCSK9 cause autosomal dominant hypercholesterolemia. *Nat Genet.* 2003;34(2):154-156.
16. Maxwell KN, Breslow JL. Proprotein convertase subtilisin kexin 9: the third locus implicated in autosomal dominant hypercholesterolemia. *Curr Opin Lipidol.* 2005;16(2):167-172.
17. Allard D, Amsellem S, Abifadel M, et al. Novel mutations of the PCSK9 gene cause variable phenotype of autosomal dominant hypercholesterolemia. *Hum Mutat.* 2005;26(5):497.
18. Hallman DM, Srinivasan SR, Chen W, Boerwinkle E, Berenson GS. Relation of PCSK9 mutations to serum low-density lipoprotein cholesterol in childhood and adulthood (from The Bogalusa Heart Study). *Am J Cardiol.* 2007;100(1):69-72.
19. Verma DR, Brinton EA. Management of hypercholesterolemia for prevention of atherosclerotic cardiovascular disease: focus on the potential role of recombinant anti-PCSK9 monoclonal antibodies. *Rev Cardiovasc Med.* 2014;15(2):86-101; quiz 101.
20. Cohen JC, Boerwinkle E, Mosley TH, Hobbs HH. Sequence variations in PCSK9, low LDL, and protection against coronary heart disease. *N Engl J Med.* 2006;354(12):1264-1272.
21. Navab M, Ananthramaiah GM, Reddy ST, et al. The oxidation hypothesis of atherogenesis: the role of oxidized phospholipids and HDL. *J Lipid Res.* 2004;45(6):993-1007.
22. Miller YI, Choi S-H, Philipp Wiesner P, et al. Oxidation-specific epitopes are danger-associated molecular patterns recognized by pattern recognition receptors of innate immunity. *Circ Res.* 2011;108(2):235-248.
23. Borén J, Williams KJ. The central role of arterial retention of cholesterol-rich apolipoprotein-B-containing lipoproteins in the pathogenesis of atherosclerosis: a triumph of simplicity. *Curr Opin Lipidol.* 2016;27(5):473-483.
24. Llorente-Cortés V, Badimon L. LDL receptor-related protein and the vascular wall: implications for atherothrombosis. *Arterioscler Thromb Vasc Biol.* 2005;25(3):497-504.
25. Burgess S, Ference BA, Staley JR, et al. Association of LPA variants with risk of coronary disease and the implications for lipoprotein(a)-lowering therapies: a mendelian randomization analysis. *JAMA Cardiol.* 2018;3(7):619-627.
26. McMaster WG, Kirabo A, Madhur MS, Harrison DG. Inflammation, immunity, and hypertensive end-organ damage. *Circ Res.* 2015;116(6):1022-1033.
27. Ketelhuth DFJ, Hansson GK. Adaptive response of T and B cells in atherosclerosis. *Circ Res.* 2016;118(4):668-678.
28. Ridker PM. A test in context: high-sensitivity c-reactive protein. *J Am Coll Cardiol.* 2016;67(6):712-23.
29. Ignarro LJ, Napoli C. Novel features of nitric oxide, endothelial nitric oxide synthase, and atherosclerosis. *Curr Diab Rep.* 2005;5(1):17-23.
30. Cybulsky MI, Gimbrone MA. Endothelial expression of a mononuclear leukocyte adhesion molecule during atherogenesis. *Science.* 1991;251(4995):788-791.
31. Li H, Cybulsky MI, Gimbrone MA, Libby P. An atherogenic diet rapidly induces VCAM-1, a cytokine-regulatable mononuclear leukocyte adhesion molecule, in rabbit aortic endothelium. *Arterioscler Thromb.* 1993;13(2):197-204.
32. Gimbrone MA, García-Cardeña G. Endothelial cell dysfunction and the pathobiology of atherosclerosis. *Circ Res.* 2016;118(4):620-636.
33. Lawrence PF, Wallis C, Dobrin PB, et al. Peripheral aneurysms and arteriomegaly: is there a familial pattern? *J Vasc Surg.* 1998;28(4):599-605.
34. Michel JB. Contrasting outcomes of atheroma evolution: intimal accumulation versus medial destruction. *Arterioscler Thromb Vasc Biol.* 2001;21(9):1389-1392.
35. Biros E, Gäbel G, Moran CS, et al. Differential gene expression in human abdominal aortic aneurysm and aortic occlusive disease. *Oncotarget.* 2015;6(15):12984-12996.
36. Bobadilla JL, Kent KC. Screening for abdominal aortic aneurysms. *Adv Surg.* 2012;46:101-109.
37. Larsson E, Granath F, Swedenborg J, Hultgren R. A population-based case-control study of the familial risk of abdominal aortic aneurysm. *J Vasc Surg.* 2009;49(1):47-50; discussion 51.
38. Sakalihasan N, Defraigne J-O, Kerstenne M-A, et al. Family members of patients with abdominal aortic aneurysms are at increased risk for aneurysms: analysis of 618 probands and their families from the liege AAA family study. *Ann Vasc Surg.* 2014;28(4):787-797.
39. Delbosc S, Alsac JM, Journe C, et al. *Porphyromonas gingivalis* participates in pathogenesis of human abdominal aortic aneurysm by neutrophil activation. Proof of concept in rats. *PLoS One.* 2011;6(4):e18679.
40. Martinez-Pinna R, Lindholt JS, Madrigal-Matute J, et al. From tissue iron retention to low systemic haemoglobin levels, new pathophysiological biomarkers of human abdominal aortic aneurysm. *Thromb Haemost.* 2014;112(1):87-95.
41. Clement M, Guedj K, Andreata F, et al. Control of the T follicular helper-germinal center B-cell axis by $CD8^+$ regulatory T cells limits atherosclerosis and tertiary

lymphoid organ development. *Circulation*. 2015;131(6):560-570.
42. Michel JB. Anoikis in the cardiovascular system: known and unknown extracellular mediators. *Arterioscler Thromb Vasc Biol*. 2003;23(12):2146-2154.
43. Wang Q, Liu Z, Ren J, Morgan S, Assa C, Liu B. Receptor-interacting protein kinase 3 contributes to abdominal aortic aneurysms via smooth muscle cell necrosis and inflammation. *Circ Res*. 2015;116(4):600-611.
44. Hagan PG, Nienaber CA, Isselbacher EM, et al. The international registry of acute aortic dissection (IRAD): new insights into an old disease. *JAMA*. 2000;283(7):897-903.
45. Landenhed M, Engström G, Gottsäter A, et al. Risk profiles for aortic dissection and ruptured or surgically treated aneurysms: a prospective cohort study. *J Am Heart Assoc*. 2015;4(1):e001513.
46. Yin H, Pickering JG. Cellular senescence and vascular disease: novel routes to better understanding and therapy. *Can J Cardiol*. 2016; 32(5):612-623.
47. Milewicz DM, Regalado ES. Use of genetics for personalized management of heritable thoracic aortic disease: how do we get there? *J Thorac Cardiovasc Surg*. 2015;149(Suppl 2):S3-S5.
48. Ziganshin BA, Bailey AE, Coons C, et al. Routine genetic testing for thoracic aortic aneurysm and dissection in a clinical setting. *Ann Thorac Surg*. 2015;100(5):1604-1611.
49. Pyeritz RE. Recent progress in understanding the natural and clinical histories of the Marfan syndrome. *Trends Cardiovasc Med*. 2016;26(5):423-428.
50. Deng H, Lu Q, Xu H, et al. Identification of a novel missense FBN2 mutation in a Chinese family with congenital contractural arachnodactyly using exome sequencing. *PLoS One*. 2016;11(5):e0155908.
51. Pyeritz RE. Heritable thoracic aortic disorders. *Curr Opin Cardiol*. 2014;29(1):97-102.
52. Pyeritz RE, McKusick VA. The Marfan syndrome: diagnosis and management. *N Engl J Med*. 1979;300(14):772-777.
53. Loeys BL, Schwarze U, Holm T, et al. Aneurysm syndromes caused by mutations in the TGF-beta receptor. *N Engl J Med*. 2006;355(8):788-798.
54. Anzai A, Masayuki S, Jin E, et al. Adventitial CXCL1/G-CSF expression in response to acute aortic dissection triggers local neutrophil recruitment and activation leading to aortic rupture. *Circ Res*. 2015;116(4):612-623.
55. Boyle JJ, Weissberg PL, Bennett MR. Tumor necrosis factor-alpha promotes macrophage-induced vascular smooth muscle cell apoptosis by direct and autocrine mechanisms. *Arterioscler Thromb Vasc Biol*. 2003;23(9):1553-1558.
56. LoGerfo FW, Quist WC, Nowak MD, Crawshaw HM, Haudenschild CC. Downstream anastomotic hyperplasia. A mechanism of failure in dacron arterial grafts. *Ann Surg*. 1983;197(4):479-483.
57. Kocher O, Gabbiani G. Expression of actin MRNAs in rat aortic smooth muscle cells during development, experimental intimal thickening, and culture. *Differentiation*. 1986;32(3):245-251.
58. Clowes AW, Reidy MA, Clowes MM. Kinetics of cellular proliferation after arterial injury. I. Smooth muscle growth in the absence of endothelium. *Lab Invest*. 1983;49(3):327-333.
59. Clowes AW, Schwartz SM. Significance of quiescent smooth muscle migration in the injured rat carotid artery. *Circ Res*. 1985;56(1):139-145.
60. Hanke H, Strohschneider T, Oberhoff M, Betz E, Karsch KR. Time course of smooth muscle cell proliferation in the intima and media of arteries following experimental angioplasty. *Circ Res*. 1990;67(3):651-659.
61. Majesky MW, Schwartz SM, Clowes MM, Clowes AW. Heparin regulates smooth muscle S phase entry in the injured rat carotid artery. *Circ Res*. 1987;61(2):296-300.
62. More RS, Rutty G, Underwood MJ, Brack MJ, Gershlick AH. Assessment of myointimal cellular kinetics in a model of angioplasty by means of proliferating cell nuclear antigen expression. *Am Heart J*. 1994;128(4):681-686.
63. Bates ER, McGillem MJ, Mickelson JK, Pitt B, Mancini GB. A monoclonal antibody against the platelet glycoprotein IIb/IIIa receptor complex prevents platelet aggregation and thrombosis in a canine model of coronary angioplasty. *Circulation*. 1991;84(6):2463-2469.
64. Bates ER, Walsh DG, Mu D-X, Abrams GD, Lucchesi BR. Sustained inhibition of the vessel wall-platelet interaction after deep coronary artery injury by temporary inhibition of the platelet glycoprotein Llb/Llla receptor. *Coron Artery Dis*. 1992;3(1):67-76.

SELF-ASSESSMENT STUDY QUESTIONS AND ANSWERS

Questions

1. Endothelial cells on the luminal surface of the intima contribute to all of the following functions except:
A. Hemostasis
B. Vasomotor tone
C. Immunity
D. Respond to physical stress
E. Align perpendicular to shear

2. Of the following clinical risk factors, all contribute to atherosclerotic disease except:
A. Male gender
B. Dyslipidemia
C. Hypertension
D. Older age
E. Obesity

3. The following risk factors contribute to the development of arterial aneurysmal disease except:
A. Family history
B. Connective tissue disorders
C. Smoking
D. Diabetes
E. Chronic inflammation

4. The tunic media of arteries:
A. Serves as a barrier to macromolecules
B. Consists mostly of smooth muscle cells
C. Has more elastic fibers in peripheral vessels
D. Contains nerves to maintain muscle tone
E. Consists primarily of fibrous connective tissues

5. Of the lipid moieties thought to contribute to atherogenesis, the most causative is thought to be:
A. Total cholesterol
B. Triglycerides
C. Low-density lipoprotein (LDL)
D. Medium-density lipoprotein (MDL)
E. High-density lipoprotein (HDL)

6. For a focal arterial dilatation to be defined as an aneurysm, it must increase in diameter an additional:
A. 25%
B. 50%
C. 75%
D. 100%
E. 150%

7. Aortic dissections are causally associated with all of the following clinical conditions *except*:
A. Marfan's Syndrome
B. Loeys–Dietz Syndrome
C. Ehler–Danlos Syndrome
D. Steven–Sjogren Syndrome
E. Atherosclerosis

8. The process of intimal hyperplasia includes all of the following except:
A. Intimal thickening
B. Proliferating endothelial cells
C. Increased extracellular matrix
D. Smooth muscle hypertrophy
E. Adventitial fibrosis

9. Which of the following does not induce intimal hyperplasia:
A. Surgical bypass
B. Surgical endarterectomy
C. Balloon angioplasty
D. Endovascular stenting
E. None of the above

10. Which of the following is a true statement:
A. Longitudinal stress on the vessel wall induces endothelial cell proliferation.
B. The luminal surface of arteries is coated with a glycocalyx layer.
C. The internal elastic lamina contributes to intimal hyperplasia.
D. The external elastic lamina separates the intima from the media.
E. The vasa vasorum is located in the tunica media layer of arteries.

SELF-ASSESSMENT STUDY QUESTIONS AND ANSWERS

Answers

1. E.
2. A.
3. D.
4. B.
5. C.
6. B.
7. D.
8. E.
9. E.
10. B.

25 Abdominal Aortic Aneurysmal Disease

Richard A. Meena and Yazan Duwayri

OUTLINE

GENERAL CONSIDERATION AND HISTORY
- History of Aortic Aneurysm Disease
- Anatomy of Aortic Aneurysm Disease
- Pathophysiology of Aortic Aneurysm Disease

CLINICAL FINDINGS
- Signs and Symptoms

DIFFERENTIAL DIAGNOSIS

DIAGNOSIS

MANAGEMENT
- Indications for Repair
- Methods of Repair of AAA
- Open versus Endovascular Repair of AAA
- Postoperative Surveillance

GENERAL CONSIDERATION AND HISTORY

Aneurysmal degeneration of the aorta is defined as dilation of the blood vessel 1.5 times of or greater than its normal diameter.[1] Aortic aneurysms carry a significant risk of morbidity and mortality. The UK Small Aneurysms Study found that of 103 recorded ruptured abdominal aortic aneurysm (AAA), 25% died without even reaching the hospital.[2] Given this, understanding the etiology and diagnosis is of the utmost importance to avoid death from aneurysm rupture.

HISTORY OF AORTIC ANEURYSM DISEASE

Egyptian hieroglyphics illustrated arterial aneurysms thousands of years before year 1 A.D.[3] The Greek surgeon Antyllus was one of the first documented to have treated an aneurysm in the second century A.D.[4] John Hunter performed a successful ligation of the superficial femoral artery to repair a popliteal artery aneurysm in 1785.[5] In 1817, British surgeon Astley Cooper performed a successful aortic ligation, and on March 6, 1888, the first successful endoaneurysmorrhaphy was first described when Rudolph Matas repaired a brachial artery aneurysm.[4,6] Endoaneurysmorrhaphy involves opening the aneurysmal sac, removing clot, and suturing together the vessel walls to create a more normal arterial lumen. Roughly 60 years later, Charles Dubost successfully resected an AAA and replaced it with a homograft.[7] In the United States, Denton Cooley and Michael DeBakey performed a similar AAA surgery just months later.[4] In 1990, Juan Parodi and Julio Palmaz performed what we believe to be the first minimally invasive endovascular approach to repair an AAA in Argentina.[8] Endovascular techniques have since evolved to allow for complex aortic aneurysm repairs through sub-centimeter incisions in a patient's groins and/or arm.

ANATOMY OF AORTIC ANEURYSM DISEASE

The aorta is defined by its relation to the aortic arch and its branches. The ascending thoracic aorta refers to the aortic arch as it begins from the aortic valve to the takeoff of the innominate artery. The descending thoracic aorta refers to the thoracic aorta distal to the left subclavian artery and continues toward the diaphragm. The supraceliac aorta refers to the aortic segment between the diaphragmatic hiatus and the celiac axis. The aorta below the diaphragmatic hiatus is referred to as the abdominal aorta. The suprarenal aorta, or visceral aorta, refers to the aortic segment between the celiac axis and the renal arteries, including the superior mesenteric artery (SMA). Finally, the infrarenal aorta refers to the segment between the renal arteries and aortic bifurcation. Of note, the infrarenal aorta includes the origin of the inferior mesenteric artery (IMA), which arises around the level of the third lumbar vertebra. Normal measurements of the aorta are given in Table 25-1.[9]

In general, aortic aneurysms are often classified as the following: ascending, descending, suprarenal, pararenal, juxtarenal, and infrarenal. The locations of these aneurysms coincide with the aortic segments. Juxtarenal aneurysms, which comprise approximately 15% of AAAs, have their proximal extent next to the origin of the renal arteries but do not involve them and traditionally require at least suprarenal aortic cross-clamping during open repair to gain proximal control.[10] Pararenal aortic aneurysms involve the origins of the renal arteries and typically require supraceliac clamping for proximal control of the aorta.

Aneurysmal degeneration can occur in the setting of aortic dissection. Aortic dissection involves a tear in the intimal layer of the aorta that propagates along the length of the aorta. This creates a true lumen where blood is supposed to flow, and a new false lumen, or channel created by the intimal tear that allows blood to flow in a space where it did not previously flow. Given this weakened state of the aortic wall, subsequent degeneration can occur and create an aneurysm. The repair of these aneurysms is often more complex, as aberrant blood flow to branch vessels and multiple entry tears must frequently be addressed.[11]

TABLE 25-1 Normal Diameters of the Aorta, in Male and Female Patients

Aortic Segments	Average Diameter in Female and Male Patients (female/male, mm)
Ascending aorta	34/40
Descending aorta	28/32
Supraceliac artery	27/30
Suprarenal artery	27/28
Infrarenal artery	22/24
Aortic bifurcation	20/23

PATHOPHYSIOLOGY OF AORTIC ANEURYSM DISEASE

Several cellular processes have been identified as causative factors in the development and, potentially, rupture of aortic aneurysms. Many of these processes are associated with inflammatory changes. Inflammation contributes to degeneration of both smooth muscle cells in the aortic media and the connective tissue matrix that provides structure and support to vessel walls. Angiotensin II has been associated with monocyte mobilization, particularly in the suprarenal aortic segment, and neutrophils have been reported to augment elastase activity, promoting wall weakening and aneurysmal degeneration.[12] Proteolytic degeneration via macrophage-produced matrix metalloproteinases (MMP) has further been associated with aneurysm formation. In particular, MMP-2 and MMP-9 have been identified in higher concentrations in human tissue from aortic aneurysms.[13] Oxidative stress has long been considered a factor promoting aneurysmal degeneration, as has proteolytic inhibition of transforming growth factor (TGF)-beta.[12]

Several clinical risk factors have also been associated with aortic aneurysm development. As demonstrated in the Aneurysm Detection and Management (ADAM) trial, male birth sex is associated with aortic aneurysm formation, particularly AAAs.[14] Older age has further been associated with increased AAA risk; with each decade after 55 years of age, the risk of AAA diagnosis increases up to 4%.[15] Smoking has been associated with aortic aneurysm formation, given its association with inflammation and endothelial dysfunction.[16] In the aforementioned ADAM trial, "ever smoking" status was associated with an odds ratio of 5.1 for incidence of AAA.[14] Further, the relative risk for aortic aneurysm development in current smokers versus nonsmokers has been calculated anywhere from 2.5 to 8.9.[17] Family history of aortic aneurysm, particularly AAAs, is a strong clinical risk factor,[15] as arehypertension and obesity. White race has been associated with the development of AAAs, although it should be noted that many of the early studies evaluating the pathophysiology of AAAs included largely Caucasian cohorts.[18]

Several connective tissue disorders have been implicated in aortic aneurysm formation. Marfan syndrome is associated with defects in the fibrillin-1 protein.[19] Loeys–Dietz syndrome is associated with mutations causing overregulation of the TGF-beta signaling pathway. Ehlers–Danlos syndrome type 4, the vascular type, is associated with defects in collagen type III; up to 25% of patients with type 4 Ehlers–Danlos have aortic aneurysm disease.[20] These connective tissue disorders are particularly important, given their early presentation, potential familial implications, and impact on intervention of choice in these populations toward long-term durability.

CLINICAL FINDINGS

Because of their often-asymptomatic state, aortic aneurysms are frequently found incidentally on imaging obtained for an unrelated reason. One institution reports that AAAs were discovered incidentally in 1.0% of their abdominal computed tomography (CT) scans, abdominal magnetic resonance imaging (MRI) scans, and abdominal ultrasounds.[21] Further, some aneurysms have even been found incidentally on plain radiographic films due to calcific deposits in the walls of more chronic aortic aneurysms.[22]

Physical examination can also be used to diagnose aortic aneurysms. AAAs are more easily palpated on examination than thoracic aortic aneurysms, due to the rib cage. Unfortunately, physical examination is not reliable for the diagnosis of AAAs. Studies have shown that the pooled sensitivity of abdominal palpation for AAAs is quite poor (39% overall; 29% for AAA between 3.0- and 3.9-cm diameter, 50% for AAA between 4.0- and 4.9-cm diameter, and 76% for AAA greater than 5.0-cm diameter).[23] Specificity is also poor, estimated to be 75%.[24] Physical examination of the aorta in a lower BMI patient can be misleading, as well, as thinner patients' vasculature may be more easily palpated regardless of vessel diameter.

SIGNS AND SYMPTOMS

The spectrum of signs and symptoms associated with aortic aneurysms is large. The majority of patients with AAAs are asymptomatic at the time of presentation. However, because AAA can be clinically silent, patients can present with rupture.[25] This broad spectrum can make the diagnosis of AAA challenging.

In a large study of those undergoing open surgery, less than 20% of patients presented with a symptomatic AAA.[26] When symptomatic, patients with AAAs classically report abdominal, back, and/or flank pain. Tenderness over the aneurysm has also been described.[27] These symptoms can result from enlarging aneurysms compressing nearby tissue, including nervous tissue which can produce referred pain.[28]

DIFFERENTIAL DIAGNOSIS

The differential diagnosis for an AAA can be delineated based on a patient's hemodynamic stability. For patients who are hemodynamically unstable, life threatening diagnoses must be ruled out immediately. These diagnoses can include myocardial infarction, pulmonary embolism, and perforated viscus, particularly if the patient presents with abdominal, back, or flank pain. For the hemodynamically stable patient, the possible conditions are much broader (Table 25-2). Gastrointestinal diagnoses such as mesenteric bowel ischemia, bowel obstruction, pancreatitis, cholecystitis, and gastritis can present with similar symptoms. Musculoskeletal pain can also mimic the clinical presentation of an AAA.[18] Genitourinary diagnoses such as pyelonephritis, cystitis, and nephrolithiasis can further present with abdominal, flank, or back pain. Thus, a focused history, physical examination, and rapid decision-making are all important when an AAA is high on one's differential (Figure 25-1).

TABLE 25-2 Differential Diagnosis for the Hemodynamically Normal Patient with Abdominal Pain and Known Abdominal Aortic Aneurysm

Body System	Other Possible Diagnoses
Gastrointestinal	• Pancreatitis • Gastritis • Cholecystitis • Bowel obstruction • Mesenteric bowel ischemia • Large tumor overlying aorta
Genitourinary	• Cystitis • Pyelonephritis • Nephrolithiasis
Musculoskeletal	• Abdominal muscle strain • Disc herniation

DIAGNOSIS

If a clinician identifies a pulsatile abdominal mass on physical examination, especially a midline supraumbilical mass or one just lateral to midline in the left upper quadrant, there should be heightened concern for an AAA. Studies report that nearly 20% of patients with AAA also have popliteal artery aneurysms; therefore, a thorough lower extremity pulse examination should be performed in the same setting.[29]

Imaging should subsequently be obtained to assess if an aneurysm is present. Ultrasonography is an appropriate first choice in the hemodynamically stable outpatient to assess for the presence of an AAA in most circumstances, given its relatively low cost, ease of access, and noninvasive nature. Abdominal ultrasound has excellent sensitivity and specificity in diagnosing AAA (98.9% and 99.9%, respectively).[30] Even ultrasounds performed by non-radiologists have good pooled diagnostic sensitivity and specificity on systematic review (97.5% and 98.9%, respectively).[31] However, ultrasound does have its limitations. Not all segments of the aorta can be easily visualized. Additionally, if a patient is not fasting, bowel gas may obscure visualization of the aorta.[30]

Cross-sectional imaging can also be used to diagnose an AAA. Particularly when contrast-enhanced CT imaging has better spatial resolution and reproducibility than ultrasound. CT imaging does utilize ionizing radiation, however, and contrast should be used cautiously or avoided completely in patients with significant renal insufficiency.[32] Additionally, if patients have metallic implants in the abdomen or pelvis, streak artifact may impede visualization of the surrounding tissues.

MRI is another form of cross-sectional imaging that can be used to evaluate the aorta. Providers can use MRI if they desire better visualization of the aneurysm with a less nephrotoxic contrast agent, gadolinium. MRI is particularly beneficial in characterizing thrombus burden within an aneurysm. It should not be used in patients with large metallic implants, however, and both CT and MRI imaging cost significantly more than ultrasound.[32]

Given the concern for perioperative cardiac events in this patient population, there remains a great deal of debate as to the ideal preoperative assessment of these patients. Early data from the 1990s suggested that preoperative cardiac workup may not be necessary for this patient population.[33] Subsequent studies explored this controversial topic and suggested that routine use of transthoracic echocardiography (TTE) might reduce postoperative mortality in this cohort.[34] Follow-up publications have declared that TTE may be beneficial in intermediate- or high-risk patients, but it should not be used routinely for cardiac risk stratification.[35] Thus, standard practice today suggests that routine electrocardiography with or without TTE may be used in the preoperative assessment of intermediate- or high-risk patients (i.e., history of myocardial infarction, congestive heart failure, or known structural abnormality), both to establish a baseline for these patients prior to surgical intervention and to determine if additional workup is necessary.

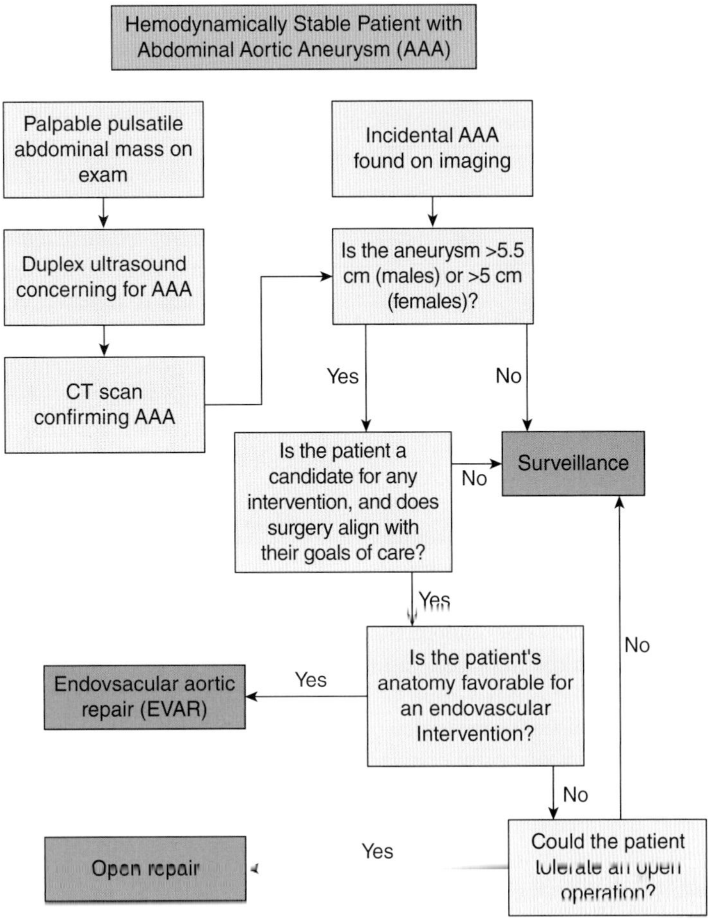

FIGURE 25-1 Flowchart describing potential workup algorithms for hemodynamically stable patients with abdominal aortic aneurysms.

MANAGEMENT

Unfortunately, there is no approved pharmacotherapy to slow aneurysm growth in humans. Initial animal models suggested beta-blockers, such as propranolol, could be used to stunt the growth of AAAs, but randomized controlled trials in humans with asymptomatic AAAs did not demonstrate the same effect.[36] Angiotensin-converting enzyme (ACE) inhibitors have also been studied, without beneficial effect on aneurysm size in humans.[37] Statins were associated with decreased major cardiovascular events after aneurysm repair, but they were associated neither with decreased AAA size nor with reduced need for AAA repair.[38,39] Doxycycline seemed to have significant promise, considering that it inhibits MMPs, but it did not definitively reduce aortic aneurysm growth in a randomized controlled trial.[40]

INDICATIONS FOR REPAIR

When determining whether a patient is an appropriate candidate for an elective AAA repair, the clinician must evaluate several clinical factors. Risk calculators have been established to assist providers in determining the appropriateness of surgery in these patients. The American College of Surgeons (ACS) National Surgical Quality Improvement Program (NSQIP)

TABLE 25-3 Risk of Rupture of Abdominal Aortic Aneurysms, Based on Diameter

Diameter of Abdominal Aortic Aneurysm (cm)	Annual Risk of Rupture
<4.0	0%
4.0–5.0	0.5%–5%
5.0–6.0	3%–15%
6.0–7.0	10%–20%
7.0–8.0	20%–40%
>8.0	30%–50%

has published a risk calculator for general operative intervention, considering demographic factors, comorbidities, disease severity, and current clinical status. Data have emerged suggesting generalized surgical risk calculators such as this one underestimate cardiac event occurrence in the high-risk vascular surgery patient. The Vascular Study Group of New England (VSGNE) has published a risk calculator that better estimates the risk of postoperative myocardial infarction in these patients, with calculators for both endovascular and open repair of AAA.[41] In general, aortic aneurysms have increased the risk of rupture with increasing diameter, which affects decision-making (Table 25-3). [42,43]

Determining when surgical intervention should be offered for AAA requires a risk-benefit analysis that balances risk of rupture with risk of repair. Based on consensus guidelines for asymptomatic AAA, size criteria for operative repair are the following: 5.5 cm or greater in maximal diameter in male patients, at least 5 cm in maximal diameter in female patients, and growth rate exceeding 1 cm in one year. As with other aneurysms, there is heightened concern for symptomatic AAA due to high risk of impending rupture, prompting more urgent repair for all symptomatic AAA.[44,45]

METHODS OF REPAIR OF AAA

For open AAA repair, the two most common approaches are transperitoneal and retroperitoneal. In the *transperitoneal approach*, the patient is positioned supine, and the abdomen is entered via a midline abdominal laparotomy. The distal infrarenal aorta and both iliac systems can be accessed easily via this approach; however, the bowel must be retracted and packed for more proximal access. For patients who have not had prior abdominal surgical intervention, the transperitoneal approach is a sound option. The *retroperitoneal approach* involves placing the patient in a right lateral decubitus position. The retroperitoneum is accessed via a left flank excision extended parallel to the rectus abdominus muscle. Once retroperitoneal contents are moved anteromedially, the surgeon can visualize the entire length of the aorta and the left common iliac artery. It is more difficult to access the right common or external iliac artery via this approach, however, and caution must be taken when attempting to expose the right common iliac artery and aortic bifurcation given the presence of the inferior vena cava and caval confluence. There is no difference in mortality between the transperitoneal and retroperitoneal approaches, but entering the intraperitoneal space can leave the patient more prone to bowel injury, prolonged ileus, bowel obstruction, and future hernias.[44]

Once dissection is complete, the aorta has been freed from surrounding tissue, and the patient is properly anticoagulated. Proximal and distal aortic clamps are subsequently placed. If a suprarenal clamp is needed, great effort should be made to limit clamp time, given risks associated with prolonged renovisceral ischemia and coagulopathy. If distal control cannot be obtained via clamping, balloon occlusion can be used. The aneurysm sac is opened, thrombus is removed, and lumbar vessels suture ligated. The aneurysmal segment is replaced, typically with prosthetic conduit (Figure 25-2). Once complete, the aneurysm sac can be enclosed around the new conduit.[44]

Open surgical repair of AAA does carry with it an increased risk of procedural morbidity and mortality. Incisional hernias are the most common postoperative complication after open surgery.[46] Postoperative renal injury and distal ischemia should be monitored, particularly after cases necessitating prolonged clamp time. Pneumonia can occur postoperatively, due to ventilator requirements in the operating room and decreased air movement in the

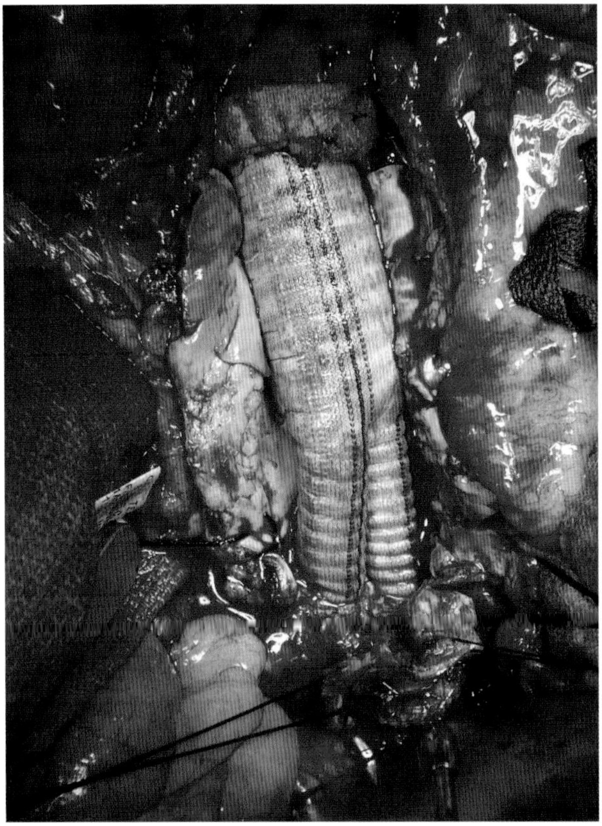

FIGURE 25-2 **Open aortic repair of abdominal aortic aneurysm with prosthetic graft.**

lungs secondary to postoperative discomfort.[44] The recovery process after open repair can be burdensome, so patients should be of adequate fitness prior to undergoing an open surgery.

Endovascular aortic repair (EVAR) utilizes stent grafts to redirect blood flow through the graft and thus exclude flow from the aneurysmal aorta. In order to obtain vascular access, either open exposure or percutaneous access of the femoral arteries can be used. Percutaneous access has been proven to be noninferior to open exposure,[47] but cutdowns may be needed in the setting of deep femoral arteries, circumferential calcification of the access vessel, if there is a need for concurrent endarterectomy, or if there is significant scar tissue in the groin. Proximal seal is necessary to prevent a type of IA endoleak (continued blood flow into the aneurysm around the proximal seal zone of the stent graft), as well as migration of the graft. Other pertinent endoleaks include type IB (via the distal seal zone), type II (via collateral vessels, such as lumbar vessels or the inferior mesenteric artery), type III (via a separation in graft components), and type IV (via fabric porosity). Continued surveillance postoperatively is imperative because sac expansion after endograft implantation can result in aneurysm rupture if not promptly addressed. If the distal components of the stent graft are not sized appropriately or kink, the graft could occlude, resulting in distal ischemia. Graft infection is a feared complication that typically requires an open explant of the stent graft with aortic replacement.

As the endovascular era progressed, endovascular techniques evolved. For a standard EVAR to be performed in an infrarenal AAA, certain anatomic criteria must be met to increase chances of deployment success and decrease chances of endoleak. First,

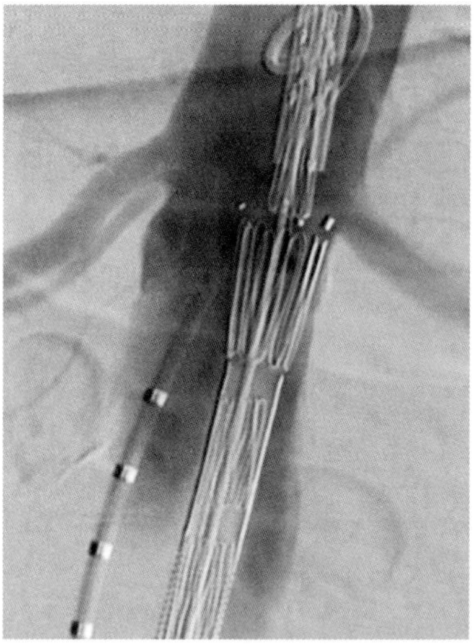

FIGURE 25-3 Endovascular aortic aneurysm repair with healthy neck.

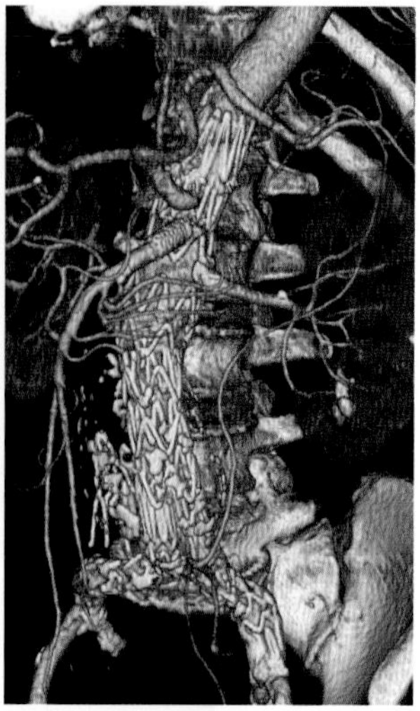

FIGURE 25-4 Fenestrated endovascular aortic repair with fenestrations in the main endograft and stents into each visceral and renal artery.

the neck of the aneurysm (the segment of the normal aorta between the renal arteries and proximal aneurysm) must be of sufficient length (Figure 25-3). Ideally, the infrarenal aneurysm neck should be 10 mm or greater, have minimal angulation (less than 60°), and must measure less than 32 mm in diameter to accommodate the largest abdominal endograft (36 mm) and to form an adequate proximal seal zone.[48] Newer endograft generations can seal in shorter infrarenal necks or in more angulated aortic anatomy. However, the high-risk features of hostile seal zones can lead to later graft migration or proximal endoleaks.

In order to address more challenging anatomy, including short neck lengths and juxtarenal aneurysms, surgeons can offer open repair or complex endovascular procedures that allow sealing within the visceral aorta. In these cases, aortic branches are accommodated in an endovascular fashion with customized graft fenestrations (Figure 25-4). Alternatively, parallel renal and visceral branch grafts, alongside a standard aortic endograft, can be used to extend the aortic seal zones more proximally. Customized fenestrated endografts delay aneurysm repair due to the need for individual graft design and manufacturing, which can take approximately 4 to 6 weeks and carries the risk of interval aneurysm rupture.[49] Fenestrated and branched endografts are available for the repair of complex aortic aneurysms but are not as widely utilized.

OPEN VERSUS ENDOVASCULAR REPAIR OF AAA

As technology in the endovascular era has advanced, numerous studies have been performed to compare open versus endovascular techniques. Four randomized controlled trials in particular have emerged as landmark studies comparing these techniques: OVER, DREAM, EVAR-1, and ACE.[44]

The OVER trial, published in 2019, randomized 881 patients with AAAs, 444 into the EVAR cohort, and 437 into the open repair cohort. There were no statistically significant differences in mortality between the two groups, although interestingly there was a trend toward improved survival for the EVAR cohort in the first 4 years of follow-up, versus improved survival for the open repair cohort between 4 to 8 years of follow-up. Patients undergoing EVAR required more secondary interventions.[50]

The DREAM trial randomized 351 patients with AAAs at least 5 cm in maximal diameter. Of these patients, 178 underwent an open repair while 173 underwent EVAR. After 6 years of follow-up, there were no significant differences in mortality, but

EVAR required more secondary interventions, similar to the OVER trial.[51]

The EVAR-1 trial randomized 1,252 patients in the United Kingdom with AAAs at least 5.5 cm in maximal diameter. A total of 626 patients were assigned to each cohort. Open repair was associated with a higher operative mortality, but there were no significant differences in long-term aneurysm-related or overall mortality between the two cohorts. EVAR was more costly, associated with more graft-related complications, and again required more secondary interventions.[52]

The ACE trial randomized 316 patients with AAAs greater than 5 cm in maximal diameter. Follow-up was 5 years in duration. There were no significant differences in survival, in-hospital mortality, or minor complications (which included minor cardiac complications, incisional complications, and buttock claudication). Again, as with the other studies, those patients in the EVAR cohort required more secondary interventions.[53]

As the endovascular technology continues to progress, and as more time passes with endografts implanted in patients, providers will accrue even more data to compare the long-term durability of the two techniques. Ultimately, clinicians must carefully review a patient's past medical and surgical history, current clinical status, anatomy, and goals of care before determining which technique to employ.

POSTOPERATIVE SURVEILLANCE

Equally important to a surgeon's perioperative care of a patient undergoing AAA repair is the surgeon's postoperative surveillance of the patient. After EVAR, surveillance is lifelong. The Society for Vascular Surgery (SVS) currently recommends that patients undergo CT imaging at 1 month and 1 year after surgery. If the 1 month imaging demonstrates an endoleak, a 6-month CT scan is recommended. After 1 year, if there is no evidence of endoleak on CT imaging, and if aneurysm sac size is stable, providers can consider duplex ultrasonography rather than CT imaging for surveillance, continuing at 1-year intervals. After open repair, noncontrast-enhanced CT imaging of the entire aorta at 5-year intervals is sufficient, given no need to surveil for endoleak.[45]

REFERENCES

1. Johnston K, Rutherford R, Tilson M, Shah M, Hollier L, Stanley J. Suggested standards for reporting on arterial aneurysms. Subcommittee on reporting standards for arterial aneurysms, ad hoc committee on reporting standards, society for vascular surgery and North American chapter, international society for cardiovascular surgery. *J Vasc Surg*. 1991;13:452-458.
2. Brown L, Powell J. Risk factors for aneurysm rupture in patients kept under ultrasound surveillance. UK small aneurysm trial participants. *Ann Surg*. 1999;230:289-296; discussion 296-297.
3. Cooley D. A brief history of aortic aneurysm surgery. *Aorta (Stamford)*. 2013;1:1-3.
4. Livesay J, Messner G, Vaughn W. Milestones in the treatment of aortic aneurysm: Denton A. Cooley, MD, and the Texas Heart Institute. *Tex Heart Inst J*. 2005;32:130-134.
5. Perry M. John Hunter—triumph and tragedy. *J Vasc Surg*. 1993;17:7-14.
6. Trotter MC. Rudolph Matas and the first endoaneurysmorrhaphy: 'A Fine Account of this Operation'. *J Vasc Surg*. 2010;51:1569-1571.
7. Dubost C, Allary M, Oeconomos N. Resection of an aneurysm of the abdominal aorta: reestablishment of the continuity by a preserved human arterial graft, with result after five months. *AMA Arch Surg*. 1952;64:405-408.
8. Ivancev K, Vogelzang R. A 35 year history of stent grafting, and how EVAR conquered the world. *Eur J Vasc Endovasc Surg*. 2020;59:685-695.
9. Wanhainen A, Themudo R, Ahlstrom H, Lind L, Johansson L. Thoracic and abdominal aortic dimension in 70-year-old men and women—a population-based whole-body magnetic resonance imaging (MRI) study. *J Vasc Surg*. 2008;47:504-512.
10. Jongkind V, Yeung K, Akkersdijk G, et al. Juxtarenal aortic aneurysm repair. *J Vasc Surg*. 2010;52:760-767.
11. Bannazadeh M, Adeyemo A, Munoz Y, et al. Aneurysmal degeneration in patients with type B aortic dissection. *Ann Vasc Surg*. 2016;36:121-126.
12. Hong L, Daughtery A. Aortic aneurysms. *Arterioscler Thromb Vasc Biol*. 2017;37:e59-e65.
13. Longo G, Xiong W, Greiner T, Zhao Y, Fiotti N, Baxter T. Matrix metalloproteinases 2 and 9 work in concert to produce aortic aneurysms. *J Clin Invest*. 2002;110:625-632.
14. Lederle F, Johnson G, Wilson S. Abdominal aortic aneurysm in women. *J Vasc Surg*. 2001;34:122-126.

15. Singh K, Bonaa K, Jacobsen B, Bjork L, Solberg S. Prevalence of and risk factors for abdominal aortic aneurysms in a population-based study: the Tromsø study. *Am J Epidemiol.* 2001;154:236-244.
16. Kakafika A, Mikhailidis D. Smoking and aortic diseases. *Circ.* 2007;71:1173-1180.
17. Lederle F, Nelson D, Joseph A. Smokers' relative risk for aortic aneurysm compared with other smoking-related diseases: a systematic review. *J Vasc Surg.* 2003;38: 329-334.
18. Moxon J, Parr A, Emeto T, Walker P, Norman P, Golledge J. Diagnosis and monitoring of abdominal aortic aneurysm: current status and future prospects. *Curr Probl Cardiol.* 2010;35:512-548.
19. Radke R, Baumgartner H. Diagnosis and treatment of Marfan syndrome: an update. *Heart.* 2014;100: 1382-1391.
20. Meester J, Verstraeten A, Schepers D, Alaerts M, Laer LV, Loeys B. Differences in manifestations of Marfan syndrome, Ehlers-Danlos syndrome, and Loeys-Dietz syndrome. *Ann Cardiothorac Surg.* 2017;6:582-594.
21. Walraven C, Wong J, Morant K, Jennings A, Jetty P, Forster A. Incidence, follow-up, and outcomes of incidental abdominal aortic aneurysms. *J Vasc Surg.* 2010; 52:282-289.e1-2.
22. Buijs R, Willems T, Tio R, et al. Calcification as a risk factor for rupture of abdominal aortic aneurysm. *Eur J Vasc Endovasc Surg.* 2013;46:542-548.
23. Silverstein M, Pitts S, Chaikof E, Ballard D. Abdominal aortic aneurysm (AAA): cost-effectiveness of screening, surveillance of intermediate-sized AAA, and management of symptomatic AAA. *Proceedings.* 2005;18: 345-367.
24. Fink H, Lederle F, Roth C, Bowles C, Nelson D, Haas M. The accuracy of physical examination to detect abdominal aortic aneurysm. *Arch Intern Med.* 2000; 160:833-836.
25. Shreibati J, Baker L, Hlatky M, Mell M. Impact of the screening abdominal aortic aneurysms very efficiently (SAAAVE) act on abdominal ultrasonography use among medicare beneficiaries. *Arch Intern Med.* 2012;172: 1456-1462.
26. Biancari F, Heikkinen M, Lepantolo M, Salenius J. Glasgow aneurysm score in patients undergoing elective open repair of abdominal aortic aneurysm: a Finnvasc study. *Eur J Vasc Endovasc Surg.* 2003;26:612-617.
27. Nevala T, Perala J, Aho P, et al. Outcome of symptomatic, unruptured abdominal aortic aneurysms after endovascular repair with the Zenith stent-graft system. *Scand Cardiovasc J.* 2008;42:178-181.
28. Booher A, Eagle K. Diagnosis and management issues in thoracic aortic aneurysm. *Am Heart.* 2011;162:38-46.
29. Tuveson V, Lofdahl H, Hultgren R. Patients with abdominal aortic aneurysm have a high prevalence of popliteal arter aneurysms. *Vasc Med.* 2016;21:369-375.
30. Lindholt J, Vammen S, Juul S, Henneberg E, Fasting H. The validity of ultrasonographic scanning as screening method for abdominal aortic aneurysm. *Eur J Vasc Endovasc Surg.* 1999;17:472-475.
31. Concannon E, McHugh S, Healy D, et al. Diagnostic accuracy of non-radiologist performed ultrasound for abdominal aortic aneurysm: systematic review and meta-analysis. *Int J Clin Pract.* 2014;68:1122-1129.
32. Hong H, Yang Y, Liu B, Cai W. Imaging of abdominal aortic aneurysm: the present and the future. *Curr Vasc Pharmacol.* 2010;8:808-819.
33. D'Angelo A, Puppala D, Farber A, Murphy A, Faust G, Cohen J. Is preoperative cardiac evaluation for abdominal aortic aneurysm repair necessary? *J Vasc Surg.* 1997;25:152-156.
34. O'Driscoll J, Bahia S, Gravina A, et al. Transthoracic echocardiography provides important long-term prognostic information in selected patients undergoing endovascular abdominal aortic repair. *Circ Cardiovasc Imaging.* 2016;9:e003557.
35. Munoz D, Beckman J. Preoperative transthoracic echocardiography in abdominal aortic aneurysm. *Circ Cardiovasc Imaging.* 2016;9:e004505.
36. Propanolol Aneurysm Trial Investigators. Propranolol for small abdominal aortic aneurysms: results of a randomized trial. *J Vasc Surg.* 2002;35:72-79.
37. Bicknell C, Kiru G, Falaschetti E, Powell J, Poulter N; AARDVARK Collaborators. An evaluation of the effect of an angiotensin-converting enzyme inhibitor on the growth rate of small abdominal aortic aneurysms: a randomized placebo-controlled trial (AARDVARK). *Eur Heart J.* 2016;37:3213-3221.
38. Heart Protection Study Collaborative Group. Randomized trial of the effects of cholesterol-lowering with simvastatin on peripheral vascular and other major vascular outcomes in 20,536 people with peripheral arterial disease and other high-risk conditions. *J Vasc Surg.* 2007;45:645-654.
39. Ferguson C, Clancy P, Bourke B, et al. Association of statin prescription with small abdominal aortic aneursym progression. *Am Heart J.* 2010;159:307-313.
40. Mosorin M, Juvonen J, Biancari F, et al. Use of doxycycline to decrease the growth rate of abdominal aortic aneurysms: a randomized, double-blind, placebo-controlled pilot study. *J Vasc Surg.* 2001;34:606-610.

41. Moses DA, Johnston LE, Tracci MC, et al. Estimating risk of adverse cardiac event after vascular surgery using currently available online calculators. *J Vasc Surg.* 2018;67:272-278.
42. Brewster DC, Cronenwett JL, Hallett JW Jr, et al. Guidelines for the treatment of abdominal aortic aneurysms: report of a subcommittee of the joint council of the American Association for vascular surgery and society for vascular surgery. *J Vasc surg.* 2003;37:1106-1117.
43. Hiratzka J, Bakris G, Beckman J, et al. 2010 ACCF/AHA/AATS/ACR/ASA/SCA/SCAI/SIR/STS/SVM guidelines for the diagnosis and management of patients with Thoracic Aortic Disease: a report of the American College of Cardiology Foundation/American Heart Association Task Force on Practice Guidelines, American Association for Thoracic Surgery, American College of Radiology, American Stroke Association, Society of Cardiovascular Anesthesiologists, Society for Cardiovascular Angiography and Interventions, Society of Interventional Radiology, Society of Thoracic Surgeons, and Society for Vascular Medicine. *Circulation.* 2010;121:e266-e369.
44. Swerdlow N, Wu W, Schermerhorn M. Open and endovascular management of aortic aneurysms. *Circ Res.* 2019;124:647-661.
45. Chaikof E, Dalman R, Eskandari M, et al. The society for vascular surgery practice guidelines on the care of patients with an abdominal aortic aneurysm. *J Vasc Surg.* 2018;67:2-77.e2.
46. Lederle F, Freischlag J, Kyriakides T, et al. Long-term comparison of endovascular and open repair of abdominal aortic aneurysm. *N Engl J Med.* 2012;367:1988-1997.
47. Nelson P, Kracjer Z, Kansal N, et al. A multicenter, randomized, controlled trial of totally percutaneous access versus open femoral exposure for endovascular aortic aneurysm repair (the PEVAR trial). *J Vasc Surg.* 2014;59:1181-1193.
48. AbuRahma AF, Campbell JE, Mousa AY, et al. Clinical outcomes for hostile versus favorable aortic neck anatomy in endovascular aortic aneurysm repair using modular devices. *J Vasc Surg.* 2011;54:13-21.
49. Graves H, Jackson B. The current state of fenestrated and branched devices for abdominal aortic aneurysm repair. *Semin Intervent Radiol.* 2015;32:304-310.
50. Lederle F, Kyriakides T, Stroupe K, et al. Open versus endovascular repair of abdominal aortic aneurysm. *N Engl J Med.* 2019;380:2126-2135.
51. Bruin JD, Baas A, Buth J, et al. Long-term outcome of open or endovascular repair of abdominal aortic aneurysm. *N Engl J Med.* 2010;362:1881-1889.
52. United Kingdom EVAR Trial Investigators; Greenhalgh RM, Brown LC, et al. Endovascular versus open repair of abdominal aortic aneurysm. *N Engl J Med.* 2010;362:1863-1871.
53. Becquemin J, Pillet J, Lescalie F, et al. A randomized controlled trial of endovascular aneurysm repair versus open surgery for abdominal aortic aneurysms in low- to moderate-risk patients. *J Vasc Surg.* 2011;53:1167-1173.

SELF-ASSESSMENT STUDY QUESTIONS AND ANSWERS

Questions

1. From which segment of the aorta does the inferior mesenteric artery typically arise?
   A. Descending thoracic aorta
   B. Supraceliac aorta
   C. Suprarenal aorta
   D. Infrarenal aorta

2. Approximately what percentage of abdominal aortic aneurysms can be classified as juxtarenal?
   A. 5%
   B. 10%
   C. 15%
   D. 20%

3. Which of the following is not associated with increased likelihood of aortic aneurysm development?
   A. African American race
   B. Smoking
   C. Hypertension
   D. Male birth sex

4. Which connective tissue disorder associated with aortic aneurysm development is associated with a collagen type III defect?
   A. Marfan syndrome
   B. Ehler–Danlos syndrome
   C. Loeys–Dietz syndrome
   D. Churg–Strauss syndrome

5. The overall sensitivity of abdominal palpation in diagnosis of an abdominal aortic aneurysm is approximately which of the following:
   A. 40%
   B. 60%
   C. 80%
   D. 95%

6. The estimated annual rupture risk of abdominal aortic aneurysms between 5 cm and 6 cm in maximal diameter is the following:
   A. 0.5%–5%
   B. 3%–15%
   C. 10%–20%
   D. 20%–40%

7. Which of the following is *not* a criterion supporting intervention on an abdominal aortic aneurysm?
   A. 6-cm diameter in female patient
   B. Growth of rate 1.3 cm in the last 12 months
   C. Back pain attributed to aneurysm
   D. 4.2-cm diameter in female patient

8. A type II endoleak is blood flow into the aneurysmal sac from which of the following?
   A. Distal seal zone
   B. Fabric porosity
   C. Small aortic branch arteries
   D. Separation of stent graft components

9. In the ACE trial, open repair and endovascular aortic repair (EVAR) were found to have similar rates of all the below outcomes, except for one. Which of the following was higher in patients undergoing EVAR?
   A. In-hospital mortality
   B. Number of secondary interventions
   C. Overall survival
   D. Overall minor complication rate

10. Per the Society for Vascular Surgery guidelines on the care of a patient with an abdominal aortic aneurysm, when should you consider performing a 6-month computed tomography (CT) scan in the postoperative period?
    A. Always obtain a 6-month CT.
    B. Consider a 6-month CT if the standard 3-month CT is abnormal.
    C. Consider a 6-month CT if the 1-month CT demonstrated an endoleak.
    D. You do not need to obtain CT scans after an EVAR.

SELF-ASSESSMENT STUDY QUESTIONS AND ANSWERS

Answers

1. D.
2. C.
3. A.
4. B.
5. A.
6. B.
7. D.
8. C.
9. B.
10. C.

CHAPTER

26 Aortic Dissection

Charles DeCarlo and Matthew J. Eagleton

OUTLINE

GENERAL CONSIDERATIONS AND HISTORY
- Historical Background
- Anatomy and Classification
- Epidemiology
- Risk Factors
  - Hypertension
  - Inheritable Conditions
  - Pregnancy
  - Cocaine Abuse
- Genetic and Molecular Basis for Aortic Dissection
- Pathophysiology of Malperfusion

CLINICAL FINDINGS
- Signs and Symptoms of Acute Aortic Dissection
- Signs and Symptoms of Malperfusion

DIFFERENTIAL DIAGNOSIS

DIAGNOSIS
- Computed Tomography Angiography
- Magnetic Resonance Angiography
- Intravascular Ultrasound
- Other Imaging Studies
- Limitations

MANAGEMENT OF THE CLINICAL PROBLEM
- Uncomplicated Aortic Dissection
  - Medical Management
  - Endovascular Management
- General Techniques
  - Graft Selection and Sizing
  - Left Subclavian Coverage
  - Procedural Adjuncts, Access Considerations, and Timing
  - Procedural Steps
- Postoperative Complications

OPEN SURGICAL MANAGEMENT

COMPLICATED TYPE B AORTIC DISSECTION—RUPTURED

COMPLICATED TYPE B AORTIC DISSECTION—MALPERFUSION

ENDOVASCULAR MANAGEMENT
- Tevar
- Mesenteric/Renal/Iliac Stenting
- Percutaneous Fenestration
  - Operative Technique
  - Outcomes and Complications
- Emerging Endovascular Techniques: Stable (Petticoat) and Stabilise

OPEN MANAGEMENT
  - Open Fenestration
  - Operative Technique
  - Complications and Outcomes
- Open Bypass

CHRONIC AORTIC DISSECTION
- Tevar
- Open Thoracoabdominal Aneurysm Repair
- Branched and Fenestrated Endovascular Aortic Repair (B/Fevar)

GENERAL CONSIDERATIONS AND HISTORY

HISTORICAL BACKGROUND

Aortic dissection is not a new disease process. While accounts prior to its initial reporting have been retrospectively identified, aortic dissection was first described by Maunoir in 1802, as blood "dissecting throughout the circumference of the aorta."[1] The inception of the concept, however, is often attributed to Laennec, much due to his fame throughout Europe garnered by inventing the stethoscope, as he coined the term "Aneurysme dissequant"—i.e., dissecting aneurysm—in 1819.[1-3] It would not be until 150 years after being originally described that the first major milestone in the treatment of aortic dissection would be achieved by Michael DeBakey and his team, who described the surgical treatment of dissecting aneurysms.[4] The superiority of medical therapy for aortic dissection in patients who were not rapidly deteriorating was established by Wheat et al. in 1965.[5] Medical therapy soon became the standard of care for patients with Type B Aortic Dissections. The modern era of treatment for aortic dissection began in 1999 when two landmark papers published in the *New England Journal of Medicine* described the use, safety, and feasibility of thoracic endovascular aortic repair (TEVAR), along with other endovascular techniques, in acute, subacute, and chronic aortic dissections.[6,7] The history of aortic dissection has been defined by major treatment advances separated by long periods of time. However, with the recent surge in new technology and techniques, it is clear that the current era is one where treatment paradigms for aortic dissection are rapidly changing and will continue to do so.

ANATOMY AND CLASSIFICATION

Under normal circumstances, the lumen of the aorta is beset by the three concentric layers of the aortic wall: the intima, the innermost layer, the media, and the outer adventitia. Dissection occurs when a false lumen, that is blood flow between the intimal and adventitial layers, is formed, giving the aorta a "double barrel" appearance (Figure 26-1). This usually occurs via a tear in the intima followed by shearing of the aortic wall layers for a variable distance.

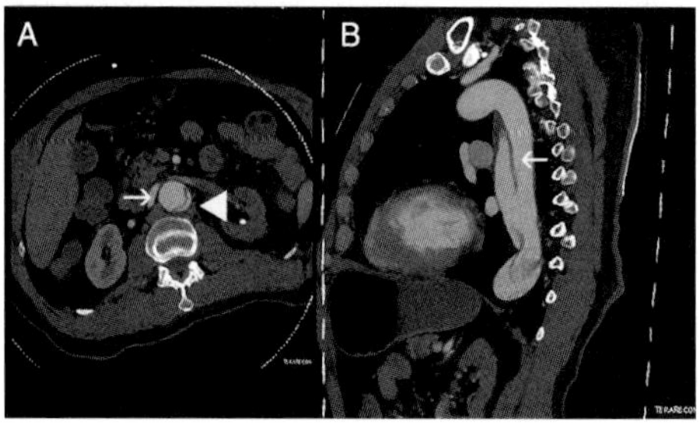

FIGURE 26-1 Computed tomographic (CT) images from a patient with an acute type B aortic dissection. (**A**) Note the false lumen (arrow) and true lumen (triangle). (**B**) The dissection flap (arrow) extends along the length of the aorta.

An alternative etiologic mechanism that has been postulated is the rupture of vasa vasorum causing an intramural hematoma, which subsequently ruptures into the aortic true lumen.[8]

Multiple anatomic classification systems have been developed to streamline communication between providers. The most common are the DeBakey and the Stanford Classifications (Table 26-1). The Society for Vascular Surgery (SVS) and the Society of Thoracic Surgeons (STS) have recently updated their reporting standards for aortic dissection with a new classification scheme.[9]

Noting the clear difference in outcomes between patients with ascending aortic involvement and those without, Daily et al. described the Stanford

TABLE 26-1 Classification Systems for Aortic Dissection

Stanford Classification
• Type A: Dissection involves the ascending aorta
• Type B: Dissection is confined to the descending aorta
DeBakey Classification
• Type I: Originating in the ascending aorta and continuing into the descending aorta
• Type II: Originating in the ascending aorta but confined to the ascending aorta
• Type IIIa: Originating distal to the left subclavian and confined to the descending thoracic aorta
• Type IIIb: Originating distal to the left subclavian and continuing into the abdominal aorta

Classification, based on the proximal extent of the dissection.[10] Given the proclivity for rupture into the pericardium, Daily et el. suggested prompt surgical treatment for type A dissections, with medical therapy reserved for type B dissections, as described by Wheat et al.[5] The Stanford Classification is the simplest and most widely used classification as it triages patients down two district treatment algorithms. While the scope of this chapter will be limited to type B aortic dissections, most of the concepts discussed herein also apply to type A dissections with involvement of the descending aorta (DeBakey Type I). The care of these patients is often undertaken by a multidisciplinary care team including both cardiac and vascular surgeons.

Debakey et al. described the first major classification system of aortic dissection in 1965.[11] Type I and II correspond to Stanford type A dissection and type IIIa and IIIb dissections correspond to Stanford type B dissections. An important and often overlooked flaw of the Stanford and the Debakey classification is that no classification scheme accounts for involvement of the aortic arch, between the innominate and the left subclavian artery. This scenario, best described as "type B dissection with arch involvement," has been shown to have similar outcomes as type B dissections, although complications from arch involvement can occur in up to 10% of patients.[12,13]

Published in March 2020, the Society for Vascular Surgery and the Society for Thoracic Surgery updated reporting standards to create a unified method to report on aortic dissection in detail, based on improved understanding of factors affecting outcomes and aforementioned limitations of other classification systems.[9] Dissections are expressed by a letter to describe the location of entry tear and one or two numbers as subscripts that describe the proximal and distal aortic involvement. The numbers correspond to zones of the aorta. A type A dissection is one with an entry tear in zone 0. Type A dissections are accompanied by a single numeric subscript given that the proximal extent must be zone 0. For example, a dissection with entry tear in the ascending aorta (zone 0) with extension into the infrarenal aorta (zone 9) would be denoted A_9. Type B dissections are ones with an entry tear in zone 1 or more distal and are accompanied by two numeric subscripts. For instance, a dissection extending from the ascending aorta to the infrarenal aorta with an entry tear just distal to the origin of the subclavian (zone 3) would be expressed as $B_{0,9}$. This example was used to illustrate that type A and B dissections within this classification scheme do not parallel Stanford type A and B dissections, as an SVS/STS $B_{0,9}$ is a Stanford type A dissection. When the location of the entry tear cannot be determined and the proximal extent is zone 0, the dissection is designated I with one numeric subscript. The goal of this classification scheme is to allow clinicians to visualize a precise image of the dissection. It is intended for research reporting and comparative effectiveness studies, not to replace the Stanford or Debakey classifications.

In addition to anatomic classification, dissections are also categorized by temporal classification, which plays an important role in prognosis and treatment:

- The **hyperacute** period is <24 hours, postdissection.[9]
- The **acute** period is the time period with the highest mortality rate after the hyperacute period and lasts up to 14 days after dissection.[9,14,15]
- The **subacute** corresponds to 15 to 90 days, postdissection. At this time, the rate of mortality drops, and remodeling of the aorta has not occurred, leaving the intimal flap pliable.[9,16,17]
- After 90 days, a dissection is deemed **chronic**. This is when mortality is the lowest and favorable or unfavorable remodeling of the aorta and intimal flap occur.[9,15]

A dissection can also be designated as complicated or uncomplicated. This is arguably the most important classification for type B dissection, as it determines prognosis and treatment algorithms. Specific complications are addressed below.

EPIDEMIOLOGY

Aortic dissection is the most common acute aortic syndrome, with an incidence of around 3 per 100,000 per year.[18–20] It is generally accepted that this is an underestimation of the true incidence, as comprehensive data on patients dying prior to receiving medical care does not exist.[21] Type B dissections account for 25% to 40% of all dissections.[22,23] Of type B dissections, about 25% are complicated dissections, associated with malperfusion or hemodynamic instability.[16] Males are disproportionally affected, with a ratio between 2:1 and 5:1.[23,24] The peak incidences of type B dissections are between ages 60 and 70 years, as opposed to type A dissections which most often occur between 50 and 55.[24]

RISK FACTORS

Hypertension

From the earliest series, hypertension is highly prevalent in patients presenting with aortic dissection.[11,23,25,26] A recent Swedish prospective cohort study, which measured outcomes over 20 years, found that patients with hypertension at initial evaluation had a significantly higher risk of aortic dissection; hypertension displayed an attributable risk of 54% within the population.[26] Hyperlipidemia and smoking also increase the risk of aortic dissection.[26]

Inheritable Conditions

Syndromes associated with aortic dissection include Marfan syndrome, Loeys–Dietz syndrome and vascular Ehlers–Danlos syndrome (EDS). Marfan syndrome accounts for 5% of all dissections and 50% of dissections in patients younger than 40 years.[27,28] Cardiac complications account for the majority of deaths in patients with Marfan syndrome and the risk of dissection increases as the aorta dilates.[29] Through surveillance and prophylactic aortic root replacement in the setting of dilation, life expectancy with Marfan syndrome has significantly improved since the 1970s.[30]

Loeys–Dietz syndrome is defined by aortopathy and characteristic craniofacial abnormality of a bifid uvula or cleft palate and hypertelorism.[31] Diffuse arterial tortuosity is the hallmark of the disease.[32] The threshold for aortic root replacement is generally 4.0 cm (as opposed to 5.0 in Marfan syndrome), as dissection has been reported at lower aortic diameters.[32]

Vascular EDS most often presents with arterial rupture, but aortic dissection does occur in a small proportion of patients.[33] Dissection has been demonstrated to occur in Turner's syndrome, but usually with underlying coarctation, bicuspid aortic valve, or both.[34] Nonsyndromic abnormalities associated with dissection include bicuspid aortic valve and familial thoracic aneurysms and dissections (FTAAD).[35] Bicuspid aortic valve, present in 0.5% to 1% of the population, is associated with aortic root dilation in 40% to 50% of cases and is present in 7% to 14% of aortic dissections.[23,35]

Pregnancy

The incidence of aortic dissection during pregnancy is four times the incidence in women who are not pregnant; however, the absolute risk is very low, affecting only 5.5 per million patients.[36] While the mechanism of this is not entirely understood, it is natural to postulate that it is related to the well-documented hemodynamic changes, such as increased heart rate, stroke volume, and cardiac output, that occur in pregnancy.

Cocaine Abuse

The use of cocaine has been associated with aortic dissection, although there is a paucity of research investigating it. Between 1% and 10% of aortic dissections occur in patients who have used cocaine.[37,38] Cocaine-associated aortic dissection usually occurs in younger, predominantly male patients. Dissection is likely mediated by the catecholamine-mediated rise in myocardial contractility and blood pressure, resulting in significantly increased first derivative of blood pressure (dP/dt) and shearing forces on the aortic wall.

GENETIC AND MOLECULAR BASIS FOR AORTIC DISSECTION

Via the study of genetically triggered aortic disease, several molecules have been found to play a role in aortic dissection. Marfan Syndrome displays autosomal dominant inheritance and is caused by a loss-of-function mutation of the *FBN1* gene, resulting in loss of functional fibrillin-1.[35] Fibrillin-1 plays an important regulatory role in the extracellular matrix, directing cellular functions and production of other matric elements.[39,40] It also normally binds transforming growth factor-beta (TGF-β); the mutation of fibrillin-1 results in an increase in bioavailable TGF-β and subsequent TGF-β signaling.[35] Mutations in the genes encoding TGF-β receptors 1 and 2 (*TGFBR1* and *TGFBR2*) and downstream signaling molecules have been shown to cause Loeys–Dietz syndrome, further supporting role of TGF-β in dissection and aneurysm formation.[41]

PATHOPHYSIOLOGY OF MALPERFUSION

Malperfusion is end-organ ischemia in the setting of aortic dissection; it can affect all vascular beds including those supplying the brain, spinal cord, viscera, kidneys, and lower extremities.[25,42] Prompt recognition and treatment are necessary as malperfusion significantly increases the mortality associated with aortic dissection due to the potentially catastrophic consequences.[43] Knowledge of the mechanism of malperfusion is critical to understanding the treatment algorithms. There are two types of obstruction that cause malperfusion: dynamic and static.

As it is pushed forward into the aorta by the left ventricle, blood flows into both the true and false lumen. The anatomy of the false lumen is the lumen enclosed on one side by the intimomedial flap and the other by the adventitia-bound outer aortic wall. The majority of the elastin in the aortic wall is contained in the intimomedial flap, making the flap compliant and the outer wall noncompliant.[44] According to the law of Laplace, in order to accommodate the wall tension produced by aortic blood pressure, the false lumen must dilate due to its lack of compliance.[44] This, along with elastic recoil of the intimomedial flap, results in variable compression of the true lumen. True lumen compression is also dependent on the proportion of aortic circumference that is dissected and the presence of a distal reentry fenestration in the flap.[45,46]

Dynamic obstruction can occur in two ways. First, severe compression of the true lumen by the false lumen due to a pressure gradient across the intimomedial flap; this limits flow from the true lumen to branch vessels. The second is related to the mobility of the intimomedial flap. The forces from variable expansion of the false lumen related to the cardiac cycle cause the flap to prolase into branch vessels, intermittently occluding flow.[45,47] As the name implies, dynamic obstruction is obstruction that fluctuates; pulse deficits may reflect that. It is the most common type, accounting for 80% of malperfusion.[48]

Static obstruction, formally defined as a pressure gradient between the aorta and a branch vessel, occurs with narrowing or occlusion of branch vessels.[47] This is usually facilitated by extension of the dissection plane into branch vessels. When branch vessel extension occurs, a few things may happen. First, the continuation of the aortic intimal flap into the branch vessel flap may be disrupted by shearing forces; this occurrence allows for perfusion of the branch vessel by the false lumen and is usually not associated with each organ ischemia.[45] Second, the extension of the false lumen into the branch vessel thromboses, leading to static narrowing or occlusion of the branch vessel.[44,49] The false lumen of the branch vessel is particularly susceptible to thrombosis due to exposed medio-adventitia and stasis in the blind end of the false lumen.[47] Third, reduced flow beyond the compromised branch ostium may result in thrombosis of the branch vessel. This can occur from a severely narrowed branch vessel lumen from false lumen thrombosis, a narrowed branch vessel lumen with concomitant dynamic obstruction, or obliteration of the branch vessel true lumen from false lumen forces. Malperfusion from static obstruction will often require direct revascularization as it is unlikely to resolve with true lumen expansion alone.

CLINICAL FINDINGS

SIGNS AND SYMPTOMS OF ACUTE AORTIC DISSECTION

The cardinal symptom of acute aortic dissection is pain, which is present in 95% of patients.[23,50] It is most often chest or back pain, but can also be accompanied by abdominal pain. It is classically described as ripping or tearing in quality but is more often reported by patients as sharp pain. The onset of pain is abrupt 85% of the time which can differentiate it from myocardial ischemia, which is often more gradual in onset.[23,51] Syncope can also be a presenting symptom and is more common in patients with tamponade and cerebral ischemia.[52] Patients with uncomplicated aortic dissection often have no appreciable signs on physical examination. The most common physical examination finding, when present, is a pulse deficit, which can be present in 15% to 20% of patients.[23,50] Type B aortic dissection patients are hypertensive 70% of the time, although patients can also present with hemodynamic instability, which portends worse outcomes.[50]

SIGNS AND SYMPTOMS OF MALPERFUSION

Malperfusion is a devastating complication of aortic dissection, and early recognition of its presence is essential. A malperfused vascular bed can often be identified with a thorough history and physical. Stroke, altered mental status, or syncope may indicate compromised arch vessels. Patients with malperfusion of the spinal cord can present with lower extremity neurologic deficits.[50] A comprehensive neurologic examination is mandatory: while full lower extremity paralysis can occur, the deficit can be limited to mild or moderate proximal muscle weakness. Abdominal pain, especially out of proportion of physical examination, can suggest mesenteric ischemia. Peritonitis may indicate compromised bowel. Renal malperfusion is mostly diagnosed from laboratory abnormalities and imaging. Pulselessness, pain, pallor, paresthesias, or poikilothermia indicates lower extremity malperfusion.[45,50] Signs and symptoms are key to diagnosing malperfusion, especially early malperfusion, as it may be missed by other diagnostic modalities. Aortic rupture is a rare but lethal complication of dissection.[50] Hemodynamic instability, altered mental status, and cardiovascular collapse can be associated with aortic rupture.

DIFFERENTIAL DIAGNOSIS

As chest pain is the most common symptom associated with aortic dissection, the differential should include myocardial infarction, pulmonary embolism, pneumothorax, pneumonia, myocarditis, and pericarditis. The probability of dissection is high in patients with chest pain (immediate onset, tearing character, or both), mediastinal/aortic widening on chest radiograph, and pulse/blood pressure discrepancy.[53] Axial aortic imaging is the gold standard for diagnosis of aortic dissection and should be pursued in any patient with the aforementioned symptoms or risk factors.[54] Other tests, such as EKG, chest radiograph, serum cardiac markers, arterial blood gas, echocardiography, and venous imaging can suggest alternative diagnoses, but none of them reliably rules out aortic dissection or should discourage aortic imaging when there is a high degree of clinical suspicion for aortic dissection.

It should be reemphasized that aortic dissection is a life-threatening condition and requires prompt evaluation and diagnostics. Delays in diagnosis and treatment can be fatal: It has been estimated that up 1% to 2% of patients die every hour until treatment is initiated for those patients presenting with type A aortic dissection.[23,55] Factors associated with delays in treatment include female gender, patients with atypical symptoms such as fever or lack of pain, patients who did not have a pulse discrepancy, or patients who did not initially present to a tertiary care center.[56] It is important to keep these factors in mind while evaluating patients with acute chest pain to prevent potentially life-threatening delays in treatment.

DIAGNOSIS

As no single sign or symptom is highly sensitive and specific for aortic dissection, imaging is required to confirm the diagnosis. Axial imaging is also able to demonstrate the extent of the dissection, the anatomic details and configuration of the dissection flap, the involvement of branch vessels, and the presence of complications such as thrombosis or rupture. Imaging modalities with the capability to diagnose aortic dissection include computed tomography angiography (CTA), magnetic resonance angiography (MRA), intravascular ultrasound (IVUS), transesophageal echocardiography (TEE), and aortic angiography. CTA is the most common and current "gold standard" for diagnosis, and MRA can be used when there are contraindications to CTA in highly stable patients. IVUS, TEE, and aortic angiography are most commonly used as an adjunct to intervention.

COMPUTED TOMOGRAPHY ANGIOGRAPHY

CTA is currently the modality of choice for imaging aortic dissections due to its fast acquisition times, ready availability in emergency rooms, high diagnostic accuracy, and ability to provide highly detailed images of the dissection flap and potential branch involvement. Sensitivity ranges from 83% to 94% and specificity ranges from 87% to 100% based on studies from the 1990s.[57] A modern meta-analysis, however, reported the sensitivity and specificity to be 100% and 98%, respectively, reflecting the improvement in technology over the past two decades.[58] The capability of standard CTA to detect aortic dissection in the ascending aorta is lower due to motion artifact. Classically, this was overcome through concurrent use of TEE; however, with modern ECG gating of CTA's which allow for precise imaging of the ascending aorta, this is no longer necessary.[59] Modern protocols, such as the Triple-Rule-out CTA, make CTA an even more useful imaging modality, as it can simultaneously exonerate other causes of chest pain by evaluating the coronary and pulmonary arteries.[60]

Important anatomic factors that prognosticate aortic dissection can be ascertained from CTA. The extent of the dissection, true lumen conformation, perfusion of branch vessels by true vs false lumen, extension of dissection into branch vessels, patency of false lumen, and aortic diameter are all important anatomic factors that should be considered on initial CTA. Concave formation of the true lumen is a sensitive finding for a pressure gradient across the dissection flap and is associated with a higher risk of dynamic obstruction.[47] Initial aortic size is associated with long-term complications and need for reintervention.[61,62] Patency of the false lumen is associated need for long-term reintervention, but partial false lumen thrombosis has also been shown to be a predictor of postdischarge mortality.[61–63] When the dissection plane extends into branch vessels, especially when associated with false lumen thrombosis, static obstruction is possible secondary to branch ostia narrowing.[44,47] Branches arising from the false lumen, however, are usually well perfused.[47] Patients with a concave, slit-like true lumen and/or narrowed branch ostia should be thoroughly evaluated for mesenteric, renal, and lower extremity malperfusion (Figure 26-2).

MAGNETIC RESONANCE ANGIOGRAPHY

The use of contrast-enhanced MRA in the acute setting is limited. The acquisition times are significantly longer, and patient monitoring is limited during acquisition. It also cannot be used in patients with implanted medical devices. It should be reserved for patients with severe contrast allergies who are stable and without signs of malperfusion in the acute setting.[59] MRA can be worthwhile for long-term surveillance, as it offers some advantages over CTA. The most notable advantage is the lack of ionizing radiation. As dissection can affect patients of any age, long-term monitoring for aneurysmal degeneration with MRA may be preferred in patients who develop aortic dissection at a young age to avoid excessive radiation exposure. While gadolinium-containing contrast agents are not appropriate for patients with renal failure due to the risk of nephrogenic systemic fibrosis, ferumoxytol, an iron-based contrast agent, is non-nephrotoxic and can be administered to patients with severe renal failure.[64–66] This may make MRA the preferred modality for long-term surveillance in renal failure patients to avoid administration of iodinated contrast.

INTRAVASCULAR ULTRASOUND

IVUS is a vital intraoperative adjunct (Figure 26-3). The ability of IVUS to identify entry tears, confirm wire position throughout the length of the true lumen, and confirm successful deployment of TEVAR is superior to angiography alone.[67] Multiple studies have reported on the potential benefits of IVUS, extending into the long-term, where the use of IVUS is associated with improved survival and aortic remodeling.[68,69] The ability of IVUS to confirm true lumen wire path and ensure safe graft deployment makes it the generally accepted standard of care for imaging prior to graft deployment.

OTHER IMAGING STUDIES

Transthoracic echocardiography can diagnose aortic dissection of the proximal ascending aorta but cannot adequately image the distal ascending aorta, aortic arch, or descending thoracic aorta.[70] Transesophageal echocardiography (TEE) can image more of the aorta and has a sensitivity and specificity of 99% and 89%, respectively.[71] TEE also has an excellent ability to detect complications of aortic dissection: it is the best modality to detect aortic regurgitation and gives a

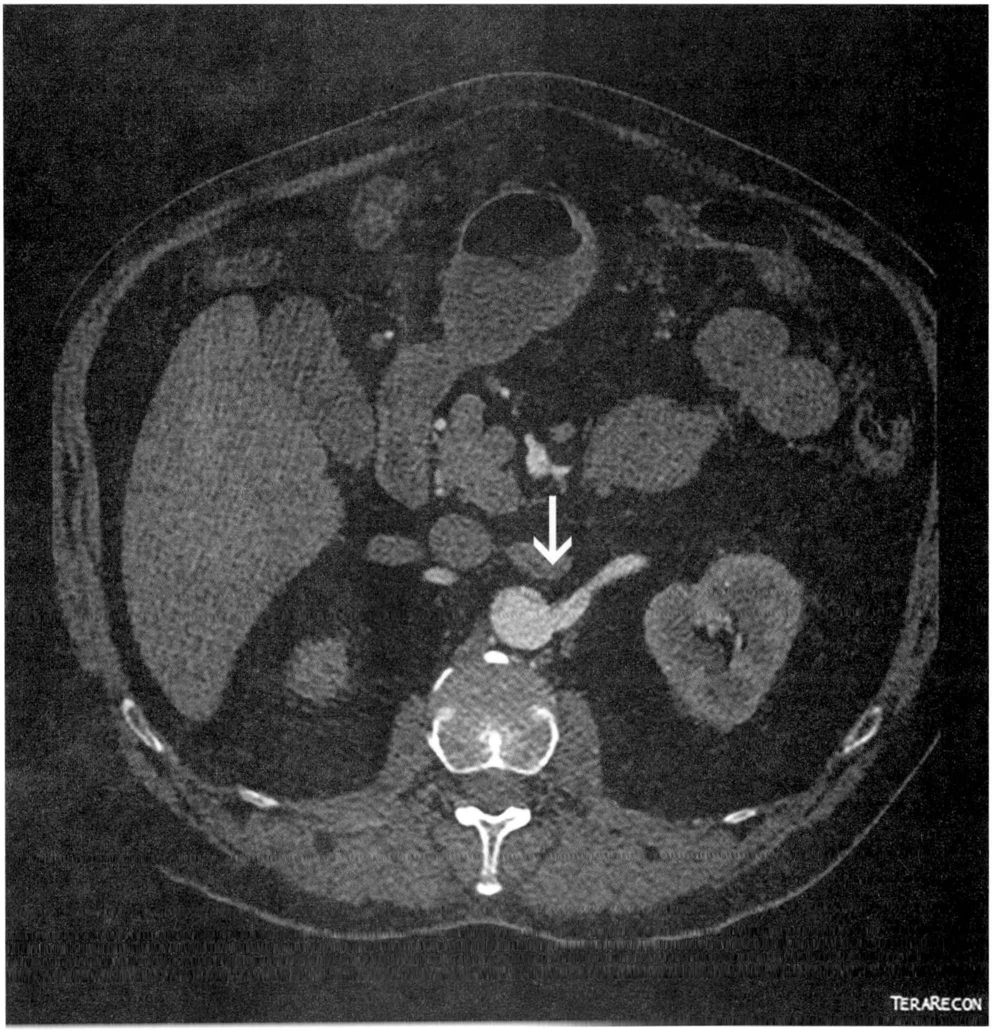

FIGURE 26-2 Computed tomographic (CT) images from a patient with a type B aortic dissection and clinical signs and symptoms of malperfusion. Note the collapsed true lumen at the level of the renal arteries with perfusion of the left renal artery by both the true and the false lumen (arrow).

dynamic picture of the heart, allowing for the identification and quantification of cardiac tamponade.[70] However, in the era of modern CTA technology, the limitations of TEE are more apparent. The images can be acquired at bedside; however, TEE generally requires esophageal intubation and sedation. The procedural nature of TEE means that it is an operator-dependent study, where operators and the necessary infrastructure to perform the procedure have to be readily available, which is often not the case. Gastrointestinal procedural complications are also possible.[70] While TEE can reliably make the diagnosis of aortic dissection, it cannot completely image the aorta: TEE cannot image the infra-diaphragmatic aorta or the aortic arch and arch vessels.[71] TEE can be utilized to diagnose patients who are already intubated and sedated in an ICU setting, who are too unstable to undergo a CTA. It can also be used as an adjunct in surgery to identify entry tears and image the proximal aorta.[67]

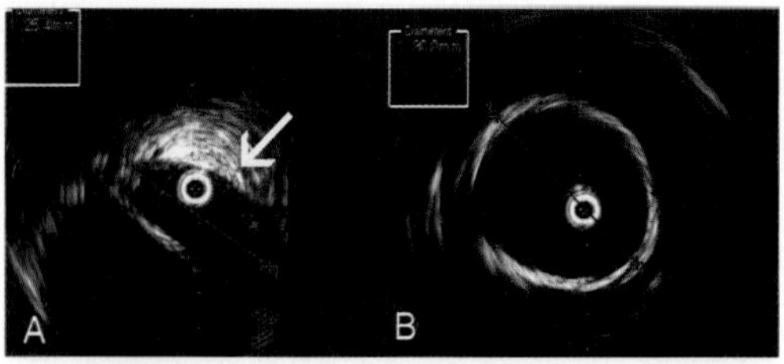

FIGURE 26-3 Example of IVUS image from a patient undergoing treatment for a type B aortic dissection. (**A**) IVUS of the proximal aspect of the aorta demonstrates the IVUS catheter is in the true lumen (arrow). The true lumen is crescentic in shape. (**B**) Further caudal in the aorta, after placement of a thoracic aortic endograft, is the full expansion of the true lumen. The dissection takes a more classic shape with the IVUS catheter in the true lumen. IVUS, intravascular ultrasound.

Chest radiography (CXR) is often obtained in the workup of acute chest pain, but findings on CXR are never diagnostic. A widen mediastinum or aortic knob can be seen with type A dissections.[23] A pleural effusion is more often seen with type B aortic dissection, due to the inflammation associated with the dissecting process.[72]

LIMITATIONS

Understanding the limitations of diagnostics is of critical importance in recognizing and treating aortic dissection, and two major limitations of imaging should be addressed. First, malperfusion is a clinical syndrome that cannot be reliably ruled out based on imaging. While previously mentioned factors can suggest that malperfusion may be present (size and shape of the true lumen, narrowed branch vessel ostia, thrombosed branch vessels), the presence of contrast in a given vessel does not affirm vessel adequate flow. Malperfusion should be diagnosed based on signs and symptoms; laboratory values such as lactic acid, creatinine, and creatine kinase can add clarity to a clinical picture when abnormal, but, again, do not reliably rule out malperfusion.

The second is that aortic dissection is a dynamic process. Subtle intimal tears can be missed on routine imaging and can progress to complicated aortic dissections over short periods.[73] Patients without malperfusion and favorable dissection anatomy can progress to malperfusion with severe anatomic changes with little or no warning. It is imperative to not be falsely reassured by any single laboratory or imaging result.

MANAGEMENT OF THE CLINICAL PROBLEM

UNCOMPLICATED AORTIC DISSECTION

Medical Management

Since Wheat et al. described their experience, medical management has been the standard of care for type B aortic dissections.[5] Medical therapy consists of reducing the hemodynamic forces acting on the dissected aorta to prevent rupture of the weakened aortic wall extension of the dissection plane, or forces across the intimal flap. Patients should be admitted to and monitored in an intensive care unit (ICU). An arterial line should be placed for continuous blood pressure monitoring. Opioids can be used to control pain.

Anti-impulse therapy is the main pharmacologic therapy for patients with acute aortic dissection. The dP/dT is the first derivative of blood pressure and is often referred to as the impulse force. The cornerstone of medical therapy is to reduce the impulse force by controlling both systolic blood pressure and heart rate. Intravenous agents should be used initially. Systolic blood pressure should be maintained between 100 and 120 mmHg, and heart rate should be kept below 60 beats per minute, if obtainable.[74,75] These goals should be achieved within the first 12 hours at the latest, but as soon as possible.[9]

Beta-blockers are the first-line agents. It is imperative to start with an agent to reduce heart rate as a vasodilator may cause reflex tachycardia and prevent a reduction of the impulse force.[76] Other agents such as calcium channel blockers, nitrate agents, or renin-angiotensin inhibitors can be added if the blood pressure cannot be controlled with a single agent.[77] In patients who are intolerant to beta-blockers, non-dihydropyridine calcium channel blockers such as verapamil and diltiazem can be used for rate control. Once pain has resolved, patients can be transitioned to oral antihypertensives. Patients can be transferred out of the ICU once blood pressure can be controlled without intravenous agents.

Blood pressure control should be continued into the subacute and chronic periods to reduce the risk of long-term degeneration and complications. Blood pressure goal can be liberalized to 140/90 mmHg as remodeling begins and the mobility of the intimal flap decreases.[74] Antihypertensive agents should be tailored to individual patients; it is reasonable to employ whichever agents achieve goal blood pressure. Beta-blockers and angiotensin II receptor blockers are ideal for patients with Marfan syndrome as they have shown potential benefits in terms of aortic disease progression.[78,79]

The mortality benefit of medical therapy, compared to open resection of the dissected aorta, was recognized in the 1960s and has remained the standard of care.[5] Recent reports describing the outcomes of medical therapy have to be interpreted in this context, as patients who undergo interventions for acute type B aortic dissection are almost uniformly complicated and will have a significantly increased rate of morbidity and mortality. For patients who can be maintained on medical therapy, in-hospital mortality ranges from 8% to 10%.[50,80] In contemporary data, patients who require an intervention have significantly higher mortality, ranging from 16% to 32%; however, some data have suggested that TEVAR does not increase in-hospital mortality.[50,80,81]

Early reports of medical therapy have focused on mortality and complications in the acute period. However, it has been more recently recognized that 30% to 50% medically managed patients will undergo aneurysmal degeneration.[61,82,83] Durham et al. reported that 29% of patients required an intervention for type B aortic dissection; 66% of these interventions were for aneurysmal degeneration at an average of 2.3 years, postdissection.[82] Given the significant morbidity and mortality associated with aortic interventions for aneurysmal aortic dissections, interventions to prevent this long-term degeneration have been a focus of interest in this last decade.

Endovascular Management

Soon after TEVAR was established, observation studies reported that thrombosis of the false lumen was associated with improved long-term outcomes. Specifically, patients with a thrombosed false lumen had lower long-term need for reintervention, dissection-related death, and change in aortic diameter.[71,84–86] It was hypothesized that inducing false lumen thrombosis via TEVAR would improve prognosis after aortic dissection by preventing long-term adverse aortic events. This was subsequently evaluated in two randomized controlled trials. The INSTEAD trial randomized clinically stable patients to best medical therapy (BMT) or BMT plus TEVAR placed between 2 weeks to 1 year postdissection with the primary endpoint of all-cause mortality at 2 years postdissection.[87] There was no difference in mortality at 2 years, postdissection, between the treatment groups. However, it did support the hypothesis that TEVAR can induce false lumen thrombosis, as 91% of TEVAR patients had favorable aortic remodeling, compared to only 19% of the BMT group. This finding was further supported by the ADDSORB trial, which randomized patients to similar treatment arms as the INSTEAD trial but evaluated aortic remodeling.[88] Patients in the TEVAR group had more false lumen thrombosis and regression, true lumen expansion, and a trend toward smaller aortic diameters.

However, beyond randomized controlled trials, there is a plethora of evidence suggesting that TEVAR conveys mortality benefits. Most notably, continued follow-up of the INSTEAD cohort to 5 years, postdissection, showed that TEVAR was associated with lower aortic specific mortality and anatomic progression.[89] Similar findings were reported from the IRAD database, as only 15% of patients treated with TEVAR were dead at 5 years, compared to 30% treatment with medical therapy.[81] Experiences from large single-centers and state-wide administrative databases have reported similar results as well.[82,90,91]

With the current body of evidence, there are no formal societal recommendations on when to perform TEVAR for uncomplicated type B aortic dissection. Most surgeons agree that it is reasonable to perform TEVAR on patients with uncomplicated type B aortic dissection who are at high risk for progression to aneurysmal degeneration. Institutional data from Massachusetts General Hospital reported anatomic factors associated with long-term aneurysmal degeneration include an entry larger than 10 mm, aortic diameter greater than 40 mm, false lumen diameter greater than 20 mm, an increase in aortic diameter more than 5 mm between imaging studies.[61] Other experiences have shown similar results, with other anatomic predictive factors including proximal location, true lumen/false lumen diameter ratio, and involvement of visceral vessels.[91,92] Beyond anatomic considerations, refractory pain and hypertension are associated with higher in-hospital mortality.[93] Connective tissue disease is generally considered a contraindication to TEVAR in uncomplicated type B aortic dissections given poor long-term outcomes.[94] Endovascular treatment should be considered in select patients with the aforementioned risk factors to prevent long-term aortic-related adverse events.

GENERAL TECHNIQUES

Graft Selection and Sizing

All commercially available TEVAR devices have been used to treat aortic dissection, but recently few have been evaluated and gained specific approval for use in aortic dissections. Important factors to consider when selecting a graft are graft diameter, graft length, and proximal bare-metal stents. While TEVAR for aneurysmal disease is oversized by 10% to 20%, TEVAR grafts for aortic dissection should be oversized by 0% to 5%, given the increased risk of retrograde type A aortic dissection with a greater degree of oversizing.[95,96] Proximal bare-metal stents may also convey an increased risk of retrograde type A aortic dissection and are avoided if suitable alternatives are available.[97]

There are varying opinions about the ideal length of the endograft for aortic dissections. Longer grafts result in better true lumen expansion and false lumen thrombosis but increase the risk of spinal cord ischemia. The goal of TEVAR for uncomplicated type B aortic dissection is to cover the proximal entry tear, redirect flow preferentially into the true lumen, and ultimately promote thrombosis of the false lumen (Figure 26-4). Expansion of the true lumen and coverage of secondary tears improves remodeling and should also be considered. While some believe that these goals can be met using a short (10 cm) endograft, most believe that longer endografts result in better remodeling. All devices in the INSTEAD and ADSORB trials were longer than 15 cm.[87,88] Grafts longer than 20 cm usually are not necessary and increase the risk of spinal cord ischemia.[98]

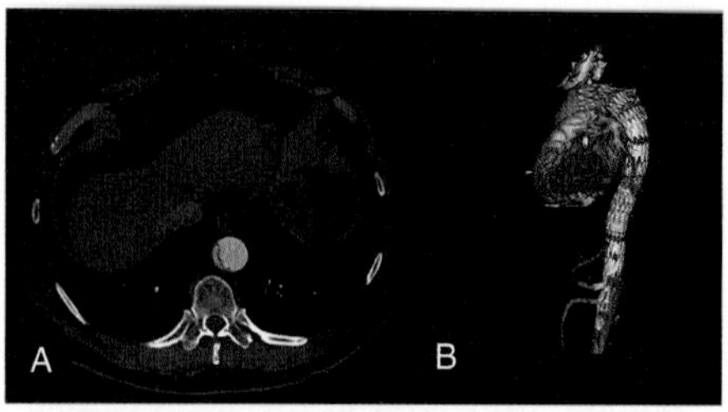

FIGURE 26-4 CT images from patient undergoing treatment for type B aortic dissection with malperfusion. (**A**) On preoperative cross-sectional CT imaging, note the complete collapse of the true lumen (arrow). (**B**) Three-dimensional reconstruction from CT images performed postoperatively. Note changes with placement of a TEVAR to cover the entry tear with re-expansion of the true lumen. CT, computed tomographic; TEVAR, thoracic endovascular aortic repair.

Left Subclavian Coverage

Given the angulation of the aorta as the aortic arch transitions to the descending thoracic aorta and the desire to have a healthy segment of the aorta as the proximal landing zone, it is usually preferable to land the proximal edge of the stent graft just distal to the left subclavian. As most type B aortic dissections originate around the origin of the left subclavian, consideration should be given to left subclavian artery revascularization. Given the elective nature of TEVAR for uncomplicated type B aortic dissection, societal recommendations suggest routine left subclavian artery revascularization.[99] Certain anatomic factors necessitate left subclavian artery revascularization (Table 26-2). Carotid-subclavian transposition AND bypass are both acceptable options for revascularization.

Procedural Adjuncts, Access Considerations, and Timing

Given the relatively small amount of aortic coverage, most vascular surgeons do not favor routine cerebrospinal fluid (CSF); the majority of studies report a low rate of spinal cord ischemia (0%–5%).[16] If coverage >20 cm is necessary, CSF drainage should be considered.[98]

Commercially available TEVAR devices range from 18 Fr to 26 Fr. Percutaneous placement has been shown to have benefits compared to open arterial

TABLE 26-2 Anatomic Factors that Necessitate Left Subclavian Artery Revascularization

Presence of a patent left internal mammary artery to coronary artery bypass graft
Termination of the left vertebral artery at the posterior inferior cerebellar artery or other discontinuity of the vertebrobasilar collaterals
Absent or diminutive or occluded right vertebral artery
A functioning arteriovenous shunt in the left arm
Prior infrarenal aortic repair with ligation of lumbar and middle sacral arteries
Planned long-segment (20 cm) coverage of the descending thoracic aorta where critical intercostal arteries originate
Hypogastric artery occlusion
Presence of early aneurysmal changes that may require subsequent therapy involving the distal thoracic aorta

exposure including shorter operative time, earlier ambulation, fewer incisional complications, and shorter length of stay. Open exposure is favorable in the setting of small or diseased common femoral arteries. Ultimately, surgeon preference and comfort should take priority. Patients with aortic dissection are less likely to have atherosclerotic and calcific iliac vessels and rarely require iliac conduits. An iliac conduit should be considered in patients with iliac vessels smaller than 6 mm in diameter or excessively calcific or tortuous iliac vessels, while taking device diameter into account.

In patients who are stable and can wait, delaying the procedure until after 2 weeks postdissection is associated with fewer perioperative complications.[100] TEVAR should be performed before 3 to 6 months, postdissection, prior to unfavorable remodeling taking place.

Procedural Steps

The procedure should be performed in a room with fluoroscopic capability. The patient should be placed in the supine position. The patient should be prepped from the nipples to mid-thighs. Access can be obtained percutaneously or by open femoral exposure on the device side. In the case of percutaneous access, a 7/8 Fr sheath should be placed, and two suture-based closure devices should be deployed without securing the knots. True lumen wire access should be obtained and confirmed using IVUS. If it is difficult to direct the wire into the true lumen, left brachial access can facilitate this in most cases. Through a 5-Fr sheath on the nondevice side, a pigtail catheter is then placed in the ascending aorta for imaging purposes and thoracic aortogram is performed. Glide wires should direct angled catheters into the thoracic aorta. A stiff wire should be placed into the ascending aorta and the endograft of choice should be brought into the field. An appropriate sheath can be placed on the device side or the device can be delivered without a sheath. Using a combination of angiography and IVUS, the graft should be placed into the desired deployment location and deployed according to manufacturer specifications. Completion angiography, and IVUS if used preplacement, should be performed to confirm good positioning and branch vessel patency. All wires, catheters, and sheaths should be removed, and the access arteries should be closed in an appropriate fashion.

POSTOPERATIVE COMPLICATIONS

Standard complications such as adverse cardiac, pulmonary, renal, and access complications can all occur. The following complications deserve further explanation:

- Spinal Cord Ischemia—As previously mentioned, spinal cord ischemia is a relatively uncommon complication with TEVAR for aortic dissection; however, it is devastating when it does occur. It can present with partial weakness that may be isolated to the proximal muscle groups or full paralysis. It can be transient or permanent. A lower extremity neurologic examination should be performed each time the patient is evaluated in the immediate postoperative period. Spinal cord ischemia can be reversible if recognized early and proper interventions are undertaken. Interventions to improve spinal cord perfusion include insertion of a spinal drain, targeting a mean arterial pressure above 90 mmHg, maximizing oxygen delivery by targeting a hemoglobin above 10 g/dL and optimizing cardiac output, and administration of naloxone or steroids.[38]

- Retrograde type A dissection—A potentially catastrophic complication that can go unnoticed intraoperatively. The ascending aorta should be imaged in a patient with severe chest pain, hemodynamic instability, or EKG or lab findings consistent with a myocardial infarction. Emergent operative repair is indicated.
- Endoleaks and Persistent False Lumen Flow—Persistent false lumen flow is common, especially when distal intimal tears are present.[39] Most endoleaks do not require urgent intervention and can be followed with serial CT scans.

OPEN SURGICAL MANAGEMENT

For uncomplicated type B aortic dissection, open surgical repair is of historical interest only. Details of open surgical repair of abdominal, thoracic, and thoracoabdominal aorta are given in Chapters 29.

COMPLICATED TYPE B AORTIC DISSECTION—RUPTURED

Rupture of acute type B aortic dissection is a rare but life-threatening complication. Mortality is certain without emergent surgical intervention. TEVAR is a feasible therapeutic option with acceptable outcomes given the prognosis.[101,102] It can be performed in a similar fashion as in an uncomplicated type B dissection. Most ruptures are supplied by false lumen flow. Small series have reported that similar lengths of coverage (130-150 mm) can achieve seal of the ruptured segment.[103,104] False lumen flow should be evaluated intraoperatively with TEE or IVUS. If false lumen flow is persistent after initial stent graft placement, aortic coverage should be extended proximally or distally, depending on IVUS/TEE finding. In the setting of inadequate landing zone for TEVAR, open repair is indicated. A key principle of open repair is to resect and reconstruct the ruptured segment, not the entire dissected segment of aorta given the risk of spinal cord ischemia and the substantial added operative time and complexity. Rupture of type B aortic dissection presents a complex clinical problem in which outcomes are generally poor.[50,105]

COMPLICATED TYPE B AORTIC DISSECTION—MALPERFUSION

Understanding the mechanism of malperfusion is critical in terms of treatment selection. Dynamic and static obstructions cause ischemia in different ways and are approached accordingly in terms of treatment. The goal of treatment in dynamic obstruction is expansion of aortic true lumen. This can be achieved by stenting the lumen open or eliminating the pressure gradient across the intimomedial flap. Static obstruction is treated by stenting or bypassing the obstructive lesion. A secondary goal of treatment is to eliminate false lumen flow to prevent long-term adverse events, but treatment of malperfusion takes precedence. Medical management should be instituted as described in the uncomplicated type B aortic dissection section; however, patients with malperfusion require urgent intervention.

ENDOVASCULAR MANAGEMENT

TEVAR

TEVAR has proven to be an effective treatment for complicated type B aortic dissection (Figure 26-5).[7] It achieves the true lumen expansion by stenting

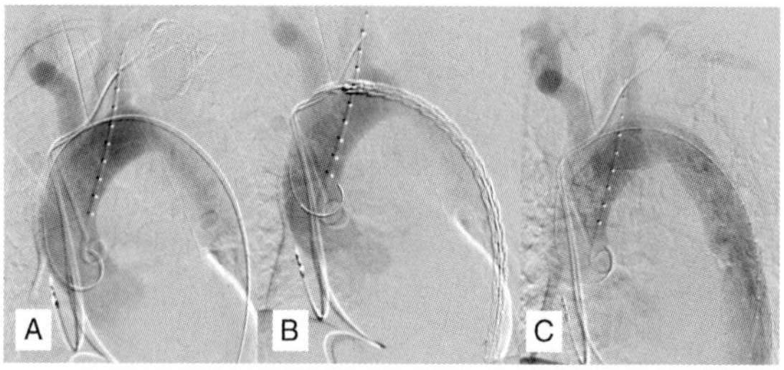

FIGURE 26-5 Angiographic demonstration. (**A**) Type B dissection with collapse of true lumen. (**B**) Positioning of a TEVAR device to land at the level of the left subclavian artery. (**C**) Expansion of the true lumen in the proximal aorta and (**D**) perfusion of the visceral vessels distal to the stent graft. TEVAR, thoracic endovascular aortic repair.

open the true lumen and eliminating the pressure gradient across the intimomedial flap by reducing or excluding false lumen flow.[63] As such, it is an effective tool to treat dynamic obstruction from a compressed true lumen. The principles of treatment are the same as in uncomplicated type B aortic dissection, with certain points deserving further emphasis. IVUS is an important adjunct to confirm true access and assess the mobility of the intimomedial flap and degree of true lumen compression.[67] Repeat IVUS, postendograft deployment, can reevaluate the intimomedial flap and be used to determine the need for further endografting. Angiography pre- and postendografting is essential to evaluate visceral arterial flow. Cessation of false lumen flow can sometimes worsen renovisceral arterial flow when the target vessels are receiving significant flow from the aortic false lumen.

TEVAR for malperfusion has shown excellent results, with resolution of malperfusion occurring in 75% to 80% of patients.[7,106] Observational data from the IRAD database have shown that patients who are managed with TEVAR had similar short-term mortality as medically managed patients, despite a significantly higher proportion of them having malperfusion.[81] For patients in whom malperfusion is not corrected with TEVAR alone, other adjunctive procedures, which are described below, are indicated. Postoperative complications are similar as TEVAR for uncomplicated type B aortic dissection.

MESENTERIC/RENAL/ILIAC STENTING

In the case of a narrow mesenteric or renal artery ostium, stenting of the ostium may be necessary in order to alleviate malperfusion. As previously stated, this usually occurs when the dissection plane extends into an aortic branch vessel and narrows the ostium. After initial identification by signs, symptoms, and axial imaging, static obstruction can be confirmed using aortography, IVUS, or pressure manometry, intraoperatively.[47] Stenting can successfully relieve ostial narrowing in the majority of cases.[48] The decision to treat can be difficult in the setting of a moderate degree of narrowing, especially in the presence of concomitant dynamic obstruction; there are no formal guidelines addressing the issue. After the relief of dynamic obstruction, the renoviseral and lower extremity vessels should be evaluated with angiography and/or IVUS. If doubt persists, the pressure gradient across the vessel narrowing can be measured. An aorto-branch gradient greater than 10 mmHg is considered significant stenosis and justifies treatment.

For acute limb ischemia from malperfusion of the iliac vessels, revascularization can be achieved by either iliac stenting or femorofemoral bypass. Flow is best assessed by angiography and pulse examination; however, IVUS and manometry can be used as adjuncts as well.

These endovascular procedures are performed in a standard fashion. As with TEVAR, true lumen wire position is essential and can be confirmed with IVUS. Access can be femoral, but left-arm access often facilitates true lumen access with more ease. See respective chapters for step-by-step guide to mesenteric, renal, and iliac stenting.

An endovascular approach to static obstruction is widely considered first-line treatment for narrowed and obstructed branch vessels; however, there is a paucity of data comparing endovascular approaches to open revascularization. The feasibility of these procedures is well established, and the technical success rate is above 90%.[107,108] Open approaches are reserved for vessels in which an endovascular intervention has failed.

PERCUTANEOUS FENESTRATION

In the 1990s, percutaneous techniques, namely bare-metal stenting of the true lumen in the mesenteric segment with flap fenestration, were described as a potential treatment for type B aortic dissection with malperfusion.[48,109] While TEVAR has replaced bare-metal stenting of the true lumen, flap fenestration remains a valuable tool to treat malperfusion. It can be utilized in conjunction with TEVAR to avoid excessive aortic coverage or in patients with poor landing zones for TEVAR.[49] In anatomically suitable patients, TEVAR is generally preferred due to the improved long-term outcomes. The risk of long-term aneurysmal degeneration, rupture, and intervention remains after percutaneous fenestration.[110]

Operative Technique

A variety of techniques have been described. Percutaneous access is achieved into the true lumen. A wire, catheter, and sheath system are placed at the desired level of fenestration, usually at the mesenteric segment. The intimomedial flap is then crossed via desired means. This can be done using a stiff wire and directional catheter (usually the back end of an 0.014-in wire works well to cross the flap), a transjugular biopsy needle, or a reentry device. Alternatively, a natural fenestration can be selected to be enlarged. Once a true-to-false lumen wire is achieved and confirmed by IVUS, a balloon is advanced to the flap and dilated to 15 mm to create a large fenestration. The dissection should then be reevaluated with IVUS and aortography to confirm adequate branch vessel flow.

Alternatively, another technique, commonly referred to as the "cheese wire" technique, can be used to achieve significant flap disruption. Percutaneous access is obtained bilaterally; a wire is placed in the true lumen from one side and in the false lumen from the other side. The flap is crossed from the true to the false lumen using the aforementioned techniques and the crossing wire is snared to the contralateral groin to achieve a through-and-through wire. At this point, each sheath is counter punctured and buddy wires are placed up the iliac arteries and into the aorta. Then, the through-and-through wire is pulled caudally to tear the dissection flap. While the "cheese wire" name is fitting, the act of fenestrating the flap is not as precise as slicing a piece of cheddar off the block: often, the entire flap with rip and embolize, occluding an iliac artery. This is why placing bilateral buddy wires is a key step; should the flap embolize, it can be jailed against the arterial wall with iliac stents placed over the buddy wires. The dissection should then be reevaluated with IVUS and aortography to confirm adequate branch vessel flow. All wires and catheters should be removed and the arteriotomies should be closed appropriately.

Outcomes and Complications

Patients should be monitored postoperatively for persistent malperfusion and access complications in the perioperative period. Percutaneous fenestration is effective in relieving malperfusion but peri-dissection mortality remains high, ranging from 17% to 25%.[48,110] None of the perioperative deaths in those two series were attributed to the procedure. There is minimal data comparing percutaneous fenestration to other techniques. Furthermore, the small amount of long-term data available suggests that the long-term risk of adverse aortic events is high; only 54% of patients did not experience an adverse aortic event, 8 years postdissection.[110]

EMERGING ENDOVASCULAR TECHNIQUES: STABLE (PETTICOAT) AND STABILISE

The STABLE trial examined the use of a composite dissection device. The device consisted of a proximal TEVAR device and bare-metal stents that extend distally through the mesenteric segment. The bare-metal stents provide true lumen expansion through the mesenteric segment without excessive aortic coverage or the need for renoviseral branches.[111,112] STABLE II, which included only complicated aortic dissection, reported an impressive 30-day mortality of 6.8%. However, the issue of delayed aortic degeneration remained, as 38% of patients experienced a diameter increase of >5 mm at 1 year postdissection.

The Stent-Assisted Balloon-Induced Intimal Disruption and Relamination in Aortic Dissection Repair (STABILISE) technique has shown the potential to decrease long-term unfavorable aortic remodeling. The procedure is similar to that used in the STABLE trial; however, the bare-metal stent portion is aggressively ballooned to disrupt the dissection flap and relaminate the aorta (Figure 26-6).[113] At 12 months, postdissection, only 5% of patients had an increase in maximum diameter. While early results are promising, the literature consists mainly of small, single-arm prospective studies. Comparative studies are necessary to further evaluate these techniques.

OPEN MANAGEMENT

Open Fenestration

Prior to percutaneous techniques, open fenestration was the most common technique employed to relieve malperfusion in type B aortic dissection. This technique has largely been replaced by percutaneous

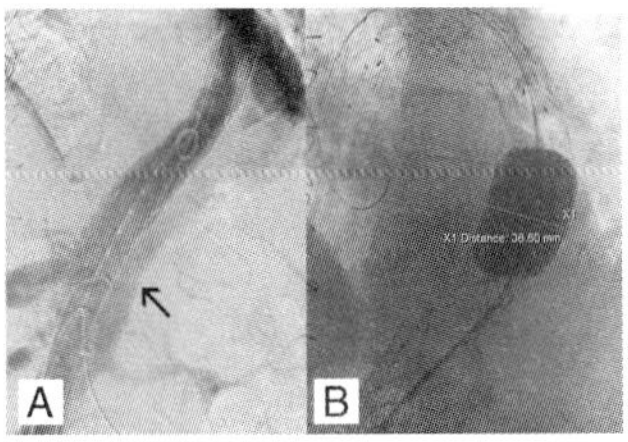

FIGURE 26-6 Angiographic demonstration. (**A**) Persistent false lumen flow into a thoracic aneurysm after initial placement of a TEVAR for aortic dissection (arrow). (**B**) After balloon dilation of TEVAR to allow it to abut the outer wall of the aorta in a fashion similar to STABILISE. Note the stent graft is against the outer wall of the aortic wall preventing retrograde flow into the more proximal thoracic component of the false lumen. TEVAR, thoracic endovascular aortic repair.

interventions; however, open fenestration should remain in the toolbox of vascular surgeons as an important and proven technique to relieve malperfusion. Open fenestration can be used in patients in whom percutaneous fenestration has failed, in patients who require an open bypass, or patients with a chronic dissection presenting with malperfusion who likely have a fibrotic flap that would be difficult to cross percutaneously.

Operative Technique

The fenestration can be confined to the infrarenal level or extend into the mesenteric segment. An infrarenal fenestration can be performed via either a transabdominal or a retroperitoneal approach; the retroperitoneal approach provides better access to the mesenteric segment. Extension into the mesenteric segment is recommended with mesenteric or renal branches appearing to be compromised, as it allows for direct examination of the vessel ostia. The dissection flap should be resected as widely as possible.

For the transabdominal approach, the patient is placed in the supine position and a midline laparotomy is performed. A standard inframesocolic infrarenal aortic exposure is performed. The small bowel is wrapped in a towel and packed in the right lower quadrant of the abdomen and the transverse colon is wrapped in a towel and eviscerated. Exposure is facilitated using a fixed retractor system. The retroperitoneal tissue overlying the aorta is incised and the aorta is dissected away from the surrounding tissue to obtain proximal and distal control. Proximal and distal clamps are placed after systemic heparinization. The fenestration can be performed through an aortotomy; however, many surgeons endorse that wide resection of dissection flap and interposition graft of a segment of infrarenal aorta is simpler and more effective.[114] The anastomosis should be reinforced with Teflon felt or bovine pericardium given the friable nature of the dissected aortic wall. The graft should be sewn to the false lumen wall—the flap should not be reapproximated.

Should the fenestration be extended up through the mesenteric segment, a retroperitoneal approach is superior. The patient is placed into the thoracoabdominal position. A thoracoabdominal incision is made over the nineth or tenth rib and extended inferiorly in the left rectus sheath. After the incision is deepened through the muscular and fascial layers of the abdominal wall, the retroperitoneal space is entered by peeling away the peritoneum from the transversalis fascia. The plane should be extended deep and posterior to Gerota's fascia, mobilizing the left kidney anteriorly. The left renal lumbar vein can be identified and followed to the left renal vein to identify the left renal artery. The left renal artery can be traced down to the aorta which is subsequently dissected away from the surrounding retroperitoneal tissue. Supraceliac control is usually utilized for a mesenteric segment fenestration. Mesenteric and renal branch can be controlled prior to clamping or controlled intraluminally, depending on the dissection anatomy. Proximal and distal clamps are placed after systemic heparinization. The aorta is opened, and the dissection flap is resected. If the aortotomy is extended into the mesenteric segment, it can be closed with a running suture, reinforced with Teflon felt. The proximal anastomosis is completed using Teflon felt or bovine pericardium and the clamp is moved onto the interposition graft and the distal anastomosis is completed. The abdomen is closed in standard fashion.

Complications and Outcomes

The literature on this procedure is quite limited. It is an uncommon but effective procedure. In two small series, open fenestration was 100% effective in relieving malperfusion.[115,116] It is a significant open aortic operation and cardiac, pulmonary, and gastrointestinal complications are not unexpected. With all complicated type B aortic dissections, patients should be monitored for new or ongoing malperfusion.

OPEN BYPASS

Aortomesenteric or aortorenal bypass can be used in the setting of static obstruction where endovascular techniques have failed. It is often performed in conjunction with open aortic fenestration and interposition graft of the infrarenal aorta to have a stable inflow segment. Femorofemoral bypass can be used for unilateral lower extremity malperfusion from a compromised iliac vessel. These techniques can be performed in a standard fashion; see Chapters 31 and 32.

CHRONIC AORTIC DISSECTION

As previously stated, medical therapy for type B aortic dissection often fails in the long term via aneurysmal degeneration and subsequent intervention. Continued medical management and serial imaging encompasses long-term management of chronic dissections; however, 30% to 50% of dissections will ultimately degenerate.[61,82,83] In a series of thoracoabdominal aortic aneurysm repairs, chronically degenerated aortic dissections account for 25% to 40% of repairs.[117-119] Traditionally, open aortic repair was the only option for repair of thoracoabdominal aneurysms; however, branched and fenestrated endografts have emerged as an enticing option for less-then-ideal surgical candidates. Aneurysms in chronically degenerated type B aortic dissections are repaired when they grow to at least 5.5 cm in diameter. For more information on preoperative preparation, operative technique, complications, and outcomes, see chapter on thoracoabdominal aneurysms.

TEVAR

If the descending thoracic aorta is aneurysmal with adequate landing zones, TEVAR can be used. The procedural has an acceptable technical success rate at 90%.[120] However, the mid-term results are guarded. At mean follow-up times ranging from 2 to 4.5 years, the reintervention rate varied from 10% to 40%. Furthermore, the underlying problem persists in the uncovered aorta, as up to 21% of patients will develop aneurysmal degeneration distal to the TEVAR. While these results are inferior to TEVAR results for nondissecting aneurysms, it does suggest that TEVAR is sufficient treatment in a proportion of patients. Placement of a TEVAR does not negatively impact further treatment strategies and should be employed in anatomically appropriate patients.

OPEN THORACOABDOMINAL ANEURYSM REPAIR

When the mesenteric segment of the aorta is aneurysmal, open repair has been the traditional standard of care; this is a common occurrence with type B aortic dissections, given their thoracoabdominal nature. The desire to prevent long-term aneurysmal degeneration is based on the outcomes of subsequent thoracoabdominal aortic aneurysm repairs. The majority of series on these repairs come from centers of excellence which report an operative mortality of 3% to 15% since 2000.[121] However, population-based data, which is a better representation of "real world" data, suggest that the operative mortality ranges from 19% to 22% with similar paraplegia rates.[122,123] While these data are inclusive of nondissecting aneurysms, the outcomes are similar for chronic dissections. Although open repair is a reasonable choice and durable option for excellent surgical candidates, operative mortality can be as high as 40% for patients older than 80 years.[123] Need to reduce perioperative morbidity and mortality for repair of these aneurysms has brought branches and fenestrated endografting to the forefront of vascular surgery research.

BRANCHED AND FENESTRATED ENDOVASCULAR AORTIC REPAIR (B/FEVAR)

The first B/FEVAR was implanted in 2001 for a contained rupture of a Crawford Extent IV thoracoabdominal aortic aneurysm.[124] Since then, published reports have shown favorable 30-day mortality, ranging from 4% to 8%.[125,126] Devices were designed to cover the entire mesenteric segment as only available in the United States through physician-sponsored investigational device exemption studies (Figure 26-7).

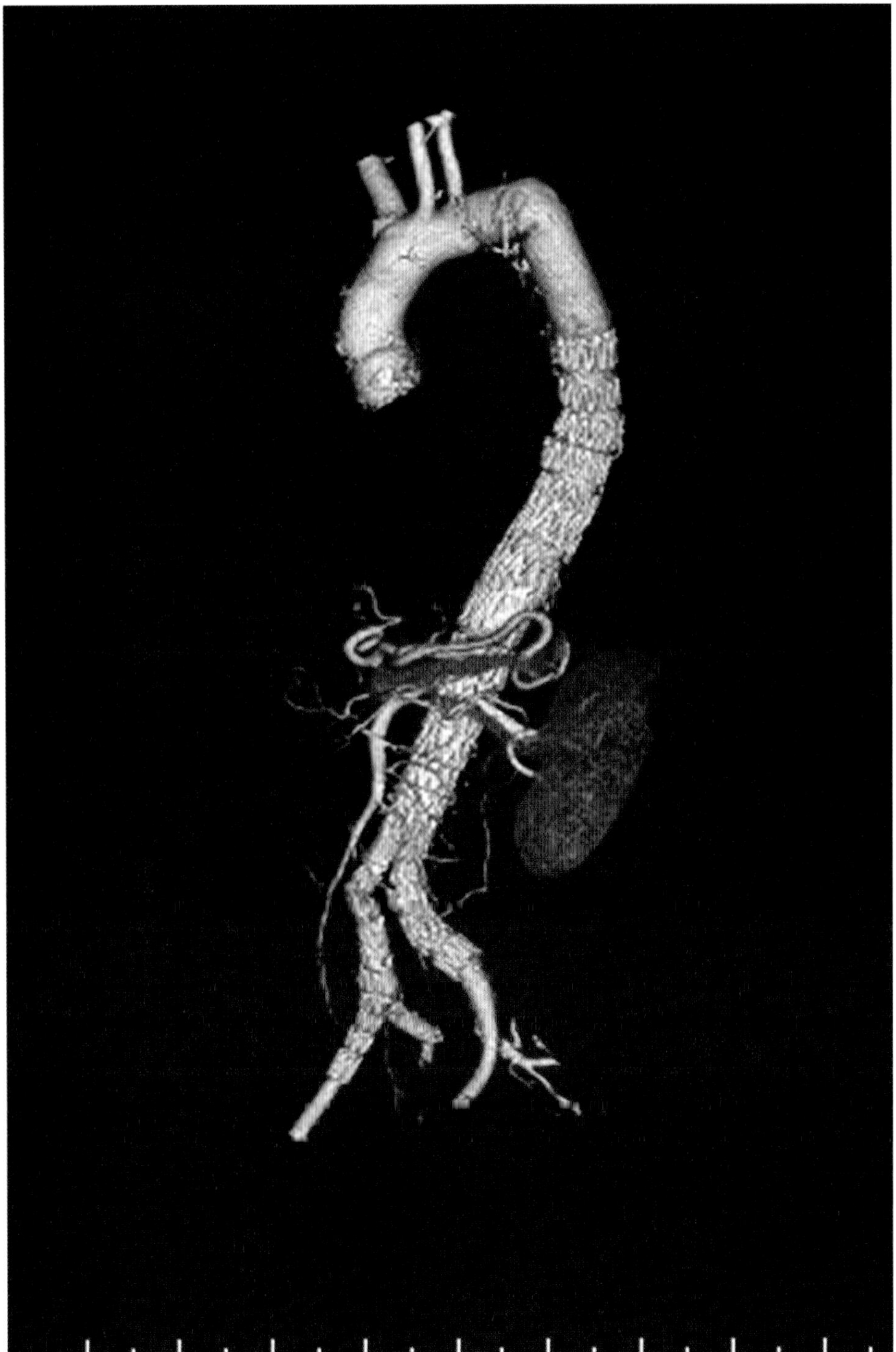

FIGURE 26-7 Three-dimensional reconstruction from a postoperative CT scan from a patient with a chronic aortic dissection with aneurysmal degeneration that was treated with a fenestrated/branched aortic endograft.

The capability of these devices is constantly improving. With current investigation devices, treatment can extend from the ascending aorta to the external iliac artery and can accommodate significant anatomic variation. These studies are restricted to patients who are deemed poor surgical candidates. As such, there is a paucity of data comparing B/FEVAR to open thoracoabdominal aneurysm repair. Again, these data are inclusive of nondissecting aneurysms. Data specific to chronic aortic dissection suggest that extensive aortic dissections are more likely to require reintervention after index procedure.[127] While the availability of these devices remains limited, the potential to reduce perioperative morbidity and mortality is significant.

REFERENCES

1. Leonard JC. Thomas Bevill Peacock and the early history of dissecting aneurysm. *BMJ.* 1979;2:260-262.
2. Criado FJ. 8th current trends in aorti and cardiothoracic surgery. *Tex Heart Inst J.* 2011;38.
3. DeSanctis RW, Doroghazi RM, Austen WG, et al. Aortic dissection. *N Engl J Med.* 1987;317:1060-1067.
4. De Bakey ME, Cooley DA, Creech O. Surgical considerations of dissecting aneurysm of the aorta. *Ann Surg.* 1955;142:586-612.
5. Wheat MW, Palmer RF, Bartley TD, et al. Treatment of dissecting aneurysms of the aorta without surgery. *J Thorac Cardiovasc Surg.* 1965;50:364-373.
6. Nienaber CA, Fattori R, Lund G, et al. Nonsurgical reconstruction of thoracic aortic dissection by stent-graft placement. *N Engl J Med.* 1999;340:1539-1545.
7. Dake MD, Kato N, Mitchell RS, et al. Endovascular stent-graft placement for the treatment of acute aortic dissection. *N Engl J Med.* 1999;340:1546-1552.
8. Vilacosta I, San Roman JA. Acute aortic syndrome. *Heart.* 2001;85:365-368.
9. Lombardi JV, Hughes GC, Appoo JJ, et al. Society for vascular surgery (SVS) and society of thoracic surgeons (STS) reporting standards for type B aortic dissections. *Ann Thorac Surg.* 2020;109:959-981.
10. Daily PO, Trueblood HW, Stinson EB, et al. Management of acute aortic dissections. *Ann Thorac Surg.* 1970; 10:237-247.
11. De Bakey ME, Henly WS, Cooley DA, et al. Surgical management of dissecting aneurysms of the aorta. *J Thorac Cardiovasc Surg.* 1965;49:130-149.
12. Tsai TT, Isselbacher EM, Trimarchi S, et al. Acute type B aortic dissection: does aortic arch involvement affect management and outcomes? Insights from the international registry of acute aortic dissection (IRAD). *Circulation.* 2007;116:I150-I156.
13. Kim JB, Sundt TM 3rd. Best surgical option for arch extension of type B aortic dissection: the open approach. *Ann Cardiothorac Surg.* 2014;3:406-412.
14. Crawford ES. The diagnosis and management of aortic dissection. *JAMA.* 1990;264:2537-2541.
15. Booher AM, Isselbacher EM, Nienaber CA, et al. The IRAD classification system for characterizing survival after aortic dissection. *Am J Med.* 2013;126:730.e719-e724.
16. Fattori R, Cao P, De Rango P, et al. Interdisciplinary expert consensus document on management of type B aortic dissection. *J Am Coll Cardiol.* 2013;61:1661-1678.
17. Desai AS, Solomon SD, Shah AM, et al. Effect of sacubitril-valsartan vs enalapril on aortic stiffness in patients with heart failure and reduced ejection fraction: a randomized clinical trial. *JAMA.* 2019:1-10.
18. Ramanath VS, Oh JK, Sundt TM 3rd, et al. Acute aortic syndromes and thoracic aortic aneurysm. *Mayo Clin Proc.* 2009;84:465-481.
19. Clouse WD, Hallett JW Jr, Schaff HV, et al. Acute aortic dissection: population-based incidence compared with degenerative aortic aneurysm rupture. *Mayo Clin Proc.* 2004;79:176-180.
20. Meszaros I, Morocz J, Szlavi J, et al. Epidemiology and clinicopathology of aortic dissection. *Chest.* 2000; 117:1271-1278.
21. Nienaber CA, Clough RE, Sakalihasan N, et al. Aortic dissection. *Nat Rev Dis Primers.* 2016;2:16053.
22. Hughes GC, Andersen ND, McCann RL. Management of acute type B aortic dissection. *J Thorac Cardiovasc Surg.* 2013;145:S202-S207.
23. Hagan PG, Nienaber CA, Isselbacher EM, et al. The International Registry of Acute Aortic Dissection (IRAD): new insights into an old disease. *JAMA.* 2000; 283:897-903.
24. Khan IA, Nair CK. Clinical, diagnostic, and management perspectives of aortic dissection. *Chest.* 2002;122: 311-328.
25. Lauterbach SR, Cambria RP, Brewster DC, et al. Contemporary management of aortic branch compromise resulting from acute aortic dissection. *J Vasc Surg.* 2001;33:1185-1192.
26. Landenhed M, Engstrom G, Gottsater A, et al. Risk profiles for aortic dissection and ruptured or surgically treated aneurysms: a prospective cohort study. *J Am Heart Assoc.* 2015;4:e001513.
27. Januzzi JL, Isselbacher EM, Fattori R, et al. Characterizing the young patient with aortic dissection:

results from the international registry of aortic dissection (IRAD). *J Am Coll Cardiol*. 2004;43:665-669.

28. Pape LA, Awais M, Woznicki EM, et al. Presentation, diagnosis, and outcomes of acute aortic dissection: 17-year trends from the international registry of acute aortic dissection. *J Am Coll Cardiol*. 2015;66:350-358.
29. Murdoch JL, Walker BA, Halpern BL, et al. Life expectancy and causes of death in the Marfan syndrome. *N Engl J Med*. 1972;286:804-808.
30. Silverman DI, Burton KJ, Gray J, et al. Life expectancy in the Marfan syndrome. *Am J Cardiol*. 1995;75:157-160.
31. Loeys BL, Schwarze U, Holm T, et al. Aneurysm syndromes caused by mutations in the TGF-beta receptor. *N Engl J Med*. 2006;355:788-798.
32. MacCarrick G, Black JH 3rd, Bowdin S, et al. Loeys-Dietz syndrome: a primer for diagnosis and management. *Genet Med*. 2014;16:576-587.
33. Leier CV, Call TD, Fulkerson PK, et al. The spectrum of cardiac defects in the Ehlers-Danlos syndrome, types I and III. *Ann Intern Med*. 1980;92:171-178.
34. Larson EW, Edwards WD. Risk factors for aortic dissection: a necropsy study of 161 cases. *Am J Cardiol*. 1984;53:849-855.
35. Isselbacher EM, Lino Cardenas CL, Lindsay ME. Hereditary influence in thoracic aortic aneurysm and dissection. *Circulation*. 2016;133:2516-2528.
36. Kamel H, Roman MJ, Pitcher A, et al. Pregnancy and the risk of aortic dissection or rupture: a cohort-crossover analysis. *Circulation*. 2016;134:527-533.
37. Daniel JC, Huynh TT, Zhou W, et al. Acute aortic dissection associated with use of cocaine. *J Vasc Surg*. 2007;46:427-433.
38. Dean JH, Woznicki EM, O'Gara P, et al. Cocaine-related aortic dissection: lessons from the International Registry of Acute Aortic Dissection. *Am J Med*. 2014;127:878-885.
39. Ramirez F, Dietz HC. Therapy insight: aortic aneurysm and dissection in Marfan's syndrome. *Nat Clin Pract Cardiovasc Med*. 2004;1:31-36.
40. Golledge J, Eagle KA. Acute aortic dissection. *Lancet*. 2008;372:55-66.
41. Loeys BL, Chen J, Neptune ER, et al. A syndrome of altered cardiovascular, craniofacial, neurocognitive and skeletal development caused by mutations in TGFBR1 or TGFBR2. *Nat Genet*. 2005;37:275-281.
42. Cambria RP, Brewster DC, Gertler J, et al. Vascular complications associated with spontaneous aortic dissection. *J Vasc Surg*. 1988;7:199-209.
43. Patel AY, Eagle KA, Vaishnava P. Acute type B aortic dissection: insights from the international registry of acute aortic dissection. *Ann Cardiothorac Surg*. 2014;3:368-374.
44. Williams DM, LePage MA, Lee DY. The dissected aorta: part I. Early anatomic changes in an in vitro model. *Radiology*. 1997;203:23-31.
45. Crawford TC, Beaulieu RJ, Ehlert BA, et al. Malperfusion syndromes in aortic dissections. *Vasc Med*. 2016;21:264-273.
46. Chung JW, Elkins C, Sakai T, et al. True-lumen collapse in aortic dissection: part II. Evaluation of treatment methods in phantoms with pulsatile flow. *Radiology*. 2000;214:99-106.
47. Williams DM, Lee DY, Hamilton BH, et al. The dissected aorta: part III. Anatomy and radiologic diagnosis of branch-vessel compromise. *Radiology*. 1997;203:37-44.
48. Williams DM, Lee DY, Hamilton BH, et al. The dissected aorta: percutaneous treatment of ischemic complications--principles and results. *J Vasc Interv Radiol*. 1997;8:605-625.
49. Kamman AV, Yang B, Kim KM, et al. Visceral malperfusion in aortic dissection: the michigan experience. *Semin Thorac Cardiovasc Surg*. 2017;29:173-178.
50. Suzuki T, Mehta RH, Ince H, et al. Clinical profiles and outcomes of acute type B aortic dissection in the current era: lessons from the international registry of aortic dissection (IRAD). *Circulation*. 2003;108(Suppl 1):II312-II317.
51. Tsai TT, Trimarchi S, Nienaber CA. Acute aortic dissection: perspectives from the international registry of acute aortic dissection (IRAD). *Eur J Vasc Endovasc Surg*. 2009;37:149-159.
52. Nallamothu BK, Mehta RH, Saint S, et al. Syncope in acute aortic dissection: diagnostic, prognostic, and clinical implications. *Am J Med*. 2002;113:468-471.
53. von Kodolitsch Y, Schwartz AG, Nienaber CA. Clinical prediction of acute aortic dissection. *Arch Intern Med*. 2000;160:2977-2982.
54. Clinical policy for the initial approach to adults presenting with a chief complaint of chest pain, with no history of trauma. American college of emergency physicians. *Ann Emerg Med*. [illegible].
55. Salmasi MY, Al Saadi N, Hartley P, et al. The risk of misdiagnosis in acute thoracic aortic dissection: a review of current guidelines. *Heart*. 2020;106:885-891.
56. Harris KM, Strauss CE, Eagle KA, et al. Correlates of delayed recognition and treatment of acute type a aortic dissection: the international registry of acute aortic dissection (IRAD). *Circulation*. 2011;124:1911-1918.
57. Erbel R, Alfonso F, Boileau C, et al. Diagnosis and management of aortic dissection. *Eur Heart J*. 2001;22:1642-1681.

58. Shiga T, Wajima Z, Apfel CC, et al. Diagnostic accuracy of transesophageal echocardiography, helical computed tomography, and magnetic resonance imaging for suspected thoracic aortic dissection: systematic review and meta-analysis. *Arch Intern Med.* 2006;166:1350-1356.
59. McMahon MA, Squirrell CA. Multidetector CT of aortic dissection: a pictorial review. *Radiographics.* 2010; 30:445-460.
60. Halpern EJ. Triple-rule-out CT angiography for evaluation of acute chest pain and possible acute coronary syndrome. *Radiology.* 2009;252:332-345.
61. Schwartz SI, Durham C, Clouse WD, et al. Predictors of late aortic intervention in patients with medically treated type B aortic dissection. *J Vasc Surg.* 2018; 67:78-84.
62. Fattouch K, Sampognaro R, Navarra E, et al. Long-term results after repair of type a acute aortic dissection according to false lumen patency. *Ann Thorac Surg.* 2009;88:1244-1250.
63. Tsai TT, Evangelista A, Nienaber CA, et al. Partial thrombosis of the false lumen in patients with acute type B aortic dissection. *N Engl J Med.* 2007;357:349-359.
64. Othersen JB, Maize JC, Woolson RF, et al. Nephrogenic systemic fibrosis after exposure to gadolinium in patients with renal failure. *Nephrol Dial Transplant.* 2007;22: 3179-3185.
65. Hope MD, Hope TA, Zhu C, et al. Vascular imaging with ferumoxytol as a contrast agent. *AJR Am J Roentgenol.* 2015;205:W366-W373.
66. Bashir MR, Bhatti L, Marin D, et al. Emerging applications for ferumoxytol as a contrast agent in MRI. *J Magn Reson Imaging.* 2015;41:884-898.
67. Koschyk DH, Nienaber CA, Knap M, et al. How to guide stent-graft implantation in type B aortic dissection? Comparison of angiography, transesophageal echocardiography, and intravascular ultrasound. *Circulation.* 2005;112:I260-I264.
68. Belkin N, Jackson BM, Foley PJ, et al. The use of intravascular ultrasound in the treatment of type B aortic dissection with thoracic endovascular aneurysm repair is associated with improved long-term survival. *J Vasc Surg.* 2020;72(2):490-497.
69. Lortz J, Tsagakis K, Rammos C, et al. Intravascular ultrasound assisted sizing in thoracic endovascular aortic repair improves aortic remodeling in type B aortic dissection. *PLoS One.* 2018;13:e0196180.
70. Baliga RR, Nienaber CA, Bossone E, et al. The role of imaging in aortic dissection and related syndromes. *JACC Cardiovasc Imaging.* 2014;7:406-424.
71. Erbel R, Oelert H, Meyer J, et al. Effect of medical and surgical therapy on aortic dissection evaluated by transesophageal echocardiography. Implications for prognosis and therapy. The European Cooperative Study Group on Echocardiography. *Circulation.* 1993; 87:1604-1615.
72. Hata N, Tanaka K, Imaizumi T, et al. Clinical significance of pleural effusion in acute aortic dissection. *Chest.* 2002;121:825-830.
73. Svensson LG, Labib SB, Eisenhauer AC, et al. Intimal tear without hematoma: an important variant of aortic dissection that can elude current imaging techniques. *Circulation.* 1999;99:1331-1336.
74. Erbel R, Aboyans V, Boileau C, et al. 2014 ESC Guidelines on the diagnosis and treatment of aortic diseases: document covering acute and chronic aortic diseases of the thoracic and abdominal aorta of the adult. The task force for the diagnosis and treatment of aortic diseases of the european society of cardiology (ESC). *Eur Heart J.* 2014;35:2873-2926.
75. Tsai TT, Nienaber CA, Eagle KA. Acute aortic syndromes. *Circulation.* 2005;112:3802-3813.
76. Khoynezhad A, Plestis KA. Managing emergency hypertension in aortic dissection and aortic aneurysm surgery. *J Card Surg.* 2006;21(suppl 1):S3-S7.
77. Nauta FJ, Trimarchi S, Kamman AV, et al. Update in the management of type B aortic dissection. *Vasc Med.* 2016;21:251-263.
78. Shores J, Berger KR, Murphy EA, et al. Progression of aortic dilatation and the benefit of long-term beta-adrenergic blockade in Marfan's syndrome. *N Engl J Med.* 1994;330:1335-1341.
79. den Hartog AW, Franken R, Zwinderman AH, et al. The risk for type B aortic dissection in Marfan syndrome. *J Am Coll Cardiol.* 2015;65:246-254.
80. Estrera AL, Miller CC 3rd, Safi HJ, et al. Outcomes of medical management of acute type B aortic dissection. *Circulation.* 2006;114:I384-I389.
81. Fattori R, Montgomery D, Lovato L, et al. Survival after endovascular therapy in patients with type B aortic dissection: a report from the international registry of acute aortic dissection (IRAD). *JACC Cardiovasc Interv.* 2013;6:876-882.
82. Durham CA, Cambria RP, Wang LJ, et al. The natural history of medically managed acute type B aortic dissection. *J Vasc Surg.* 2015;61:1192-1198.
83. Durham CA, Aranson NJ, Ergul EA, et al. Aneurysmal degeneration of the thoracoabdominal aorta after medical management of type B aortic dissections. *J Vasc Surg.* 2015;62:900-906.
84. Kato K, Nishio A, Kato N, et al. Uptake of 18F-FDG in acute aortic dissection: a determinant of unfavorable outcome. *J Nucl Med.* 2010;51:674-681.

85. Akutsu K, Nejima J, Kiuchi K, et al. Effects of the patent false lumen on the long-term outcome of type B acute aortic dissection. *Eur J Cardiothorac Surg*. 2004;26:359-366.
86. Schoder M, Czerny M, Cejna M, et al. Endovascular repair of acute type B aortic dissection: long-term follow-up of true and false lumen diameter changes. *Ann Thorac Surg*. 2007;83:1059-1066.
87. Nienaber CA, Rousseau H, Eggebrecht H, et al. Randomized comparison of strategies for type B aortic dissection: the INvestigation of STEnt grafts in aortic dissection (INSTEAD) trial. *Circulation*. 2009;120: 2519-2528.
88. Brunkwall J, Kasprzak P, Verhoeven E, et al. Endovascular repair of acute uncomplicated aortic type B dissection promotes aortic remodelling: 1 year results of the ADSORB trial. *Eur J Vasc Endovasc Surg*. 2014;48:285-291.
89. Nienaber CA, Kische S, Rousseau H, et al. Endovascular repair of type B aortic dissection: long-term results of the randomized investigation of stent grafts in aortic dissection trial. *Circ Cardiovasc Interv*. 2013;6:407-416.
90. Iannuzzi JC, Stapleton SM, Bababekov YJ, et al. Favorable impact of thoracic endovascular aortic repair on survival of patients with acute uncomplicated type B aortic dissection. *J Vasc Surg*. 2018;68:1649-1655.
91. Song C, Lu Q, Zhou J, et al. The new indication of TEVAR for uncomplicated type B aortic dissection. *Medicine (Baltimore)*. 2016;95:e3919.
92. Evangelista A, Salas A, Ribera A, et al. Long-term outcome of aortic dissection with patent false lumen: predictive role of entry tear size and location. *Circulation*. 2012;125:3133-3141.
93. Trimarchi S, Eagle KA, Nienaber CA, et al. Importance of refractory pain and hypertension in acute type B aortic dissection: insights from the international registry of acute aortic dissection (IRAD). *Circulation*. 2010;122:1283-1289.
94. Geisbüsch P, Kotelis D, von Tengg-Kobligk H, et al. Thoracic aortic endografting in patients with connective tissue diseases. *J Endovasc Ther*. 2008;15:144-149.
95. Liu L, Zhang S, Lu Q, et al. Impact of oversizing on the risk of retrograde dissection after TEVAR for acute and chronic type B dissection. *J Endovasc Ther*. 2016; 23:620-625.
96. Canaud L, Ozdemir BA, Patterson BO, et al. Retrograde aortic dissection after thoracic endovascular aortic repair. *Ann Surg*. 2014;260:389-395.
97. Chen Y, Zhang S, Liu L, et al. Retrograde type A aortic dissection after thoracic endovascular aortic repair: a systematic review and meta-analysis. *J Am Heart Assoc*. 2017;6(9):e004649.
98. Feezor RJ, Martin TD, Hess PJ Jr, et al. Extent of aortic coverage and incidence of spinal cord ischemia after thoracic endovascular aneurysm repair. *Ann Thorac Surg*. 2008;86:1809-1814; discussion 1814.
99. Matsumura JS, Lee WA, Mitchell RS, et al. The society for vascular surgery practice guidelines: management of the left subclavian artery with thoracic endovascular aortic repair. *J Vasc Surg*. 2009;50:1155-1158.
100. Desai ND, Gottret JP, Szeto WY, et al. Impact of timing on major complications after thoracic endovascular aortic repair for acute type B aortic dissection. *J Thorac Cardiovasc Surg*. 2015;149:S151-S156.
101. Wilkinson DA, Patel HJ, Williams DM, et al. Early open and endovascular thoracic aortic repair for complicated type B aortic dissection. *Ann Thorac Surg*. 2013;96:23-30; discussion 230.
102. Duebener LF, Lorenzen P, Richardt G, et al. Emergency endovascular stent-grafting for life-threatening acute type B aortic dissections. *Ann Thorac Surg*. 2004;78; 1261-1266; discussion 1266-1267.
103. Faure EM, Canaud L, Marty-Ane C, et al. Endovascular management of rupture in acute type B aortic dissections. *Eur J Vasc Endovasc Surg*. 2015;49:655-660.
104. Nienaber CA, Ince H, Weber F, et al. Emergency stent-graft placement in thoracic aortic dissection and evolving rupture. *J Card Surg*. 2003;18:464-470.
105. Fann JI, Smith JA, Miller DC, et al. Surgical management of aortic dissection during a 30-year period. *Circulation*. 1995;92:II113-II121.
106. Pearce BJ, Passman MA, Patterson MA, et al. Early outcomes of thoracic endovascular stent-graft repair for acute complicated type B dissection using the Gore TAG endoprosthesis. *Ann Vasc Surg*. 2008;22:742-749.
107. Henke PK, Williams DM, Upchurch GR Jr, et al. Acute limb ischemia associated with type B aortic dissection: clinical relevance and therapy. *Surgery*. 2006;140:532-539; discussion 539-540.
108. Barnes DM, Williams DM, Dasika NL, et al. A single-center experience treating renal malperfusion after aortic dissection with central aortic fenestration and renal artery stenting. *J Vasc Surg*. 2008;47:903-910; discussion 910-901.
109. Williams DM, Andrews JC, Marx MV, et al. Creation of reentry tears in aortic dissection by means of percutaneous balloon fenestration: gross anatomic and histologic considerations. *J Vasc Interv Radiol*. 1993;4:75-83.
110. Patel HJ, Williams DM, Meerkov M, et al. Long-term results of percutaneous management of malperfusion

in acute type B aortic dissection: implications for thoracic aortic endovascular repair. *J Thorac Cardiovasc Surg*. 2009;138:300-308.
111. Lombardi JV, Cambria RP, Nienaber CA, et al. Prospective multicenter clinical trial (STABLE) on the endovascular treatment of complicated type B aortic dissection using a composite device design. *J Vasc Surg*. 2012;55:629-640 e622.
112. Lombardi JV, Gleason TG, Panneton JM, et al. STABLE II clinical trial on endovascular treatment of acute, complicated type B aortic dissection with a composite device design. *J Vasc Surg*. 2020;71:1077-1087 e1072.
113. Faure EM, El Batti S, Abou Rjeili M, et al. Mid-term outcomes of stent assisted balloon induced intimal disruption and relamination in aortic dissection repair (STABILISE) in acute type B aortic dissection. *Eur J Vasc Endovasc Surg*. 2018;56:209-215.
114. Cambria RP. Surgical treatment of complicated distal aortic dissection. *Semin Vasc Surg*. 2002;15:97-107.
115. Panneton JM, Teh SH, Cherry KJ Jr, et al. Aortic fenestration for acute or chronic aortic dissection: an uncommon but effective procedure. *J Vasc Surg*. 2000;32:711-721.
116. Webb TH, Williams GM. Abdominal aortic tailoring for renal, visceral, and lower extremity malperfusion resulting from acute aortic dissection. *J Vasc Surg*. 1997;26:474-480; discussion 480-471.
117. Bashir M, Shaw M, Fok M, et al. Long-term outcomes in thoracoabdominal aortic aneurysm repair for chronic type B dissection. *Ann Cardiothorac Surg*. 2014;3:385-392.
118. Conway AM, Sadek M, Lugo J, et al. Outcomes of open surgical repair for chronic type B aortic dissections. *J Vasc Surg*. 2014;59:1217-1223.
119. Coselli JS, Bozinovski J, LeMaire SA. Open surgical repair of 2286 thoracoabdominal aortic aneurysms. *Ann Thorac Surg*. 2007;83:S862-S864; discussion S890-862.
120. Thrumurthy SG, Karthikesalingam A, Patterson BO, et al. A systematic review of mid-term outcomes of thoracic endovascular repair (TEVAR) of chronic type B aortic dissection. *Eur J Vasc Endovasc Surg*. 2011;42:632-647.
121. Acher C, Wynn M. Outcomes in open repair of the thoracic and thoracoabdominal aorta. *J Vasc Surg*. 2010;52:3S-9S.
122. Cowan JA Jr, Dimick JB, Henke PK, et al. Surgical treatment of intact thoracoabdominal aortic aneurysms in the United States: hospital and surgeon volume-related outcomes. *J Vasc Surg*. 2003;37:1169-1174.
123. Rigberg DA, McGory ML, Zingmond DS, et al. Thirty-day mortality statistics underestimate the risk of repair of thoracoabdominal aortic aneurysms: a statewide experience. *J Vasc Surg*. 2006;43:217-222; discussion 223.
124. Chuter TA, Gordon RL, Reilly LM, et al. An endovascular system for thoracoabdominal aortic aneurysm repair. *J Endovasc Ther*. 2001;8:25-33.
125. Verhoeven EL, Katsargyris A, Bekkema F, et al. Editor's choice—ten-year experience with endovascular repair of thoracoabdominal aortic aneurysms: results from 166 consecutive patients. *Eur J Vasc Endovasc Surg*. 2015;49:524-531.
126. Eagleton MJ, Follansbee M, Wolski K, et al. Fenestrated and branched endovascular aneurysm repair outcomes for type II and III thoracoabdominal aortic aneurysms. *J Vasc Surg*. 2016;63:930-942.
127. Kitagawa A, Greenberg RK, Eagleton MJ, et al. Fenestrated and branched endovascular aortic repair for chronic type B aortic dissection with thoracoabdominal aneurysms. *J Vasc Surg*. 2013;58:625-634.

SELF-ASSESSMENT STUDY QUESTIONS AND ANSWERS

Questions

1. A 55-year-old man is admitted to the ICU with an uncomplicated type B aortic dissection 5 days prior to evaluation. At that time, he was admitted to the ICU for blood pressure control and close monitoring. Despite adequate pain medication, he still has severe chest pain that is similar to the pain he had on admission. His systolic blood pressure has been well controlled and has been ranging from 100 to 110 mmHg; his heart rate has been in the 50s. His labs are normal, and all pulses are palpable. A repeat CTA chest, abdomen, and pelvis is performed, and it shows a stable type B aortic dissection without signs of organ malperfusion or severe compression of the true lumen. What is the next most appropriate move?

A. Move him to the floor since his blood pressure is well controlled
B. Keep him in the ICU for monitoring
C. Keep him in the ICU for monitoring but plan to repeat a CTA in 2 days
D. TEVAR

2. A 32-year-old woman with Marfan syndrome presents to the emergency room with tearing chest pain and is found to have an uncomplicated type B aortic dissection. She is admitted to the ICU for medical management. On day 4 in the ICU, she is transferred to the floor as her pain has resolved and her blood pressure is controlled on oral antihypertensives. Prior to discharge on hospital day 7, a CTA is repeated, which shows that her thoracic aorta has enlarged by 5 mm, making her total aortic diameter 42 mm. The false lumen is patent. What is the next most appropriate intervention?

A. Discharge the patient with a plan to repeat the CTA in 1 month
B. Keep the patient in the hospital for continued monitoring
C. Increase the doses of her antihypertensives
D. Place TEVAR to prevent further degeneration

3. A 49-year-old man presents to the hospital with severe back, abdominal, and bilateral lower extremity pain. He has nonpalpable femoral pulses and abdominal pain out of proportion to physical examination. He undergoes a CTA which is notable for a type B aortic dissection with severe true lumen compression starting in the descending thoracic aorta and poor enhancement of the bowel and bilateral kidneys. The dissection does not extend into any visceral vessels. Zones 2 and 3 of the aorta are dilated to 4.4 cm and are lined with intramural hematoma. What is the most appropriate intervention for this patient?

A. TEVAR
B. Open repair of the descending thoracic aorta
C. Percutaneous flap fenestration
D. Mesenteric, renal artery stenting, and femorofemoral bypass

4. A 65-year-old woman undergoes TEVAR for a complicated aortic dissection. The total length of covered aorta was 240 mm. Her initial postoperative examination is normal, however, you are paged to the bedside 4 hours later because the patient cannot move her legs. The rest of her neurologic examination is intact What is the next most appropriate action?

A. Obtain a STAT CTA to evaluate for endograft migration
B. Obtain a STAT head CT and neurology consult for consideration of tPA administration
C. Place a spinal drain, increase target mean arterial pressure to 90 mmHg, draw labs, and transfuse packed red blood cells to a goal hemoglobin of 10 g/dL
D. Emergently return to the operating room

SELF-ASSESSMENT STUDY QUESTIONS AND ANSWERS

5. A 44-year-old woman presents with a type B aortic dissection with a severely compressed true lumen that is causing mesenteric malperfusion. The plan is to place a TEVAR to alleviate her malperfusion. When reviewing the scan, you notice that the dissection originates at the left subclavian origin. Her vertebral arteries are the same size and she has no other medical problems or prior surgeries. What is the best course of action?

A. Perform an open repair instead of a TEVAR
B. Perform a left carotid-subclavian bypass prior to TEVAR
C. Perform a TEVAR; cover the left subclavian artery without additional procedures
D. Snorkel the left subclavian from the left arm and place TEVAR

6. What is the role of stent-assisted balloon-induced intimal disruption with TEVAR?

A. Normalize pressure in the visceral aortic true and false lumen
B. Prevent distal abdominal aortic dilation
C. Prevent retrograde dissection
D. Prevent retrograde false lumen flow

7. A 50-year-old man presents with mesenteric ischemia from a type B aortic dissection causing malperfusion. The true lumen is significantly compressed in the descending thoracic aorta. The dissection plane extends into the SMA, where the false lumen is thrombosed and narrows the ostium. The patient is taken to the operating room and a TEVAR is placed. After endograft deployment, an angiogram is performed which shows minimal flow through the SMA. What is the next most appropriate action?

A. Select and stent the SMA ostium
B. Perform a percutaneous fenestration
C. Perform a retrograde aorta-SMA
D. Start a heparin drip and transfer the patient to the ICU

8. A patient is being admitted to the ICU for medical management of an uncomplicated type B aortic dissection. An arterial catheter is placed for blood pressure management. What is the most appropriate first agent to initiate?

A. Nicardipine
B. Esmolol
C. Nitroprusside
D. Hydralazine

9. A patient undergoing a TEVAR for an uncomplicated type B aortic dissection, originating at the origin of the left subclavian artery.

A. Dominant right vertebral artery
B. Thrombosed left upper extremity arteriovenous fistula
C. Patent left internal mammary artery to LAD coronary artery bypass graft
D. Bovine aortic arch anatomy

10. Select the correct Stanford, Debakey, and STS/SVS designation for a dissection with the following conformation: Entry tear in the ascending aorta with extension of the dissection into the descending thoracic aorta, just above the diaphragm.

A. Stanford A, Debakey IIIb, STS/SVS A_5
B. Stanford A, Debakey I, STS/SVS A_5
C. Stanford B, Debakey II, STS/SVS $B_{0,5}$
D. Stanford A, Debakey I, STS/SVS $B_{0,5}$

SELF-ASSESSMENT STUDY QUESTIONS AND ANSWERS

Answers

1. D.
2. A.
3. C.
4. C.
5. C.
6. D.
7. A.
8. B.
9. C.
10. B.

CHAPTER

27 Penetrating Aortic Ulcerations and Intramural Hematomas

Matthew B. Schneck and Behzad S. Farivar

OUTLINE

BACKGROUND
PENETRATING AORTIC ULCER (PAU)
INTRAMURAL HEMATOMA (IMH)
CLINICAL FINDINGS
LABORATORY EVALUATION
Imaging
NATURAL HISTORY AND DISEASE PROGRESSION
TREATMENT
Medical Management
Surgical Management
Overview
Ascending Aorta
Descending Aorta
SUMMARY

BACKGROUND

Acute aortic syndromes (AAS) are constellation of potentially life-threatening pathologies characterized by disruption of tunica media layer of the aortic wall. It includes a spectrum of disease entities consisting of aortic dissection (AD), penetrating aortic ulcers (PAUs), and intramural hematomas (IMH). Age and sex-adjusted incidence of AAS is reported to be 7.7 cases per 100,000 person-years.[1,2] In this chapter, we will focus on pathophysiology, epidemiology, natural history, and treatment of PAU and IMH.

PENETRATING AORTIC ULCER (PAU)

PAU is a focal disruption in the intima and internal elastic lamina of the aorta typically caused by erosion of an atherosclerotic plaque and corresponding inflammatory changes in the aortic wall. PAUs can present as an isolated entity or concomitantly with IMH and ADs. Similar to ADs, PAUs are classified using the Stanford classification. Type A PAUs occur in the ascending aorta, whereas type B PAUs occur in the descending aorta. PAUs are located in the aortic arch in 7% of cases, descending thoracic aortic in 63% of cases, and abdominal aorta in 30%.[3] In patients with symptomatic PAU on presentation, rupture rates of up to 45% have been reported.[3]

First described by Shennan in 1934, PAUs are responsible for 2% to 10% of AAS and are disproportionately found in older patients with advanced atherosclerotic disease as opposed to ADs, which are more prevalent in young hypertensive patients.[1,4] The incidence of PAU is 2.1 per 100,000 person-years. It most commonly affects older patients with diffuse atherosclerosis and significant cardiovascular risk factors; however, young patients with connective tissue diseases are also at high risk.[2]

INTRAMURAL HEMATOMA (IMH)

IMH, identified by Krukenberg in 1920, is defined as an accumulation of hemorrhage in the tunica media without an identifiable intimal tear on imaging. Classically, IMH was thought to be due to vasa vasorum rupture. However, new theories suggest that a transient intimal tear allowing for accumulation of blood in the media layer of the aortic with subsequent thromboses of blood may be responsible.[5] Interestingly, these tears seem to occur in a plane closer to the adventitia than classic dissections which may explain IMH's propensity for rupture.[6] The accumulated hemorrhage can then infarct the aortic wall predisposing the patient to AD, pseudoaneurysm development, and aneurysmal degeneration.[1,7-9] While IMH may present with symptoms similar to an AD, they occur in the absence of false lumen flow and are most commonly localized to the descending thoracic aorta in 50% to 85% of cases.[5]

The precise prevalence of IMH in AAS remains unclear, with reported rates ranging from the low-single digits to as high as one-third of all AAS cases. The International Registry of Acute Aortic Dissection (IRAD), comprising 30 aortic centers in 10 countries, reported a rate of only 6.3% while several Asian studies report rates of greater than 30%.[7,8] Similar to the PAU population cohort, IMHs are typically found in elderly patients with extensive cardiovascular risk factors. The reported incidence of IMH is slightly lower than that of PAU at 1.2 cases per 100,000 person-years.[2]

CLINICAL FINDINGS

In the acute setting, the most common presentation of symptomatic AAS, including IMH and PAU, is a sudden and intense tearing pain that radiates down the chest or toward the back. Type A AAS is more commonly associated with chest pain, whereas type B AAS is more commonly associated with back pain.[7] Corresponding signs and symptoms are highly dependent on aortic branch involvement. Aortic branch vessel compromise can cause malperfusion syndromes when there is end-organ ischemia. It is important to recognize that AAS can cause symptoms and electrocardiogram (ECG) changes (i.e., T-wave inversions) that mimic acute coronary syndrome (ACS) and therefore should be kept on the differential for all patients presenting with chest pain.[10] In the chronic setting, these lesions might be asymptomatic and incidentally discovered on cross-sectional imaging.

LABORATORY EVALUATION

While nonspecific for AAS, biomarker evaluation may offer prognostic data and guide treatment. All patients who present with symptoms concerning for AAS should have a comprehensive biomarker evaluation to aid in differential diagnosis and identification of complications. Comprehensive blood counts should be used to evaluate for anemia, infection, and inflammatory response. Liver function tests, creatinine, and troponins should be collected to evaluate hepatic, renal, and myocardial ischemia, respectively. The negative predictive value of a D-dimer has been proven useful in detecting IMH (but not PAUs) when a cutoff of 500 ng/mL is applied.[7] D-dimer can be trended through admission and following the diagnosis of AAS. A level greater than 9000 ng/mL is an independent predictor of mortality.[11]

IMAGING

Computed tomography angiography (CTA) is the mainstay of AAS diagnosis, providing excellent visualization of the entire aorta. In IMH, the sensitivity of CT is nearly 100%. In equivocal cases, MRI can be used to confirm the diagnosis in stable patients.[12] To effectively diagnose IMH, both nonenhanced and contrast-enhanced imaging must be performed. On nonenhanced CT, IMH is characterized by crescentic hyperattenuated thickening in the aortic wall usually greater than 5 to 7 mm with Hounsfield units of 60 to 70. When contrast is administered, the aortic wall thickening characteristic of IMH should not enhance. IMH can be differentiated from mural thrombus by identifying the presence of medially displaced intimal calcification.[7] IMH also typically does not narrow the lumen like a mural thrombus.[4] PAUs, on the other hand, tend to demonstrate crater-like ulcerations with a thickened aortic wall in a diffusely atherosclerotic aorta. When evaluating for aortic pathology, utilization of ECG-gated CT scans can be useful in eliminating heart pulsation-induced motion artifact.[9] This is especially important for the identification of type A AAS.

Recent reports have highlighted the potential role of transesophageal echocardiography (TEE) in IMH diagnosis, particularly when hemodynamic instability prevents preoperative CT. IMH can be visualized as a crescentic thickening of the aortic wall to >7 mm, with corresponding mixed echogenicity in the wall and a smooth intimal surface. This can be distinguished from atheromatous plaques, which appear echo-dense and exhibit a cobblestone shape with an uneven surface. Thrombosed false lumens are also different in the appearance on TEE, demonstrating irregular intimal surfaces and often a spiral pattern.[13,14]

NATURAL HISTORY AND DISEASE PROGRESSION

Successful treatment of PAU and IMH depends on understanding their natural history. Compared to classic ADs, the natural history of PAU and IMH is neither well known nor well understood. The clinical course of PAUs is highly variable, ranging from indefinite stability to aortic rupture if the adventitia is penetrated. Major risk factors for PAU progression are symptomatic presentation, depth greater than 10 mm, diameter greater than 20 mm, accompanying IMH, or presence of a pleural effusion.[5,15] In patients with refractory symptoms, it must be assumed that there is adventitia involvement and rupture is impending.[16] A single institution study of 63 symptomatic PAU patients specifically identified a depth of greater than 15 mm as an independent predictor of mortality.[17] Risk of rupture in PAU is related to ulcer depth. Multiple retrospective single-institution studies examining PAUs have found that the natural course of small, isolated, and uncomplicated PAUs is relatively benign, thus warranting conservative management alongside best medical therapy (BMT). In a study of 43 consecutive patients with PAU with a mean follow-up of 4 years, overall mortality was 30%, while mortality for those who eventually required surgery was 39%.[4] Annual CTA surveillance to evaluate PAU progression is recommended due to its associated high mortality of 17% to 30%.[3,4,18] In a large, single-center study, asymptomatic PAUs with a baseline aortic diameter of >42 mm enlarged more rapidly and required more frequent surveillance.[19]

Similar to PAUs, the natural history of IMH is also highly variable. When untreated, IMH can progress to dissection in 28% to 47% of patients and aneurysmal degeneration or contained rupture in 20% to 45% of patients.[1,2] Fewer than 10% of cases will resolve without intervention.[8] Predictors of IMH-related complications are involvement of the ascending aorta, aortic diameter > 50 mm, progressive maximum aortic wall thickness > 11 mm, recurrent pleural effusion, association with a PAU, and presence of ulcer-like projections.[20,21] Younger patients and hematoma thickness of <10 mm portend a better prognosis. Concomitant presence of PAUs with IMHs portends a worse prognosis and carries a higher risk of rupture.

In a 10-year retrospective study based on the Rochester Epidemiology Project comprising 133 AAS patients with a mean follow-up of 10 years, aortic-related mortality was 32% with over half of aortic-related deaths attributed to rupture. Following AAS, freedom from aortic-related mortality at 5, 10, and 15 years was 84%, 80%, and 77%, respectively.[22]

After an AAS event and surviving to the 14-day time-point (subacute phase), patients are at 2.4 times higher risk of nonaortic cardiovascular death and a threefold higher risk of nonfatal cardiovascular event (stroke, myocardial infarct, or heart failure). Therefore, lifelong cardiovascular care with cardiovascular risk factor modification and long-term surveillance and follow-up are paramount in these patients.[23]

TREATMENT

MEDICAL MANAGEMENT

Anti-impulse therapy remains the cornerstone of medical treatment for AAS management. This results in the reduction of left ventricular contraction velocity, thereby reducing sheer stress and lesion propagation. Antihypertensive agents are initiated with the goal of reducing the systolic blood pressure to 100 to 120 mmHg and heart rate to <60 beats per minute, if tolerable.[21] This can be accomplished with initiation of beta-blockers first followed by sodium nitroprusside.[16,24] Calcium channel blockers and renin–angiotensin inhibitors can be used when patients are unable to tolerate beta blockers. Beta-blockade remains the first-line medical therapy considering its benefit of improved 1-year mortality regardless of the lesion's anatomic location. Opioid pain control is also an essential component of BMT in AAS.[21]

Aortic replacement remains the gold standard treatment of type A IMH, even though best practice management continues to be debated. Multiple meta-analyses have demonstrated superiority of surgical management, although several Asian studies—a region with higher frequency of IMH among AAS cases—advocate for initial medical management.[8,25] A North American-based study analyzing BMT demonstrated a high failure rate when used in isolation, particularly within 14 days of presentation. Type B IMH is generally more responsive to initial medical therapy and less likely to require surgical intervention. Although there are no well-established guidelines, treatment indications parallel that of type B AD. In a single institution retrospective analysis of 92 IMH cases with 67 initially treated with BMT alone, 32 patients underwent thoracic endovascular aortic repair (TEVAR) within 14 days for early BMT failure and another 11 underwent TEVAR following late BMT failure. In this study, medical management alone was successful in only 19 patients.[26] IMH thickness of >8 mm was shown to be an independent risk factor for BMT failure.[26] Regardless of management strategy, referral of IMH patients upon initial presentation to a comprehensive aortic center with cardiovascular expertise has been shown to reduce the likelihood of disease progression by 40%.[18]

SURGICAL MANAGEMENT

Overview

Historically, open surgical repair (OSR) has demonstrated durable success in the management of PAU and IMH with an operative mortality of nearly 16%.[27] PAUs and IMHs present in patients with severe diffuse atherosclerotic disease, and therefore might have limited aortic clamp site availability.[19] If OSR of IMH is indicated, particularly in cases involving the ascending aorta, clamps should not be placed across hematoma to prevent inadvertent conversion to a dissection when the contained IMH is dislodged.[28] A large-scale review comprising 310 PAU patients involving the descending thoracic aorta resulted in a 30-day mortality rate of 4.8% and 1-year survival of 91.1% in the setting of minimal complications and excellent technical success. In the current era, endovascular therapy offers significantly reduced morbidity and mortality for the treatment of descending aortic pathologies.

Ascending Aorta

Symptomatic Stanford type A IMHs warrant urgent surgical intervention, justified by an early mortality rate of 55% when using medical management alone versus 8% following surgical intervention.[24] Ascending aortic PAUs also warrant urgent surgical repair.[1] In cases of PAU along the arch, success has been achieved using a hybrid approach consisting of cervical debranching procedures followed by TEVAR deployment just distal to the innominate artery. The ability to repair arch lesions without the need for cardiopulmonary bypass and hypothermic circulatory arrest is essential for a pathology that presents frequently in the patients unable to tolerate extreme physiologic stress.[29] For PAUs that occur proximal to the innominate, custom stent-graft deployment has also achieved success without the need for cervical debranching in high-risk patients where open surgery is contraindicated.[30] These custom stent-grafts are currently only available as investigational devices at select centers in the United States.

Descending Aorta

Current optimal management of Stanford Type B PAU and IMH parallels that of Type B dissections. Provided the lesion is uncomplicated, medical treatment as described previously is warranted.[1] Symptomatic descending aortic PAUs and IMHs in hemodynamically stable patients should be initially medically optimized, usually in the intensive care environment, while a definitive repair is planned. Hemodynamic instability is an indication for urgent operative repair with the European Society for Vascular Surgery recommending endovascular repair as first-line treatment in complicated Type B PAU and IMH.[15]

Other indications for type B PAU repair include the presence of saccular aneurysms, periaortic hematoma, associated enlarging IMH, intimal disruption, or refractory pain despite optimal medical therapy. Indications for type B IMH repair include failed optimal medical management, aortic diameter greater than 50 to 55 mm, or signs of contained rupture.[1,20] Based on a recent meta-analysis, the small intimal disruptions that can be seen in advanced imaging, are not associated with higher complication rates and should not be a standalone indication for surgery.[31]

Utilization of TEVAR in PAU patients has been successful with excellent technical success, low complication rates, and minimal need for repeat intervention.[17] In circumstances where standard TEVAR is not anatomically feasible, several groups have achieved success using physician-modified endografts. For paraceliac PAUs, exclusion and adequate landing zones have been achieved with a celiac fenestration and an Superior mesenteric artery scallop on a thoracic stent graft.[32]

It is important to recognize that PAU in the descending aorta, particularly along the free lateral wall or at the concavity of the distal arch, can result in IMH of the entire thoracic aorta. In these locations, the natural barrier of the supra-aortic branches does not prevent retrograde extension. When this pathology presents, it can be successfully treated with TEVAR exclusion of the PAU site in isolation based on the results of a small retrospective study demonstrating complete remodeling of the ascending aorta in all patients with uneventful follow-up to a mean duration of 16 months.[9]

A useful decision tree for PAU management has been published by Janosi et al.[17] In summary, patients exhibiting hemodynamic instability, rupture, refractory pain, aortic diameter > 55 mm, large pseudoaneurysms, or an IMH were immediately referred for TEVAR. Patients not meeting these criteria were followed-up and received TEVAR only if they developed the previously described signs or had an increase in aortic diameter or PAU depth of >5 mm per year.[17]

Recent reports also highlight the potential for intravascular ultrasound (IVUS) guided exclusion of PAUs in a series of 13 consecutive patients, significantly decreasing radiation and contrast exposure while at the same time demonstrating excellent technical success, morbidity, and mortality at a mean follow-up of 25 months. Long-term data of IVUS-based PAU repair are not currently available.[33]

SUMMARY

IMH and PAU are distinct yet interlinked complex pathologies and along with AD comprise AAS. IMH and PAUs are prevalent in elderly patients with significant comorbidity, thus early diagnosis and treatment are key for preventing aortic-related mortality. Early diagnosis is facilitated by cross-sectional imaging in stable patients and TEE in unstable patients. Type A IMH and PAU are less responsive to medical management and warrant a lower threshold for surgical intervention. Surgical treatment with graft replacement of the involved aortic segment remains the gold standard treatment of type A IMH and PAU. Type B IMH and PAU are more responsive to medical therapy. Complicated, symptomatic, rapid disease progression or ruptured type B IMH and PAUs should undergo TEVAR if anatomically amenable to endovascular repair. Lifelong aortic care with long-term follow-up, optimal medical therapy with cardiovascular risk factor modification, and imaging surveillance are critical in preventing complications and identifying the need for further intervention.

REFERENCES

1. Oderich GS, Kärkkäinen JM, Reed NR, Tenorio ER, Sandri GA. Penetrating aortic ulcer and intramural hematoma. *Cardiovasc Intervent Radiol.* 2019;42(3): 321-334.
2. Demartino RR, Sen I, Huang Y, et al. Population-based assessment of the incidence of aortic dissection, intramural hematoma, and penetrating ulcer, and its associated mortality from 1995 to 2015. *Circ Cardiovasc Qual Outcomes.* 2018;11(8):e004689.
3. Nathan DP, Boonn W, Lai E, et al. Presentation, complications, and natural history of penetrating atherosclerotic ulcer disease. *J Vasc Surg.* 2012;55(1):10-15.
4. Salim S, Locci R, Martin G, et al. Short- and long-term outcomes in isolated penetrating aortic ulcer disease. *J Vasc Surg.* 2020;72(1):84-91.
5. Riambau V, Böckler D, Brunkwall J, et al. Editor's choice—management of descending thoracic aorta diseases. *Eur J Vasc Endovasc Surg.* 2017;53(1):4-52.
6. Uchida K, Imoto K, Takahashi M, et al. Pathologic characteristics and surgical indications of superacute type a intramural hematoma. *Ann Thorac Surg.* 2005;79(5):1518-1521.
7. Ferrera C, Vilacosta I, Cabeza B, et al. Diagnosing aortic intramural hematoma: current perspectives. *Vasc Health Risk Manag.* 2020;16:203-213.
8. Harris KM, Braverman AC, Eagle KA, et al. Acute aortic intramural hematoma: an analysis from the International Registry of Acute Aortic Dissection. *Circulation.* 2012;126(11 Suppl 1):S91-S96.

9. Grimm M, Loewe C, Gottardi R, et al. Novel insights into the mechanisms and treatment of intramural hematoma affecting the entire thoracic aorta. *Ann Thorac Surg*. 2008;86(2):453-456.
10. Mishra AK, Nadadur S, Sahu KK, Lal A. Penetrating aortic ulcer masquerading as acute coronary syndrome *Am J Med Sci*. 2019;358(4):e15-e16.
11. Gorla R, Erbel R, Kahlert P, et al. Diagnostic role and prognostic implications of D-dimer in different classes of acute aortic syndromes. *Eur Heart J: Acute Cardiovascular Care*. 2017;6(5):379-388.
12. Alomari IB, Hamirani YS, Madera G, Tabe C, Akhtar N, Raizada V. Aortic intramural hematoma and its complications. *Circulation*. 2014;129(6):711-716.
13. Makhija N, Magoon R, Sarkar S. Transesophageal echocardiographic imaging of an aortic intramural hematoma: characterizing the crescent. *Can J Anaesth*. 2019;66(11):1415-1416.
14. Ivascu NS, Skubas NJ. Aortic intramural hematoma: echocardiographic characteristics. *Anesth Analg*. 2012; 114(2):286-288.
15. Evangelista A, Czerny M, Nienaber C, et al. Interdisciplinary expert consensus on management of type B intramural haematoma and penetrating aortic ulcer. *Eur J Cardiothorac Surg*. February 2015;47(2): 209-217.
16. Soyama A, Kono T, Matsuoka T, et al. A case of penetrating atherosclerotic ulcer treated with thoracic endovascular aortic repair. *Circulation*. 2015;132(24): 2352-2353.
17. Janosi RA, Gorla R, Tsagakis K, et al. Thoracic endovascular repair of complicated penetrating aortic ulcer: an 11-year single-center experience. *J Endovasc Ther*. 2016;23(1):150-159.
18. Gabel JA, Tomihama RT, Abou-Zamzam AM Jr, et al. Early surgical referral for penetrating aortic ulcer leads to improved outcome and overall survival. *Ann Vasc Surg*. May 2019;57:29-34.
19. Gifford SM, Duncan AA, Greiten LE, et al. The natural history and outcomes for thoracic and abdominal penetrating aortic ulcers. *J Vasc Surg*. 2016;63(5):1182-1188.
20. Li Z, Liu C, Wu R, et al. Prognostic value of clinical and morphologic findings in patients with type B aortic intramural hematoma. *J Cardiothorac Surg*. 2020;15(1):49.
21. Piffaretti G, Lomazzi C, Benedetto F, et al. Best medical treatment and selective stent graft repair for acute type B aortic intramural hematoma. Multicenter study observational study. *Semin Thorac Cardiovasc Surg*. Autumn 2018;30(3):279-287.
22. Weiss S, Sen I, Huang Y, et al. Population-based assessment of aortic-related outcomes in aortic dissection, intramural hematoma, and penetrating aortic ulcer. *Ann Vasc Surg*. 2020;69:62-73.
23. Weiss S, Sen I, Huang Y, et al. Cardiovascular morbidity and mortality after aortic dissection, intramural hematoma, and penetrating aortic ulcer. *J Vasc Surg*. 2019;70(3):724-731.e1.
24. Von Kodolitsch Y, CsöSz SK, Koschyk DH, et al. Intramural hematoma of the aorta. *Circulation*. 2003; 107(8):1158-1163.
25. Maraj R, Rerkpattanapipat P, Jacobs LE, Makornwattana P, Kotler MN. Meta-analysis of 143 reported cases of aortic intramural hematoma. *Am J Cardiol*. 2000;86(6): 664-668.
26. Mesar T, Lin MJ, Kabir I, Dexter DJ, Rathore A, Panneton JM. Medical therapy in type B aortic intramural hematoma is associated with a high failure rate. *J Vasc Surg*. 2020;71(4):1088-1096.
27. D'Annoville T, Ozdemir BA, Alric P, Marty-Ane CH, Canaud L. Thoracic endovascular aortic repair for penetrating aortic ulcer: literature review. *Ann Thorac Surg*. 2016;101(6):2272-2278.
28. Beckmann E, Dalia AA, Jelly CA, Melnitchouk S. Type A intramural haematoma secondary to penetrating atherosclerotic ulcer of the ascending aorta. *Interact Cardiovasc Thorac Surg*. 2019;28(3):491-492.
29. Canaud L, Hireche K, D'Annoville T, Alric P. Hybrid aortic arch repair for a ruptured and infected penetrating atherosclerotic ulcer of the aortic arch. *Ann Vasc Surg*. 2011;25(2):266.e5-266.e7.
30. Kratimenos T, Baikoussis NG, Tomais D, Argiriou M. Ascending aorta endovascular repair of a symptomatic penetrating atherosclerotic ulcer with a custom-made endograft. *Ann Vasc Surg*. 2018;47:280.e1-280.e4.
31. Moral S, Ballesteros E, Roque M, et al. Intimal disruption in type B aortic intramural hematoma. Does size matter? A systematic review and meta-analysis. *Int J Cardiol*. 2018;269:298-303.
32. Natalicchio G, Biello A, Castriotta G, La Marca MG, Sorino G, Salcuni M. Endovascular repair of a penetrating aortic ulcer with a custom-made relay stent graft featuring a single celiac trunk fenestration and a superior mesenteric artery scallop. *Ann Vasc Surg*. 2018;52:314.e1-314.e5.
33. Illuminati G, Pasqua R, Nardi P, Fratini C, Calio FG, Ricco J-B. Intravascular ultrasound-assisted endovascular exclusion of penetrating aortic ulcers. *Ann Vasc Surg*. 2021;70:467-473.

SELF-ASSESSMENT STUDY QUESTIONS AND ANSWERS

Questions

1. When performing transesophageal echocardiography (TEE) in a patient with symptoms concerning for an acute aortic syndrome, a crescentic thickening of the aortic wall is visualized. This finding is associated with mixed echogenicity in the wall with a maintained smooth intimal surface. The likely diagnosis based on the TEE findings in this patient is:
   A. Penetrating aortic ulcer
   B. Intramural hematoma
   C. Contained rupture
   D. Aortic dissection

2. Multiple retrospective single-institution studies have demonstrated that the natural course of small, isolated, and uncomplicated PAUs is relatively benign, although CT surveillance is essential. At which interval is surveillance of PAUs recommended?
   A. Every 6 months
   B. Every 6 months for the first 2 years, annually thereafter
   C. Every 1 year
   D. Every 2 years

3. Anti-impulse control is the cornerstone of medical treatment for acute aortic syndromes. The goal hemodynamic parameters for anti-impulse control are SBP from 100 to 120 mmHg and HR < 60. The first-line medications to achieve these parameters are:
   A. Beta-blockers and systemic vasodilators
   B. Calcium channel blockers
   C. ACE inhibitors
   D. Thiazide diuretics

4. Which one of the following findings on imaging has the greatest association with risk of rupture in penetrating aortic ulcerations?
   A. Ulcer width
   B. Ulcer depth
   C. Ulcer calcification
   D. Thrombus burden

5. Compared to patient with acute aortic dissections, patients with intramural hematomas and penetrating aortic ulceration are typically
   A. Younger and have risk factors for atherosclerosis
   B. Younger and have risk factors for long-standing hypertension
   C. Older and have risk factors for connective tissue disorders
   D. Older and have risk factors for atherosclerosis and hypertension

SELF-ASSESSMENT STUDY QUESTIONS AND ANSWERS

Answers

1. B.
2. C.
3. A.
4. B.
5. D.

CHAPTER

28 Visceral Aneurysms

Rachael Nicholson

OUTLINE

GENERAL CONSIDERATION AND HISTORY
- Splenic Artery Aneurysms
- Hepatic Artery Aneurysms
- Superior Mesenteric Artery Aneurysms
- Celiac Artery Aneurysms
- Gastric, Gastroepiploic Arteries, Pancreaticoduodenal, and Gastroduodenal Artery Aneurysms
- Inferior Mesenteric Artery Aneurysms
- Ileal, Jejunal, and Colic Artery Aneurysms

CLINICAL FINDINGS
- Splenic Artery Aneurysms
- Hepatic Artery Aneurysms
- Celiac Artery Aneurysms
- Superior Mesenteric Artery Aneurysms
- Gastroduodenal/Pancreaticoduodenal
- Jejunal, Ileal, Colic, and Inferior Mesenteric Artery Aneurysms

DIFFERENTIAL DIAGNOSIS

DIAGNOSIS

MANAGEMENT OF THE CLINICAL PROBLEM
- General Considerations of Endovascular Management
- Endovascular Treatment of Splenic Artery Aneurysms
- Endovascular Treatment of Hepatic Artery Aneurysms
- Endovascular Treatment of Superior Mesenteric Artery Aneurysms
- Endovascular Treatment of Celiac Artery Aneurysms
- Endovascular Treatment of Gastric, Gastroepiploic, Gastroduodenal, and Pancreaticoduodenal Aneurysms
- Endovascular Treatment of Jejunal, Ileal, and Colic Artery Aneurysms

OPEN REPAIR
- General Considerations
- Open Repair of Splenic Artery Aneurysms
- Open Repair of Hepatic Artery Aneurysms
- Open Repair of Superior Mesenteric Artery Aneurysms
- Open Repair of Celiac Artery Aneurysms
- Open Repair of Gastric, Gastroepiploic, Gastroduodenal, and Pancreaticoduodenal Artery Aneurysms
- Open Repair of Jejunal, Ileal, and Colic Artery Aneurysms

GENERAL CONSIDERATION AND HISTORY

Visceral artery aneurysms (VAAs) include aneurysms affecting the celiac, superior mesenteric, and inferior mesenteric arteries and their branches. VAAs are rare with a reported incidence of 0.01% to 2% based on autopsy results, but the incidence has been reported as high as 10% in the elderly population.[1,2] They comprise only 5% of aneurysms within the abdominal cavity. Of those who present with a VAA, 45% have aneurysms in other locations, such as the aorta, iliac renal, lower extremity, intracranial, and other visceral vessels.[3]

VAA was first reported by Beaussier in 1770, who described a splenic artery aneurysm found on autopsy of a 60-year-old woman.[4] The first hepatic artery aneurysm (HAA) was described in 1809 by Wilson after a postmortem examination demonstrated a ruptured left HAA. In 1903, Kehr described the first repair of a VAA by ligating a proper HAA.[5] De Bakey reported the repair of a mycotic superior mesenteric artery aneurysm (SMAA) in 1953.[6]

VAAs include both true and false aneurysms. Atherosclerosis is the most common cause of true visceral aneurysms, although they can be associated with medial degeneration, connective tissue diseases, such as Ehlers–Danlos syndrome and Marfan syndrome, fibromuscular dysplasia, pregnancy, portal hypertension, and posttransplant status. Visceral pseudoaneurysms are a result of trauma, infection, inflammation, and iatrogenic causes. VAAs are also associated with some rare conditions, such as Von Recklinghausen disease, polyarteritis nodosa, and Behcet disease.[1,7,8]

Most visceral aneurysms are found in the splenic artery (40%–60%). This is followed by the hepatic artery (19%–25%), the superior mesenteric artery (SMA, 4%–9%), and the celiac trunk (3%–4%). Aneurysms of the gastroduodenal and pancreaticoduodenal arteries along with other visceral branches are even rarer (Table 28-1).[1,2,9,10]

TABLE 28-1 Distribution of Visceral Artery Aneurysms

Splenic artery	40%–60%
Hepatic artery	19%–25%
Superior mesenteric artery	4%–9%
Celiac trunk	3%–4%
Gastroduodenal and pancreaticoduodenal arteries	2%–9%
Gastric or gastroepiploic arteries	2%–4%
Jejunal, ileal, inferior mesenteric, colic arteries	1%–3%

SPLENIC ARTERY ANEURYSMS

Splenic artery aneurysms (SAAs) are the most common type of VAA accounting for 60% of all visceral aneurysms.[1] Autopsy studies have shown an incidence of 0.01% to 0.23% in the general population, with the incidence rising as high as 10.4% in autopsies performed when specific attention was paid to evaluate the splenic artery for aneurysms as they can often be missed in their nonruptured, relatively small states on routine autopsy.[11] Most SAAs are located in the distal third of the artery and are saccular in morphology. Women are more affected than men by a ratio 4 to 1. Underlying etiologies include atherosclerosis, arterial fibrodysplasia, and arteritis. Additionally, female gender, multiparty, and portal hypertension are associated risks. In a 20-year review of 100 cases of splenic artery aneurysms, 92% of the women in the study had been pregnant with the average number of pregnancies being 4.5. Furthermore, 24.1% of the women had been pregnant six or more times.[12,13] Most reported ruptures during pregnancy are in the third trimester, although there are three case reports of first-trimester rupture.[14] Even though an association between pregnancy and ruptured SAA has been demonstrated, the mechanisms behind the relationship are not completely understood. The combined insult of increased splenic blood flow along with the effects of hormonal changes of pregnancy on the vessel wall is thought to play a role.[13] Similarly, increased pressures are thought to explain the 10% to 20% incidence of SAA seen in patients with portal hypertension. Chronic pancreatitis and trauma are common causes of pseudoaneurysm formation of the splenic artery.[15]

HEPATIC ARTERY ANEURYSMS

Hepatic artery aneurysms (HAA) are the second most common visceral aneurysm. Nearly half of HAAs are pseudoaneurysms, likely a result of an increase in hepatobiliary procedures and the use of CT scans for blunt liver trauma.[16] Most of these are found in the extrahepatic arteries (66%–80%).[1,16] Unlike splenic artery aneurysms, HAAs affect men more commonly than women, present later in the fifth or sixth decade of life, and are not associated with pregnancy. Atherosclerosis, arterial dysplasia, medial degeneration, and vasculitis (such as polyarteritis nodosa) are often causes of extrahepatic aneurysms. Mycotic etiologies have decreased over time likely due to the availability of antibiotics. Intrahepatic lesions are commonly caused by trauma or iatrogenic reasons.[17,18]

SUPERIOR MESENTERIC ARTERY ANEURYSMS

Superior mesenteric artery aneurysms (SMAAs) are rare and comprise a small number of visceral aneurysms.[1] They typically involve the proximal 5 cm of the vessel and occur more frequently in men than women. Aside from the risk of rupture and hemorrhage, SMAAs also pose a risk of intestinal ischemia. One-third of SMAAs are the result of infection. Many patients have a history of bacterial endocarditis and intravenous drug use. *Streptococcal* and *Staphylococcal* organisms are common culprit organisms.[19] The size of the vessel and the angle of its takeoff relative to the aorta are proposed reasons for its increased vulnerability to mycotic aneurysm formation. Other mechanisms include degeneration and dysplasia from atherosclerosis, fibrodysplasia, pancreatitis, dissection, connective tissue diseases (such as neurofibromatosis and Ehlers–Danlos syndrome), Behcet's disease, polyarteritis nodosa, and blunt trauma.[20–22]

CELIAC ARTERY ANEURYSMS

Celiac artery aneurysms (CAA) also represent only a small portion of VAAs. Men are more commonly affected than women and are mostly present in the sixth decade of life. Historically, many of these were associated with infection (often luetic), some with trauma, and over half were from undetermined causes. More contemporary reports suggest that atherosclerosis and medial defects of the arterial wall are the most common etiologies.[23,24]

GASTRIC, GASTROEPIPLOIC ARTERIES, PANCREATICODUODENAL, AND GASTRODUODENAL ARTERY ANEURYSMS

Gastric and gastroepiploic artery aneurysms are extremely rare and makeup only 1% to 2% of all reported VAAs. They are associated with peptic ulcer disease, pancreatitis, vasculitis (such as polyangiitis), and segmental arterial mediolysis.[25]

Most pancreaticoduodenal artery aneurysms and gastroduodenal artery aneurysms (GAAs) are present in the fifth or sixth decade of life. Men are more affected than women by a ratio of 3 or 4 to 1. The most common etiologies are infection and inflammation as well as fibromuscular dysplasia and cystic medial necrosis. They are often associated with pancreatitis, biliary disease, alcohol use, peptic ulcer disease, and a history of cholecystectomy.[26]

INFERIOR MESENTERIC ARTERY ANEURYSMS

Inferior mesenteric artery (IMA) aneurysms are rare. Those that have been reported are commonly in the sixth decade of life. Men are affected more often than women by a ratio of more than 4 to 1. Infection, fibromuscular dysplasia, and cystic medial necrosis are reported etiologies. Additional associated conditions include peptic ulcer disease, abdominal trauma, coronary disease, aortic aneurysms, and pancreatitis.[26]

ILEAL, JEJUNAL, AND COLIC ARTERY ANEURYSMS

Ileal and jejunal artery aneurysms are also extremely rare. Pseudoaneurysms have been reported after bowel resection with stapled anastomosis.[27] More common causes include atherosclerosis and medial degeneration.[28]

Colic artery aneurysms are extremely rare as well, accounting for less than 2% of reported visceral aneurysms. As with many other visceral aneurysms, colic artery aneurysms are often present in the sixth decade. Men are nearly equally affected as women. Most involve the mid and right colic arteries. Associated conditions include cholecystitis, peptic ulcer disease, endocarditis, and pancreatitis.[26]

CLINICAL FINDINGS

In early reports, 87% of patients with visceral aneurysms presented ruptured and were often diagnosed in the postmortem state (95%). In more contemporary data, only 13% of patients with visceral aneurysms present ruptured. The majority of VAAs are now discovered in asymptomatic patients during a workup for unrelated reasons.[29] When patients are symptomatic, the most common presenting complaint is abdominal pain which can initially be tolerable. The specific location of the aneurysms affects their clinical presentations.[9,24]

SPLENIC ARTERY ANEURYSMS

Splenic artery aneurysms are usually asymptomatic, but when symptomatic, they present with epigastric or left upper quadrant pain. If ruptured, patients have severe abdominal pain and hypovolemic shock. Often, a "double-rupture" phenomenon is witnessed in which the rupture is initially contained within the lesser sac and the patient stabilizes. This is then followed by rupture through the foramen of Winslow or rupture of the pars flaccida into the peritoneal cavity and severe hypotension ensues. Splenic aneurysms can also erode through the pancreatic duct presenting with hemosuccus pancreaticus or erode into the bowel or stomach presenting with a gastrointestinal (GI) bleed.[16] Overall mortality associated with rupture is 25%, but rupture during pregnancy carries an exceptionally high maternal mortality rate of 80% and fetal mortality rate of 90%.[30]

HEPATIC ARTERY ANEURYSMS

Patients with hepatic artery pseudoaneurysms will usually report a history of iatrogenic injury or liver trauma. These pseudoaneurysms are symptomatic with GI bleeding or hemobilia.[31] Most true HAAs are asymptomatic and found incidentally. When they are symptomatic, common symptoms and signs are pain in the right upper quadrant radiating to the back (55%), GI hemorrhage (46%), and hemobilia (46%). Extrahepatic aneurysms can rupture into the peritoneal cavity causing hypotension. Intrahepatic aneurysms can rupture into the biliary tree causing Quincke's triad of epigastric pain, hemobilia, and obstructive jaundice. A wide range of rupture rates have been reported for HAAs (14%-80%) with an associated mortality of 20% to 40%.[16,17,30]

CELIAC ARTERY ANEURYSMS

Symptomatic CAAs most commonly present with epigastric pain or upper GI hemorrhage. Dysphagia from esophageal compression has been described. Other presentations include a palpable mass, jaundice, bleeding gastric varices as a result of splenic vein compression, and hepatic and portal obstruction as a result of extrinsic compression.[27,32,33] The risk of rupture is 10% to 20% with rupture associated with mortality as high as 100%.[16,23]

SUPERIOR MESENTERIC ARTERY ANEURYSMS

Unlike other VAAs, SMAAs are often symptomatic (60%-90%). Pain is the predominant symptom (68%) and is usually progressive and moderate-to-severe in nature.[34] Often there is a palpable mass (50%). Up to half of the patients will present ruptured with a mortality ranging from 30% to 90%.[9] Other symptoms include nausea and vomiting (19%), GI hemorrhage (15%), hemobilia (15%), jaundice (15%), anemia (12%), and shock (12%).[23,26]

GASTRODUODENAL/ PANCREATICODUODENAL

Most gastroduodenal and pancreaticoduodenal aneurysms are symptomatic at presentation (80%). Many have associated pancreatic or biliary diseases. Those with GAAs present with abdominal pain (64%), GI bleed or hemobilia (56%), jaundice (31%), abdominal mass (28%), nausea and/or vomiting (25%), and shock (11%) with an overall mortality of 11%. Patients with pancreaticoduodenal aneurysms present with pain (71%), GI bleeding or hemobilia (39%), jaundice (14%), or shock (9%) with an overall mortality of 30%.[26]

JEJUNAL, ILEAL, COLIC, AND INFERIOR MESENTERIC ARTERY ANEURYSMS

Jejunal and ileal aneurysms are often asymptomatic and have an estimated rupture risk of 30%. Colic aneurysms are usually symptomatic (90%) with the primary complaint of abdominal pain. Colic aneurysms carry a high risk of rupture (70%). Overall mortality for these rare aneurysms is 20% to 50%.[30] Pain is the presenting symptom (87%), along with shock (52%) and a palpable mass (17%). Nausea and vomiting (17%), GI bleeding (14%), and jaundice (13%) have also been reported.[26]

Aneurysms of the IMA are extremely rare and present with pain and palpable mass (50%).[26]

DIFFERENTIAL DIAGNOSIS

Because of the rarity of VAAs and the nonspecific nature of the usual presenting complaint of abdominal pain, they are difficult to diagnose. The differential diagnosis for abdominal pain is exhaustive. Symptomatology of biliary colic, pancreatitis, gastroesophageal reflux, peptic ulcer disease, and ruptured abdominal aortic aneurysms often overlap with those of VAAs. Clinical history, laboratory values, and imaging can be used to differentiate the cause of the abdominal pain.

DIAGNOSIS

Evaluation should begin by obtaining a relevant history and performing physical examination. Information regarding any known history of infection, pancreatitis, trauma, GI bleed, abdominal procedures, or personal and/or family history of connective tissue disorders should be obtained. On examination, patients may be in extremis if presenting ruptured. A mass can sometimes be palpated.[26]

Plain radiographs are not a definitive tool for the diagnosis of VAA, but when obtained they can demonstrate curvilinear calcifications suggestive of VAAs. Large splenic artery aneurysms are sometimes detected by classic signet ring-shaped calcifications in the left upper quadrant on x-ray.

Duplex ultrasonography can be helpful in the evaluation of a patient with suspected VAA. It has the advantages of being readily available, noninvasive, and inexpensive. It can demonstrate a dilated artery, thickened wall, atherosclerotic plaque, hemodynamic evaluation of blood flow, or thrombus. The study is technician-dependent. Sensitivity to detect VAAs less than 3 cm is poor. Other limitations include obesity, vascular calcifications, and the presence of bowel gas.[35]

Contrast-enhanced CT angiography is the diagnostic tool of choice when a VAA is suspected. It provides information about location, surrounding structures, aneurysm size, wall inflammation, hematoma, dissection, underlying disease processes, and rupture. It also can demonstrate the presence of other aneurysms. CTA also serves as a procedural planning tool for open and endovascular aneurysm repair. Use in patients with renal insufficiency or contrast allergy should be avoided. Sensitivity and specificity can be as high as 100%.[35,36]

Magnetic resonance angiography (MRA) provides good spatial resolution. It is not readily available for emergent presentations. It has limitations in patients with pacemakers, those unable to lie still and those with claustrophobia. After coil embolization, it can be useful to assess for flow within the aneurysm sac.[37,38] In children, pregnant patients, and those with contrast allergies or renal insufficiency, noncontrast-enhanced MRA can be used.[30]

Digital subtraction angiography is more invasive and costly but does provide the opportunity for intervention along with the diagnosis. It only provides an evaluation of the lumen and not the entire vessel and is not the diagnostic tool of choice for VAAs.

MANAGEMENT OF THE CLINICAL PROBLEM

GENERAL CONSIDERATIONS OF ENDOVASCULAR MANAGEMENT

Because of their rarity, most recommendations for the management of VAAs are based on published data from small series. Patient factors such as age, gender, and comorbidities along with aneurysm type, morphology, location, and collateral circulation play a role in determining the need for intervention and the options for endovascular and open repair. As a general rule, any pseudoaneurysm or symptomatic aneurysm should be treated regardless of size due to the high propensity for rupture. An endovascular first approach should be considered for all visceral aneurysms if the anatomy is appropriate and if the etiology is not mycotic (Figure 28-1).[30]

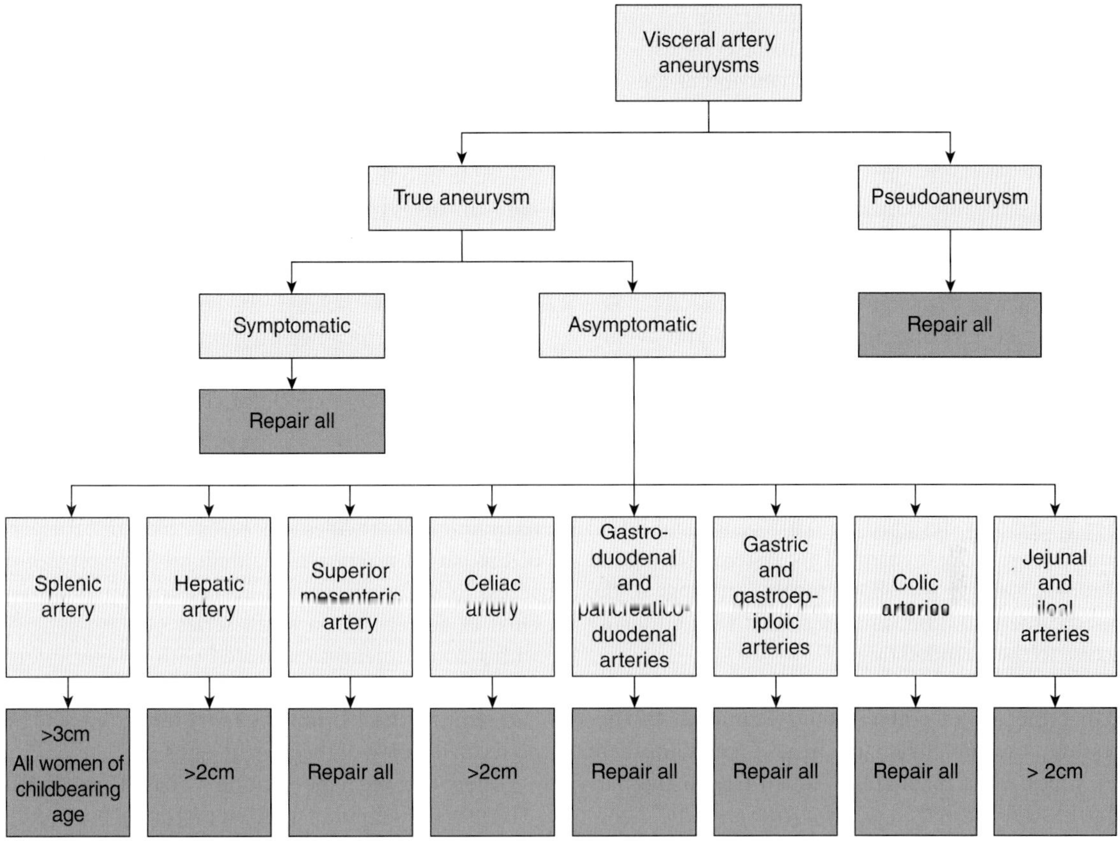

FIGURE 28-1 Algorithm for the treatment of visceral artery aneurysms.

Endovascular strategies for the treatment of VAAs include occluding the affected vessel or maintaining patency of the vessel while excluding only the aneurysm from flow. The former approach employs the use of coils, vascular plugs, and liquid embolic agents when collateral circulation can prevent distal ischemia. Efforts to maintain patency of the parent vessel while excluding the aneurysm from flow can be achieved with covered stents, assisted sac embolization, and flow diversion. These treatment modalities offer the benefits of being less invasive, having shorter recovery times, and lower morbidity and mortality than open repair.[39] One downside to these techniques is the higher rate of reintervention (3.2% per year) compared to open procedures (0.5% per year).[39,40] Often endovascular therapy can be done with local anesthetic providing advantages to patients with multiple comorbidities or hostile abdomens. Risks include access site complications, target vessel rupture, distal embolization, contrast toxicity, and the need for long-term surveillance. Recent guidelines from the Society of Vascular Surgery recommend periodic or annual follow-up with CTA for most VAAs treated with endovascular methods due to the possibility of recanalization or continued perfusion that could lead to growth and late rupture.[30]

Many options exist for embolization. A common technique includes the use of coils to first embolize the distal native artery, followed by coil packing of the aneurysm and finally embolizing the proximal vessel. This can be done with a 5-Fr sheath in the ostium and a 4-Fr catheter for the delivery of 0.035″ metal coils. Vascular plugs are an alternative to coils and are particularly useful in large vessels with high flow. They do require a larger delivery system but provide effective occlusion with excellent deployment accuracy. At times, they can be more economical when a large number of coils would otherwise be necessary to occlude the artery. Detachable coils also offer predictable and controlled deployment, but they are more expensive than standard metal coils.

Liquid embolic agents including cyanoacrylate glue and ethylene–vinyl alcohol copolymer with dimethyl sulfoxide (Onyx) can be used alone or as adjuncts to coiling and are particularly helpful in aneurysms that develop in a terminal branch where the inflow vessel can be embolized directly.[41] For embolization utilizing both coils and liquid agents, a triaxial system with a 5 or 6-Fr sheath at the access site with the end of the sheath or a guiding catheter placed into the target visceral vessel is used. A 4 or 5-Fr catheter is advanced through the sheath near the aneurysm. This is followed by a 3-Fr microcatheter, specifically designed for 0.018″ coils and liquid embolic agent deployment. This system offers good platform stability and allows for the exchange of the microcatheter if it becomes occluded without losing access to the intended target.[42]

Although collateral flow to end organs often allows the use of embolization techniques to successfully exclude aneurysms from circulation, there are times when maintaining flow through the parent vessel is desired in order to preserve end-organ perfusion. The use of stent-grafts, balloon- and stent-assisted coiling, and flow-diverting stents provide a means to achieve this goal. Stent grafts are available in both balloon-expandable and self-expanding options, and their major challenge is their rigid delivery systems. If a vessel is small (<4 mm), heavily calcified, highly angled, or tortuous, success is less likely, and there is a high risk of rupture of the vessel during an attempt to position the stent graft. A large discrepancy between the diameters of the proximal and distal landing zones can also be a limiting factor for stent-grafts. Technical success with stent-grafts for VAAs has been reported at 80% or greater.[43,44] Morality has been reported as high as 10.6% at 30 days and 21.2% at 12 months. Patency has been noted to be 82% and sac thrombosis at 100% at 28 months.[44]

Balloon- or stent-assisted embolization are other endovascular methods employed to preserve flow through the parent vessel while treating a saccular VAA. With these techniques, a low-profile balloon or bare metal stent is positioned within the parent artery to prevent migration and distal embolization of coils or liquid embolic agents. Balloon-assisted aneurysm exclusion can be considered if an aneurysm has a neck narrow enough to retain formed coils, but there is a concern that during placement, part of the coil will protrude into the parent vessel or migrate. This technique involves placing a microcatheter into the aneurysm sac and positioning a hypercompliant balloon in the parent vessel spanning the neck of the aneurysm. With the balloon inflated, the coils can be deployed through the microcatheter limiting the risk of protrusion or distal embolization. The balloon can be intermittently deflated to check for coil pack stability and to allow for distal perfusion. Balloon assistance has been described with the use of liquid embolic agents as well.[45] A double-lumen balloon can be useful with this technique as it provides wire access to the distal aspect of the parent artery while simultaneously providing access to the aneurysm sac for coils or liquid agents. Onal et al. reported a small series of nine patients with visceral aneurysms treated with this technique and followed up at 6 months with MRA. Two SMAAs had remnant necks, and the remaining patients had no recanalization of their aneurysm sacs.[46]

Stent-assisted embolization is based on similar principles as balloon-assisted embolization but utilizes a bare stent positioned proximal and distal to the neck of the aneurysm to prevent stray coil deployment. This technique is useful if the aneurysm has a wide neck and a higher risk of a coil protruding into the lumen. A microcatheter is placed parallel to the stent or through the struts of the stent and into the sac.[47] There are also retrievable stents and scaffolds which protect the parent vessel during coil deployment while allowing flow to be maintained to the target organ.[48,49]

Flow-diverting stent technology has been adapted from the treatment of intracerebral aneurysms to the management of VAAs. These multilayered stents have a large metallic surface area and tightly spaced nonocclusive interstices. This induces gradual aneurysm thrombosis by lowering the flow velocity with aneurysm vortices, reducing stress on the wall of the vessel while at the same time improving laminar flow in the lumen of the main artery. Branches can be preserved despite ostial coverage if the struts occlude less than 50% and a pressure gradient exists.[50] Flow diversion thereby offers the potential to maintain patency of the parent artery and side branches as well. An additional advantage of this technique is that the sac does not need to be entered and intraprocedural rupture risk is lower. One downside to stent-assisted and flow-diverting stents is the need for dual antiplatelet therapy following the procedure. In a series of 54 patients with visceral and peripheral aneurysms treated with this technique, sac occlusion at 1 year was 93.3%. The primary stent patency was 86.9%. Side branch patency was 96.1%, and 91.1% of aneurysms demonstrated size reduction.[51]

ENDOVASCULAR TREATMENT OF SPLENIC ARTERY ANEURYSMS

For splenic artery aneurysms, current recommendations are to repair all pseudoaneurysms, any symptomatic aneurysms, true aneurysms greater than 3 cm, and aneurysms of any size in women of childbearing age.[30] Endovascular interventions on SAAs have a high technical success rate (>95%). In the proximal splenic artery, stent-grafts can be used. The farther distal the lesion, the more difficult it is to obtain enough support to advance the stent-grafts through the tortuous splenic artery. Techniques that facilitate stent-graft placement have been described and include the use of open brachial access for a 10-or 12-Fr sheath advanced to the visceral aorta. Through and through access from the femoral artery with a 0.014″ wire can eliminate challenges of arch tortuosity when placing this large sheath. A 7-or 8-Fr hydrophilic sheath is then placed through the larger sheath and into the distal splenic artery. This can be facilitated by progressively stiffening the working platform from a floppy wire and microcatheter to a stiff 0.035″ wire and catheter. The use of an undersized angioplasty balloon can also be helpful to advance the sheath through the tortuous artery. Nitroglycerin can be given to prevent vessel spasms. Once in position, the stent-graft can then be deployed. If there are any kinks after deployment, a bare stent can be overlapped with it to negate them. Success with this technique has been reported at 80%.[43] Because the tortuous course of the splenic is so challenging, embolization is often the procedure of choice for mid and distal SAAs. Risks include access site complications, target vessel rupture, splenic infarction, splenic abscess, and postembolization syndrome.

ENDOVASCULAR TREATMENT OF HEPATIC ARTERY ANEURYSMS

Hepatic artery aneurysms should be treated if symptomatic, greater than 2 cm, or demonstrate a growth rate greater than 0.5 cm per year.[30] Endovascular management offers significant advantages to open repair in terms of reduced morbidity and mortality.[52] HAAs proximal to the gastroduodenal artery (GDA) can be embolized or potentially treated with stent-grafts. Hepatic aneurysms involving the GDA or more distal extrahepatic circulation should be considered for open repair in order to preserve arterial flow. Intrahepatic lesions are better treated by embolization (either with coils and/or liquid embolic agents) as open access is extremely difficult and would likely require hepatic resection.[30]

ENDOVASCULAR TREATMENT OF SUPERIOR MESENTERIC ARTERY ANEURYSMS

Because the mortality associated with rupture of SMAAs is between 30% and 90% and the mortality associated with elective repair is less than 15%, these aneurysms should be repaired at any size.[30] The limiting factor for endovascular treatment options is the inability to cover branches of the SMA without significant ischemic consequences. If there is a good landing zone proximal and distal to the aneurysm without the need to cover branches exists, a stent-graft can be considered. Also, if the aneurysm is saccular and has an appropriate neck, coil embolization or assisted coil embolization can be performed. Many aneurysms of the SMA are mycotic in nature and these are better treated with open surgery. Risks of endovascular repair include dissection, rupture, thrombosis, distal embolization, and dissemination of infection.[41]

ENDOVASCULAR TREATMENT OF CELIAC ARTERY ANEURYSMS

Repair of all pseudoaneurysms and any CAA greater than 2 cm is recommended. Endovascular repair is often limited by the lack of a proximal landing zone but if the anatomy is appropriate, an endovascular first approach is not unreasonable.[30]

ENDOVASCULAR TREATMENT OF GASTRIC, GASTROEPIPLOIC, GASTRODUODENAL, AND PANCREATICODUODENAL ANEURYSMS

Aneurysms of the gastric, gastroepiploic, gastroduodenal, and pancreaticoduodenal should be repaired at any size due to the high mortality associated with rupture. For GDA and pancreaticoduodenal aneurysm (PDA) aneurysms, size does not seem to correlate with the risk of rupture. Endovascular methods should be attempted first if anatomically suitable. Coil embolization is often the procedure of choice with a technical success rate >90%.[30]

ENDOVASCULAR TREATMENT OF JEJUNAL, ILEAL, AND COLIC ARTERY ANEURYSMS

Jejunal and ileal artery aneurysms are indicated for repair when greater than 2 cm. Colic artery aneurysms seem to have a higher risk of rupture (70%) associated with high mortality of 20% to 50%. Therefore, it is recommended that colic aneurysms are repaired regardless of size. For elective repair, an endovascular first strategy should be considered and embolization is the most common way these aneurysms are managed. An exception to these criteria is when asymptomatic ileal, jejunal, and colic artery aneurysms are associated with polyarteritis nodosa in which case, medical management is recommended with repeat imaging in 3 to 4 months to assess for regression.[30]

OPEN REPAIR

GENERAL CONSIDERATIONS

With advances in endovascular therapy, open repair is generally not the first-line treatment for most VAAs. It is often reserved for when endovascular options have been attempted or are too difficult to perform. Options for open management include proximal and distal ligation of the aneurysm without arterial reconstruction, resection, or exclusion of the aneurysm with arterial reconstruction via bypass or end-to-end anastomosis, and aneurysmorrhaphy with or without patch angioplasty. Ligation proximal and distal to the VAA without arterial reconstruction is one option widely used in emergencies, such as rupture. It is also an acceptable method in elective cases if collateral circulation is adequate. Thorough inspection intraoperatively for ischemia and close monitoring postoperatively must be done if revascularization is not pursued. Outcomes from elective open repair have acceptable with 1-, 5- and 10-year survival rates of 98%, 98%, and 79.5%, respectively, with no aneurysm-related deaths.[29] Reintervention rates are low with open repair at 0.5% per year compared to the endovascular group at 3.2% per year. In the setting of rupture, open repair carries significantly higher mortality.[40] Recently published guidelines from the Society of Vascular Surgery suggest one-time screening patients with VAAs for other intrathoracic, intracranial, and peripheral aneurysms with CT, MRA, or ultrasound.[30] For patients with segmental medial arteriolysis, interval surveillance (i.e., every 12–24 months) with CTA or MRA is recommended due to reports of rapid arterial transformation and to monitor for regression in patients with polyarteritis nodosa.[30] There is not a consensus on postoperative imaging follow-up after open treatment, but it can be done at intervals to evaluate for patency of any revascularization and the development of aneurysmal changes.

OPEN REPAIR OF SPLENIC ARTERY ANEURYSMS

Options for open repair of splenic aneurysms depend on their location along the artery and can be exposed via a subcostal or midline incision. In the proximal two-thirds of the artery, the vessel can be ligated proximally and distally and the spleen will maintain perfusion through the short gastric. Aneurysms in this location can also be treated with resection and end-to-end anastomosis or aneurysmorrhaphy with low morbidity and mortality.[29] Aneurysms involving the distal third of the splenic artery or hilum often require splenectomy. In this latter scenario, splenectomy vaccinations need to be given to reduce the chance of overwhelming post-splenectomy infection.

OPEN REPAIR OF HEPATIC ARTERY ANEURYSMS

Hepatic artery aneurysms (HAAs) can be approached via a right subcostal or midline incision to enter the lesser sac. For extrahepatic aneurysms, aneurysmorrhaphy with or without patch angioplasty, ligation with or without revascularization, are surgical options. If endovascular techniques are not possible for intrahepatic aneurysms, hepatic resection might be necessary. Ligation of HAAs can be considered if the diseased segment does not involve the GDA and the patient does not have liver disease. Lee et al. reported a large common HAA that involved the origins of the GDA and proper hepatic artery repaired with aneurysmectomy including the dilated origins of the two branches followed by anastomosis of the proper hepatic artery to the GDA.[53] Although this is an elegant solution, it might not be always possible to mobilize enough length of the proper hepatic and GDA to be able to perform this anastomosis. More commonly, when the HAA involves the GDA, resection and bypass are performed.[52,54] The conduit for this can be autogenous vein or prosthetic grafts with 5-year patency rates of 86%. Elective repair has a morbidity of 29% and mortality of 6%. In the setting of rupture, mortality is 40%.[52]

OPEN REPAIR OF SUPERIOR MESENTERIC ARTERY ANEURYSMS

Aneurysms of the SMA can be approached through a midline or retroperitoneal flank incision. These aneurysms can be treated with aneurysmectomy or aneurysmorrhaphy with arterial reconstruction and rarely simple ligation if the celiac artery and pancreatic arcades are intact. Because SMAAs more often have a mycotic or inflammatory etiology, autogenous vein should be considered for conduit rather than prosthetic grafts. Rupture carries a high mortality (30%–90%). Even in the elective setting, mortality has been reported as high as 15%.[55] If a patient presents with aneurysm thrombosis and intestinal ischemia, bypass should be performed along with ligation of the aneurysm as later recanalization and rupture have been reported after revascularization alone in this setting.[56]

OPEN REPAIR OF CELIAC ARTERY ANEURYSMS

Endovascular management of CAAs is sometimes not possible when the aneurysm involves the origin of the vessel and no zone for proximal seal is available. CAAs can be approached through the midline or from a retroperitoneal flank incision. Aneurysm ligation with or without reconstruction, aneurysmorrhaphy, and aneurysmectomy have been described. Ligation without revascularization with close monitoring for ischemia is often reserved for emergent presentations. In patients with underlying liver disease, ligation alone should be avoided. In the elective setting, ligation with bypass from the aorta using vein or prosthetic graft is usually the procedure of choice.[8]

OPEN REPAIR OF GASTRIC, GASTROEPIPLOIC, GASTRODUODENAL, AND PANCREATICODUODENAL ARTERY ANEURYSMS

Aneurysms of gastric, gastroepiploic, gastroduodenal, and pancreaticoduodenal are often best treated by endovascular means. For gastric and gastroepiploic arteries, ligation or excision is done without revascularization. If the aneurysm is intramural, involving the gastric wall, a wedge excision of the involved portion of the stomach may be necessary. Open repair of aneurysms of the pancreaticoduodenal and gastroduodenal arteries typically involves excision with end-to-end anastomosis. Morbidity and mortality for this in the elective setting are 9.4% and 1.3%, respectively. If performed in a ruptured setting, mortality can be as high as 30%.[30] In some cases, partial pancreatectomy or pancreaticoduodenectomy may need to be performed.[57,58]

OPEN REPAIR OF JEJUNAL, ILEAL, AND COLIC ARTERY ANEURYSMS

Most jejunal, ileal, and colic artery aneurysms are treated electively with embolization. Open repair options typically include ligation or aneurysm excision without reconstruction. For those who present ruptured and there is a concern for bowel compromise, exploratory laparotomy allows for hematoma evacuation, bowel assessment, treatment of the aneurysm, and possible bowel resection if not viable.[30]

REFERENCES

1. Stanley JC, Thompson NW, Fry WJ. Splanchnic artery aneurysms. *Arch Surg*. 1970;101(6):689-697.
2. Park S, Jang L. The incidence of visceral artery aneruysms based on abdominal CT. *Eur J Vasc Endovasc Surg*. 2019;58(6 Suppl 2):E429.
3. Erben Y, Brownstein AJ, Rajaee S, et al. Natural history and management of splanchnic artery aneurysms in a single tertiary referral center. *J Vasc Surg*. 2018;68(4): 1079-1087.
4. Beaussier M. Sur un aneurisme de l'artère splénique dont les parois se sont ossifiées. *J Med Chir Pharm (Paris)*. 1770;32: 157-162.
5. Rolland W. Aneurysm of the hepatic artery; clinical and pathological notes of a case with a review of the previously reported cases. *Glosgow Med J*. 1908:342-358.
6. De Bakey ME, Cooley DA. Successful resection of mycotic aneurysm of superior mesenteric artery; case report and review of literature. *Am Surg*. 1953;19(2): 202-212.
7. Parfitt J. Visceral aneurysms in Ehlers-Danlos syndrome: case report and review of the literature *J Vasc Surg*. 2000;31(6) 1248-1251.
8. Obara H, Kentaro M, Inoue M, et al. Current management strategies for visceral artery aneurysms: an overview. *Surg Today*. 2020;50:38-49.
9. Pitton MB, Dappa E, Jungmann F, et al. Visceral artery aneurysms: incidence, management, and outcome analysis in a tertiary care center over one decade. *Eur Radiol*. 2015;25(7):2004-2014.
10. Martinelli O, Giglio A, Irace L, et al. Single-center experience in the treatment of visceral artery aneurysms. *Ann Vasc Surg*. 2019;60:447-454.
11. Bedford PD, Lodge B. Aneurysms of the splenic artery. *Gut*. 1960;1(4):312-320.
12. Stanley JC, Fry WJ. Pathogenesis and clinical significance of splenic artery aneurysms. *Surgery*. 1974;76(6): 898-905.
13. Trastek VF, Pairolero PC, Joyce JW, et al. Splenic artery aneurysms. *Surgery*. 1982;91(6):694-699.
14. Gourgiotis S, Alfaras P, Salemis NS. Spontaneous rupture of splenic artery aneurysm in pregnancy: a case report. *Adv Med Sci*. 2008;53(2):344-347.
15. Tessier DJ, Stone WM, Fowl RJ, et al. Clinical features and management of splenic artery pseudoaneurysm: case series and cumulative review of literature. *J Vasc Surg*. 2003;38(5):969-974.
16. Shanley CJ, Shah NL, Messina LM. Common splanchnic artery aneurysms: splenic, hepatic, and celiac. *Ann Vasc Surg*. 1996;10(3):315-322.
17. O'Driscoll D, Olliff SP, Olliff JF. Hepatic artery aneurysm. *Br J Radiol*. 1999;72(862):1018-1025.
18. Pasha SF, Gloviczki P, Stanson AW, et al. Splanchnic artery aneurysms. *Mayo Clin Proc*. 2007;82(4):472-479.
19. Sharma G, Semel ME, McGillicuddy EA, et al. Ruptured and unruptured mycotic superior mesenteric artery aneurysms. *Ann Vasc Surg*. 2014;28(8):1931.e5-1931.e8.
20. de Troia A, Mottini F, Biasi L, et al. Superior mesenteric artery aneurysm caused by aortic valve endocarditis: the case report and review of the literature. *Vasc Endovascular Surg*. 2016;50(2):88-93.
21. Cormier F, Ferry J, Artru B, et al. Dissecting aneurysms of the main trunk of the superior mesenteric artery. *J Vasc Surg*. 1992;15:424-430.
22. Olsen AB, Ralhan T, Harris JH Jr, et al. Superior mesenteric artery pseudoaneurysm after blunt abdominal trauma. *Ann Vasc Surg*. 2013;27(5):674-678.
23. Messina LM, Shanley CJ. Visceral artery aneurysms. *Surg Clin North Am*. 1997;77(2):425-442.
24. Graham LM, Stanley JC, Whitehouse WM Jr, et al. Celiac artery aneurysms: historic (1945-1949) versus contemporary (1950-1984) differences in etiology and clinical importance. *J Vasc Surg*. 1985;2(5):757-764.
25. Kohara Y, Fujimoto K, Katsura H, et al. Biphasic clinical course of a ruptured right gastric artery aneurysm caused by segmental arterial mediolysis: a case report. *BMC Surg*. 2020;20(1):191.
26. Shanley CJ, Shah NL, Messina LM. Uncommon splanchnic artery aneurysms: pancreaticoduodenal, gastroduodenal, superior mesenteric, inferior mesenteric, and colic. *Ann Vasc Surg*. 1996;10(5):506-515.
27. Kimura H, Sato O, Miyata T, et al. Bleeding gastric varices as a result of splenic vein compression by a celiac arterial aneurysm. *Surgery*. 1996;120(1):106-110.
28. Roche-Nagle G, O'Donnell D, O'Hanrahan T. Visceral artery aneurysms: a symptomatic aneurysm of the ileocolic artery. *Vascular*. 2007;15(3):162-166.
29. Pulli R, Dorigo W, Troisi N, et al. Surgical treatment of visceral artery aneurysms: a 25-year experience. *J Vasc Surg*. 2008;48(2):334-342.
30. Chaer RA, Abularrage CJ, Coleman DM, et al. The Society for Vascular Surgery clinical practice guidelines on the management of visceral aneurysms. *J Vasc Surg*. 2020;72(1S):3S-39S.

31. Wagner ML, Streit S, Makley AT, et al. Hepatic pseudoaneurysm incidence after liver trauma. *J Surg Res.* 2020;256:623-628.
32. Kamran A, Yaqoob N, Soomro R, et al. Coeliac artery aneurysm. *J Pak Med Assoc.* 2009;59(1):51-53.
33. McMullan DM, McBride M, Livesay JJ, et al. Celiac artery aneurysm: a case report. *Tex Heart Inst J.* 2006;33(2): 235-240.
34. Zilun L, Henghui Y, Yang Z, et al. The management of superior mesenteric artery aneurysm: experience with 16 cases in a single center. *Ann Vasc Surg.* 2017;42: 120-127.
35. Saba L, Anzidei M, Lucatelli P, et al. The multidetector computed tomography angiography (MDCTA) in the diagnosis of splenic artery aneurysm and pseudoaneurysm. *Acta Radiol.* 2011;52(5):488-498.
36. Ming WD, Li XG, Xue HD, et al. Role of multi-slice computed tomography angiography in the diagnosis of visceral artery aneurysms. *Zhongguo Yi Xue Ke Xue Yuan Xue Bao.* 2014;36(3):296-299.
37. Kawai T, Shimohira M, Suzuki K, et al. Time-resolved magnetic resonance angiography as a follow-up method for visceral artery aneurysm treated with coil-embolisation. *Pol J Radiol.* 2018;83:e137-e142.
38. Kurosaka K, Kawai T, Shimohira M, et al. Time-resolved magnetic resonance angiography for assessment of recanalization after coil embolization of visceral artery aneurysms. *Pol J Radiol.* 2013;78(1):64-68.
39. Chin JA, Heib A, Ochoa Chaar CI, et al. Trends and outcomes in endovascular and open surgical treatment of visceral aneurysms. *J Vasc Surg.* 2017;66(1):195-201.e1.
40. Hogendoorn W, Lavida A, Hunink MG, et al. Open repair, endovascular repair, and conservative management of true splenic artery aneurysms. *J Vasc Surg.* 2014;60(6):1667-1676.e1.
41. Sousa J, Costa D, Mansilha A. Visceral artery aneurysms: review on indications and current treatment strategies. *Int Angiol.* 2019;38(5):381-394.
42. Chadha M, Ahuja C. Visceral artery aneurysms: diagnosis and percutaneous management. *Semin Intervent Radiol.* 2009;26(3):196-206.
43. Reed NR, Oderich GS, Manunga J, et al. Feasibility of endovascular repair of splenic artery aneurysms using stent grafts. *J Vasc Surg.* 2015;62(6):1504-1510.
44. Künzle S, Glenck M, Puippe G, et al. Stent-graft repairs of visceral and renal artery aneurysms are effective and result in long-term patency. *J Vasc Interv Radiol.* 2013;24(7):989-996.
45. Bratby MJ, Lehmann ED, Bottomley J, et al. Endovascular embolization of visceral artery aneurysms with ethylene-vinyl alcohol (Onyx): a case series. *Cardiovasc Intervent Radiol.* 2006;29:1125-1128.
46. Onal Y, Samanci C, Cicek ED. Double-lumen balloons, are they only useful in neurointerventions? Preliminary outcomes of double-lumen balloon-assisted embolization of visceral artery aneurysms. *Vasc Endovascular Surg.* 2020;54(3):214-219.
47. Etezadi V, Gandhi RT, Benenati JF, et al. Endovascular treatment of visceral and renal artery aneurysms. *J Vasc Interv Radiol.* 2011;22:1246-1253.
48. Maingard J, Kok HK, Phelan E, et al. Endovascular treatment of wide-necked visceral artery aneurysms using the neurovascular Comaneci neck-bridging device: a technical report. *Cardiovasc Intervent Radiol.* 2017;40: 1784-1791.
49. Murray TE, Brennan P, Maingard JT, et al. Treatment of visceral artery aneurysms using novel neurointerventional devices and techniques. *J Vasc Interv Radiol.* 2019;30(9):1407-1417.
50. Seshadhri S, Janiga G, Beuing O, et al. Impact of stents and flow diverters on hemodynamics in idealized aneurysm models. *J Biomech Eng.* 2011;133:071005-071009.
51. Ruffino MA, Rabbia C. Endovascular repair of peripheral and visceral aneurysms with the cardiatis multilayer flow modulator: one-year results from the Italian multicenter registry. *J Endovasc Ther.* 2012; 19:599-610.
52. Erben Y, De Martino RR, Bjarnason H, et al. Operative management of hepatic artery aneurysms. *J Vasc Surg.* 2015;62(3):610-615.
53. Lee D, Chung BH, Heo SH, et al. Case report of a large common hepatic artery aneurysm. *Ann Vasc Surg.* 2018;52:316.e11-316.e13.
54. Abbas MA, Fowl RJ, Stone WM, et al. Hepatic artery aneurysm: factors that predict complications. *J Vasc Surg.* 2003;38(1):41-45.
55. Lorelli DR, Cambria RA, Seabrook GR, et al. Diagnosis and management of aneurysms involving the superior mesenteric artery and its branches—a report of four cases. *Vasc Endovascular Surg.* 2003;37(1):59-66.
56. van Rijn MJ, Ten Raa S, Hendriks JM, et al. Visceral aneurysms: old paradigms, new insights? *Best Pract Res Clin Gastroenterol.* 2017;31(1):97-104.
57. Vandy FC, Sell KA, Eliason JL, et al. Pancreaticoduodenal and gastroduodenal artery aneurysms associated with celiac artery occlusive disease. *Ann Vasc Surg.* 2017;41: 32-40.
58. Barrionuevo P, Malas MB, Nejim B, et al. A systematic review and meta-analysis of the management of visceral artery aneurysms. *J Vasc Surg.* 2020;72(1S):40S-45S.

SELF-ASSESSMENT STUDY QUESTIONS AND ANSWERS

Questions

1. An 87-year-old male presents to the emergency room after sudden onset of severe left upper quadrant pain, followed by a syncopal episode. He is now alert and answers questions appropriately but does appear to be in significant pain. His systolic blood pressure is 100 mm Hg and his heart rate is 60 beats per minute. A CT scan is obtained demonstrating a splenic artery aneurysm in the distal 1/3 of the splenic artery. Obvious contrast extravasation is not seen, but there is significant fat stranding in the surrounding tissues. What is the best management for this patient?
A. Admission to the intensive care unit for beta-blockade and pain control followed by delayed open repair
B. Admission to the intensive care unit for beta-blockade and pain control followed by delayed endovascular treatment
C. Immediate endovascular treatment
D. Immediate open repair
E. Discharge to home with pain medicine and outpatient follow-up in 1 week

2. What percentage of patients who present with a visceral artery aneurysm have an aneurysm in another location?
A. 5%
B. 15%
C. 45%
D. 70%
E. 90%

3. What is the most common cause of visceral aneurysms?
A. Atherosclerosis
B. Ehlers–Danlos syndrome
C. Vasculitis
D. Portal hypertension
E. Fibromuscular dysplasia

4. What is the most common location for visceral artery aneurysms?
A. Celiac artery
B. Superior mesenteric artery
C. Hepatic artery
D. Gastroduodenal artery
E. Splenic artery

5. A 56-year-old female presents with an incidentally found large splenic artery aneurysm. During attempted stent-graft placement to exclude the aneurysm, the artery proximal and distal to the aneurysm was successfully crossed with a wire and small catheter. However, while attempting to position a stent graft to bridge the proximal and distal targets, the vessel ruptured just distal to the aneurysm. Which of the following anatomical factors increase the risk of this complication?
A. Proximal location of a splenic artery aneurysm
B. Extremely tortuous turn in the splenic artery just distal to the aneurysm
C. Securing distal wire access into the hilum of the spleen
D. Lack of significant calcifications in the splenic artery wall
E. Normal diameter size of the artery (6 mm) proximal and distal to the aneurysm

6. Prior to the widespread use of antibiotics, what was the most common etiology for celiac artery aneurysms?
A. Atherosclerosis
B. Trauma
C. Fibromuscular dysplasia
D. Syphilis
E. Pancreatitis

SELF-ASSESSMENT STUDY QUESTIONS AND ANSWERS

7. An otherwise healthy 60-year-old male presents to the clinic with a superior mesenteric artery aneurysm found incidentally during a screening chest CT. A CT scan of the abdomen and pelvis demonstrates a 2.5 × 2.6 × 2.6 cm aneurysm in the mid portion of the superior mesenteric artery with several jejunal branches coming off the aneurysm. What is the best management strategy for this aneurysm?

A. Coiling of the artery proximal and distal to the aneurysm
B. Coiling the origins of each branch coming off the aneurysm followed by stent-graft placement to exclude the aneurysm
C. Observation with yearly follow-up until the aneurysm is over 3 cm
D. Nonoperative management due to the patient's age
E. Open surgical repair

8. A 50-year-old male with a recent history of endocarditis presents to the emergency room with abdominal pain and fever. A CT scan demonstrates a superior mesenteric artery aneurysm. What is the most likely culprit organism?

A. Salmonella
B. Candida
C. Enterococcus
D. Pseudomonas
E. Staphylococcus

9. An otherwise healthy 45-year-old male presents with an incidentally found 3-cm nonruptured hepatic artery aneurysm that extends beyond the origin of the gastroduodenal artery (GDA) up to the origins of the right and left hepatic arteries. He is asymptomatic with no abdominal pain, fevers, chills, or malaise. He has no history of GI procedures or surgeries. What is the best management for this lesion?

A. Observation with yearly CT scan
B. Coil embolization of the left hepatic artery origin followed by stent graft placement from the common hepatic artery into the right hepatic artery
C. Open replacement of the aneurysmal hepatic artery with autogenous vein graft
D. Coil embolization of the entire aneurysm
E. Palliative care consult

10. A 40-year-old male patient recently left the hospital 3 weeks ago against medical advice after undergoing splenectomy performed during an open repair of a distal splenic artery aneurysm. He now presents to the emergency room with 24 hours of worsening fevers, chills, diarrhea, and malaise. On examination, he is febrile, hypotensive, tachycardic, and in distress. His hemoglobin and hematocrit are stable from discharge. His white blood cell count is significantly elevated. What is the next best step in the management of this patient?

A. Administer 1 L of normal saline and discharge home with seven days of amoxicillin and clavulanate
B. Administer pneumococcal, Hemophilus influenza type b, and meningococcal vaccines immediately
C. CT angiography to evaluate intra-abdominal hemorrhage and intra-abdominal abscess
D. Expeditiously draw blood cultures, commence fluid resuscitation, and administer broad-spectrum antibiotics
E. Rapidly obtain an electrocardiography, troponins, and trans thoracic echo

SELF-ASSESSMENT STUDY QUESTIONS AND ANSWERS

Answers

1. C.
2. C.
3. A.
4. E.
5. B.
6. D.
7. E.
8. E.
9. C.
10. D.

CHAPTER

29 Thoracoabdominal Aortic Aneurysms

Tanvi Subramanian and Ross Milner

OUTLINE

GENERAL CONSIDERATIONS AND HISTORY
CLINICAL FINDINGS
DIFFERENTIAL DIAGNOSIS
DIAGNOSIS
MANAGEMENT

GENERAL CONSIDERATIONS AND HISTORY

Aortic aneurysm disease overall leads to 10,000 deaths annually, much of which is likely secondary to the failure to identify and diagnose disease in these patients. Aortic aneurysms are the ninth overall cause of death in the United States.[1] These are defined as localized, full-thickness arterial dilations measuring ≥50% of the normal diameter. Descending thoracic aortic aneurysms (TAAs) and thoracoabdominal aortic aneurysms (TAAAs) account only for 2% to 5% of these, as the vast majority are abdominal.

The descending thoracic aorta is defined as beginning distal to the aortic arch, at the origin of the left subclavian artery, and continuing down until just proximal to the takeoff of the celiac axis. Thoracoabdominal aneurysms account for ~10% of thoracic aneurysms and include any portion of the descending thoracic aorta as well as the visceral and/or infrarenal segments.[2]

The pathogenesis of most TAAs is degenerative in nature, characterized by a loss of elastic fibers from the medial layer, as well as loss of smooth muscle and proteoglycan deposition. This is thought to be secondary to increased activity of matrix metalloproteinases (MMP-2, MMP-9), leading to lysis of elastic fibers and medial remodeling. TGF-b is also involved in regulation of these matrix metalloproteinases, and mutations or dysregulation of this cytokine is often seen in associated diseases.[3]

A small fraction of TAAs is secondary to genetic and connective tissue disorders, inflammatory vasculitides, or infection (mycotic). Genetic disorders include Marfan syndrome, Loeys-Dietz syndrome, Ehlers-Danlos syndrome, Turner syndrome, bicuspid aortic valve, and familial TAA and dissection syndrome. Inflammatory conditions include Takayasu arteritis, giant cell arteritis, and Behcet's disease.

Associated risk factors include hypertension, smoking, cocaine use, COPD, large initial diameter, female gender, history of cardiac/renal transplant, and certain patterns of wall stress. Rupture risk is most closely correlated with the maximal cross sectional diameter of the aneurysm but is also associated with the development of a dissection within the aneurysm. The annual rupture risk when the aneurysm size is <5 cm is 1.5%, but this increases sharply when aneurysm size is >6 cm, with risk of dissection, rupture, or death occurring in ~15%.[4,5] Thoracic aneurysms, on average, tend to grow ~0.1 cm/year.[2]

CLINICAL FINDINGS

Most TAA are discovered incidentally during workup for an unrelated diagnosis. These patients are usually asymptomatic. For those who are symptomatic, this is usually secondary to local compression on surrounding

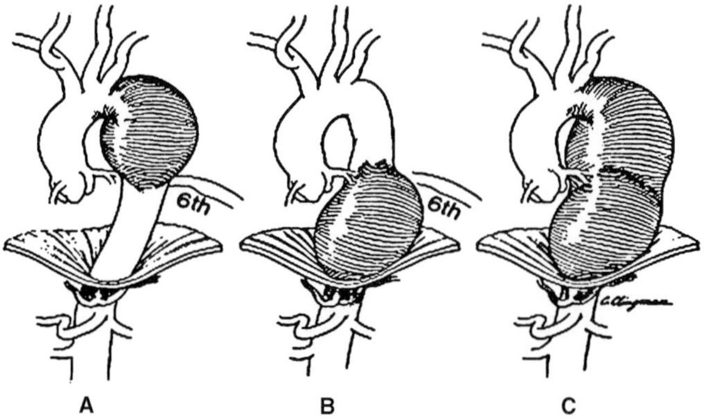

FIGURE 29-1 **DTAA classification**. (Reproduced with permission from Estrera AL, Miller CC 3rd, Chen EP, et al. Descending thoracic aortic aneurysm repair: 12-year experience using distal aortic perfusion and cerebrospinal fluid drainage. *Ann Thorac Surg.* 2005;80(4):1290-1296.)

structures, including the esophagus, recurrent laryngeal nerve, trachea, or vertebral bodies, or from mediastinal pleural inflammation. Back pain is the most commonly experienced symptom. Symptomatic TAA are associated with an increased risk of rupture.

Descending thoracic aortic aneurysms (DTAA) are classified by location within the aorta (Figure 29-1).[6] Type A DTAAs extend from distal to the left subclavian to the sixth intercostal space. Type B extend from the sixth intercostal space to the twelfth intercostal space, or above the diaphragm. Type C involve the entire descending aorta, from distal to the left subclavian to above the diaphragm.

TAAAs are described according to the Crawford classification, again based on location (Figure 29-2).[7] Type I TAAAs extend from distal to the left subclavian to above the renal arteries. Type II extend from distal to the left subclavian to the infrarenal aorta. Type III extend from the sixth intercostal space to the infrarenal aorta. Type IV extend from the twelfth intercostal space to the aortic bifurcation (total AAA). Type V extend from below the sixth intercostal space to just above the renal arteries.

DIFFERENTIAL DIAGNOSIS

True aneurysms are defined as dilation within the arterial wall to ≥50% normal diameter that includes all three layers (intima, media, adventitia) of the vessel wall. However, these may be confused with other

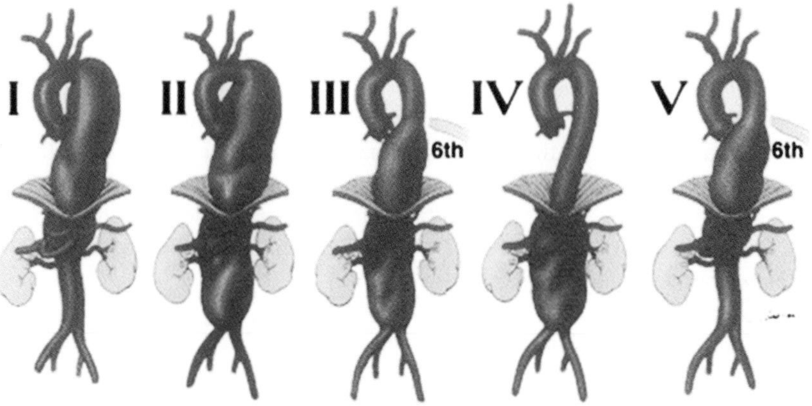

FIGURE 29-2 **Crawford classification of TAAA**. (Reproduced with permission from Safi HJ, Winnerkvist A, Miller CC 3rd, et al. Effect of extended cross-clamp time during thoracoabdominal aortic aneurysm repair. *Ann Thorac Surg.* 1998;66(4):1204-1209.)

thoracic aortic pathologies, including pseudoaneurysm and dissection.

Pseudoaneurysms do not involve all three layers of vessel wall. These can occur in the thoracic aorta as the result of a contained aortic rupture. Etiologies also include ulcerated aortic plaque, aortic dissection, and blunt aortic injury.

Dissection will present with severe, sharp, ripping back pain. Based on location in the thoracic aorta, this may involve extension of the dissection flap into nearby vessels, leading to cerebral embolic symptoms and upper extremity ischemia. This may also occur in the setting of aneurysmal disease.

Thoracic and abdominal aortic imaging in conjunction with clinical correlation can be used to distinguish these diagnoses from true aneurysms.

DIAGNOSIS

As mentioned previously, many TAAs are diagnosed incidentally on imaging for other conditions. However, once these are identified, several diagnostic tests must be performed to determine if surgical intervention is necessary, and if so, what type of surgical intervention is most appropriate (Figure 29-3).

Computed tomography angiography (Figure 29-4) is necessary to evaluate the entire aorta and is considered the gold standard for aortic imaging (sensitivity 100%, specificity 98%).[5] Magnetic resonance angiography is appropriate in the setting of renal insufficiency. These imaging studies will help to determine the size and extent of the aneurysm, which guides decision-making for whether surgery is indicated, based on the risk-benefit analysis for any given patient. Additionally, this elucidates the patient's aortic anatomy, which is crucial in determining whether an endovascular repair versus an open repair is most appropriate. There must be clear proximal and distal landing zones for the stent graft in order to prevent a postoperative endoleak. An adequate proximal seal zone may require coverage of supra-aortic vessels, most commonly the origin of the left subclavian artery (LSA). Coverage of the LSA will usually require extra-anatomic reconstruction to preserve blood flow. The distal seal zone is typically proximal to the celiac axis for a true DTAA, but will extend into the abdomen and may involve coverage of visceral arteries for TAAA. Additionally, increased tortuosity of the aorta will make placement of certain stent grafts difficult, though there are some newer devices that are better able to accommodate tortuosity. It is also important to assess the femoral and iliac arterial access pathways, in order to allow for safe passage of the stent graft. Risk of iliac artery disruption is approximately 1 in 200, and placement of iliac conduits may be required depending on the extent of iliac occlusive disease, tortuosity, and calcification.[8]

Cardiac testing may be necessary to evaluate a patient's fitness prior to elective repair. This includes an echocardiogram to assess ventricular and valvular function, with further testing/intervention with nuclear stress testing or cardiac catheterization as necessary. Poor cardiac function may preclude open surgical repair. In addition, carotid duplex imaging is frequently completed. The carotid duplex is especially important when there is great vessel involvement.

Determination of preoperative renal function is crucial in the case of TAAAs. This can be assessed by baseline serum creatinine levels. Up to 15% of patients with TAAA have been shown to have significant preoperative renal insufficiency (Cr $\geq$1.8), which has been shown to be associated with postoperative renal failure and mortality. These patients may require preoperative renal revascularization via percutaneous stenting or a surgical bypass or endarterectomy to preserve renal blood flow. Severe renal insufficiency may preclude open surgical repair.

Pulmonary function testing may also be required if a large part of the thoracic aorta is involved, as single-lung ventilation may be required in the case of open surgical repair. Appropriate preoperative findings include FEV1 $\geq$1.0, PCO2 $\leq$45. If these are not met, patient will require preoperative medical therapy, or endovascular repair.

MANAGEMENT

Repair is indicated for any symptomatic patient who does not have specific contraindications (unacceptable pulmonary or cardiac risk or very limited life expectancy due to other issues, such as recurrent or metastatic cancer). For asymptomatic patients, management is based mainly on aneurysm size. The current consensus mandates repair if aneurysmal

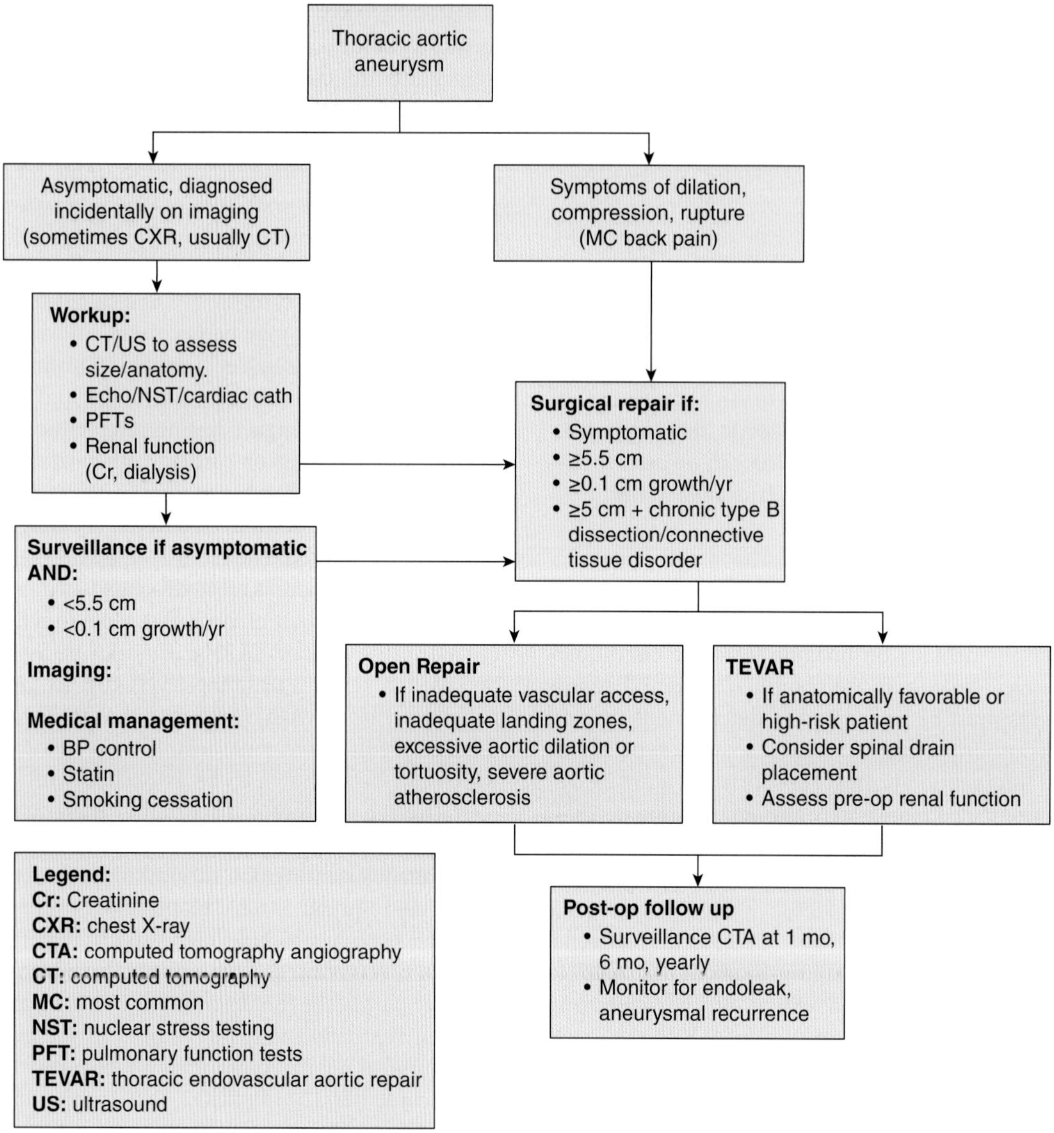

FIGURE 29-3 **Flowchart depicting diagnosis and treatment algorithms for TAAA.**

diameter is ≥5.5 cm. This cutoff is adjusted to ≥5 cm if the patient has a known connective tissue disorder causing their aneurysmal disease (Figure 29-3). Workup as mentioned in the previous section must be performed to determine aortic anatomy, cardiac and renal function, and fitness for surgery.

Conservative therapy with medical management may be appropriate in patients who are asymptomatic without known connective tissue disorder with aneurysmal sizes <5.5 cm. This includes blood pressure control to <120 systolic, smoking cessation, and cessation of illicit drug use. These patients require close surveillance imaging, with time between scans based on aneurysm size, to follow for growth.[2]

Thoracic endovascular aortic repair (TEVAR) is the recommended treatment option for high-risk

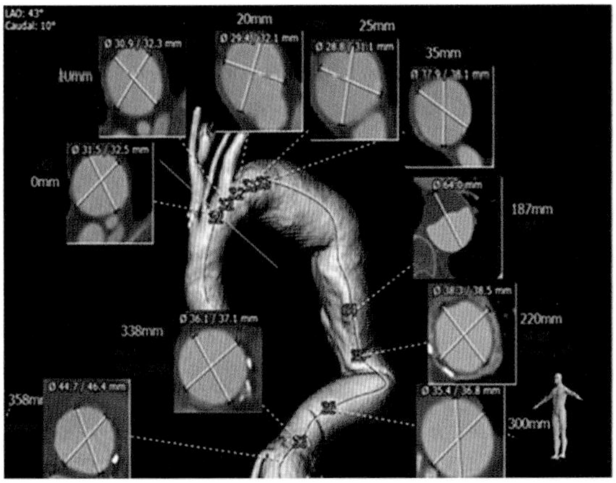

FIGURE 29-4 CTA reconstruction demonstrating thoracic aortic aneurysm >6 cm.

patients or with favorable aortic anatomy, and may soon be the first-line treatment recommended for all patients. Open repair is still indicated in patients with densely calcified vessels, infection, trauma, anatomical challenges, or previously failed endografts.

Open repair of the thoracic aorta was first described by Bahnson in 1952, later refined and mastered by Crawford. This approach has historically been rife with high rates of renovisceral and spinal cord complications due to ischemia. Typically, this involves positioning the patient in right lateral decubitus position with a thoracoretroperitoneal approach, as well as additional thoracotomy as needed for exposure depending on the proximal extent of the aneurysm. The recurrent laryngeal and vagus nerves are identified, and proximal and distal control are obtained prior to aortotomy, with sequential aortic cross-clamping to minimize the risk of end-organ ischemia. The graft is then implanted with reconstruction of visceral vasculature as indicated.

In 2005, the FDA approved the GORE TAG Thoracic Endoprosthesis.[9] Since then, TEVAR has become the preferred form of repair for thoracic aneurysms, with significantly lower rates of short-term morbidity and mortality compared to open repair (30-day mortality, 5.57% vs 16.5%).[5] TEVAR involves placing the patient supine. A groin cut-down or percutaneous access is performed on the intended access vessel, and vascular access is obtained on the contralateral common femoral artery with placement of a 5Fr sheath. A catheter is introduced into the thoracic aorta over a guidewire and the device introduced over this. The stent graft is then deployed, with a balloon used to ensure fixation to the aortic wall at the proximal and distal landing zones; overlapping stent grafts may be placed depending on the size and anatomical configuration of the aneurysm. The access sheaths are removed with closure of the arteriotomy. Figure 29-5 demonstrates the successful placement of a graft within the thoracic aorta.

Limitations of TEVAR use are defined by anatomy and patient comorbidity. The size and configuration of the aneurysm, as well as the location within and tortuosity of the aorta, must be determined preoperatively via imaging to determine whether a graft may appropriately be placed. Available endograft diameters range from 21 mm to 46 mm, which limits use in aneurysms with large proximal necks or small-caliber aortas. There are new graft models allowing for some flexibility of use in these situations, including the use of branched

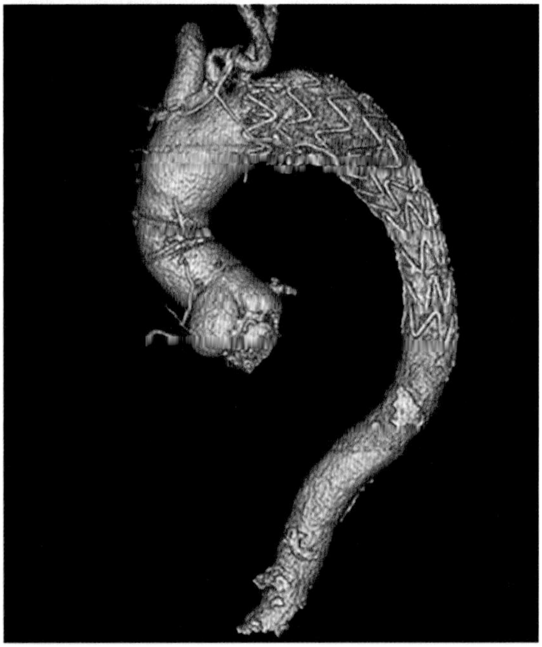

FIGURE 29-5 Postoperative CTA reconstruction after placement of a Medtronic Valiant Navion device.

or fenestrated devices as well as snorkel or chimney techniques that are used in off-label approaches to aneurysm care. Additionally, the location of the aneurysm within the thoracic aorta may require coverage of the supra-aortic vessels to ensure adequate landing and seal zones proximally. This most commonly entails the origin of the left subclavian artery, which requires extra-anatomic reconstruction via a carotid-subclavian bypass or subclavian artery transposition in order to preserve flow to the left vertebral artery as well as the left arm.

One severe complication of aneurysm repair is spinal cord ischemia (SCI). In the setting of TEVAR, SCI occurs in 2% to 10% of patients, often in a delayed fashion.[10] Etiology of SCI is multifactorial, but graft coverage of the artery of Adamkiewicz, which originates from the distal thoracic aorta usually between T8 and L1, and provides a majority of blood flow to the lumbosacral cord, is thought to play a large role. The exact location of this artery in individual patients is determined by the preoperative CTA. Preoperative placement of lumbar spinal drains to decrease risk of ischemia secondary to cord compression from elevated CSF pressure has demonstrated efficacy following open repair; however, there is no evidence-based consensus for their use in the setting of TEVAR and is institution-dependent. Use of neurophysiologic monitoring has also been demonstrated to detect ischemia intraoperatively. If detected, SCI should be managed by maintaining MAP >90 mmHg using fluids or vasopressors as indicated, and reducing CSF pressure to 0 mmHg.[11]

Another serious complication is acute renal failure. Preoperative renal failure is the strongest predictor of the development of postoperative renal failure, which is an independent risk factor for mortality. Need for postoperative dialysis must be discussed as a possible complication during the consent process, as dialysis-dependent renal failure has been reported in 1.5% to 10.7% of patients after elective TAAA repair, and in even higher numbers after emergent repair.[10,12]

Close follow-up with surveillance imaging at 1 month, 6 months, and then annually is indicated for detection of endoleak.

REFERENCES

1. Centers for Disease Control and Prevention. Leading Causes of Death. https://www.cdc.gov/nchs/fastats/leading-causes-of-death.htm. Accessed on August 24, 2020.
2. Isselbacher EM. Thoracic and abdominal aortic aneurysms. *Circulation*. 2005;111(6):816-828.
3. Goldfinger JZ, Halperin JL, Marin ML, Stewart AS, Eagle KA, Fuster V.Thoracic aortic aneurysm and dissection. *J Am Coll Cardiol*. 2014;64(16):1725-1739.
4. Trimarchi S, Jonker FH, Hutchison S, et al. Descending aortic diameter of 5.5 cm or greater is not an accurate predictor of acute type B aortic dissection. *J Thorac Cardiovasc Surg*. 2011;142(3):e101-e107.
5. Riambau V, Böckler D, Brunkwall J, et al. Editor's choice: management of descending thoracic aorta diseases: clinical practice guidelines of the European Society for vascular surgery (ESVS). *Eur J Vasc Endovasc Surg*. 2017;53(1):4-52.
6. Estrera AL, Miller CC 3rd, Chen EP, et al. Descending thoracic aortic aneurysm repair: 12-year experience using distal aortic perfusion and cerebrospinal fluid drainage. *Ann Thorac Surg*. 2005;80(4):1290-1296; discussion 1296.
7. Safi HJ, Winnerkvist A, Miller CC 3rd, et al. Effect of extended cross-clamp time during thoracoabdominal aortic aneurysm repair. *Ann Thorac Surg*. 1998;66(4):1204-1209.
8. Fernandez JD, Craig JM, Garrett HE Jr, Burgar SR, Bush AJ.Endovascular management of iliac rupture during endovascular aneurysm repair. *J Vasc Surg*. 2009;50(6):1293-1299; discussion 1299-1300.
9. WL Gore & Associates. Conformable GORE® TAG® Thoracic Endoprosthesis. https://www.goremedical.com/products/ctag. Accessed on August 24, 2022.
10. Wong CS, Healy D, Canning C, Coffey JC, Boyle JR, Walsh SR.A systematic review of spinal cord injury and cerebrospinal fluid drainage after thoracic aortic endografting. *J Vasc Surg*. 2012;56(5):1438-1447.
11. Bobadilla JL, Wynn M, Tefera G, Acher CW. Low incidence of paraplegia after thoracic endovascular aneurysm repair with proactive spinal cord protective protocols. *J Vasc Surg*. 2013;57(6):1537-1542.
12. Wynn MM, Acher C, Marks E, Engelbert T, Acher CW.Postoperative renal failure in thoracoabdominal aortic aneurysm repair with simple cross-clamp technique and 4°C renal perfusion. *J Vasc Surg*. 2015;61(3):611-622.

SELF-ASSESSMENT STUDY QUESTIONS AND ANSWERS

Questions

1. Which of the following is most closely correlated with increased rupture risk?
   A. Connective tissue disorder
   B. Uncontrolled hypertension
   C. Aneurysm diameter
   D. History of smoking and cocaine use

2. Per the Crawford classification, a type II TAAA is defined as:
   A. 6th intercostal space to above renal arteries
   B. 6th intercostal space to infrarenal aorta
   C. 12th intercostal space to aortic bifurcation
   D. Distal to LSA to infrarenal aorta

3. Gold standard for preoperative imaging workup is:
   A. CT angiography
   B. MR angiography
   C. Transthoracic echocardiogram
   D. Intravascular ultrasound

4. Preoperative testing prior to aneurysm repair may include all of the following except:
   A. PFTs
   B. Baseline Cr
   C. Echocardiogram
   D. MRI T/L spine

5. Indications for open repair over TEVAR include:
   A. Extensive comorbidities
   B. History of previous TEVAR
   C. Favorable aortic anatomy
   D. Pre-existing renal failure

6. Which of the following is NOT a known etiology for thoracic aneurysmal disease?
   A. Sarcoidosis
   B. Bicuspid aortic valve
   C. Behcet's disease
   D. Hypertension

7. A genetic defect in which of the following is *most commonly* associated with aneurysmal disease?
   A. COL5A1 (Ehlers-Danlos)
   B. TGF-b (Loeys-Dietz)
   C. FBN-1 (Marfan's)
   D. ACTA2 (familial TAAD)

8. Surgical repair of aneurysm is mandated for patients with:
   A. Aneurysmal diameter >4 cm
   B. Symptoms
   C. Growth of 0.5 mm/year
   D. Known connective tissue disorder

9. Followup after TEVAR should include surveillance imaging at:
   A. 2 weeks, 4 weeks, 8 weeks
   B. 1 month, 3 months, 6 months
   C. 1 month, 6 months, 12 months
   D. 6 months, 1 year, 5 years

10. All of the following are important to assess on imaging prior to operative repair of a TAAA except:
   A. Celiac artery
   B. Right iliac artery
   C. Left renal artery
   D. Right subclavian artery

SELF-ASSESSMENT STUDY QUESTIONS AND ANSWERS

Answers

1. C.
2. D.
3. A.
4. D.
5. B.
6. A.
7. C.
8. B.
9. C.
10. D.

CHAPTER

30 Peripheral Arterial Aneurysms

Ahmed A. Sorour and Levester Kirksey

OUTLINE

PERIPHERAL ARTERIAL ANEURYSMS
LOWER EXTREMITY ANEURYSMS
Common Femoral Aneurysm
Epidemiology and Etiology
Clinical Presentation and Diagnosis
Treatment
Indications
Surgical repair
Endovascular repair
Femoral Artery False Aneurysm
Epidemiology and Etiology
Clinical Presentation and Diagnosis
Treatment
Observation
Ultrasound-guided-thrombin injection (UGTI)
Ultrasound guided compression (UGC)
Open surgical repair
Superficial Femoral Artery Aneurysm
Profunda Femoral Artery Aneurysm
Popliteal Artery Aneurysm
Epidemiology
Pathogenesis and Clinical Presentation
Diagnosis
Treatment
Indications
Open Treatment
Medial approach
Posterior approach
Medial versus posterior outcome
Endovascular and Hybrid Treatment
Open versus endovascular outcome
Thrombolysis
Infrapopliteal Aneurysm
UPPER EXTREMITY ANEURYSMS
Axillary Artery Aneurysms
Etiology and Clinical Presentation
Diagnosis and Treatment
Open surgical treatment
Endovascular treatment
Brachial Artery Aneurysm
Epidemiology and Etiology
Clinical Presentation and Diagnosis
Treatment
Brachial Artery False Aneurysm
Infected Peripheral Arterial Aneurysms
Etiology and Risk Factors
Diagnosis and Treatment
Lower Extremity Infected Aneurysm
Upper Extremity Infected Aneurysm
PERIPHERAL VENOUS ANEURYSM
Popliteal Venous Aneurysm
Jugular Venous Aneurysm

PERIPHERAL ARTERIAL ANEURYSMS

Peripheral aneurysms can be broadly categorized, based on location, into upper and lower extremity aneurysms. In any artery, the Society for Vascular Surgery clinical practice guidelines defines an aneurysm as a focal dilation 1.5 times the normal diameter of the disease-free proximal adjacent segment.[1] True aneurysms consist of the outpouching of all three layers of the vessel wall including tunica intima, media, and adventitia. False aneurysms (pseudoaneurysms), on the other hand, include dilation of one or two layers of the vessel wall (Figure 30-1a-b). The most common false aneurysms will be discussed separately after the corresponding artery.

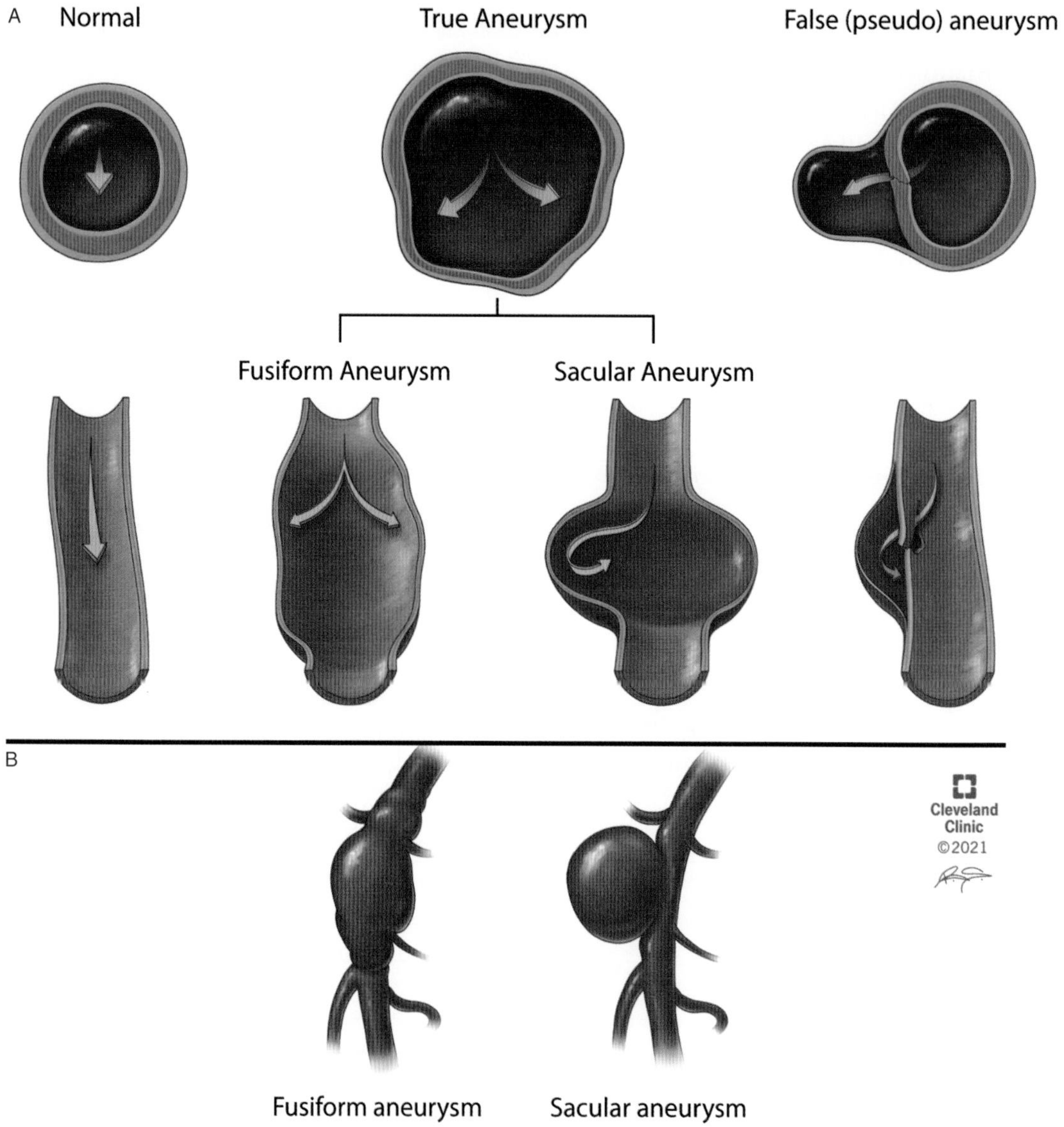

FIGURE 30-1 True aneurysm and false aneurysm. (**A**) Depicts transverse and longitudinal illustrations of a normal, true aneurysm, and false aneurysm vessel. (**B**) Schematic representation of fusiform and saccular aneurysms. (Reprinted with permission, Cleveland Clinic Foundation ©2022. All Rights Reserved.)

The incidence of aneurysms in peripheral arteries is rare in comparison to that of abdominal aortic aneurysms (AAA).[2] Hence, diagnosis of a peripheral aneurysm warrants screening in other vascular beds due to the high incidence of concomitant diseases. The most common underlying pathology of peripheral aneurysm formation is a degenerative or atherosclerotic disease (Table 30-1). In order of frequency, the most common peripheral aneurysm locations are the popliteal/superficial femoral, common femoral, and axillary arteries. Reports on distal aneurysms involving profunda femoral, tibial, peroneal, brachial, and ulnar arteries are limited to case reports.

Peripheral aneurysms may be asymptomatic or lead to local/end-organ complications. Local compression of surrounding venous or neurologic structures and thromboembolic complications are the most common presenting symptoms. Unlike the aorta, peripheral aneurysms are less prone to rupture. The decision to repair peripheral aneurysms depends on the size of the aneurysm, rate of expansion, presence of symptoms, and the patient's overall medical condition. Treatment may be initiated through open, endovascular, or hybrid surgical techniques, with two primary goals: (1) to exclude the aneurysm and (2) to restore arterial continuity.

TABLE 30-1 Etiology of Peripheral Artery Aneurysms

Atherosclerotic
Iatrogenic
Main etiology for false aneurysm
Mycotic
Bacterial, fungal, spirochetal
Inflammatory
Behçet's disease, Parkes Weber syndrome, Granulomatosis with polyangiitis
Congenital
Ehlers-Danolas, Marfan's syndrome
Traumatic
Blunt or penetrating trauma
Mechanical
Atriovenous fistula associated, poststenotic

Data from Johnston KW, Rutherford RB, Tilson MD, et al. Suggested standards for reporting on arterial aneurysms. Subcommittee on Reporting Standards for Arterial Aneurysms, Ad Hoc Committee on Reporting Standards, Society for Vascular Surgery and North American Chapter, International Society for Cardiovascular Surgery. *J Vasc Surg*. 1991;13(3):452-458.

LOWER EXTREMITY ANEURYSMS

COMMON FEMORAL ANEURYSM

The common femoral artery (CFA) is a continuation of the external iliac artery as it passes deep to the inguinal ligament and ends by bifurcating into superficial femoral (SFA) and profunda femoral (PFA) arteries. The normal diameter of CFA is approximately 1 cm and 0.8 cm in men and women respectively.[3] The CFA is a site for both true and false aneurysms. With the increased utilization of percutaneous therapies for the heart and peripheral vasculature, false aneurysms are encountered more frequently.[4]

Epidemiology and Etiology

CFA aneurysms are the second most commonly occurring peripheral aneurysm only after popliteal aneurysms. Historically, Cutler and Darling classified aneurysms into the following: the more common *type 1* which involved the CFA up to the level of the bifurcation and a less encountered *type 2* which extends into Profunda femoris (PFA).[5] Degenerative disease is the main pathoetiology of CFA aneurysms; hence, the risk factors include age (70 years or older), men, smoking, and hypertension.[2,6] Other rarely encountered causes include Behçet's disease, arteriomegaly, and acromegaly.[7–9]

The majority of patients with CFA aneurysms have aneurysms within other vascular beds including aorto-iliac aneurysms in 40% to 92%, popliteal aneurysms in 27% to 44%, and contralateral CFAs in 41% to 72%.[10] This strong association is not reciprocally seen in patients with AAA, as only 2.8% to 6.7% of patients with AAA have concurrent CFA.[2] This leads to the conclusion that isolated CFA is a rare entity and once CFA is diagnosed active search for concomitant aneurysms should be undertaken.

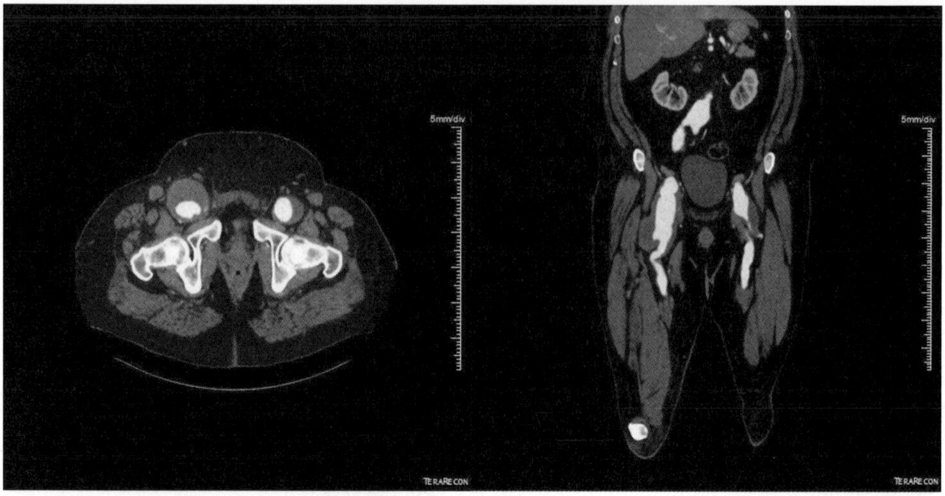

FIGURE 30-2 Common femoral artery aneurysm. CT angiography showing bilateral common femoral on the axial and coronal plane.

Clinical Presentation and Diagnosis

About one-third of patients with CFA aneurysms are asymptomatic, with the aneurysm found incidentally during physical examination or as a part of evaluation for a suspected aorto-iliac and popliteal aneurysmal disease. The other one-third present with mass effect symptoms, including but not limited to tenderness, pain, femoral nerve compression, deep venous thromboses, and phlebitis (due to femoral vein compression). The final one-third present with complications associated with the aneurysm. Thrombosis, the most common complication, may be acute presenting as a limb-threatening ischemia or chronic with symptoms of claudication (more common). Other complications include embolization and rupture. The existing literature is controversial as to whether CFA aneurysms are a definitive source of thromboembolic complications, as many of these patients have concurrent AAA and popliteal artery aneurysms (PAA).

Duplex ultrasound (DUS), which is noninvasive, inexpensive, widely available, and accurate, is the first-line modality of choice for diagnosing and characterizing CFA aneurysms. It is also the best method of surveilling the pathology over time. Computed tomography angiography (CTA) and/or magnetic resonance angiography (MRA) may be helpful at the time of preoperative planning to determine the size and morphologic detail which influences the feasibility of open or endovascular repair (Figure 30-2). Moreover, CTA and MRA are valuable to look for additional aneurysms (AAA, PAA, and contralateral CFA).

Treatment

Indications All symptomatic femoral artery aneurysm (FAA) should be treated. Asymptomatic FAAS were conventionally indicated for treatment if their size was larger than 2.5 cm in diameter.[10] This was challenged by Lawerence et al.[11] With data pooled from eight institutions, the authors recommended surgery to be undertaken if the size of the aneurysm was 3.5 cm or more. One exception to this notion was the presence of intraluminal thrombus, which was a predictor of symptomatic progression and should be an indication by itself even at a smaller aneurysm diameter.[11]

Surgical repair Treatment of CFA aneurysms is mainly done with open surgical repair by excluding the aneurysmal segment with an interposition graft. Open repair is the preferred procedure in elective and emergency settings as the treatment has minimal morbidity and excellent long-term patency.[6,10] Studies have shown that prosthetic grafts have equivalent patency and better size match in comparison with vein grafts in this area.[6] The graft material used is either polytetrafluoroethylene (PTFE) or Dacron.

Proximal control could be achieved by one of the following mechanisms:

1. Clamping the distal external iliac artery or proximal CFA via a longitudinal or oblique groin incision.
2. Balloon occlusion placed via contralateral approach (preferred in large aneurysms or reoperative fields).
3. Suprainguinal retroperitoneal exposure of the external iliac artery (if 1 and 2 are not possible).

Type 1 aneurysm could be treated with an interposition graft, while type 2 requires a complex reconstruction and reimplantation of the SFA to the graft (Figures 30-3 and 30-4). To prevent injury to surrounding structures, the aneurysm sac is usually not resected. It is essential to preserve flow to the PFA to prevent future severe ischemia. In cases of chronic superficial artery occlusion, the PFA may be the sole runoff for femoral reconstruction. The open aneurysm sac may be used to wrap the repaired artery and graft to mitigate infection and close the surgical dead space (Figure 30-5).

Endovascular repair Endovascular treatment of CFA is limited due to the possibility of stent fracture or dislodgement at the inguinal ligament. This approach should be preserved for those patients in whom medical comorbidities are prohibitive for open repair and anatomic features permit reliable exclusion of the aneurysm sac. Endovascular techniques have also been described as a temporizing measure in an emergency situation, with a contralateral common femoral access, distal superficial femoral access, or brachial artery access required for delivery of a covered stent graft.[12] The use of a hybrid approach to either establish proximal control via a balloon or to deploy multiple stent grafts has been described in case reports.[13] Like other endovascular approaches, lifelong surveillance of the repair is necessary (CT or US) to evaluate the integrity of the repair including the seal zone and stent patency and the presence of stent strut fracture (maximal intensity projection or multiview oblique plain film radiograph).

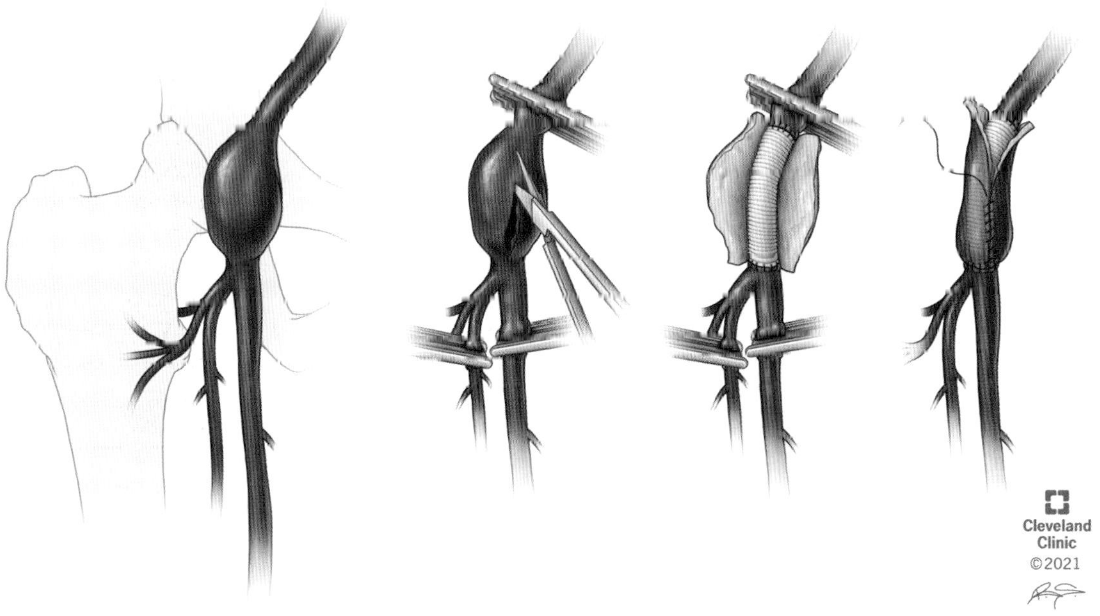

FIGURE 30-3 Repair of type 1 CFA. (Reprinted with permission, Cleveland Clinic Foundation ©2022. All Rights Reserved.)

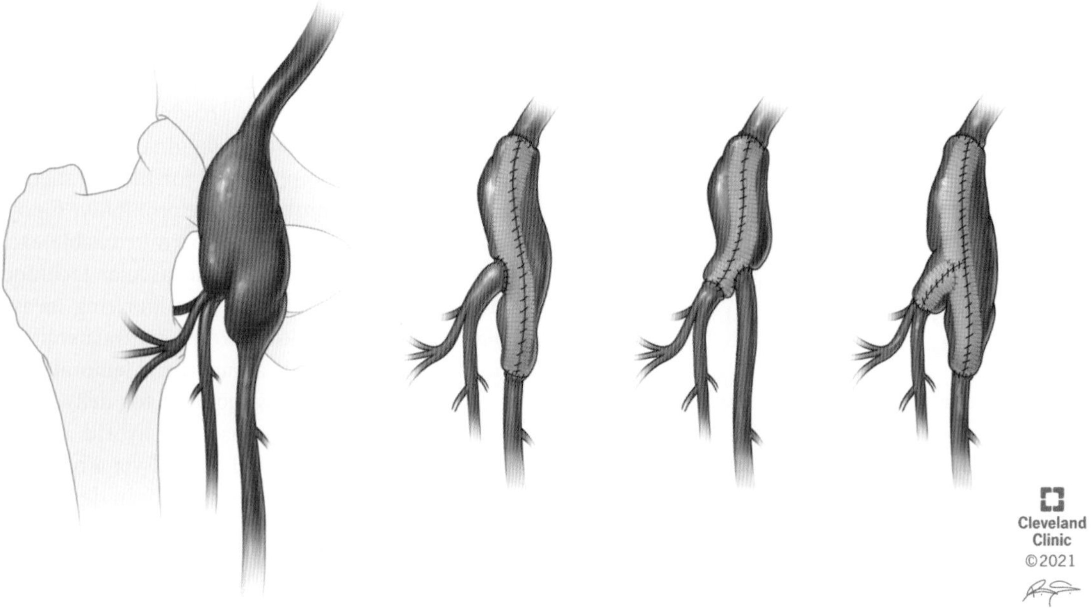

FIGURE 30-4 Repair of type 2 CFA. Multiple reconstruction possibilities presented. (Reprinted with permission, Cleveland Clinic Foundation ©2022. All Rights Reserved.)

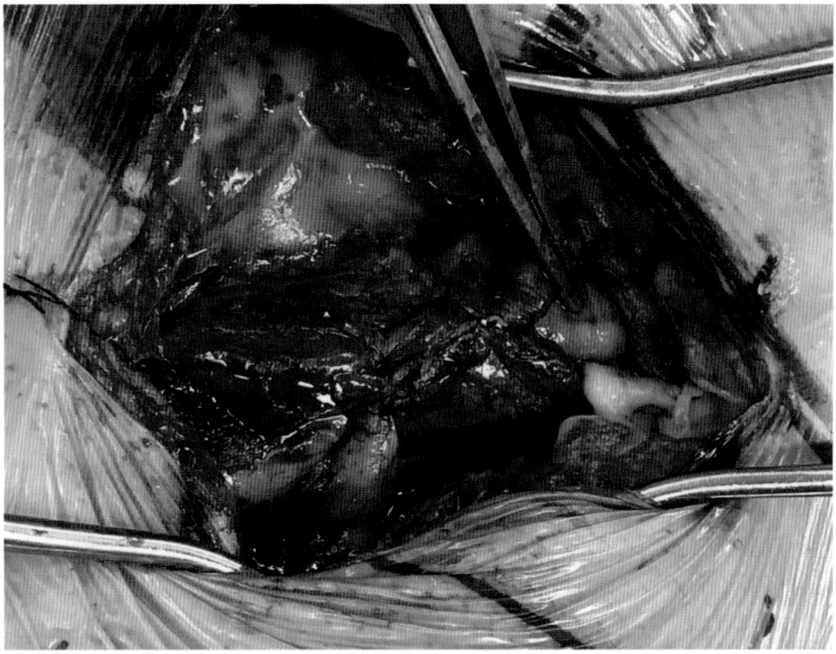

FIGURE 30-5 CFA repair. Intraoperative view of aneurysm sac used to wrap the repaired CFA.

FEMORAL ARTERY FALSE ANEURYSM

Epidemiology and Etiology

Femoral false aneurysm (FFA) is a common entity. It results when a leak from an arterial defect is contained by the surrounding soft tissue or adventitia, forming a thin fibrous capsule enclosing the defect. The most common etiology is femoral artery puncture done for percutaneous-based diagnostic and interventional procedures. The incidence of FFA after femoral catheterization ranges from 0.6% to 6%.[14,15] Risk factors predictive of the development of FFA formation postcatheterization are summarized in Table 30-2. Anastomotic leakage, noniatrogenic trauma, and infection are other causes of FFA.[10]

Clinical Presentation and Diagnosis

The most common clinical manifestation of FFA is a painful pulsatile mass. Femoral bruit, palpable thrill, edema, and femoral neuropathic symptoms are all possible manifestations. Complications of FFA include progressive enlargement leading to rupture, bleeding, overlying skin ischemia or necrosis, and distal embolization. The rupture of FFA is regarded as a surgical emergency as it could lead to hemorrhagic shock and death.[17] Bleeding from FFA could be occult if it occurred in the retroperitoneal space; thus, CTA or MRA is advised whenever clinical suspicion exists.

TABLE 30-2 Risk Factors Associated with Increased FFA in Percutaneous Procedures

Patient-related	Procedure-related
Age (75+)	Emergency procedures
Female	Femoral puncture at an incorrect location (below bifurcation or above inguinal ligament)
Obesity	
Medical history of Hypertension	Sheath size > 7 French
Platelet count < 200,000 cells/mm^3	Use of peri-procedural platelet inhibitors
Arterial calcification	

Data from Madia C. Management trends for postcatheterization femoral artery pseudoaneurysms. *JAAPA*. 2019;32(6):15-18.[16]

DUS is the modality of choice. The sensitivity and specificity to detect FFA are 94% and 97%, respectively.[18] The FFA presents as a hypoechoic cyst adjacent to the artery, in grey scale sonography (B mode). While in the color flow mode, blood flow could be seen entering via the "neck" of the sac. The whirling of blood flow inside the FFA, also known as the ying-yang sign, has been historically regarded as a characteristic feature of pseudoanuerysms. However, this phenomenon is observed due to turbulent flow and could be present in a true aneurysm sac. Thus to differentiate FFA from true aneurysm, hematomas, or cysts, the detection of the communicating neck with a "to-and-fro" waveform is pathognomonic. The "to" refers to the blood flow that occurs during systole (shorter in duration) while the "fro" is the blood flow that occurs during diastole (longer in duration)[19] (Figure 30-6).

Treatment

FFA could be managed with observation, ultrasound guided-thrombin injection, ultrasound-guided compression or open surgical repair. Aneurysm size, presence of anticoagulation and patient profile determines the choice of management.

Observation FFA less than 3 cm in diameter are typically managed with observation as they undergo spontaneous thrombosis. Patients who are not on anticoagulation with an aneurysm size of < 3 cm have a 88% chance of spontaneous thrombosis, with a time average of 3 weeks.[20] Surveillance with DUS every 1 to 2 weeks is performed while patients are advised to limit their activity.

Ultrasound-guided-thrombin injection (UGTI) UGTI is the preferred method of treatment today due to its ease of application, rapid result, success rate and effectiveness in patients on anticoagulation and/or antiplatelet agents. In this procedure, thrombin is injected into the aneurysm cavity percutaneously and under ultrasound guidance, to achieve immediate thrombosis. Thrombin potentiates the coagulation cascade via the conversion of soluble fibrinogen into insoluble fibrin. After confirming successful thrombus formation by the absence of a Doppler flow signal within the FFA, patients are prescribed bed rest from

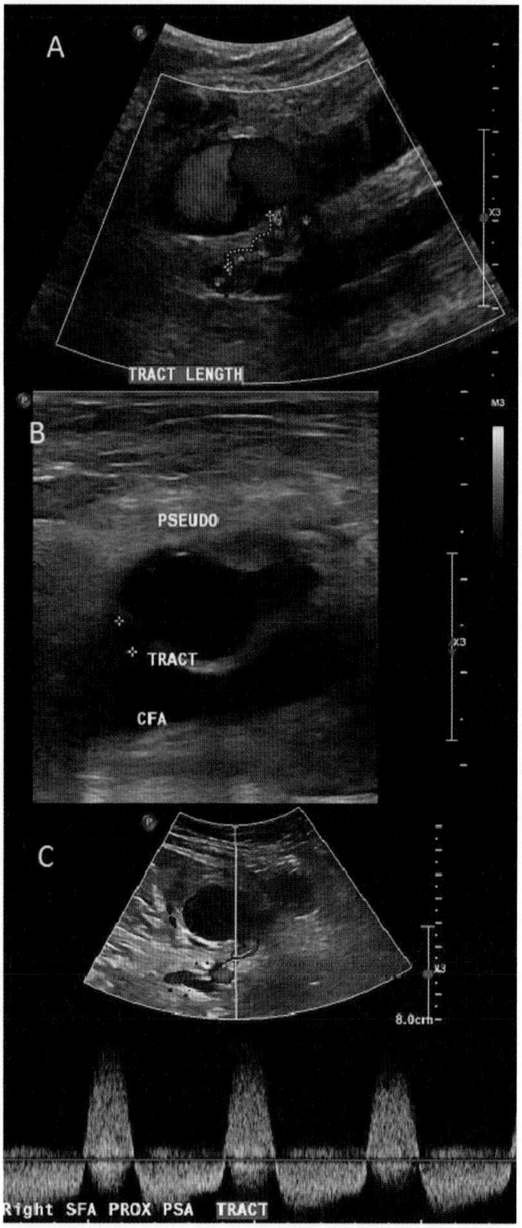

FIGURE 30-6 Duplex ultrasound of femoral false aneurysm. (**A**) Color flow image depicting the neck (tract) between the vessel and false aneurysm. (**B**) Image without color flow, and (**C**) depicts the to-and-fro sign.

1 to 24 hours depending on the practice. Pedal pulses should be assessed before and after the procedure, with any changes noted. The success rate of UGTI is about 96%, with a second injection required in up to 7% of cases.[21,22] The complications of UGTI are rare but serious. Thrombosis and distal arterial embolization are the most feared sequelae. This may be prevented by ensuring needle location within the false aneurysm cavity with saline injection, injecting thrombin slowly, and stopping immediately when thrombosis occurs. Controversy exists over the FFA neck size and length that is amenable to safe UGTI therapy. This led many clinicians to avoid UGTI in necks shorter than 0.5 cm and/or wider than 1 cm. This notion was challenged by a recent study that demonstrated 100% efficacy of UGTI without complication in a cohort that compromised 31% of subjects with an FFA neck length < 0.5 cm.[23] Thus, currently, no definitive guidelines exist for neck size in UGTI therapy.

Ultrasound-guided compression (UGC) UGC was once the gold standard for the treatment of FFA before the initiation of UGTI; it provided a noninvasive alternative to open repair. In UGC the neck of the FFA is located with DUS, and pressure is applied by the ultrasound transducer until flow to the sac ceases. Compression is applied for 10 to 20 minutes, after which flow is reassessed. If complete thrombosis has not been achieved, the process is repeated. The minimum amount of pressure needed to cease flow to the FFA must be applied to prevent potential femoral artery thrombosis. After the procedure, the patient is kept on bed rest for 6 hours, and reassessment with DUS at 24 and 48 hours is done to rule out recurrence. UGC has a success rate of 66% to 86%, with a compression time averaging 44 minutes.[10] The use of UGC is limited by long compression time, which may be painful for the patient and physically exhausting for the operator. Moreover, a Cochrane review conferred that UGTI was more effective than a single session of UGC.[24] Complications associated with UGC are rare. The rupture of FFA has been reported at a rate of 0.3%.[19] Other mentioned complications include femoral vein thrombosis, limb ischemia from femoral artery thrombosis, and vasovagal events leading to hypotension.[19]

Open surgical repair This was the preferred method of treatment before the introduction of

UGTI and UGC. Surgical repair is reserved today for complicated FFA. False aneurysms that are ruptured, infected, causing mass effect with ischemia of overlying skin, associated with the arteriovenous fistula or those that failed UGTI and UGC should be surgically corrected. Direct repair with polypropylene sutures is an effective method of repair. Patch angioplasty could be justified in cases with extensive damage to the arterial wall. For cases, in which infection is suspected, femoral reconstruction should be performed with autologous tissue such as greater saphenous or femoral vein with or without muscle flap coverage. Of special mention, FFA associated with the recent placement of a femoral artery closure device represents an absolute indication for surgical repair with debridement, foreign body removal, and reconstruction of the involved artery.

SUPERFICIAL FEMORAL ARTERY ANEURYSM

Aneurysms confined to SFA territory are relatively rare. The majority of SFA aneurysms (SFAA) (Figure 30-7) are encountered as an extension of PA and CFA aneurysms, with the former being more common. Two of the largest studies focusing on true femoral artery aneurysms reported the frequency of the disease to be 14% to 26% in SFA compared to 57% to 81%, and 5% to 17%, in CFA and PFA, respectively.[4,11] Leon et al.[25] identified 61 reported cases of isolated SFA in a comprehensive all-language literature review in 2007. They reported a male predominance (87%). SFAA were often located in the middle third of the artery and were large in diameter at presentation (mean 8.4 cm, range 3-24 cm).[25] The large

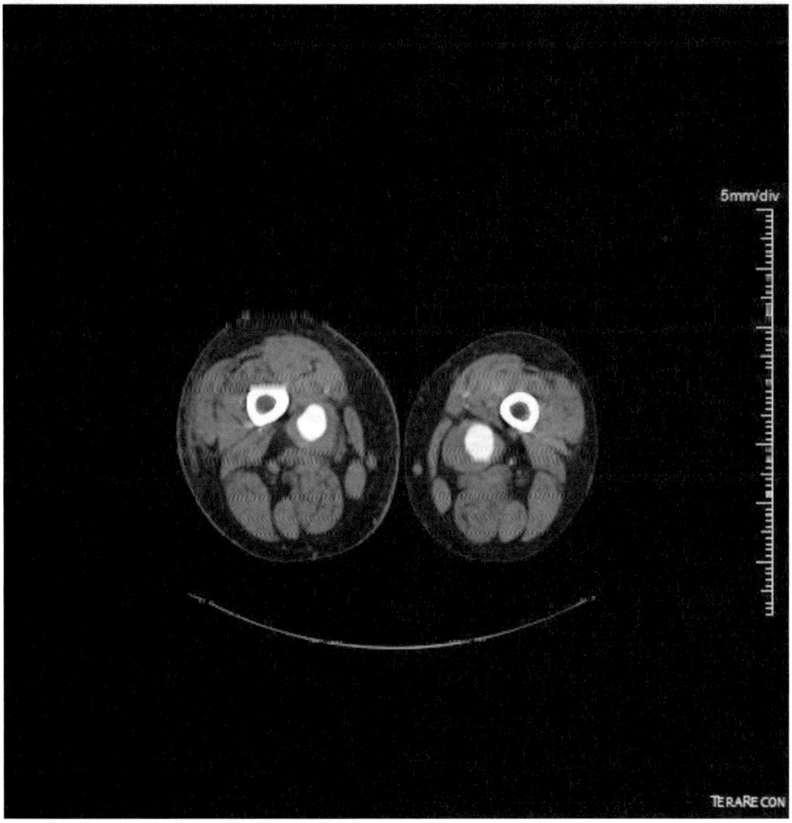

FIGURE 30-7 CTA of bilateral SFA aneurysm.

size is explained by the deeper anatomical location of the artery. The most common clinical presentation is a pulsatile thigh mass, although it was reported that SFAA is not palpable on physical exam in up to 69% of cases.[26] Contrary to other peripheral aneurysms complications, SFAA have a higher tendency to rupture than to embolize or thrombose.[25]

DUS is an accurate modality for both diagnosis and surveilling asymptomatic patients. No specific aneurysm diameter has been identified as an indication for repair, but several publications suggest a threshold of 2.5 cm similar to the indication for CFA aneurysm. SFAA are frequently amenable to both surgical and endovascular repair. CTA is used preprocedurally to evaluate inflow/outflow vessels or to identify a target landing zone if endovascular therapy is planned. Multiple surgical procedures could be performed, in order of preference:

1. Aneurysm resection and placement of interposition graft—The most common procedure performed, graft choice could be prosthetic or venous. Venous grafts are used for any reconstruction crossing the knee joint.
2. Aneurysm ligation and reconstruction with a femoropopliteal bypass—Used in cases of a diffuse aneurysm morphology.
3. Simple ligation—Described in high surgical risk patients who present in an emergency context (ruptured aneurysm). Viable limbs after the procedure have been reported due to the presence of collaterals more likely in patients who suffer from a chronic occlusive process.[27]

Endovascular repair is limited to a few case reports in the literature (Figure 30-8).[28–30] But we believe it is becoming a frequent approach to manage

A

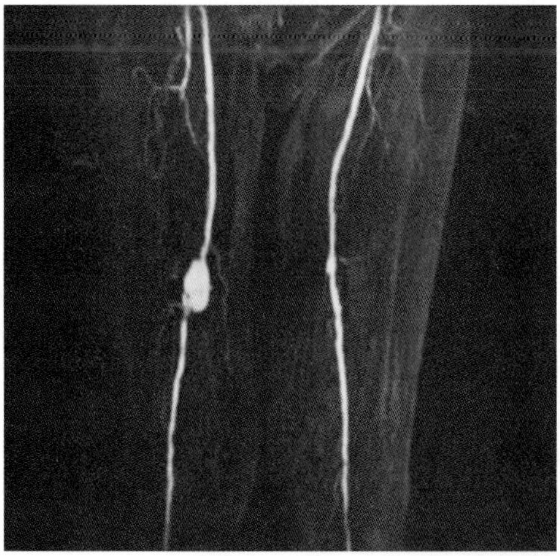

B

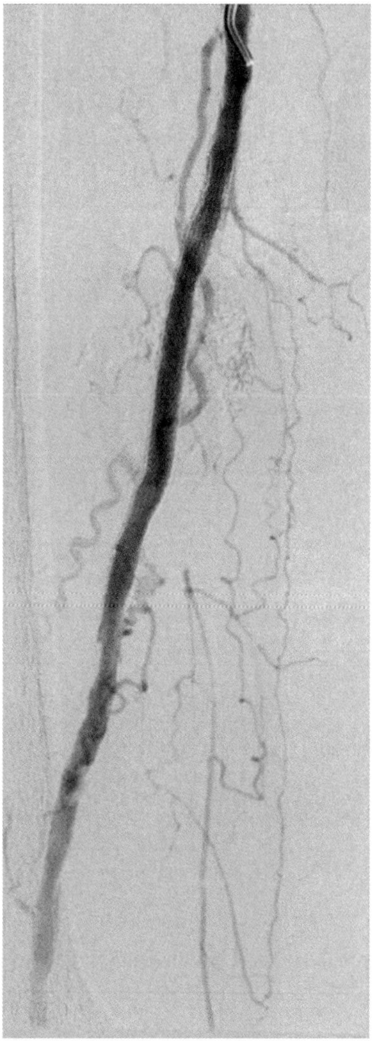

FIGURE 30-8 SFA aneurysm. (**A**) MRA demonstrating right SFAA. (**B**) Angiogram after endovascular repair. (Reproduced with permission from Mufty H, Daenens K, Houthoofd S, et al. Endovascular Treatment of Isolated Degenerative Superficial Femoral Artery Aneurysm. *Ann Vasc Surg*. 2018;49:311.e11-311.e14.)

the pathology, although long-term follow-up data are still lacking.

PROFUNDA FEMORAL ARTERY ANEURYSM

PFA aneurysms (PFAA) are rare, approximated to be 0.5% of all peripheral aneurysms.[31] Synchronous aneurysms are common and occur up to 73%, with popliteal aneurysms being the most common associated pathology.[32] The mean average size of the PFAA at presentation is 5.4 cm (range 2-18 cm).[33] Kibrik et al.[34] did a recent literature review in 2020, including data from 2002 till the publication date; they summarized the presentation of PFAA to be 30% asymptomatic, 38% presented as painful unruptured swelling, and 18% presented with rupture. They also reported a rise of CTA in diagnosing PFAA in the recent years compared to DUS, 71% versus 46%.[34] This observation does not imply the inferiority of DUS in detecting the pathology, but rather emphasizes the fact that PFAA are usually diagnosed incidentally during workup for another aneurysm (Figure 30-9).

Exclusion of PFAA may be achieved via surgical and endovascular procedures. In open surgery, two procedures are commonly performed. In order of preference:

1. *Aneurysm resection and placement of interposition graft*: Either saphenous vein or prosthetic graft should be used. Large branches of PFA should be preserved when constructing the interposition graft. Dissection is approached with care to prevent injury to crossing branches of the deep femoral vein and branches of the femoral nerve.
2. *Simple ligation*: Although the previously mentioned method is the preferred approach, simple ligation is justified in a ruptured aneurysm or if the aneurysm is confined to the distal branches of PFA. This approach may put the patient at a risk of future limb ischemia, thus clinicians should outlay the risks over the benefits when considering such an approach. If proximal ligation of a previously patent PFAA is emergently performed in an unstable patient, consideration should be given to stage revascularization to preserve this important structure.

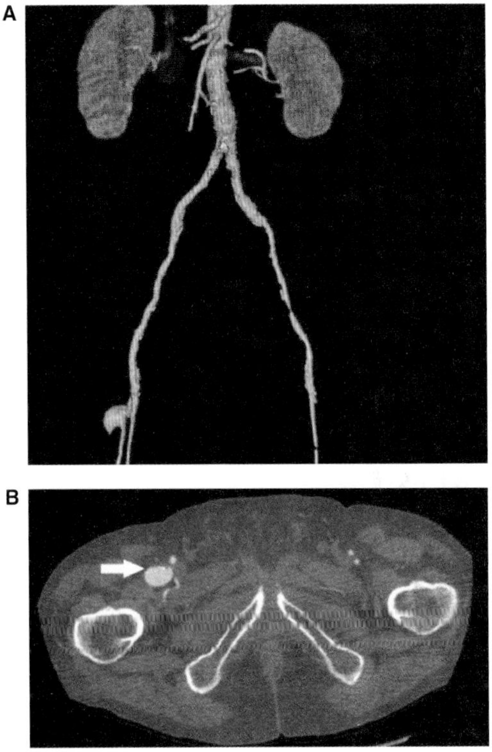

FIGURE 30-9 PFA aneurysm. (**A**) Three-dimensional reconstruction showing the aneurysm of the distal right profunda femoris artery PFA and aortoiliac calcification. (**B**) A contrast-enhanced computed tomography (CT) image showing a right profunda femoris artery aneurysm (white arrow). (Reproduced with permission from Parsa P, Cantu K, Eldt J, Gable D, Pearl G. Case report: a durable open repair of a rare profunda aneurysm. Ann Vasc Surg. 2017;44:424.e7-424.e10.)

Endovascular treatment of PFAA is limited to a few case reports. This may be due to the rarity of the disease making it difficult to assess the efficacy of such procedures in comparison to open surgery. Stent grafting and coil embolization have been presented as potential methods of successful endovascular treatment of PFAA.[35,36]

POPLITEAL ARTERY ANEURYSM

The popliteal artery (PA) is the continuation of the SFA as it exits the adductor canal; it extends to the origin of the anterior tibial artery. The normal diameter of PA ranges from 0.7 to 1.1 cm.[37] The diameter varies with gender, patient size, and portion of the vessel (proximal portion > distal portion).[37,38] This formerly led to controversy in diagnosing popliteal artery aneurysm (PAA), but the previously mentioned aneurysm definition of 1.5 times the adjacent segment of the artery is acceptably used here. PAA is mainly true aneurysms with false aneurysms of the popliteal artery a rarely encountered entity. The following excerpt will focus on the degenerative PAA, which is the most commonly observed etiology of the disease. Trauma and rare congenital disorder will not be discussed.

Epidemiology

Although PAAs are quite rare, they are the most common peripheral artery aneurysm, accounting for at least 70%.[39] It is predominantly found in men, with a study on hospitalized patients reporting the incidence of PAA and FAA to be 7.4 per 100,000 in males and 1.0 per 100,000 females.[39] Like other peripheral aneurysms PAA are usually synchronous, with about 50% of patients having bilateral PAAs while 37% may have an associated AAA (Figure 30-10).[40] On the contrary, only 14% of patients with AAA have coexisting PAA.[41] These data were obtained from a recent screening study, in which about 20,000 men older than 65 years were screened, the authors reported that the diameter of the popliteal artery did not correlate with the aortic diameter. Surprisingly, there was a positive correlation between the popliteal and common iliac artery diameter.[41] It must be noted that patients undergoing treatment for isolated PAA should be apprised of the need for lifelong surveillance of the aneurysmal disease development/progression in other vascular beds, as it is estimated that 50% of these patients will develop another aneurysm at a different site over a 10-year period.[42]

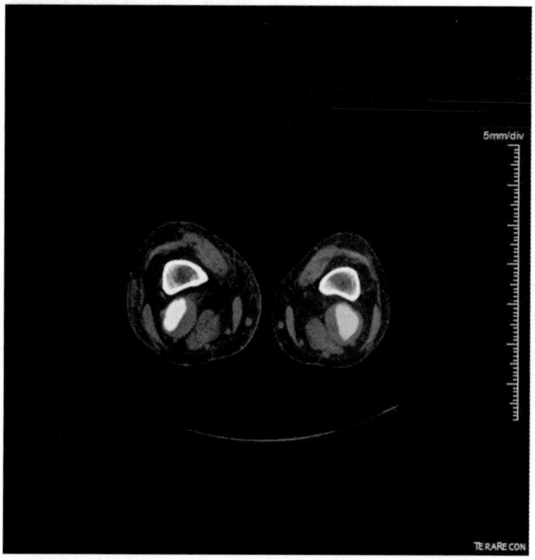

FIGURE 30-10 Popliteal artery aneurysm. CTA demonstrating bilateral popliteal aneurysm.

Pathogenesis and Clinical Presentation

The pathogenesis of PAA like other aneurysmal diseases is multifactorial, but certain differences exist. The etiology of PAAs is regarded as degenerative rather than atherosclerotic in origin. PAA formation occurs due to the loss of mechanical integrity of the vessel wall and altered balance between production and degradation of vessel wall constituents.[43] This process involves both inflammatory and immunological components. Another important pathogenesis difference between PAA and other aneurysmal disease is its anatomical location, and repeated flexion and extension of the knee have been regarded as an additional causative factor.[40] The growth rate of PAA is size-dependent. PAAs <20 mm grow by 1.5 mm/year, while of PAAs measuring 20 to 30 mm and >30-mm growth rate is 3 and 4 mm/year, respectively.[44]

Up to 40% of patients are asymptomatic at the time of diagnosis.[40,45] The most common symptomatic presentation is thromboembolism leading to ischemic symptoms (60%)[45]:

- *Claudication:* The most common symptom, presenting similarly to atherosclerotic disease.
- *Acute limb ischemia:* The most dramatic ischemic presentation, results from abrupt PA thrombosis
- *Digital thromboembolism:* The least common of the three may occur due to distal embolization

Less frequently patients present with mass effect, with the aneurysm compressing surrounding structures including the popliteal vein (swelling, phlebitis, and development of varicose veins) and surrounding nerves (motor and sensory deficiencies). Rupture is a rare, limb-threatening complication that occurs only in 2.5% of cases, but up to 9% will require amputation (Figure 30-5).[46]

Diagnosis

The diagnosis of PAA should be suspected in any patient with a prominent and widened popliteal artery pulse on physical examination. PAA can be incidentally seen on plain radiography as a calcified mass in the popliteal fossa. The diagnosis of PAA should be made before symptoms of limb ischemia develop, as surgical treatment outcomes are better in asymptomatic patients.[47] The main imaging modalities used for the diagnosis of PAA are DUS, CTA, and MRA. DUS, as mentioned before, is not only cheap and does not require contrast agent but also has the ability to detect thrombin burden in the pathology. CTA/MRA is useful in confirming the diagnoses, planning the treatment, and characterizing the inflow and outflow vessels. Digital subtraction angiography (DSA), previously the "gold standard" modality, has been slowly replaced by CTA and MRA. DSA is still beneficial in patients presenting with acute symptoms, as it provides an opportunity for thrombolytic therapy.

Treatment

Indications Repair of PAA could be achieved via an open, endovascular, or hybrid approach. Recommendations for the repair of PAA from the American College of Cardiology and American Heart Association practice guidelines include[48]:

- All symptomatic patients regardless of the aneurysm size should be treated.
- Patients with popliteal aneurysms 2.0 cm in diameter or larger should undergo repair to reduce the risk of thromboembolic complications and limb loss.

These recommendations are not without controversy. Some advocate that all popliteal aneurysms should be repaired, regardless of the size, because of the high ischemic complication rate.[49] Other authors have advocated for a more conservative approach, suggesting that asymptomatic patients with PAA less than 3 cm may be safely observed.[50] Another variable that the previously mentioned criteria do not consider is the volume and morphology of the intraluminal thrombus. Thrombus in PAA has been shown to augment the development of symptoms and cause aneurysm expansion.[51]

Accepting each of these valid factors, the decision to repair PAA should be individualized. The physician should tailor the approach based on the patient's operative risk, presence of symptoms, size of the aneurysm, presence of autologous conduit, and adequacy of run-off vessels. A special comment regarding the asymptomatic patient with a completely thrombosed PAA. Consideration should be given to managing these patients expectantly unless chronic limb-threatening ischemia or lifestyle-limiting claudication is present.

Open Treatment

Two approaches are the mainstay today for open surgery. The more common medial approach involves ligation of the inflow/outflow aneurysm and construction of an arterial bypass. While the posterior approach involves direct endoaneurysmorrhaphy repair with placement of an interposition graft.

Medial approach In this approach, the PAA is left in situ, ligated and bypassed using autologous vein (preferred) as a conduit. In cases where autologous vein is unavailable, externally supported polytetrafluoroethylene performs well since the arteries are generally larger in caliber for this patient population.

The procedure begins with exposing the ipsilateral saphenous vein. The conduit may be harvested and used as either reversed or nonreversed, while in situ bypass is possible for more distal targets (tibial and pedal vessels). The popliteal artery is ligated proximally and distally. Ligation should be done as close to the PAA as possible to promote thrombosis and prevent continued expansion from collateral geniculate vessels. The arterial bypass is performed in an end-to-side fashion to optimize hemodynamic

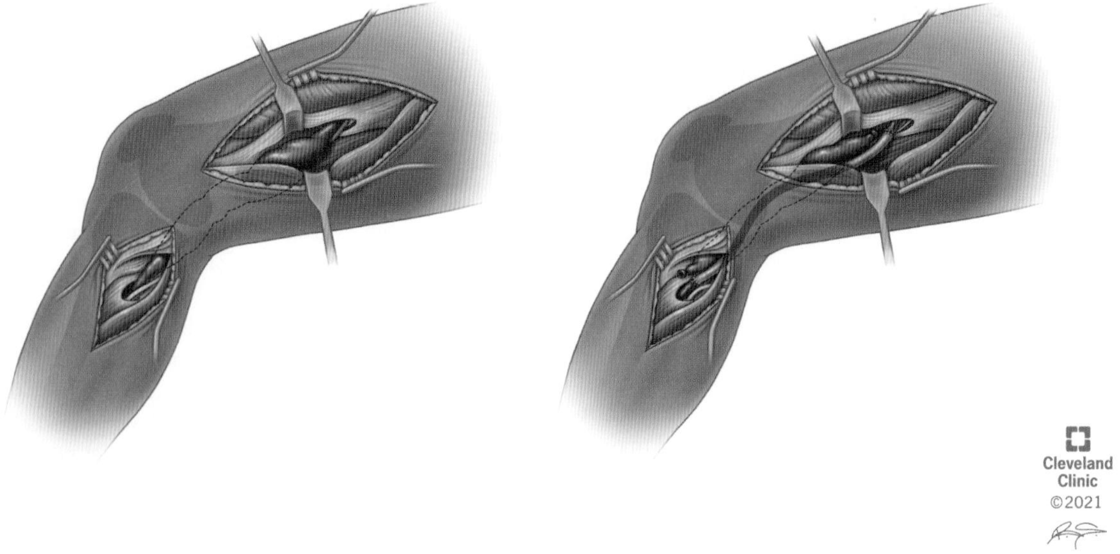

FIGURE 30-11 Medial approach for popliteal artery aneurysm. Exposure is performed via two incisions above and below the knee. Popliteal artery is ligated proximally and distally. Bypass is performed in end-to-side fashion. (Reprinted with permission, Cleveland Clinic Foundation ©2022. All Rights Reserved.)

flow. The size difference between the conduit and inflow femoral artery may be accommodated by spatulating the vein. The graft can be positioned adjacent to the popliteal artery (anatomically between the gastrocnemius heads) or tunneled subcutaneously through the medial aspect of the knee (Figure 30-11). Completion arteriography or DUS is performed. The medial approach is the preferred technique for PAA repair when fusiform morphology is present. The disadvantage of the approach is the inability to imbricate or decompress the aneurysm which may allow progressive aneurysm enlargement. This may occur in 10% to 15% of bypass PAA. Hence, surveillance of the reconstruction should include imaging of the dimensions of the residual aneurysm sac for residual flow and expansion.

Posterior approach In this approach, a vein or prosthetic graft is used to construct the popliteal artery. The procedure begins with the patient in a prone position. The popliteal fossa is exposed through an S-shaped incision, in an effort to minimize the postprocedural scar contracture. Proximal and distal control of PAA is obtained, and the aneurysm sac is opened. Thrombus is removed and collateral vessels are ligated in the opened sac. Continuity is restored through an interposition graft or a bypass. Because of the short length of bypass, vein grafts and PTFE grafts have been shown to have similar 1 year patency rates (85% and 81%, respectively).[52]

The posterior approach is preferred for saccular aneurysms confined to the popliteal fossa, especially if they are large and compressing surrounding structures. This approach is not possible for PAA extending proximally to the popliteal fossa. It also limits embolectomy of distal vessels in cases in which outflow is compromised (Figure 30-12).

Medial versus posterior outcome In a retrospective study analyzing the Swedish Vascular Registry containing 571 patients with 717 PAA, Ravn et al. reported the use of medial and posterior approaches in 87% and 8.4%, respectively.[52] With a mean follow-up of 7.2 years, postoperative aneurysm expansion was 33% when the medial approach was used compared to only 8.3% in the posterior approach. There was no difference in patency between vein and prosthetic graft in the posterior approach, but better patency with veins in the medial approach

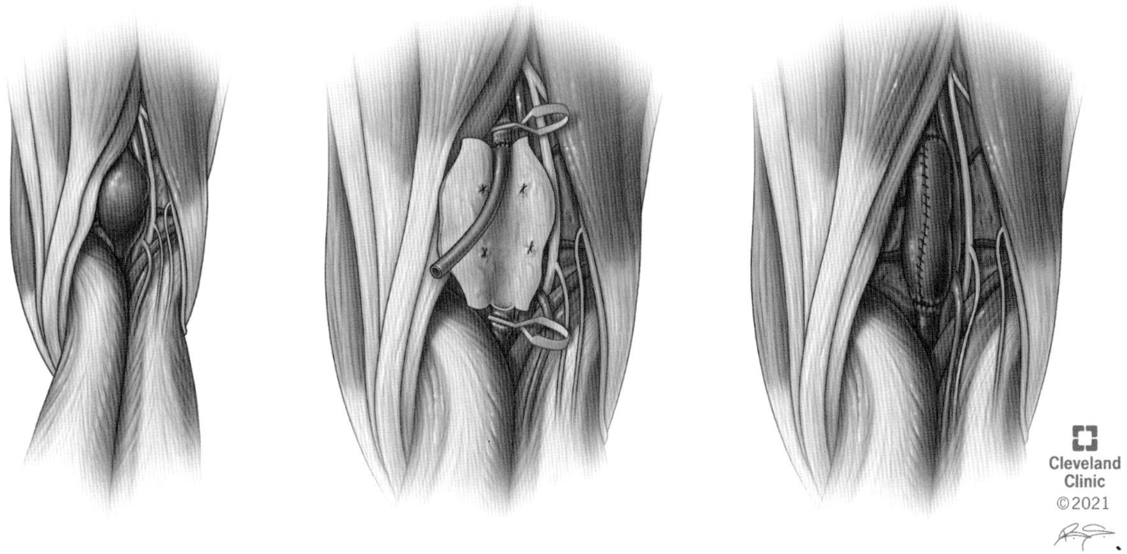

FIGURE 30-12 Posterior approach for popliteal artery aneurysm. Aneurysm is opened, thrombus removed and genicular vessels ligated. Interposition graft is then used for reconstruction, and finally, the aneurysm sac can be wrapped around the anastomosis. (Reprinted with permission, Cleveland Clinic Foundation ©2022. All Rights Reserved.)

(90% vs 72%).[52] In another meta-analysis, aimed to compare primary outcomes of both procedures, a total of 1427 patients were included. Seventy-six percent underwent the procedure via a medial approach, while 24% had a posterior approach. There was no difference in the two groups in terms of postoperative nerve damage (odds ratio [OR], 1.01; 95% confidence interval [CI], 0.24–4.2), and 30-day postoperative complications (OR, 0.87; 95% CI, 0.43–1.77). The 30-day primary patency was not statistically different between groups (RD, −0.01; 95% CI, −0.04 to 0.02), but the 30-day secondary patency suggested superiority of the posterior approach (RD, 0.05; 95% CI, 0.02–0.07). Long-term primary and secondary patency both favored the posterior approach (OR, 1.61 [95% CI, 1.06–2.43] and OR, 1.73 [95% CI, 0.91–3.30], respectively).[53]

These results favoring the posterior approach should not be taken out of context, as many patients are not amenable to the procedure in the first place. While no randomized clinical trials are available to compare both methods. Therefore, the procedure choice should depend on the pathology extent (size and location) and the surgeon's expertise.

Endovascular and Hybrid Treatment

The most suitable PAA characteristics for endovascular repair are summarized (Table 30-3). The procedure can be approached either percutaneously or via a small cut-down to expose either CFA or SFA.

TABLE 30-3 Anatomical and Patient Characteristics Suited for Endovascular Repair.

- Focal popliteal aneurysms that don't extend to into distal popliteal artery
- A safe landing zone of at least 2 cm both proximally and distally.
- Lack of extensive vessel tortuosity.
- Patient with two or three-vessel outflow.
- Patient is able to receive antiplatelet therapy.
- Patient does not frequently flex their knee to more than 90 degrees, such as gardeners and auto mechanics, due to the risk of stent deformation and stenosis

Data from Sidawy AN, Saltz LB. *Rutherford's Vascular Surgery and Endovascular Therapy*, 9th ed. Philadelphia PA: Elsevier; 2019.

SFA is preferred in the latter, as it avoids the extra step of directing the wire.

Before the procedure patients are prescribed clopidogrel. CTA imaging provides the necessary measurements for covered stent sizing. Femoral puncture with a delivery of an appropriately sized sheath can be obtained in a retrograde or antegrade fashion. Once access is obtained, an angiogram is performed to visualize landing zones and runoff vessels. The patient is subsequently heparinized to an activated clotting time (ACT) exceeding 250 seconds. Patients with an acute presentation from infrapopliteal vessel thrombosis may benefit from thrombolysis (discussed later) prior to definitive stent grafting of PAA pathology. The covered stent is delivered to the target vessel and deployed and molded with a balloon. A completion angiogram is then performed to evaluate for endoleaks, kinks, and runoff vessel patency. The angiogram should be done in both an extended and flexed knee, to identify potential areas of kinking. Following the procedure, the patients are prescribed clopidogrel indefinitely (Figure 30-13).

Open versus endovascular outcome Results of both open and endovascular repair of PAA have been shown to have worse outcomes in patients presenting with severe symptoms.[54,55] Hence, the strong advocates of early PAA repair before symptoms develop. Comparing open and endovascular treatment for PAA is difficult due to the rarity of the condition. Excluding hospital stay and length of operation, which endovascular surgery will be superior in, three major endpoints will be used to compare open and endovascular treatment outcomes.

1. *Primary patency* refers to the revascularized region that did not require re-intervention. In open repair, the observed 5-year patency ranges between 76% and 95%. Smaller series for endovascular primary patency exist with rates ranging 80% to 92% in 1 year.[56]
2. *Secondary patency* refers to a revascularized region that has occluded at some point but revascularization was restored with some form of re-intervention. Secondary patency rates range between 87% and 95% versus 75% and 88%, in open and endovascular, respectively.[56]
3. *Peri-operative limb loss following intervention.* In open repair, limb loss could reach up to 2% in elective procedures and 6.5% after emergent repair (until discharge/30 days).[57] While the limb loss following endovascular repair for the same period is reported to be around 1%.[57]

These data support the conclusion that endovascular therapy is a reasonable option for the medically compromised patient or for patients in whom autologous alternative conduit is absent.

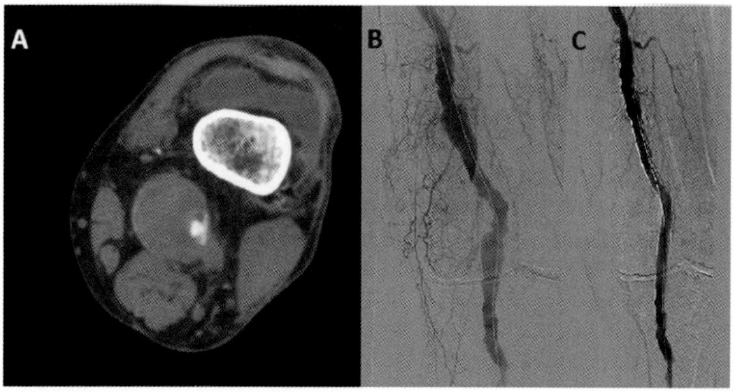

FIGURE 30-13 Endovascular repair of popliteal artery aneurysm. (**A**) CTA showing left popliteal aneurysm. (**B**) Preprocedural angiography. (**C**) Postprocedural angiography showing complete exclusion of the aneurysm. (Reproduced with permission from Guzzardi G, Natrella M, Del Sette B, et al. Endovascular repair of popliteal artery aneurysms: an Italian multicenter study. *Radiol Med.* 2019;124:79-85.)

Thrombolysis

Patients presenting with acute thromboembolic complications of the popliteal artery usually have poor outflow vessels. Thrombosis also involves microcirculation, leading to a high failure rate of treatment. In such patients, the use of prerepair thrombolysis can establish a patent outflow allowing successful open or endovascular repair. Studies have shown that following acute thrombosis of PAA, initial thrombolysis followed by repair is superior to operative intervention alone in graft patency and limb salvage rates.[45,58] It is important to realize that thrombolysis may delay surgery and for that reason should only be considered in patients without immediate threat to limb. In such cases, surgical embolectomy and thrombectomy provide a viable alternative to achieve outflow vessel patency.

INFRAPOPLITEAL ANEURYSM

Infrapopliteal aneurysms, including tibial, peroneal, and pedal arteries, are very rare. True aneurysms of infrapopliteal vessels are limited to a few case reports.[59,60] The majority of the aneurysms reported are due to trauma and iatrogenic injuries during peripheral interventions or orthopedic procedures.[61] Indication for repair is not defined but for symptomatic aneurysms or large aneurysms (two times the size of a normal adjacent artery) repair is preferred. If other tibial arteries are patent, ligation or coil embolization will suffice. In the absence of adequate collateral flow, repair with an autologous vein bypass graft is recommended.

UPPER EXTREMITY ANEURYSMS

AXILLARY ARTERY ANEURYSMS

The axillary artery begins at the outer border of the first rib as a continuation of the subclavian artery and ends at the lower border of teres major by becoming the brachial artery. Axillary artery aneurysms are rare. Both true and false aneurysms have been reported in the literature, but since both pathologies have similar etiology and management, they will be discussed together.

Etiology and Clinical Presentation

Axillary aneurysms are mainly caused by blunt and penetrating trauma. The typical patient would be a young male athlete involved in the sport that involves repetitive, forceful movement of the shoulder. Thoracic outlet compression of the artery leads to endothelial injury with subsequent degenerative aneurysmal changes. Case reports on baseball pitchers with axillary aneurysms have been published.[62,63]

Axillary aneurysms may be asymptomatic, present as a mass in the upper extremity or cause neurovascular complications. The axillary artery runs in the vascular sheath along with the cords of the brachial plexus, thus expansion could lead to neurological deficit.[64] The commonly associated complication is distal embolization leading to tissue ischemia and loss; rupture is infrequently encountered.[64]

Diagnosis and Treatment

Axillary artery aneurysm should be suspected in any patient presenting with an abnormal pulse examination and/or brachial nerve palsy after upper extremity trauma. DUS may allow accurate diagnosis. Angiography in form of CT, MR, or digital is all effective in detecting the pathology.

Management of nontraumatic axillary aneurysms, such as other aneurysms, could be achieved through open or endovascular techniques. Open surgery is still the preferred method of treatment today and has the additional benefit of permitting decompression of Thoracic Outlet compression at the time of aneurysm ligation and bypass. This is often accomplished by removal of any associated cervical rib or spinous process, first rib, and fibrous structures along with the anterior and medial scalene muscle. The patency of this short bypass performed with externally supported PTFE is greater than 90% at 5 years. When technically feasible, endovascular therapy is the method of choice for traumatic injury resulting in axillary artery aneurysms.

Open surgical treatment The main procedure performed is aneurysm resection with interposition reconstruction. Since the conduit often crosses the subscapular space with the risk of compression, externally supported PTFE is often used. For reconstructions lateral to the thoracic inlet, autologous conduit may be an option. Careful dissection should be performed during the surgery to prevent injury to the brachial plexus.

Endovascular treatment The procedure involves complete exclusion of the aneurysm cavity by a stent graft. DuBose et al.[65] conducted review of literature, describing endovascular treatment for 160 patients with axillo-subclavian injuries. Only 10 of the patients had the axillary injury, but they reported a technical success in 97% of all patients and 84% overall patency during follow-up period.[65]

BRACHIAL ARTERY ANEURYSM

Epidemiology and Etiology

True aneurysms of the brachial artery (BAA) are extremely rare. In a retrospective outlook of all the brachial artery procedures done at the Cleveland clinic between 1989 and 2000, only 1 out of 581 procedures (0.17%) was for a BAA repair.[66] Since the atherosclerotic disease is not commonly observed in the brachial artery, the etiology of BAA includes trauma, complication of ateriovenous access, and connective tissue abnormalities.[67,68] In many instances, no cause could be attributed rendering the pathology to be idiopathic in origin.[66]

Clinical Presentation and Diagnosis

Most patients present with symptoms of median nerve compression due to the proximity of both structures. Distal digital embolization has also been reported as a potential complication.[67] On physical examination, BAA presents as a pulsatile mass. But as in previously mentioned peripheral aneurysms, DUS and CTA are used to confirm diagnoses and plan treatment.

Treatment

Management of BAA is mainly through open surgical treatment. The brachial artery is easily accessible and the operation is associated with minimal morbidity. The procedure often involves resection with end-to-end anastomosis or the use of an interposition vein graft. Endovascular therapy has been mentioned in a few case reports.[69] But the main limitations to the endovascular approach include mismatch of the artery diameter between the proximal and distal end of the aneurysm and the possibility of stent fracture with flexion of the extremity.

Brachial Artery False Aneurysm

Brachial artery false aneurysms could be due to iatrogenic or traumatic injury to the vessel (Figure 30-14). Iatrogenically, the brachial artery could be injured during peripheral angiography, cardiac catheterization, and endovascular interventions. The brachial artery is the third preferred access site after femoral and radial arteries. In a recent study comparing the incidence of false aneurysms in femoral and brachial arteries postcardiac catheterization, Tamanha et al. reported that the incidence of false aneurysms was significantly higher in brachial access than in femoral access (odds ratio: 4.16, 95% confidence interval: 1.80–9.65; $P < 0.001$).[70] The authors followed this by emphasizing that the complication itself is quite rare in both procedures.[70] Traumatic causes of BAA include penetrating and blunt injuries, orthopedic fractures and intravenous drug abuse (a common cause of infected false aneurysm).

Symptomatic brachial artery false aneurysms should be surgically managed with open surgery with direct suture repair mostly preferred. Thrombin injection of the false aneurysm has been described, but limited as the false aneurysm's short neck is a potential source of complication.[71]

INFECTED PERIPHERAL ARTERIAL ANEURYSMS

Infected peripheral aneurysms are associated with different causes, require different management, and have worse outcomes than degenerative or traumatic peripheral aneurysms per se. The term "mycotic aneurysm" is a misnomer, used initially to describe aneurysms associated with bacterial endocarditis, while other clinicians used the term to specifically refer to aneurysms caused by fungi. Nevertheless, many clinicians today refer to any infected aneurysm regardless of its etiology as a "mycotic aneurysm".[72] To prevent confusion, we will use the term infected aneurysm.

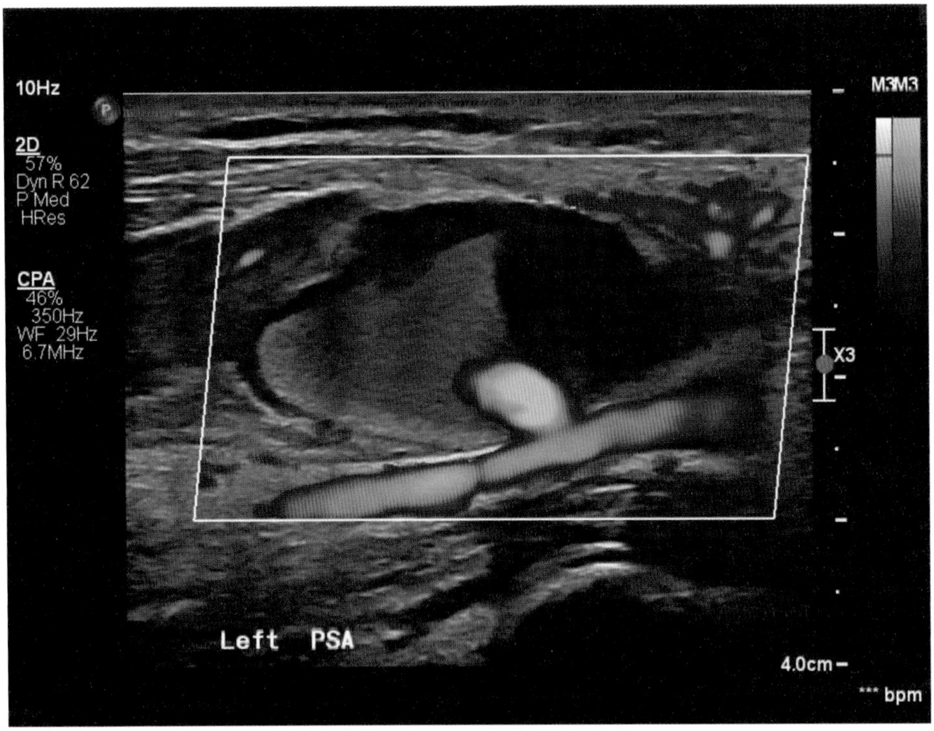

FIGURE 30-14 Duplex ultrasound of brachial false aneurysm. Color flow Doppler depicts blood entering the aneurysm sac.

Etiology and Risk Factors

Theoretically peripheral aneurysms provide a nidus for pathogens to seed and proliferate. Pathogens lodging into healthy peripheral vessels can result in an inflammatory response, transmural necrosis, and finally aneurysm formation. Conversely, a pre-existing aneurysm may be a host site for hematogenous wall seeding. Hence, peripheral aneurysms could be the cause or an effect of vessel infection. Infected peripheral aneurysms could be classified based on the source of infection and the pre-existing status of the artery.[73] The source of infection could be endogenous or exogenous in origin. While a normal vessel pre-existing condition is least likely to become primarily infected compared to atherosclerotic, aneurysmal degenerative, and prosthetic vessels. The microorganism depends on the infection source, vessel type, patient's immunity, and geographic location. Pathogens range from bacterial gram-positive and gram-negative infections to mycobacterium to fungi. Currently, the most common pathogen is *Staphylococcus aureus*, many of which are methicillin-resistant.[74]

Diagnosis and Treatment

Diagnosing infected peripheral aneurysm requires a combination of history, clinical findings, laboratory studies, and imaging. A history of trauma or recent infectious disease should raise suspicion. General symptoms can include malaise and fever. Locally, the aneurysm may have signs of overlying skin erythema, warmth, and pain. Leukocytosis, elevated sedimentation rate and positive blood cultures are usually present. Negative blood cultures are not sufficient to rule out infected peripheral aneurysm, as patients are reported to have sterile blood cultures in 18% to 50% of the cases.[74]

Ultrasonography, CTA, and MRA are all used to diagnose an infected peripheral aneurysm. Contrary to an infected aortic aneurysm, DUS is useful in diagnosing peripheral infected aneurysms. CTA has an advantage of being able to delineate surrounding inflammation, fluid, or air. Positron emission tomography (PET) offers an effective modality usually in combination with CT.[75]

Medical treatment alone with antibiotics rarely eradicates the infection. Surgical intervention is mandatory in nearly all cases. Surgery involves the removal of all infected tissue followed by preservation of continuity of circulation preferentially with either autologous vessels. When a primary autologous conduit is not available, the use of a femoral vein is appropriate.

Lower Extremity Infected Aneurysm

The most common location for lower extremity infected peripheral artery aneurysms is the femoral artery, while popliteal and infrapopliteal infected aneurysms are limited to a few case reports.[76,77] Infected femoral artery aneurysm is most commonly caused by endovascular access and drug abuse. The development of a femoral peripheral infected aneurysm in a setting of drug abuse has a high rate of limb loss, and definitive treatment should be addressed quickly.[78] Surgical revascularization options include ligation with the formation of an obturator bypass, interposition bypass, lateral femoral bypass, or extra anatomical axillary to the femoral artery or a lateral profunda arterial exposure. Treatment involves antibiotics for at least 6 weeks following surgical intervention.

Upper Extremity Infected Aneurysm

Upper extremity infected aneurysms are very rare. Endocarditis is the most commonly reported etiology in the literature.[79] Recently peripheral catheterization led to an increased incidence of radial and brachial peripheral aneurysms, while drug abuse remains an important etiology of infected brachial artery aneurysms.[79,80] Due to rich collateral in the forearm, infected aneurysms of radial and ulnar vessels are amenable to just ligation and debridement of infected tissue. The brachial artery usually requires a revascularization procedure, preferably with an autologous vein (preferred).

PERIPHERAL VENOUS ANEURYSM

A venous aneurysm (VA) is a localized area of venous dilatation that occurs in a nonvaricose vein that is not associated with a false aneurysm or arteriovenous communication. Peripheral venous aneurysms (PVAs) are rare, rendering their true incidence unknown.[81] VAs have been reported throughout the body including extremities, head and neck, and abdominal veins.[82] VA could be primary or secondary in origin. Primary VAs are seen in inherited conditions such as Klippel–Trénaunay syndrome and neurofirbomatosis type 1.[83,84] Secondary VA is encountered due to trauma, degenerative process, inflammation, and venous hypertension. PVA could occur in both superficial and deep venous systems of upper and lower extremity veins, but we will discuss only popliteal and jugular VAs.

POPLITEAL VENOUS ANEURYSM

Popliteal venous aneurysms are the most reported PVAs in literature. The importance of popliteal venous aneurysms lies in their high rate of thrombosis and risk of thromboembolic disease. Pulmonary embolism associated with popliteal venous aneurysm range from 40% to 70%.[85,86] Surgical reconstruction is the preferred treatment for the pathology. Tangential aneurysmectomy with lateral venorrhaphy is the preferred procedure.

Jugular Venous Aneurysm

Venous aneurysms of the jugular veins are usually asymptomatic and are not associated with thromboembolic disease. Intervention is usually performed due to cosmetic purposes (Figure 30-15).[82] Depending on the caliber of the vessel, both ligation and plication of jugular veins aneurysms have been described in case reports.[87]

REFERENCES

1. Hirsch AT, Haskal ZJ, Hertzer NR, et al. ACC/AHA guidelines for the management of patients with peripheral arterial disease (lower extremity, renal, mesenteric, and abdominal aortic). *J Vasc Interv Radiol*. 2006;17(9):1383-1398.

A

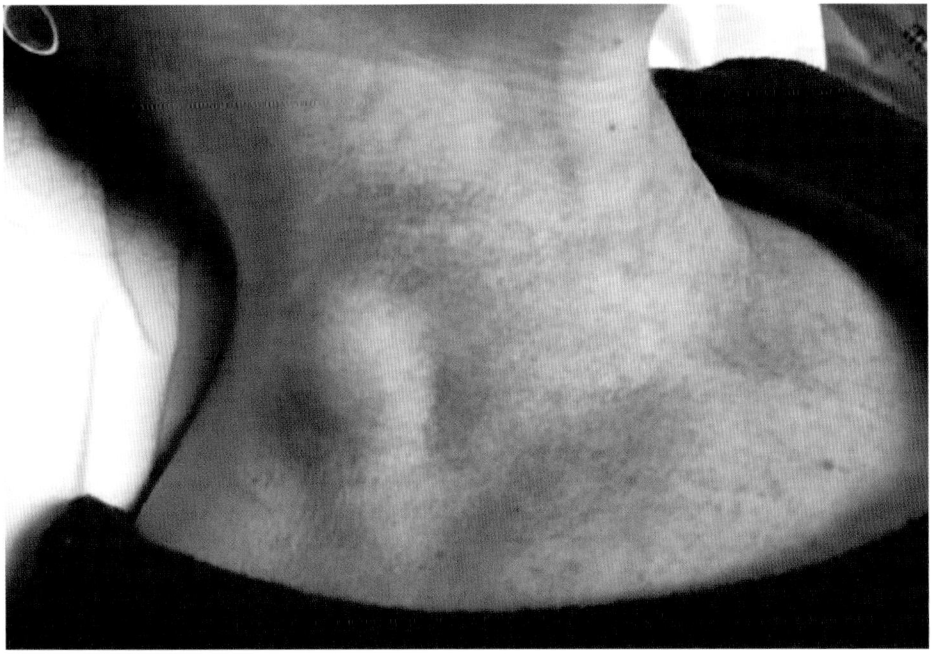

B

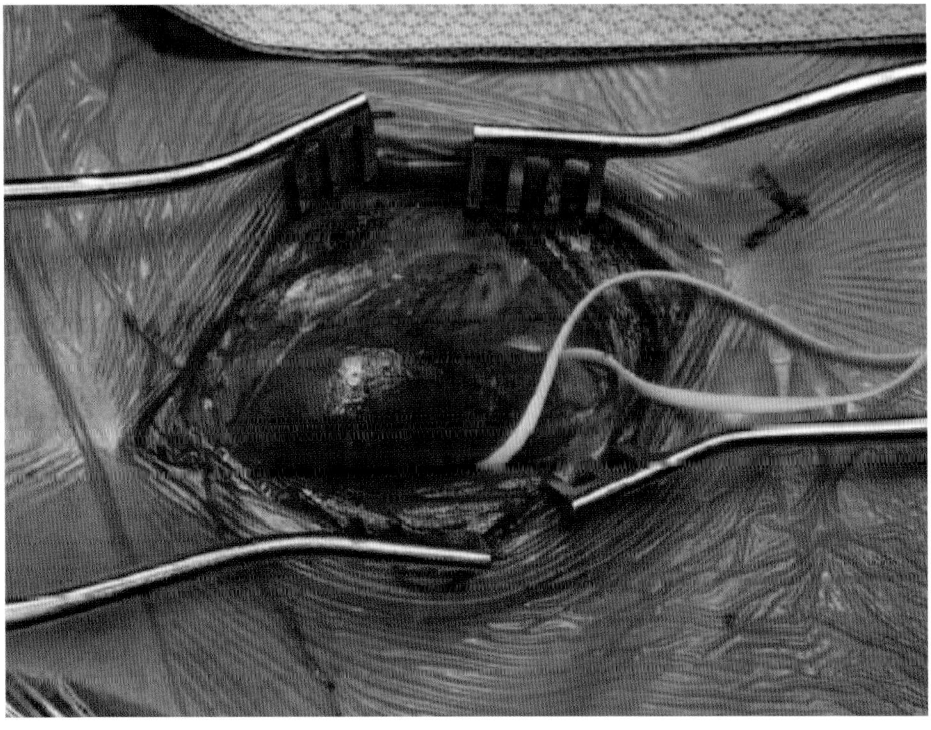

FIGURE 30-15 **Jugular venous aneurysm.** (**A**) Nonpulsatile mass on the right neck due to the jugular venous aneurysm. (**B**) Intraoperative depiction of the right jugular venous aneurysm. (Reproduced with permission from Bartholomew JR, et al. *Ann Vasc Surg*. 2020;68:567.e5-567.e9.)

2. Graham LM. Clinical significance of arteriosclerotic femoral artery aneurysms. *Arch Surg*. 1980;115(4):502.
3. Sandgren T, Sonesson B, Ryden-Ahlgren Å, Länne T. Arterial dimensions in the lower extremities of patients with abdominal aortic aneurysms—no indications of a generalized dilating diathesis. *J Vasc Surg*. 2001;34(6):1079-1084.
4. Piffaretti G, Mariscalco G, Tozzi M, Rivolta N, Annoni M, Castelli P. Twenty-year experience of femoral artery aneurysms. *J Vasc Surg*. 2011;53(5):1230-1236.
5. Cutler BS, Darling RC. Surgical management of arteriosclerotic femoral aneurysms. *Surgery*. 1973;74(5):764-773.
6. Sapienza P, Mingoli A, Feldhaus RJ, di Marzo L, Cavallari N, Cavallaro A. Femoral artery aneurysms: long-term follow-up and results of surgical treatment. *Cardiovasc Surg Lond Engl*. 1996;4(2):181-184.
7. Yamamoto T, Kurosaka M, Sugimoto T. A true aneurysm of the femoral artery in acromegaly. *Clin Imaging*. 2001;25(2):126-129.
8. D'Andrea V, Malinovsky L, Cavallotti C, et al. Angiomegaly. *J Cardiovasc Surg (Torino)*. 1997;38(5):447-455.
9. Chung SW, Bae M, Lee CW, et al. Surgical Experience of Behcet's Disease Involving the Peripheral Artery. *Ann Vasc Surg*. 2020;69:246-253.
10. Corriere MA, Guzman RJ. True and false aneurysms of the femoral artery. *Semin Vasc Surg*. 2005;18(4):216-223.
11. Lawrence PF, Harlander-Locke MP, Oderich GS, et al. The current management of isolated degenerative femoral artery aneurysms is too aggressive for their natural history. *J Vasc Surg*. 2014;59(2):343-349.
12. Jacobowitz G, Cayne NS. Lower extremity aneurysms. In: *Rutherford's Vascular Surgery and Endovascular Therapy*. 9th ed. Phaldelphia, PA: Elsevier; 2019:1078-1094.e3. Accessed October 26, 2020. https://www.clinicalkey.com/#!/content/book/3-s2.0-B9780323427913000839.
13. Bakoyiannis CN, Tsekouras NS, Economopoulos KP, Bastounis EA. A hybrid approach using a composite endovascular and open graft procedure for a symptomatic common femoral aneurysm extending well above the inguinal ligament. *J Vasc Surg*. 2008;48(2):461-464.
14. Kresowik TF, Khoury MD, Miller BV, et al. A prospective study of the incidence and natural history of femoral vascular complications after percutaneous transluminal coronary angioplasty. 1991;13(2):328-355.
15. Hessel SJ, Adams DF, Abrams HL. Complications of angiography. Accessed October 20, 2020. https://pubs.rsna.org/doi/pdf/10.1148/radiology.138.2.7455105
16. Madia C. Management trends for postcatheterization femoral artery pseudoaneurysms. *J Am Acad Physician Assist*. 2019;32(6):15-18.
17. McCann RL, Schwartz LB, Pieper KS. Vascular complications of cardiac catheterization. *J Vasc Surg*. 1991;14(3):375-381.
18. Coughlin BF, Paushter DM. Peripheral pseudoaneurysms: evaluation with duplex US. *Radiology*. 1988;168(2):339-342.
19. Stolt M, Braun-Dullaeus R, Herold J. Do not underestimate the femoral pseudoaneurysm. *Vasa*. 2018;47(3):177-186.
20. Toursarkissian B, Allen BT, Petrinec D, et al. Spontaneous closure of selected iatrogenic pseudoaneurysms and arteriovenous fistulae. *J Vasc Surg*. 1997;25(5):803-809.
21. Khoury M, Rebecca A, Greene K, et al. Duplex scanning–guided thrombin injection for the treatment of iatrogenic pseudoaneurysms. *J Vasc Surg*. 2002;35(3):517-521.
22. Gurel K, Gur S, Ozkan U, Tekbas G, Onder H, Oguzkurt L. Ultrasonography guided percutaneous thrombin injection of postcatheterization pseudoaneurysms. *Diagn Interv Radiol*. 2012;18(3):319-25.
23. Yang EY, Tabbara MM, Sanchez PG, et al. Comparison of ultrasound-guided thrombin injection of iatrogenic pseudoaneurysms based on neck dimension. *Ann Vasc Surg*. 2018;47:121-127.
24. Tisi PV, Callam MJ. Treatment for femoral pseudoaneurysms. *Cochrane Database Syst Rev*. 2013;(11):CD004981.
25. Leon LR, Taylor Z, Psalms SB, Mills JL. Degenerative aneurysms of the superficial femoral artery. *Eur J Vasc Endovasc Surg*. 2008;35(3):332-340.
26. Jarrett F, Makaroun MS, Rhee RY, Bertges DJ. Superficial femoral artery aneurysms: an unusual entity? *J Vasc Surg*. 2002;36(3):571-574.
27. Perini P, Jean-Baptiste E, Vezzosi M, et al. Surgical management of isolated superficial femoral artery degenerative aneurysms. *J Vasc Surg*. 2014;59(1):152-158.
28. Chung S, Jang J-Y, Kim D-K. Rare case of isolated true aneurysm in the superficial femoral artery treated with endovascular intervention: a case report. *Eur Heart J - Case Rep*. 2020;4(1):1-4.
29. Mufty H, Daenens K, Houthoofd S, Fourneau I. Endovascular treatment of isolated degenerative superficial femoral artery aneurysm. *Ann Vasc Surg*. 2018;49:311.e11-311.e14.
30. Lyazidi Y, Abissegue Y, Chtata H, Taberkant M. Endovascular treatment of 2 true degenerative aneurysms of superficial femoral arteries. *Ann Vasc Surg*. 2016;30:307.e1-307.e5.
31. Ruslan OM, Sundick S, Razayat C, Brener BJ, Raffetto JD. Rupture of a true profunda femoris artery aneurysm:

two case reports and review of the English language literature. *Ann Vasc Surg*. 2017;39:290.e1-290.e9.

32. Harbuzariu C, Duncan AA, Bower TC, Kalra M, Gloviczki P. Profunda femoris artery aneurysms: association with aneurysmal disease and limb ischemia. *J Vasc Surg*. 2008;47(1):31-35.
33. Tsilimparis N, Faber E, Zindler K, et al. Aneurysms of the deep femoral artery–a systematic review of literature. *Zentralblatt Chir - Z Allg Visz Gefasschirurgie*. 2012;137(5):430-435.
34. Kibrik P, Arustamyan M, Stern JR, Dua A. A systematic review of the diagnosis, management, and outcomes of true profunda femoris artery aneurysm. *J Vasc Surg*. 2020;71(6):2145-2151.
35. Lewszuk A, Madycki G. Endovascular management of a giant true aneurysm of the deep femoral artery in a patient with a history of internal diseases. *World J Surg Surgical Res*. 2019;2:1120
36. Keskin S, Koc O, Keskin Z, Erol S. Radiological findings and endovascular treatment in giant deep femoral artery aneurysms. *BMJ Case Rep*. 2014;2014:bcr2013201201.
37. Wolf YG, Kobzantsev Z, Zelmanovich L. Size of normal and aneurysmal popliteal arteries: a duplex ultrasound study. *J Vasc Surg*. 2006;43(3):488-492.
38. Johnston KW, Rutherford RB, Tilson MD, Shah DM, Hollier L, Stanley JC. Suggested standards for reporting on arterial aneurysms. Subcommittee on reporting standards for arterial aneurysms, Ad Hoc Committee on Reporting Standards, Society for vascular surgery and north american chapter, international society for cardiovascular surgery. *J Vasc Surg*. 1991;13(3):452-458.
39. Lawrence PF, Lorenzo-Rivero S, Lyon JL. The incidence of iliac, femoral, and popliteal artery aneurysms in hospitalized patients. *J Vasc Surg*. 1995;22(4):409-416.
40. Dawson I, Sie RB, van Bockel JH Atherosclerotic popliteal aneurysm. *BJS Br J Surg*. 1997;84(3):293-299.
41. Cervin A, Wanhainen A, Björck M. Popliteal aneurysms are common among men with screening detected abdominal aortic aneurysms, and prevalence correlates with the diameters of the common iliac arteries. *Eur J Vasc Endovasc Surg*. 2020;59(1):67-72.
42. Dawson I, van Bockel JH, Brand R, Terpstra JL. Popliteal artery aneurysms. Long-term follow-up of aneurysmal disease and results of surgical treatment. *J Vasc Surg*. 1991;13(3):398-407.
43. Jacob T, Hingorani A, Ascher E. Examination of the apoptotic pathway and proteolysis in the pathogenesis of popliteal artery aneurysms. *Eur J Vasc Endovasc Surg*. 2001;22(1):77-85.
44. Pittathankal AA, Dattani R, Magee TR, Galland RB. Expansion rates of asymptomatic popliteal artery aneurysms. *Eur J Vasc Endovasc Surg*. 2004;27(4):382-384.
45. Varga ZA, Locke-Edmunds JC, Baird RN, Joint Vascular Research Group. A multicenter study of popliteal aneurysms. *J Vasc Surg*. 1994;20(2):171-177.
46. Cervin A, Ravn H, Björck M. Ruptured popliteal artery aneurysm. *Br J Surg*. 2018;105(13):1753-1758.
47. Huang Y, Gloviczki P, Noel AA, et al. Early complications and long-term outcome after open surgical treatment of popliteal artery aneurysms: is exclusion with saphenous vein bypass still the gold standard? *J Vasc Surg*. 2007;45(4):706-715.e1.
48. Hirsch Alan T., Haskal Ziv J., Hertzer Norman R., et al. ACC/AHA 2005 Practice guidelines for the management of patients with peripheral arterial disease (lower extremity, renal, mesenteric, and abdominal aortic). *Circulation*. 2006;113(11):e463-e654.
49. Ascher E, Markevich N, Schutzer RW, Kallakuri S, Jacob T, Hingorani AP. Small popliteal artery aneurysms: are they clinically significant? *J Vasc Surg*. 2003;37(4):755-760.
50. Galland RB, Magee TR. Management of popliteal aneurysm. *Br J Surg*. 2002;89(11):1382-1385.
51. Lowell RC, Gloviczki P, Hallett JW, et al. Popliteal artery aneurysms: the risk of nonoperative management. *Ann Vasc Surg*. 1994;8(1):14-23.
52. Ravn H, Wanhainen A, Björck M. Surgical technique and long-term results after popliteal artery aneurysm repair: results from 717 legs. *J Vasc Surg*. 2007;46(2):236-243.
53. Phair A, Hajibandeh S, Hajibandeh S, Kelleher D, Ibrahim R, Antoniou GA. Meta-analysis of posterior versus medial approach for popliteal artery aneurysm repair. *J Vasc Surg*. 2016;64(4):1141-1150.e1.
54. Shortell CK, DeWeese JA, Ouriel K, Green RM. Popliteal artery aneurysms: a 25-year surgical experience. *J Vasc Surg*. 1991;14(6):771-779.
55. Garg K, Rockman CB, Kim BJ, et al. Outcome of endovascular repair of popliteal artery aneurysm using the Viabahn endoprosthesis. *J Vasc Surg*. 2012;55(6):1647-1653.
56. Moore RD, Hill AB. Open versus endovascular repair of popliteal artery aneurysms. *J Vasc Surg*. 2010;51(1):271-276.
57. Björck M, Beiles B, Menyhei G, et al. Editor's choice: contemporary treatment of popliteal artery aneurysm in eight countries: a report from the vascunet collaboration of registries. *Eur J Vasc Endovasc Surg*. 2014;47(2):164-171.
58. Ravn H, Björck M. Popliteal artery aneurysm with acute ischemia in 229 patients. outcome after

thrombolytic and surgical therapy. *Eur J Vasc Endovasc Surg*. 2007;33(6):690-695.
59. Murakami H, Izawa N, Miyahara S: A true aneurysm of posterior tibial artery. *Ann Vasc Surg*. 2011;25(7): 980.e1-2. doi: 10.1016/j.avsg./2011.02.038. Epub 21011, May 31.
60. Tshomba Y, Papa M, Marone EM, Kahlberg A, Rizzo N, Chiesa R. A true posterior tibial artery aneurysm: a case report. *Vasc Endovascular Surg*. 2006;40(3):243-249.
61. Sagar J, Button M. Posterior tibial artery aneurysm: a case report with review of literature. *BMC Surg*. 2014;14:37.
62. Schneider K, Kasparyan NG, Altchek DW, Fantini GA, Weiland AJ. An aneurysm involving the axillary artery and its branch vessels in a major league baseball pitcher. *Am J Sports Med*. 1999;27(3):370-375.
63. Baumgarten KM, Dines JS, Winchester PA, et al. Axillary artery aneurysm with distal embolization in a major league baseball pitcher. *Am J Sports Med*. 2007;35(4):650-653.
64. Tham S, Guo Y, Pang MC-Y, Chng JK. Surgical management of axillary artery aneurysms with endovascular stenting versus open repair: a report of two cases and literature review. *Ann Vasc Surg*. 2019;58:385.e11-385.e16.
65. DuBose JJ, Rajani R, Gilani R, et al. Endovascular management of axillo-subclavian arterial injury: a review of published experience. *Injury*. 2012;43(11):1785-1792.
66. Schunn CD, Sullivan TM. Brachial arteriomegaly and true aneurysmal degeneration: case report and literature review. *Vasc Med*. 2002;7(1):25-27.
67. Senarslan DA, Yildirim F, Tetik O. Three cases of large-diameter true brachial and axillary artery aneurysm and a review of the literature. *Ann Vasc Surg*. 2019;57:273.e11 273.e15.
68. Fendri J, Palcau L, Cameliere L, et al. True brachial artery aneurysm after arteriovenous fistula for hemodialysis: five cases and literature review. *Ann Vasc Surg*. 2017;39:228-235.
69. Buda SJ, Johanning JM. Brachial, radial, and ulnar arteries in the endovascular era: choice of intervention. *Semin Vasc Surg*. 2005;18(4):191-195.
70. Tamanaha Y, Sakakura K, Taniguchi Y, et al. Comparison of postcatheterization pseudoaneurysm between brachial access and femoral access. *Int Heart J*. 2019;60(5):1030-1036.
71. Sheiman RG, Brophy DP, Perry LJ, Akbari C. Thrombin injection for the repair of brachial artery pseudoaneurysms. *Am J Roentgenol*. 1999;173(4):1029-1030.
72. Bisdas T, Teebken OE. Mycotic or infected aneurysm? Time to change the term. *Eur J Vasc Endovasc Surg*. 2011;41(4):570.
73. Patel S, Johnston KW. Classification and management of mycotic aneurysms. *Surg Gynecol Obstet*. 1977; 144(5):691-694.
74. Lee W-K, Mossop PJ, Little AF, et al. Infected (Mycotic) aneurysms: spectrum of imaging appearances and management. *RadioGraphics*. 2008;28(7):1853-1868.
75. Mikail N, Benali K, Mahida B, et al. 18F-FDG-PET/CT imaging to diagnose septic emboli and mycotic aneurysms in patients with endocarditis and cardiac device infections. *Curr Cardiol Rep*. 2018;20(3):14.
76. Silver J, Ferranti K, Radtka J. Open surgical ligation of a symptomatic mycotic aneurysm of the peroneal artery. *J Vasc Surg Cases Innov Tech*. 2019;5(1):68-70.
77. Killeen SD, O'Brien N, O'Sullivan MJ, Karr G, Redmond HP, Fulton GJ. Mycotic aneurysm of the popliteal artery secondary to Streptococus pneumoniae: a case report and review of the literature. *J Med Case Reports*. 2009;3:117.
78. Reddy DJ, Smith RF, Elliott JP, Haddad GK, Wanek EA. Infected femoral artery false aneurysms in drug addicts: Evolution of selective vascular reconstruction. *J Vasc Surg*. 1986;3(5):718-724.
79. Leon LR, Psalms SB, Labropoulos N, Mills JL. Infected upper extremity aneurysms: a review. *Eur J Vasc Endovasc Surg*. 2008;35(3):320-331.
80. Garg K, Howell BW, Saltzberg SS, et al. Open surgical management of complications from indwelling radial artery catheters. *J Vasc Surg*. 2013;58(5):1325-1330.
81. Gillespie DL, Villavicencio JL, Gallagher C, et al. Presentation and management of venous aneurysms. *J Vasc Surg*. 1997;26(5):845-852.
82. Teter KA, Maldonado TM, Adelman MA. A systematic review of venous aneurysms by anatomic location. *J Vasc Surg Venous Lymphat Disord*. 2018;6(3):408-413.
83. Beaulieu RJ, Boniakowski AM, Coleman DM, Vemuri C, Obi AT, Wakefield TW. Closed plication is a safe and effective method for treating popliteal vein aneurysm. *J Vasc Surg Venous Lymphat Disord*. 2021;9(1):187-192.
84. Delvecchio K, Moghul F, Patel B, Seman S. Surgical resection of rare internal jugular vein aneurysm in neurofibromatosis type 1. *World J Clin Cases*. 2017;5(12): 419-422.
85. Aldridge SC, Comerota AJ, Katz ML, Wolk JH, Goldman BI, White JV. Popliteal venous aneurysm: report of two cases and review of the world literature. *J Vasc Surg*. 1993;18(4):708-715.
86. Johnstone JK, Fleming MD, Gloviczki P, et al. Surgical treatment of popliteal venous aneurysms. *Ann Vasc Surg*. 2015;29(6):1084-1089.
87. Bartholomew JR, Smolock CJ, Kirksey L, et al. Jugular venous aneurysm. *Ann Vasc Surg*. 2020;68:567.e5-567.e9.

SELF-ASSESSMENT STUDY QUESTIONS AND ANSWERS

Questions

1. The most common presenting complication related to peripheral arterial aneurysm include:
   A. Rupture
   B. Bleeding
   C. Thromboembolic event
   D. Dissection

2. The second most common true peripheral arterial aneurysm encountered after popliteal aneurysm is:
   A. Axillary artery aneurysm
   B. Common femoral artery aneurysm
   C. Superficial femoral artery aneurysm
   D. Deep femoral artery aneurysm

3. What percentage of patients who have popliteal artery aneurysm will have abdominal artery aneurysm?
   A. 15%
   B. 35%
   C. 55%
   D. 75%

4. What percentage of patients with abdominal artery aneurysm will have popliteal artery aneurysm?
   A. 15%
   B. 35%
   C. 55%
   D. 75%

5. The most common organism associated with infected peripheral artery aneurysm include:
   A. *Escherichia coli*
   B. *Candida albicans*
   C. *Streptococcus pyogenes*
   D. *Staphylococcus aureus*

SELF-ASSESSMENT STUDY QUESTIONS AND ANSWERS

Answers

1. C.
2. B.
3. B.
4. A.
5. D.

CHAPTER

31 Acute Limb Ischemia

Nicolas J. Mouawad and Abdullah Nasif

OUTLINE

ETIOLOGY
- Embolism
- Thrombosis

CLINICAL PRESENTATION
- Medical History
- Physical Examination

CLASSIFICATION OF ACUTE LIMB ISCHEMIA

DIAGNOSIS AND DIFFERENTIALS
- Aortic Occlusion
- Iliac Occlusion
- Femoropopliteal Occlusion
- Infragenicular Occlusion

EVALUATION & INVESTIGATION
- Noninvasive Physiologic Tests
- Ultrasound
- Computed Tomography Angiography
- Catheter-Based Angiography

INITIAL MANAGEMENT AND TREATMENT
- Anticoagulation
- Treatment Selection

MANAGEMENT OPTIONS
- Open Revascularization
- Endovascular Approaches
- Comparing Open Versus Endovascular Options
- Fasciotomy

CONCLUSIONS

The history of the recognition and surgical treatment of lower limb ischemia dates back to the Middle Ages. The twin Saints Comas and Damian were ascribed to have saved a gangrenous limb in the thirteenth century and became patrons of future surgeons. The physicians who followed developed the theories of blood flow, anatomy of the arterial circulation, and recognition that occlusive disease was the cause of limb ischemia and gangrene. Innovative physicians developed the techniques of arterial surgery and bypass grafting to restore limb blood flow and allow the healing of lesions. In the 1960s, the era of endovascular intervention began through the pioneering work of Charles Dotter who developed techniques to image diseased arteries during a recanalization procedure. The development of guide wires, angioplasty balloons, and stents quickly followed. Management of lower limb ischemia and the diabetic foot will continue to evolve, building on the history and passion of proceeding physicians and surgeons.[1]

Acute limb ischemia (ALI) is defined as a sudden decrease in limb perfusion that threatens the viability of the limb. Diagnosis of acute ischemia of a limb can be a challenging clinical concern for vascular surgeons and interventionalists. Compounded with the degree of potential ischemia is the need for a timely and accurate diagnosis to best determine the urgent course of revascularization as significant delays risk limb loss resulting in amputation or even death, with historic rates ranging from 10% to 25%.[2]

This chapter will discuss basic etiology, clinical presentation, differential diagnosis, evaluation, and treatment options. With the continued advancement of endovascular techniques, multiple interventional modalities are available but as with other vascular conditions, they are predicated on appropriate and accurate initial diagnosis.

ETIOLOGY

Complete or major partial occlusion of the arterial supply to a limb can lead to rapid ischemia and poor functional outcomes within hours. ALI has an incidence of about 1.5 per 10,000 years.[3] The two main causes of ALI are arterial embolism and thrombosis. Other nonvascular causes include trauma and iatrogenic injury. Other than understanding the precipitating cause for ALI in an effort to reduce or eliminate it from recurring, the acute management of limb occlusion is essentially independent of its cause—restoring perfusion to the limb urgently is crucial.

EMBOLISM

Embolism is whereby a thrombus from a more proximal source travels to a distal segment and obstructs a peripheral vessel. The usual source is the heart or thoracic aorta where embolization can affect any segment of the arterial tree. These emboli generally lodge at bifurcations as the vessels naturally narrow. In the upper extremity, this includes the brachial bifurcation. In the lower extremity, it is generally at the common femoral artery or popliteal trifurcation.

Arterial embolic ischemia generally has a dramatic presentation due to an acute occlusion of otherwise normal vessels, where the body has not had an opportunity to develop a satisfactory collateral network to maintain perfusion. Patients present with an acute white limb with significant pain including profound sensorimotor deficits.

Emboli can be divided into cardiac and noncardiac sources and are listed in Table 31-1.

TABLE 31-1 Sources of Emboli

Cardiac Emboli	Noncardiac Emboli
Atrial	Aortic Mural thrombus
Ventricular	
Endocarditis and valve-related	Atheroembolism
Cardiac tumor (atrial myxoma)	

THROMBOSIS

Thrombosis results from blood clotting within an artery and is usually secondary to progressive atherosclerotic narrowing and subsequent occlusion of already severely diseased vessels, notably in the lower extremity. Once the stenosis becomes critical, a platelet thrombus forms ultimately leading to vessel obstruction and limb ischemia. Other causes of thrombosis include a hypercoagulable state, vessel dissection, vasospasm, and poor cardiac output resulting in a global reduction in limb perfusion.

Acute limb ischemia secondary to in situ thrombosis is rarely as profound as embolic ischemia because the gradual process of atherosclerotic narrowing has already stimulated the formation of a robust collateral arterial network. The presence of these rich collaterals lessens the severity and rapidity of the ischemic symptoms.

Due to advances in cardiac surgery, the use of anticoagulation, and the reduction of rheumatic heart disease, progressive atherosclerosis with an incident in situ thrombosis is the most common cause of the acute limb ischemia as compared to historically where cardiac embolic sources were the most common.

CLINICAL PRESENTATION

The symptoms and clinical presentation of acute limb ischemia (Figure 31-1) are dependent on the vascular territory, the size of the vessel occluded, and whether or not a collateral network of perfusion is present. Therefore, in patients with acute embolic ischemia, the limb may be painful and white whereas patients presenting with in situ thrombosis of their entire superficial femoral artery with robust collaterals may be completely asymptomatic. Importantly, ischemia affects sensory nerves first and as such, numbness and tingling are the earliest signs of arterial ischemia.

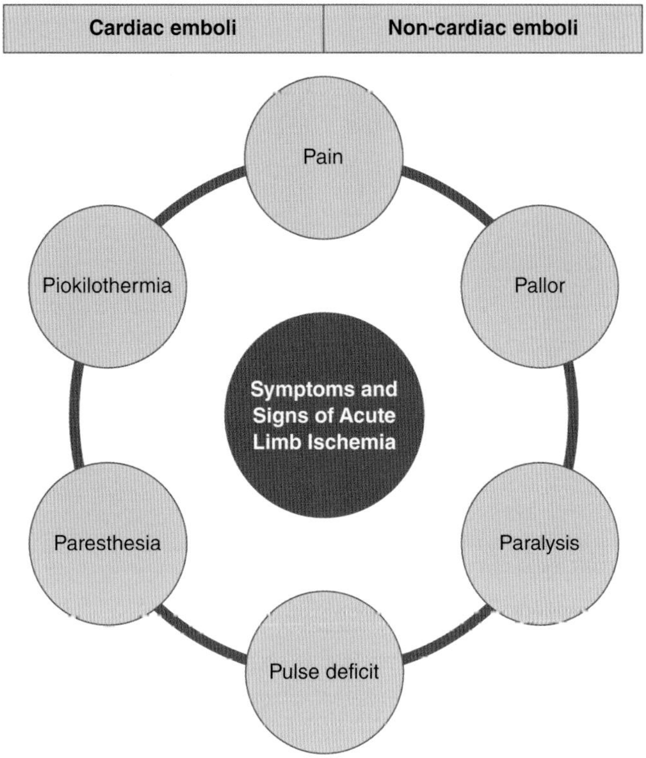

FIGURE 31-1 **Classic clinical signs of acute limb ischemia.**

As this becomes more progressive, motor fibers are affected presenting with muscle weakness.

MEDICAL HISTORY

As with any medical evaluation, a full detailed assessment is mandatory. The more severe the symptoms, the faster the patient will seek medical attention. The duration of symptoms is the most important aspect of the history as it helps determine options for therapy and the urgency of intervention. A previous history of peripheral arterial disease and intermittent claudication may point to a more longstanding vascular disease with developed collaterals as opposed to an acute arterial occlusion from a cardioembolic source. In fact, patients presenting with acute emboli remember almost exactly when the pain started and what they were doing and present for evaluation emergently. History should include the location, intensity, duration, and character of pain as well as any changes over time.

An investigation into risk factors should also be sought, including hypertension, hyperlipidemia, diabetes mellitus, tobacco use, coronary artery disease, arrhythmias, and use of anticoagulation. Medicine compliance is important as many times patients with atrial fibrillation hold their medications for procedures such as cataract surgery or colonoscopies at which point they are at risk for an arterial embolus and present with acute limb ischemia. Furthermore, documentation of a history of vascular interventions and procedures, such as previous lower extremity bypass, is essential.

PHYSICAL EXAMINATION

Examination of both extremities is mandatory and fundamental to define the severity of ischemia and assist in understanding the etiology. The color of the skin will depict its vascular supply and specific focus should be spent on it. Once ischemia is established, the skin may initially be white with pallor

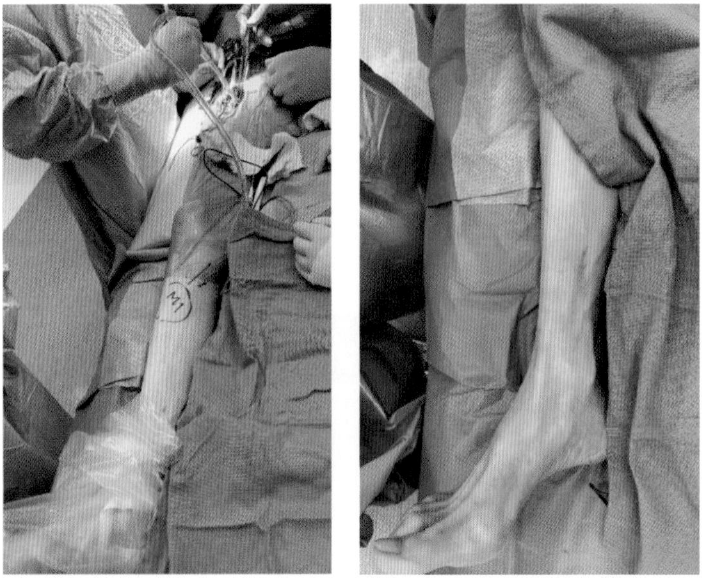

FIGURE 31-2 **Cold white ischemic foot.**

(Figure 31-2) but then becomes dusky blue as capillary venodilation occurs. Manual pressure over the skin at this point leaves the skin white because no new blood fills the vessel. Late stages of skin ischemia note capillary disruption with extravasation of blood making it blotchy.

Paresthesia and sensory changes are common early signs. The dorsal columns are affected first specifically with changes in fine touch and proprioception. Muscle weakness ensues and muscle pain is an advanced finding in acute limb ischemia due to the reduction in muscle perfusion. A detailed vascular pulse examination will help identify the level of occlusion. Normal pulses on the contralateral side suggest an embolic cause for occlusion. Handheld Doppler evaluation (Figure 31-3) is very helpful and easy to perform at the bedside. The presence of multiphasic arterial Doppler signals excludes the diagnosis. Monophasic signals are indicative of continuous flow with proximal obstruction. Absent Doppler signals note complete occlusion with no distal perfusion and are a poor prognostic sign. The Doppler probe may also be used to evaluate venous flow where lack of a venous signal as well in a patient with acute limb ischemia usually points to irreversible and end-stage presentation.

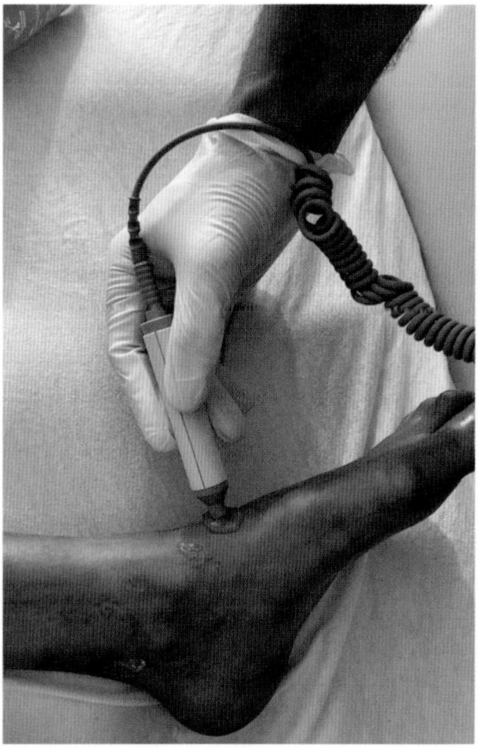

FIGURE 31-3 **Use of bedside handheld Doppler interrogation.**

CLASSIFICATION OF ACUTE LIMB ISCHEMIA

The classification of acute limb ischemia (Table 31-2) is based on the severity of arterial ischemia as this is helpful in determining the urgency of intervention and can prognosticate outcomes.[5,6] The Society for Vascular Surgery and the International Society for Cardiovascular Surgery have published definitions of acute limb ischemia that have withstood the test of time thus far and have been a valuable guide to direct treatment.[4,6]

Class I ischemia refers to patients with acute onset claudication. The limb is viable, and both arterial and venous Doppler signals are present although reproducible discomfort with activity is present and is relieved at rest. On the other hand, Class III ischemia refers to irreversibly and permanently damaged limbs, usually presenting after multiple hours of ischemia where profound sensory and motor loss is noted with Doppler signals; in this situation, there is no indication for revascularization.

Most patients present with Class II ischemia, where the limb is threatened. In Class IIA, the limb is marginally threatened and as such, there is an opportunity for further investigations and imaging after anticoagulation. The patient will have some mild sensory abnormality but will maintain the motor function of the limb despite so appreciable arterial Doppler signals. When the motor function is affected, this is a later sign of arterial ischemia and denotes Class IIB ischemia where the limb is immediately threatened and prompt intervention and revascularization are necessary in order to avoid permanent damage and potential limb loss.

DIAGNOSIS AND DIFFERENTIALS

The differential diagnosis for acute limb ischemia includes critical chronic limb-threatening ischemia, acute extensive deep vein thrombosis with phlegmasia, or spinal cord or peripheral nerve compression and neurologic syndromes. The pulse examination, however, will be key and will assist in determining the level of occlusion.

AORTIC OCCLUSION

Occlusion of the aorta is rather obvious with profound lower extremity symptoms including a lack of femoral and infrainguinal pulses. There is usually associated with significant paresthesia if not lower extremity paralysis. Mottling of the skin usually occurs above the inguinal ligament on the inferior abdomen and extends distally. The emergent treatment is indicated but importantly, postoperative critical care management is essential as restoration of flow to such a large muscle mass following limb hypoperfusion results in electrolyte abnormalities and systemic acid-base changes that affect the heart and renal function.

TABLE 31-2 Rutherford Classification of Acute Limb Ischemia

Category	Description	Sensory Loss	Muscle Weakness	Arterial Signal	Venous Signal
I Viable	No immediate threat	None	None	Audible	Audible
II Threatened					
II A Marginally Threatened	Salvageable if promptly treated	Minimal	None	Inaudible	Audible
II B Immediately Threatened	Salvageable if immediately revascularized	Rest pain	Mild, moderate	Inaudible	Audible
III Irreversible	Major tissue loss, permanent nerve damage	Significant	Profound, paralysis	Inaudible	Inaudible

Reproduced with permission from Rutherford RB, Baker JD, Ernst C, et al. Recommended standards for reports dealing with lower extremity ischemia: revised version. *J Vasc Surg*. 1997;26(3):517-538.

ILIAC OCCLUSION

This presentation is similar to that of an aortic occlusion except that it is unilateral. Emergent revascularization is imperative. The femoral and distal pulses are absent on the affected side. If normal pulses are present on the contralateral side, embolism is the cause.

FEMOROPOPLITEAL OCCLUSION

This is the most common type of presentation as most patients tend to already have peripheral arterial disease with established atherosclerosis. The femoral pulse may be present; however, they will complain of pain primarily in the calf. The severity of ischemia will depend primarily on whether the profunda femoris is involved; it is more profound if the profunda is occluded.

INFRAGENICULAR OCCLUSION

These patients present with a palpable femoral pulse but complain of pain in the calf. Tibial occlusions tend to not be very symptomatic unless the distal popliteal artery is occluded at the level of the trifurcation. With three tibial vessels present, occlusion of one vessel is rarely a cause of patient presentation. Tibial emboli are infrequent as most emboli lodge in larger vessels and generally do not reach the small caliber tibial vessels although chronic tibial occlusions from popliteal entrapment, adventitial cystic disease, or popliteal aneurysms do pose a poorer prognosis.

EVALUATION & INVESTIGATION

There are multiple modalities available for the evaluation of the acutely ischemic limb. Importantly, intervention should not be delayed for further imaging if the limb is immediately threatened. Intraoperative imaging may be employed in such cases to allow the best possibility for limb salvage.

NONINVASIVE PHYSIOLOGIC TESTS

Noninvasive imaging with segmental pressure evaluation and pulse volume recording waveform analysis may be helpful in confirming the lack of distal flow as well as the level of occlusion. These can be performed relatively quickly and will supplement the clinical evaluation although sometimes patients may not tolerate the cuffs due to muscle tenderness from the ischemia.

ULTRASOUND

Duplex ultrasonography is the mainstay of treatment for the evaluation of patients with peripheral arterial disease and chronic limb-threatening ischemia. It is operator dependent and not always available after hours. It does not use ionizing radiation which is protective for patients who may have significant ischemia and concerns for nephrotoxicity with revascularization. It can be performed quickly at the bedside to identify the segment or level of occlusion.

COMPUTED TOMOGRAPHY ANGIOGRAPHY

The use of computed tomography angiography (CTA) has essentially become the imaging modality of choice for the arterial vasculature. It can be acquired very rapidly, is available in all emergency departments, and is noninvasive avoiding the inherent risks of catheter-based angiography. The images can be rendered three-dimensionally and reconstructed with available software. Disadvantages include the use of ionizing radiation that is nephrotoxic as well as the inability to intervene as it is diagnostic.

CATHETER-BASED ANGIOGRAPHY

The catheter-based angiogram is the gold standard evaluation of the arterial vasculature. It may not be as readily available as a CTA as an operating suite or catheterization laboratory is necessary for it as well as equipped staff; however, it is both diagnostic and therapeutic if an intervention is conducted. Through angiography, endovascular interventions can be conducted including thrombolytics, percutaneous mechanical thrombectomy, angioplasty, and stenting.

INITIAL MANAGEMENT AND TREATMENT

Once the diagnosis of acute limb ischemia is confirmed and its severity classified, several immediate interventions are necessary to optimize patient outcomes.

ANTICOAGULATION

Systemic anticoagulation with intravenous unfractionated heparin should be instituted immediately to help prevent further clot propagation and to minimize thrombosis of distal, small under-perfused vessels. This was first introduced by Blaisdell and colleagues in 1978 and is the mainstay of treatment prior to intervention.[7] An initial bolus dose of 100U/kg is administered followed by a weight-based dose titrated per heparin nomogram to achieve an activated partial thromboplastin time between 50 and 80 seconds or 2.0 to 3.0 times normal values. Immediate full dose heparinization can result in symptomatic improvement in many patients. For those with heparin allergies, other anticoagulants such as argatroban or bivalirudin can be used.

Ancillary support measures such as volume resuscitation, intravenous fluid hydration, supplemental oxygen, analgesia, and laboratory investigations are also important.

TREATMENT SELECTION

Treatment for acute limb ischemia depends on the severity of ischemia presenting clinically and graded by the classification established by Rutherford and colleagues.[4]

Class I acute limb ischemia may only require medical therapy with anticoagulation. There is no sensory or motor compromise, and an addition to optimizing medical therapy, any intervention (if planned) may be performed on an elective basis. The type of intervention will be based on the location and extent of the disease and the patient's underlying medical comorbidities.

Class II acute limb ischemia tends to encompass the majority of patients, and all will require revascularization. The timing and urgency of intervention depend on the clinical examination of the patient.

Class IIA acute limb ischemia presents with sensory deficits without motor involvement. The patients have a marginally threatened limb. Immediate revascularization is not necessary and therefore either an endovascular approach or an open approach may be utilized. The duration of symptoms is key—endovascular approaches are more effective if instituted within 2 weeks of symptoms, whereas open surgical revascularization is preferred in patients with symptoms greater than 2 weeks duration.[8] Therefore, most would offer endovascular approaches and thrombolytic therapy for patients presenting with 14 days of ischemic symptoms and reserving open surgery for those limbs that do not respond to lytic therapy. Revascularization in Class IIA is performed on an urgent, not emergent, basis.

Class IIB acute limb ischemia presents with both sensory and motor deficits, and immediate revascularization is recommended for limb salvage. Because timing is critical, open surgical revascularization has been preferred although newer endovascular techniques have been gaining traction with single-session therapies such as percutaneous mechanical thrombectomy and combination aspiration/lytic options.

Class III acute limb ischemia presents with profound sensory and motor deficits, usually paralysis, with no audible arterial or venous Doppler signals. Revascularization is not indicated and is usually futile. Primary amputation should be considered before severe acid-base and electrolyte abnormalities ensue from the ischemic limb that may cause cardiopulmonary and renal collapse.

MANAGEMENT OPTIONS

The treatment options for the management of acute limb ischemia (Table 31-3) depend again on the severity of presentation and the urgency of revascularization. The options include the following.

OPEN REVASCULARIZATION

In 1963, Fogarty and colleagues described embolectomy remote from the surgical site with a balloon catheter; since then, surgery has become the cornerstone of treatment for acute limb ischemia.[9,10] Open revascularization remains the treatment of choice for Class IIB ischemia due to the need for urgent

TABLE 31-3 Treatment and Revascularization Options for ALI

Anticoagulation	Open revascularization	Endovascular
Heparin	Balloon thrombo-embolectomy	Catheter-directed thrombolysis
	Surgical bypass	Percutaneous mechanical thrombectomy
	Endarterectomy	

intervention and restoration of perfusion for the immediately threatened limb that are generally not possible with long infusion times in some endovascular procedures.

While improvements in surgical techniques have reduced the rate of limb loss with acute limb ischemia, the mortality rate remains unacceptably high.[10] This is primarily due to patients living longer while still having the concurrent significant medical comorbidities. The refinement in surgical techniques, however, truly has decreased the rate of amputation if an accurate and timely diagnosis is reached (Table 31-4).

1. **Balloon catheter thrombo-embolectomy.** This technique is routinely used to deal with an embolic event or bypass graft thrombosis. Typically, a transverse arteriotomy is performed just proximal to the vessel bifurcation (femoral, popliteal, brachial, etc.) in order to allow direct visualization of the origins of the branches, and ultimately direct the embolectomy catheter to the designated vessel. Embolectomy (Figure 31-4) is performed in both antegrade and retrograde fashions until a "clean" pass is obtained with adequate inflow and satisfactory back-bleeding.
2. **Surgical bypass procedures.** Over the years, the pattern of disease has changed with more people suffering from peripheral arterial disease. Therefore, balloon catheter embolectomy has become much more complicated than trying to pass the catheter through severely diseased or stenotic arterial segments. In such patients, or failed balloon embolectomy, surgical bypass is becoming more prominent. Satisfactory inflow and outflow vessel targets are identified by preprocedural or intraprocedural imaging. The ideal bypass target is a single-segment great saphenous vein of adequate caliber. Otherwise, small saphenous veins, arm veins, spliced segments, or even prosthetic conduits may be used.
3. **Endarterectomy**. Formal endarterectomy is used at times due to in-situ thrombosis of a vessel with preexisting severe atherosclerotic burden. A longitudinal arteriotomy is performed with the extraction of thrombus and a standard endarterectomy of plaque with appropriate distal endpoints. Patch reconstruction (Figure 31-5) is mandatory to maintain vessel luminal size.

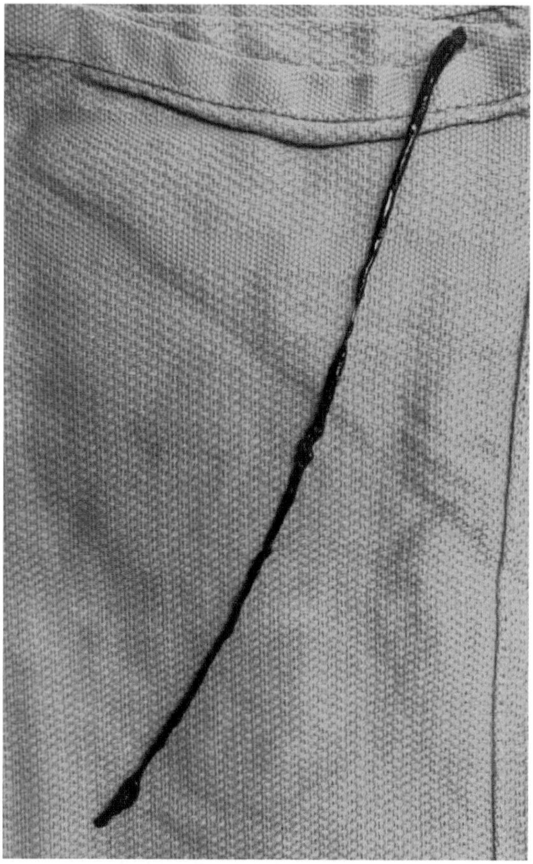

FIGURE 31-4 Extracted fresh single-segment embolus.

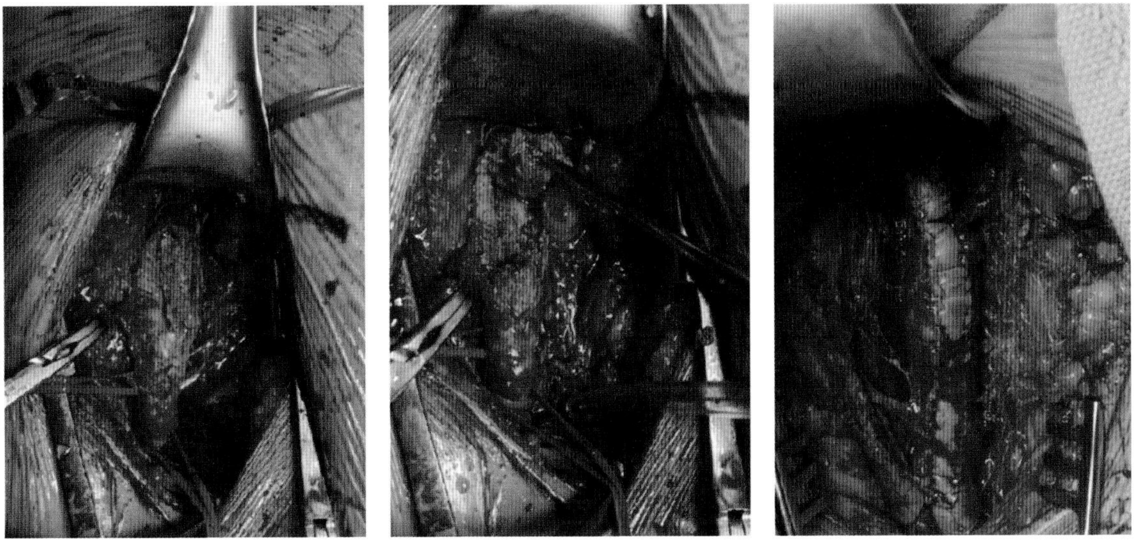

FIGURE 31-5 **In-situ thrombosis with patch angioplasty reconstruction and revascularization.**

ENDOVASCULAR APPROACHES

The search for less invasive revascularization options has continued as patients with acute limb ischemia have multiple comorbidities that place them generally at higher surgical risk. The goal of decreasing revascularization morbidity without compromising the rates of limb salvage has been challenging but with new endovascular approaches, there has been a promise. The use of catheter-directed thrombolysis (CDT) and percutaneous mechanical thrombectomy (PMT) have the potential to clear the occluding thrombus from the peripheral vessel in a minimally invasive approach, restore blood flow and capillary perfusion, and identify the culprit lesion that can then be managed by standard endovascular techniques such as balloon angioplasty, atherectomy and/or stenting.

1. **Catheter-Directed Thrombolysis.** The use of CDT has become the preferred method of revascularization for viable or marginally threatened limbs, as these limbs "allow" an infusion time for thrombolytic therapy. In the United States, only tissue Plasminogen Activator (tPA) is used. The standard angiographic technique is used in imaging and ultimately crossing the thrombosed segment or lesion with wires and catheters. Contrast injection is then performed to confirm true lumen and then a thrombolytic infusion catheter is advanced over the wire to the lesion in question. At this point, tPA is slowly instilled within the thrombus for a variable amount of time. Such thrombolytic therapy is predicated on the activation of plasmin

TABLE 31-4 **Amputation, Mortality, and Long-Term Limb Salvage for Open Revascularization in Acute Limb Ischemia**

Series	Year	N	Amputation %	Mortality %	Limb Salvage
Campbell et al.[11]	1998	474	16	22	Not reported
Nypaver et al.[12]	1998	71	7	10	62% at 1 year
Pemberton et al.[13]	1999	107	12	25	75% at 2 years

from the precursor zymogen plasminogen, which ultimately cleaves fibrin to cause dissolution of the thrombus. By directing the thrombolysis at the level of the thrombus, regional thrombus dissolution is achieved with minimal systemic fibrinolysis. Despite these efforts, a modest systemic proteolytic state may occur from these thrombolytic agents, and most would continue to check fibrinogen levels, and limit the use of thrombolytics to patients with no contraindications or concerns for bleeding diathesis.

2. **Percutaneous Mechanical Thrombectomy.** There exist multiple devices that promote mechanical clot removal with and without the use of thrombolysis. These PMT devices range from pure aspiration such as with the Penumbra® catheter to rheolytic mechanisms such as the AngioJet® device. A stream of fluid and hydrodynamic forces is instituted to extract the thrombotic material from the lumen.[14,15]

Mechanical aspiration offers the opportunity for faster thrombus removal without the long infusion times that are sometimes necessary with CDT. Partial reperfusion of the extremity may provide sufficient improvement in ischemia to allow more complete removal of thrombus with thrombolytic therapy later. Furthermore, initial debulking of significant thrombus may reduce the number of thrombolytic agents needed, thereby further decreasing the risks of hemorrhagic complications from lytic agents. PMT devices may be the only endovascular option in patients who cannot undergo lytic therapy due to recent surgery or other contraindications.

It is unlikely that mechanical thrombectomy will completely eliminate the need for thrombolytic therapy or open revascularization. The added benefits of thrombolysis include not only removal of the large occluding clot burden but also breaking-up of the clot in the smaller vessels and arteriolar and capillary beds, maintaining distal perfusion.

COMPARING OPEN VERSUS ENDOVASCULAR OPTIONS

In the 1990s, three multicenter, randomized trials were published (Table 31-5) comparing thrombolysis versus primary open revascularization for patients presenting with acute limb ischemia.

The first trial, performed at the University of Rochester,[16] randomly assigned 114 patients with acute limb-threatening ischemia to revascularization with thrombolysis using urokinase in 57 patients or to immediate operation in 57 patients. At 1 year, the amputation-free survival rates were 75% and 52%, respectively, a statistically significant difference. Further analysis identified that this result was secondary to a higher rate of death in the operative group—deaths occurring in association with perioperative cardiopulmonary complications. It seemed that taking patients with severe ischemia to open surgery without adequate preoperative preparation resulted in a high complication and death rate.

The second trial was the landmark surgery versus thrombolysis for ischemia of the lower extremity (STILE) trial, a large multicenter evaluation randomly assigning 393 patients to surgery or thrombolysis with either rt-PA or urokinase.[17] The clinical outcomes between both thrombolytic groups were similar, so their data were combined for analysis. Post

TABLE 31-5 Randomized Trials Comparing Open versus Endovascular Revascularization in ALI

			Thrombolytic		Operative	
Series	**N**	**Period (months)**	**Amputation (%)**	**Death (%)**	**Amputation (%)**	**Death (%)**
Rochester Study	114	12	18	16	18	42
SITLE Trial	393	6	12	6.5	11	8.5
TOPAS Trial	544	12	15	20	13.1	17

hoc stratification placed patients in two subgroups based on the duration of symptoms prior to enrollment (<14 days vs >14 days). Results noted that patients with shorter duration of symptoms (<14 days) assigned to thrombolysis had lower amputation rates than did the surgical patients (11% vs 30%) and for those patients with longer duration of symptoms (>14 days), the surgical group had a lower rate of amputation at 6 months compared to the thrombolysis group (3% vs 12%).

The third multicenter trial to evaluate thrombolytic therapy versus open surgery was the Thrombolysis or Peripheral Arterial Surgery (TOPAS) trial.[18] In 544 patients, recombinant urokinase was compared to primary operation for patients with lower extremity native artery or bypass graft occlusions of 14 days' duration or less. The amputation-free survival rates at 6 months following randomization were not significantly different: 71.8% in the thrombolysis group and 74.8% in the operative group. There were also no significant differences in rates of amputation-free survival or death at discharge. Importantly, however, at the end of 6 months, 31.5% of patients in the thrombolysis group had avoided amputation or death without the need for more than a percutaneous procedure.

In patients with acute limb ischemia, thrombolytic therapy leads to resolution of the thrombus with good clinical results in 75% to 92% of patients.[3] Factors for successful endovascular results include short duration of presenting symptoms (within 14 days); ability to cross the lesion successfully; the presence of an identifiable culprit lesion that can be treated; and patency of the bypass graft for at least a year prior to occlusion.

It is important to note that the use of thrombolytics predisposes to hemorrhagic complications that are not unnoticed. Major hemorrhagic complications were noted in 12.5% of the thrombolytic group as compared to 5.5% in the operative group within TOPAS. Furthermore, wire and catheter manipulation also can cause distal embolization of thrombus during attempted endovascular therapy.

FASCIOTOMY

Multiple studies have demonstrated that muscle poorly tolerates ischemia. When the ischemic state is unduly prolonged, the successfully replanted or revascularized limb undergoes deleterious biochemical reactions that cascade to vessel intimal damage, increased vessel permeability, and lowering of pH. The resultant tissue edema leads to increasing compartment pressures, which not only impede the recovery of function but also can lead to irreversible muscle necrosis, increased risk of infection, and sepsis if not reversed in a timely fashion. The development of compartment syndrome jeopardizes not only the injured limb but life itself secondary to the biochemical toxins produced by the ischemic extremity.[19]

Compartment syndrome (CS) is a feared complication after revascularization for acute limb ischemia (ALI), and patients often undergo prophylactic four-compartment fasciotomy at the time of revascularization to avoid developing CS (Figure 31-6) and its associated complications. However, fasciotomy carries its own morbidity and surgeons may opt against this initially. The subsequent development of CS would mandate fasciotomy in a delayed fashion. The development of CS requiring delayed fasciotomy was associated with an increased risk of major amputation at 30 days compared to patients who underwent prophylactic fasciotomy. Although the decision to perform prophylactic fasciotomy in the setting of ALI is complex, a liberal approach to prophylactic fasciotomy at the time of revascularization may improve limb salvage rates.[20]

The diagnosis of CS is usually based on clinical symptoms and signs; however, they have poor sensitivity, which may result in delayed diagnosis. Pain is usually present and is often severe, but it is an unreliable indicator as its intensity can be variable. Pain may be minimal in CS associated with nerve injury. Swelling and tenderness of the muscle compartments are signs, which should suggest the diagnosis, although a hematoma may be an alternative explanation. Sensory symptoms and signs are often present in the extremity at an early stage, but by the time, a motor deficit develops, full recovery is unusual, being reported in only 13% of patients. Compartment pressure measurement is straightforward using a needle manometer, but there is little consensus about the threshold value for diagnosis and treatment of CS. Elevated compartment pressure

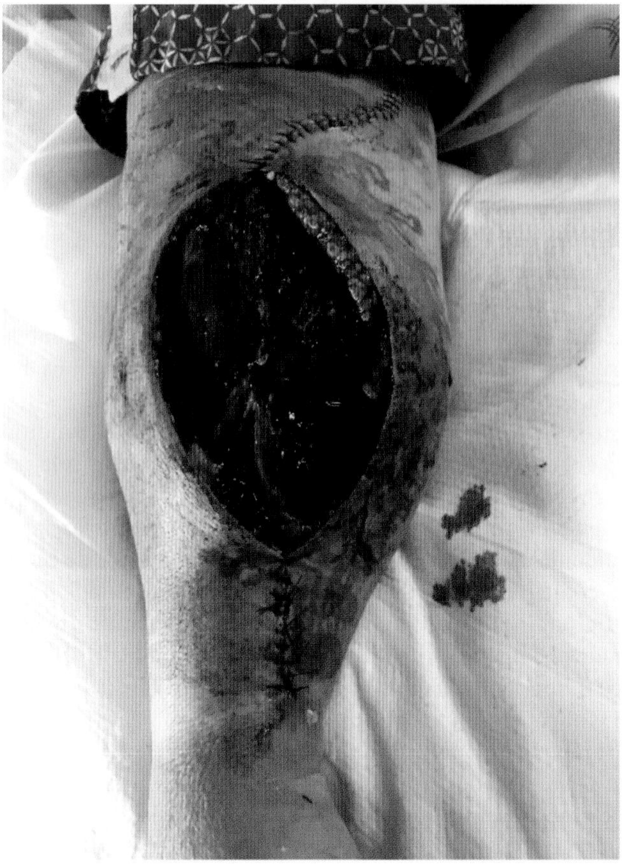

FIGURE 31-6 Compartment syndrome of the arm.

above 20 to 30 mmHg has high sensitivity and specificity (94%–98%) for CS. Several authors have attempted to identify risk factors for the development of CS, including ischemia duration > 6 hours, young age, previous history of ALI, and hypotension. Others found that elevated serum CK, the severity of acute ischemia (Rutherford IIb), inadequate intraoperative backflow, and positive fluid balance were associated with CS after ALI treatment. The importance of these findings lies in the possibility of identifying patients who would benefit from immediate fasciotomy after revascularization for ALI, or at least undergo close monitoring postoperatively, and delayed fasciotomy if necessary. The main way to prevent CS is to conduct prophylactic fasciotomy after revascularization. Obviously, this is an easier option for patients who have had surgical treatment, but must be considered after all urgent revascularization procedures. Decisions will be individualized for each patient but should take into account the risk factors mentioned above. Fasciotomy is the treatment for both established CS and prophylaxis against possible IRI. The lower leg is the most common location of CS. A single incision technique over the anterior compartment was advocated, but this risk leaving the posterior compartments untreated and ischemic. A full four-compartment Fasciotomy is needed less often in the arm. The timing of fasciotomy is critically important in patients who develop CS. Untreated CS compounds ischemic muscle damage and risks myoglobinuria and renal failure. Fasciotomy should usually be done within 2 hours of diagnosis; waiting longer than 6 hours is not acceptable. Fasciotomy should be done within 8 hours of the development of CS, but even that may be too late in some patients.[21]

CONCLUSIONS

Acute limb ischemia results from the sudden decrease in limb perfusion that threatens the viability of the limb. Complete or even partial occlusion can lead to rapid ischemia that can lead to poor functional outcomes within hours. The etiology is usually embolization or in-situ thrombosis of progressive atherosclerosis. Most patients have significant medical comorbidities and medical optimization and risk factor control are essential in the treatment algorithm.

Management options are based on the accurate and rapid diagnosis of the clinical severity of the presenting ischemic limb (Figure 31-7). Both endovascular and open techniques are available and should not be viewed as competitive, but rather, symbiotic in an effort to restore perfusion as quick as possible understanding their advantages and disadvantages.

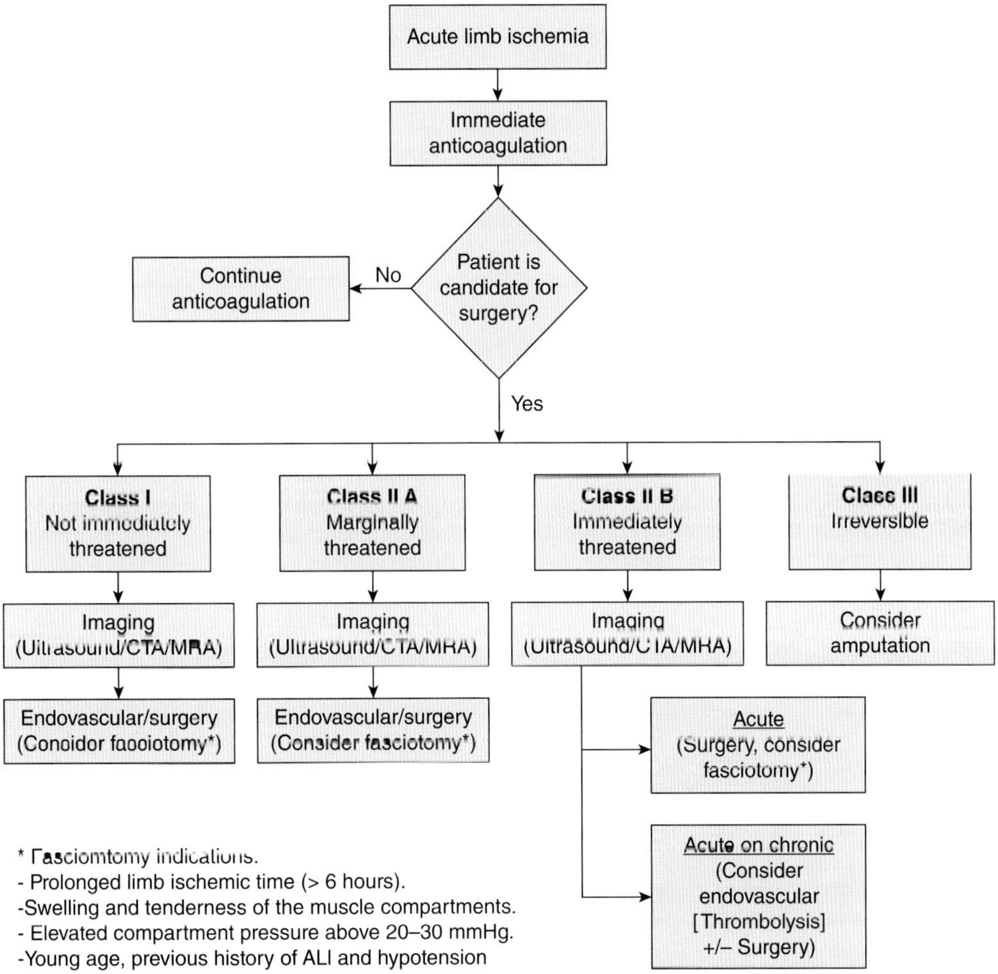

FIGURE 31-7 Algorithm for management of ALI.

REFERENCES

1. Argenteri A, de Donato G, Setacci F, et al. History of the diagnosis and treatment of critical limb ischemia and diabetic foot. *Semin Vasc Surg*. 2018;31:25-42.
2. Norgren L, Hiatt WR, Dormandy JA, Nehler MR, Harris KA, Fowkes FG; TASC II Working Group. Intersociety consensus for the management of peripheral arterial disease (TASC II). *J Vasc Surg*. 2007;45(Suppl):S5-S67.
3. Creager MA, Kaufman JA, Conte MS. Acute limb ischemia. *N Engl J Med*. 2012;366:2198-2206.
4. Rutherford RB, Baker JD, Ernst C, et al. Recommended standards for reports dealing with lower extremity ischemia: revised version. *J Vasc Surg*. 1997;26:517-538.
5. Jivegård L, Bergqvist D, Holm J. When is urgent revascularization unnecessary for acute lower limb ischaemia? *Eur J Vasc Endovasc Surg*. 1995;9:448-453.
6. Suggested standards for reports dealing with lower extremity ischemia. Prepared by the Ad Hoc Committee on Reporting Standards, Society for Vascular Surgery/North American Chapter, International Society for Cardiovascular Surgery. *J Vasc Surg*. 1986;4:80-94.
7. Blaisdell FW, Steele M, Allen RE. Management of acute lower extremity arterial ischemia due to embolism and thrombosis. *Surgery*. 1978;84:822-834.
8. Creager MA, Kaufman JA, Conte MS. Acute limb ischemia. *N Eng J Med*. 2012;366(23):2198-2206.
9. Fogarty TJ, Cranley JJ, Krause RJ, Strasser ES, Hafner CD. A method for extraction of arterial emboli and thrombi. *Surg Gynecol Obstet*. 1963;116:241-244
10. Kasirajan K, Ouriel K. Management of acute lower extremity ischemia: treatment strategies and outcomes. *Curr Interv Cardiol Rep*. 2000;2:119-129.
11. Campbell WB, Ridler BM, Szymanska TH. Current management of acute leg ischemia: results of audit by the Vascular Surgical Society of Great Britain and Ireland. *Br J Surg*. 1998;85:1498-1503.
12. Nypaver TJ, Whyte BR, Endean ED, Schwarcz TH, Hyde GL. Nontraumatic lower-extremity acute arterial ischemia. *Am J Surg*. 1998;176:147-152.
13. Pemberton N, Varty K, Nydahl S, Bell PR. The surgical management of acute limb ischemia due to native vessel occlusion. *Eur J Vasc Endovasc Surg*. 1999;17:72-76.
14. Silva JA, Ramee SR, Collins TJ, et al. Rheolytic thrombectomy in the treatment of acute limb-threatening ischemia: immediate results and six-month follow-up of the multicenter Angiojet registry. *Cathet Cardiovasc Diagn*. 1998;45:386-393.
15. WagneHJ,Muler-HulsbeckS,PittonMB,etal.Rapidthromecxtomy with a hydrodynamic catheter: results from a prospective, multicenter trial. *Radiology*. 1997;205:675-681.
16. Ouriel K, Shortell CK, DeWeese JA, et al. A comparison of a thrombolytic therapy with operative revascularization in the initial treatment of acute peripheral arterial ischemia. *J Vasc Surg*. 1994;19:1021-1030.
17. The STILE Trial: results of a prospective randomized trial evaluating surgery versus thrombolysis for ischemia of the lower extremity. *Ann Surg*. 1994;220:251-266.
18. Ouriel K, Veith FJ, Sasahara AA. A comparison of recombinant urokinase with vascular surgery as initial treatment for acute arterial occlusion of the legs. Thrombolysis or Peripheral Arterial Surgery (TOPAS) investigators. *N Engl J Med*. 1998;338:1105-1111.
19. Hofmeister EP, Shin AY. The role of prophylactic fasciotomy and medical treatment in limb ischemia and revascularization. *Hand Clin*. 1998;14(3):457-465.
20. Rothenberg KA, George EL, Trickey AW, Chandra V, Stern JR. Delayed fasciotomy is associated with higher risk of major amputation in patients with acute limb ischemia. *Ann Vasc Surg*. 1989;10:343-350.
21. Björck M, Earnshaw JJ, Acosta S, et al. Clinical practice guidelines on the management of acute limb ischemia. *Eur J Vasc Endovasc Surg*. 2020; 59:198-199.

SELF-ASSESSMENT STUDY QUESTIONS AND ANSWERS

Questions

1. A 74-year-old female with a history of atrial fibrillation presents with 2 hours of acute onset right lower extremity pain. She is scheduled to undergo a screening colonoscopy this week and was asked to hold her medications. Her examination notes absent right lower extremity pulses but palpable left pedal pulses. The most probable cause of her ischemia is:
A. In-situ thrombosis of peripheral arterial disease
B. Atrial embolus
C. Raynaud's syndrome
D. Cardiac myxoma
E. Vessel dissection

2. Which of the following is not a clinical sign of acute limb ischemia?
A. Pulselessness
B. Poikilothermia
C. Paralysis
D. Pallor
E. Pigmentation

3. A 69-year-old male presents with left lower extremity discomfort of 4 hours duration. On assessment, he denies pain on passive or active flexion, and he is able to move the foot with normal motor function. He does endorse numbness along the dorsum of the foot. You cannot identify pulses or signals in the left foot. What is his class of acute limb ischemia?
A. Class I
B. Class IIA
C. Class IIB
D. Class III

4. In acute limb ischemia, the earliest signs of sensory dysfunction are noted in:
A. Temperature
B. Pain fibers
C. Proprioception
D. Vibration
E. Crude touch

5. All the following are factors for successful endovascular outcomes in acute limb ischemia using thrombolytic therapy except:
A. Crossing the lesion
B. Duration of symptoms of greater than 2 weeks
C. Identifying a culprit lesion
D. Patency of the bypass graft for greater than 1 year prior to presentation
E. Duration of symptoms of less than 2 weeks

6. A 79-year-old male with a history of peripheral arterial disease and baseline ABIs of 0.6 bilaterally presents to the emergency room with new onset left leg pain that he can not handle anymore at home. It has been ongoing for the last 6 days. You cannot identify a pulse or signal in the affected leg. He has a normal sensory and motor functions. Noninvasive imaging demonstrates occlusion of his left superficial femoral artery with reconstitution at the P2 segment of the popliteal artery. What is your management strategy?
A. Anticoagulation alone
B. Aspirin and clopidogrel alone
C. Open thrombo embolectomy
D. Left femoral to popliteal artery bypass with prosthetic conduit
E. Endovascular therapy with thrombolytics or PMT

7. The STILE trial randomized 393 patients to thrombolytic therapy versus open surgery. The results noted that at 6 months in the shorter duration group (less than 14 days):
A. Open surgery had a higher mortality
B. The open surgery amputation rate was 11%
C. The thrombolytic therapy amputation rate was 11%
D. Open surgery is recommended in patients with shorter symptom duration

SELF-ASSESSMENT STUDY QUESTIONS AND ANSWERS

8. Patients presenting with Class IIB ischemia have a limb that is:

A. Viable
B. Nonfunctional
C. Irreversibly ischemic
D. Immediately threatened
E. Marginally threatened

9. A 65-year-old male presents with acute right lower extremity pain. Physical examination reveals a white limb with poor capillary refill and no pulses in the affected limb. He has chronic kidney disease and an elevated creatinine at 2.3 g/dL. He is able to move the foot but has sensory changes. What initial imaging will you obtain?

A. CT angiogram
B. MR angiogram
C. Lower extremity ultrasound
D. Echocardiogram

10. A 65-year-old male presents with 2 hours of acute right lower extremity pain. He has no previous medical history. Physical examination reveals a white limb with poor capillary refill and no pulses in the affected limb. The contralateral limb has palpable pulses. He has sensory and motor deficits. You decide to proceed emergently to the operating room and perform:

A. Open embolectomy via a transverse arteriotomy
B. Endovascular therapy with thrombolytics and planned 12-hour infusion
C. Surgical tibial bypass
D. Open embolectomy via a longitudinal arteriotomy
E. Endarterectomy

SELF-ASSESSMENT STUDY QUESTIONS AND ANSWERS

Answers

1. B.
2. E.
3. B.
4. C.
5. B.
6. E.
7. C.
8. D.
9. C.
10. A.

CHAPTER

32 Chronic Lower Extremity Ischemia

Steven Scoville and Timur Sarac

OUTLINE

GENERAL CONSIDERATION AND HISTORY
CLINICAL FINDINGS
DIFFERENTIAL DIAGNOSIS
DIAGNOSIS
MANAGEMENT OF CLI

GENERAL CONSIDERATION AND HISTORY

Worldwide, more than 200 million people are affected by peripheral artery disease (PAD). The definition of PAD is variable, but in general consists of a disease state characterized by compromised arterial perfusion to meet the oxygen and metabolic needs of organs. PAD overwhelmingly involves the lower extremities and to a much less extent upper extremities. Approximately 5% to 10% of patients with PAD of the lower extremities will progress to develop critical limb ischemia (CLI) over a 5-year period characterized by rest pain and/or the presence of nonhealing wounds or gangrene.[1] If left untreated, rates of limb loss are nearly 40% over the first year.[2] Despite a variety of available limb sparing open and minimally invasive surgical options, amputation rates among patients who are not candidates for treatment are as high as approximately 70%.[3] Furthermore, it is reported that patients presenting with CLI have as high as 20% mortality rate in the first year after presentation.[4] Risk factors for progression to CLI include advanced age, smoking, diabetes, hypertension, age, renal disease, and hypercholesterolemia.[4] Due to increased prevalence of uncontrolled tobacco use and diabetes, the number of people affected is only expected to increase. In addition, nearly 90% of patients with CLI also have concomitant coronary artery disease of which two-thirds require treatment.[5] Therefore, the clinical knowledge required for appropriate prevention, diagnosis, and treatment are critical to allow for concise evaluation, workup, and treatment.

CLINICAL FINDINGS

CLI typically occurs in the lower extremities with the most distal foot being the most symptomatic. However, it is a systemic disease, and atherosclerosis is common in other arterial beds. Most commonly, the disease process is secondary to atherosclerotic changes that affect arteries from the aortoiliac region to the terminal lower extremity vessels. Regardless of the etiology, the resulting disease process is caused by a mismatch of arterial perfusion to tissue dependent oxygen and nutrient requirements resulting in ischemia, vasodilation, inflammation, and angiogenesis.[6] Early symptoms of PAD consist of calf, gluteal, thigh, or foot pain, discomfort, or fatigue induced with activity that ultimately subsides with rest, commonly referred to as claudication. Progression of the disease to CLI as opposed to an acute process must have been present for greater than 2 weeks, and pain is experienced at rest with limb elevation or dependent positioning.[7] Classically, patients will complain of waking up at night with foot pain relieved by hanging their feet over the edge of the bed, and hyperemic-dependent rubror. Physical exam findings consistent with CLI include diminished or absent palpable distal pulses, elevation pallor or dependent rubror, thin and shiny skin, absence of hair, and increased capillary refill time.[8] Chronic ulceration, typically seen as well-demarcated punched-out lesions involving the lower extremity, can also be pathognomonic of the disease process and should heighten suspicion for ongoing vascular compromise.[9] Progression to gangrene indicates an advanced stage. Physical exam findings are corroborated by imaging studies to finalize the diagnosis and are discussed further in the diagnosis section.

DIFFERENTIAL DIAGNOSIS

The symptoms and clinical findings of CLI, though specific, can be caused by alternative disease processes, and therefore a thorough physical exam and differential diagnosis should be applied to patients being worked up for CLI. Diabetic neuropathy, for example, can present with decreased lower extremity function, skin changes, paresthesia and even disabling foot pain that can also be worse at night. It is generally bilateral with similar distributions and can be further confirmed with monofilament testing and with vibratory changes that would not be present in neuropathy strictly from CLI.[10] Nerve root compression originates in the nerves as it leaves the spinal column and generally follows dermatome distributions that can include the feet and lower extremities. L4 involves the knee and big toe, L5 involves the medial edge of the foot, and S1 includes the extensor surface of the foot. L4 and S1 deficits result in diminished reflexes of the knee and ankle. Furthermore, straight leg raising would be limited in nerve root compression. These findings including pain along dermatomes and reflex changes are not present in CLI. Peripheral neuropathy can also be caused by vitamin B12 deficiency. Night cramps and arthritis are also common nonvascular etiologies for lower extremity pain and may be difficult to discern from CLI. However, one way CLI may be realized is that the time from recumbent positioning to symptomatic pain would be consistent, whereas night cramps and arthritis are more likely to be more sporadic.

Lower extremity ulcers can be due to several types of disease processes, and a comprehensive understanding of these will assist in diagnosis of the vascular or nonvascular etiologies. Causes include venous ulcers, diabetic ulcers, vasculitis, Buerger's disease, sickle cells, pyoderma gangrenosum, and even malignancy.[9] Key findings with arterial ulcers are involvement of the distal foot with the toes being most common and there is minimal collateral circulation. The ulcers themselves are in general dry, with necrotic and poor granulating wound bases.[9] The location of symptoms can also be predictive of the level of occlusion. For example, usually for tissue loss, there is obstruction at two levels, inflow (including the iliacs common and profunda femoral arteries) and outflow (superficial femoral, popliteal, and tibials). Ischemic rest pain can develop with just one level of blockage, and also always has a degree of tibial disease.

DIAGNOSIS

Patients presenting with symptoms, risk factors, and history concerning for arterial insufficiency require further focused vascular exam and workup (Figure 32-1). Beginning with physical exam, patients with CLI are often found to have absent distal dorsalis pedis and posterior tibial artery pulses. Other findings including ulcerations, absence of hair, rubror, and thin or shiny skin are generally indicators of vascular insufficiency. Several noninvasive testing can further be performed for objective evidence regarding arterial occlusion. Ankle brachial index (ABI) is one of the most utilized tests that compares systolic ankle pressure to systolic brachial pressure.[8] ABIs, however, are less reliable in patients with diabetes, chronic kidney disease, or advanced age due to reduced vessel compliance and calcification resulting in falsely elevated reported pressures.[11] ABI values less than 0.9 are consistent with PAD, while less than 0.4 are indicative of CLI. In patients with noncompressible vessels due to compliance or calcification, the ABIs may be artificially elevated. Therefore, toe pressures can be obtained as these are usually spared from the noncompressible disease process that may be present in the DP and PT vessels. Transcutaneous oxygen measurements,

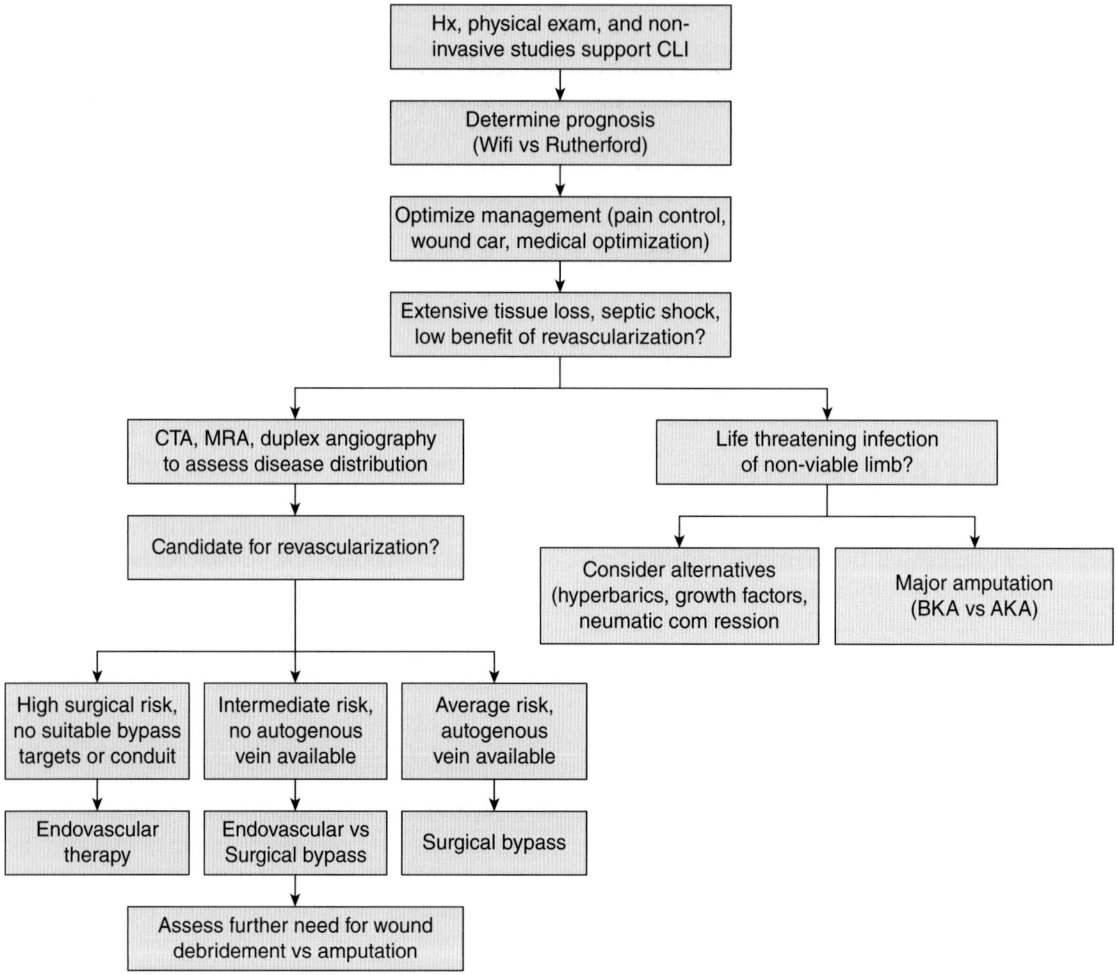

FIGURE 32-1 Algorithm for the management of CLI. (Reproduced with permission from Levin SR, Arinze N, Siracuse JJ. Lower extremity critical limb ischemia: A review of clinical features and management. *Trends Cardiovasc Med.* 2020;30(3):125-130.)

pulse volume recordings, and the characteristic wave forms on Doppler have also been shown to be useful in evaluating CLI and even determine potential for wound healing.[12] Though CLI is a clinical diagnosis, the Trans-Atlantic Inter-Society consensus (TASC II) for diagnosis of CLI in patients with noncompressible vessels require patients have ischemic rest pain or tissue loss and ankle systolic pressure $\leq$50 mmHg, toe pressure of $\leq$30 mmHg in a nondiabetic and 60 mmHg in a diabetic, transcutaneous oxygen pressure of <30 mmHg, or flat-line transtarsal pulse volume recordings.[13]

Once CLI has been diagnosed, the decisions must be made regarding whether or not patients are candidates for revascularization. To this end, several classification guides exist to assist in stratifying patients as that the optimal treatment and outcomes vary according to the severity of the disease. The Rutherford classification consists of 1-3 grades and 0-6 categories based on clinical description and degree of symptoms with objective findings such as exertional activity, ankle pressures, pulse volume recordings, or toe pressures (Table 32-1).[4] One downside, however, is that the Rutherford classification tool excludes

TABLE 32-1 Rutherford Classification for Chronic Limb Ischemia

Grade	Category	Clinical Description	Objective Criteria
0	0	Asymptomatic, no occlusive disease	Normal treadmill or reactive hyperemia test
	1	Mild claudication	Able to complete treadmill test
			AP after exercise >50 mmHg but at least 20 mmHg lower than resting
I	2	Moderate claudication	Between categories 1-3
	3	Severe claudication	Cannot complete treadmill exercise
			AP after exercise <50 mmHg
II	4	Ischemic foot rest	Resting AP <40 mmHg
			Flat or barely pulsatile ankle or metatarsal PVR
			TP <30
III	5	Minor tissue loss	Resting AP <60 mmHg
		Nonhealing ulcer	Ankle or metatarsal PVR flat or barely pulsatile
		Focal gangrene and pedal ischemia	TP <40 mmHg
	6	Major tissue loss extending above transmetatarsa 1 level	Same as 5
		Functional foot is no longer	
		Salvageable	

AP, Ankle Pressure; PVR pulse volume recording; TM, Transmetatarsal; TP, toe pressure.

Data from Brunicardi FC, Andersen DK, Billiar TR, et al. *Schwartz's Principles of Surgery*, 11th ed. New York, NY: McGraw Hill; 2019.

patients with underlying diabetes and therefore a significant portion of patients with CLI. Recently, the Society for Vascular Surgery wound, ischemia, and foot infection (WIfI) classification system devised a scoring system that can account for diabetic patients and infection, and while it is still being verified, early studies have shown it is effective and in particular is useful in evaluation of patients with underlying diabetes (Table 32-2).[14,15]

If endovascular or open interventional treatment is being considered, anatomic imaging is utilized to prepare for definitive treatment with digital subtraction angiography considered the gold standard of imaging modalities with computed tomographic and magnetic resonance angiography can also be useful studies.[16] Enhanced preprocedural imaging allows for identification of the source lesion. The TASC II publication identified four different classes of lesions based on the extent, type, and location of where the abnormalities are (Figure 32-2).[4]

These were first created to assist in the disease management decisions that are discussed below.

MANAGEMENT OF CLI

The goals of CLI treatment and intervention are to relieve ischemic pain, heal wounds, maintain ability to ambulate, and preserve functional limbs whenever possible. Critical to this overall goal when CLI truly is identified is time to revascularization—the sooner the better. When it comes to revascularization there are many different modalities that can be utilized including open or endovascular approaches. Relevant open surgical repair includes lower extremity bypass (LEB) and endarterectomy. Aortoiliac occlusive disease can be bypassed through anatomic

TABLE 32-2 The Society for Vascular Surgery Wound, Ischemia, and Foot Infection (WIfI) Classification System

	Wound Grade		Ischemia Grade		Infection Grade
0	No wound, No gangrene	0	TP >60 mmHg ABI >0.8 ASP >100 mmHg	0	No infection, erythema, pain, purulence
1	Small shallow ulcer No exposed bone No gangrene	1	TP 40–59 mmHg ABI 0.6–0.79 ASP 70–100 mmHg	1	Local infection involving only skin or soft tissue
2	Deeper ulcer with exposed bone joint, tendon. Does not involve heal Shallow heel ulcer without calcaneal involvement Gangrene limited to digits	2	TP 30–39 mmHg ABI 0.4–0.59 ASP 50–70 mmHg	2	Local infection and erythema >2 cm, involves structures deeper than subcutaneous tissue (osteomyelitis, abscess), no SIRS criteria
3	Extensive Deep ulcer involving forefoot/midfoot Depp, full thickness heel ulcer with calcaneal involvement Extensive gangrene involving forefoot, midfoot Full thickness necrosis and calcaneal involvement	3	TP <30 mmHg ABI < 0.39 ASP < 30 mmHg	3	Local infection with at least 2 SIRS response (fever, tachycardia, heart rate, leukocytosis or leukopenia, increased respiratory rate)

Data from Hardman RL, Jazaeri O, Yi J, et al. Overview of classification systems in peripheral artery disease. *Semin Intervent Radiol.* 2014;31(4):378-388.

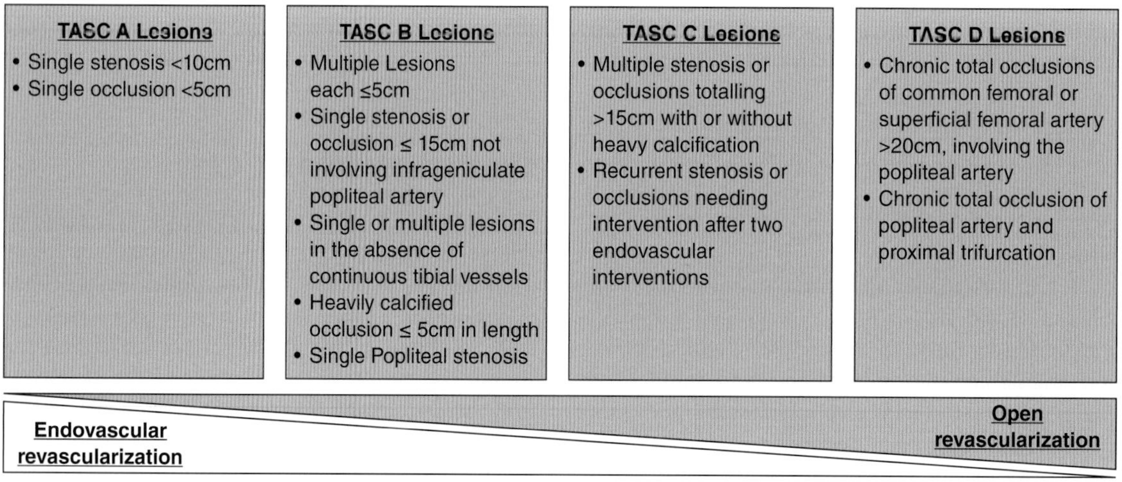

TASC A Lesions
• Single stenosis <10cm
• Single occlusion <5cm
TASC B Lesions
• Multiple Lesions each ≤5cm
• Single stenosis or occlusion ≤ 15cm not involving infrageniculate popliteal artery
• Single or multiple lesions in the absence of continuous tibial vessels
• Heavily calcified occlusion ≤ 5cm in length
• Single Popliteal stenosis
TASC C Lesions
• Multiple stenosis or occlusions totalling >15cm with or without heavy calcification
• Recurrent stenosis or occlusions needing intervention after two endovascular interventions
TASC D Lesions
• Chronic total occlusions of common femoral or superficial femoral artery >20cm, involving the popliteal artery
• Chronic total occlusion of popliteal artery and proximal trifurcation
Endovascular revascularization
Open revascularization

FIGURE 32-2 The Trans-Atlantic Inter-Society Consensus (TASC II) of femoral popliteal lesions. (Reproduced with permission from Brunicardi FC, Andersen DK, Billiar TR, et al. *Schwartz's Principles of Surgery,* 11th ed. New York, NY: McGraw Hill; 2019.)

and extra-anatomic approaches including aortobifemoral bypass, aortoiliac endarterectomy, or femorofemoral and axillary femoral bypass grafts, respectively. Aortobifemoral bypass has a high 5-year patency rate of 90% and 10-year patency of 80% compared to the axillary bifemoral or femoral-femoral grafts which both have approximately 70% 5-year patency rates.[17,18] Aortobifemoral, though superior in patency, is a taxing operation with higher morbidity (16%) and mortality (4%).[19] However, this has changed with technologic improvements which added circumferential rings to the graft to prevent external compression, and Samson et al. have demonstrated improved 5-year patency nearing 90%.[20] Therefore, axillary bifemoral or femoral-femoral is typically reserved for high-risk patients who may not otherwise tolerate a larger operation. Occlusion at the common femoral artery is typically addressed through open endarterectomy with patch angioplasty, and have been shown to have 5-year patency rates of approximately 90%, though wound complications can be common and sometimes require further surgical interventions.[21] Downstream, infrainguinal, arterial occlusions can be repaired through bypass procedures utilizing autogenous (preferable), or prosthetic (polytetrafluoro ethylene (ePTFE), or polyester), or cryopreserved saphenous vein. Autogenous greater saphenous vein bypass grafts are associated with the best primary patency with over 80% after 1 year and a 1-year limb salvage rate over 90%.[22,23] ePTFE bypass grafts for above knee bypass have comparable patency to vein grafts; however, a substantial decrease in long-term patency exists for below knee grafts (20% for 4-year patency for ePTFE vs 75% for vein bypass).[24] Furthermore, thrombosis of prosthetic grafts has been shown to have a higher risk of embolization with resultant risk of acute limb ischemia and possible threatened limb. In comparison, when vein grafts fail, it is typically from a chronic scarring process of neointimal hyperplasia with less likelihood of limb loss.[24] Though durability remains high, open procedures are associated with higher morbidity with wound infection (11%).[19,25]

Endovascular revascularization utilizes minimally invasive percutaneous delivery of a balloon, stent or debulking atherectomy device over a wire for effective treatment of CLI. Its use as an alternative to surgery has been expanded rapidly for the past several decades.[6] More recent advances in endovascular therapy include the development of drug coated balloons, drug eluting stents, and improvements to allow for crossing long occlusions. Overall, endovascular strategies have been shown to have high early success rates without even the need for general anesthesia leading to lower admission rates, morbidity, and mortality.[8] Stents for example are known to be superior to angioplasty alone with patency rates of 58% to 68% out to 5 years with limb salvage rate as high as 75% at 3 years.[26] Newer drug eluting stents and coated balloons also show superior results when compared to bare stents and balloons alone in certain anatomic sites.[27,28] Despite clinical effectiveness in certain settings, the long-term durability and cost of these approaches have yet to equal open surgery beyond 2 years.[29]

The effectiveness of both open and endovascular revascularization has led to significant variability in the approach to CLI treatment, without level one data to support one versus the other except in certain situations. However, current trials are under way to provide more guidance.[30] Disease patterns, and availability of suitable donor vein, comorbidities, socioeconomic factors, and providers' experience are primary factors that drive the observed variability. The TASC II guidelines published in 2007 identified type A lesions are best treated with endovascular repair as first-line treatment, while type D lesions are best treated through open repair (Figure 32-2).[4] Type B and C lesions did not have sufficient evidence to support one approach versus the other; however, B lesions were favored to be endovascular first while C was favored to be revascularized through an open approach. While these guidelines have been hotly debated, clinical experience continues to dictate practice patterns. To date, one randomized control trial has been performed known as the multicenter comparing bypass versus angioplasty in severe ischemia of the leg (BASIL) trial.[31,32] This trial was based in the United Kingdom and focused on the clinical and cost-effectiveness of treatments of angioplasty alone compared to open bypass for infrainguinal disease. Overall, it showed no difference in endpoint amputation-free survival (AFS) based on treatment modality. Based on this study, patients with a life expectancy of greater than 2 years with an available vein would best benefit from open repair first approach, while those with life expectancy of less than 2 years are best treated through angioplasty first. In instances where a suitable vein is not available, angioplasty is the recommended next alternative before prosthetic grafts should be considered. Finally, the BASIL trial showed that patients who underwent LEB after a failed angioplasty often had worse outcomes compared to the patients who underwent LEB as their original procedure.[33,34] The best endovascular versus best surgical therapy in patients with critical limb ischemia (BEST-CLI) trial is an ongoing large-scale multispecialty and multi-institution randomized control trial comparing treatment outcomes for patients with Rutherford category 4-6 CLI undergoing essentially all available endovascular and open techniques.[30,35] Its primary endpoint is to measure major adverse limb event (MALE)–free survival that is a new metric meant encompassing functionality, quality of life, and cost as opposed to just limb survival in AFS. Once completed, these new resources will be a resource to guide evidence-based practice for optimal patient outcomes.

Despite best attempts especially in the setting of multiple comorbidities, not all patients will improve or are candidates for any revascularization efforts. For example, in patients with extensive foot necrosis, with no viable sites for bypass, and who are not candidates for angioplasty or stent placement or who present with severe life-threatening foot sepsis, above the ankle amputation is most appropriate and definitive treatment.[6] Furthermore, patients who are nonambulatory with secondary severe flexion contractures are similarly appropriate candidates for primary amputation.[4]

Medical optimization of patients with CLI remains a critical component of patient care, as the 4-year risk of myocardial infarction and ischemic strokes have previously been reported as high as 10% and 8%.[3] Antiplatelet, lipid-lowering medications, β-blockers, angiotensin-converting enzyme inhibitors are critical in this patient population.[36] Smoking remains the most preventable risk factor associated with disease onset, and also with failure of treatment after interventions are performed; therefore, its importance cannot be overstated.[37] For the many patients also with diagnosis of diabetes, strict consistent blood glucose management has been shown to improve limb outcomes after revascularization.[38]

REFERENCES

1. Nehler MR, Duval S, Diao L, et al. Epidemiology of peripheral arterial disease and critical limb ischemia in an insured national population. *J Vasc Surg.* 2014;60(3):686-695.e2.
2. Hirsch AT, Haskal ZJ, Hertzer NR, et al. ACC/AHA 2005 Practice Guidelines for the management of patients with peripheral arterial disease (lower extremity, renal, mesenteric, and abdominal aortic): a collaborative report from the American Association for Vascular Surgery/Society for Vascular Surgery, Society for Cardiovascular Angiography and Interventions, Society for Vascular Medicine and Biology, Society of Interventional Radiology, and the ACC/AHA Task Force on Practice Guidelines (Writing Committee to Develop Guidelines for the Management of Patients With Peripheral Arterial Disease): endorsed by the American Association of Cardiovascular and Pulmonary Rehabilitation; National Heart, Lung, and Blood Institute; Society for Vascular Nursing; TransAtlantic Inter-Society Consensus; and Vascular Disease Foundation. *Circulation.* 2006;113(11):e463-e654.
3. Reinecke H, Unrath M, Freisinger E, et al. Peripheral arterial disease and critical limb ischaemia: still poor outcomes and lack of guideline adherence. *Eur Heart J.* 2015;36(15):932-938.
4. Norgren L, Hiatt WR, Dormandy JA, et al. Inter-society consensus for the management of peripheral arterial disease. *Int Angiol.* 2007;26(2):81-157.
5. Hertzer NR, Beven EG, Young JR, et al. Coronary artery disease in peripheral vascular patients. A classification of 1000 coronary angiograms and results of surgical management. *Ann Surg.* 1984;199(2):223-233.
6. Farber A, Eberhardt RT. The current state of critical limb ischemia: a systematic review. *JAMA Surg.* 2016;151(11):1070-1077.
7. Rutherford RB, Baker JD, Ernst C, et al. Recommended standards for reports dealing with lower extremity ischemia: revised version. *J Vasc Surg.* 1997;26(3):517-538.
8. Farber A. Chronic limb-threatening ischemia. *N Engl J Med.* 2018;379(2):171-180.
9. Kirsner RS, Vivas AC. Lower-extremity ulcers: diagnosis and management. *Br J Dermatol.* 2015;173(2):379-390.

10. Perkins BA, Olaleye D, Zinman B, Bril V. Simple screening tests for peripheral neuropathy in the diabetes clinic. *Diabetes Care.* 2001;24(2):250-256.
11. Williams DT, Harding KG, Price P. An evaluation of the efficacy of methods used in screening for lower-limb arterial disease in diabetes. *Diabetes Care.* 2005;28(9):2206-2210.
12. Cao P, Eckstein HH, De Rango P, et al. Chapter II: diagnostic methods. *Eur J Vasc Endovasc Surg.* 2011;42(Suppl 2):S13-S32.
13. Patel MR, Conte MS, Cutlip DE, et al. Evaluation and treatment of patients with lower extremity peripheral artery disease: consensus definitions from peripheral academic research consortium (PARC). *J Am Coll Cardiol.* 2015;65(9):931-941.
14. Mills JL, Conte MS, Armstrong DG, et al. The society for vascular surgery lower extremity threatened limb classification system: risk stratification based on wound, ischemia, and foot infection (WIfI). *J Vasc Surg.* 2014;59(1):220-234.e1-2.
15. Darling JD, McCallum JC, Soden PA, et al. Predictive ability of the society for vascular surgery wound, ischemia, and foot infection (WIfI) classification system following infrapopliteal endovascular interventions for critical limb ischemia. *J Vasc Surg.* 2016;64(3):616-622.
16. Iglesias J, Peña C. Computed tomography angiography and magnetic resonance angiography imaging in critical limb ischemia: an overview. *Tech Vasc Interv Radiol.* 2014;17(3):147-154.
17. Schneider JR, Besso SR, Walsh DB, Zwolak RM, Cronenwett JL. Femorofemoral versus aortobifemoral bypass: outcome and hemodynamic results. *J Vasc Surg.* 1994;19(1):43-55; discussion 55-7.
18. Brewster DC, Cambria RP, Darling RC, et al. Long-term results of combined iliac balloon angioplasty and distal surgical revascularization. *Ann Surg.* 1989;210(3):324-330; discussion 331.
19. Chiu KW, Davies RS, Nightingale PG, Bradbury AW, Adam DJ. Review of direct anatomical open surgical management of atherosclerotic aorto-iliac occlusive disease. *Eur J Vasc Endovasc Surg.* 2010;39(4):460-471.
20. Samson RH, Morales R, Showalter DP, Lepore MR, Nair DG. Heparin-bonded expanded polytetrafluoroethylene femoropopliteal bypass grafts outperform expanded polytetrafluoroethylene grafts without heparin in a long-term comparison. *J Vasc Surg.* 2016;64(3):638-647.
21. Kang JL, Patel VI, Conrad MF, Lamuraglia GM, Chung TK, Cambria RP. Common femoral artery occlusive disease: contemporary results following surgical endarterectomy. *J Vasc Surg.* 2008;48(4):872-877.
22. Schanzer A, Hevelone N, Owens CD, et al. Technical factors affecting autogenous vein graft failure: observations from a large multicenter trial. *J Vasc Surg.* 2007;46(6):1180-1190; discussion 1190.
23. Sarac TP, Huber TS, Back MR, et al. Warfarin improves the outcome of infrainguinal vein bypass grafting at high risk for failure. *J Vasc Surg.* 1998;28(3):446-457.
24. Mills J. *Infrainguinal Disease: Surgical Treatment.* Philadelphia, PA: Saunders; 2010: 1682-1703.
25. Greenblatt DY, Rajamanickam V, Mell MW. Predictors of surgical site infection after open lower extremity revascularization. *J Vasc Surg.* 2011;54(2):433-439.
26. Setacci C, de Donato G, Teraa M, et al. Chapter IV: treatment of critical limb ischaemia. *Eur J Vasc Endovasc Surg.* 2011;42(Suppl 2):S43-S59.
27. Dake MD, Ansel GM, Jaff MR, et al. Durable clinical effectiveness with paclitaxel-eluting stents in the femoropopliteal artery: 5-year results of the zilver PTX randomized trial. *Circulation.* 2016;133(15):1472-1483; discussion 1483.
28. Rosenfield K, Jaff MR, White CJ, et al. Trial of a paclitaxel-coated balloon for femoropopliteal artery disease. *N Engl J Med.* 2015;373(2):145-153.
29. Popplewell MA, Davies H, Jarrett H, et al. Bypass versus angio plasty in severe ischaemia of the leg – 2 (BASIL-2) trial: study protocol for a randomised controlled trial. *Trials.* 2016;17:11.
30. Menard MT, Farber A. The BEST-CLI trial: a multidisciplinary effort to assess whether surgical or endovascular therapy is better for patients with critical limb ischemia. *Semin Vasc Surg.* 2014;27(1):82-84.
31. Adam DJ, Beard JD, Cleveland T, et al. Bypass versus angioplasty in severe ischaemia of the leg (BASIL): multicentre, randomised controlled trial. *Lancet.* 2005;366(9501):1925-1934.
32. Bradbury AW, Adam DJ, Bell J, et al. Bypass versus angioplasty in severe ischaemia of the leg (BASIL) trial: a survival prediction model to facilitate clinical decision making. *J Vasc Surg.* 2010;51(Suppl 5):52S-68S.
33. Nolan BW, De Martino RR, Stone DH, et al. Prior failed ipsilateral percutaneous endovascular intervention in patients with critical limb ischemia predicts poor outcome after lower extremity bypass. *J Vasc Surg.* 2011;54(3):730-735; discussion 735-6.
34. Jones DW, Schanzer A, Zhao Y, et al. Growing impact of restenosis on the surgical treatment of peripheral arterial disease. *J Am Heart Assoc.* 2013;2(6):e000345.
35. Farber A, Rosenfield K, Menard M. The BEST-CLI trial: a multidisciplinary effort to assess which therapy is best for patients with critical limb ischemia. *Tech Vasc Interv Radiol.* 2014;17(3):221-224.

36. Das JR, Eberhardt RT. Contemporary risk assessment and cardiovascular outcomes in peripheral arterial disease. *Cardiovasc Hematol Disord Drug Targets.* 2013;13(3):185-196.
37. Armstrong EJ, Wu J, Singh GD, et al. Smoking cessation is associated with decreased mortality and improved amputation-free survival among patients with symptomatic peripheral artery disease. *J Vasc Surg.* 2014;60(6):1565-1571.
38. Rooke TW, Hirsch AT, Misra S, et al. 2011 ACCF/AHA focused update of the guideline for the management of patients with peripheral artery disease (updating the 2005 guideline): a report of the American college of cardiology foundation/american heart association task force on practice guidelines. *J Am Coll Cardiol.* 2011;58(19):2020-2045.

SELF-ASSESSMENT STUDY QUESTIONS AND ANSWERS

Questions

1. Key findings that distinguish lower extremity ulcers as being from PAD as opposed to other causes include all of the following except:
A. Dry wound
B. Necrotic base with poor granulation
C. Tibial disease
D. Hemorrhagic bullae
E. Gangrene

2. Ankle brachial index is of limited utility due to reduced vessel compliance in patients with the following comorbidities except:
A. Acute kidney injury
B. Advanced age
C. Chronic kidney injury
D. Diabetes

3. The Rutherford Classification tool excludes patients with what underlying disorder?
A. Chronic obstructive pulmonary disease
B. Seizures
C. Diabetes
D. Current smoker
E. Coronary artery disease

4. TASC B lesions include all of the following except:
A. >20 cm, involving the popliteal artery
B. Heavily calcified occlusion ≤5 cm
C. Single Popliteal Stenosis
D. Single Stenosis ≤15 cm not involving infrageniculate popliteal artery
E. Multiple lesions each <5 cm

5. Under the wound, ischemia, and foot infection (WIfI) classification model, a grade 2 infection grade is defined as which of the following:
A. Local infection with at least 2 systemic inflammatory response syndrome (SIRS) responses
B. Local infection involving only skin or soft tissue
C. No infection, erythema, pain, purulence
D. Local infection and erythema >2 cm, involves structures deeper than subcutaneous tissue, No SIRS criteria

6. According to the bypass versus angioplasty in severe ischemia of the leg (BASIL) trial which of the following is true:
A. Patients with life expectancy <2 years and available vein would best benefit from open repair first.
B. Patients with life expectancy >2 years and available vein would benefit from angioplasty first.
C. Patients with life expectancy >2 years and available vein would benefit from open repair first.
D. In instances of where vein is not available, prosthetics should be considered first over angioplasty.

7. The most preventable risk factor associated with CLI is:
A. Hypertension
B. Diabetes
C. Smoking
D. Obesity
E. Hypercholesterolemia

SELF-ASSESSMENT STUDY QUESTIONS AND ANSWERS

8. The preferable source of bypass material for infrainguinal arterial occlusions is which of the following:
A. ePTFE
B. Cryopreserved saphenous vein
C. Autogenous vein
D. Dacron

9. 5-year limb-salvage rates for people who are able to undergo stent placement for arterial insufficiency in general around:
A. 55%
B. 65%
C. 75%
D. 85%

10. Which of the following provides a correct pairing between the category, clinical description, and objective criteria, respectively, found in Rutherford classification system:
A. Category 5; minor tissue loss; cannot complete treadmill exercise
B. Category 4; ischemic foot rest; flat or barely pulsatile ankle or metatarsal PVR
C. Category 1; mild claudication; normal treadmill or reactive hyperemia
D. Category 2; moderate claudication; resting AP <40 mmHg
E. Category 3; severe claudication; able to complete treadmill exercise

SELF-ASSESSMENT STUDY QUESTIONS AND ANSWERS

Answers

1. D.
2. A.
3. C.
4. A.
5. D.
6. C.
7. C.
8. C.
9. C.
10. B.

CHAPTER

33 Chronic Upper Extremity Ischemia

Joseph P. Hart and Mark G. Davies

OUTLINE

INTRODUCTION
PATHOLOGY
Differential Diagnosis
Presentation and Symptoms
Workup
Treatment
Outcomes
CONCLUSION

INTRODUCTION

Chronic limb-threatening ischemia in the upper extremity, and in particular, chronic hand ischemia is relatively unusual and arterial occlusions are often an incidental finding on physical, ultrasonic, or arteriographic examination.[1] The presence of rich collateral networks, small muscle mass, and ease of adaptation of activity of the upper extremity mitigates against symptomatic disease. For management purposes of, occlusive disease of the upper limb arteries can be classified as above-the-elbow arteries (innominate, subclavian, axillary, and humeral) or below-the-elbow arteries (radial, ulnar, interosseous, and hand arteries).[2,3] Compared with lower extremity ischemia, direct reconstruction of upper extremity arterial occlusive disease constitutes less than 4% of all vascular bypass procedures and as a result, there is limited data available on outcomes.[4,5] It has been estimated that only 5% of patients with limb ischemia have symptomatic involvement of the upper extremity.[6] Chronic critical ischemia of the hand due to atherosclerotic disease is rare but is a disabling condition.[1] Below elbow disease is a frequent problem in diabetics mirroring the problem in the lower extremities. The majority of the literature on digital ischemia has concentrated on nonatherosclerotic occlusive disease of the hand. Porter and Taylor[7] demonstrated that small arterial occlusive disease of the palmar and digital arteries due to diverse causes, is a frequent cause of upper extremity ischemia.

PATHOLOGY

Several disease processes involve the upper extremity and many are shared with the lower extremity.

- Atherosclerosis: Atherosclerotic occlusive disease is common etiology of above elbow disease[8] and most commonly presents with arm claudication or distal embolism. Its most common location is in the proximal subclavian artery.
- Diabetes: The increasing incidence of diabetes mellitus is leading to an increasing prevalence of below elbow disease and increasing small vessel disease of the hand.[9] This has led to more common presentations with armrest pain and/or distal gangrene. Its most common location is in the distal radial and ulnar arteries and the metacarpal and digital arteries of the hand.
- Vasculitides: Giant cell arteritis of the arm is referred to as large vessel vasculitis and patients with predominant large vessel vasculitis are

usually affected at a younger age and often have nonspecific manifestations such as constitutional syndrome, fever of unknown origin, or refractory/ atypical polymyalgia rheumatica.[10] The condition is seen in the above elbow vasculature and leads to claudication or rest pain.

- Autoimmune digital diseases: Ischemic finger ulceration due to digital occlusive disease has an autoimmune disease etiology in 54% of cases: hypersensitivity angiitis in 22%, Buerger's disease in 9%, arteriosclerosis obliterans in 9%, and miscellaneous diseases in remaining 6%.[11,12]
- Chronic thromboembolism: An upstream source of intermittent but continuous atheroembolism to the forearm and hand is recognized as a contributing pathology to hand ischemia and arm claudication. These situations require treatment of the culprit lesion in addition to the treatment of the presenting hand issues.

DIFFERENTIAL DIAGNOSIS

The differential diagnosis of chronic upper extremity ischemia is dependent on the gender and age of the patient and their pre-existing comorbidities.

PRESENTATION AND SYMPTOMS

In general, many patients will be asymptomatic in the presence of chronic upper extremity ischemia and many may have adapted to the restrictions placed on them by the symptoms which they have experienced. In those presenting with symptoms, the constellation is similar to the lower extremity except neurological and cardiac symptoms induced by inflow disease before the vertebral artery or internal mammary artery in the setting of a Coronary Artery Bypass Surgery (CABG).

- Claudication: Patients will complain of tiredness in the arm with activity, which is reproducible and dissipates with rest.
- Critical ischemia: Patients will complain of digital and hand rest pain relieved by dependency, but this can be intermittent in nature. They will complain of weakness and inability to complete tasks with the arm in question. Many will present with digital ulcers which can be painless or painful similar to rest pain. Many of these ulcers will progress over time.
- Vertebral Steal Syndrome. A unique feature of chronic upper extremity ischemia is proximal subclavian disease.[13] In this setting, patients may develop vertebral steal which is often asymptomatic but with arm exertion can lead to syncopal symptoms as the steal is exacerbated.
- Coronary Subclavian Steal Syndrome. A rare but important phenomenon in the setting of a prior CABG with IMA is the development of proximal subclavian disease leading to exertional angina and upper extremity symptoms.[14]

WORKUP

- Blood tests: Given the range of pathology that can present in the upper extremity, standard laboratory workup is appropriate and should include measure of renal function, Hb_{AiC}, and a lipid panel. However, serology testing for vasculitis and possible hypercoagulability may be required, if imaging suggests the features of vasculitis or chronic thromboembolism.
- Noninvasive imaging: The first test to perform is to examine the blood pressure between the arms of the patient, which can identify inflow diseases. Segmental pressures and finger brachial indices allow for a determination of perfusion and potential localization of a culprit lesion If there is a 20 mmHg drop between segments. Finally, duplex ultrasound of the upper extremity can provide information on the size, location, acoustic characteristics, and extent of vascular disease present and also allow for vein mapping for potential bypass conduit. In the case of proximal subclavian disease, direct imaging of the vertebral artery and using provocative testing can identify vertebral steal physiology.
- Computed tomography angiogram (CTA): It is now the most common next step imaging to illustrate pertinent anatomy and allow for preoperative planning. The technique does expose the patient to ionizing radiation and

requires intravenous contrast. It can be considered redundant if based on noninvasive imaging; the plan is to proceed with percutaneous intervention and contrast angiography.

- Magnetic resonance angiography: It requires no ionizing radiation, does not induce vasospasm, and has no renal side effects. It can demonstrate the fine detail of small and diseased vessels when enhanced by the administration of gadolinium (with the caveat of its renal toxicity warnings) or alternatives such as superparamagnetic iron oxide MR contrast agents.
- Contrast angiography: It remains a gold standard for much of upper extremity imaging. Access can be retrograde femoral to the upper extremity in question, retrograde from the radial or brachial in the ipsilateral upper extremity, and finally, antegrade axillary or brachial in the ipsilateral upper extremity. With percutaneous access obtained, endovascular intervention can be performed using the wire platform and treatment system with which the operator is most comfortable.
- Ancillary imaging: If there is a concern of a vertebral steal syndrome, then a carotid vertebral duplex is indicated. In the setting of coronary subclavian steal syndrome, transthoracic echocardiography, cardiac stress testing, and invasive coronary imaging may be required.

TREATMENT

The treatment algorithm for the patient should be designed to treat the systemic issues of underlying pathology, and then address the local issues manifesting in the upper extremity based on presenting symptoms of claudication (Figure 33-1) or critical ischemia (Figure 33-2).

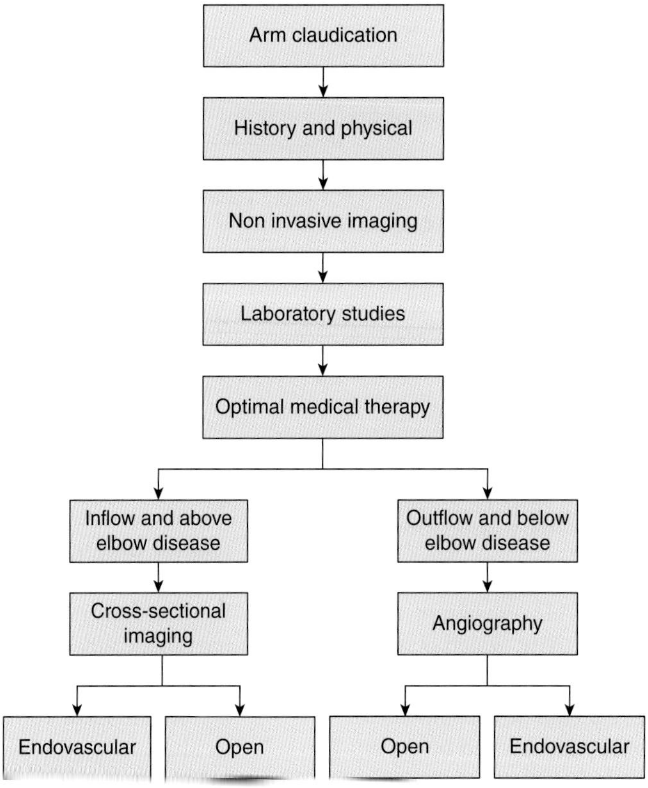

FIGURE 33-1 A treatment algorithm for the treatment of patients with arm claudication.

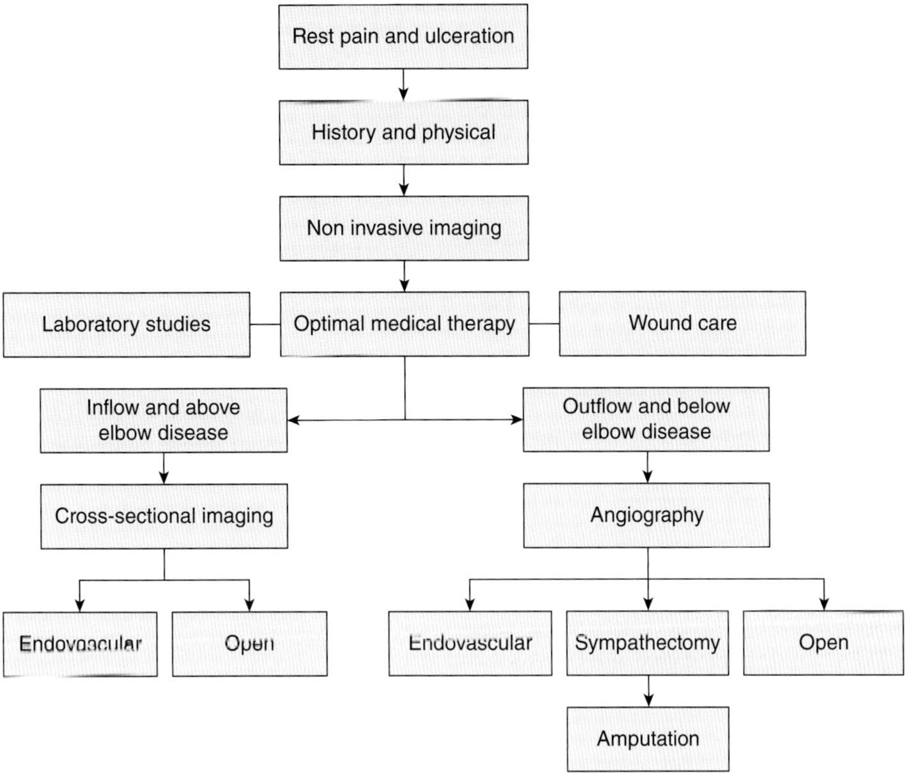

FIGURE 33-2 **A treatment algorithm for the treatment of patients with critical ischemia of the arm.**

- Medical: Medical management should seek to mitigate all cardiovascular risk factors in those presenting with atherosclerosis and diabetes. The vascular surgeon should follow the current national guidelines and engage the appropriate PCP for longitudinal care.[15] First line management for vasospastic disease begins with lifestyle modification in combination with medications (antiplatelet or vasodilator therapy). In cases of vasculitis, immunosuppression will be important, and acute and long-term case management should be coordinated with rheumatology faculty.
- Wound care: Local wound care with or without adjunctive appropriate hyperbaric oxygen therapy should be aggressively pursued to manage digital and hand wounds. Antimicrobial therapy should be guided by cultures, bone biopsies, and imaging that can assess for osteomyelitis.
- Infusion therapy: In some centers, intravenous prostaglandin E_1 is offered, when there is small vessel disease. Prostaglandin E_1 used as its synthetic form, alprostadil, is a vasodilator and smooth muscle relaxant. It is often used off-label to treat ulceration from Raynaud's phenomenon due to systemic sclerosis after standard oral therapies such as calcium-channel blockers and phosphodiesterase (PDE-5) inhibitors have proven insufficient. However, some studies indicate alprostadil has the same efficacy as a placebo. Active cardiovascular disease can be a contraindication or a clinical caution to the use of intravenous prostaglandin E_1.
- Cervico-thoracic sympathectomy: Cervico-thoracic sympathetic ablation was historically indicated for ischemia, but its use has declined to a few selected cases of thromboangiitis obliterans (Buerger's disease), micro-emboli, primary Raynaud's phenomenon and Raynaud's

phenomenon secondary to collagen diseases, paraneoplastic syndrome, frostbite, and vibration syndrome with either rest pain or ulceration.[16] A preliminary chemical sympathetic block is advised as it should suggest what benefit could be expected from the procedure. Using a VATS procedure with the patient in a semiseated position at 45° to 60° and with both arms abducted to 90°, the sympathetic chain is identified between T2 and T4 levels. The sympathetic chain is fully mobilized, and a resection is performed from the lower level of the second rib to the upper level of the fourth rib.

- Palmar sympathectomy and BOTOX therapy. In a palmar sympathectomy, the adventitia of the proper and common digital arteries is excised, removing sympathetic fibers contained in the adventitia and some of the media.[17] The aim of the intervention is to increase vessel dilation by interrupting the sympathetic tome to the digital and by removing the constrictive cuff of periadventitial fibrosis surrounding the arteries that is inherent to the pathophysiology. Local injection of botulinum toxin (100 units of botulinum toxin A per hand) around the relevant neurovascular bundle has also been shown to have a beneficial effect.[18]
- Endovascular procedures: Endovascular interventions are more frequent in above elbow disease than in below elbow disease. In general, angioplasty and balloon expandable stenting are used within the axillo-subclavian segments, and angioplasty with optional self-expanding stenting is used in the brachial and forearm vessels. Choice of access and technology is diverse in the literature and is operator-dependent.
- Open procedures: Open surgery is common for the treatment of above and below elbow disease. Synthetic grafts can be used to bypass the axillo-subclavian segments with the carotid artery being the most common inflow vessel, while autologous vein is preferred when the target outflow vessel is below the elbow with the brachial artery being the most common inflow vessel.

OUTCOMES

- Wound care: Advanced wound care, antibiotics, and local resection/debridement resulted in long-term healing without recurrence in 88% of patients with digital ulceration studied. In comparative studies, patients receiving wound care, where no open or endovascular intervention could be performed but with some having a palmar sympathectomy, had similar outcomes to the patients reported in the cohorts with nonatherosclerotic disease (80% healing rate). The arterial anatomy in these patients who are moved to wound care is similar to that found in autoimmune disease with palmar arch disease and poor digital runoff.
- Infusion therapy: A 75% healing rate followed treatment with intravenous prostaglandin E_1 infusion in selected patients with digital ischemia has been reported.[19] Most of this data is related to patients with collagen vascular disease.
- Cervico-thoracic sympathectomy: In very selected patients, a 75% healing rate has been attributed to the performance of cervicothoracic sympathectomy for digital ischemia.[20,21] The general consensus is that there is a very limited role for cervicothoracic sympathectomy in digital ulceration.
- Palmar sympathectomy: Surgery can result in 68% improvement through both healed amputations and ulcer healing.
- BOTOX therapy: Local injection of botulinum toxin has been reported to provide a 70% recovery from ulceration and rest pain in selected patients.
- Endovascular procedures: Endovascular interventions are usually the first-line treatment in patients with high risk who have stenotic disease. Multiple reports have demonstrated the success and durability of above-elbow endovascular interventions for ischemia,[22–26] but there is very limited data on the outcomes of interventions for chronic critical hand ischemia due to below-the-elbow atherosclerotic occlusive disease.[27] In a recent retrospective report, where patients with critical ischemia

(tissue loss and rest pain) who underwent endovascular revascularization, the secondary patencies at 5 years were 54% ± 9% at 5 years.[28] Forty-four percent of the patients in the Endo underwent additional endovascular interventions for restenosis or occlusion of one vessel to maintain patency.

- Open procedures: Open surgical repair is usually the first-line treatment in patients with low risk who have occlusive disease. A recent meta-analysis of patients with subclavian artery disease demonstrated that outcomes were equivalent for open and endovascular reconstructions in the above elbow disease.[29] In below elbow disease, McCarthy et al.[30] have demonstrated a 2-year patency rate of 53% for bypasses distal to the brachial bifurcation. However, major amputation was not required in any case, even after graft occlusion.[30] Kleene et al. reported that at a single center, an aggressive forearm bypass strategy with vein will yield effective hand salvage and that the bypasses have a cumulative patency of 90% at 18 months.[31] At 18 months, they saw an 8% major amputation rate with 40% occurring despite a patent bypass. In a recent retrospective report by Cheun et al., where patients with critical ischemia (tissue loss and rest pain) underwent open revascularization by bypass with a secondary patency of 69% ± 9% at 5 years.[28] Fifty percent of patients undergoing bypass underwent open or endovascular intervention to maintain patency with 20% in the inflow tract, 50% in the body of the graft, and the remainder in the outflow tract.
- Functional outcomes: One study examined the functional outcomes after surgery for upper extremity ischemia using Patient-Reported Outcomes Measurement Information System (PROMIS) Physical Function (PF), Upper Extremity(UE), Pain Interference (PI), and Depression domains.[32] Patients undergoing surgical treatment for upper extremity ischemia experience a worsening of functional symptoms initially within 3 weeks of surgery, as expected, followed by a notable improvement in the mid-term defined as greater than 3 weeks and up to 1 year (52 weeks) after surgery.

CONCLUSION

The local outcome of severe upper extremity ischemia is generally favorable, with good response to both medical management and/or digital amputation. Conservative therapy in patients with no revascularization options shows results in lower wound healing rates compared to both endovascular and bypass interventions but does not result in major amputation. The predictors of wound healing are technical success of the revascularization, the presence of an intact palmar arch, and presence of digital run-off. It is important to keep in mind that the life expectancy of patients with upper extremity ischemia from true atherosclerotic disease is dismal. Therefore, surgical intervention should be reserved for infection control or pain relief only in selected patients.

REFERENCES

1. Higgins JP, McClinton MA. Vascular insufficiency of the upper extremity. *J Hand Surg*. 2010;35(9):1545-1553.
2. McNamara MF, Takaki HS, Yao J, Bergan JJ. A systematic approach to severe hand ischemia. *Surgery*. 1978;83(1):1-11.
3. Bingham HG. A systematic approach to severe hand ischemia. *Plast Reconstr Surg*. 1978;62(5):814.
4. Harris RW, Andros G, Dulawa LB, Oblath RW, Salles-Cunha SX, Apyan R. Large-vessel arterial occlusive disease in symptomatic upper extremity. *Arch Surg*. 1984;119(11):1277-1282.
5. Bergqvist D, Ericsson B, Konrad P, Bergentz S-E. Arterial surgery of the upper extremity. *World J Surg*. 1983;7(6):786-791.
6. Welling RE, Cranley JJ, Krause RJ, Hafner CD. Obliterative arterial disease of the upper extremity. *Arch Surg*. 1981;116(12):1593-1596.
7. Porter JM, Taylor LM. Limb ischemia caused by small artery disease. *World J Surg*. 1983;7(3):326-333.
8. Narula N, Dannenberg AJ, Olin JW, et al. Pathology of peripheral artery disease in patients with critical limb ischemia. *J Am Coll Cardiol*. 2018;72(18):2152-2163.

9. Soyoye DO, Abiodun OO, Ikem RT, Kolawole BA, Akintomide AO. Diabetes and peripheral artery disease: a review. *World J Diabetes.* 2021;12(6):827-838.
10. González-Gay MA, Prieto-Peña D, Martínez-Rodríguez I, et al. Early large vessel systemic vasculitis in adults. *Best Prac Res Clin Rheumatol.* 2019;33(4):101424.
11. Mills JL, Friedman EI, Taylor L Jr, Porter JM. Upper extremity ischemia caused by small artery disease. *Ann Surg.* 1987;206(4):521-528.
12. Edwards JM. Upper extremity ischemia: small artery occlusive disease. In: Hallett JW Jr, Mills JL Sr, Earnshaw JJ, et al, eds. *Comprehensive Vascular and Endovascular Surgery.* 2nd ed. Philadelphia, PA: Elsevier; 2009: 309-317.
13. Kikkeri NS, Nagalli S. *Subclavian Steal Syndrome.* StatPearls [Internet]: StatPearls Publishing; 2021.
14. Lak HM, Shah R, Verma BR, Roselli E, Caputo F, Xu B. Coronary subclavian steal syndrome: a contemporary review. *Cardiol.* 2020;145(9):601-607.
15. Kinoshita M, Yokote K, Arai H, et al. Japan atherosclerosis society (JAS) guidelines for prevention of atherosclerotic cardiovascular diseases 2017. *J Atheroscler Thromb.* 2018;25(9):846-984.
16. Hashmonai M, Cameron AE, Licht PB, Hensman C, Schick CH. Thoracic sympathectomy: a review of current indications. *Surg Endosc.* 2016;30(4):1255-1269.
17. Sampson CE. Periarterial sympathectomy in the treatment of upper extremity peripheral vascular disease. In: Hyam JA, Pereira EAC, Green AL, eds. *Surgery of the Autonomic Nervous System.* Oxford: Oxford University Press; 2016: 129-141.
18. Van Beek AL, Lim PK, Gear AJ, Pritzker MR. Management of vasospastic disorders with botulinum toxin A. *Plast Reconstr Surg.* 2007;119(1):217-226.
19. Pardy BJ, Lewis JD, Eastcott H. Preliminary experience with prostaglandins E1 and I2 in peripheral vascular disease. In: Bircks W, Ostermeyer J, Schulte HD, eds. *Cardiovascular Surgery 1980.* Berlin, Heidelberg: Springer; 1981:720.
20. Dale WA. Occlusive arterial lesions of the wrist and hand. *J Tenn Med Assoc.* 1964;57:402-406.
21. Wheeler E, Barker WF, Machleder H. Treatment of upper extremity ischemia by cervico-dorsal sympathectomy. *Vasc Surg.* 1979;13(6):399-404.
22. Byrne C, Tawfick W, Hynes N, Sultan S. Ten-year experience in subclavian revascularisation. A parallel comparative observational study. *Vascular.* 2016;24(4): 378-382.
23. Bakken AM, Palchik E, Saad WE, et al. Outcomes of endoluminal therapy for ostial disease of the major branches of the aortic arch. *Ann Vasc Surg.* 2008;22(3): 388-394.
24. Palchik E, Bakken AM, Wolford HY, Saad WE, Davies MG. Subclavian artery revascularization: an outcome analysis based on mode of therapy and presenting symptoms. *Anna Vasc Surg.* 2008;22(1):70-78.
25. Palchik E, Bakken AM, Wolford HY, Waldman DL, Davies MG. Evolving strategies in treatment of isolated symptomatic innominate artery disease. *Vasc Endovasc Surg.* 2008;42(5):440-445.
26. Benhammamia M, Mazzaccaro D, Mrad MB, Denguir R, Nano G. Endovascular and surgical management of subclavian artery occlusive disease: early and long-term outcomes. *Ann Vasc Surg.* 2020;66:462-469.
27. Jones NF. Acute and chronic ischemia of the hand: pathophysiology, treatment, and prognosis. *J Hand Surg Am.* 1991;16(6):1074-1083.
28. Cheun TJ, Jayakumar L, Sheehan MK, Sideman MJ, Pounds LL, Davies MG. Outcomes of upper extremity interventions for chronic critical ischemia. *J Vasc Surg.* 2019;69(1):120-128. e2.
29. Galyfos GC, Kakisis I, Maltezos C, Geroulakos G. Open versus endovascular treatment of subclavian artery atherosclerotic disease. *J Vasc Surg.* 2019;69(1):269-279. e7.
30. McCarthy WJ, Flinn WR, Yao JS, Williams LR, Bergan JJ. Result of bypass grafting for upper limb ischemia. *J Vasc Surg.* 1986;3(5):741-746.
31. Kleene J, Shaw R, Hnath J, Chang B, Darling HC. Distal upper extremity bypass for hand salvage. Annual Meeting of the Society for Clinical Vascular Surgery; Las Vegas, NV 2018.
32. Bernstein DN, Cliburn JA, Lachant DJ, White RJ, Hammert WC. Evaluation of clinical recovery after surgical treatment for hand ischemia from vasospastic and occlusive disease using PROMIS. *Hand (NY).* 2021; 1558944721999727.

SELF-ASSESSMENT STUDY QUESTIONS AND ANSWERS

Questions

1. An early 30s male with a greater than two (2) pack-per-day smoking history complains of cool feet and hands on both sides, exacerbated by exposure to cold. He has tissue loss of his left fifth toe with dry ulceration only. Catheter angiography in this patient should demonstrate:
   A. Occlusive disease of the thoracic aorta
   B. Changes consistent with fibromuscular dysplasia in multiple vascular beds
   C. Abrupt vessel cutoffs distally in upper and lower extremities with so-called "corkscrew collaterals" present.
   D. Atherosclerotic occlusive disease of the extremities
   E. Arterial spasm

2. Of the following statements, which most clearly applies to observed outcomes in the care of patients with Raynaud's syndrome?
   A. Cold and tobacco avoidance is typically ineffective.
   B. Nifedipine has greater effectiveness in the treatment of patients with the obstructive form of Raynaud's syndrome than the vasospastic variant.
   C. Major amputation above the metacarpal–phalangeal joint is rare.
   D. Digital ulceration is most commonly treated by thoracic sympathectomy.

3. The greatest number of anatomic variations within upper extremity arterial vascular anatomy is observed in which of these arterial segments.
   A. Subclavian artery
   B. Axillary/brachial/radial/ulnar arteries
   C. Deep volar arch
   D. Superficial volar arch
   E. Innominate artery

4. Of the following connective tissue disorders, which is most frequently seen in Raynaud's syndrome patients?
   A. Rheumatoid arthritis
   B. Systemic lupus erythematosus
   C. Sjögren's syndrome
   D. Scleroderma

5. A male patient in their late 40s with a history of radiation therapy following neck surgery complains of left arm exertional pain with numbness over the past 6 months. CT angiogram demonstrates a critical (>80%) stenosis, 1.8 cm in length at the left subclavian artery origin. This is best treated in this case by:
   A. Carotid to subclavian bypass
   B. Plain old balloon angioplasty
   C. Subclavian to carotid bypass
   D. Angioplasty with balloon expandable stent placement
   E. Nonoperative management

6. The presentation of a cool, moist, blue hand that is exquisitely painful to touch most of the time correlates best with which of the following? (No hemodialysis access, catheter access, or other upper extremity invasive procedures have previously occurred in the limb.)
   A. Secondary Raynaud's phenomenon
   B. Scleroderma
   C. Primary Raynaud's disease
   D. Arterial embolus
   E. Reflex sympathetic dystrophy (causalgia)

SELF-ASSESSMENT STUDY QUESTIONS AND ANSWERS

7. Concerning arteriography for patients with unexplained digital artery occlusion, which of the following statements is TRUE?
   A. Arteriography is mandatory in any patient with suspicion for digital artery occlusion by noninvasive examination.
   B. The affected side *only* needs to be studied.
   C. Primarily patients suffering from unilateral disease will benefit from catheter arteriography.
   D. Computed tomography angiography (CTA) is adequate, and catheter angiography should be avoided considering possible embolic and access-site-related adverse events.

8. Nonatherosclerotic diseases typically impacting the great vessels proximal include all but:
   A. Giant cell arteritis
   B. Radiation arteritis
   C. Syphilitic aneurysms
   D. Takayasu's arteritis
   E. All of the above

9. In patients referred for evaluation of "subclavian steal" syndrome, which of the following are most likely?
   A. Objective and disabling neurologic symptoms
   B. Effort-induced muscle arm pain and fatigue ("upper extremity claudication")
   C. Roughly equivalent systolic blood pressures in bilateral arms
   D. Flow reversal in the ipsilateral vertebral artery
   E. Ultimately come to surgical or endovascular intervention

10. An early 70s female reports a history of diabetes and tobacco abuse complains of right arm pain and right middle finger gangrene is evident on examination. Also on examination, they have nonpalpable right brachial and radial pulses with only a Doppler signal present at the radial and ulnar arteries. A right upper extremity angiogram shows severe occlusive disease with brachial artery occlusion and reconstitution of the radial artery. The optimal treatment for this patient is:
   A. Antiplatelet agent, best medical therapy, and stop smoking
   B. Percutaneous angioplasty with stent placement
   C. Bypass from brachial to radial artery with GSV
   D. Bypass from brachial to radial artery with ipsilateral cephalic vein
   E. Bypass from brachial to radial artery with PTFE

SELF-ASSESSMENT STUDY QUESTIONS AND ANSWERS

Answers

1. C.
2. C.
3. B.
4. D.
5. D.
6. E.
7. C.
8. A.
9. D.
10. C.

CHAPTER

34 Atherosclerotic Carotid Disease

Rebecca A. Marmor and Mahmoud Malas

OUTLINE

BACKGROUND AND HISTORY
CLINICAL FINDINGS
DIFFERENTIAL DIAGNOSIS
Diseases Affecting the Extracranial Carotid Territory
DIAGNOSIS
MANAGEMENT OF THE CLINICAL PROBLEM
Symptomatic Carotid Stenosis
Asymptomatic Carotid Stenosis
Carotid Endarterectomy (CEA)
Perioperative Considerations
Intraoperative Considerations
Standard Endarterectomy
Eversion Endarterectomy
CEA Technical Pearls
CEA Complications
Transfemoral Carotid Stenting (TFCAS)
Perioperative Considerations
Stent Selection
Intraoperative Considerations
TFCAS Technical Pearls
Complications
Transcarotid Artery Revascularization (TCAR)
Perioperative Considerations
Intraoperative Considerations
TCAR Technical Pearls
Complications
Choosing a Carotid Intervention
CONCLUSION
ACKNOWLEDGMENT

BACKGROUND AND HISTORY

Stroke remains a major cause of morbidity and mortality both in the United States and abroad. Worldwide, stroke is currently the second leading cause of death, after ischemic heart disease, accounting for 11.8% of total deaths.[1] In the United States, stroke is the fifth leading cause of death and the leading cause of disability.[2] Among stroke survivors, quality of life continues to decline for an average of 5 years following the event.[3]

Eighty-seven percent of strokes in the United States are ischemic, with the remainder related to intracerebral and subarachoid hemorrhage.[4] Carotid atherosclerotic disease has been implicated as the cause of stroke (cerebral vascular accident [CVA]) via three major pathways:

1. **Embolic:** Unstable plaque embolization to the middle or anterior cerebral artery leads to transient ischemic attack (TIA) or stroke. This is the most common etiology of ischemic stroke secondary to carotid stenosis. High-risk plaques are soft and often radiolucent on cross-sectional imaging. They are fibrous ridges that have continuous penetration of lipids into the arterial wall. This results in an inflammatory cascade ultimately leading to lysis of

proteolytic enzymes resulting in necrotic debris and an unstable plaque.[5] Unstable plaques are rich with neovasculature that can rupture and lead to Intraplaque hemorrhage. This can increase the stenosis exponentially. Embolization occurs when the fibrous cap of the plaque ruptures. The underlying ulcer, which is exposed once the cap ruptures, serves as a nidus for platelet aggregation and puts the patient at risk for further embolic events.

2. **Hypoperfusion:** Less commonly, low flow state through a highly stenotic extracranial carotid artery can lead to hypoperfusion. In patients with poor collateralization, this can result in stroke.
3. **In-situ-thrombosis:** Acute thrombosis from dissection and/or atherosclerosis can lead to obstruction and stroke.

The carotid bifurcation is a high-risk location for atherosclerotic disease. The separation of flow between the high-resistance external carotid artery and the low-resistance internal-carotid artery leads to turbulent flow and plaque formation on the walls opposite the flow divider. Turbulent flow, coupled with an intimal injury, results in the inflammatory cascade leading to atherosclerotic plaque formation and eventual luminal narrowing. Luminal narrowing, in turn, leads to both increasing flow velocities and more turbulent flow. This resultant increased turbulence is a risk factor for embolic events.

Other risk factors for atherosclerotic carotid artery disease include hypertension, diabetes, hypercholesterolemia, obesity, genetics, and smoking.

CLINICAL FINDINGS

Atherosclerotic carotid disease classically manifests symptoms as:

1. **Transient ischemic attack (TIA):** Although traditionally defined as acute onset neurologic events with symptoms lasting less than 24 hours, the most recent American Heart Association guidelines define TIAs as "brief episodes of neurological dysfunction resulting from focal cerebral ischemia not associated with permanent cerebral infarction."[6] This new definition dispenses of the somewhat arbitrary time-threshold which prior studies have found was too broad and resulted in 30% to 50% of classically defined TIAs actually showing evidence of brain injury on diffusion-weighted magnetic resonance imaging (MRI). TIAs can portend stroke, with many studies demonstrating long-term elevated stroke risk.[7,8] Most studies find the risk of stroke in the first 90 days following TIA to be close to 10%.[9]
2. **Amaurosis fugax:** Amaurosis fugax is temporary monocular blindness from cholesterol embolization to the retinal artery via the ophthalmic artery. Patients may complain of sudden monocular vision loss lasting between 2 and 30 minutes. Classically described as a "shade coming down" in front of their eye, the episode resolves spontaneously. The symptoms occur on the ipsilateral side of the carotid stenosis. On retinal examination, there may be evidence of a cholesterol plaque lodged in a retinal vessel (i.e., Hollenhorst plaque).[10] Patients may also have persistent monocular blindness.
3. **Stroke (CVA):** Stroke symptoms can manifest as either sensory or motor changes. Sensory changes include numbness or paresthesias of the extremities. Motor deficits include dysarthria, dysphasia, aphasia, monoparesis, hemiparesis, and/or hemiplegia. When resulting from carotid disease, these symptoms occur on the contralateral side of the carotid stenosis due to the ipsilateral cerebral embolization. The American Heart Association (AHA) recommends utilizing a stroke severity rating scale, such as the NIH Stroke Scale/Score (NIHSS) to help describe the degree of neurologic deficit, identify changes to neurologic status, and identify patients who may benefit from thrombolytic or mechanical intervention.[11]
4. **Chronic ocular ischemic syndrome:** Chronic ocular ischemic syndrome is a severe chronic monocular visual deterioration resulting from critical ipsilateral carotid stenosis. It is the least common of the aforementioned

presentations. Patients may complain of gradual reduction of vision in one eye or frequent amaurosis fugax.[12] Carotid stenosis has been implicated in the pathophysiology of this disease process, and the surgical treatment of carotid stenosis has been shown to ameliorate symptoms.[13]

Just as important as recognizing what symptoms may be attributed to atherosclerotic disease is being able to recognize what symptoms are unlikely related to this disease process. Although the vascular surgeon may be asked to evaluate patients for carotid intervention whose primary symptoms include dizziness, syncope, vertigo, seizures, migraines, and scintillating scotomas, these are most commonly unrelated to carotid stenosis and warrant further evaluation to ascertain their etiology.

DIFFERENTIAL DIAGNOSIS

Atherosclerotic carotid artery disease is a potential cause of ischemic stroke.[14] However, other causes should be carefully assessed in a patient with carotid atherosclerotic plaque and TIA or stroke (Table 34-1). A thorough neurological evaluation is mandated prior to carotid intervention to exclude these etiologies.

DISEASES AFFECTING THE EXTRACRANIAL CAROTID TERRITORY

Various vasculopathies other than atherosclerosis can affect carotid arteries. Dissection, fibromuscular dysplasia (FMD) and vasculitides are among the most common differential diagnoses of atherosclerotic carotid disease (Table 34-2).[15–17] Differentiating the disease which affects the carotid artery requires precise clinical suspicion and evidence-based diagnostic evaluation. Diagnostic imaging with duplex, CTA, MRA, and conventional angiography is necessary based on the presenting symptoms. Diagnosis of vasculitis necessitates specific antibody testing and human leukocyte antigen (HLA) typing. Giant cell arteritis (GCA) and Takayasu disease are among the most common vasculitides which affect the extracranial carotid arteries.

TABLE 34-1 Differential Diagnosis of TIA and Stroke

Stroke	TIA
Ischemic Stroke	Extracranial carotid artery plaque
Atherosclerotic plaque	Seizures
Carotid artery dissection	Migraine headache
FMD	Syncope
Ischemic stroke: Small vessel	Transient global amnesia
Lacunar infarction	Carotid sinus hypersensitivity
Ischemic stroke: Embolus	Metabolic abnormalities
Cardiac embolus	Drug toxicity
Embolus from carotid plaque	Other causes of stroke with symptoms persisting less than 24 hours
Embolus from aortic arch	
Ischemic stroke: Hypoperfusion	
Cardiac failure	
Pulmonary embolism	
Hemorrhagic stroke	
Intracerebral hemorrhage	
Subarachnoid hemorrhage	
Other causes	
Metabolic causes	
Infectious causes	
Toxic causes	
Brain tumors	
Vasculitides	

FMD, fibromuscular dysplasia; TIA, transient ischemic attack.

DIAGNOSIS

As current US Preventative Services Task Force (USPTF) and Society for Vascular Surgery (SVS) guidelines recommend against screening asymptomatic patients for carotid stenosis,[18,19] most carotid stenosis is detected upon onset of neurologic symptoms. The SVS, however, does recommend screening for select patient populations (Table 34-3).[19] A carotid bruit may be the only indication of carotid stenosis on history or physical examination. Prior research

TABLE 34-2 Differential Diagnosis of Atherosclerotic Carotid Artery Disease

Differential Diagnosis	Common Location	Neurologic Findings	Diagnostic Evaluation	Key Point
Radiation-induced carotid stenosis	Similar to ACAD (longer plaque; maximal area of stenosis at the end of the plaque)	Similar to ACAD	DUS and CTA	History of radiation
Carotid artery dissection (Spontaneous)	ICA	Headache, Horner syndrome, hemispheric symptoms	CTA and CA	Absence of atherosclerotic risk factors except HTN
Carotid artery dissection (Traumatic)	ICA	Asymptomatic to lateralizing symptoms	CTA and CA	Head and neck trauma
Carotid artery aneurysm	Bifurcation, proximal, and distal ICA	Asymptomatic, pulsatile mass, lateralizing symptoms	DUS and CTA	High clinical suspicion
Carotid sinus hypersensitivity	Carotid sinus	Dizziness or syncope	Carotid sinus massage	High clinical suspicion
Moyamoya disease	ICA	Vary according to pediatric or adult-onset types	MRA and CA	High clinical suspicion; Japanese/East Asians
Carotid artery kinks and coils	ICA	Kinks are more symptomatic than coils	DUS, CTA, MRA, CA	High clinical suspicion
Lacunar infarcts	Intracranial small vessels	Depends on involved anatomic territory	CT, MRI	History of HTN and DM
Vertebral artery disease	Posterior circulation	Depends on involved anatomic territory	CTA, MAR, CA	Posterior circulation symptoms
Brachiocephalic artery atherosclerosis	LSCA, IA	Subclavian steal syndrome, stroke, TIA, thromboembolic events	CTA, MAR, CA	High clinical suspicion
Vasculitis	CCA, ICA	Vary according to disease type, stage, and anatomical territory	DUS, CTA, MRA, CA	Specific antibody testing and HLA typing
FMD	ICA	Asymptomatic, TIA, stroke	DUS, CTA, CA	High clinical suspicion; absence of atherosclerotic risk factors except smoking

ACAD, atherosclerotic carotid artery disease; CA, conventional angiography; CCA, common carotid artery; CT, computed tomography; CTA, commuted tomography angiography; DM, diabetes mellitus; DUS, duplex ultrasound; FMD, fibromuscular dysplasia; HLA, human-leukocyte antigen; HTN, hypertension; IA, innominate artery; ICA, internal carotid artery; LSCA, left subclavian artery; MRA, magnetic resonance angiography; MRI, magnetic resonance imaging; TIA, transient ischemic attack.

has demonstrated that the presence of carotid bruit is associated with an increased risk of both TIA and stroke[20]; however, the sensitivity and positive predictive value are low for detection of severe carotid stenosis.[21]

Once the specter of carotid stenosis has been raised, either based on risk factors identification and physical examination findings or presenting symptoms, duplex ultrasonography (DUS) is the primary diagnostic modality for identifying hemodynamically

TABLE 34-3 Society for Vascular Surgery (SVS) Indications of Screening for Asymptomatic Clinically Significant Carotid Bifurcation Stenosis

Patients with multiple risk factors who are fit for and willing to consider intervention+
Grade 1, Level of Evidence B
1 Patients with clinically significant PAD regardless of age
2 Patients ≥65 years of age with at least one of these risk factors:
CAD, smoking, hypercholesterolemia
Before CABG
Grade 2, Level of Evidence B
Most useful in three groups of patients:
1 Patients ≥65 years of age
2 Patients with left main disease
3 Patients with history of PAD

CABG, coronary artery bypass graft, CAD, coronary artery disease, PAD, peripheral arterial disease.

+The presence of bruit increases the likelihood of a significant stenosis in this group of patients.

Data from Ricotta JJ, Aburahma A, Ascher E, et al. Updated Society for Vascular Surgery guidelines for management of extracranial carotid disease. *J Vasc Surg.* 2011;54(3):e1-e31.

significant stenosis. DUS is a favored imaging modality because it offers excellent sensitivity and specificity, is low cost, and avoids radiation.[22] Current SVS guidelines suggest that in the setting of unequivocal identification of stenosis of 50% to 90% in asymptomatic patients, DUS is sufficient to make decisions regarding intervention.[19]

Estimations of the degree of stenosis are determined by measuring the peak systolic velocity (PSV), end-diastolic velocity (EDV), and the ratio of PSV of the internal carotid artery to common carotid artery (ICA/CCA). The two major DUS criteria for determining carotid stenosis are the modified University of Washington (UW) criteria and the Carotid Consensus Panel (CCP) duplex criteria (Tables 34-4 and 34-5). The CCP criteria incorporate ICA/CCA ratio and have higher thresholds for a given percentage of stenosis, whereas the UW criteria do not incorporate ratios. Prior research has demonstrated that CCP criteria have a higher concordance rate with CTA measurements and may be more sensitive as compared with UW criteria with sensitivity and specificity of 73% and 82%, respectively.[23]

Although DUS is an ideal study to evaluate carotid stenosis, there are a few limitations to the technique which should be mentioned. The quality of DUS is both technology- and operator-dependent.[24] Prior research has demonstrated that DUS results from nonaccredited vascular laboratories may be unreliable.[25] Additionally, high bifurcations, proximal

TABLE 34-4 Modified UW (Strandness) Criteria for Carotid Stenosis

Stenosis Severity (%)	ICA PSV (cm/s)	ICA EDV (cm/s)	Spectral Broadening
1%–14%	<125	N/A	None
15%–49%	<125	N/A	Present and minimal
50%–79%	>125	<140	Present
80%–99%	>125	>140	Diffuse and marked
Occluded	0	0	N/A

EDV, end-diastolic velocity; ICA, internal carotid artery; PSV, peak systolic velocity.

TABLE 34-5 Carotid Consensus Panel Duplex Criteria (CCPC) Duplex Ultrasound Criteria for Carotid Artery Stenosis

Degree of Stenosis (%)	ICA PSV (cm/s)	ICA EDV (cm/s)	ICA/CCA ratio	Carotid Plaque (%)
Normal	<125	<40	<2.0	None
<50	<125	<40	<2.0	<50
50–69	125–230	40–100	2.0–4.0	>50
70–99	>230	>100	>4.0	>70

CCA, common carotid artery; EDV, end-diastolic velocity; ICA, internal carotid artery; PSV, peak systolic velocity.

common carotid artery lesions leading to dampened waveforms, and extensive calcification causing acoustic shadowing can limit the ability of DUS to detect carotid stenosis.

Although decisions regarding surgical intervention for carotid stenosis can often be made based on DUS results, there are certain circumstances when corroborative imaging may be necessary. The SVS recommends obtaining adjunctive imaging for those with nondiagnostic DUS, asymptomatic patients with 50% to 69% stenosis, and/ or when evaluation of the proximal or distal vessels is needed to plan therapy.[19] Adjunctive imaging can include magnetic resonance angiography (MRA), computed tomographic angiography (CTA), or digital subtraction angiography (DSA).

MRA and CTA provide important anatomical information regarding the aortic arch, vessel tortuosity, presence of brachiocephalic or common carotid disease, location of the carotid bifurcation, and information regarding intracerebral collateralization. CTA is highly accurate for diagnosing carotid stenosis with overall sensitivity and specificity values of 97% and 99%, respectively.[26] Contrast-enhanced MRA has a sensitivity of 94% and specificity of 93% for high-grade stenosis.[22]

DSA remains the gold standard for diagnosing atherosclerotic carotid disease, however, carries with it an approximately 1% risk of stroke.[27] The majority of strokes during DSA are thought to be related to aggressive injection of contrast and air emboli. Just as with transfemoral carotid stenting, microemboli can occur during carotid angiogram; however, these are usually asymptomatic and not seen on follow-up MRI.[28]

MANAGEMENT OF THE CLINICAL PROBLEM

The management of atherosclerotic disease is based, in part, on patients' symptomatic status. Symptomatic patients are those who have suffered TIA within 6 months, stroke, and/ or amaurosis fugax. Extensive research has demonstrated that symptomatic patients achieve more benefit from carotid intervention than asymptomatic patients. However, there is a strong evidence that asymptomatic patients with severe stenosis will benefit from intervention. Management strategies for atherosclerotic carotid disease include medical management, carotid endarterectomy (CEA), transfemoral carotid stent (TFCAS), and transcarotid artery revascularization (TCAR). Below, we will elucidate management options given a patient's symptomatic status and discuss indications for the aforementioned approaches.

SYMPTOMATIC CAROTID STENOSIS

Patients with symptomatic carotid stenosis are at highest risk of ipsilateral stroke. Both the North American Symptomatic Carotid Endarterectomy Trial (NASCET) and the European Carotid Surgery Trial (ECST) demonstrated a direct relationship between the degree of stenosis and the risk of ipsilateral stroke if the disease goes untreated.[29,30] These landmark trials also validated the benefit of CEA over medical management for the treatment of carotid stenosis. The NASCET study was a randomized controlled trial comparing symptomatic patients treated with medical therapy (with aspirin) with those who underwent CEA for a >50% ipsilateral stenosis. Patients with severe stenosis (70%–99%) achieved a 2-year absolute risk reduction (ARR) of 6.7% for death or major disabling stroke as compared with patients treated with medical therapy.[29] Patients with mild-moderate (50%–69%) stenosis achieved a 5-year ARR of 4.7%.[29] The European trial confirmed NASCET findings with high-grade (>70%) stenosis, however, found no benefit for surgery over medical management for moderate (50%–69%) stenosis.[30]

The literature clearly demonstrates that patients with symptomatic, high-grade stenosis are best managed with intervention. However, the timing of intervention remains somewhat controversial. Traditionally, surgeons would wait at least 6 weeks prior to intervention to allow for resolution of the ischemic penumbra. However, much prior research has demonstrated that the 30-day risk of recurrent ipsilateral stroke is not insignificant, with a large meta-analysis demonstrating a 5.2% risk of ipsilateral stroke at 7 days in patients who had TIA.[31] Based on this literature, many advocated for early (<48 hours) intervention to maximize benefits of stroke prevention. However, research has demonstrated that patients undergoing CEA <48 hours from onset of symptoms have higher risk of perioperative stroke and death.[32] Current recommendations for patients with a mild-moderate stroke or TIA who have returned to their baseline is to undergo carotid intervention between 2 and 14 days following the event.[19] Patients with rapidly fluctuating neurologic status (i.e., both crescendo TIAs and stroke in evolution) should be considered for urgent or emergent intervention to reverse ischemia or salvage brain at risk.[33]

ASYMPTOMATIC CAROTID STENOSIS

Although intervention for high-grade symptomatic stenosis is clearly an evidence-based practice, intervention for asymptomatic disease remains controversial. The asymptomatic carotid atherosclerosis study (ACAS) is the seminal North American randomized control trial comparing outcomes of asymptomatic patients with >60% stenosis managed with CEA versus medical management. At 5 years, patients treated with medical management had an increased risk of ipsilateral stroke (11% for medical therapy versus 5.1% for CEA).[34] These findings were confirmed in the European Asymptomatic Carotid Surgery Trial (ACST), with a benefit for CEA in patients undergoing surgery over BMT with >60% carotid stenosis.[35] Both trials showed a significant relative risk reduction of stroke when undergoing CEA (53% in ACAS and 46% in ACST). Although these trials garnered enthusiasm for CEA in the asymptomatic patient, it is important to remember that when they were performed, optimal medical management consisted primarily of antiplatelet therapy with aspirin. In the ensuing decades since the publication of these trials, however, medical management of carotid stenosis has evolved with the use of statins, dual antiplatelet therapy, aggressive glycemic control, and increased uptake of smoking cessation. Risk reduction of stroke from these new regimens has been purported to be at or below levels achieved with carotid intervention. The medical community is eagerly awaiting results from the Carotid Revascularization and Medical Management for Asymptomatic Carotid Stenosis Trial (CREST-2) comparing current standards of optimal medical management with carotid intervention with CEA or CAS for asymptomatic patients with >80% stenosis.[36]

CAROTID ENDARTERECTOMY (CEA)

The first CEA was performed by Dr. Michael Debakey in 1953.[37] Since that time, the procedure has been one of the most common operations performed by vascular surgeons and has served as the "gold standard" by which other management strategies for carotid stenosis are evaluated. Numerous randomized trials have demonstrated its efficacy in preventing strokes in both symptomatic and asymptomatic patients.

Perioperative Considerations

When planning for CEA, the surgeon must consider what type of anesthesia is desired. CEA may be safely performed under general anesthesia (GA), regional anesthesia (RA) with a deep or superficial cervical block, or local anesthesia (LA). The impact of anesthetic choice on perioperative outcomes remains a matter of debate with our studies, suggesting that RA/LA is associated with decreased risk of MI[38,39] and others find no association.[40] Surgeon, patient, and anesthesiologist preference, local resources, and patient's medical risk may influence decisions regarding anesthetic choices. Additionally, the surgeon must determine what, if any, intraoperative cerebral monitoring s/he wishes to utilize. This decision is closely related to the anesthetic choice as patients who undergo CEA under LA/RA can undergo periodic neurologic examinations throughout the procedure, which are a surrogate for determining the adequacy of collateral flow during clamping. Patients undergoing CEA under GA, however, may be considered for cerebral monitoring to inform the decision regarding shunting. There are currently a variety of options available which include:

1. **Electroencephalogram (EEG) with somatosensory evoked potentials (SSEPs)**: The most widely utilized form of neuromonitoring which measures brain activity with 10 to 16 leads. A 50% drop in fast background activity indicates possible cerebral ischemia and may be considered an indication for shunting.
2. **Transcranial Dopplers (TCD):** It evaluates primarily the middle cerebral artery for changes in flow with clamping.
3. **Stump pressure measurement:** It requires clamping the common and external carotid artery while keeping the internal carotid open and using a transducer to measure back pressure. A mean pressure <40 mmHg is considered the standard threshold to indicate lack of clamp tolerance and indication for shunting.
4. **Cerebral pulse oximetry (Near Infrared Spectroscopy)** is a continuous, trans-cutaneous, noninvasive, optical-based method of measurement used to estimate cerebral tissue oxygen saturation.

Shunting is a hotly debated topic among vascular surgeons who exhibit a wide variety of practice patterns. A large study performed by our group looking at nationwide data found that 41% of surgeons routinely performed shunting, 46% selectively shunted based on intraoperative neuromonitoring techniques, and the remainder never shunting.[41] The data regarding the impact of the approach to shunting on perioperative outcomes are mixed and our recent work suggests that the impact of shunting may be related to anesthetic choice.[42]

Intraoperative Considerations

Patient position is of the utmost importance during CEA, especially for high lesions. The patient is placed in a supine position with a shoulder roll allowing for hyperextension of the neck. The neck is rotated away from the operative side. The patient is placed in a "beach chair" position, with a slight reverse Trendelenburg allowing for decreased jugular venous pressure.

Intraoperative ultrasound to mark the level of the bifurcation may be helpful and allow for smaller incisions centered on the lesion, a longitudinal incision is made along the anterior border of the sternocleidomastoid muscle (SCM). The dissection continues through the platysma muscle, and the medial border of the SCM is retracted laterally, exposing the internal jugular vein. The facial vein is the gateway to the carotid bifurcation and is usually doubly ligated and divided. The inferior boundary of the dissection is the omohyoid muscle. The carotid sheath is entered carefully to avoid injury to the vagus nerve. The common carotid artery is dissected circumferentially at the base of the incision and controlled with a vessel loop, followed by the external carotid and the internal carotid. The ICA dissection proceeds very carefully, avoiding excessive manipulation to prevent distal embolization. The hypoglossal nerve is identified and preserved in the superior aspect of the incision. After complete vascular control of the CCA, ECA, and ICA is obtained, intravenous heparin (80 mg/kg) is given and allowed to circulate for 3 to 5 minutes prior to clamping. The ICA is clamped first in an area free of atherosclerosis to allow for safe clamp placement, followed by the CCA and ECA. Depending on surgeon preference and results of neuromonitoring, shunting is next performed if indicated. Endarterectomy is next performed in either a standard fashion or by eversion endarterectomy.

Standard Endarterectomy

With standard endarterectomy, the surgeon, carefully separates the plaque from the intima with a freer elevator. The intima is irrigated and closely inspected to ensure small flaps or debris are removed. Not uncommonly, the area of the distal endpoint on the ICA has soft intimal flap that is tacked down with interrupted 6.0 prolene or silk sutures to prevent dissection when antegrade flow is restored. If the distal endpoint is not secured, the patient is at risk for acute carotid occlusion following CEA which can be a devastating complication.

Prior research by our senior author and others has demonstrated that the arteriotomy should be repaired with patch angioplasty.[43–45] Commonly used patch materials include bovine pericardium, dacron, and autogenous materials. Arteriotomies repaired via patch angioplasty have a decreased risk of perioperative death or stroke, as well as long-term risk for restenosis and ipsilateral ischemic stroke. No difference in outcomes between different patch materials has been observed.

If a shunt was used, the patch is almost completed prior to its removal and resumption of clamping. Prior to completing the patch, the ICA is back-bled and any debris which may have accumulated is cleared. Once patch is completed, the ECA and ICA clamps are removed first to ensure any remaining debris of thrombus does not proceed into the anterior cerebral circulation.

Eversion Endarterectomy

Eversion endarterectomy requires transection of the ICA at the carotid bulb with a small portion of CCA. The edges of the ICA are peeled back allowing for exposure of a cleavage plane between the intimal and medial layers. The atherosclerotic plaque is removed as it proceeds distally until a clean portion is encountered. Closure is accomplished primarily by anastomosing the ICA onto the CCA without compromising the lumen of the ICA. Eversion endarterectomy is advantageous as it does not require a patch closure with the potential need for prosthetic material. However, it can be very difficult to shunt and place distal tacking sutures with this technique. The EVERsion carotid Endarterectomy versus Standard Trial (EVEREST) demonstrated that there were no significant differences in the cumulative risks of ipsilateral stroke and death between patients repaired with standard CEA when compared with those repaired via eversion endarterectomy.[46] Interestingly, our study of the national vascular quality initiative showed that when eversion endarterectomy is compared with standard endarterectomy performed with patch angioplasty closure, there were no differences in postoperative outcomes. However, when eversion endarterectomy is compared with endarterectomy performed with primary closure, eversion endarterectomy is superior with a 30% reduction in risk of death and stroke at 30 days.[47]

After unclamping, the surgeon may consider the use of completion study to assess for technical issues. Commonly utilized completion studies include continuous waveform Doppler, intraoperative duplex, and intraoperative angiogram. Continuous waveform Doppler is inexpensive and readily available. It can confirm patency of the carotid vessels and indicate if there are potential issues based on the resistance heard or a high pitch Doppler sound indicating possible stenosis. However, it is not a sensitive technique for detecting small flaps or more subtle stenoses. Duplex ultrasound provides detailed anatomic imaging and can demonstrate the presence of intimal flaps or high-grade stenosis. Intraoperative angiogram is the gold standard of completion studies and requires the injection of contrast directly into the CCA. Completion imaging studies are certainly not a uniform practice among surgeons. Our group recent study looking at the practice patterns of vascular surgeons found that 45% never perform completion imaging.[48] Completion imaging is associated with higher rates of immediate re-exploration, return to the operating room, and longer operating times.[48] There is little evidence that completion imaging leads to lower rates of 30-day stroke or death.[49]

Following the completion study, meticulous hemostasis is obtained and protamine is given. Administration of protamine has been shown to decrease the need for re-exploration secondary to hematoma formation and has not been shown to increase the risk of periprocedural stroke.[50] Although many surgeons routinely utilize drains following CEA, a large analysis of Vascular Quality Initiative data demonstrated that drain placement did not reduce the return to OR for bleeding or reduce the risk of perioperative stroke or death. Drain placement was associated with increased length of stay, however.[51] Once the wound is closed, a full neurologic examination is performed prior to extubation if possible or immediately thereafter in the OR to ensure that there are no deficits.

CEA Technical Pearls

1. Dissection at the carotid bifurcation may result in bradycardia due to stimulation of the carotid body. This can be relieved by the administration of less than 0.5 mL of 1% lidocaine into the adventitia and directly into the carotid body.
2. Techniques to gain access to high lesions include careful division of the posterior belly of the digastric, subluxation of the mandible, removal of the styloid process, and nasotracheal intubation.

CEA Complications

The most common cause of perioperative death following CEA is MI. MI is responsible for 25% to 50% of all perioperative deaths after CEA in the early perioperative period as well as later on.[52] Stroke is one of the most feared complications following CEA. It can be the result of embolization during the procedure, hypoperfusion in the setting of an incomplete Circle of Willis, hyperfusion, and rarely, acute occlusion. The CREST trial demonstrated a 0.3% risk of periprocedural death, a 2.3% risk of CVA, and a 2.3% risk of MI for patients undergoing CEA, with a higher risk of all outcomes for symptomatic patients.[53]

TRANSFEMORAL CAROTID STENTING (TFCAS)

The first report of balloon angioplasty for carotid stenosis was published by Kerber et al. in 1980 but it was not until 2004 when TFCAS with distal embolic protection device (EPD) was approved by the FDA.[54] Indications for TFCAS are similar to those for CEA; symptomatic patients with >50% stenosis and asymptomatic patients with >80% stenosis may be considered for the procedure.

In its early phase, TFCAS was reserved for high-risk, elderly patients deemed to be too high risk for CEA. However, our group work demonstrated that octogenarians have double the risk of stroke with TFCAS compared to CEA.[55,56] An extensive literature has demonstrated that TFCAS confers a higher risk of periprocedural stroke as compared with CEA, however, still may be advantageous for medically and anatomically high-risk patients. The Stent-Supported Percutaneous Angioplasty of the Carotid Artery versus Endarterectomy (SPACE) trial is a noninferiority trial that randomized patients with >70% symptomatic stenosis to TFCAS or CEA. The study failed to prove the noninferiority of TFCAS at 30 days and concluded that the results "do not justify the widespread use in the short-term of carotid-artery stenting for treatment of carotid-artery stenoses."[57] Analysis of 2-year data, however, found that the rate of recurrent ipsilateral strokes did not differ between CEA and TFCAS, although patients treated with stenting had higher risk of recurrent stenoses.[58] Similarly, the European Endarterectomy Versus Angioplasty in Patients with Symptomatic Severe Carotid Stenosis (EVA-3S) randomized symptomatic patients with >60% carotid stenosis to TFCAS or CEA. The trial was stopped early secondary to a 2.5-fold higher risk for 30-day stroke and death in the unprotected TFCAS group.[59] Most recently, the Carotid Revascularization Endarterectomy versus Stenting Trial (CREST) randomized standard-risk symptomatic and asymptomatic patients with carotid stenosis to TFCAS or CEA. Although long-term follow-up data did not show a difference in risk of stroke and death between TFCAS and CEA at 10 years.[60] 30-day outcomes showed significantly higher rates of stroke among patients treated with TFCAS.[53]

Based on these data, most vascular surgeons currently reserve TFCAS for patients who are medically or anatomically high-risk for CEA (Table 34-6). Currently, the Center for Medicare and Medicaid Services (CMS) will only reimburse high-risk patients with symptomatic >70% carotid artery stenosis, thus also impacting surgeon selection for the procedure.

Perioperative Considerations

Careful review of preoperative imaging is essential prior to embarking on TFCAS. MRA or CTA with thin cuts are performed and include images from the aortic arch to the Circle of Willis. The surgeon must closely study the images to identify a diseased arch or tortuous anatomy, both of which can make

TABLE 34-6 High Risk Medical and Surgical Patients for CEA.

Clinical Criteria	Anatomic Criteria
Unstable angina	High lesion above C2
NYHA class III or IV CHF	CEA restenosis
LVEF <35%	Prior neck irradiation
MI <6 weeks	Cervical immobility
Severe pulmonary disease	Tracheostomy
Contralateral recurrent laryngeal nerve injury	Previous neck surgery

CHF, congestive heart failure; LVEF, left ventricular ejection fraction; NYHA, New York Heart Association.

cannulation of the carotid with wires or catheters challenging, and lead to higher risk of periprocedural stroke from excessive manipulation of the arch.

Aortic arches are classified based on anatomical criteria and tortuosity (Figure 34-1). Type III arches are the most difficult to navigate and are commonly considered a contraindication to TFCAS as they confer an increased risk of intraprocedural embolization.[61] The surgeon must also review imaging for additional possible contraindications to TFCAS including fresh thrombus, circumferential calcification, unstable plaque, and others (Table 34-7).

All patients planned for TFCAS should be started on dual antiplatelet therapy (DAPT) with aspirin and clopidogrel at least 7 days prior to surgery. Patients should also be on a statin, as our senior author's prior research has demonstrated a significant reduction in risk of death among patients on statins undergoing TFCAS.[62]

Ideally, carotid stenting should be performed in an angiographic suite or hybrid operating room with excellent imaging quality. Preoperative arterial line placement is preferred for close heart rate and blood

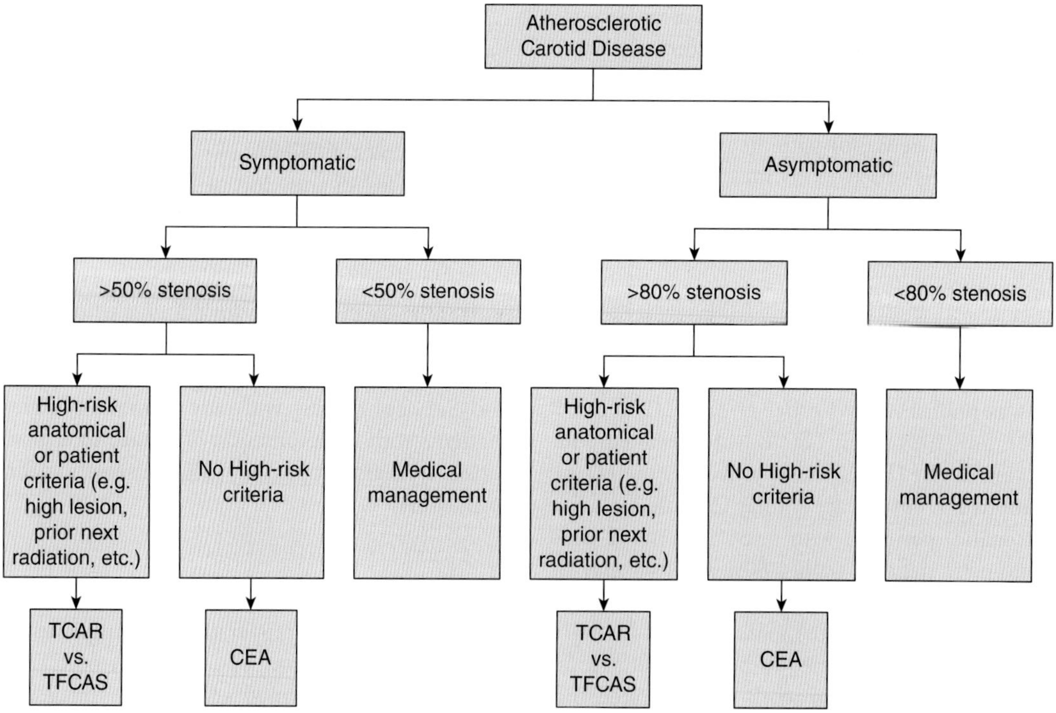

FIGURE 34-1 Arch types based on tortuosity. Type I allows easiest access to arch vessels. Type III arches require navigation of two 90-degree bends to access the common carotid arteries. This increases the risk of TFCAS leading to more manipulation of the arch and a lack of sheath stability. TFCAS, transfemoral carotid stent.

TABLE 34-7 Contraindications and High-Risk Features for Carotid Artery Stenting

Carotid Artery Stenting Contraindications
Severe ICA kinking
Unstable plaque
Fresh thrombus
Brachiocephalic vessel tortuosity
Brachiocephalic vessel severe stenosis or occlusion
Acute aortic arch angle or anomalous aortic arch (type III arch)
Significant aortic arch plaque or thrombus
Circumferential calcification
Poor arterial access

pressure measurement during and following the procedure. Because bradycardia and hypotension may occur with ballooning of the lesion, many surgeons prophylactically administer glycopyrrolate at the outset of the operation. Vasopressor agents including dopamine and phenylephrine should be readily available to be given if needed. Carotid stenting should be done under local anesthesia only in order to be able to adequately and frequently assess neurologic function, as well as to minimize the risk of cardiac complications.[63]

Stent Selection

Stents are sized based on the ICA and CCA. They come in straight and tapered configurations and are self-expanding. Most surgeons oversize the stent by 1 or 2 mm over the diameter of the CCA for straight stent. Both open and closed cell designs are utilized in the carotid. Open cell stents are more flexible and may be advantageous in a tortuous ICA. Closed cell stents are less flexible but may be used in symptomatic disease to lessen plaque embolization or extrusion. The evidence regarding the benefits of stent design is mixed,[64] and the decision about which type of stent to utilize is up to the discretion of the interventionalist.

Intraoperative Considerations

The patient is placed in a supine position with bilateral groins prepped. Standard ultrasound-guided retrograde femoral access is obtained. The patient is systemically heparinized in order to maintain activated clotting time (ACT) between 250 and 300 seconds. Arch angiogram is performed with a long diagnostic catheter placed through 90 cm, 6F shuttle select sheath parked in the proximal descending thoracic aorta, to evaluate the anatomy. The carotid artery is selected and the catheter is placed just proximal to the carotid bifurcation. Multiple catheter types are available for selection (e.g., H1, JB1, JB2, Vert, VTK, and SIM). In our experience, the majority of CCA can be selected with JB1 or vertebral catheters. VTK catheter is helpful in tortuous and bovine arches. Angiogram is performed to confirm carotid stenosis location and severity, assess external carotid artery patency and evaluate distal carotid artery flow and evaluate ipsilateral intracerebral circulation.

The 6 Fr shuttle select sheath is telescoped over the catheter and wire into the mid-CCA. It is imperative to avoid inadvertently manipulating the lesion and risk distal embolization. In difficult access anatomy, the ECA can be selected and stiff wire placed with the advancement of the sheath in a nontelescoped manner. Repeat angiogram through the sheath is performed with magnification and obliques views to mark bifurcation and ICA anatomy in anticipation of ICA cannulation and EPD placement. It is our practice to open and prepare balloon stents and wires prior to crossing the lesion. The lesion is crossed with EPD to place in the distal ICA. The remainder of the procedure is performed over the EPD wire via rapid exchange platform. The lesion is gently predilated with an undersized 3- to 4-mm balloon at low atmosphere pressure. Next, the preselected stent is advanced and carefully deployed to encompass the entire lesion. The proximal part of the stent is deployed in the CCA to stabilize the plaque. Our senior author's research was the first to demonstrate that postdilation of the stent is associated with an increased risk of stroke and death and hemodynamic compromise and thus should not be performed routinely, however, may be necessary in select cases.[65,66] After completion angiogram is performed, the EPD is removed. The femora sheath is removed and closure device is deployed. Our practice is to administer protamine to reduce the risk of access complications, and we had never encountered an increased risk of stroke with protamine.

TFCAS Technical Pearls

1. In difficult access anatomy, the ECA can be cannulated and stiff wire placed with the advancement of the sheath into the common carotid artery in a nontelescoped manner.
2. In order to minimize the time from predilation to completion stenting, it is ideal to open and flush the appropriate predilation balloon, stent, and EPD prior to crossing the lesion.
3. Postdilation should only be performed in very select cases as it has been associated with an increased risk of periprocedural stroke, death, and hemodynamic instability.

Complications

Stroke is the most serious and feared complication following TFCAS as it can have devastating consequences for patients. Etiologies of periprocedural stroke can include arch embolization, thrombosed EPD, acute stent thrombosis, stent kinking, carotid dissection, and hyperperfusion. Acute stent thrombosis is most commonly related failure of a stent to adequately expand in a dense plaque or circumferentially dense calcification. It usually requires immediate stent explantation and conversion to CEA. We have recently performed stent salvage procedures with TCAR under cerebral flow reversal.

EPDs can lead to their own set of complications. EPD filters can dissect the distal ICA and can also thrombose if they fill up with plaque or thrombus. It is our senior author's practice to have a rapid exchange suction catheter (Export catheter, Medtronic, Dublin, Ireland) to salvage acute thrombosis of distal EPD. Distal embolization may require neuro-rescue techniques including aspiration thrombectomy, catheter-directed thrombolysis, or stent retrieval. MI is another serious complication following TFCAS. CREST described a 1.1% rate of periprocedural MI with TFCAS, which was lower than that of CEA (2.3%, $P = 0.03$).[53] Access site complications including hematoma, pseudoaneurysm formation, arteriovenous fistula, thrombosis, and/ or infection can occur after TFCAS with or without the use of a closure device.

TRANSCAROTID ARTERY REVASCULARIZATION (TCAR)

TCAR is an innovative hybrid procedure that offers a minimally invasive approach to treating carotid stenosis by direct trans-carotid placement of the stent, thus avoiding arch cannulation and its attendant risks of embolization and utilizes a novel flow reversal technique in the carotid and ipsilateral cerebrum. Early results from the pivotal TCAR Roadster trial showed similar perioperative stroke rates as CEA in high-risk patients with a 30-day all-stroke rate of 1.4% and combined 30-day stroke and death rate of 2.8%.[67] Additionally, MI rates of TCAR are similar to those seen with CEA, and rates of cranial nerve injury are much lower. The initial ROADSTER trial reported a 0.7% rate of cranial nerve injury, with only one patient suffering from hoarseness from a potential injury to the vagus nerve which had completely resolved by the 6-month postoperative visit.[67] Our study of 1-year outcomes showed a 4.2% mortality rate (no deaths attributed to neurologic issues) following TCAR.[68] Importantly, the postapproval ROADSTER-2 trial has demonstrated an acceptably low rate of 1.7% for composite endpoint of stroke, death, and MI.[69] In our large analyses of several thousand patients undergoing TCAR in the Surveillance Project (TCP), performed by less-experienced operators, the risk of stroke and death was half that of TFCAS and similar to CEA.[70–73] The risk of CNI and MI was significantly lower than CEA.

Perioperative Considerations

Currently, TCAR is approved for high-risk patients with >50% symptomatic carotid stenosis or >80% asymptomatic stenosis. CMS mandates that hospitals participate in the Vascular Quality Initiative (VQI) Carotid Artery Stent Registry for the Society for Vascular Surgery (SVS). As compared to previous

TABLE 34-8 High Risk Medical and Anatomic Inclusion Criteria for TCAR

Clinical Criteria	Anatomic Criteria
Patient >75 years of age	Contralateral carotid artery occlusion
Patient with >2-vessel CAD and history of angina	Tandem stenosis >70%
History of unstable angina	High cervical carotid artery stenosis
NYHA functional class III or IV	Restenosis after CEA
LVEF <30%	Bilateral carotid artery stenosis
MI >72 hours and <6 weeks prior to procedure	Hostile neck but amenable to transcarotid access
Severe COPD w/ FEV1 <50% predicted	
Permanent contralateral cranial nerve injury	
Chronic renal insufficiency (>2.5 mg/dL)	

CHF, congestive heart failure; LVEF, left ventricular ejection fraction; NYHA, New York Heart Association.

high-risk criteria used for standard TFCAS, TCAR has wider high risk inclusion criteria (Table 34-8). Anatomic criteria for successful TCAR include ≥6-mm diameter CCA, CCA puncture site at the base of neck free of calcified plaque, ≥5-cm clavicle to carotid bifurcation distance (landing zone), and ICA diameter of 4 to 9 mm. Similar to TFCAS, patients must be treated with dual antiplatelet therapy for a minimum of 5 days prior to TCAR and should be started on a statin as well.

Intraoperative Considerations

TCAR is performed in a standard OR or hybrid operating suite. The procedure may be performed under general, regional, or local anesthesia. A radial arterial line is placed for continuous blood pressure monitoring. Patients are positioned similar to CEA, supine on the operating room table with a shoulder roll and the neck turned to the contralateral side. Ultrasound is performed to confirm adequate clavicle to bifurcation distance, that the CCA is free of atherosclerotic disease, and that the ICA remains patent.

A small incision is made at the base of the neck (transverse or longitudinal) in order to isolate the CCA in between the two heads of the sternocleidomastoid muscle. A 3- to 4-cm segment of CCA is circumferentially controlled and an umbilical tape with a Rummel tourniquet is placed proximally as possible under direct vision. A purse string 5-0 prolene suture is placed on the anterior adventitial surface of the CCA to facilitate arterial closure. Standard femoral venous access is then obtained under ultrasound guidance with the insertion of an 8 Fr sheath for flow reversal.[74]

The patient is then systemically heparinized with 100 units/kg of heparin for a goal ACT > 250 seconds. Micropuncture needle and wire are inserted into the carotid artery, and the micropuncture sheath is advanced in the carotid artery. A diagnostic angiogram maps out the carotid bifurcation. It is preferable to engage the ECA if patent is with microwire and sheath. Stiff wire is parked into the ECA and the EnRoute 8 Fr sheath (Silk Road Medical, Sunnyvale, CA) is advanced into the CCA and secured into place with silk sutures at two points on the skin. The arterial and venous sheaths are then connected initiating passive flow reversal via the dynamic flow controller and integrated 200 μL filter.

Next, TCAR time-out is performed confirming: (1) adequate anticoagulation with acceptable ACT level, (2) prophylactic administration of glycopyrrolate, (3) adequate mean arterial pressure (MAP) to allow significant delta between the arterial and venous pressure, and (4) the wire, balloon, and stent are open, flushed, and ready for use.

The CCA is clamped and active flow reversal is initiated. Debris that accumulates during the intervention is flushed out of the carotid and into the circuit where it is trapped in the filter. Blood is returned to the venous system. Next, the ICA lesion is crossed with 0.014 wire. As in TFCAS, predilation with a short 3- or 4-mm balloon is performed. The EnRoute stent is delivered and deployed via standard technique. Completion angiogram is performed to confirm adequate treatment. Poststent balloon dilation is reserved for severe residual stenosis, as it has been associated with severe hemodynamic issues and persistent poststenting hypotension.[66] Our recent study showed that poststent ballooning might not increase the risk of stroke with TCAR as we have shown in prior research on TFCAS.[75] Flow reversal is maintained for an additional 1 to 2 minutes to ensure no further accumulation of debris. The CCA is then unclamped and flow reversal is stopped. The carotid sheath is removed and the purse-string suture tied down. The venous sheath is removed and manual pressure held.

Meticulous hemostasis is obtained in the neck; drain placement is left to the surgeon's discretion. The wound is closed in multiple layers. Protamine is given to reduce the risk of bleeding with no evidence on increasing the risk of stroke.[76] Prior to leaving the OR, a good neurologic examination is obtained as is the case for all carotid interventions.

TCAR Technical Pearls

1. Some have suggested more aggressive pre-stent balloon dilation of the carotid lesion with a 5- or 6-mm diameter balloon, as the flow-reversal is more protective for atheroembolic lesions occurring during pre-stent dilation.
2. Many have moved toward systemic heparinization shortly after incision due to the quick dissection times, so the need for additional boluses does not delay the operation.

Complications

Risks of TCAR are similar to those for CEA and TFCAS. A large propensity-matched analysis of 5251 patients who underwent TCAR in VQI described an in-hospital 1.3% stroke rate for TCAR patients, similar to that of CEA.[72] More recently, our group has demonstrated a similar risk of stroke and death between TCAR and CEA with a larger propensity score-matched analysis including 6384 patients in each arm.[73] Importantly, however, TCAR has been shown to have decreased risk of periprocedural stroke as compared with TFCAS (50% reduction in stroke rate).[72] Additionally, the series described a low risk of MI (approximately 0.3%), similar to that of TFCAS. TCAR is associated with a >90% reduction in risk of cranial nerve injury and >50% reduction in risk of MI as compared with CEA.[73] Other associated complications include wound complications, postoperative hematoma, and access site complications at the femoral sheath site. Administration of protamine can significantly reduce that risk.[76]

Choosing a Carotid Intervention

Carotid interventions for patients with symptomatic (>50%) and asymptomatic (>80%) carotid artery stenosis are widely accepted practice.[77] Choosing which intervention to perform is the next step in the decision-making algorithm (Flowchart). CEA is the gold-standard treatment for atherosclerotic carotid artery disease. In multiple randomized trials, TFCAS has been associated with an increased risk of periprocedural stroke and death[53,59]; however, it may still be considered a viable option for revascularization in a subset of patients who are considered too high risk for CEA. TCAR has added an additional powerful tool to the vascular surgeon's armamentarium for treated atherosclerotic carotid artery disease. A multi-institutional analysis comparing TCAR and CEA outcomes showed similar 30-day and 1-year stroke rates (1.0% vs 1.1%; 2.8% vs 3.05%, $P > 0.05$, respectively) in spite of TCAR patients having higher rates of diabetes, hyperlipidemia, CAD, and renal insufficiency. TCAR was also associated with a decreased rate of cranial nerve injury (0.3% vs 3.8%; $P = 0.01$).[78] Additionally, although TCAR patients were older than CEA patients, they did not experience an increased incidence of stroke. This is especially important as prior research has demonstrated, whereas the risk of stroke following CEA remains constant across the age spectrum,[55] increased age is associated with an increased risk of stroke following TFCAS. Data comparing TFCAS directly to TCAR also shows the advantages of TCAR as well. In-hospital stroke and mortality rates are lower for TCAR, and there is no statistically significant difference in perioperative MI rates between the procedures. Long-term data is emerging to demonstrate the benefits of TCAR; at 1-year, TCAR is associated with a lower rate of stroke or death as compared to TFCAS.[71] Although TCAR has shown substantial advantages over TFCAS with decreased risk of stroke and death, not all patients may be suitable candidates for TCAR based on anatomical constraints (Table 34-8). Therefore, TFCAS will likely retain an important place in the toolkit of the vascular surgeon for the foreseeable future.

CONCLUSION

Atherosclerotic carotid artery disease remains a major source of morbidity and mortality in the United States as well as worldwide. Although there are no current recommendations for widespread screening protocols, any symptomatic disease warrants prompt evaluation by a vascular surgeon for consideration of possible intervention. High-grade asymptomatic disease warrants consideration as well.

Vascular surgeons currently have a wide range of tools in their arsenal to manage atherosclerotic carotid disease. Recent advances in medical management including statins, dual antiplatelet therapy, monitored smoking cessation program, and tight glycemic control have made a significant impact on the management algorithms for atherosclerotic carotid disease.[79] The result of the ongoing CREST-2 trial will help reestablish the indications for intervention among asymptomatic patients which will change with these advances. Additionally, although CEA remains the gold-standard approach to surgical management of carotid disease, TCAR represents an important paradigm shift conferring the benefits of a minimally invasive approach with a stroke risk similar to that of CEA. Finally, TFCAS remains an important part of the management algorithm for patients who may not be TCAR candidates based on anatomical constraints.

ACKNOWLEDGMENT

The authors wish to thank Sina Zarrintan, MD, MS, MPH for his invaluable contributions to the preparation of this manuscript.

REFERENCES

1. Collaborators GBDRF. Global, regional, and national comparative risk assessment of 84 behavioural, environmental and occupational, and metabolic risks or clusters of risks, 1990-2016: a systematic analysis for the global burden of disease study 2016. *Lancet*. 2017;390:1345-422.
2. Centers for Disease Control and Prevention (CDC): Stroke. Available at: https://www.cdc.gov/stroke/index.htm.
3. Dhamoon MS, Moon YP, Paik MC, et al. Quality of life declines after first ischemic stroke. The Northern Manhattan study. *Neurology*. 2010;75:328-334.
4. Benjamin EJ, Blaha MJ, Chiuve SE, et al. Heart disease and stroke statistics-2017 update: a report from the American heart association. *Circulation*. 2017;135: e146-e603.
5. Ross R. The pathogenesis of atherosclerosis: a perspective for the 1990s. *Nature*. 1993;362:801-809.
6. Easton JD, Saver JL, Albers GW, et al. Definition and evaluation of transient ischemic attack: a scientific statement for healthcare professionals from the American Heart Association/American Stroke Association Stroke Council; Council on Cardiovascular Surgery and Anesthesia; Council on Cardiovascular Radiology and Intervention; Council on Cardiovascular Nursing; and the Interdisciplinary Council on Peripheral Vascular Disease. The American Academy of Neurology affirms the value of this statement as an educational tool for neurologists. *Stroke*. 2009;40:2276-2293.
7. Kernan WN, Horwitz RI, Brass LM, Viscoli CM, Taylor KJ. A prognostic system for transient ischemia or minor stroke. *Ann Intern Med*. 1991;114:552-557.
8. Muuronen A, Kaste M. Outcome of 314 patients with transient ischemic attacks. *Stroke*. 1982;13:24-31.
9. Johnston SC, Gress DR, Browner WS, Sidney S. Short-term prognosis after emergency department diagnosis of TIA. *JAMA*. 2000;284:2901-2906.
10. Pula JH, Yuen CA. Eyes and stroke: the visual aspects of cerebrovascular disease. *Stroke Vasc Neurol*. 2017;2: 210-20.
11. Powers WJ, Rabinstein AA, Ackerson T, et al. 2018 Guidelines for the early management of patients with

acute ischemic stroke: a guideline for healthcare professionals from the American heart association/American stroke association. *Stroke.* 2018;49:e46-e110.

12. Costa VP, Kuzniec S, Molnar LJ, Cerri GG, Puech-Leao P, Carvalho CA. Clinical findings and hemodynamic changes associated with severe occlusive carotid artery disease. *Ophthalmology.* 1997;104:1994-2002.
13. Kawaguchi S, Iida J, Uchiyama Y. Ocular circulation and chronic ocular ischemic syndrome before and after carotid artery revascularization surgery. *J Ophthalmol.* 2012;2012:350475.
14. Conrad MF, Michalczyk MJ, Opalacz A, Patel VI, LaMuraglia GM, Cambria RP. The natural history of asymptomatic severe carotid artery stenosis. *J Vasc Surg.* 2014;60:1218-26.
15. Touze E, Southerland AM, Boulanger M, et al. Fibromuscular dysplasia and its neurologic manifestations: a systematic review. *JAMA Neurol.* 2019;76: 217-226.
16. Weyand CM, Goronzy JJ. Medium- and large-vessel vasculitis. *N Engl J Med.* 2003;349:160-169.
17. Lee VH, Brown RD Jr, Mandrekar JN, Mokri B. Incidence and outcome of cervical artery dissection: a population-based study. *Neurology.* 2006;67:1809-1812.
18. LeFevre ML, Force USPST. Screening for asymptomatic carotid artery stenosis: U.S. Preventive Services Task Force recommendation statement. *Ann Intern Med.* 2014;161:356-362.
19. Ricotta JJ, Aburahma A, Ascher E, et al. Updated society for vascular surgery guidelines for management of extracranial carotid disease. *J Vasc Surg.* 2011;54: e1-e31.
20. Pickett CA, Jackson JL, Hemann BA, Atwood JE. Carotid bruits and cerebrovascular disease risk: a meta-analysis. *Stroke.* 2010;41:2295-2302.
21. Ratchford EV, Jin Z, Di Tullio MR, et al. Carotid bruit for detection of hemodynamically significant carotid stenosis: the Northern manhattan study. *Neurol Res.* 2009;31:748-752.
22. Wardlaw JM, Chappell FM, Stevenson M, et al. Accurate, practical and cost-effective assessment of carotid stenosis in the UK. *Health Technol Assess.* 2006;10:iii-iv, ix-x, 1-182.
23. Kim AH, Augustin G, Shevitz A, et al. Carotid consensus panel duplex criteria can replace modified university of Washington criteria without affecting accuracy. *Vasc Med.* 2018;23:126-133.
24. Fillinger MF, Baker RJ Jr, Zwolak RM, et al. Carotid duplex criteria for a 60% or greater angiographic stenosis: variation according to equipment. *J Vasc Surg.* 1996;24:856-864.
25. Brown OW, Bendick PJ, Bove PG, et al. Reliability of extracranial carotid artery duplex ultrasound scanning: value of vascular laboratory accreditation. *J Vasc Surg.* 2004;39:366-371; discussion 71.
26. van Prehn J, Muhs BE, Pramanik B, et al. Multidimensional characterization of carotid artery stenosis using CT imaging: a comparison with ultrasound grading and peak flow measurement. *Eur J Vasc Endovasc Surg.* 2008;36:267-272.
27. Davies KN, Humphrey PR. Complications of cerebral angiography in patients with symptomatic carotid territory ischaemia screened by carotid ultrasound. *J Neurol Neurosurg Psychiatry.* 1993;56:967-972.
28. Gerraty RP, Bowser DN, Infeld B, Mitchell PJ, Davis SM. Microemboli during carotid angiography. Association with stroke risk factors or subsequent magnetic resonance imaging changes? *Stroke.* 1996;27:1543-1547.
29. Barnett HJ, Taylor DW, Eliasziw M, et al. Benefit of carotid endarterectomy in patients with symptomatic moderate or severe stenosis. North American symptomatic carotid endarterectomy trial collaborators. *N Engl J Med.* 1998;339:1415-1425.
30. Warlow CP. Symptomatic patients: the European carotid surgery trial (ECST). *J Mal Vasc.* 1993;18:198-201.
31. Giles MF, Rothwell PM. Risk of stroke early after transient ischaemic attack: a systematic review and meta-analysis. *Lancet Neurol.* 2007;6:1063-1072.
32. Tanious A, Pothof AB, Boitano LT, et al. Timing of carotid endarterectomy after stroke: retrospective review of prospectively collected national database. *Ann Surg.* 2018;268:449-456.
33. Karkos CD, McMahon G, McCarthy MJ, et al. The value of urgent carotid surgery for crescendo transient ischemic attacks. *J Vasc Surg.* 2007;45:1148-1154.
34. Endarterectomy for asymptomatic carotid artery stenosis. Executive committee for the asymptomatic carotid atherosclerosis study. *JAMA.* 1995;273:1421-1428.
35. Halliday A, Mansfield A, Marro J, et al. Prevention of disabling and fatal strokes by successful carotid endarterectomy in patients without recent neurological symptoms: randomised controlled trial. *Lancet.* 2004; 363:1491-1502.
36. Howard VJ, Meschia JF, Lal BK, et al. Carotid revascularization and medical management for asymptomatic carotid stenosis: protocol of the CREST-2 clinical trials. *Int J Stroke.* 2017;12:770-778.
37. Easton JD. History of carotid endarterectomy then and now: personal perspective. *Stroke.* 2014;45:e101-e103.
38. Hye RJ, Voeks JH, Malas MB, et al. Anesthetic type and risk of myocardial infarction after carotid endarterectomy in the carotid revascularization endarterectomy

versus stenting trial (CREST). *J Vasc Surg*. 2016;64:3-8 e1.
39. Dakour Aridi H, Paracha N, Nejim B, Locham S, Malas MB. Anesthetic type and hospital outcomes after carotid endarterectomy from the vascular quality initiative database. *J Vasc Surg*. 2018;67:1419-1428.
40. Group GTC, Lewis SC, Warlow CP, et al. General anaesthesia versus local anaesthesia for carotid surgery (GALA): a multicentre, randomised controlled trial. *Lancet*. 2008;372:2132-2142.
41. Wiske C, Arhuidese I, Malas M, Patterson R. Comparing the efficacy of shunting approaches and cerebral monitoring during carotid endarterectomy using a national database. *J Vasc Surg*. 2018;68:416-425.
42. Dakour-Aridi H, Gaber MG, Khalid M, Patterson R, Malas MB. Examination of the interaction between method of anesthesia and shunting with carotid endarterectomy. *J Vasc Surg*. 2020;71:1964-1971.
43. AbuRahma AF, Robinson PA, Saiedy S, Richmond BK, Khan J. Prospective randomized trial of bilateral carotid endarterectomies: primary closure versus patching. *Stroke*. 1999;30:1185-1189.
44. Bond R, Rerkasem K, Naylor AR, Aburahma AF, Rothwell PM. Systematic review of randomized controlled trials of patch angioplasty versus primary closure and different types of patch materials during carotid endarterectomy. *J Vasc Surg*. 2004;40:1126-1135.
45. Malas M, Glebova NO, Hughes SE, et al. Effect of patching on reducing restenosis in the carotid revascularization endarterectomy versus stenting trial. *Stroke*. 2015;46:757-761.
46. Cao P, Giordano G, De Rango P, et al. Eversion versus conventional carotid endarterectomy: late results of a prospective multicenter randomized trial. *J Vasc Surg*. 2000;31:19-30.
47. Dakour-Aridi H, Ou M, Locham S, AbuRahma A, Schneider JR, Malas M. Outcomes following eversion versus conventional endarterectomy in the vascular quality initiative database. *Ann Vasc Surg*. 2020;65:1-9.
48. Dakour-Aridi H, Ibrahim EA, Mathlouthi A, Naazie I, Cronenwett JL, Malas MB. Practice patterns in the use of completion imaging after carotid endarterectomy. *J Vasc Surg*. 2021;73(1):151-160.e2.
49. Wallaert JB, Goodney PP, Vignati JJ, et al. Completion imaging after carotid endarterectomy in the vascular study group of New England. *J Vasc Surg*. 2011;54:376-385, 385 e1-3.
50. Kakisis JD, Antonopoulos CN, Moulakakis KG, Schneider F, Geroulakos G, Ricco JB. Protamine reduces bleeding complications without increasing the risk of stroke after carotid endarterectomy: a meta-analysis. *Eur J Vasc Endovasc Surg*. 2016;52:296-307.
51. Smolock CJ, Morrow KL, Kang J, Kelso RL, Bena JF, Clair DG. Drain placement confers no benefit after carotid endarterectomy in the vascular quality initiative. *J Vasc Surg*. 2020;72:204-208 e1.
52. Hertzer NR, Lees CD. Fatal myocardial infarction following carotid endarterectomy: three hundred thirty-five patients followed 6-11 years after operation. *Ann Surg*. 1981;194:212-218.
53. Brott TG, Hobson RW 2nd, Howard G, et al. Stenting versus endarterectomy for treatment of carotid-artery stenosis. *N Engl J Med*. 2010;363:11-23.
54. Kerber CW, Cromwell LD, Loehden OL. Catheter dilatation of proximal carotid stenosis during distal bifurcation endarterectomy. *AJNR Am J Neuroradiol*. 1980;1:348-349.
55. Voeks JH, Howard G, Roubin GS, et al. Age and outcomes after carotid stenting and endarterectomy: the carotid revascularization endarterectomy versus stenting trial. *Stroke*. 2011;42:3484-3490.
56. Nejim B, Alshwaily W, Dakour-Aridi H, Locham S, Goodney P, Malas MB. Age modifies the efficacy and safety of carotid artery revascularization procedures. *J Vasc Surg*. 2019;69:1490-1503 e3.
57. Group SC, Ringleb PA, Allenberg J, et al. 30 day results from the SPACE trial of stent-protected angioplasty versus carotid endarterectomy in symptomatic patients: a randomised non-inferiority trial. *Lancet*. 2006;368:1239-1247.
58. Eckstein HH, Ringleb P, Allenberg JR, et al. Results of the stent-protected angioplasty versus carotid endarterectomy (SPACE) study to treat symptomatic stenoses at 2 years, a multinational, prospective, randomised trial. *Lancet Neurol*. 2008;7:893-902.
59. Mas JL, Chatellier G, Beyssen B, Investigators E-S. Carotid angioplasty and stenting with and without cerebral protection: clinical alert from the endarterectomy versus angioplasty in patients with symptomatic severe carotid stenosis (EVA 3S) trial. *Stroke*. 2004;35:e18-e20.
60. Brott TG, Howard G, Roubin GS, et al. Long-term results of stenting versus endarterectomy for carotid-artery stenosis. *N Engl J Med*. 2016;374:1021-1031.
61. Bijuklic K, Wandler A, Varnakov Y, Tuebler T, Schofer J. Risk factors for cerebral embolization after carotid artery stenting with embolic protection: a diffusion-weighted magnetic resonance imaging study in 837 consecutive patients. *Circ Cardiovasc Interv*. 2013;6:311-316.

62. Rizwan M, Faateh M, Dakour-Aridi H, Nejim B, Alshwaily W, Malas MB. Statins reduce mortality and failure to rescue after carotid artery stenting. *J Vasc Surg*. 2019;69:112-119.
63. Dakour-Aridi H, Rizwan M, Nejim B, Locham S, Malas MB. Association between the choice of anesthesia and in-hospital outcomes after carotid artery stenting. *J Vasc Surg*. 2019;69:1461-1470 e4.
64. Faateh M, Dakour-Aridi H, Mathlouthi A, Locham S, Naazie I, Malas M. Comparison of open and closed-cell stent design outcomes after carotid artery stenting in the vascular quality initiative. *J Vasc Surg*. 2021;73(5):1639-1648.
65. Obeid T, Arnaoutakis DJ, Arhuidese I, et al. Poststent ballooning is associated with increased periprocedural stroke and death rate in carotid artery stenting. *J Vasc Surg*. 2015;62:616-623 e1.
66. Qazi U, Obeid TE, Enwerem N, et al. The effect of ballooning following carotid stent deployment on hemodynamic stability. *J Vasc Surg*. 2014;59:756-760.
67. Kwolek CJ, Jaff MR, Leal JI, et al. Results of the ROADSTER multicenter trial of transcarotid stenting with dynamic flow reversal. *J Vasc Surg*. 2015;62:1227-1234.
68. Malas MB, Leal Lorenzo JI, Nejim B, et al. Analysis of the ROADSTER pivotal and extended-access cohorts shows excellent 1-year durability of transcarotid stenting with dynamic flow reversal. *J Vasc Surg*. 2019;69:1786-1796.
69. Kashyap VS, Schneider PA, Foteh M, et al. Early outcomes in the ROADSTER 2 study of transcarotid artery revascularization in patients with significant carotid artery disease. *Stroke*. 2020;51:2620-2629.
70. Schermerhorn ML, Liang P, Dakour-Aridi H, et al. In-hospital outcomes of transcarotid artery revascularization and carotid endarterectomy in the society for vascular surgery vascular quality initiative. *J Vasc Surg*. 2020;71:87-95.
71. Malas MB, Dakour-Aridi H, Wang GJ, et al. Transcarotid artery revascularization versus transfemoral carotid artery stenting in the Society for vascular surgery vascular quality initiative. *J Vasc Surg*. 2019;69:92-103 e2.
72. Schermerhorn ML, Liang P, Eldrup-Jorgensen J, et al. Association of transcarotid artery revascularization vs transfemoral carotid artery stenting with stroke or death among patients with carotid artery stenosis. *JAMA*. 2019;322:2313-2322.
73. Malas MB, Dakour-Aridi H, Kashyap VS, et al. Transcarotid revascularization with dynamic flow reversal versus carotid endarterectomy in the Vascular Quality Initiative surveillance project. *Ann Surg*. 2022; 276:398-403.
74. Malas MB, Leal J, Kashyap V, Cambria RP, Kwolek CJ, Criado E. Technical aspects of transcarotid artery revascularization using the ENROUTE transcarotid neuroprotection and stent system. *J Vasc Surg*. 2017;65: 916-920.
75. Dakour-Aridi H, Cui CL, Barleben A, Schermerhorn ML, Eldrup-Jorgensen J, Malas MB. Post-stent ballooning during transcarotid artery revascularization. *J Vasc Surg*. 2021;73(6):2041-2049.e1.
76. Liang P, Motaganahalli RL, Malas MB, et al. Protamine use in transcarotid artery revascularization is associated with lower risk of bleeding complications without higher risk of thromboembolic events. *J Vasc Surg*. 2020;72:2079-2087.
77. Kernan WN, Ovbiagele B, Black HR, et al. Guidelines for the prevention of stroke in patients with stroke and transient ischemic attack: a guideline for healthcare professionals from the American Heart Association/American Stroke Association [published correction appears in *Stroke*. 2015 Feb;46(2):e54]. *Stroke*. 2014; 45(7):2160-2236.
78. Kashyap VS, King AH, Foteh MI, et al. A multi-institutional analysis of transcarotid artery revascularization compared to carotid endarterectomy. *J Vasc Surg*. 2019;70:123-129.
79. Katsanos AH, Hart RG. New horizons in pharmacologic therapy for secondary stroke prevention. *JAMA Neurol*. 2020;77(10):1308-1317.

SELF-ASSESSMENT STUDY QUESTIONS AND ANSWERS

Questions

1. According to the Society of Vascular Surgery guidelines, screening for carotid stenosis is mandatory for which patient?
A. A 55-year-old male with ABI of 0.3 and left foot arterial ulcer
B. A 67-year-old male with 5.8-cm infrarenal AAA and no history of CAD, smoking, or hyperlipidemia
C. A 62-year-old female with 3 vessel CAD planned for CABG
D. A 52-year-old male with history of left neck radiation for squamous cell cancer 10 years ago
E. A 61-year-old female with history of hyperlipidemia

2. All of the following are examples of improvements in medical management which occurred since the publication of ACAS and NASCET except:
A. Increased uptake of recommendations to stop smoking among patients
B. Push for improved glycemic control in patients with carotid stenosis
C. Widespread availability of dual antiplatelet therapy
D. Statins
E. Increased screening for carotid stenosis and earlier detection of lesions

3. Maneuvers to gain distal control during CEA include all of the following except:
A. Division of the posterior belly of the digastric muscle
B. Subluxation of the mandible
C. Division of the omohyoid muscle
D. Nasotracheal intubation
E. Resection of the styloid process

4. Postdilation of carotid stent with balloon angioplasty has been shown to:
A. Improve long-term stent patency
B. Prevent stent thrombosis
C. Decrease risk of hemodynamic stability following the procedure
D. Increase periprocedural risk of hemodynamic instability, death, and stroke
E. Have no impact on periprocedural outcomes

SELF-ASSESSMENT STUDY QUESTIONS AND ANSWERS

Answers

1. A.
2. E.
3. C.
4. D.

CHAPTER

35 Vertebrobasilar Insufficiency

Mouhammad Jumaa and Diana Slawski

OUTLINE

ANATOMY AND PATHOPHYSIOLOGY OF VERTEBROBASILAR INSUFFICIENCY
- **Anatomy of the Vertebrobasilar System**
- **Vascular Supply to the Brainstem and Cerebellum**
- **Mechanisms of Vertebrobasilar Insufficiency**
  - Atherosclerosis
  - Acute Embolic Events
  - Vertebral Artery Dissection
  - Small Vessel Disease
  - Vertebrobasilar Dolichoectasia
  - Subclavian Stenosis
  - Bow Hunter's Syndrome

CLINICAL FEATURES OF VERTEBROBASILAR INSUFFICIENCY
- **Neurologic Symptoms**
- **Physical Exam Findings**

VERTEBROBASILAR SYNDROMES
- **Lateral Medullary (Wallenburg) Syndrome**
- **Medial Medullary (Dejerine) Syndrome**
- **Lateral Pontine Syndrome**
- **Ventral Pontine (Locked-In) Syndrome**
- **Top of the Basilar Syndrome**

DIFFERENTIAL DIAGNOSIS
- **Dizziness, Nausea, and Vomiting**
- **Double Vision or Diplopia**
- **Syncope and Coma**

DIAGNOSTIC MEASURES
- **Computed Tomography**
- **Magnetic Resonance Imaging**
- **Catheter-Based Angiography**
- **Ultrasound**

MANAGEMENT OF VERTEBROBASILAR INSUFFICIENCY
- **Acute Thrombotic Occlusion**
  - Medical Management
  - Surgical Management
- **Chronic High-Grade Stenosis or Occlusion**
  - Transient Ischemic Attack and Mild Strokes
  - Vertebral Artery Stenting
  - Acute Dissection
  - Bow Hunter's Syndrome
  - Subclavian Stenosis
- **Vertebrobasilar Dolichoectasia**
  - Medical Management
  - Surgical Management

ANATOMY AND PATHOPHYSIOLOGY OF VERTEBROBASILAR INSUFFICIENCY

ANATOMY OF THE VERTEBROBASILAR SYSTEM

Understanding vertebrobasilar anatomy is essential for accurate diagnosis and management of posterior circulation ischemia and stroke. The brachiocephalic trunk (also called the innominate artery) ascends within the thorax and divides into the right common carotid and the right subclavian at the level of the sternoclavicular joint, while the left subclavian artery arises directly from the arch of the aorta. The subclavian artery crosses the dome of the cervical pleura below its summit, immediately superior to the subclavian vein.

The right vertebral artery arises from the subclavian artery and tracks posteriorly toward the cervical vertebrae. On the left side, the left vertebral artery is the first branch of the left subclavian artery. Less commonly, in 5% of the population, a nondominant left vertebral artery can arise directly from the aortic arch, between the origin of the left common carotid artery and the left subclavian artery (Figure 35-1).

Vertebral artery usually arises from the posterior superior aspect of the subclavian artery; other anatomic variants include direct origin from the superior aspect, the anterior superior aspect, or the proximal subclavian artery.

The vertebral artery has four named segments (Figure 35-2). V1 begins at the takeoff from the subclavian. The V2 segment begins when the artery enters the first transverse foramen at the C6 cervical vertebra. V2 continues to ascend cephalad throughout the foramina and becomes V3 upon exiting C2. Medial and lateral segmental arteries arise from V2 at the level of each vertebral body. Medial segmental arteries can supply the cervical cord in a watershed distribution, and the lateral segmental arteries supply the soft tissue. Several anastomoses to this segment can become prominent

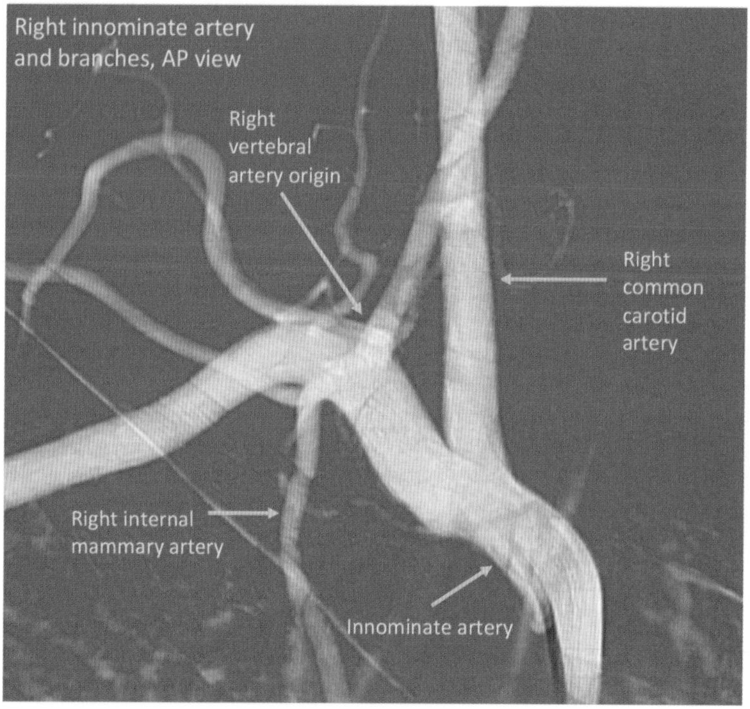

FIGURE 35-1 Catheter is positioned in the innominate artery. This roadmap demonstrates the right common carotid most medially, followed by the vertebral artery arising from the superior-anterior aspect of the subclavian artery.

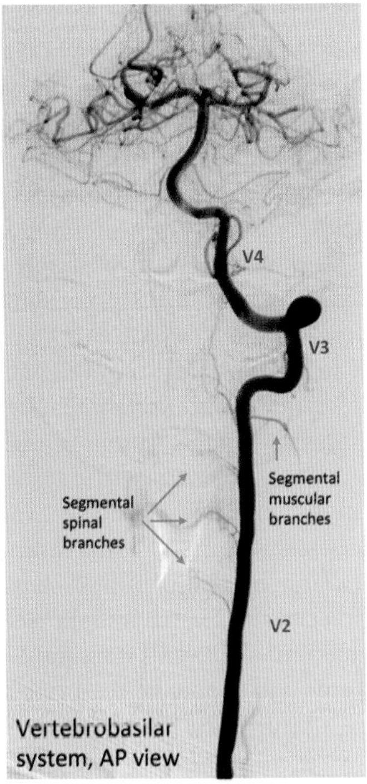

FIGURE 35-2 Segments of the vertebral artery.

in cases of cervical artery occlusive disease, with deep cervical artery and occipital artery anastomoses being the most common. The V3 segment is the last extradural segment. It passes through the C1 foramen and courses posteriorly in its groove along the C1 spinous process before looping around the occipital condyle. Posterior meningeal artery arises from this segment and supplies the dura around the foramen magnum. The V4 segment begins when the vessel pierces the dura. It passes through the foramen magnum and into the skull. The V4 segment gives rise to the posterior inferior cerebellar artery (PICA) and the anterior spinal artery (ASA). The left and right vertebral arteries meet at the lower border of the pons to form the basilar artery. It is not unusual for one vertebral artery (typically the left) to be larger and, therefore, the dominant supply to the basilar. The size of the transverse foramen usually correlates well to the size of the vertebral artery.

The basilar artery typically runs a linear, midline course along the ventral surface of the pons. Its first major branches are the anterior inferior cerebellar arteries (AICA), followed by the small labyrinthine arteries and perforating pontine arteries. The basilar continues to ascend and gives off its last branches, the superior cerebellar arteries (SCA), at the superior margin of the pons. Then, the basilar divides into bilateral posterior cerebral arteries (PCA) that give off small branches to the ventral midbrain before circling posteriorly (Figure 35-3). Ultimately the basilar is joined to the anterior circulation when the posterior cerebral artery intersects with the posterior communicating artery, forming the posterior half of the circle of Willis.

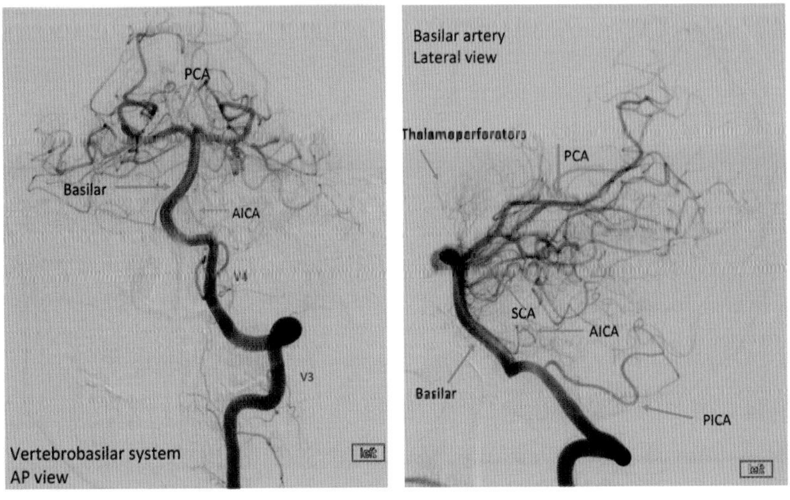

FIGURE 35-3 Intracranial posterior circulation. (AP [anterio-posterior] and lateral views.)

The vertebrobasilar system provides blood supply to brain areas controlling some of our most basic functions such as level of arousal, swallowing, hearing, balance, and eye movements. The symptoms of vertebrobasilar insufficiency (VBI) can present as classic syndromes based on the affected artery, but oftentimes vascular anatomy is variable and so too are symptoms. One important note is that VBI rarely causes one symptom in isolation, which is simply due to the density of functions represented in the brainstem.

VASCULAR SUPPLY TO THE BRAINSTEM AND CEREBELLUM

The PICA is the first branch of the vertebral artery and feeds the lateral medulla on its way toward the lower half of the cerebellum. Its major territories include cranial nerves IX and X, in addition to cerebellar function. Next, the ASA provides for a portion of the anterior medulla, which notably controls cranial nerve XII and the motor tracts within the pyramids. Once formed, the basilar feeds the ventral pons with small perforating branches that go to cranial nerves VI and VII, as well as the motor tracts and reticular formation that is responsible for arousal. The small AICA is responsible for the dorsal pons and portions of the cerebellum, areas that govern hearing and balance. Moving upward, the SCA covers the dorsal pons and midbrain as well as the superior cerebellum. Finally, the PCA sends branches to the ventral midbrain where cranial nerve III and motor tracts reside before it heads for the occipital lobes and the visual cortex.

MECHANISMS OF VERTEBROBASILAR INSUFFICIENCY

In this section, we will discuss the major factors underlying VBI. The majority of causes fall under the category of vasculopathy, where inflammatory or noninflammatory factors lead to disrupted vessel architecture. We will also discuss cardiac sources and compressive lesions that can cause VBI.

Atherosclerosis

The deposition of intimal and subintimal atherosclerotic plaque has major implications for VBI. Atherosclerotic plaque buildup can affect any level of the vertebrobasilar system, although it is most commonly seen at the origin of the vertebral artery or in the mid-V4 segment. Risk factors for atherosclerosis include hypertension, hyperlipidemia, and smoking. Aside from these modifiable risks, intracranial atherosclerosis is much more prevalent in Asian populations for unclear reasons. The most common locations for plaque accumulation in the posterior circulation are V1, V4, lower-mid basilar, and proximal posterior cerebral artery.[1] In the New England Medical Center Posterior Circulation Registry (NEMC-PCR) of patients with symptomatic vertebrobasilar ischemia, large artery hemodynamic compromise accounted for 32% of all posterior circulation strokes.[2] This could be due to an episode of acute hypoperfusion across a stenosed vessel or in situ thrombosis of a vessel with a large burden of atherosclerosis. Plaque fragmentation can also lead to embolic occlusion (see section "Acute Embolic Events"). In the NEMC-PCR 18% of patients had moderate-to-severe atherosclerotic disease affecting the basilar artery specifically, and, in many cases, it was the only vessel affected by atherosclerosis in the entire posterior circulation.[3]

Chronic VBI may occur in patients with critical vessel stenosis of 70% or more. These individuals may be highly susceptible to hemodynamic changes that reduce flow across the area of critical stenosis and often present with recurrent symptoms over months or even years. Patients may present with transient ischemic attacks (TIAs) without permanent injury or may suffer recurrent infarctions, leading to significant morbidity and mortality. Ischemia may be avoided in patients who have developed extensive collateral supply over time and in those with robust posterior communicating arteries.

Ostial and V1 segment stenosis account for approximately 20% of posterior circulation strokes. An artery-to-artery embolus is the most common etiology and is usually seen when the stenosis reaches a critical degree. VBI is rarely encountered due to the rich collateralization of the upper V2 segment from deep cervical branches.

Acute Embolic Events

Embolic events are common in the posterior circulation: approximately 40% of all posterior circulation strokes in the NEMC-PCR were attributed to embolism, most of which were cardiogenic.

The two most common sources of emboli in the brain are large vessels or the heart. Proximal vessels such as the aortic arch or subclavian arteries may harbor atherosclerotic plaque with overlying thrombus, which can fragment and embolize toward the vertebral arteries or the basilar artery. This is termed thromboembolism, and these types of emboli have a distinct composition, usually containing 50% red blood cells, 40% fibrin, and the remaining percentage a mix of inflammatory components (Sporns). Thrombosis occurs over unstable plaques in large vessels and can also be triggered by focal areas of vessel dissection or aneurysmal dilation. These areas of endothelial and flow disruption may act as a nidus for thrombus formation.

Cardiogenic emboli may form in the atria secondary to atrial fibrillation or on diseased valves (most commonly mitral and aortic). Atrial thrombus formation occurs in a different environment compared to arterial thrombus: the low-pressure atrium generates thrombi with higher ratios of fibrin (60%) in addition to red blood cells (30%) and other inflammatory components (10%).[4]

Embolic occlusion of the posterior circulation characteristically causes quite an abrupt onset of symptoms and more often occurs in younger patients.[3] The vascular territories affected and the laterality of the lesions can provide helpful information for the etiology of stroke. When multiple vascular territories and/or bilateral hemispheres are affected, this suggests a cardiogenic source for emboli. If the ischemia occurs distal to an artery with extracranial or intracranial atherosclerosis, it is reasonable to conclude an artery-to-artery embolic event.

Lastly, instrumentation to the vasculature can trigger embolic events that are distinct from cardiogenic and large-vessel emboli. Procedures such as cardiac catheterization or coronary artery bypass grafting may disturb fragments of cholesterol plaque causing cholesterol crystal embolization (atheroembolus) in the brain. This debris scatters widely and causes multiple, small infarcts throughout the brain and other organs as well.

Vertebral Artery Dissection

Vessel dissection occurs when the intimal layer is torn away from the media, creating a space for high pressure blood to fill. This process creates a false lumen that is generally situated within the media itself. Expansion of the media can cause the narrowing of the true lumen or bulging of the outer vessel wall (pseudoaneurysm) (Figure 35-4). The disrupted vessel wall is thrombogenic, and subsequent thromboembolus can lead to posterior circulation stroke. Within the vertebral artery, dissection is most likely to occur at V1/V2 junction, where the vessel transitions into the transverse foramen, and at V3 where the vessel exits the C1 foramen and is susceptible to injury from neck torsion, minor innocuous physical activities, or major trauma (Figure 35-5).

Spontaneous dissection can also occur as a complication of connective tissue disorders such as Ehlers–Danlos syndrome, Marfan syndrome, fibromuscular dysplasia, and autosomal dominant polycystic kidney disease. In these disorders, the

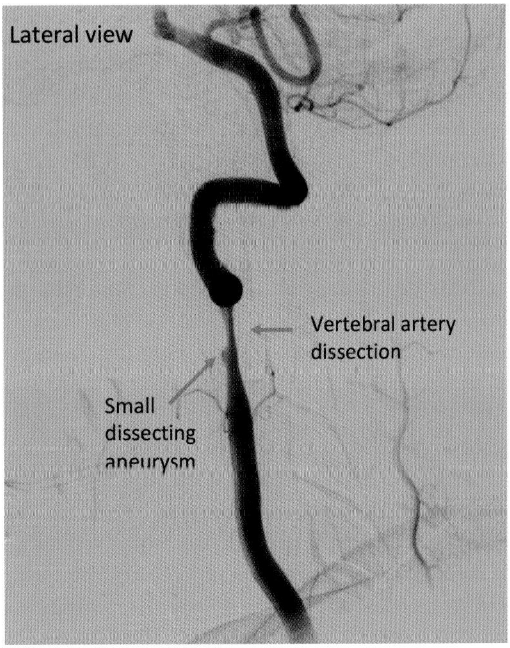

FIGURE 35-4 This image shows the dissection of the vertebral artery at the distal V2 segment with a small dissecting aneurysm.

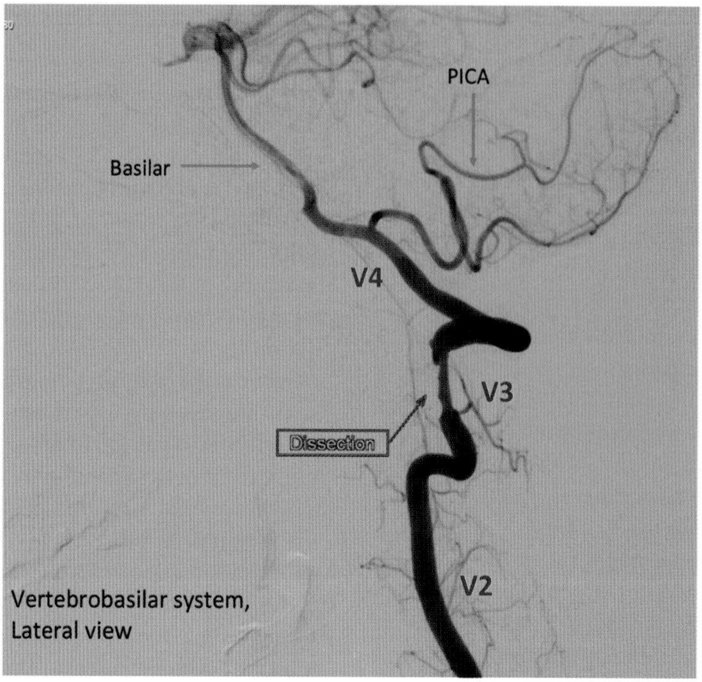

FIGURE 35-5 **Vertebral artery dissection most commonly occurs in the V3 segment.**

structures of the vessel wall are compromised and thus susceptible to injury. Spontaneous dissections may be triggered by small, nontraumatic events like coughing, yoga, or throwing back a few drinks ("bottoms up" dissection). The overall incidence of nontraumatic dissection is approximately 1 in 100,000.[5]

Athletic maneuvers involving sudden neck movements, neck hyperextension, or a blow to the mastoid bone where the underlying V3 is unprotected were all reported as inciting factors for traumatic vertebral artery dissection.[6] Sports involving high-impact physical contact, including football, hockey, and martial arts, have been implicated, but so too have individual sports like golf and running. Outside of sports, other causes such as motor vehicle collision or falls can produce blunt force trauma to the head and neck, leading to vertebral artery dissection. In many cases, there is associated cervical vertebrae fracture as well. The overall incidence of traumatic dissection is quite low, however, with one estimate demonstrating that only 0.01% of all head and neck traumas will have vertebral artery dissection.[7]

Regardless of whether the dissection is spontaneous or traumatic, the usual presenting features include posterior head and neck pain. It is not unusual for patients to be asymptomatic initially, which can make early diagnosis challenging. Subsequent ischemic symptoms can occur within minutes to weeks but are usually concentrated within the first month. Therefore, early recognition and treatment are crucial in preventing adverse events.

Intracranial dissection in the vertebral artery or the basilar artery is rare to occur but very difficult to manage. While an extracranial dissection in the V3 segment can propagate to the V4 segment, spontaneous dissections due to hypertension, trauma, or vasculopathy can also occur in an isolated intracranial distribution. Intracranial dissections present the added risk of subarachnoid hemorrhage and should be managed with a single antiplatelet medication and tight blood pressure control unless stenting or flow diversion is needed.

Small Vessel Disease

The small vessels of the intracranial vasculature can be affected by many different disease processes that are heritable (such as CADASIL) or sporadic. The sporadic form is generally referred to as cerebral small vessel disease and is thought to occur from longstanding hypertension. The vessels that tend to be affected are those that branch off major arteries like the basilar, which are less vulnerable to hypertensive injury. Over time, increased pressure within the small perforating vessels leads to thickening of the smooth muscle layer and/or increased collagen deposition within the vessel wall. These changes are termed hyperplastic or hyaline arteriolosclerosis and can become severe enough that the vessel wall narrows to the point of complete obstruction. Newer theories suggest that the failure of the endothelium and leakage of the blood–brain barrier leads to inflammatory infiltration of small vessel walls, which can also lead to wall thickening and obstruction. The overall effect is ischemia to tissue that is supplied by these perforating branches. This small portion of ischemic tissue undergoes degenerative changes after a few weeks and becomes a round, fluid-filled cavity called a "lacune." This is an important disease mechanism when considering VBI because small vessel disease is responsible for approximately one-fifth of all strokes.[8] Within the posterior circulation, lacunar infarcts are commonly seen in the pons secondary to the occlusion of basilar perforating branches. The thalamus can be affected when small branches of the posterior cerebral artery are occluded. Cerebral small vessel disease has other manifestations as well, such as microhemorrhage. The presentation of lacunar stroke can be unique from other presentations of VBI. Some patients are completely asymptomatic, and the lesion may be discovered incidentally. Others will have an acute onset of symptoms, and others may have subacute, fluctuating symptoms that can progress over several days. This latter presentation is sometimes referred to as a "stuttering lacune" and may be the result of a small vessel under severe compromise before succumbing to complete occlusion.

Vertebrobasilar Dolichoectasia

This condition is a dilative arteriopathy where changes to vessel composition lead to lengthening (dolicho) and widening (ectasia) of intracranial arteries, often lending a tortuous appearance to the vessels. It most commonly affects the vertebrobasilar system rather than the anterior circulation and can be seen in approximately 10% of patients presenting with stroke.[9] Pathological analysis reveals an overall decomposition of the tunica media, where thinning of the elastic layer and atrophy of the muscular layer cause widening of the vessel diameter and a more fragile arterial wall. One potential cause for this degradation is excess secretion of matrix metalloproteinases from the vascular endothelium with an associated lack of proteinase inhibitor activity. Risk factors include advanced age, male sex, and hypertension. Atherosclerosis is not a risk factor but is more likely to occur subsequent to these vessel wall disruptions. Vertebrobasilar dolichoectasia (VBD) is often comorbid with abdominal aortic aneurysm due to shared risk factors and similar underlying pathology.

There are no universal criteria for diagnosis of VBD, but the Smoker criteria can be used as a guideline. This score is based on three aspects of the basilar artery: laterality, height of bifurcation, and diameter. A basilar that is lateral to the clivus or dorsum sellae is abnormal, as is bifurcation above the dorsum sellae (Figure 35-6). Lastly, a diameter > 4.5 mm measured at the mid-pons on computed tomography (CT) qualifies as atypical enlargement.

The two most common presentations of VBD are stroke (both ischemic and hemorrhagic) and brainstem compression. Ischemic stroke can occur in several ways: intraluminal thrombus formation with in situ thrombosis, thrombus formation with subsequent embolization, distortion of smaller branch vessels emanating from the basilar, and reduced anterograde flow. A widened and irregular vessel wall disrupts the laminar flow and promotes intraluminal thrombus formation. Over time this may lead to complete vessel occlusion, perforating branch obstruction, or thromboembolic events in more distal areas. The small perforating branches that originate off the basilar and feed the midline brainstem structures can be distorted by severe basilar curvature and digression from the midline, which is another discrete mechanism to cause ischemic stroke. Lastly, vessel lengthening can cause reduced anterograde flow leading to hypoperfusion and infarction of more distal territories such as the thalamus. One study reported a stroke incidence rate of 48% in patients with this condition over a median 11-year period (Passero).

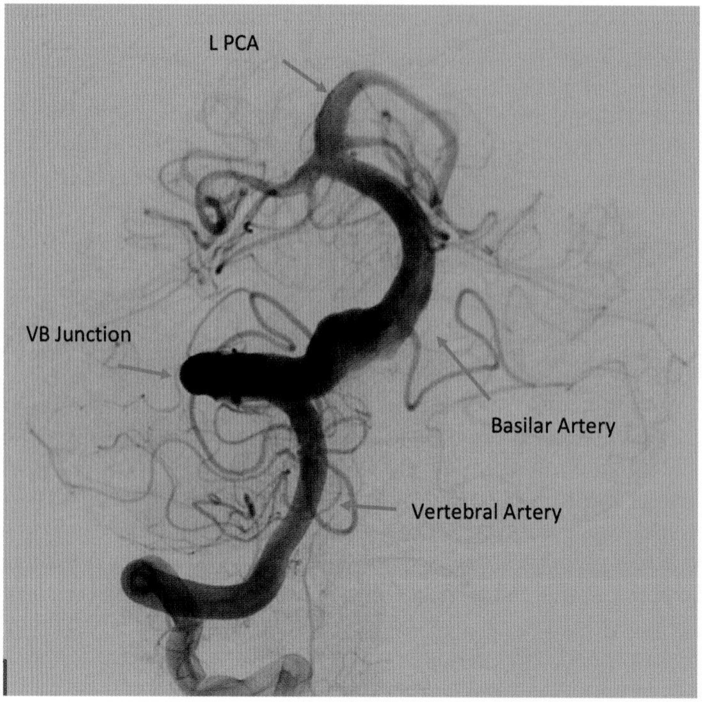

FIGURE 35-6 Dolichoectasia of the vertebral and basilar artery and left posterior cerebral artery. Notice how the vertebrobasilar junction shifted significantly to the right side.

Patients who presented with stroke were more likely to have recurrent strokes, with a cumulative risk of first recurrent stroke reaching 56% at 10 years.[10] This high rate of recurrent events is thought to be linked to the progression of dolichoectasia, for which there is no modifying therapy. One meta-analysis reported an aneurysm growth rate of 6% or 1.3 mm per year.[11,12]

Alternatively, enlargement of the basilar can itself cause compression of the brainstem and thus focal neurologic symptoms. This is a less common presenting feature of VBD and composes approximately 25% of symptomatic cases.[11] Patients are most likely to present with weakness or vertigo as the ectatic artery tends to compress the ventrolateral structures. The symptoms are unlikely to present acutely as the compression will gradually progress over time.

Rupture of an enlarged and fragile basilar artery is uncommon, with some estimates of an annual rupture rate <1% per year.[13] Furthermore, this tends to occur in patients with severe disease-causing vessel dilation to 10 mm or more in diameter.

Subclavian Stenosis

Aside from conditions that cause vessel occlusion, VBI can also be caused by redirection of blood flow. Subclavian steal syndrome occurs when there is stenosis or occlusion of the subclavian artery proximal to the takeoff of the vertebral artery. The stenosis is most commonly caused by atherosclerosis but can also be from an accessory rib, radiation vasculopathy, or large-vessel vasculitis, among other causes. As the stenosis becomes increasingly severe, the intravascular pressure distal to the lesion drops significantly. When the pressure drops below the level of the intracranial circulation, blood flow reverses within the vertebral artery and instead moves toward the low-pressure subclavian artery (Figures 35-7 and 35-8). Thus, the path of least resistance will "steal" flow from the vertebral artery. Some degree of flow reversal starts to occur when the subclavian stenosis reaches about 50%, though patients may not become symptomatic until later in this disease. Symptoms involve the ipsilateral limb, posterior circulation, and even the heart in patients with left internal mammary artery bypass grafting. The most common presentation of subclavian stenosis is weakness and pain in the ipsilateral arm that is worsened with activity and relieved with rest. VBI is a rare presentation of subclavian

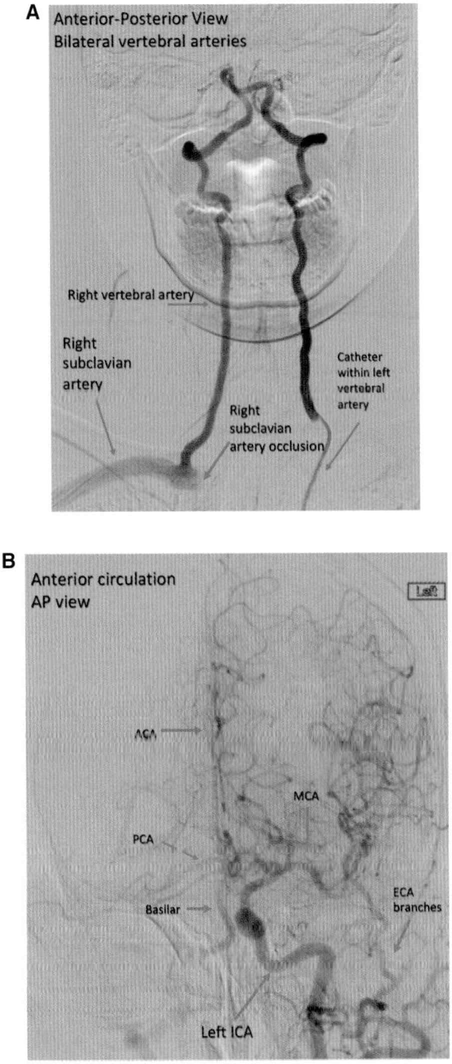

FIGURE 35-7 **(A–B) Patient with subclavian steal syndrome due to occlusion of the right subclavian artery proximal to the vertebral artery origin.** Catheter injection of the left vertebral artery shows flow reversal from the right vertebral artery toward the right subclavian. In image **A**, the basilar artery does not opacify as it fills from the left internal carotid artery through the posterior communicating artery (**B**).

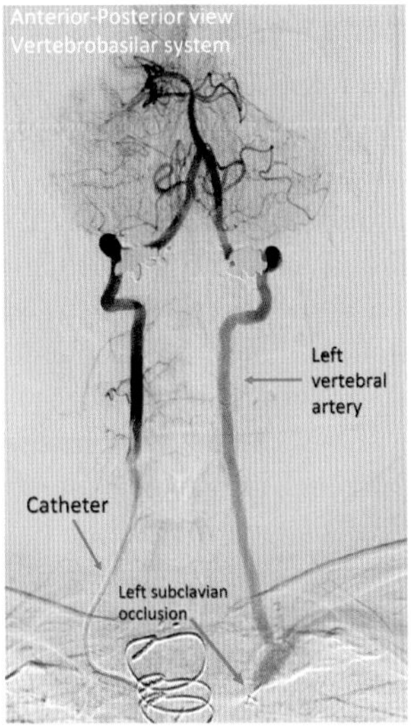

FIGURE 35-8 **This patient has subclavian steal syndrome.** There is occlusion of the left subclavian artery proximal to the left vertebral artery origin. Contrast injection of the unaffected right side demonstrates flow reversal from the left vertebral artery into the left subclavian artery.

steal and is most likely to occur when there are additional exacerbating factors. For example, engaging the affected limb in vigorous physical activity will reduce arterial resistance and create a larger pressure gradient for flow reversal in the vertebral artery. Or, if a patient has preexisting compromise to the posterior circulation and poor collateral flow, they may be less able to sustain flow diversion from the affected vertebral artery with the contralateral vertebral artery. Under these circumstances, patients with severe subclavian stenosis may develop signs of VBI. The symptoms may resolve if the exacerbating factor (such as a vigorous activity) is removed. This creates a clinical picture of transient neurologic deficits. In addition to the neurologic symptoms discussed in detail in section "Clinical Features of Vertebrobasilar Insufficiency," subclavian stenosis may have unique physical exam findings. Measurement of blood pressure in both arms may reveal a difference between the extremities owing to the drop in pressure distal to the stenosis in the affected limb. A difference of 15 mmHg between the limbs is considered clinically significant. Diminished pulses in the affected limb and auscultation of a bruit in the supraclavicular fossa may be additional clues suggesting subclavian stenosis.[14]

Bow Hunter's Syndrome

Reversible flow obstruction can occur in a condition termed Bow Hunter's syndrome. This rare condition is also known as rotational VBI, where a structural abnormality causes transient compression of the vertebral artery with neck rotation or extension. The name comes from a student who suffered a medullary stroke from this syndrome during archery practice. There are numerous causes including osteophytes at the uncovertebral joint, intervertebral disc herniation, thickened atlantoaxial membrane, and, in children, bony malformation at the atlantoaxial joint.

In one review of the case series, 58% of patients had obstruction of the V2 segment and 36% at the V3 segment.[15] The typical age of symptom onset is 50 years old, and the syndrome is overall more common in males. There are numerous pediatric case reports as well.

Symptoms are elicited by head turn or head extension, and the most commonly reported symptom is syncope, vertigo, and vision loss. The pathophysiology involves flow-limiting compression that leads to tissue ischemia. Symptomatic patients typically have insufficient collateral flow due to contralateral vertebral artery hypoplasia or stenosis.[16]

CLINICAL FEATURES OF VERTEBROBASILAR INSUFFICIENCY

NEUROLOGIC SYMPTOMS

It is challenging to diagnose VBI because the symptoms are often nonspecific and can lead to the workup of other etiologies. Nausea, vomiting, and dizziness, in particular, have a large differential and can make zeroing in on the diagnosis of VBI more difficult.

When considering a diagnosis of VBI, it is helpful to think about symptoms in the context of anatomy. Any symptom relating to a cranial nerve, including double vision, difficulty swallowing, facial weakness, hearing loss, dizziness, vertigo, hoarse voice, or loss of facial sensation, can be a clue to VBI affecting the brainstem. The brainstem also carries descending motor and ascending sensory fibers; therefore, weakness or sensory loss on one side can also be a sign of VBI. Symptoms such as unsteady gait, falls, nausea, and vomiting suggest the involvement of the cerebellum. The most worrisome symptom is an altered level of consciousness or coma. This, too, can be a consequence of VBI as the basilar supplies arousal centers in the brainstem and thalamus, and therefore VBI should be on the differential for any patient presenting with an acutely decreased level of consciousness.

The NEMC-PCR evaluated over 400 patients with stroke or TIA involving the posterior circulation. Within this group of patients, the most common symptoms and signs were documented. The most common symptom of posterior circulation insufficiency is dizziness (47%), followed by unilateral weakness (40%) and slurred speech or dysarthria (30%). The most worrisome symptoms of lethargy and reduced level of consciousness were evident in 15% and 10% of patients, respectively. This may represent injury to wakefulness centers or a large stroke, causing edema and elevated intracranial pressure. These statistics account for all presentations of posterior circulation ischemia, and the evaluating provider should expect variation based on the location of the injury. It is important for non-neurologists to recognize that VBI almost never presents with one sign or symptom in isolation. In the NEMC-PCR, <1% of patients with confirmed VBI had just one presenting feature.[17]

PHYSICAL EXAM FINDINGS

All practitioners should be comfortable with a gross assessment of VBI; however, it would be appropriate to consult a neurologist for a detailed exam as well. As mentioned in section "Clinical Features of Vertebrobasilar Insufficiency," the most critical physical exam finding is an altered level of consciousness. This can present acutely and maximally at the onset in the case of basilar artery occlusion, or it can develop over time from drowsiness to coma as perfusion is impaired.

A basic assessment of cranial nerves can yield important findings. Impaired eye movements, facial numbness and weakness, decreased hearing, nystagmus, and tongue and palatal deviation are relatively straightforward to evaluate. Nystagmus may be one of the more challenging physical exam findings to identify. Recall that nystagmus is a type of eye movement associated with a slow and fast phase and appears as repetitive beating movements of the eye. Ask the patient to look in all cardinal directions of gaze and check for these quick beating movements. Any vertical nystagmus or nystagmus that alternates (beats to the left and to the right) is concerning for VBI.

Additional findings on physical exams may include weakness or loss of sensation on one side of the body. The simple finger-to-nose test evaluates coordination and is abnormal when the patient misses the target (either by overshoot or undershoot). Similarly, asking the patient to slide the heel of one leg straight down the shin of the other leg can pinpoint coordination problems. Look to see whether the patient can maintain a straight path without the heel sliding off the shin bone. If the patient is able to safely stand and walk, then gait assessment is also helpful. A widened stance, swaying trunk, and inability to tandem walk are all signs concerning VBI affecting the cerebellum.

In the New England posterior circulation registry, the most common physical exam findings in all posterior circulation strokes include unilateral limb weakness (39%), ataxia in gait or limb (30%), and dysarthria (29%).[17]

VERTEBROBASILAR SYNDROMES

The following section reviews classic syndromes of VBI. They describe a collection of symptoms that reliably occur with the obstruction of a particular vascular segment. Due to variable individual anatomy, it is not necessary for patients to have all components of the syndrome, but the identification of two or more features can be helpful in identifying the region of injury.

LATERAL MEDULLARY (WALLENBURG) SYNDROME

The lateral medulla is supplied by small perforating branches of the vertebral artery or the premedullary segment of the PICA. The syndrome is usually caused by thrombosis of the vertebral artery and is most common among all brainstem stroke syndromes. The most prominent features of this syndrome include vertigo, ataxia, hoarseness, and dysphagia, which reflects the involvement of cranial nerves IX–X as well as the inferior cerebellar peduncle. The ataxia is more prominent in the limbs rather than the trunk and may be associated with nausea and vomiting.

MEDIAL MEDULLARY (DEJERINE) SYNDROME

This region carries motor fibers from the cortex to the spinal motor neurons, and therefore lesions of the medial medulla will cause weakness. Sensory fibers and cranial nerve XII can also be affected, leading to sensory symptoms and tongue deviation, respectively. This syndrome is often the result of atherothrombotic occlusion of the vertebral artery or the ASA. It is not uncommon for one vertebral artery or the ASA to supply the entire medial medulla, which can lead to bilateral weakness in the event of occlusion.

LATERAL PONTINE SYNDROME

Ischemia to the lateral pons shares the features of vertigo and ataxia seen in lateral medullary syndrome due to the involvement of the middle cerebellar peduncle. Uniquely, this syndrome results in ipsilateral hearing loss, which reflects the involvement of the labyrinthine artery. The lateral pons is mostly supplied by the AICA, which is an early branch of the basilar artery.

VENTRAL PONTINE (LOCKED-IN) SYNDROME

One of the most well-known and disabling brainstem strokes is the locked-in syndrome that occurs with bilateral pontine infarcts. The ventral pons is supplied by small perforating branches of the basilar artery that are susceptible to arteriolosclerosis from longstanding hypertension, in addition to thrombosis and occlusion by an embolus. Symptoms involve weakness in all four extremities and nearly all of the cranial nerve nuclei, which impairs essentially all movement. Consciousness and vertical eye movements are spared; therefore, it is important to evaluate eye movements in all seemingly comatose patients to rule out locked-in syndrome. Many patients with large pontine strokes also develop respiratory failure requiring mechanical ventilation and dysphagia requiring artificial nutrition. Patients may be severely disabled for days to weeks before showing any signs of recovery.

TOP OF THE BASILAR SYNDROME

Occlusion of the distal basilar artery affects the midbrain as well as territories supplied by the posterior cerebral artery, including the thalamus and occipital cortex. Symptoms corresponding with these territories include ophthalmoplegia, lethargy or coma, hallucinations, and cortical blindness. Various pupillary abnormalities may appear based on the affected area: thalamic lesions can cause pinpoint pupils, while midbrain lesions can produce dilated pupils. Occlusion of the distal basilar could affect both PCA to cause infarction of the bilateral occipital lobes. This particular scenario leads to Anton syndrome, where the patient is cortically blind yet denies vision loss.

DIFFERENTIAL DIAGNOSIS

The symptoms of VBI can occur in many different combinations, which will influence the differential diagnosis. We will go through the most common pairs and determine how to distinguish these symptoms from non-VBI etiologies. As mentioned previously, the presence of only one symptom or sign makes VBI unlikely.

DIZZINESS, NAUSEA, AND VOMITING

Patients often describe a feeling of dizziness or "room spinning" that is accompanied by nausea. They may have difficulty walking straight or keeping their eyes open due to the discomfort. The most important differentiating feature from the history is the duration of symptoms. If the symptoms are intermittent and last seconds to minutes, consider benign paroxysmal positional vertigo or vestibular migraine. Symptoms that are continuous over many hours should raise suspicion for posterior circulation ischemia, intracranial mass lesion, vestibular neuritis, or medication effects. Physical exam findings such as the presence and direction of nystagmus, skew deviation, and corrective saccades can help narrow the differential.

DOUBLE VISION OR DIPLOPIA

This is another symptom common to VBI and is caused by weakness of extraocular muscles that impairs conjugate gaze. Patients may inaccurately relay what they are experiencing and may report blurry vision instead of double vision. Therefore, it is important to specifically ask whether the patient sees two objects stacked horizontally or vertically. Assessment of extraocular movements in all cardinal directions of gaze may reveal palsy of one or more extraocular muscles. Testing each eye individually can be helpful as well; if there is monocular diplopia, the problem may be better explained by intraocular pathology.

SYNCOPE AND COMA

Transient loss of consciousness has a broad differential, and vertebrobasilar disease is much less common than alternative etiologies such as cardiogenic syncope, vasovagal syncope, and even seizure. VBI may be higher on the differential when the patient has vascular risk factors and when the syncope is associated with other symptoms that also localize to the brainstem. Patients who are comatose will require a broad diagnostic workup to rule out intracranial hemorrhage, seizure, or a systemic metabolic or infectious process.

DIAGNOSTIC MEASURES

COMPUTED TOMOGRAPHY

The use of non-contrast CT is helpful but often insufficient for the evaluation of VBI. In the acute setting, it may provide enough information to rule out intracranial hemorrhage and to administer tPA, but it often does not capture the posterior fossa in adequate detail due to skull base artifact. It is important to recognize that CT may not show findings of acute stroke until 6 or more hours after symptom onset; therefore, if suspicion of an acute stroke is high and CT is negative, further imaging should be pursued.

In addition to plain CT, the use of CT angiography (CTA) of the head and neck is ideal for evaluating atherosclerotic burden, dissection, and occlusion.

CTA is a useful first study in a suspected case of Bow Hunter's syndrome because it allows evaluation of the vasculature and potential bony abnormalities that may cause transient compression. When evaluating subclavian stenosis, duplex ultrasound is an appropriate first-tier approach but may be followed by CTA for surgical planning.

CT brain perfusion is usually used for anterior circulation ischemia, but it has limited utility in posterior circulation disease.

MAGNETIC RESONANCE IMAGING

Magnetic resonance imaging (MRI) is the optimal imaging method for the assessment of stroke. The diffusion-weighted imaging sequences often show diffusion restriction (indicating acute stroke) in as little as 30 minutes from symptom onset. Unlike CT, there is no significant skull base artifact. MR angiography and MR perfusion are also available and are roughly equivalent to their CT-based counterparts. The disadvantage of MRI is that it is more time-consuming and therefore can delay acute treatment. Patients with pacemakers or left ventricular assist devices may also be ineligible for MRI.

CATHETER-BASED ANGIOGRAPHY

The endovascular approach to visualizing the vertebrobasilar system is typically pursued when intervention is planned. In the case of a suspected acute occlusion where perfusion imaging demonstrates salvageable tissue, the patient may be taken for intervention. Catheter angiography may also be helpful if there is suspected vasculitis or vasculopathy that is poorly visualized on MRI or CT. In Bow Hunter's syndrome, catheter angiography is the gold standard because it allows for real-time assessment of vessel compression when asking the patient to perform certain exacerbating maneuvers.

Aortic arch injection is essential for the evaluation of the proximal left subclavian artery and the brachiocephalic trunk. In a patient with recent TIA or ischemic stroke, selective catheterization of the vertebral artery should be performed only after the V1 and V2 segments are evaluated through subclavian artery injections. As anatomic variants are commonly seen, multiple angiographic projections are usually needed to evaluate the ostium of the vertebral artery. In patients with contralateral vertebral artery occlusion or severe stenosis, the operator should try to avoid selective catheterization of the patent vertebral artery, if possible. It is common for the patient to experience transient vertigo and nausea during selective vertebral artery injections. Several projections of the intracranial circulation are recommended to evaluate contrast transit times, tandem lesions, and the completeness of the circle of Willis. In cases of subclavian steal syndrome, prolonged filming from the healthy subclavian artery is needed to delineate the angiographic steal and the subclavian lesion.

ULTRASOUND

This is best used for specific conditions. In the workup for Bow Hunter's syndrome, transcranial Doppler can measure the velocity of flow within the intracranial vasculature during certain maneuvers to help identify provocative causes of VBI. Similarly, transcranial Doppler can be helpful in the diagnosis of subclavian steal syndrome when neurologic symptoms are involved. Duplex ultrasound of the upper limb is an efficient method for the evaluation of subclavian stenosis, but its accuracy may be operator dependent.[11]

MANAGEMENT OF VERTEBROBASILAR INSUFFICIENCY

ACUTE THROMBOTIC OCCLUSION

Acute obstruction of the vertebrobasilar system can range from the extracranial vertebral artery to the intracranial posterior circulation and is an emergency. Patients will usually present with abrupt onset of symptoms and physical exam findings, as described earlier in this chapter. The time of last known well should be obtained, as well as imaging with CT, CTA head and neck, and/or CT perfusion. The physical exam findings should be scored according to the National Institutes of Health Stroke Scale (NIHSS).

Medical Management

In the setting of acute vessel occlusion, where history and physical exam findings are concerning for ischemic stroke, treatment with a tissue plasminogen activator needs to be considered. Current practice requires that the patient must have a last known well within 4.5 hours to be eligible for tPA. This is rapidly evolving with the rise of diffusion-weighted MRI (DWI) and fluid-attenuated inversion recovery (FLAIR) MRI (DWI-FLAIR mismatch) mismatch to identify stroke with unknown time of onset and CT perfusion for tissue-based (rather than time-based) patient selection. However, these options have not yet been widely adopted and so the current recommendation is to limit tPA administration to within 4.5 hours of last known well. If the patient is within the time window, the provider must first rule out absolute contraindications: active treatment with anticoagulation therapy, including warfarin and novel anticoagulants, intracranial hemorrhage on CT scan, recent or active internal bleeding, recent major surgery, and blood pressure > 185/110. Blood pressure can be treated prior to the administration of tPA, if needed. If the patient is deemed eligible, the next step is to consider whether the symptoms are severe enough to warrant treatment. The NIHSS is helpful in this assessment, and usually scores of 3–4 or higher would prompt treatment. This scoring system is not so representative of posterior circulation symptoms, however, and may be low in highly symptomatic patients. It is, therefore, reasonable to treat patients with low NIHSS who have disabling symptoms due to posterior circulation stroke. Prior to administration of tPA, you must consent to the patient or if possible a close contact who can speak for the patient. It is important to outline the risks and benefits of this medication. The risk of symptomatic intracranial hemorrhage is often quoted as 6% based on trial data[18] but is usually lower in real-life practice. If consent is obtained, then the next step is to administer a total dose of 0.9 mg/kg with 10% of the total dose administered as a bolus over 1 to 2 minutes, followed by the remainder of the dose as a continuous IV infusion over 60 minutes.

Generally speaking, patients treated with tPA are likely to have better outcomes: 40% reach minimal or no disability at 1 year compared to 28% in the placebo group.[18,19] However, when examining a subset of patients with large-vessel occlusion, it is clear that these patients are far less likely to have a good outcome because tPA is less effective at dissolving large thrombi. Even with tPA, acute basilar occlusion only has a successful rate of recanalization of 33%. The outcomes are highly polarized: 25% of patients with basilar artery occlusion will survive and have few deficits, while the remaining 75% will die.[20] The dismal prognosis of an acute basilar artery occlusion has led to an interest in trying mechanical thrombectomy, which is now a well-established treatment for anterior circulation large-vessel occlusions.

Surgical Management

Endovascular management of acute stroke is now widely adopted based on a number of randomized trials that were published in 2015. However, these studies were limited to patients presenting with ischemic stroke in the anterior circulation only. Up until recently, the practice of treating posterior circulation large-vessel occlusion (i.e., basilar occlusion) with mechanical thrombectomy was based on small, unrandomized studies.

The ENDOSTROKE study was published in 2015. This was an observational cohort of patients who underwent mechanical thrombolysis with or without intravenous thrombolysis for a basilar artery occlusion. With a recanalization rate of nearly 80%, a moderately good outcome (mRS 0-3) was reached in 42% of patients. These were encouraging results, but still many patients who were adequately recanalized did not achieve a good outcome.[21]

Randomized studies of basilar occlusion have been hampered by low recruitment and high rates of crossover to the treatment arm. The acute basilar artery occlusion: Endovascular Interventions versus Standard Medical Treatment (BEST) trial randomized 131 patients in China to receive either medical therapy or medical and interventional treatment for an acute basilar occlusion within 8 hours of symptom onset. The rate of crossover to the interventional group was 22%. The study did not show any significant difference in the primary endpoint of good functional outcome (mRS 0-3) between groups. However, patients who underwent mechanical thrombectomy did have higher rates of a good outcome: 44% versus 25% in the interventional and medical arms, respectively. Early termination of the trial and crossover led to an underpowered study.[22]

Our approach to the treatment of acute basilar artery occlusion includes emergent mechanical thrombectomy with aspiration catheters or stentrievers. A base 6 to 7 French sheath is advanced into the dominant vertebral artery, and a triaxial system of a distal access catheter (usually 0.0815 in/2.1 mm) over a microcatheter over a microwire is then advanced to the basilar artery. Aspiration through the distal access catheter is performed with a 20cc syringe or an aspiration pump. Alternatively, a stentriever can be deployed across the site of the occlusion before aspiration is applied.

CHRONIC HIGH-GRADE STENOSIS OR OCCLUSION

Transient Ischemic Attack and Mild Strokes

Transient neurologic symptoms involving the posterior circulation that self-resolve and do not cause diffusion restriction on MRI can be considered TIA. In the New England posterior circulation registry, 24% of patients had a TIA prior to the onset of stroke. These transient events serve as an opportunity to prevent future episodes. When a patient presents with TIA or mild ischemic stroke, it is appropriate to administer aspirin 81 mg. The next steps involve assessing the likely cause of the event, which usually includes a transthoracic echocardiogram with bubble study, serum lipids, and hemoglobin A1C. MRI brain with vessel imaging is helpful to look for any radiographic evidence of acute or old infarcts, as well as to assess the degree of the atherosclerotic burden, if any. Currently, patients with anterior circulation TIA or mild strokes are started on a 3-week course of dual antiplatelet therapy with aspirin and clopidogrel. This practice arose from the POINT and CHANCE trials, which found that the highest risk of recurrent events occurred in the first month after the primary event, and dual antiplatelet therapy reduces this risk.[23,24] There is no such trial for posterior circulation TIA or mild strokes; therefore, treatment with dual antiplatelet therapy is not an evidence-based practice. However, some propose that the spirit of the POINT and CHANCE trials could apply to posterior circulation minor stroke or TIA as well.

Vertebral Artery Stenting

There is enough evidence to support revascularization of internal carotid artery stenosis after a correlating ischemic event. Although the mechanism of stroke (artery-to-artery embolism and/or hypoperfusion) is similar in most cases of vertebral artery stenosis and posterior circulation TIAs or strokes, evidence for vertebral artery revascularization remains limited. Vertebral artery origin stenosis (VAOS) represents a relatively easy target for endovascular treatment. Several studies have demonstrated that stenting of VAOS, with or without distal protection devices, is feasible and has a good safety profile. However, a randomized trial from the UK (VIST) was published in 2017 and failed to show the superiority of angioplasty and stenting when compared to the best medical treatment. It is important to note that this trial was stopped early due to a lack of funding after the enrollment of 182 patients, which could have resulted in an underpower bias. Among patients who underwent stenting, 79% had extracranial stenosis, and 21% had intracranial stents. During follow-up (median, 3.5 years), five strokes occurred in the stenting group compared with 12 in the BMT-alone group (hazard ratio, 0.40; $P = 0.08$). Authors also performed a meta-analysis that did not demonstrate any added benefit to stenting.

Intracranial vertebral artery stenosis is usually treated similar to other intracranial vasculature lesions. Following the completion of the SAMMPRIS trial, most practitioners would maximize medical therapy before stenting is considered in refractory cases.

Acute Dissection

Vertebral artery dissection is treated medically. The CADISS trial sought to answer whether anticoagulation or antiplatelet therapy was more effective at reducing the risk of stroke from dissection.[25] The trial showed no difference in the rate of stroke recurrence in either group. Once medical treatment is initiated, follow-up imaging at 3 to 6 months should be obtained to assess whether the vessel has recanalized and whether the dissection remains stable. If the lesion is stable, discontinuation of aspirin or anticoagulation is reasonable given the low risk of future thrombotic events. In patients with an expanding pseudoaneurysm, worsening dissection, or persistent symptoms from limited flow, escalation to endovascular treatment may be warranted. There are no randomized studies evaluating endovascular treatment for vertebral artery dissection, but retrospective reviews suggest that stenting of a stenotic lesion or coiling of a pseudoaneurysm can be helpful in select patients in addition to medical therapy. Periprocedural morbidity is low, and in one study, 21% of patients felt improvement after stenting or coiling.[26] Intracranial dissections can be managed with flow diversion devices or vessel sacrifice if the contralateral side is patent. It is crucial to identify the origin of the ASA before this procedure is undertaken.

Bow Hunter's Syndrome

Treatment of this condition should begin with conservative measures. This includes the use of a c-collar to stabilize the neck, aspirin, and avoidance of triggering activities. Vertebral artery stenting is rarely performed but can be helpful in patients with ostial atherosclerosis. The most commonly performed procedure is decompression and/or fusion, which involves removing the anterior border of the vertebral foramen ("unroofing") and clearing any adhesive membrane or tissue. This technique yielded symptomatic improvement or complete relief in 87% of patients.[15]

Subclavian Stenosis

When caused by atherosclerosis, subclavian stenosis is indicative of advanced cardiovascular disease and thus carries with it greater morbidity and mortality. Regardless of whether the patient is symptomatic or not, the underlying cardiovascular disease should be managed aggressively with statin therapy, antihypertensives (particularly Angiotensin-converting enzyme inhibitors and beta blockers), and antiplatelet therapy with aspirin. Patients who are mildly symptomatic may be started on medical management only and observed. For patients with disabling symptoms or those who are planning for coronary artery bypass grafting, surgical management in addition to medical therapy is appropriate. In one cohort, approximately 70% of patients who were surgically treated had symptomatic VBI.[27]

Endovascular options include percutaneous angioplasty and/or stenting; however, evidence for their use is based on observational studies only. Henry et al. presented data for 407 patients, of which 59 were treated with balloon angioplasty only and 348 were treated with stenting, with an overall recanalization success rate of 95%. Over a mean follow-up period of about 6 years, the rate of restenosis was 10%. Patients treated with angioplasty alone had higher rates of restenosis (18.8%), compared to patients who underwent stenting (7.8%). The mean lesion length was about 24 mm. The authors concluded that stenting yielded more durable results with fewer cases of restenosis.

The open surgical approach for subclavian stenosis involves bypassing the lesion. The most common techniques are carotid-subclavian bypass, subclavian-carotid transposition, and axilloaxillary bypass. In one study, the 5-year patency rate was 73%, with most of the success driven by the use of the common carotid artery as the donor vessel instead of the contralateral subclavian or axillary arteries.[28] Many patients with subclavian stenosis also have extensive extracranial carotid artery disease and therefore would require carotid endarterectomy first.

There are no randomized trials comparing open and endovascular approaches for subclavian stenosis. Both methods have reasonably good patency rates and low surgical morbidity and mortality. Endovascular treatment is generally preferred in patients with shorter lesions that are located more proximally; stenting across more distal lesions may compromise the origin of the vertebral artery.

VERTEBROBASILAR DOLICHOECTASIA

As of this time, there is no treatment that can reverse the destruction of the media in VBD. Management of hypertension, the only modifiable risk factor in most cases, may be helpful in reducing disease progression. Patients should be treated with antihypertensives to a standard goal of 140/80 or less. Brain MRI and magnetic resonance angiography (MRA) should be completed 6 months after the first presentation and yearly thereafter to monitor for progression.[29]

The secondary aim of treatment for VBD is to prevent adverse outcomes such as hemorrhagic and ischemic stroke. This can be achieved with both medical and surgical options.

Overall there is very little high-quality evidence for treatment recommendations for this condition.

Medical Management

In patients presenting with ischemic stroke, the preferred medical therapy is antiplatelet agents. Anticoagulation has been described in the literature, but due to concern for intracranial hemorrhage, the current practice is to avoid this class of medications. Unfortunately, even despite antiplatelet therapy, over half of the patients will go on to have a recurrent stroke, with the highest risk of recurrence in the first 5 years after the initial event.[10]

Surgical Management

Pico et al propose surgical management for patients with a basilar measuring 10 mm in diameter or diameter growth of 2 mm or more in a 1-year period. One of the oldest described methods involves occlusion of the upper and lower limits of the ectatic portion of the artery. This reduces flow through the lumen and decreases pressure on the arterial wall. This method is limited by the availability of collateral flow to support the structures maintained by the diseased portion of the vessel. Newer techniques employ stents with or without coils to reconstruct the vessel. One method involves placing a stent in a nondiseased distal target vessel and then arranging multiple consecutive stents proximally into the diseased vessel in an overlapping fashion. The use of a stent may alter the geometry of the vessel, thereby reducing its curvature.[30]

REFERENCES

1. Kim JS, Caplan LR, Wong KS eds. *Intracranial Atherosclerosis: Pathophysiology, Diagnosis and Treatment.* Front Neurol Neurosci. Vol. 40. Basel, Switzerland: Karger; 2016:72-92.
2. Caplan L, Chung CS, Wityk R, et al. New England medical center posterior circulation stroke registry: I. Methods, data base, distribution of brain lesions, stroke mechanisms, and outcomes. *J Clin Neurol.* 2005;1(1): 14-30.
3. Voetsch B, DeWitt D, Pessin M, Caplan LR. Basilar artery occlusive disease in the New England Medical Center Posterior Circulation Registry. *Arch Neurol.* 2004;61:496-504.
4. Sporns PB, Hanning U, Schwindt W, et al. Ischemic stroke: what does the histological composition tell us about the origin of the thrombus? *Stroke.* 2017;48(8): 2206-2210.
5. Schievink W. Spontaneous dissection of the carotid and vertebral arteries. *N Engl J Med.* 2001;344:898-906.
6. Saw AE, McIntosh AS, Kountouris A. Vertebral artery dissection in sport: expert opinion of mechanisms and risk-reduction strategies. *J Clin Neurosci.* 2019;68: 28-32.
7. Majidi S, Hassan AE, Adil MM, et al. Incidence and outcome of vertebral artery dissection in trauma setting: analysis of national trauma data base. *Neurocrit Care.* 2014;21: 253-258.
8. Sudlow CLM, Warlow CP. Comparable studies of the incidence of stroke and its pathological types. Results from an international collaboration. *Stroke.* 1997;28: 491-499.
9. Lou M, Caplan LR. Vertebrobasilar dilatative arteriopathy (dolichoectasia). *Ann N Y Acad Sci.* 2010; 1184:121 133.
10. Passero SG, Rossi S. Natural history of vertebrobasilar dolichoectasia. *Neurology.* 2008;70:66-72.
11. Nasr DM, Flemming KD, Lanzino G, et al. Natural history of vertebrobasilar dolichoectatic and fusiform aneurysms: a systematic review and meta-analysis. *Cerebrovasc Dis.* 2018;45(1-2):68-77.
12. Mangrum WI, Huston J 3rd, Link MJ, et al. Enlarging vertebrobasilar nonsaccular intracranial aneurysms: frequency, predictors, and clinical outcome of growth. *J Neurosurg.* 2005;102:72-79.
13. Flemming KD, Wiebers DO, Brown RD Jr, et al. The natural history of radiographically defined vertebrobasilar nonsaccular intracranial aneurysms. *Cerebrovasc Dis.* 2005;20:270-279.

14. Potter BJ, Pinto DS. Subclavian steal syndrome. *Circulation*. 2014;129(22):2320-2323.
15. Jost GF, Dailey AT. Bow Hunter's syndrome revisited: 2 New cases and literature review of 124 cases (2015). *Neurosurgical Focus*. 2015;38(4): E7.
16. Duan G, Xu J, Shi J, Cao Y. Advances in the pathogenesis, diagnosis, and treatment of Bow Hunter's syndrome: a comprehensive review of the literature. *Interve Neurol*. 2016;5:29-38.
17. Searls DE, Pazdera L, Korbel E, et al. Symptoms and signs of posterior circulation ischemia in the New England Medical Center Posterior Circulation Registry. *Arch Neurol*. 2012;69(3):346-351.
18. National Institute of Neurological Disorders and Stroke rt-PA Stroke Study Group. Tissue plasminogen activator for acute ischemic stroke. *N Engl J Med*. 1995;333(24):1581-1587.
19. Kwiatkowski TG, Libman RB, Frankel M, et al. Effects of tissue plasminogen activator for acute ischemic stroke at one year. National Institute of Neurological Disorders and Stroke Recombinant Tissue Plasminogen Activator Stroke Study Group. *N Engl J Med*. 1999; 340(23):1781-1787.
20. Saqqur M, Uchino K, Demchuk AM, et al. Site of arterial occlusion identified by transcranial Doppler predicts the response to intravenous thrombolysis for stroke. *Stroke*. 2007;38(3):948-954.
21. Singer O, Berkefeld J, Nolte C, et al. Mechanical recanalization in basilar artery occlusion: the ENDOSTROKE study. *Ann Neurol*. 2015;77:415-424.
22. Liu X, Dai Q, Ye R, et al. Endovascular treatment versus standard medical treatment for vertebrobasilar artery occlusion (BEST): an open-label, randomized controlled trial. *Lancet Neurol*. 2020;19:115-122.
23. Caliborne Johnston S, Easton JD, Farrant M, et al. Clopidogrel and aspirin in acute ischemic stroke and high-risk TIA. *N Engl J Med*. 2018;379:215-225.
24. Wang Y, Wang Y, Zhao X, et al. Clopidogrel with aspirin in acute minor stroke or transient ischemic attack. *N Engl J Med*. 2013;369:11-19.
25. Markus HS, Hayter E, Levi C. Antiplatelet treatment compared with anticoagulation treatment for cervical artery dissection (CADISS): a randomized trial. *Lancet Neurol*. 2015;14(4):361-367.
26. Moon K, Albuquerque FC, Cole T, et al. Stroke prevention by endovascular treatment of carotid and vertebral artery dissections. *J Neurointerv Surg*. 2017;9:952-957.
27. Henry I, Henry MC, Benjelloun A. TCT-780 Percutaneous transluminal angioplasty of the subclavian arteries: long-term follow up. *J Am Coll Cardiol*. 2015; 66(Suppl 5):B317.
28. Salam TA, Lumsden AB, Smith RB III Subclavian artery revascularization: a decade of experience with extrathoracic bypass procedures. *J Surg Res*. 1994;56(5): 387-392.
29. Pico F, Labreuche J, Amarenco P. Pathophysiology, presentation, prognosis, and management of intracranial arterial dolichoectasia. *Lancet Neurol*. 2015; 14(8):833-845.
30. Wu X, Xu Y, Hong B, et al. Endovascular reconstruction for treatment of vertebrobasilar dolichoectasia: long-term outcomes. *Am J Neuroradiol*. 2013;34(3): 583-588.

SELF-ASSESSMENT STUDY QUESTIONS AND ANSWERS

Questions

1. A 68-year-old woman with a history of smoking, hypertension, and poorly controlled type II diabetes mellitus presents with acute onset vertigo and ataxia. Exam is notable for gaze-evoked nystagmus, dysmetria in the right arm, and unsteady gait. CT imaging reveals no early ischemic changes, and she is subsequently treated with tPA. Vessel imaging shows a severe right vertebral artery stenosis at the V4 segment. Follow-up MRI shows scattered areas of increased diffusion restriction within the right cerebellar hemisphere. What is the most likely mechanism of stroke?
   A. Small vessel disease with lacunar stroke
   B. Cardioembolic
   C. Vessel-to-vessel atheroembolic event
   D. In situ thrombosis

2. Suppose this patient's transthoracic echocardiogram and cardiac rhythm monitoring are unremarkable, and you feel confident that the stroke is caused by symptomatic internal carotid artery dissection (ICAD) from the vertebral artery. What would be the next most appropriate treatment option?
   A. Lifestyle modification, aspirin, and high-dose statin
   B. Lifestyle modification and dual antiplatelet therapy with aspirin and clopidogrel
   C. Lifestyle modification, dual antiplatelet therapy, and high-dose statin
   D. Lifestyle modification, single antiplatelet therapy, high-dose statin, and stenting

3. This patient quits smoking with the aid of nicotine patches and tries to exercise about once per week. She starts atorvastatin 80 mg, aspirin 81 mg, and clopidogrel 75 mg. She is compliant with her medications. About 1 year after her initial event, she suffered a second ischemic stroke, this time in the distribution of the posterior cerebral artery. Vessel imaging reveals worsening right V4 segment severe stenosis. She suffers from hemiparesis and requires short-term rehabilitation. What would be your recommendation for the next steps in treatment?
   A. Continue current maximal medical therapy
   B. Switch from aspirin + clopidogrel to aspirin + ticagrelor
   C. Add ticagrelor to existing dual antiplatelet therapy
   D. Stent the stenotic vertebral artery

4. A 35-year-old man is involved in a biking accident. He suffers a loss of consciousness for 5 minutes. He is brought to the ED. Within a few hours, he develops unilateral neck pain on the right side and a headache. Initial trauma survey, including CT head and spine, is unremarkable. The ED team decides to scan for vertebral artery dissection, and the CT angiogram of the neck reveals a right-sided vertebral artery dissection at the V3 segment. What is the evidence-based treatment for traumatic vertebral artery dissection?
   A. Urgent angioplasty with or without stenting
   B. Start aspirin and follow-up imaging in 6 months
   C. Start anticoagulation and follow-up imaging in 6 months
   D. Either B or C

5. A 70-year-old woman with hypertension and dyslipidemia presents to the emergency department with recurrent episodes of vertigo, diplopia, and dysarthria. Episodes were initially sporadic but then became frequent. Cervical artery ultrasound demonstrates flow reversal in the left vertebral artery. The patient has a faint radial pulse on the left side. What is her most likely diagnosis?
   A. Subclavian steal syndrome
   B. Left vertebral artery occlusion
   C. Left brachial artery stenosis
   D. Basilar artery stenosis

SELF-ASSESSMENT STUDY QUESTIONS AND ANSWERS

6. A 79-year-old woman with hypertension, hyperlipidemia, and type II diabetes mellitus is found unresponsive at her nursing home. She went to bed in her usual state of health at 11 pm the night before. At 6 am the next morning, her nurse came to check on her and found her unresponsive. On arrival at the ER, she has a glasgow coma scale/score (GCS) of 3. Her pupils are dilated bilaterally and poorly responsive to light. She is found to be in atrial fibrillation, which is not previously documented in her history. Non-contrast head CT and basic labs are unremarkable. What would be a reasonable next step for the evaluation of a possible cerebrovascular event? Where would you localize the vascular abnormality?
A. Take the patient to the cath lab for DSA
B. Obtain CTA and CT perfusion
C. Obtain MRA and MR perfusion
D. Either B or C

7. The patient is found to have an occlusion of the upper basilar artery segment, with associated occlusion of the left superior cerebellar artery and the bilateral PCA. What therapies should be considered for this patient?
A. Intravenous thrombolysis with tPA.
B. Mechanical thrombectomy
C. The patient is beyond all treatment windows.
D. Both A and B.

8. A 64-year-old man with hypertension and alcohol abuse develops recurrent dizziness and presyncope over a period of 1 month. He is evaluated by his primary care doctor and later a cardiologist with unremarkable workup. After another such episode, the patient decided to present to the emergency room. A brain MRI and MRA are obtained to rule out stroke. MRI shows no acute ischemic event, but vessel imaging reveals critical stenosis of the basilar artery. The patient is currently asymptomatic with a normal neurologic exam. What should be your next step?
A. Start maximum medical therapy with aspirin, clopidogrel, and high-dose statin
B. Perform a diagnostic angiogram to determine the degree of stenosis
C. Schedule the patient for angioplasty and stenting immediately
D. Both A and B

9. A 72-year-old man with a history of coronary artery disease and multiple cardiac stents now on high-intensity statin, aspirin, and clopidogrel developed sudden right leg weakness and dysarthria. His family brought him to the emergency room within 1 hour of symptom onset, but by that time the weakness and dysarthria had resolved. CT head was unremarkable. Vessel imaging showed a widened and tortuous basilar artery measuring 7.5 mm at its widest diameter. What are the criteria for the diagnosis of vertebrobasilar dolichoectasia?
A. Bifurcation above the dorsum sellae, vessel situated lateral to dorsum sellae, and a vessel diameter > 4.5 mm
B. Vessel diameter > 4.5 mm only
C. Bifurcation above the dorsum sellae and vessel diameter > 4.5 mm

10. What steps can be taken to prevent this patient from experiencing a recurrent stroke or TIA? At what point should surgical intervention be considered?
A. Cautiously manage blood pressure; intervene if symptoms develop
B. Cautiously manage blood pressure, start antiplatelet therapy; intervene if the lesion enlarges by 2 mm or more within 1 year
C. Cautiously manage blood pressure, start antiplatelet therapy; intervene if the lesion enlarges by 4 mm or more within 1 year

SELF-ASSESSMENT STUDY QUESTIONS AND ANSWERS

Answers

1. C.
2. C.
3. D.
4. D.
5. A.
6. B.
7. B.
8. D.
9. A.
10. B.

CHAPTER

36 Chronic Mesenteric Ischemia

Tania A. Torres-Ruiz and Mohamed F. Osman

OUTLINE

GENERAL CONSIDERATIONS AND HISTORY
CLINICAL FINDINGS
DIFFERENTIAL DIAGNOSIS
DIAGNOSIS
Noninvasive Modalities
Invasive Modalities
MANAGEMENT
Endovascular Intervention
Surgical Management
Antegrade Aortoceliac to Superior Mesenteric Artery Bypass
Retrograde Aorta to Superior Mesenteric Artery Bypass
CONSIDERATIONS
Mesenteric Infarction
Aortic Reconstruction and Mesenteric Revascularization
Remedial Procedures after Open Surgical Mesenteric Revascularization
Nonatherosclerotic Causes of Chronic Mesenteric Ischemia
OUTCOMES

GENERAL CONSIDERATIONS AND HISTORY

Chronic mesenteric ischemia (CMI), also known as intestinal angina, is characterized by abdominal pain after meals due to low mesenteric blood flow as a result of mesenteric occlusive disease. Although atherosclerotic disease in the mesenteric vascular bed is quite common, intenstinal angina is rare.[1,2] The prevalence of CMI is estimated to be 1 in 100,000 of the annual US hospital admissions and accounts for 2% of admissions for gastrointestinal (GI) conditions.[3] CMI is more commonly seen in females compared to males and atherosclerotic disease in the most common underlying pathology.[3,4] The majority of the clinical presentation of this disease process can be attributed to the decreased blood flow. After ingestion of a meal, blood flow increases to around 2000 cc/hr over the following 3 to 6 hours in order to provide adequate oxygenation to the GI system.[4,5] Patients with mesenteric ischemia are unable to mount this postprandial hyperemic response that is required for adequate oxygenation and energy to proceed with the metabolic processes of secretion and absorption as well as peristalsis. As such, intestinal angina results from visceral organs failing to meet the regular metabolic requirements. However, the mesenteric circulation is a complex network involving multiple collateral, and due to this, one may not develop symptoms until at least two of the three major mesenteric vessels—the superior mesenteric artery, inferior mesenteric artery, or celiac axis (SMA, IMA, or celiac axis)—are completely occluded or severely narrowed.[6]

Mesenteric ischemia can be characterized as either acute or chronic based on the acuity and duration of the symptoms. Chronic mesenteric ischemia progresses over weeks or months, and the most common cause being occlusive disease secondary to atherosclerotic disease process. This chapter will discuss the clinical findings, differential diagnosis, the surgical and endovascular management of chronic mesenteric ischemia.[4]

CLINICAL FINDINGS

When approaching a patient with suspected mesenteric ischemia, it is imperative to obtain a thorough history and physical exam as symptoms of mesenteric ischemia can sometimes mimic other disease processes and vice versa. Frequently, patients will complain of postprandial abdominal pain which is seen 15 to 60 minutes after a meal. The pain is quite reproducible and described as dull and cramp-like in nature and located in the epigastric region. This can be attributed to the lack of energy and nutritional support from decreased blood flow to the mesenteric vessels. This lack of nutritional support can lead to failure of smooth muscle relaxation that intensifies the cramping experienced.[3–5]

Patients will also complain of progressive involuntary weight loss which is attributed to "food aversion, food fear" due to anticipation of postprandial pain. The intensified abdominal pain after eating leads patients to associate the pain with eating and will modify their oral intake in order to prevent as much abdominal pain as possible. The modified diet will preferentially include liquids. Not uncommonly the patient may maintain normal weight with high caloric liquid diet. Frequently, patients will also describe symptoms from decreased blood flow to other vascular beds, that is, coronary, cerebral, or peripheral arteries with symptoms such as claudication, angina, and symptoms consistent with TIA. This can be attributed to associated atherosclerosis in these regions as well.[1] Nausea, emesis, and changes in bowel habit may be present; however, these are less common findings and are less specific to mesenteric ischemia. The physical exam will include non specific findings, but the patient will appear severely undernourished with evidence of cachexia. Guarding and rebound tenderness are usually absent and an abdominal bruit may be present; however, it is not specific for mesenteric ischemia.[7,8]

Additionally, it is important to screen patients for risk factors that are associated with atherosclerotic disease as this seems to be the major cause of mesenteric ischemia. Common risk factors include history of hypertension, hyperlipidemia, diabetes, heavy smoking history, family history of hyperlipidemia. Hansen et al. in their population-based prevalence study found mesenteric atheroscoertic disease in 17.5 percent among those over 65.[1] In the same study, a multivariate analysis identified renal artery stenosis was significantly associated with celiac or mesenteric artery stenosis or occlusion.[1]

DIFFERENTIAL DIAGNOSIS

The diagnosis for CMI is rarely blatant and often requires further workup to rule out other pathologies that could cause the typical presenting symptoms. It is imperative to eliminate other pathological processes such as gastroparesis, gastric ulceration, gastroduodenitis, gallbladder dysfunction, and intra-abdominal malignancy from the differential diagnosis prior to proceeding with further workup for mesenteric ischemia. Recent SVS guidelines recommended an expedited workup to exclude gastrointestinal malignancies and other potential causes. The expedited workup may include an esophagogastroduodenoscopy, a colonoscopy, an abdominal computed tomography (CT) scan and an abdominal ultrasound.[9]

DIAGNOSIS

A high index of clinical suspicion is critical for making a timely diagnosis of chronic mesenteric ischemia. A presumptive diagnosis of CMI in patients with typical symptoms (postprandial pain, food aversion, weight loss) should be further investigated with appropriate imaging to demonstrate high-grade stenosis (>70%) or occlusion of at least two mesenteric vessels. Celiac axis or superior mesteric artery occlusion, particulaly light of prior surgical disruption of collateral circulation, may result in intestinal angina.[10] Frequently patients will undergo an esophagogastroduodenoscopy (EGD), colonoscopy, barium studies of the upper and lower GI tract, abdominal ultrasound which includes gallbladder visualization, and finally CT imaging for evaluation of the hepatobiliary disease and to exclude any occult tumors before CMI diagnosis is confirmed.[3] The diagnosis of mesenteric ischemia can be further evaluated with noninvasive and invasive modalities which are described below.[3,4]

NONINVASIVE MODALITIES

A mesenteric duplex aids in interrogating blood flow patterns within the mesenteric vessels and for the identification of stenosis within a vessel. One of the major advantages of this modality is that it is also able to determine any changes in the blood flow through the mesenteric vessels before and after a meal. It is important to note that the IMA is difficult to visualize with a mesenteric duplex and will rarely be included in the examination.[11] General findings of a duplex that indicate 70% or greater stenosis can be seen in Table 36-1; however, one must take into consideration that the values may vary based on the criteria between different institutions.[6] The sensitivities and specificities of this modality are known to be greater than 80%, and MRA and arteriography findings have shown good correlation with the mesenteric duplex findings. The SVS guidelines recommended using the mesenteric duplex ultrasound (DUS) examination as the preferred screening test for mesenteric artery occlusive disease.[9]

The disadvantage of the mesenteric duplex is that it is a fairly difficult modality to technically master and it is user-dependent accounting for both false positives and negatives. Also, while the examination is being performed, there is respiratory variation in the velocities and the deep locations of the mesenteric vessels which could be overshadowed by intra-abdominal gas making it fairly difficult to obtain adequate visualization of the vessels of interest.

CT arteriography and magnetic resonance arteriography have recently replaced mesenteric duplex ultrasound and catheter-based contrast arteriography as the imaging of choice for suspected chronic mesenteric ischemia.[2,5] The advantages of these imaging modalities are that they can accurately identify significant stenosis in the major vessels while simultaneously excluding additional potential intra-abdominal processes which may be causing the symptoms in the patient. Recent guidelines by the Society for Vascular Surgery recommended computed tomographic (CT) angiography of the abdomen and pelvis as the best imaging modality since it reliably identifies or excludes the presence of atherosclerotic vascular disease as the most likely etiology, and concurrently rules out other potential abdominal pathologies as the source of symptoms.[9]

TABLE 36-1 Arterial Mesenteric Duplex Findings Consistent with >70% Stenosis

Celiac trunk	PSV > 200 cm/s	EDV > 55 cm/s
SMA	PSV > 275 cm/s	EDV > 45 cm/s

INVASIVE MODALITIES

Catheter-based contrast arteriography is done by gaining access to the vessels via femoral or brachial access. Contrast is shot through a catheter and views of the aorta including the mesenteric vessels are visualised. Lateral views of the aorta should be obtained to allow for evaluation of the mesenteric vessels at the origin. Selective catheterization of each artery is done for better evaluation of the arteries and in some case to measure the pressure gradient in the arteries compared to the aort. Angiography of the celiac trunk, SMA, and IMA remains the "gold standard" in the diagnosis and evaluation for mesenteric ischemia.[1] Not only is arteriography advantageous because it identifies a lesion and its specific location, but also allows for endovascular treatment once a lesion is identified either by angioplasty with or without stenting although in most cases stenting of the lesions is done. In addition to endovascular intervention, angiography can help identify, and plan open surgical intervention. It is important to note that mesenteric atherosclerosis is usually considered an extension "spill over" of aortic disease. The lesions seen on arteriography will primarily be at the origins of the celiac trunk and SMA, whereas the distal branches of these major vessels might appear patent, with well-developed collaterals between the visceral vessels.

MANAGEMENT

The aim toward treatment of symptomatic chronic mesenteric ischemia is correction of the occlusive disease and restoration of flow in timely amnner. Unfortunately, there is no role for noninterventional therapies in this setting. Although parenteral nutrition may be used in the perioperative setting to aid in nutritional optimization, it is not practical as a long-term solution and any delay may be associated with acute on chronic ischemia and worse outcomes.[12,13] Patients who are identified as having chronic mesenteric ischemia should undergo revascularization for symptomatic relief, to prevent bowel infarction and to help restore nutritional status of the patient.

Endovascular, open surgical and hybrid techniques are well established in mesenteric revascularization. Endovascularization revascularization with primary stenting has become the first choice of treatment in the majority of patients.[9,14] The recent SVS guidelines recommended reserving open surgical revascularization for patients with CMI who have lesions that are not amenable to endovascular therapy, endovascular failures, and a select group of younger, healthier patients for whom the long-term benefits may offset the increased perioperative risks.[9]

ENDOVASCULAR INTERVENTION

Endovascular intervention has its advantages compared to open surgical repair. It is associated with shorter hospital stay, reduced morbidity and mortality, and improvement in the quality of life. However, despite the advantages, it has been noted that the long-term patency rates for the vessels are inferior compared to the open surgical revascularization. The SMA is the recommended primary target for revascularization. The ideal lesion for endovascularization revascularization is a short, focal stenosis or occlusion with minimal to moderate calcification or thrombus (Figure 36-1).[14] Preoperative considerations in planning endovascular repair include contrast allergy which can be treated with steroid preparation. Preoperative creatinine levels that are considered to be elevated (above 1.5 mg/dL) should be prehydrated prior to endovascular intervention.[3,15]

Percutaneous access should be set up through the femoral, brachial artery or radial artery depending on whether there is planned therapeutic intervention during the angiography. If planning intervention, it should be noted that if catheters are used through the femoral approach, intervention may pose a difficult challenge due to the anatomy of the mesenteric vessels in relation to the aorta. The angle of the mesenteric vessels is notably acute and directed caudad which would make the vectors from the femoral approach opposite the angles. Once the arteriogram

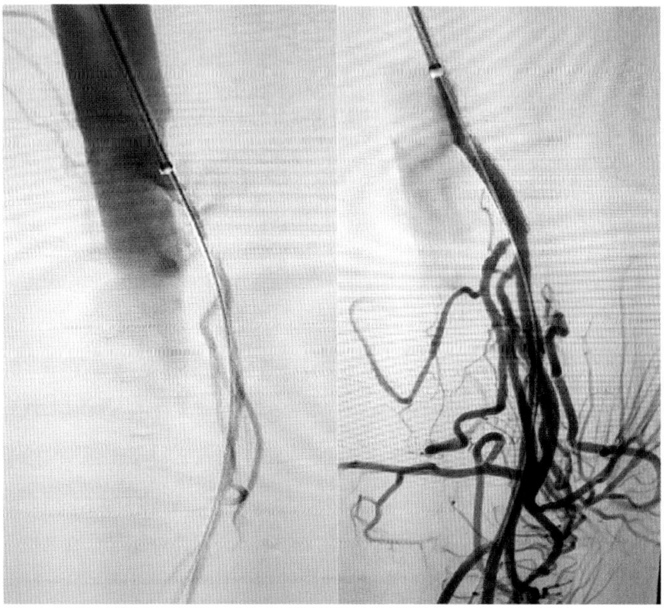

FIGURE 36-1 Sagittal view of an SMA with high grade stenosis, before and after stenting.

is shot and adequate visualization of the lesion is obtained, there is a chance that the symptomatic stenosis can be treated at the time of the diagnostic arteriogram. Ideally, multivessel revascularization is optimal given the decreased incidence of refractory symptoms. However, it must be noted that orificial stenosis at the mesenteric vessels is refractory to angioplasty alone and angioplasty with primary stenting is recommended with balloon-expanding stents.[5] Retrograde stenting of the superior mesenteric artery can be achieved through an open abdomen by dissecting a disal segment of the SMA then accessing this segment retrogradely toward the orifice of the SMA which can be treated through balloon angioplasty and stenting. This approach can be used in a flush occluded SMA at the origin that is difficult to negotiate through the femoral or arm approach.

Owing to the high recurrence rate, patients undergoing revascularization for CMI should be educated and counseled about recurrent symptoms. Patients should be followed in the outpatient setting after revascularization within 1 month of the procedure and then biannually for the first 2 years, and then annually thereafter. The SVS guidelines suggest surveillance with mesenteric DUS examination to identify recurrent stenoses and recommended CTA or catheter-based arteriograms to confirm any restenosis detected by DUS examination. The remedial treatment should be guided by similar principles of the de novo lesions. The choice of revascularization for recurrent stenoses should be similar to the de novo lesions with the endovascular approach recommended as the initial option and open revascularization reserved for lesions not amenable to the endovascular approach.[9]

SURGICAL MANAGEMENT

Prior to open revascularization, a patient should be medically optimized and preoperative planning should be done with a CT angiogram or catheter-based angiography. Bypass grafting can be done in multiple ways including an antegrade aorto celiac and aorto superior mesenteric artery bypass or retrograde infrarenal aorta to superior mesenteric artery bypass. It should be noted that multivessel reconstructions have not been shown to have a significant clinical advantage compared to single vessel reconstructions.

ANTEGRADE AORTOCELIAC TO SUPERIOR MESENTERIC ARTERY BYPASS

The antegrade bypass is performed by exposing and dissecting free an adequate length of supraceliac aorta followed by adequate exposure of the celiac axis for facilitation of the anastomosis. The SMA should be inspected thoroughly and an adequate segment of the SMA measuring approximately 2 to 3 cm should be identified and dissected for the distal anastomosis. It is important to note that the SMA sits within retroperitoneal tissue and fat which can cause confusion of the SMA for collaterals.[3] Identification of the superior mesenteric vein (SMV) can sometimes aid in the identification of the SMA. The anastomosis is then performed by partially occluding the aorta with a side-biting clamp or by two straight aortic clamps depending on the degree of calcification. Prior to clamping, it should be noted that the patient should undergo systemic heparinization with 100 units/kg. A bifurcated Dacron graft with a body diameter measuring 12 mm and limb diameter of 7 mm has been a popular graft option; however, this graft can be substituted for grafts measuring 12 by 6 mm or 14 by 7 mm.[3,16] The cephalic limb of the graft is used to perform the celiac axis anastomosis in an end-to-end fashion and the caudal limb is carefully tunneled deep to the pancreas with the anastomosis to the SMA done in an end-to-side fashion.[16] After the procedure, a doppler should be used to interrogate the completed bypass. Some of the advantages of this bypass are that the segments used for the bypass are usually uninvolved with atherosclerosis and the limbs of the graft itself follow a direct path.

RETROGRADE AORTA TO SUPERIOR MESENTERIC ARTERY BYPASS

The principles for the retrograde aorto-SMA bypass remain similar to the antegrade bypass; however, the proximal anastomosis has multiple variations in terms of location. In the case of the retrograde bypass, the proximal anastomosis can arise from the proximal right common iliac artery, the infrarenal aorta, or the proximal left common iliac artery. The adequacy of the anastomosis is contingent on various factors including the configuration of the graft as well as the extent of the atherosclerotic disease in the respective vessels. The distal anastomosis to the SMA graft may be done in an end-to-end or end-to-side fashion and can be done using a 6 or 8 mm in diameter Dacron graft or reinforced walled PTFE graft that is similar in diameter.[3,5] It is important to gently curve the graft between the two anastomoses in a C loop manner to avoid kinking of the graft and to provide a tension-free anastomosis. Some of the advantages of the retrograde bypass include an easier and faster exposure given the vessels used. There is also a decrease in the risk of embolization when distal clamping is used. However, one of the major disadvantages of this technique is the positioning of the graft as it increases the risk of kinking.

CONSIDERATIONS

MESENTERIC INFARCTION

At times, patients can be noted to have evidence of compromised bowel at the time of open revascularization. This is more frequently noted in a subset of patients who have evidence of acute changes to the chronic symptoms that they have been experiencing. It is recommended that when approaching this subset of patients, revascularization should proceed definitive bowel resection with the exception of frank necrotic bowel. A second-look operation should be done 24 to 48 hours after the index procedure to re-evaluate the bowel after the revascularization.[3,4] This will help determine definite resection points and may lead to the preservation of bowel that was judged as having compromised blood flow before intervention but undoubtedly appears to have survived after the revascularization. Determining the viability of bowel can pose a challenge; however, there are additional techniques which can be used in addition to visual inspection. For example, intraoperative Doppler to detect arterial signals, intravenous fluorescein in combination with Wood's lamp may be used.

Surgical revascularization in the setting of necrotic bowel should be performed using an autogenous conduit with the saphenous and femoral veins being adequate options. Cadaveric femoral veins have also been considered an option in this setting and the bypass itself can be formed in either the antegrade or the retrograde fashion which was explained above.

AORTIC RECONSTRUCTION AND MESENTERIC REVASCULARIZATION

Patients with occlusive visceral artery disease who require aortic reconstruction present a high risk for postoperative complications. In patients who are to undergo aortic reconstruction, it is important to proceed with revascularization of the visceral vessels prior to the aortic reconstruction. Studies have shown that simultaneous open aortic reconstruction and mesenteric revascularization have a higher complication rate including mortality. Therefore, a staged approach should be considered with either an initial endovascular or open mesenteric revascularization procedure followed by the aortic reconstruction. If it is imperative that both procedures be done simultaneously, a retrograde technique of open revascularization is preferred as it is a simpler procedure and requires minimal dissection.

REMEDIAL PROCEDURES AFTER OPEN SURGICAL MESENTERIC REVASCULARIZATION

Recurrent symptoms after open surgical revascularization for chronic mesenteric ischemia are rare; however, if necessary both antegrade and retrograde bypasses should be considered. Additionally, if a bypass is failing, it is imperative to identify the anastomotic problem of the bypass and to correct it by either thrombectomy, revision of the anastomosis with a vein patch, or a new interposition graft. In case that an antegrade and retrograde bypass is not feasible, the axillary artery, ascending thoracic aorta, and descending thoracic aorta can all be considered as an alternative inflow source.[3,5] Alternative distal targets include the hepatic artery, the splenic artery, the distal SMA, and its branches.

NONATHEROSCLEROTIC CAUSES OF CHRONIC MESENTERIC ISCHEMIA

In rare occasions, nonatherosclerotic causes of chronic mesenteric ischemia may be encountered.

Fibromuscular dysplasia can sometimes involve visceral vessels and cause symptomatic stenosis which are amenable to endovascular treatment with balloon angioplasty. There are also other inflammatory arterial diseases which involve the visceral vessels which can cause chronic mesenteric ischemia. In these instances, the most effective treatment would include controlling the inflammatory process which may include a multidisciplinary approach with the help of a rheumatologist . In these rare cases, revascularization should be delayed until the underlying disease is controlled.

OUTCOMES

Review of literature has shown that the perioperative morbidity and mortality rates for the endovascular approach have been significantly lower than open surgical approaches reporting results less than 20% for each compared to the morbidity rates of around 5% to 65% and mortality rates of 2% to 15% for the open revascularization approach.[2] The types of complications differ depending on the approach. For example, the endovascular approach is associated with predominantly access-related complications (i.e., pseudoaneurysms, hematomas) or contrast-related complications. It should be noted, however, that both approaches are very successful in symptomatic relief exceeding 88% and long-term survival for both endovascular and open revascularization appear to be comparable with an average of approximately 70% at 5 years.[3,5,17]

REFERENCES

1. Hansen KJ, Wilson DB, Craven TE, et al. Mesenteric artery disease in the elderly. *J Vasc Surg.* 2004; 40(1):45-52.
2. Thomas JH, Blake K, Pierce GE, Hermreck AS, Seigel E. The clinical course of asymptomatic mesenteric arterial stenosis. *J Vasc Surg.* 1998;27(5):840-844.
3. Mitchell EL, Moneta GL. Mesenteric duplex scanning. *Perspect Vasc Surg Endovasc Ther.* 2006;18(2):175-183.
4. Fara JW, Rubinstein EH, Sonnenschein RR. Intestinal hormones in mesenteric vasodilation after intraduodenal agents. *Am J Physiol.* 1972;223(5):1058-1067.
5. Sardar P, White CJ. Chronic mesenteric ischemia: diagnosis and management. *Prog Cardiovasc Dis.* 2021; 65:71-75.
6. Mitchell EL. The Society for Vascular Surgery clinical practice guidelines define the optimal care of patients with chronic mesenteric ischemia. *J Vasc Surg.* 2021; 73(1S), 84S-86S.
7. Veenstra RP, ter Steege RW, Geelkerken RH, Huisman AB, Kolkman JJ. The cardiovascular risk profile of atherosclerotic gastrointestinal ischemia is different from other vascular beds. *Am J Med.* 2012;125(4):394-398.
8. Sreenarasimhaiah J. Chronic mesenteric ischemia. *Best Pract Res Clin Gastroenterol.* 1995;19(2):283-295.
9. Huber TS, Björck M, Chandra A. Chronic mesenteric ischemia: clinical practice guidelines from the Society for Vascular Surgery. *J Vasc Surg.* 2021;73(1S):87S-115S.
10. Zeller T, Rastan A, Sixt S. Chronic atherosclerotic mesenteric ischemia (CMI). *Vasc Med.* 2010;15(4):333-338.
11. Cronenwett JL. Mesenteric and celiac duplex scanning: a validation study. *J Vasc Surg.* 1998;27(6):1078-1087; discussion 1088.
12. Oderich GS. Current concepts in the management of chronic mesenteric ischemia. *Curr Treat Options Cardiovasc Med.* 2010;12(2):117-130.
13. Rheudasil JM, Stewart MT, Schellack JV, Smith RB 3rd, Salam AA, Perdue GD. Surgical treatment of chronic mesenteric arterial insufficiency. *J Vasc Surg.* 1998;8(4):495-500.
14. Malgor RD, Oderich GS, McKusick MA, et al. Results of single- and two-vessel mesenteric artery stents for chronic mesenteric ischemia. *Ann Vasc Surg.* 2010;24(8): 1094-1101.
15. Wolk S, Kapalla M, Ludwig S, et al. Surgical and endovascular revascularization of chronic mesenteric ischemia. *Langenbecks Arch Surg.* 2022;407:2085-2094.
16. Chaouch N, Zagzoog MM. Antegrade revascularization of the three mesenteric vessels to treat chronic mesenteric ischemia. *J Surg Case Rep.* 2021(8):rjab328.
17. van Petersen AS, Kolkman JJ; Multidisciplinary Study Group of Splanchnic Ischemia, et al. Open or percutaneous revascularization for chronic splanchnic syndrome. *J Vasc Surg.* 2010;51(5):1309-1316.

SELF-ASSESSMENT STUDY QUESTIONS AND ANSWERS

Questions

1. A 63-year-old woman presents to the clinic with complaints of abdominal pain over the past month. She has a history of hypertension, hyperlipidemia and states she smoked 1 pack per day. Over the past month she states she has developed postprandial abdominal pain in the epigastric region and a 15-lb associated weight loss. What is the next best step in management?
   A. Continue with observation and administration of pain medication as needed
   B. Proceed with a CT angiogram of the abdomen and pelvis
   C. Load the patient with aspirin and Plavix
   D. Proceed with a mesenteric duplex

2. A 35-year-old woman with a history of postprandial abdominal pain and unintentional weight loss presents to the clinic for further evaluation. She has undergone extensive workup including EGD, abdominal US, and HIDA scan for further evaluation of her abdominal pain which has thus far been unremarkable. MRA of her abdomen and pelvis was done which showed impingement of the celiac axis with no other significant lesions. What is the most appropriate next step in her management?
   A. Mesenteric angiography
   B. No further workup required at this time
   C. CTA of the abdomen and pelvis
   D. Dynamic transabdominal duplex

3. During an antegrade bypass to the superior mesenteric artery, which of the following is at risk of injury during the creation of the posterior pancreatic graft tunnel?
   A. The hepatic artery
   B. The splenic artery
   C. The splenic vein
   D. The gastroduodenal artery

4. When planning a retrograde aortomesenteric bypass for chronic mesenteric ischemia, in the absence of an infected field, which of the following would be the most appropriate conduit for the bypass?
   A. Greater saphenous vein
   B. Deep femoral vein
   C. An 8-mm standard wall nonreinforced polytetrafluoroethylene graft
   D. A 7-mm Dacron graft

5. When evaluating a patient with chronic mesenteric ischemia for intervention, which of the following findings would lead you to preferentially prefer an endovascular approach versus an open surgery?
   A. Heavily calcified lesion
   B. Aortic occlusive disease
   C. Short-segment superior mesenteric artery occlusion
   D. Aberrant anatomy

6. When comparing endovascular treatment of chronic mesenteric ischemia to open surgical revascularization, which of the following is associated with open surgery?
   A. Lower mortality rate
   B. Less extended hospital stay
   C. Higher long term patency
   D. Decreased perioperative mortality

SELF-ASSESSMENT STUDY QUESTIONS AND ANSWERS

7. A 70-year-old male with history of aortobifemoral bypass who presents with 25-lb unintentional weight loss and complaints of postprandial abdominal pain. CT angiography of the abdomen and pelvis is done which shows evidence of occlusion at the celiac artery and the superior mesenteric artery. Patient has an ejection fraction of 20% and is noted to have a heavily calcified aorta. Which of the following would be the preferred approach for revascularization?
A. Retrograde bypass from the common iliac to the SMA
B. Antegrade bypass to the celiac axis and SMA
C. SMA stenting via femoral access
D. SMA stenting via brachial access

8. Which of the following peak systolic velocities of the celiac axis is considered to represent greater than 70% stenosis?
A. PSV > 100 cm/s
B. PSV > 150 cm/s
C. PSV > 200 cm/s
D. PSV > 250 cm/s

9. What is the most common cause of chronic mesenteric ischemia?
A. Atherosclerotic disease
B. Embolic disease
C. Thrombosis
D. Dissection

10. In addition to the typical symptoms of postprandial pain and "fear of food", which of the following can be seen in patients with chronic mesenteric ischemia secondary to the nature of atherosclerotic disease?
A. Venous thromboembolism
B. Irregular heart rate
C. Claudication
D. Nausea

SELF-ASSESSMENT STUDY QUESTIONS AND ANSWERS

Answers

1. B.
2. D.
3. C.
4. D.
5. D.
6. C.
7. D.
8. C.
9. A.
10. C.

CHAPTER

37 Acute Mesenteric Ischemia

Susan Natalie Eisert and Michael R. Go

OUTLINE

GENERAL CONSIDERATIONS AND HISTORY
- **Introduction**
- **History of AMI**
- **Pathophysiology**
- **Embolic Causes**
  - Anatomy
  - Risk Factors
  - Clinical Course
- **Thrombotic Causes**
  - Anatomy
  - Risk Factors
  - Clinical Course
- **Nonocclusive Mesenteric Ischemia (NOMI)**
  - Anatomy
  - Risk Factors
  - Clinical Course
- **Mesenteric Venous Thrombosis (MVT)**
  - Anatomy
  - Risk Factors
  - Clinical Course

CLINICAL FINDINGS

DIFFERENTIAL DIAGNOSIS

DIAGNOSIS
- **Laboratory Values**
- **Abdominal X-ray**
- **Ultrasound**
- **CT Angiogram**
- **Other Assessment Modalities**
  - Magnetic Resonance Angiogram (MRA)
  - Diagnostic Laparoscopy

MANAGEMENT OF THE CLINICAL PROBLEM
- **Medical Therapies**
- **Endovascular Therapy**
  - General Considerations
  - Treatment of Embolic Causes of AMI
  - Treatment for Thrombotic Causes of AMI
  - Treatment for NOMI
- **Open Surgery**
  - General Considerations
  - Treatment for Embolic Causes of AMI
  - Treatment for Thrombotic Causes of AMI
- **Hybrid Procedure: Retrograde Open Mesenteric Stenting (ROMS)**
- **Treatment for Mesenteric Venous Thrombosis**
- **Bowel Evaluation**
- **Complications and Follow-Up**
  - Initial Postoperative Treatment, Anticoagulation, and Antiplatelet Therapy
  - Malnutrition, Malabsorption, Sort Gut Syndrome, and Strictures
  - Bypass or Stent Occlusion
- **Tips for Management and to Avoid Complications**

GENERAL CONSIDERATIONS AND HISTORY

INTRODUCTION

Acute mesenteric ischemia (AMI) is caused by a decrease in blood flow to the intestines such that perfusion no longer meets their metabolic demands.[1] This leads to gut ischemia, necrosis, sepsis, and if left untreated, certain death. The incidence of AMI is low; it occurs in 3-5 individuals per 100,000 population and accounts for only 0.09% to 0.2% of all acute admissions to the ED.[2] Yet the mortality rate is high and directly correlated to the time to diagnosis and treatment. Thus, a high index of suspicion is required. A delay in diagnosis of more than 24 hours from onset increases mortality from 50% to 70%.[3] AMI can be categorized into four types: embolic, thrombotic, nonocclusive mesenteric ischemia (NOMI), or mesenteric venous thrombosis (MVT). Rare causes of AMI include arterial dissection, vasculitis, or aneurysm. Table 37-1 provides a general overview of the four most common types of AMI, while the flow chart in Figure 37-1 depicts the general paradigms for workup and treatment for each respective category, and can be used as a visual guide throughout this chapter.

HISTORY OF AMI

While the first successful intestinal resection for bowel gangrene due to mesenteric ischemia was described by Dr. Elliot in 1895,[8] one of the earliest advances in the treatment of AMI was by Dr. Klass in 1951.[9] He was the first surgeon to focus on the restoration of blood supply to salvage ischemic bowel. Drs. Boley and Clark's innovations with the early use of angiograms and vasodilators in the 1970s decreased the mortality rate for AMI to approximately 50%.[10-13] One of the main vasodilators in use for AMI is papaverine. It is an opium alkaloid antispasmodic drug that was discovered in 1848 by Georg Merck,[14] who went on to found the German drug company. Papaverine is a phosphodiesterase inhibitor that causes increased cyclic AMP, allowing for its use in the treatment of visceral vasospasm.

PATHOPHYSIOLOGY

In a fasting state, the splanchnic circulation accounts for about 25% of the cardiac output. This increases to 35% of the cardiac output in the postprandial state. The small intestine in particular gets 10% to 15% of resting cardiac output, and up to 50% in the postprandial state. Of the blood flow to the intestine, 70% supplies the mucosa and submucosa, while the remaining 30% supplies the muscularis and serosal layers. Multiple mechanisms regulate splanchnic blood flow, including endogenous hormones, and also medications. For example, norepinephrine and high levels of epinephrine cause vasoconstriction, while vasopressin, phenylephrine, and digoxin decrease splanchnic blood flow overall. Whereas low-dose dopamine causes splanchnic vasodilation, higher doses cause vasoconstriction by activating alpha-adrenergic receptors. Though the celiac axis, the superior mesenteric artery (SMA) and the inferior mesenteric artery all supply portions of the intestines, the SMA supplies the majority of the small intestine. When it becomes compromised through arterial occlusion or vasospasm, it frequently leads to devastating small bowel necrosis if not treated.

EMBOLIC CAUSES

Anatomy

Embolic occlusion accounts for 40% to 50% of all AMI cases.[4] Thromboembolism most commonly affects the SMA due to the oblique origin off of the aorta, with lodging of the clot as the SMA tapers. While only 22% of emboli lodge at the SMA origin, most occlude just beyond the first jejunal branches with 37% lodging proximal to the middle colic artery and 41% distal to the middle colic artery.[5] When the middle colic artery is not affected, a characteristic sparing of the proximal jejunum and distal ascending colon can be seen, with ischemia affecting the distal jejunum through proximal colon.[2] Atheroemboli on the other hand are smaller and tend to lodge more distally, causing more focal areas of necrosis. In about 20% of emboli to the SMA there is an associated concurrent embolic event to another arterial bed, including the spleen or kidney.[5]

TABLE 37-1 The Four Types of Acute Mesenteric Ischemia.

	Embolic	Thrombotic	NOMI	MVT
Depiction	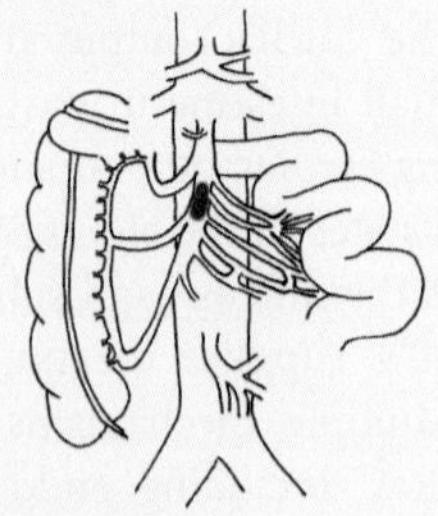	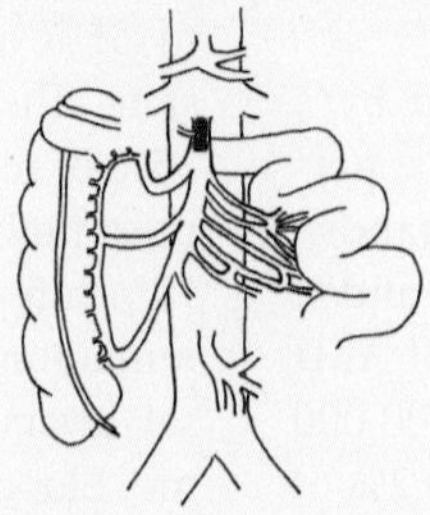	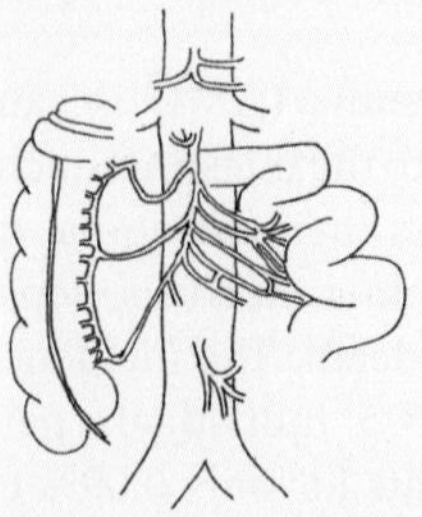	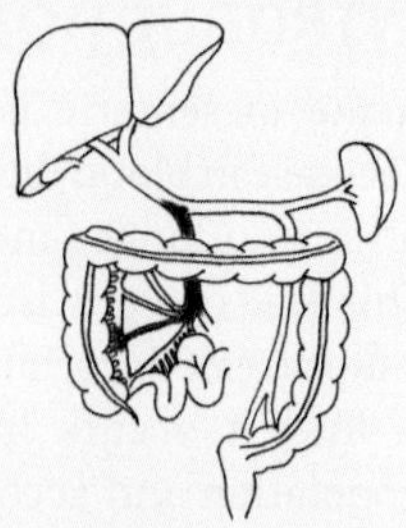
~ % of AMI cases	40%–50%[4]	20%–35%[4]	5%–15%[4]	5%–15%[4]
Description	Embolic arterial occlusion	Acute arterial thrombosis usually on preexisting severe atherosclerotic disease	Low cardiac output associated with diffuse mesenteric vasoconstriction	Venous thrombosis causing venous engorgement and in turn impaired arterial inflow
Anatomy	Most frequently affects SMA due to oblique origin. Most emboli lodge distal to middle colic artery.[5] This can lead to characteristic sparing of the first portion of small intestine and ascending colon.	Most frequently affect SMA origin, causing ischemia from midduodenum to splenic flexure. Collaterals can delay bowel infarction until critical. Stenosis/occlusion of vessel or collateral.	Paradoxical splanchnic vasoconstriction usually affects distribution of SMA. NOMI has a propensity to affect water shed areas.	Thrombi usually originate in venous arcades and propagates to SMV, ± to the portal vein. This causes bowel wall edema, sloughing, and hemorrhage, as well as ascites on imaging.
Risk factors	Most emboli are cardiac origin: Afib/aflutter, low EF (CHF, cardiomyopathy) recent MI, ventricular aneurysm, or proximal arterial source (cardiac valvular disease, endocarditis), proximal aneurysm, aortic mural thrombi, recent catheter-based angiogram.	History of chronic mesenteric ischemia (in about 20%), complication of mesenteric revascularization (stent occlusion, stent migration, distal embolization, vessel perforation/dissection), and PAD (27%).	Critically ill with significant hemodynamic insults, cardiac failure, peripheral hypoxemia, reperfusion injury, pressors causing vasoconstriction, and preexisting heavy atherosclerotic burden.	Dehydration, local infection/inflammation, hypercoagulability, thrombophilia, trauma, history of DVT, cancer, chronic liver disease, or portal thrombosis. 20% of cases remain idiopathic.
Clinical course	Rapid deterioration due to lack of collaterals. Hospital mortality is estimated to be 66%–71%.[6]	Presence of collaterals can slow deterioration; mortality is 70%–87%[6] given delay in diagnosis and large area of bowel infarction and need for complex revascularization procedure.	Insidious onset as often in critical care and hard to evaluate in sedated patients. High mortality rates due to frequent association with multisystem organ failure Overall mortality for NOMI: 70%–80%[6]	More subtle onset; 30-day mortality around 20% and the 5-year mortality is 30%.[7]

MVT, mesenteric venous thrombosis; NOMI, nonocclusive mesenteric ischemia; SMA, superior mesenteric artery; CHF, congestive heart failure; DVT, deep vein thrombosis; PAD, peripheral artery disease.

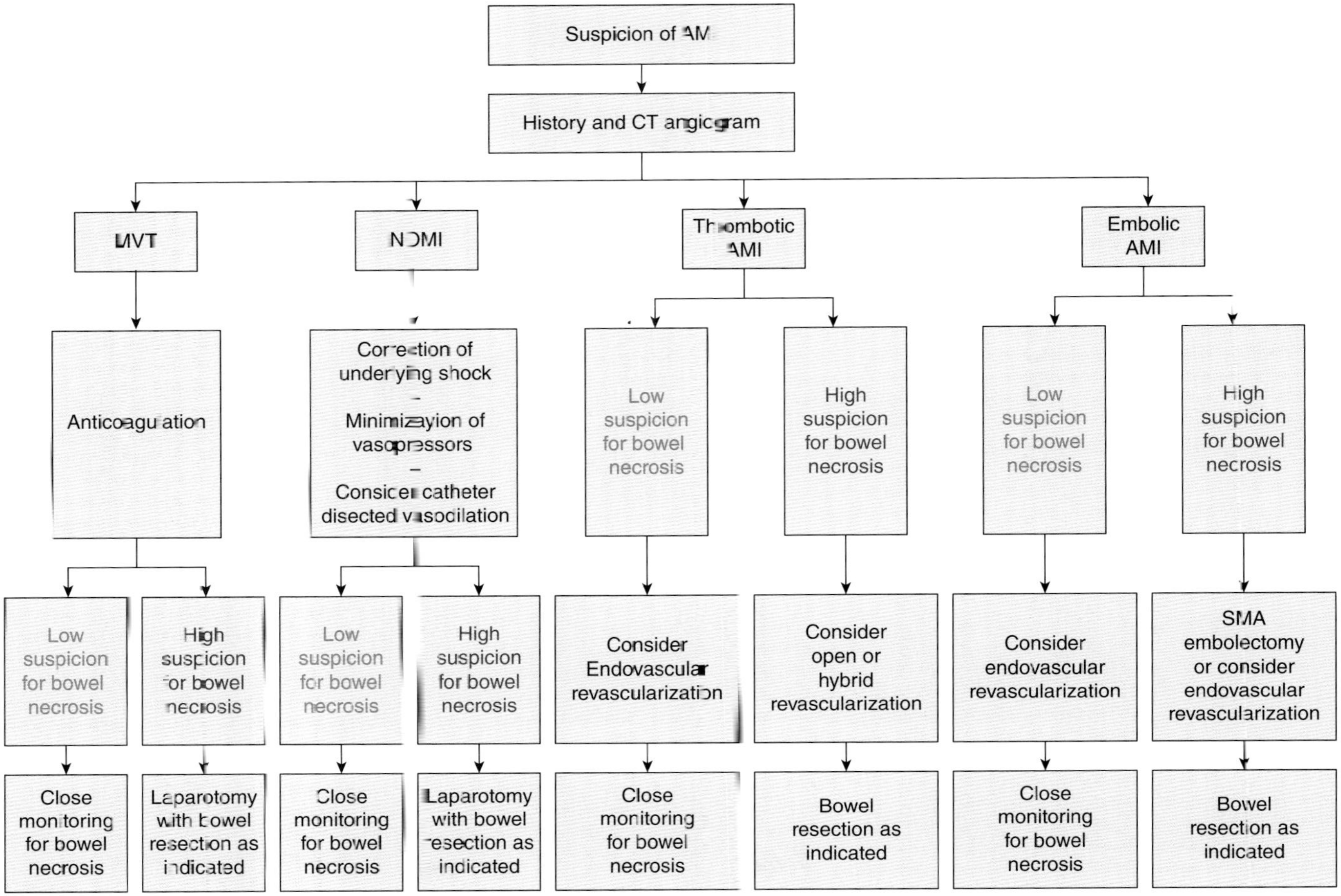

FIGURE 37-1 Work-up and treatment algorithm for AMI going from left to right. Note alternative pathways for "high suspicion for bowel necrosis" designated with the red text, as compared to "low suspicion for bowel necrosis" as designated with the green text, for each type of mesenteric ischemia. AMI, acute mesenteric ischemia; MVT, mesenteric venous thrombosis; NOMI, nonocclusive mesenteric ischemia; SMA, superior mesenteric artery.

Risk Factors

The two main risk factors in AMI overall are gender, with a 3:1 female to male incidence, and age, with most cases occurring in patient's 60s and 70s. Embolic AMI is predominantly caused by atrial fibrillation, accounting for nearly 50%[15] of all emboli. Alternative causes are atrial flutter, low ejection fraction (such as from congestive heart failure or cardiomyopathy), recent myocardial infarction, ventricular aneurysm, or proximal arterial sources including cardiac valvular disease, valvular replacement, endocarditis, proximal aneurysms, aortic mural thrombi, or recent catheter-based angiogram.[16] Of patients with AMI secondary to an embolic cause, one-third had an antecedent arterial embolism.[15]

Clinical Course

Embolic AMI can lead to rapid deterioration in patient status. This is mostly due to a lack of any preformed collaterals in this disease pathology.

THROMBOTIC CAUSES

Anatomy

Around 20% to 35% of AMI cases are caused by in situ arterial thrombosis.[4] Usually acute arterial thrombosis occurs on preexisting severe atherosclerotic disease. While 80% of patients with a thrombotic cause for AMI were asymptomatic prior to the event, 20% had chronic mesenteric ischemia symptoms prior. Atherosclerosis causing lower extremity peripheral arterial disease is concomitantly present in 27%. The SMA origin is most likely to be involved, in turn leading to less bowel sparing and a characteristic pattern of bowel ischemia from the mid-duodenum all the way to the splenic flexure of the colon. Due to the underlying atherosclerosis of the mesenteric arteries, collateralization occurs, which can delay bowel infarction until critical stenosis or occlusion of the vessel has occurred. Also because of underlying atherosclerosis, celiac occlusion is often observed at the time of acute SMA thrombosis.[17]

Risk Factors

A history of chronic mesenteric ischemia is present in 20% of thrombotic AMI patients,[18] which means that prior symptoms can include postprandial pain 30-60 minutes after eating, weight loss, or food fear. Alternatively, a history of prior mesenteric revascularization can be the cause of a complication, such as stent occlusion, restenosis, or distal embolization. A history of other atherosclerotic diseases, such as coronary artery disease, carotid disease, or peripheral vascular disease is additional risk factors.

Clinical Course

The presence of collateral blood flow can slow the course of AMI, leading to a less acute presentation. Patients with prior chronic mesenteric ischemia tend to present with acute chronic mesenteric ischemia. This typically delays diagnosis, and the usually larger area of bowel infarction and the need for complex revascularization in the setting of diffuse atherosclerosis leads to in-hospital mortality of 70% to 87% in patients with thrombotic AMI.[6]

NONOCCLUSIVE MESENTERIC ISCHEMIA (NOMI)

Anatomy

While the exact cause for NOMI remains unknown, it is thought to be caused by global hypoperfusion, with subsequent mesenteric vasospasm that can usually be observed in the distribution of the SMA. Thus, NOMI predominantly affects the watershed areas. NOMI accounts for about 5% to 15% of AMI presentations.[4] It is also associated with vasoactive drugs and digitalis due to their vasoconstrictive properties.

Risk Factors

NOMI occurs in the critically ill patients after a significant hemodynamic insult, such as cardiac surgery or hemodialysis, and also cardiac failure or peripheral hypoxemia. The resulting reperfusion injury leads to paradoxical splanchnic vasospasm, which is often further exacerbated by concomitant treatment with epinephrine, norepinephrine, vasopressin, and digoxin.[19] Current literature indicates that several short episodes of ischemia with reperfusion might cause worse reperfusion injury than a single longer insult.[20] Main risk factors are age greater than

50 years, recent myocardial infarction, congestive heart failure, aortic insufficiency, cardiopulmonary bypass, renal or hepatic disease, or major abdominal or cardiovascular surgery. Patients with a preexisting heavy atherosclerotic burden are at risk of having decreased intestinal perfusion at baseline, and may have a propensity to deteriorate to AMI with a superimposed hemodynamic insult.

Clinical Course

NOMI has a considerable mortality rate, ranging from 70% to 80%.[6] This is due to the insidious onset in a patient who is already critically ill. Detection can be hindered due to ICU sedation in the setting of their critical illness, leading to an additional delay in diagnosis. It is frequently associated with multisystem organ failure, adding to the mortality.

MESENTERIC VENOUS THROMBOSIS (MVT)

Anatomy

MVT accounts for about 5% to 15% of AMI.[4] It is caused by venous thrombi originating from the venous arcades and propagating to the SMV and portal vein, while the inferior mesenteric vein usually remains uninvolved. Unlike arterial causes of AMI where within a short segment there is a transition from normal bowel to ischemic bowel, MVT has a more gradual transition between normal and ischemic bowel. While many SMV thromboses remain asymptomatic, abdominal findings and imaging with SMV occlusion means AMI is on the differential. Often imaging also reveals a significant amount of ascites in these patients.

Risk Factors

Virchow's triad with stagnant blood flow, hypercoagulability, and vascular inflammation can explain 80% of MVT cases, while the remaining 20% are idiopathic.[2] Consequently, the main risk factors include dehydration, hypercoagulability with thrombophilia including myeloproliferative disease and hemolytic disease, as well as genetic risk factors including Factor V Leiden mutation and antithrombin deficiency, trauma, or local inflammatory changes including pancreatitis, diverticulitis, or inflammation/infection of the biliary system. A history of deep venous thrombosis, cancer, chronic liver disease or portal thrombosis, recent abdominal surgery, inflammatory disease, or thrombophilia are associated with MVT.[21]

Clinical Course

The clinical course of MVT is often more subtle than arterial occlusion such that patients usually present 1-2 weeks after onset. Long-term mortality is dependent on the underlying cause of thrombosis, but on average the 30-day mortality is 20% and the 5-year mortality is 30%.[7]

CLINICAL FINDINGS

The hallmark symptom of AMI is abdominal pain out of proportion to exam. This excruciating abdominal pain with an unrevealing abdominal exam is present in up to 95% of AMI patients.[15] It is typically unrelenting periumbilical pain with minimal additional physical findings. Accompanying symptoms include nausea (in 44% of AMI cases), vomiting (in 35% of AMI cases), and diarrhea (in 35% of AMI cases). If significant bowel ischemia is already present, blood per rectum can appear (16% of AMI cases).[15] In patients with a slower onset of AMI, there is frequent abdominal distension and diarrhea from malabsorption due to mucosal surface ischemia. Pain with palpation, on the other hand, signifies peritonitis and is indicative of transmural ischemia. With bowel necrosis, signs of sepsis are seen, such as mental confusion, tachycardia, tachypnea, circulatory collage, up to multiorgan failure.

DIFFERENTIAL DIAGNOSIS

The differential diagnosis of abdominal pain, nausea, emesis, and diarrhea is broad, and as such includes acute appendicitis, acute pancreatitis, abdominal aortic aneurysm, aortic dissection, bowel obstruction, bowel perforation, cholecystitis, gastroenteritis, and others. A high index of suspicion is required to allow for a timely diagnosis of AMI. Identifying risk factors for atherosclerosis or embolic events may help narrow the differential in patients with abdominal pain.

DIAGNOSIS

LABORATORY VALUES

The diagnosis of AMI can be made clinically and is confirmed by imaging or in the operating room. Laboratory values might demonstrate signs of dehydration, bowel ischemia or possibly sepsis, such as leukocytosis (abnormal WBC count in >90% of AMI patients[22]), hemoconcentration, metabolic acidosis with elevated anion gap, or elevated serum lactate levels, which are present in 88% of AMI patients[22]). A lactate level of >2 mmol/L has been associated with irreversible intestinal ischemia.[23] While an elevated D-dimer level is nondiagnostic, a normal D-dimer makes AMI significantly less likely. As such a level greater 0.9 m/L is only 60% sensitive, while 82% specific and 79% accurate.[24] Other lab values can also become elevated, such as lactate dehydrogenase (LDH), alanine aminotransferase (ALT), aspartate aminotransferase (AST), or creatine phosphokinase (CPK), although they all remain nonspecific findings. A rise in serum amylase occurs late in the course of the disease in about 50% of AMI cases.[25]

ABDOMINAL X-RAY

Abdominal X-rays are nonspecific and normal in 25% of AMI patients but can show ileus or intestinal wall edema with "thumbprinting," which is present in under 40% of x-rays in AMI patients. In more advanced AMI, pneumatosis might be seen.[26]

ULTRASOUND

Ultrasound, and specifically Doppler examination, is not used for the diagnosis of AMI. While it can evaluate the proximal celiac artery and SMA well, it is unable to assess flow in the more distal SMA. Due to additional technical limitations of visualization, such as lack of bowel evaluation, painfulness of examination for the patient, prolonged examination, and need for qualified sonographers and reading physicians, Doppler ultrasound examination is not routinely used for AMI. It is often used to initially diagnose chronic mesenteric ischemia. When used for chronic mesenteric ischemia, it has a sensitivity of 92% and specificity of 96% for SMA >70% stenosis.[27]

CT ANGIOGRAM

CT angiogram is the diagnostic test of choice. A sensitivity of 93%, specificity 100%, positive predictive value (PPV) 100%, and negative predictive value (NPV) 94%[28] are all a result of recent technological strides in CT imaging. With a 95% to 100% accuracy, it is now the recommended method of imaging for the diagnosis of AMI.[29] It should be performed as soon as possible in a patient with suspected AMI, even in patients with renal failure, as the benefits outweigh the risks in that population.[2] On modern CT angiogram protocols, three scans are performed with one contrast bolus. A precontrast scan is performed to detect vascular calcifications, hyperattenuating vascular thrombi, or intramural hemorrhage.[30] In the biphasic scan, the arterial phase visualizes thrombi in the mesenteric arteries, while the venous phase demonstrates any thrombi in the veins, abnormal bowel wall enhancement, as well as the presence of emboli or infarction in other organs. Depending on institutional preferences, multiplanar reconstructions (MPR) are used to assist in the visualization of the mesenteric arteries.[30] While "positive" oral contrast is thought to detract from the image quality and is consequently not recommended, "negative" oral contrast in the form of 500–750 cc of water immediately before the scan is recommended if the patient can tolerate this. The merit of CT angiogram lies in its broad availability, speed, as well as the ability to evaluate other abdominal pathologies beyond AMI. While no single CT finding is both sensitive and specific, a constellation of visceral arterial occlusion, intestinal pneumatosis, portomesenteric venous gas, or bowel wall thickening in combination with either portomesenteric thrombosis or solid organ infarction was able to give the sensitivity, specificity, PPV and NPV listed above when using contemporary technology.[28] For MVT, the most common radiographic findings are SMV thrombus, "target sign" of the bowel through increased bowel wall enhancement and thickening, as well as pneumatosis, splenomegaly, and ascites.[30]

OTHER ASSESSMENT MODALITIES

Magnetic Resonance Angiogram (MRA)

At this time MRA is too time consuming and not as precise as CT in the assessment of bowel wall thickening and mesenteric fat stranding to be of any clinical use.

Diagnostic Laparoscopy

Diagnostic laparoscopy has traditionally been considered not sensitive enough for the evaluation of bowel viability.[31] More recent case reports indicate that laparoscopic evaluation of the bowel in NOMI patients can prevent negative laparotomies.[32] The use of fluorescein dye and ultraviolet light has been promising in enhancing visualization of bowel ischemia in AMI,[33] but no studies have proven improved outcomes in humans to date.

MANAGEMENT OF THE CLINICAL PROBLEM

MEDICAL THERAPIES

When AMI is suspected or diagnosed, rapid surgical intervention with revascularization is paramount. But while the patient is being prepared for surgery, the available time should be used diligently, and timely resuscitation should be initiated. As such, the patient should immediately be placed on bowel rest, preventing exacerbation of ischemia. Nasogastric tube placement can assist.[2] Intravenous fluid resuscitation is essential due to the large volume that can be sequestered in this pathology and can be as much as 100 mL per kg. Frequent assessment is necessary to avoid extensive crystalloid overload. Initial fluid resuscitation with isotonic crystalloid solution can be followed by blood transfusion as needed. Large fluid shifts and cellular death makes correction of electrolytes from the beginning essential. Intravenous heparin should be started in all the patients who do not have a contraindication, with the goal of partial thromboplastin time (PTT) being double the normal PTT. Prompt initiation of heparin is particularly important in MVT, where this is the mainstay therapy, as systemic thrombolytic therapy is rarely indicated and only possible if there are no findings of peritonitis. Due to the mucosal breakdown in AMI leading to bacterial translocation, broad spectrum antibiotics should be initiated when AMI is suspected. As many patients present in extremis or tend to decompensate quickly, aggressive monitoring strategies are recommended with early initiation of cardiac monitoring, urinary catheter placement, continuous central venous pressure monitoring, and arterial line placement. Most patients with AMI benefit from ICU care early on, where hemodynamic instability is continuously addressed, and resuscitation can be geared to an adequate right heart filling pressure. When pressor support is needed, cardioselective drugs should be used whenever possible; this includes dobutamine, low-dose dopamine (3–8 μg/kg/min), or milrinone. Epinephrine at low doses (0.05–0.01 μg/kg/min) can also be used but is less preferred. Pure alpha-adrenergic pressors should be avoided before and after revascularization. Due to the high mortality of AMI, early goals of care discussions with the patient and family, as much as possible, are important. Ensuring adequate pre- and perioperative discussions are paramount in pursuing a plan that follows the patient's wishes. If a large amount of gut necrosis is found, the patient might require life-long total parenteral nutrition in the setting of short gut syndrome, which most—including the elderly and infirm—do not tend to tolerate well. Initial resuscitation should not delay surgical revascularization and resection of any irreversible bowel necrosis should be pursued as indicated.

ENDOVASCULAR THERAPY

General Considerations

Endovascular therapy has been successfully used as isolated treatment in patients without any concerns for bowel compromise.[34] If there are signs of peritonitis, exploration is required for bowel evaluation[34,35]; concerning imaging findings or laboratory values should lead to open exploration, laparoscopic exploration, or close clinical evaluation. Endovascular therapy for AMI accounts for 6.2% of AMI surgeries (while 5.2% are hybrid and 88.6% open revascularizations)[36] nationally, with a rise in some institutions up to 30% as of 2009,[37] and with endovascular becoming the preferred approach to open in 2004 in Sweden.[35] However, there is insufficient evidence to show a clear advantage of endovascular techniques over open surgery at this time, particularly due to the fact that patients with more advanced AMI tend to require open surgery with bowel resection, while patients who undergo total endovascular procedures have less severe disease and tend to have better outcomes.[37] Endovascular procedures are well suited to patients with mild cases of AMI and severe coexisting conditions that increase the risk of open surgery but may also be used in conjunction with laparotomy or other bowel examination in patients with more severe bowel ischemia. When the endovascular approach without bowel assessment is selected, this needs to be followed by close observation for any clinical deterioration or peritonitis requiring possible emergent laparotomy, as statistically about 40% to 70% of AMI patients will ultimately require a bowel resection.[38,39] When endovascular treatment for AMI is judiciously applied, about 60% of patients can avoid a laparotomy.[36]

In the proximal SMA at the calcified ostium a 7-8 mm diameter balloon-expandable stent is preferred as it can allow for more radial force, more accurate placement, and if placed into the aorta can treat spillover disease into the aorta. More distal SMA lesions benefit from treatment with self-expanding stents to avoid arterial dissection in areas of unfavorable arterial angulation. A residual pressure gradient of >12 mmHg across the stent requires additional treatment.[35] Covered stents were superior to bare metal stents in freedom from restenosis and patency rates when assessed in chronic mesenteric ischemia,[40] without data particular to AMI. While in general femoral access is preferred to brachial access due to the lower rate of possible complications,[41] brachial access may be preferred in certain circumstances, such as a very sharp angle between aorta and SMA and extensive calcification at the ostium or occlusive lesions below the SMA along the aorta or iliac arteries.[35]

Treatment of Embolic Causes of AMI

In the treatment of embolic AMI, mechanical thrombectomy or angioplasty and stent placement are the mainstay treatments. Thrombolysis can occasionally be used as an adjunct, particularly when restoring perfusion to occluded arterial branches, but is contraindicated in patients with suspected bowel compromise, as well as recent surgery, trauma, cerebrovascular or gastrointestinal bleeding, or uncontrolled hypertension.[2]

Treatment for Thrombotic Causes of AMI

Much like the treatment for embolic occlusions, thrombotic occlusions can be treated with mechanical thrombectomy to treat the thrombosis with angioplasty and stenting to address the underlying atherosclerosis. However, terminal occlusion of the diseased SMA is challenging to treat endovascularly and operative bypass is frequently required. This is due to the difficulty of long segment occlusion recanalization.

Treatment for NOMI

When performing an angiogram for NOMI, classic findings include "pruning" or narrowing of multiple branches of SMA vessels all the way into the mesenteric arcades and intermittent areas of vasospasm.[42] Treatment includes any arterial clot removal if present, followed by catheter directed vasodilators or heparin anticoagulation. Catheter-directed treatment options include papaverine[43] (30–60 mg/hr), alprostadil (PGE_1; 20 μg bolus with 60–80 μg over 24 hrs), or epopostenol (PGI_2; 5–6 ng/kg/min).[34] Papaverine and aloprostadil have similar potency to relax mesenteric arteries.[44] The catheter should be kept in place until the patient improves. This catheter-directed application of papaverine can also be used after arterial revascularization to improve splanchnic blood flow. It should be noted that heparin is not compatible with papaverine, and as such cannot both be given through the SMA catheter.

OPEN SURGERY

General Considerations

Emergent laparotomy with damage control and immediate revascularization should be pursued in any patient with peritonitis or signs of bowel compromise. The patient is positioned supine, with a towel roll under the costal margin to facilitate exposure of the supraceliac aorta, should bypass from there later be needed. Prep of the patient should range from "nipples to knees" to allow for possible saphenous or femoral vein harvest. A generous laparotomy is recommended, with the goals of containing any enteric spillage first, followed by arterial revascularization, and assessment of bowel viability at the end with the goal of bowel preservation. The initial containment of enteric spillage should include resection only in the setting of frank necrosis or perforation. Next, the root of the mesentery is palpated; if there is no palpable pulse, a thrombotic occlusion due to proximal plaque is more likely. On the other hand, if a pulse is palpable, this can occur due to transmission through the fresh clot from an embolic event.

Treatment for Embolic Causes of AMI

When performing a proximal SMA embolectomy, no mobilization of the duodenum or ligament of Treitz is required. Instead the SMA can be approached anteriorly and from the base of the transverse colon.

For SMA exposure, the omentum and transverse colon are elevated. The small intestine is wrapped in moist laparotomy pads and retracted to the right. A horizontal incision is performed in the peritoneum at the base of the transverse colon and one proceeds with careful division of the tributaries to the superior mesenteric vein, autonomic nerves, and small lymphatics along the SMA. The SMA lies to the left of the superior mesenteric vein. Additional careful exposure can be achieved through mobilization of the inferior pancreatic border and splenic vein for a more proximal SMA segment but should only be performed when needed due to the added risk of pancreatic irritation and leak. The proximal SMA is isolated between the middle and right colic branches, followed by circumferential dissection of the SMA for control, given the jejunal branches in this segment. Systemic heparization should be performed at that time, followed by the arteriotomy. In general, a transverse arteriotomy is preferred, but for a smaller SMA a short longitudinal arteriotomy with later patch closure is indicated. Venting the proximal SMA for clot removal or passing a 4-5 Fr balloon catheter for embolectomy is followed by a distal embolectomy using a 3-4 Fr balloon catheter as needed. Successful embolectomy should result in the return of pulsatile blood flow. For more distal SMA embolectomies, an even smaller embolectomy catheter with 2-3 Fr can be used or the thrombotic material can be "milked" back from the mesentery using one hand on either side of the mesentery. On some occasions one time use of thrombolytic agents injected through the arteriotomy into distal SMA branched has been described. The primary arteriotomy is closed using interrupted nonabsorbable polypropylene suture or with a vein patch. If embolectomy is not successful, a bypass may be needed.

Treatment for Thrombotic Causes of AMI

For bypass, the duodenum may need to be mobilized to expose the more proximal SMA under the 4th portion of the duodenum. This will allow for a smoother curve for a bypass originating from the distal aorta or iliac arteries, compared to an SMA anastomosis performed more distally. This lateral approach is followed by a longitudinal arteriotomy, allowing for bypass placement or later closure with patch angioplasty should bypass not be required. There are several bypass graft configurations: a retrograde bypass from the right common iliac artery in the "lazy C" configuration can be the most expeditious if there is no aortoiliac disease. The left iliac artery or distal infrarenal aorta are also options. The increased graft length and course of this bypass in these options can help prevent graft kinking. If distal inflow sources are diseased or unclampable, an antegrade supraceliac aorta to SMA bypass can be placed. This requires dissection of the supraceliac aorta. In addition, aortic cross-clamping can cause hemodynamic and physiological stress on the patient, and should be taken into account when performing this bypass surgery. In AMI, a single bypass may be the best choice to allow for a more expeditious surgery. In contrast, for chronic mesenteric ischemia many surgeons choose to perform two-vessel revascularization in the elective setting.

Choice of graft material is dependent on peritoneal soiling. If there is no peritoneal soiling, a 6- to 8-mm Dacron or externally supported polytetrafluoroethylene graft is preferred. Prosthetic graft is less prone to kinking and external compression than vein, and eliminates vein harvest time, making it the preferred material in this situation. If peritoneal soiling is present, a vein bypass is indicated, with the main harvest sites being great saphenous vein or thigh femoral vein. If there is no native vein available, a rifampin-soaked Dacron graft can be considered. To decrease the risk of graft infection, an omental coverage can be placed. Dr. Kazmers and colleagues describes a technique for omental coverage for a retrograde bypass by bringing omentum through the transverse mesocolon and over the bypass.[45]

HYBRID PROCEDURE: RETROGRADE OPEN MESENTERIC STENTING (ROMS)

Retrograde open mesenteric stenting (ROMS) is a newer approach in the treatment of AMI and uses a hybrid combination of open and endovascular surgery. The patient undergoes a laparotomy. The visceral peritoneum is incised at the base of the mesocolon, and the SMA inflow and outflow is controlled as in an embolectomy SMA exposure. An arteriotomy is performed, with local thromboendarterectomy of the SMA if necessary. Through the arteriotomy a 6-Fr sheath is placed in order to achieve retrograde cannulation of the SMA to the aorta and allow for recanalization of the occlusion. The recanalized SMA lesion can then be treated. This approach has been promising due to the improved angle of access to the SMA achieved through this retrograde approach, as well as the ability to assess bowel viability at the index operation, and avoid lengthy bypass procedures with possible aortic cross-clamping, though no study has been able to prove a statistically significant improvement in outcome at this time. Patency rates and reintervention are comparable to percutaneous stenting.[46]

TREATMENT FOR MESENTERIC VENOUS THROMBOSIS

Most MVT is able to be treated conservatively, but approximately 5% of patients will deteriorate and require further intervention. While any signs of peritonitis, obstruction, or GI bleeding should trigger an exploratory laparotomy with bowel assessment, additional measures including transhepatic and percutaneous mechanical thrombectomy,[47] percutaneous transhepatic thrombolysis,[48] and open intra-arterial thrombolysis[49] have been described but not adequately studied.

BOWEL EVALUATION

After successful revascularization, the bowel needs to be evaluated with resection of irreversibly damaged and necrotic bowel. Since after revascularization some bowel might recover and the goal is to preserve as much bowel as possible to prevent malabsorption and short gut, it is recommended to wait at least 20–30 min after reperfusion before proceeding with bowel evaluation and possible resection. Adjuncts in assessment can be useful, such as Doppler interrogation or fluorescein, but if there is more extensive bowel involved, many advocate resecting only frankly necrotic bowel at the first operation, leaving the bowel in discontinuity if needed, and planning a second-look operation to reevaluate any segments of questionable bowel-viability within 12–48 hours. With the placement of a temporary abdominal closure, such as a negative pressure wound closure, bowel edema can develop without causing intraabdominal pressure increases and potential additional vascular compromise, while the hemodynamics can be optimized for any bowel anastomoses during the second-look operation. The second-look operation includes re-exploration of the abdomen, reassessment of the mesenteric blood flow, resection of nonviable bowel, anastomoses of bowel, and abdominal wall closure. Occasionally, an ostomy is needed for continued observation of bowel viability. It is estimated that nearly 40% of patients who undergo a second-look operation require a bowel resection at that time.[15] Bowel can become very swollen in AMI and at high risk for anastomotic leak. While stapler technology is constantly improving, a hand sewn anastomosis should be considered when encountering swollen bowel and can be preferable to certain staplers in order to prevent anastomotic leaks.[2]

COMPLICATIONS AND FOLLOW-UP

Initial Postoperative Treatment, Anticoagulation, and Antiplatelet Therapy

Due to mesenteric capillary leak syndrome after revascularization, most patients will continue to require aggressive fluid resuscitation after surgery. Some patients require as much as 10–20 L of crystalloid resuscitation in the first 24–48 hours after surgery. Electrolytes need to be monitored closely in this phase, as revascularized bowel can lead to metabolic acidosis and hyperkalemia. In a patient with normal kidney function, additional bowel necrosis to be suspected. Continue on systemic heparin immediately post-op to minimize the risk of early occlusion of mesenteric stenting or bypass. In MVT, recurrence of thrombosis was decreased from 26% to 14% with heparinization and mortality decreased from 59% to 22%.[1] All patients should be on systemic anticoagulation, such as warfarin, for at least 6 months, especially if the patient has atrial fibrillation, MVT, or inherited or acquired thrombophilia until the underlying cause is resolved. Antiplatelet therapy should include lifelong aspirin, and clopidogrel for 1-3 months after endovascular stenting procedures. Risk management for underlying causes of AMI should be pursued. If atherosclerosis was the cause, smoking-cessation, blood pressure control, and statin therapy should be initiated.

Malnutrition, Malabsorption, Sort Gut Syndrome, and Strictures

If the patient had a history of chronic mesenteric ischemia before developing AMI, such as food fear and malnutrition, one should pay close attention to nutritional status with a low threshold for adding total parenteral nutrition until adequate oral intact can be achieved. Depending on the portion of resected bowel, vitamin supplementation might be needed, such as vitamin B12 after a terminal ileum resection. If a large amount of bowel was resected, the patient should be evaluated for diarrhea and malabsorption as signs of short gut syndrome. Strictures can form in areas of prior bowel ischemia. In NOMI, the most common sites are the descending colon and sigmoid colon.[50] Should the patient develop symptoms from these, additional treatment might be required in the future.

Bypass or Stent Occlusion

After successful revascularization with stent placement or bypass surgery, close surveillance is required with the preferred modality being duplex ultrasound or CT angiogram. Current recommendations are for the first surveillance scan 3 months postoperatively, followed by imaging examinations every 6–12 months.[35] While there are no duplex scan characteristics to predict graft thrombosis[51] and no absolute threshold velocity values in stented SMAs for reintervention at this time, it still allows for the most precise quantitative evaluation of flow over time with the assessment of recurrent stenosis. Acute thrombotic stent occlusion is a rare complication, but has a mortality of 50%.[35] Most recurrent stenoses can be treated with percutaneous intervention as an outpatient, but if the patient is a good surgical candidate, a more durable operative bypass can be discussed with the patient in clinic. While graft and stent patency rates are not readily available for AMI, in chronic mesenteric ischemia 36% of patients treated endovascularly will experience restenosis, of which half will require reintervention.[52] Conversely, open repairs for acute and chronic mesenteric ischemia have primary patency rates of 57% at 5 years and long-term survival did not differ between chronic and AMI patients when perioperative mortality is excluded.[53] Overall, primary patency and primary assisted patency were increased in patients who underwent open repair as compared to percutaneous angioplasty/stent in patients with chronic mesenteric ischemia.[54]

TIPS FOR MANAGEMENT AND TO AVOID COMPLICATIONS

- Have a high index of suspicion for AMI in a patient with abdominal pain out of proportion to exam. A CT angiogram is the best study to obtain should AMI be on the differential.
- AMI patients either arrive very ill or have a propensity to deteriorate quickly. Erring on the side of a higher level of care and more invasive monitoring is recommended.
- Prompt revascularization is paramount, but use your time wisely to resuscitate, anticoagulate, initiate broad-spectrum antibiotics, correct electrolytes, and talk to the patient and family about treatment wishes.
- Try to preserve bowel. When in doubt, perform a second-look surgery.
- Watch for metabolic disturbances once the bowel is revascularized, including metabolic acidosis and hyperkalemia. If acidemia does not correct in a patient with normal kidney function, suspect additional necrotic bowel.

REFERENCES

1. Oldenburg WA, Lau LL, Rodenberg TJ, Edmonds HJ. Acute mesenteric ischemia. *Arch Intern Med*. 2004;164(10):1054-1062.
2. Bala M, Kashuk J, Moore EE, et al. Acute mesenteric ischemia: guidelines of the World Society of Emergency Surgery. *World J Emerg Surg*. 2017;12(1):1-11.
3. Boley SJ, Feinstein FR, Sammartano R, Brandt LJ, Sprayregen S. New concepts in the management of emboli of the superior mesenteric artery. *Surg Gynecol Obstet*. 1981;153(4):561-569.
4. Clair DG, Beach JM. Mesenteric ischemia. *N Engl J Med*. 2016;374(10):959-968.
5. Acosta S, Ögren M, Sternby NH, Bergqvist D, Björck M. Clinical implications for the management of acute thromboembolic occlusion of the superior mesenteric artery: autopsy findings in 213 patients. *Ann Surg*. 2005;241(3):516-522.
6. Schoots IG, Koffeman GI, Legemate DA, Levi M, Van Gulik TM. Systematic review of survival after acute mesenteric ischaemia according to disease aetiology. *Br J Surg*. 2004;91(1):17-27.
7. Acosta S, Alhadad A, Svensson P, Ekberg O. Epidemiology, risk and prognostic factors in mesenteric venous thrombosis. *Br J Surg*. 2008;95(10):1245-1251.
8. Elliot JW. The operative relief of gangrene of intestine due to occlusion of the mesenteric vessels. *Ann Surg*. 1895;21(1):9-23.
9. KLASS AA. Embolectomy in acute mesenteric occlusion. *Ann Surg*. 1951;134(5):913-917.
10. Boley SJ, Sprayregen S, Veith FJ, Siegelman SS. An aggressive roentgenologic and surgical approach to acute mesenteric ischemia. *Surg Annu*. 1973;5:355-378.
11. Boley SJ, Brandt LJ. Selective mesenteric vasodilators. A future role in acute mesenteric ischemia? *Gastroenterology*. 1986;91:247-249.
12. Clark RA, Colley DP, Jacobson ED, Herman R, Tyler G, Stahl D. Superior mesenteric angiography and blood flow measurement following intra-arterial injection of prostaglandin E1. *Radiology*. 1980;134(2):327-333.
13. Clark RA, Gallant TE. Acute mesenteric ischemia: angiographic spectrum. *Am J Roentgenol*. 1984;142(3):555-562.
14. Merck G. Vorläufige Notiz über eine neue organische Base im Opium. *Ann der Chemie und Pharm*. 1848;66(1):125-128.
15. Park WM, Gloviczki P, Cherry KJ Jr, et al. Contemporary management of acute mesenteric ischemia. *J Vasc Surg*. 2002;35(3):445-452.
16. Batellier J, Kieny R. Superior mesenteric artery embolism: eighty-two cases. *Ann Vasc Surg*. 1990;4(2):112-116.
17. Kärkkäinen JM, Acosta S. Acute mesenteric ischemia (part I) –incidence, etiologies, and how to improve early diagnosis. *Best Pract Res Clin Gastroenterol*. 2017;31(1):15-25.
18. Savlania A, Tripathi RK. Acute mesenteric ischemia: current multidisciplinary approach. *J Cardiovasc Surg (Torino)*. 2017;58(2):339-350.
19. Boley SJ, Brandt LJ, Veith FJ. Ischemic disorders of the intestines. *Curr Probl Surg*. 1978;15(4):1-85.
20. Clark ET, Gewertz BL. Intermittent ischemia potentiates intestinal reperfusion injury. *J Vasc Surg*. 1991;13(5):601-606.
21. Kumar S, Sarr MG, Kamath PS. Mesenteric venous thrombosis. *N Engl J Med*. 2001;345(23):1683-1688.
22. Kougias P, Lau D, El Sayed HF, Zhou W, Huynh TT, Lin PH. Determinants of mortality and treatment outcome following surgical interventions for acute mesenteric ischemia. *J Vasc Surg*. 2007;46(3):467-474.

23. Nuzzo A, Maggiori L, Ronot M, et al. Predictive factors of intestinal necrosis in acute mesenteric ischemia: prospective study from an Intestinal Stroke Center. *Am J Gastroenterol.* 2017;112(4):597-605.
24. Block T, Nilsson TK, Björck M, Acosta S. Diagnostic accuracy of plasma biomarkers for intestinal ischaemia. *Scand J Clin Lab Invest.* 2008;68(3):242-248.
25. Wilson C, Imrie CW. Amylase and gut infarction. *Br J Surg.* 1986;73(3):219-221.
26. Smerud MJ, Johnson CD, Stephens DH. Diagnosis of bowel infarction: a comparison of plain films and CT scans in 23 cases. *Am J Roentgenol.* 1990;154(1):99-103.
27. Moneta GL. Screening for mesenteric vascular insufficiency and follow-up of mesenteric artery bypass procedures. *Semin Vasc Surg.* 2001;14(3):186-192.
28. Aschoff AJ, Stuber G, Becker BW, et al. Evaluation of acute mesenteric ischemia: accuracy of biphasic mesenteric multi-detector CT angiography. *Abdom Imaging.* 2009;34(3):345-357.
29. Hagspiel KD, Flors L, Hanley M, Norton PT. Computed tomography angiography and magnetic resonance angiography imaging of the [illegible] vasculature. *Tech Vasc Interv Radiol.* 2015;18(1):2-13.
30. Furukawa A, Kanasaki S, Kono N, et al. CT diagnosis of acute mesenteric ischemia from various causes. *Am J Roentgenol.* 2009;192(2):408-416.
31. Sauerland S, Agresta F, Bergamaschi R, et al. Laparoscopy for abdominal emergencies: evidence-based guidelines of the European Association for Endoscopic Surgery. *Surg Endosc Other Interv Tech.* 2006;20(1):14-29.
32. Kim SH, Hwang HY, Kim MJ, Park KJ, Kim K-B. Early laparoscopic exploration for acute mesenteric ischemia after cardiac surgery. *Acute Crit Care.* [illegible]
33. Jiri P, Alexander F, Michal P, et al. Laparoscopic diagnostics of acute bowel ischemia using ultraviolet light and fluorescein dye: an experimental study. *Surg Laparosc Endosc Percutan Tech.* 2007;17(4):291-295.
34. Luther B, Mamopoulos A, Lehmann C, Klar E. The ongoing challenge of acute mesenteric ischemia. *Visc Med.* 2018;34(3):217-223.
35. Acosta S. Surgical management of peritonitis secondary to acute superior mesenteric artery occlusion. *World J Gastroenterol.* 2014;20(29):9936-9941.
36. Branco BC, Montero-Baker MF, Aziz H, Taylor Z, Mills JL. Endovascular therapy for acute mesenteric ischemia: an NSQIP analysis. *Am Surg.* 2015;81(11):1170-1176.
37. Beaulieu RJ, Arnaoutakis KD, Abularrage CJ, Efron DT, Schneider E, Black JH. Comparison of open and endovascular treatment of acute mesenteric ischemia. *J Vasc Surg.* 2014;59(1):159-164.
38. Schermerhorn ML, Giles KA, Hamdan AD, Wyers MC, Pomposelli FB. Mesenteric revascularization: management and outcomes in the United States, 1988-2006. *J Vasc Surg.* 2009;50(2):341-348.
39. Arthurs ZM, Titus J, Bannazadeh M, et al. A comparison of endovascular revascularization with traditional therapy for the treatment of acute mesenteric ischemia. *J Vasc Surg.* 2011;53(3):698-705.
40. Oderich GS, Erdoes LS, Lesar C, et al. Comparison of covered stents versus bare metal stents for treatment of chronic atherosclerotic mesenteric arterial disease. *J Vasc Surg.* 2013;58(5):1316-1324.
41. Otsuka M, Shiode N, Nakao Y, et al. Comparison of radial, brachial, and femoral accesses using hemostatic devices for percutaneous coronary intervention. *Cardiovasc Interv Ther.* 2018;33(1):62-69.
42. Siegelman SS, Sprayregen S, Boley SJ. Angiographic diagnosis of mesenteric arterial vasoconstriction. *Radiology.* 1974;112(3):533-542.
43. Mellahn JL, Morris JB, Ceppa EP, Bulkley GB. Effect of prolonged selective intramesenteric arterial vasodilator therapy on intestinal viability after acute segmental mesenteric vascular occlusion. *Ann Surg.* 2001;234(1):107-115.
44. Mahlke C, Kühn JP, Mensel B, et al. Iloprost, prostaglandin e 1, and papaverine relax human mesenteric arteries with similar potency. *Shock.* 2017;48(3):333-339.
45. Kazmers A. Operative management of acute mesenteric ischemia. *Ann Vasc Surg.* 1998;12(2):187-197.
46. Oderich GS, Macedo R, Stone DH, et al. Multicenter study of retrograde open mesenteric artery stenting through laparotomy for treatment of acute and chronic mesenteric ischemia. *J Vasc Surg.* 2018;68(2):470-480.e1.
47. Takahashi N, Kuroki K, Yanaga K. Percutaneous transhepatic mechanical thrombectomy for acute mesenteric venous thrombosis. *J Endovasc Ther.* 2005;12(4):508-511.
48. Di Minno MND, Milone F, Milone M, et al. Endovascular thrombolysis in acute mesenteric vein thrombosis: A 3-year follow-up with the rate of short and long-term sequaelae in 32 patients. *Thromb Res.* 2010;126(4):295-298.
49. Ozdogan M, Gurer A, Gokakin AK, Kulacoglu H, Aydin R. Thrombolysis via an operatively placed mesenteric catheter for portal and superior mesenteric vein thrombosis: report of a case. *Surg Today.* 2006;36(9):846-848.

50. Sise MJ. Acute mesenteric ischemia. *Surg Clin North Am*. 2014;94(1):165-181.
51. Liem TK, Segall JA, Wei W, Landry GJ, Taylor LM, Moneta GL. Duplex scan characteristics of bypass grafts to mesenteric arteries. *J Vasc Surg*. 2007;45(5):922-928.
52. Tallarita T, Oderich GS, Macedo TA, et al. Reinterventions for stent restenosis in patients treated for atherosclerotic mesenteric artery disease. *J Vasc Surg*. 2011;54(5):1422-1429.e1.
53. Cho JS, Carr JA, Jacobsen G, Shepard AD, Nypaver TJ, Reddy DJ. Long-term outcome after mesenteric artery reconstruction: a 37-year experience. *J Vasc Surg*. 2002;35(3):453-460.
54. Atkins MD, Kwolek CJ, LaMuraglia GM, Brewster DC, Chung TK, Cambria RP. Surgical revascularization versus endovascular therapy for chronic mesenteric ischemia: a comparative experience. *J Vasc Surg*. 2007;45(6):1162-1171.

SELF-ASSESSMENT STUDY QUESTIONS AND ANSWERS

Questions

1. What percentage of the cardiac output goes to the small intestines at rest?
A. 1%–5%
B. 10%–15%
C. 30%–50%
D. 50%–80%

2. Which mesenteric artery is most frequently affected in AMI?
A. Celiac trunk
B. Superior mesenteric artery
C. Inferior mesenteric artery
D. Superior rectal artery

3. What is the most common type of AMI?
A. Embolic
B. Thrombotic
C. Nonocclusive mesenteric ischemia
D. Mesenteric venous thrombosis

4. Where does thrombotic occlusion causing AMI most frequently occur?
A. Origin of superior mesenteric artery
B. Along the superior mesenteric artery, just distal to the middle colic artery
C. Along the superior mesenteric artery, just distal to the right colic artery
D. In the mesenteric arcades

5. The most frequent source of embolic AMI is:
A. Aortic mural thrombi
B. Atrial fibrillation
C. Endocarditis
D. Recent catheter-based angiogram

6. What type of AMI is most likely to go undiagnosed?
A. Embolic
B. Thrombotic
C. Nonocclusive mesenteric ischemia
D. Mesenteric venous thrombosis

7. What is the most frequent laboratory abnormality in AMI?
A. Abnormal WBC
B. Elevated AST/ALT
C. Elevated D-dimer
D. Elevated lactate

8. The diagnostic test of choice for AMI is:
A. Abdominal X-ray
B. CT angiogram
C. Doppler ultrasound
D. MR angiogram

9. Which of the following treatments is not indicated in a patient with AMI?
A. Antifungal medication
B. Broad spectrum antibiotics
C. Fluid resuscitation
D. Intravenous heparin

10. What is a contraindication for a purely endovascular treatment for AMI?
A. Active smoking history
B. History of chronic mesenteric ischemia
C. Left groin wound
D. Peritonitis

SELF-ASSESSMENT STUDY QUESTIONS AND ANSWERS

Answers

1. B.
2. B.
3. A.
4. A.
5. B.
6. C.
7. A.
8. B.
9. A.
10. D.

CHAPTER

38 Renal Artery Stenosis

Christopher J. Cooper and Kristin Schafer

OUTLINE

GENERAL CONSIDERATION AND HISTORY
- **History**
  - Causes
  - Atherosclerotic RAS (ARAS)
  - Fibromuscular Dysplasia (FMD)
  - Anatomy
  - Pathophysiology of Renovascular Hypertension

CLINICAL FINDINGS
- Signs and Symptoms
- Screening

DIFFERENTIAL DIAGNOSIS

DIAGNOSIS
- Laboratory Evaluation
- **Noninvasive Imaging**
  - Renal Duplex Ultrasonography
  - Computerized Tomographic Angiography (CTA)
  - Magnetic Resonance Angiography (MRA)
  - Additional Tests
  - Invasive Imaging

MANAGEMENT
- Medical Therapy
- Indications for Intervention
- Endovascular Therapy
- Percutaneous Transluminal Angioplasty (PTA)
- Endovascular Stenting
- Complications
- Surveillance and Follow-up
- Open Surgery
- Aortorenal Endarterectomy
- Aortorenal Bypass
- Renal Artery Re-implantation
- Extra-anatomic Bypass
- Complications
- Surveillance and Follow-up

GENERAL CONSIDERATION AND HISTORY

HISTORY

Renal artery stenosis (RAS) is a relatively common problem that manifests in several ways, including renovascular hypertension, ischemic nephropathy and as an incidental finding during abdominal imaging for other disorders (Figure 38-1). Renovascular hypertension due to RAS, a narrowing of one or both renal arteries, is a leading cause of secondary hypertension in adults. While less than 1% of adults with mild hypertension are affected, these numbers climb dramatically in those with severe hypertension, with up to 40% of individuals affected.[1] The prevalence is increased in people with atherosclerosis, including those with coronary artery disease (CAD) and peripheral arterial disease (PAD).

Causes

The overwhelming majority of RAS cases are attributable to atherosclerotic disease (90%), followed by

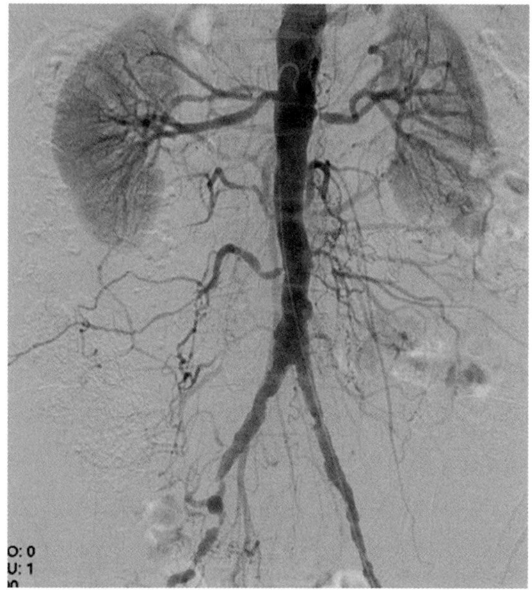

FIGURE 38-1 Unilateral stenosis of the left renal artery utilizing digital subtraction imaging of the abdominal aorta.

fibromuscular dysplasia (FMD; 8%–10%). Less frequent causes include congenital stenosis, Takayasu's arteritis, Kawasaki disease, neurofibromatosis and inherited disorders including William's Syndrome make up the remaining small percentage of cases (1%–2%).

Atherosclerotic RAS (ARAS)

Atherosclerotic RAS (ARAS) is generally a condition of the elderly, with an average age of approximately 70 years at the time of diagnosis. It most commonly affects the ostium, or aortic orifice, and proximal one-third (approximately 1–2 cm) of the renal artery. For many of these patients, the stenosis can be attributed to aortic plaque protruding into the orifice of the renal artery. As with other diseases of the abdominal aorta, the prevalence of RAS increases with traditional cardiovascular risk factors such as pre-existing hypertension, CAD, PAD, hyperlipidemia, diabetes mellitus (DM), hypercholesterolemia, tobacco use, and advanced age. Interestingly, ARAS appears to affect women and men equally, which is in clear distinction from some other atherosclerotic conditions such as CAD which tends to affect men more frequently and at a younger age. Smoking appears to have a marked effect on ARAS, occurring nearly a decade earlier than in non-smokers and resulting in a higher rate of adverse events.[2]

In the era before effective treatment of atherosclerosis, ARAS was considered a progressive disease, with 31% progression at 3 years and 51% progression at 5 years in a study of 295 kidneys followed by serial duplex ultrasonography.[3] Despite the lack of effective treatment at the time of that study, of those arteries with ≥60% stenosis, less than 15% progressed to complete occlusion at 5 years. In a more contemporary study, a elderly hypertensives demonstrated a significant change of renovascular disease (RVD) in only 14.0% of kidneys on follow-up of 8 years (annualized rate, 1.3% per year), progression to significant RVD was observed in only 4% (annualized rate, 0.5% per year), and no prevalent RVD progressed to occlusion.[4]

Many ARAS cases are identified not during workup for secondary causes of hypertension, but rather are identified incidentally on imaging studies for screening or other unrelated disease processes.[5]

Fibromuscular Dysplasia (FMD)

FMD is generally a condition of younger people, oftentimes presenting in the mid-20s and occasionally occurring in children. Whereas ARAS, tends to occur in people with other forms of atherosclerosis, FMD often presents in young women who have no other risk factor for hypertension. FMD is a non-atherosclerotic disease process affecting small and medium-sized arteries, most notably the renal and carotid arteries.[6] Of those patients affected by FMD, up to 80% will have involvement of the renal arteries. The distal two-thirds of the renal artery are affected, and extension into the intrarenal branches may occur in some people. When distal extension occurs into the branch arteries of the kidney, renal artery aneurysms are not uncommon. Histological classification of FMD divides the disease into three categories based on the layer of the arterial wall involved: (1) intimal, (2) medial, (3) adventitial or periarterial. Medial FMD is the most common category and is recognized on angiography by its "string of beads" appearance caused by alternating areas of stenotic fibrous webs and poststenotic dilatation. In all categories of FMD, women ages 20-60 are primarily affected over men in a ratio of 9:1. Adventitial FMD, though rare, may affect girls as young as 5 years old. FMD appears to have a genetic component, with studies suggesting autosomal dominant inheritance with incomplete penetrance. Other factors such as tobacco use and estrogen levels are thought to contribute to the disease process as well, though it is not known to what extent.

Anatomy

The renal arteries originate from the lateral aspect of the abdominal aorta at the L1-L2 vertebral body level, just distal to the takeoff of the superior mesenteric artery (SMA). The right renal artery arises from the anterolateral portion of the aorta and courses posterior to the head of the pancreas, descending duodenum, inferior vena cava (IVC), and right renal vein to enter the right renal hilum. The left renal artery arises from the posterolateral aorta and courses posterior to the body of the pancreas, splenic vein, and left renal vein along the left psoas muscle to enter the left renal hilum. For these reasons, it is commonplace to see a 10–20 degree tilt of the renal arteries toward the left when conventional angiography is performed. This may be critical when identifying the origin of the renal artery and the extent of ostial stenosis. Upon reaching the renal hilum, the main renal artery divides into anterior and posterior branches which further subdivide into interlobar and interlobular arteries. Approximately 25% of patients may have one or more accessory renal arteries. Identification of the main and accessory arteries becomes critical during Duplex ultrasonography and conventional angiography.

Pathophysiology of Renovascular Hypertension

The pathophysiology behind renovascular disease is complex and multi-factorial. In the early 1930s Goldblatt determined that stenosis of a renal artery resulted in increases in systemic blood pressure.[7] Furthermore, disorders of the arterial inflow to the kidneys may adversely impact renal filtration, salt and water excretion resulting in renal dysfunction or volume overload. Thus, a "find it, fix it" approach would seem logical. However, the circulation of the kidney is not as straightforward as some other vascular beds. In the cortex of the kidney, where filtration takes place in the glomerulus, renal blood flow is controlled by the afferent and efferent arterioles. In the cortex, there is minimal oxygen extraction and the function of the glomerulus is autoregulated. In addition, there is a separate medullary circulation within the kidney. As a consequence, through autoregulation, hemodynamically significant stenoses often have little if any effect on excretory renal function.

In the case of both ARAS and FMD, renovascular hypertension results from decreased perfusion pressure in the renal artery distal to the stenosis. Acutely, this perceived hypotension activates the renin–angiotensin–aldosterone system (RAAS) and renin is released from juxtaglomerular cells of the afferent arterioles. The circulating renin acts on angiotensinogen produced in the liver to create angiotensin I which is then converted to angiotensin II in pulmonary circulation by angiotensin-converting enzyme (ACE). A key mechanism of RAAS activation is vasoconstriction of the efferent arteriole that serves to maintain glomerular filtration despite reductions in afferent pressure. Angiotensin II, in addition to being a potent vasoconstrictor for arterial smooth muscle, stimulates the release of aldosterone from the adrenal cortex. Aldosterone in turn activates the Na^+/K^+ATPase pump on the distal convoluted tubule to increase Na^+ and H_2O absorption, leading to intravascular volume expansion. While a temporary and normal response to volume-depletion in the healthy adult, persistent activation of the RAAS by stenotic arteries is a hallmark of renovascular hypertension.

While the former explanation for hypertension is supported by experimental models, it is well accepted now that hypertension in people with RAS is oftentimes more complex than this simple explanation. First, many people with ARAS have had long-standing essential hypertension well before they develop a stenosis in the renal artery. In addition, the condition of the contralateral artery may be critical. In unilateral RAS the contralateral kidney has no stenosis and in the early stages of disease may moderate the hypertension by excreting excess salt and water. However, it has also been observed that the "normal" develop parenchymal injury, presumably due to the unimpeded effect of the hypertension on that kidney, and it is well demonstrated that this kidney in diabetics may develop the classic Kimmelstiel-Wilson (KW) lesions while the architecture of the stenotic kidney is spared. In contrast, bilateral RAS is not uncommon and the degree of stenosis may differentially effect each kidney (Figure 38-2). In some people the contralateral renal artery is occluded or the kidney is absent or non-functional, resulting in perfusion of a solitary kidney through a stenotic vessel. An iatrogenic example of this is an anastamotic stenosis in a transplanted kidney. Finally, it is now well recognized that several other mechanisms are responsible for the hypertensive response in people with RAS including sympathetic activation and endothelin.

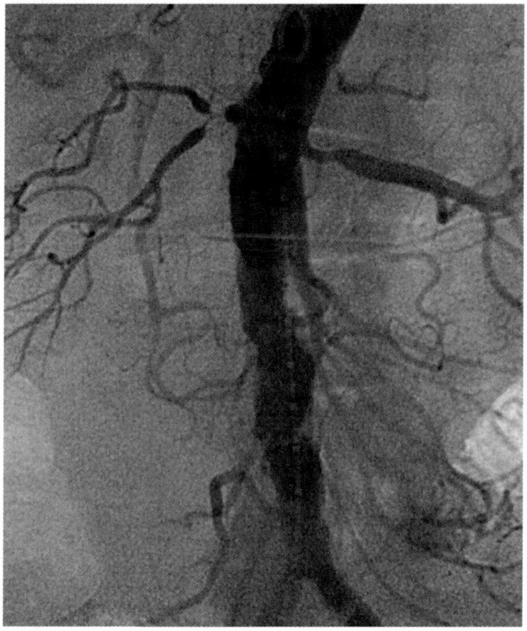

FIGURE 38-2 Bilateral renal artery stenosis as seen with digital subtraction angiography of the abdominal aorta.

CLINICAL FINDINGS

Signs and Symptoms

People with RAS rarely present with symptoms per se. However, they may present with symptoms related to uncontrolled high blood pressure or due to excessive retention of salt and water. An uncommon but concerning presentation is with pulmonary edema, the Pickering Syndrome. In those patients with symptomatic RAS, the most common presenting complaint is new or worsened hypertension, some of whom may have uncontrolled hypertension, defined as hypertension despite the effective use of three or more antihypertensive medications. The age of the patient is a pertinent consideration, as hypertension in a young female might suggest FMD while hypertension in an older adult is more suggestive of atherosclerotic disease. Relevant family history of any endocrine and cardiovascular disorders should be elicited during the interview. Review of systems must involve a detailed review of constitutional symptoms such as dizziness, syncope, and headaches in addition to more specific organ-based symptoms such as hematuria, flank pain, and endocrine disturbances that might suggest other etiologies. Physical exam should be sure to include a detailed pulse exam and assessment for abdominal and flank bruits, although the presence of bruits does not establish a diagnosis of RAS and the absence of a bruit does not exclude RAS.

Screening

Screening for RAS is warranted in people who are likely to benefit from treatment if found, such as the child with a congenital syndrome, and the younger adult with the abrupt onset of hypertension or medically-resistant hypertension. It should also be considered in people with unexplained worsening of hypertension or kidney dysfunction and known CAD or PAD, with an age greater than 55 years, recurrent episodes of pulmonary edema, or recurrent acute CHF exacerbations. An acute worsening of renal function after the initiation of an ACE-inhibitor is concerning for underlying renovascular disease and should also be investigated.

TABLE 38-1 Differential Diagnosis of Uncontrolled Hypertension

Condition	Common Features	Useful Tests
Essential HTN	CV risk factors (e.g., smoking, diabetes)	CBC, BMP, glucose, cholesterol
Endocrine disorders		
Hyperaldosteronism	Polydipsia, polyuria, weakness	Serum aldosterone, renin
Hyperthyroidism	Goiter, heat intolerance, weight loss, exophthalmos	Thyroid function tests
Pheochromocytoma	Episodic HTN; diaphoresis; palpitations	Serum and urine catecholamines
Renal parenchymal disease	Flank pain, gross hematuria	Urinalysis
Renal artery stenosis		Renal US, angiography
Atherosclerotic	Advanced age, CV risk factors	CTA
Fibromuscular Dysplasia	Young age, female gender	MRA
Vasculitis	Fever, arthralgia, weakness	CBC, CRP, ESR
neurofibromatosis	Family history, skin pigmentation	Genetic testing
Segmental arterial mediolysis	Acute abdominal pain, acute flank pain, diffuse aneurysmal disease	CTA, histology

CRP, C-reactive protein; CTA, CT angiography; CV, cardiovascular; ESR, erythrocyte sedimentation rate; HTN, hypertension; MRA, MR angiography; US, ultrasound; CBC, complete blood count; BMP, basic metabolic panel.

DIFFERENTIAL DIAGNOSIS

The differential diagnosis for new onset, worsening, and uncontrolled HTN is fairly broad (Table 38-1). Importantly, most (95%) of hypertension is attributable to essential HTN. Of the remaining five percent of cases in which a clear cause can be identified, the majority are due to RAS. Similarly, there are many causes of worsening kidney function that can be broadly categorized as prerenal, intrarenal, and postrenal causes. As described previously, it is reasonable to consider the diagnosis of RAS when other medical issues such as known atherosclerosis, advanced or young age, known congenital syndromes or other conditions are present that may raise the suspicion for co-existing RAS.

DIAGNOSIS

Laboratory Evaluation

Laboratory workup for patients with suspected renovascular disease should include a baseline measurement of blood urea nitrogen and creatinine to assess the degree of renal impairment and a measurement of urinary protein excretion, most commonly performed as a urine protein to urine creatinine ratio which may be useful in treatment planning since people with significant proteinuria appear to do poorly with revascularization.[8] Additional studies, when clinically indicated for other conditions affecting blood pressure control, may include urinalysis, and endocrine studies such as aldosterone to renin ratio to assess for primary aldosteronism, catecholamines if a pheochromocytoma is considered, and rarely thyroid hormone levels.

NONINVASIVE IMAGING

Renal Duplex Ultrasonography

Considered the first-line diagnostic test of RAS, renal duplex ultrasonography has a sensitivity of 90% to 95% and specificity of 60% to 90% and allows evaluation of both arterial size and hemodynamics.[5] While inexpensive, results are affected by operator experience, patient obesity, overlying bowel gas, and anatomic variations such as nephroptosis, multiple renal arteries, and segmental or branch stenosis. With improvements in operator technique and simple pre-test steps such as 12-hr fasting and simethicone tablets taken the night before and the morning of testing to limit gastric distention and bowel gas, complete examination is possible in 80% to 90% of patients. Direct visualization of the abdominal aorta, renal arteries, and kidneys may also show evidence of aneurysmal changes or atrophy of the kidney. Unilateral renal atrophy, defined as a difference in pole-to-pole length of greater than one centimeter, is suggestive of renal arterial disease. Poststenotic turbulence or decreased flow on Doppler indicates arterial disease for which hemodynamic measurements such as peak systolic velocity (PSV) can be obtained to better quantify the degree of disease. Normal renal artery PSV ranges from 60 to 100 cm/s. Several criteria are used to evaluate the severity of RAS, and it is generally accepted that most clinically relevant stenoses are greater than 60%. When using PSV as a criteria, greater than 180 cm/s is sensitive and detects most clinically significant stenoses. However, a PSV greater than 300 cm/s is more specific and has a higher reliability for indicating a clinically relevant stenosis. The renal-to-aortic PSV ratio can also be used and a ratio of greater than 3.5 is generally accepted. Doppler waveforms may also be useful for accessing RAS within the hilar and intralobar arteries. One such finding is the "pulsus parvus et tardus" effect, in which waveforms of prolonged systolic acceleration and small amplitude appear in the intrarenal arteries downstream of stenotic areas during ventricular systole. Absence of this effect does not exclude the presence of RAS, however, as vessel compliance in severe disease may dampen the waveform morphology. On determining the presence of RAS on Doppler, the renal resistive index (RRI) has been suggested as a criteria to predict the effectiveness of revascularization of the affected kidney in correcting renal function and controlling systemic hypertension:

$$\text{RRI} = 1 - (\text{end diastolic velocity}/\text{maximal systolic velocity}) \times 100$$

RRI values >0.80 indicate there may be little to no correction in systemic hypertension and renal function by the patient undergoing intervention for their RAS,[9] although this has been questioned in several subsequent publications. The utility of the RRI remains controversial and has not gained widespread acceptance as a criteria for determining the treatment of people with RAS.

Computerized Tomographic Angiography (CTA)

Computerized tomographic angiography (CTA) is another useful diagnostic modality that allows the collection of raw-data for subsequent 3D reconstruction, with 98% sensitivity and 94% specificity for proximal lesions. When compared to US, CTA has the added benefit of being able to visualize the entirety of the renal vasculature, including any accessory vessels. Owing to its high spatial resolution capability, CTA is also the imaging study of choice in distinguishing ARAS from FMD, with both sensitivity and specificity nearing 98%. As an iodinated contrast-based imaging study, CTA has the disadvantages of allergic reaction and potential nephrotoxicity, particularly in those with pre-existing renal disease. CTA also results in exposure to ionizing radiation. Results of CTA are highly variable in the presence of heavy calcification which commonly occurs in elderly people with suspected ARAS, and in these instances other imaging modalities may be favored.

Magnetic Resonance Angiography (MRA)

Similarly to CTA, magnetic resonance angiography (MRA) allows for detailed anatomical analysis from 2D and 3D reconstruction with 90% to 100% sensitivity and specificity for proximal lesions. Unlike CTA, MRA is not affected by calcium artifact and does not use an iodinated contrast medium. Gadolinium-enhanced MRA can be used to further improve the quality of vessel-to-tissue contrast in the proximal artery, though it is not recommended in patients with an estimated glomerular filtration rate < 30 mL/min due to a risk of nephrogenic systemic fibrosis (NSF). Though rare, NSF leads to painful thickening of the skin which can result in significant physical disability. In noncontrast and gadolinium-enhanced MRA alike, the test is limited by motion artifact and is not ideal in patients who cannot be immobile for long periods of time or in those with claustrophobia. The test is also limited by the presence of implanted metallic devices such as pacemakers, spinal cord stimulators, prostheses, vascular stents, and surgical clips which alter the magnetic field.

It should be noted that while both CTA and MRA provide excellent visualization of aneurysmal and proximal disease, both tests are limited in their ability to identify interlobar and interlobular stenosis. These modalities also benefit from their ability to identify accessory arteries and accurately depict anatomic relationships which can be useful in making treatment decisions. In contrast, Duplex ultrasonography provides functional data, since the continuous nature of the systolic velocity provides a functionally relevant understanding of the effect of the stenosis on the translesional pressure gradient.

Additional Tests

Physiologic and perfusion studies such as renal vein renin assay and renal scintigraphy have fallen out of favor in the diagnostic workup of ARAS due to low sensitivity and specificity. Such tests require the discontinuation of any antihypertensive medications that act on the RAAS, and may not be ideal in elderly patients with severe atherosclerotic disease. The usefulness of these studies is extremely limited. In clinical practice, renal vein renin is most commonly used now to determine the functional significance of a kidney with an occluded renal artery in the presence of persistent hypertension despite medical treatment. Renal scintigraphy is used in a somewhat analogous fashion, to determine the proportion of excretory renal function in an atrophic kidney that is supplied by an occluded renal artery.

Invasive Imaging

Conventional catheter angiography remains the diagnostic gold standard for RAS due to its high spatial resolution. Compared to noninvasive studies, there is unparalleled visualization of the small branch vessels. Digital subtraction angiography allows for improved resolution while limiting the volume of contrast administered to the patient. In those patients with contrast allergies or advanced renal disease, carbon dioxide angiography provides a noniodinated contrast alternative. Through the combined use of angiography with intra-arterial pressure measurements to identify hemodynamically significant stenoses (cross-sectional area > 80%), RAS can be diagnosed and treated in a single session. As an invasive procedure, catheter angiography requires an arterial puncture and carries with it the associated risks of arterial trauma and embolization of debris through manipulation of the catheter and wires. An important first step is an aortogram to visualize the ostia of the renal arteries, identify the presence and location of accessory renal arteries, and determine the nature of the aortic wall near the ostia of the renal arteries. From this, the origin can be carefully selected with a diagnostic catheter, or utilizing a "no touch technique," to minimize aortic wall contact.[10] This is critical to avoid atheroembolization and other complications.

MANAGEMENT

Medical Therapy

In order to prevent irreversible sequelae of RAS, aggressive medical treatment is required that may necessitate the use of multiple pharmacologic agents. In people with RAS of all causes, initial therapy should include an ACE inhibitors or an angiotensin receptor blockers (ARBs) in a manner that provides adequate 24-hour effects, such as a long-acting agent or twice daily dosing of shorter acting medications. Infrequently, these agents can precipitate acute renal insufficiency, particularly in patients with bilateral disease, a solitary functioning kidney, or when the contralateral kidney has severe intrarenal disease. It can at times be responsible for acute, hemodynamic reductions in kidney function. This is attributed to ACE/ARB efferent arteriolar vasodilation that results in reduction in intra-glomerular pressure leading to a rise in creatinine or blood urea nitrogen.[11] However, several lines of evidence demonstrate that ACE-I/ARB therapy is safe and effective as long as renal function is monitored and that a subsequent rise in creatinine is less than 25% rise of baseline.[12] Importantly, when there is an abrupted, sustained

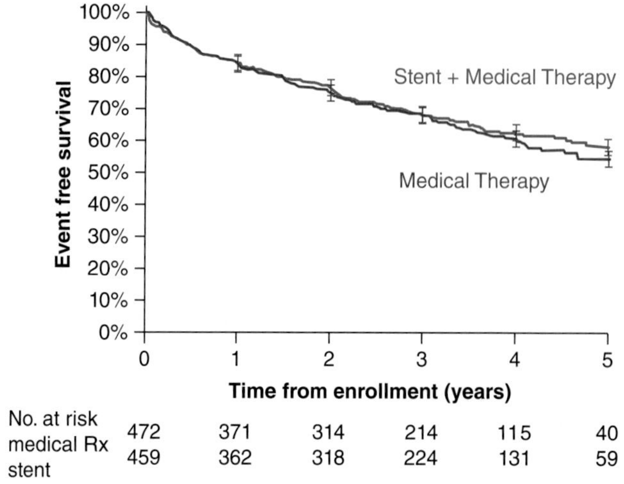

FIGURE 38-3 Composite clinical event rate comparing medical therapy alone vs. medical therapy with stenting of renal artery stenosis in the CORAL trial.

increase in serum creatinine, it is reasonable to stop the ACE/ARB and recheck the creatinine in 3–7 days.

All people undergoing medical management should be monitored with regular BUN and creatinine checks. The second line agent should be a long-acting dihydropyridine-type calcium channel antagonist such as amlodipine. Other useful antihypertensives include alpha/beta-blockers, long-acting diuretics, and aldosterone antagonists. During initiation of effective antihypertensive therapy, it is critical that patients be seen on a frequent schedule, such as every 2 weeks, to monitor for adequacy of blood pressure control and side effects. Similarly, treatment regimens should rely on long-acting medications that provide adequate control of blood pressure until the next dose is taken, which is provided in the drug package insert as the trough to peak ratio. In addition to antihypertensive therapy, optimization of cardiovascular risk factors in the form of smoking cessation counseling and treatment, effective glycemic control, cholesterol management with statins and other medications, and initiation of antiplatelet medications like aspirin should not be forgotten.

Indications for Intervention

The Atherosclerotic Ostial Stenosis of the Renal Artery Trial and the Angioplasty and Stenting for Renal Artery Lesions Trial both published in 2009 set an important precedent in the management of symptomatic ARAS, showing that medical therapy in combination with revascularization resulted in no significant clinical benefit in progression of kidney disease or hypertension control when compared to medical therapy alone.[13,14] As seen in Figure 38-3, the Cardiovascular Outcomes in Renal Atherosclerotic Lesions (CORAL) Trial which was followed in 2014 similarly showed that medical therapy in combination with renal artery stenting did not confer an advantage in preventing adverse cardiovascular and renal events when compared to medical therapy alone.[15] Based on these findings, revascularization is generally reserved for symptomatic ARAS with one of the following characteristics:

- Severe hypertension not controlled by antihypertensive medication regimen,
- Progressively worsening renal function or renal size despite optimal medical therapy,
- Recurrent pulmonary edema or congestive heart failure despite optimal medical therapy

FMD-induced RAS with the above characteristics should also be considered for revascularization. Young people with FMD and congenital causes who have newly diagnosed HTN may benefit from early revascularization which can be curative is as much as 50% and thereby prevent the need for antihypertensive medications. Of note, hypertension cure to current blood pressure guidelines is almost never achieved in people with ARAS undergoing revascularization.

Endovascular Therapy

With advances in vascular technology, technical success rates for endovascular treatments are comparable to open surgical approaches, though with significant improvements in postoperative morbidity and mortality. The first surgical treatment for RAS, when anatomically feasible, is therefore via an endovascular approach. Anatomical characteristics which may favor an open approach over endovascular therapy include congenital RAS associated with a small abdominal aorta in need of repair, an occluded renal artery that is viable and functionally significant, severe aortic pathology that obviate a safe approach to the renal artery, and the need for repair of an associated renal artery aneurysm greater than 2 cm that cannot be treated with an endovascular method.

Percutaneous Transluminal Angioplasty (PTA)

Percutaneous transluminal angioplasty (PTA), when combined with stenting, is currently the most common endovascular intervention for RAS. Arterial access may be obtained through a common femoral, brachial, or radial artery approach, depending on the anatomy of the renal artery and aorta. When a femoral approach is utilized, fluoroscopy should be employed to ensure access directly over the femoral head, which provides a bony structure against which manual pressure can be applied to achieve hemostasis following procedure completion. Brachial or radial access is appropriate for some patients with severe aortoiliac disease and those with a steeply downgoing renal artery . The next steps of the procedure are determined by the pathophysiology of the RAS and the location of stenosis. RAS secondary to FMD responds well to balloon angioplasty alone and generally does not require stenting. Trinquart and colleagues performed a meta-regression analysis that utilized a number of case series and demonstrated that hypertension cure decreased with age.[16] Stents should be avoided in these young patients to avoid late complications including restenosis and stent fracture.

To perform a balloon angioplasty, a balloon is sized based on the diameter of the nondiseased pre- or poststenotic renal artery. The balloon is advanced across the area of stenosis over a guidewire and inflated until the stenotic region is comparable in size to the native renal artery. Successful treatment of the stenosis can be confirmed with a completion angiogram and postintervention pressure measurements. For people with FMD, the mechanism of treatment with balloon angioplasty is stretching and tearing of the lesions. Extreme care is needed to balance the need to adequately stretch and tear while avoiding the complications of vessel rupture. As a consequence, it is oftentimes necessary to dilate, reassess, and redilate until an adequate result is obtained. Because these lesions can be difficult to assess angiographically, it can be useful to use a pressure sensing guidewire and remeasure pressure gradients until the desired outcome is obtained.

Endovascular Stenting

In almost all cases of ARAS where treatment is of ostial and proximal lesions, low profile balloon-inflatable endovascular stents are deployed. For ostial lesions, the stent is positioned with approximately 2 mm of overhang into the aorta to prevent encroachment of aortic plaque into the ostium of the renal artery, provide maximal bracing to the proximal renal artery, and minimize the risk of future restenosis. All stents should be long enough to adequately cover the area of stenosis with 1–3 mm of coverage on either side of the stenotic area. Technical success for both PTA and endovascular stent placement is defined as a postintervention stenosis of less than 30% and a transstenotic peak systolic gradient less than 10 mmHg. The goal of stent deployment is to match the diameter of the normal renal artery, just distal to the stenosis and any poststenotic dilation. Technical success rates of PTA and endovascular stenting range from 80% to 100%, with long-term patency rates greater in those who undergo stent placement. When directly compared to optimal medical therapy, the improvement in blood pressure is significant but modest and in the range of several mmHg.[15] Complete resolution of hypertension following PTA and stenting for ARAS is exceedingly rare but can be seen in young patients with FMD.

Complications

The most common postoperative complication of PTA and endovascular stenting is groin hematoma, occurring in approximately 5% of patients. Hemostasis should be assured following completion of the angiogram, whether by utilizing a vascular closure device or by applying manual pressure to the access site. The majority of access site hematomas can be managed conservatively with the application of pressure dressings. Duplex ultrasound should be employed to rule out an underlying pseudoaneurysm in patients with persistent or enlarging groin masses. Pseudoaneurysms smaller than 1 cm in size can be monitored with serial ultrasounds; those larger than 1 cm in size should undergo ultrasound-guided compression or thrombin injection. Any evidence of skin compromise should prompt surgical exploration. Another potential complication of endovascular intervention is renal artery dissection. Occurring at a rate of 3% to 5%, dissection most frequently occurs with passage of the wire across a particularly tight stenosis. Treatment involves placing a stent across the area of dissection. Covered stents can also be deployed across areas of iatrogenic perforation. For distal wire perforations, often caused by use of hydrophilic guide wires or lack of attention to distal wire position, embolization can be utilized. When severe arterial ruptures occur that cannot be managed with a covered stent, conversion to an open procedure can prevent significant blood loss. In these cases balloon tamponade with a slightly oversized balloon at low (1-2 atmosphere) pressure can be used to stop the hemorrhage while further treatment planning occurs. This will result in undesireable effect of warm ischemia to the kidney but is necessary to prevent severe blood loss and or tamponade of the kidney by a surrounding hematoma. In young patients with FMD, whose vasoreactivity is more pronounced than in those patients with ARAS, renal artery vasospasm is sometimes encountered. Pre-medication with calcium channel blockers such as nifedipine or intraoperative injection of nitroglycerin can prevent this complication. Finally, side branch occlusion can occur when early branches originate near the site of the stenosis and plaque is shifted into the branch. These occlusions may result in renal infarction and should be avoided. In addition, contrast nephropathy is a serious concern since many people who are indicated for treatment have pre-existing advanced kidney disease, thus necessitating meticulous attention to treatment planning. Late complications of renal artery interventions include restenosis, stent occlusion, stent fracture (Figure 38-4), and progression to end stage renal disease.

Surveillance and Follow-up

Aspirin (81 mg or 325 mg daily) and a statin are continued for the life of the patient. For PTA with stent placement, Clopidogrel (75 mg daily) is generally recommended for a minimum duration of 1-month, although success has been documented with a aspirin-only treatment regimen. Regular 6-month outpatient renal duplex US can be considered, especially for the first 2 years postoperatively, and potentially annually thereafter. Monitoring of serum creatinine is also recommended.

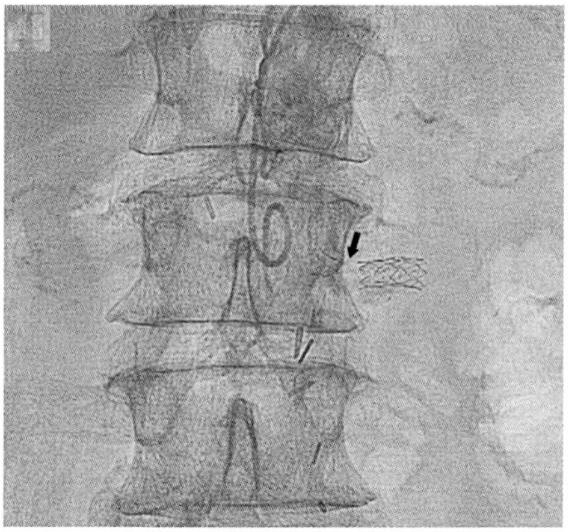

FIGURE 38-4 Fracture and separation of a left renal artery stent into two pieces, one proximal and one distal with an arrow indicating the gap between the pieces.

Open Surgery

In children, young adults, and older adult patients with otherwise unfavorable anatomy for endovascular repair of RAS, open surgery may be indicated in highly selected patients (Figure 38-5). Open surgical treatment for RAS is also preferred in those patients undergoing elective open surgery for aortic disease. Open procedures are also available as salvage procedures for failed attempts at endovascular management. In all open interventions, renal ischemia time should be closely monitored. Cold preservation solution is recommended for renal ischemia times anticipated to be greater than 1 hour. Open procedures can be divided into direct and indirect revascularization. Direct procedures (aortorenal endarterectomy, aortorenal bypass, renal artery re-implantation) involve a new, direct connection between the abdominal aorta and the renal artery, whereas indirect procedures (extra-anatomic bypasses such as hepatorenal and splenorenal) supply blood to the renal artery via an artery which itself arises from the abdominal aorta.

Aortorenal Endarterectomy

ARAS at the origin of the bilateral renal arteries may be treated with aortorenal endarterectomy via a transaortic or transrenal approach. Utilizing a midline incision, the small bowel is retracted to the right of the abdomen and the retroperitoneum is incised to expose the aorta. In the transaortic approach, a longitudinal aortotomy is made to expose the bilateral renal ostia and allow for plaque removal using eversion endarterectomy. In the transrenal approach, a transverse incision is made on the aorta and carried onto the proximal renal artery. The incisions can be closed with either a continuous suture or a patch.

Aortorenal Bypass

Aortorenal bypass is the most frequently utilized open surgery for RAS, and is particularly for multifocal or long-segment ARAS. Using the approach described above, the abdominal aorta and renal

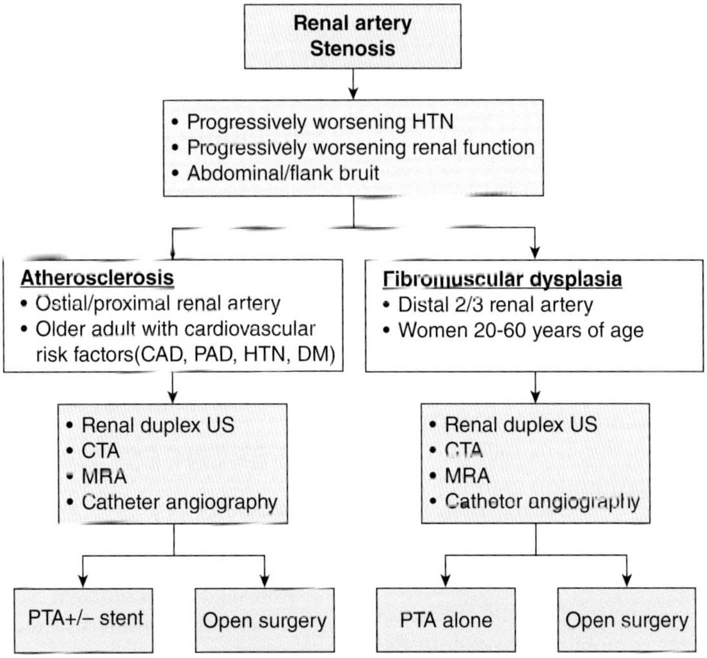

FIGURE 38-5 Flow chart for the diagnosis and management of renal artery stenosis. CAD, coronary artery disease; CTA, CT angiography; DM, diabetes mellitus; HTN, hypertension; MRA, MR angiography; PAD, peripheral arterial disease; PTA, percutaneous transluminal angioplasty; US, ultrasound.

artery origins are exposed. One of three materials is then used to create an aortorenal bypass. The most commonly used bypass material is autologous saphenous vein. To be useful for bypass, the saphenous vein should measure at minimum 4 mm in diameter and should be free of disease. Autologous hypogastric vein with similar qualifications can also be used and is the graft of choice in children, as saphenous vein may over time undergo aneurysmal changes. If no suitable autologous veins are available, synthetic Dacron and polytetrafluoroethylene (PTFE) graft are available. The graft is sewn to the infrarenal aorta in an end-to-side fashion and the distal renal artery in a spatulated end-to-end fashion, ensuring that the bypass is free of tension and redundancy. The infrarenal aorta is preferred to the suprarenal aorta as celiac and SMA stenosis are not uncommon in patients affected by RAS.

Renal Artery Re-implantation

If during open intervention there is sufficient redundancy of the renal artery, the artery can be ligated at its origin and re-implanted into an area of nondiseased infrarenal aorta. This option is most commonly used in children and young adults in whom the aorta is healthy and there may be limited durability of an venous or artificial conduit.

Extra-anatomic Bypass

In patients with severe calcific aortic disease and those who would not tolerate the hemodynamic effect of aortic cross-clamping, several extra-anatomic bypass options exist. Disease of the right renal artery can be treated with hepatorenal bypass by use of a saphenous vein or PTFE interposition graft. After creating an end-to-side proximal anastomosis with the common hepatic artery, the interposition graft is passed posterior to the portal triad and anterior to the IVC to create an end-to-end anastomosis with the right renal artery. Similarly to right-sided disease, disease of the left renal artery can be treated with splenorenal bypass. The pancreas is mobilized to expose the underlying splenic artery which is ligated distally. Unlike the hepatorenal bypass which employs the use of a bridge, the splenic artery is often of sufficient length to anastomose directly to the left renal artery in an end-to-end fashion. Splenic viability is afterward maintained by collateral circulation. The iliac-renal bypass by use of autologous vein or synthetic bypass has also been employed in the past, though care must be taken to avoid tension and redundancy in the graft.

Complications

The most common postoperative complications following open surgery are related to underlying pulmonary and cardiac comorbidities, with increased morbidity and mortality seen in those with advanced age, congestive heart failure, and chronic renal failure. Open intervention also has increased risk of distal showering of emboli, particularly if the vessels undergoing manipulation are heavily diseased. Unfortunately for people with ARAS, morbidity and mortality occur at a high frequency and for this reason surgical treatment is used sparingly. Marone showed that surgical management of ischemic nephropathy for ARAS carried a perioperative mortality and morbidity of 4% and 5%, respectively.[17] Renal function improved in 42%, worsened in 17% and 41% exhibited no significant change.

Surveillance and Follow-up

Similarly to endovascular repair, aspirin (81 mg or 325 mg daily) and a statin are continued for the life of the patient. Regular 6-month outpatient renal duplex US should be performed for 2 years postoperatively and annually thereafter to monitor for disease recurrence. Monitoring of serum creatinine is also recommended.

REFERENCES

1. Safian RD, Textor SC. Renal-artery stenosis. *N Engl J Med.* 2001;344(6):431-442.
2. Drummond CA, Brewster PS, He W, et al. Cigarette smoking and cardio-renal events in patients with atherosclerotic renal artery stenosis. *PLoS One.* 2017;12(3): e0173562.
3. Caps MT, Perissinotto C, Zierler RE, et al. Prospective study of atherosclerotic disease progression in the renal artery. *Circulation.* 1998;98(25):2866-2872.

4. Pearce JD, Craven BL, Craven TE, et al. Progression of atherosclerotic renovascular disease: a prospective population-based study. *J Vasc Surg*. 2006;44(5):955-962.
5. Lao D, Parasher P, Cho K, Yeghiazarians Y. Atherosclerotic renal artery stenosis—diagnosis and treatment. *Mayo Clin Proc*. 2011;86(7):649-657.
6. Olin JW, Sealove BA. Diagnosis, management, and future developments of fibromuscular dysplasia. *J Vasc Surg*. 2011;53(3):826-836.
7. Goldblatt H, Lynch J, Hanzal RF, Summerville WW. Studies on experimental hypertension; production of persistent elevation of systolic blood pressure by means of renal ischemia. *J Exper Med*. 1934;59:347-379.
8. Murphy TP, Cooper CJ, Pencina KM, et al. Relationship of albuminuria and renal artery stent outcomes: results from the CORAL randomized clinical trial (Cardiovascular Outcomes With Renal Artery Lesions). *Hypertension*. 2016;68(5):1145-1152.
9. Radermacher J, Chavan A, Bleck J, et al. Use of doppler ultrasonography to predict the outcome of therapy for renal-artery stenosis. *N Engl J Med*. 2001;344(6):410-417.
10. Feldman RL, Wargovich TJ, Bittl JA. No-touch technique for reducing aortic wall trauma during renal artery stenting. *Catheter Cardiovasc Interv*. 1999;46(2):245-248.
11. Khosla S, Ahmed A, Siddiqui M, et al. Safety of angiotensin-converting enzyme inhibitors in patients with bilateral renal artery stenosis following successful renal artery stent revascularization. *Am J Ther*. 2006;13(4):306-308.
12. Gupta R, Assiri S, Cooper CJ. Renal artery stenosis: new findings from the CORAL trial. *Curr Cardiol Rep*. 2017;19(9):75.
13. Bax L, Woittiez AJJ, Kouwenberg HJ, et al. Stent placement in patients with atherosclerotic renal artery stenosis and impaired renal function: a randomized trial. *Ann Intern Med*. 2009;150(12):840-848.
14. Wheatley K, Ives N, Gray R, et al. Revascularization versus medical therapy for renal-artery stenosis. *N Engl J Med*. 2009;361(20):1953-1962.
15. Cooper CJ, Murphy TP, Cutlip DE, et al. Stenting and medical therapy for atherosclerotic renal-artery stenosis. *N Engl J Med*. 2014;370(1):13-22.
16. Trinquart L, Mounier-Vehier C, Sapoval M, Gagnon N, Plouin P. Efficacy of revascularization for renal artery stenosis caused by fibromuscular dysplasia: a systematic review and meta-analysis. *Hypertension*. 2010;56:525-532.
17. Marone LK, Clouse WD, Dorer DJ, et al. Preservation of renal function with surgical revascularization in patients with atherosclerotic renovascular disease. *J Vasc Surg*. 2004;39(2):322-329.

SELF-ASSESSMENT STUDY QUESTIONS AND ANSWERS

Questions

1. A 78-year-old female presents to your office with refractory hypertension despite being on three maximally dosed antihypertensive medications. Renal ultrasound shows right renal peak systolic velocity (PSV) of 230 cm/s with a right renal-to-aortic PSV ratio of 3.7. Left renal PSV is 120 cm/s with left renal-to-aortic PSV ratio of 2.6. Which of the following statements is most likely to be true?
A. The right renal artery has a stenosis that may be greater than 60% stenosis
B. The left renal artery has a stenosis that may be greater than 60% stenosis.
C. Neither renal artery evidence suggests a hemodynamically significant stenosis
D. Both renal arteries have a stenosis that may be greater than stenosis

2. A 60-year-old male develops swelling in his right groin 24-hours after undergoing renal artery stenting via right groin access. A discrete, pulsatile mass is appreciated. The skin overlying the mass is taught and discolored. Which of the following is the best treatment option for this patient?
A. Serial examinations
B. Manual compression
C. Ultrasound-guided thrombin injection
D. Operative exploration

3. What is the most common layer of the arterial wall affected by fibromuscular dysplasia?
A. Intima
B. Media
C. Adventitia
D. All layers of the arterial wall are affected equally

4. A 29-year-old female with fibromuscular dysplasia presents for evaluation of uncontrolled hypertension despite four antihypertensive medications. Ultrasound shows left renal artery stenosis in the mid-portion of the artery with peak systolic velocity of 225 cm/s. Which of the following is the best treatment option for this patient?
A. Continue medical therapy
B. Percutaneous balloon angioplasty alone
C. Percutaneous balloon angioplasty with stenting
D. Aortorenal bypass

5. A 72-year old male undergoes open aortorenal bypass for bilateral renal artery stenosis. He asks what imaging studies he will need to undergo as an outpatient during follow-up. What is the preferred imaging study following renal artery revascularization?
A. Renal duplex ultrasound
B. CT angiography
C. MR angiography
D. No routine imaging is required

6. Which of the following is not an indication for surgical intervention in renal artery stenosis?
A. Uncontrolled hypertension on 3 or more antihypertensive medications
B. Progressively worsening renal function despite optimal medical therapy
C. Recurrent flash pulmonary edema
D. All of the above are indications for surgical intervention

7. What is the minimum diameter of saphenous vein necessary for autologous vein bypass in aortorenal bypass?
A. 2 mm
B. 3 mm
C. 4 mm
D. 5 mm

SELF-ASSESSMENT STUDY QUESTIONS AND ANSWERS

8. An 80-year-old female presents with worsening renal function and a right-sided flank bruit on physical exam. Which of the following imaging studies is considered the gold standard confirmatory test in the diagnosis of her condition?

A. Renal duplex ultrasound
B. CT angiography
C. MR angiography
D. Catheter angiography

9. Which of the following patients with renal artery stenosis is most likely to benefit from percutaneous balloon angioplasty and stenting?

A. A 73-year-old female with uncontrolled hypertension on four long-acting medications
B. A 60-year-old male with blood pressure well controlled on two antihypertensive medications
C. A 63-year-old female with uncontrolled hypertension on four medications who has previously undergone renal artery angioplasty and stenting
D. A 30-year-old female with fibromuscular dysplasia and no history of hypertension

10. Which of the following risk factors is not associated with renal artery stenosis?

A. Coronary artery disease
B. Peripheral arterial disease
C. Alcohol abuse
D. Diabetes

SELF-ASSESSMENT STUDY QUESTIONS AND ANSWERS

Answers

1. A.
2. D.
3. B.
4. C.
5. A.
6. D.
7. C.
8. D.
9. A.
10. C.

SECTION IV Special Vascular Conditions

CHAPTER

39 Thoracic Outlet Syndrome and Supraclavicular Decompression

Francis J. Caputo and John W. Perry

OUTLINE

DEFINITION
CAUSE
TYPES
- Neurogenic TOS
- Venous TOS
- Arterial TOS

PRESENTATION AND PHYSICAL FINDINGS
- Neurogenic TOS
- Venous TOS
- Arterial TOS

OPERATIVE STRATEGY
- Anatomy of the Thoracic Outlet

OPERATIVE TECHNIQUE
- Positioning and Incision
- Scalenectomy
- First Rib Resection
- Brachial Plexus Neurolysis
- Pectoralis Minor Tenotomy
- Subclavian Artery Aneurysm or Pathology Management
- Management of Subclavian Vein Occlusion, Stenosis, or other Pathologies
- Drain Placement and Closure

POSTOPERATIVE MANAGEMENT

DEFINITION

Thoracic outlet syndrome (TOS) is defined as symptomatic compression of the neurovascular structures at the thoracic outlet within an upper extremity.[1–3] This group of conditions can take three forms including neurogenic, venous, and arterial. The majority of which is comprised of neurogenic symptoms, although vascular problems may be present. The incident of TOS is reported to be approximately 0.3% to 2% in the general population, affecting an age range from 25 to 40 years typically.[4] Women are more commonly affected then men, with a ratio of 4:1.

CAUSE

The causes of TOS vary among the different forms. With neurogenic TOS, it is hypothesized to be a combination of osseous changes, soft tissue abnormalities, trauma, and inflammation.[5] In addition to congenital predisposition of anatomic structures, acquired extrinsic factors may produce further compression. The causes of arterial TOS are usually a bony abnormality, such as a cervical rib or rudimentary first rib. Venous TOS is typically due to the costoclavicular ligament and subclavius muscle compression the subclavian vein.

TYPES

NEUROGENIC TOS

The most common type of TOS is the neurogenic type constituting 94 to 97%.[5] Symptoms are caused by compression of the brachial plexus. There are typically two patterns of brachial plexus compression: lower C8 and T1 plexus involvement and upper C5 and C6 involvement. The pictures can sometimes be mixed as well.

Lower plexus compression causes sensory disturbances to the ulnar nerve distribution. Complaints of pain and paresthesias in the medial aspect of the arm from axilla, through the brachial area and the forearm, down to hand in the fourth an fifth fingers are common. There can be weakness and even muscle wasting in extreme cases within the ulnar innervated muscles such as the hypothenar and interosseous. Pain in the anterior and posterior shoulder region as well as within the side or back of the neck can be present. Patients with upper plexus compression usually show symptoms within the upper and forearm, rather than the hand.[6] This can also produce pain in the side of the neck that can radiate toward the ear, mandible, face, and temple. Typically will involve the median nerve distribution. Brachial plexus compression can cause subjective coldness of the hand and pallor. In very severe cases or in advanced cases, you may see muscle atrophy and weakness in the hand.

VENOUS TOS

Venous TOS accounts for 2% to 3% of patients.[4] Usually will see signs of venous obstruction within the upper extremity that produces swelling, edema, cyanosis, and discomfort of the extremity that is aggravated with exertion. Patients can describe a sudden onset of symptoms from subclavian vein thrombosis. Over time, venous collateralization may develop and can be evident on exam with distension of superficial veins across the shoulder and chest.

ARTERIAL TOS

Arterial involvement is the least common form of TOS and comprises 1% to 2% of case.[4] These patients will display signs of ischemia within the extremity: pain, pallor, paresthesia, pulselessness, and coolness. They can often experience arm claudication with fatigue and pain during exertion or use of the arm, particularly when the arm is elevated. Thrombosis or embolization from the subclavian artery may develop ischemic ulcerations or gangrenous changes to the fingertips. These symptoms indicate severe subclavian artery narrowing or aneurysmal changes from the compression.

PRESENTATION AND PHYSICAL FINDINGS

NEUROGENIC TOS

The diagnosis of neurogenic TOS is based on clinical evaluation and supplemented by diagnostic tools or procedures to exclude other etiologies on symptoms. Symptoms attributable to brachial plexus compression include pain, numbness, and paresthesias in the neck, shoulder, arm, or hand. The involvement in the hand usually extends beyond the median and ulnar nerve regions, involving all fingers. The symptoms of neurogenic TOS can be exacerbated or intensified by the extent of upper extremity activity involving abduction and elevation. Patients with neurogenic TOS may exhibit symptoms from compression of the pectoralis minor tendon that produce anterior chest wall and axillary pain.

The symptoms may be slow and gradual onset, with episodes of exacerbation. Others can develop steady progression leading to severe symptoms and disability. Long-terms effects and prolonged brachial plexus compression may even lead to hand muscle atrophy and weakness.

The physical exam will demonstrate localized tenderness to palpation over the supraclavicular scalene triangle and/or the infraclavicular subcoracoid space, which will reproduce the extremity symptoms. Long-standing neurogenic TOS may show muscle thinning along the thenar and hypothenar prominence or intrinsic muscle atrophy. Provocative maneuvers like the positive upper limb tension test or the 3 minutes elevated arm stress test will rapidly reproduce upper extremity symptoms. The physical exam should also include assessment for potential cervical spine degenerative disease or peripheral nerve compression, as well any arterial or venous compromise to the upper extremity. Upper extremity pulse volume recordings can be helpful in demonstrating compression, but are nonspecific. Many times these patients will have prior MRIs and electromyography studies to exclude other diagnoses.

After clinical diagnosis, almost all patients shoulder undergo an anterior scalene or pectoralis minor muscle block with short-acting local anesthetic to support the diagnosis of neurogenic TOS and to help predict the improvement of symptoms with treatment to aide as prognosis factor. A positive muscle block with provide patients with temporary relief or improvement in their presenting symptoms. Patients are also directed toward appropriate course of physical therapy with a therapist who specializes in goal direct neurogenic TOS therapy. This physical therapy is aimed to relieve scalene/pectoralis minor muscle spasm, improve postural disturbances, enhance limb mobility, strengthen associated shoulder musculature, and diminish repetitive strain exposure. Usually, patients with mild neurogenic TOS will have significant improvement in symptoms after 4–6 weeks of physical therapy. Incorrect physical therapy may exacerbate symptoms and lead to premature cessation of therapy. Patients who have continued substantial disability are often recommended surgical treatment.

VENOUS TOS

These patients (typically young) will present with axillary–subclavian vein effort thrombosis syndrome, which is the formation of a deep venous thrombus within the subclavian vein at the level of compression. Sudden onset of swelling and upper extremity pain is usually described by the patient. Occasionally can be associated with cyanotic changes to the fingers and paresthesia, as well. The arm will feel full and heavy with aching. In a chronic setting, you may see venous engorgement and collateralization along the anterior chest wall and shoulder.

Besides clinical exam evidence of a deep venous thrombosis, venous duplex imaging will demonstrate subclavian vein thrombosis, although there can be false negatives with this imaging modality. Venography is an accurate diagnostic and therapeutic step for these patients. Contrast venography is immediately followed by venous thrombolysis or thrombectomy with pharmacomechanical approaches. Completion venography will usually demonstrate focal area of stenosis or occlusion of the subclavian vein at the level of the first rib. Balloon angioplasty is usually not helpful with lese lesions until after the rib resection, and stenting is strongly discouraged.

ARTERIAL TOS

Upper extremity thromboembolisms can be the first event leading to the diagnosis of arterial TOS. These patients may present with a cold and pale hand with acute limb ischemic changes, or even frank gangrene or ulcerations to the hand and fingers. Patients may report arm and hand pain, especially with overhand motion. On physical exam, there may be reduced or discrepant pulse exams. Patient may have a supraclavicular bruit from aneurysm changes to the subclavian artery due to compression. Aneurysmal changes can then lead to embolic events. Usually computed tomographic angiography is performed in these patients to determine the presence or absence of subclavian artery aneurysm in patients with a cervical rib or first rib anomaly suspected of having arterial TOS. Surgical treatment with supraclavicular decompression is recommended for all patients with subclavian aneurysms and include arterial reconstruction.

OPERATIVE STRATEGY

ANATOMY OF THE THORACIC OUTLET

The treatment and successful decompression of all three types of TOS relies on the understanding of the anatomy and the variations to be encountered. The supraclavicular approach allows excellent exposure of this anatomy, providing a complete decompression when compared with the alternative approaches.[7–11] It is the preferred exposure by the authors of the chapter.

The anatomy of the thoracic outlet involves three critical areas: scalene triangle, costoclavicular space, and the subcoracoid space. The scalene triangle is bordered by the anterior scalene muscle (ASM), middle scalene muscle (MSM), and the first rib. The brachial plexus and the subclavian artery pass through over the first rib, whereas the subclavian vein passes over the first rib in front of this triangle (Figure 39-1A). The costoclavicular space lies between the clavicle and the first rib. It is bordered superiorly by the subclavius muscle, medially by the costoclavicular ligament and posteriorly by the ASM tendon on the first rib (Figure 39-1B). The subcoracoid space lies inferior to the clavicle and underneath the pectoralis minor muscle muscle tendon (Figure 39-1C).

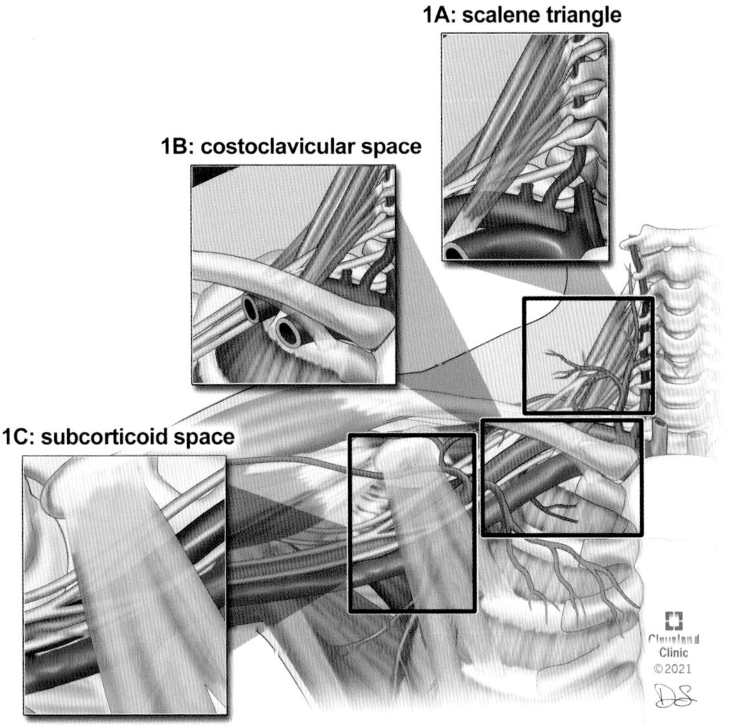

FIGURE 39-1 **(A)** The figure shows the anatomy of the thoracic outlet, **(B)** costoclavicular space, and **(C)** subarachnoid space. (Reprinted with permission, Cleveland Clinic Foundation ©2022. All Rights Reserved.)

OPERATIVE TECHNIQUE

POSITIONING AND INCISION

After induction of general anesthesia, the patient is placed supine with the head of the bed elevated to 30 degrees. The head and neck are extended and turned to the opposite side of planned intervention, an axillary or neck roll is placed behind the shoulder to further extend the neck, and the neck, chest, and affected extremity are prepped into the the field with usual sterile technique. The upper extremity is wrapped in a stockinette to allow free range of motion during the procedure and gentle held across the abdomen.

A transverse incision is made parallel to and above the clavicle, beginning at the lateral edge of the sternocleidomastoid (SCM) extending to the anterior border of the trapezius muscle. The incision is then carried through the subcutaneous layer, the platysma muscle is divided, and the subplatysmal flaps are created to expose the scalene fat pad. The SCM is then lifted and retracted medially.

One of the key steps to the supraclavicular approach is the mobilization and lateral reflection of the scalene fat pad. This begins with the dissection of the fat pad off the lateral edge of the internal jugular (IJ) vein and the superior edge of the clavicle. The small blood vessel and lymphatic tissues can be ligated and divided. A short segment of omohyoid muscle is resected and divided. The thoracic duct, located at the confluence of the IJ vein, and subclavian vein near the interomedial aspect of the fat pad on the left side are ligated and divided. Deliberate ligation and division of the lymphatics is important as a lymphatic leak is a potential complication to this exposure. The scalene fat pad is mobilized from a medial to lateral direction with gentle fingertip dissection along the surface of the ASM. Care must be taken to avoid injuring the phrenic nerve which passes from a lateral to medial direction as it descends on the muscle surface. After progressive lateral mobilization of the fat pad, the brachial plexus nerve roots (at the posterolateral aspect of the ASM) and the MSM (behind the plexus) can be visualized. The long thoracic nerve is identified as it emerges from the MSM coursing past the lateral aspect of the first rib. Silk retraction sutures can be used to hold the scalene fat pad in position. This portion of the exposure represents the first of six critical views to be obtained during the supraclavicular approach.

SCALENECTOMY

The brachial plexus and the subclavian artery are gently dissected and mobilized away from the lower lateral aspect of the ASM until a fingertip can be passed behind the muscle above the first rib, helping to displace the neurovascular bundle posteriorly. This fingertip dissection can then be carried behind the ASM toward the medial edge carefully avoiding injury to the phrenic nerve. This dissection has now freed the medial, posterior, and lateral aspect of the ASM leaving a well protected view of the ASM. After protection of the phrenic nerve, subclavian artery, and brachial plexus, the ASM can be sharply divided under direct visualization. The end of the muscle is elevated, the rest of the extrapleural attachments are freed and any muscle fibers that surround the subclavian artery are resected to full release the artery. Any scalene minimus muscle fibers passing between the plexus are divided as well. The ASM can then be passed underneath to the medial side of the phrenic nerve and lifted further to aide in the dissection toward the origin of the muscle onto C6 transverse process. The C6 process can easily be palpated and once completely freed, the ASM can be fully transected off the surgical field. Minor bleeding from the muscle edges can be controlled with suture ligation to avoid using electrocautery close to the nerve plexus. There are a wide variation of anomalous fibrofascial bands that can be observed after ASM resection, typically passing near the brachial plexus. These structures can be resected to ensure full decompression.

The brachial plexus nerve roots are separated from the front edge of the MSM, until a small malleable retractor can be placed behind the plexus in front of the MSM. Blunt fingertip dissection can be used along the lateral aspect of the plexus to facilitate further exposure deeper to the inner aspect of the first rib. Medial retraction of the plexus and posterolateral reflection of the long thoracic nerve by a second small malleable placed lateral to the MSM will expose the attachments of the MSM to the lateral first rib. The transverse cervical artery and vein should be ligated and divided as they pass through the plexus and MSM to avoid unnecessary bleeding from avulsion during retraction. Electrocautery can then be used to divide the MSM insertion off the surface of the bone, using a periosteal elevator for dissection as it progresses posteriorly, extending to a parallel point of the underlying T1 nerve root on the first rib. The bulk of the MSM anterior the long thoracic nerve is then resected off the surgical field. Any minor bleeding once again is controlled with suture ligation to avoid nerve injury with electrocautery to the C8 nerve root.

FIRST RIB RESECTION

Once complete anterior and middle scalenectomy has been performed, the intercostal muscle attachments to the lateral aspect of the first rib are divided. The exposure of the first rib is then carried posteriorly where the T1 nerve roots emerge from underneath the bone to join C8 nerve root. A right-angled clamp is passed underneath the posterior neck of the first rib to spread and dissect remaining intercostal attachments. Under direct visualization and verification of the nerve roots, a modified Stille-Giertz rib cutter is inserted around the neck of the first rib and divided. The posterior end of the bone is then smoothed to a level medial to the underlying T1 nerve root using a bone rongeur. The free end of the bone is elevated and blunt fingertip dissection is used to remove any remaining attachments to the undersurface of the bone proceeding in an anterior direction to the level of the prior ASM. The pleural space is almost always intentionally opened during the firs rib resection to allow drainage of postoperative fluid into the pleural space away from the brachial plexus, which theoretically could decrease perineural adhesions.

A small Richardson retractor is used to elevate soft tissues and subclavian vein underneath the clavicle. The posterior rib is displaced inferiorly with fingertip pressure to open the anterior costoclavicular space. A small malleable can displace the brachial plexus and subclavian artery laterally. The rib cutter is placed around the anterior first rib, immediately medial to the ASM insertion site or the scalene tubercle and divided under direct vision. The anterior end of the first rib is smoothed with a bone rongeur to a level underneath the clavicle. Hemostasis is then achieved within the resection bed.

Cervical ribs can be encountered within the plane of the MSM during the scalenectomy, where they lie behind the brachial plexus and subclavian artery. There can be ligamentous extensions to the first rib from incomplete cervical ribs, whereas complete cervical ribs attach to the lateral first rib. The posterior aspect of the cervical rib is divided in a manner similar to the posterior first rib during the MSM dissection. The anterior attachment of the cervical rib is then divided and removed prior to the first rib resection. When there is a true joint from a complete cervical rib on the first rib, the anterior attachment of the cervical rib is left until the first rib resection is completed and the specimen can be removed in whole.

BRACHIAL PLEXUS NEUROLYSIS

After the scalenectomy and the removal of the first rib, each nerve root from C5 to T1 is meticulously dissected free of perineural fibrous scar tissue that might impair nerve mobility. There is often a small fibrofascial band at the most proximal aspects of C8 and T1 nerve roots, which should be specifically sought out and resected. This aspect of the operation is not complete until each nerve root is cleared throughout its course within the operative field.

PECTORALIS MINOR TENOTOMY

When performing supraclavicular decompression for neurogenic TOS, pectoralis minor tenotomy is often performed in addition to decompression to ensure complete relief of brachial plexus nerve compression. Pectoralis minor release may also be performed for patients with persistent or recurrent nTOS who has previous had TOS decompression.

A small vertical infraclavicular incision is made in the deltopectoral groove below the coracoid process. The fascia between the deltoid and pec major muscle is divided medial to the cephalic vein. The lateral edge of the pec major muscle is retracted medially, exposing the underlying fascia. The pectoralis minor muscle is exposed and encircled close to the insertion on the coracoid process. This is then divided under direct vision within 2 cm of the coracoid. The medial edge of the muscle can be oversewn to achieve hemostasis and the clavipectoral fascia is opened to the level of the clavicle.

SUBCLAVIAN ARTERY ANEURYSM OR PATHOLOGY MANAGEMENT

Subclavian artery aneurysms which can be formed in patients with arterial TOS (usually in association with cervical ribs or anomalous first rib) usually arise within several centimeters of the scalene triangle where the artery crossed over the first rib and underneath the clavicle.[12]

After supraclavicular decompression (including removal of the cervical and first ribs), the subclavian artery is mobilized in enough length for an interposition graft repair of the aneurysmal segment. In situations where distal control cannot be achieved from the supraclavicular approach, a transverse infraclavicular incision is made with division of the pec minor muscle tendon and the axillary artery is isolated for distal control. The subclavian artery is clamped distal to the vertebral artery and distally beyond the aneurysmal segment. The aneurysmal segment is excised and replaced with an interposition graft sewn end to end. In most cases, a completion angiogram is obtained to evaluate the reconstruction in different arm positions.

MANAGEMENT OF SUBCLAVIAN VEIN OCCLUSION, STENOSIS, OR OTHER PATHOLOGIES

The operative management of venous TOS begins with the supraclavicular decompression as described, except the anterior first rib is not yet divided. Prior to the anterior division of the first rib, a second transverse incision is made one fingerbreadth below the medial clavicle or along the anterior surface of the first rib which can be palpated under the clavicle. The upper and middle portions of the pectoralis major are spread, and the anteromedial portion of the first rib is identified. Downward fingertip pressure to the divided posterior segment of the first rib from the supraclavicular incision allows the superior edge of the first rib to be dissected from its attachments from the infraclavicular incision. The subclavius muscle tendon, costoclavicular ligament, and the first intercostal muscles are all divided. The first rib is divided adjacent to the sternum with the rib cutters, after which the entire first rib can be removed from the operative field.

Through the lateral portion of the infraclavicular incision, the subclavian–axillary vein is identified and separated from the subclavius muscle, which is then resected. Further exposure of the vein can be achieved through the supraclavicular incision, continuing medially toward the junction of the subclavian and IJ vein. A collateral branch from the subclavian vein, usually located underneath the medial clavicle, is ligated and divided which allows the subclavian vein to fall away from the clavicle. Pathologic changes to the subclavian vein can be assessed at this time. Due to chronic repetitive injury, the vein can have focal areas of fibrous wall thickening. This residual scar tissue surrounding the vein is excised circumferentially to perform a venolysis. For 50% of patients with venous TOS, this results in full expansion of the prior constricted segment of the vein and no further venous reconstruction is necessary.[12] If a residual stenosis is apparent despite external venolysis, additional venous reconstruction is performed. Venography can be used postoperatively in addition to balloon angioplasty to treat the residual stenosis. A vein patch angioplasty along the full length of the affected vessel can be performed using greater saphenous vein during the rib resection. When dense fibrosis remains within the wall of the subclavian vein despite external venolysis, the affected segment of the subclavian vein can be excised and replaced by interposition bypass.

DRAIN PLACEMENT AND CLOSURE

On completions of surgical decompression, the apex of the pleural membrane is opened to allow postoperative fluid drainage as mentioned above. A closed suction drain is placed into the operative field through a separate stab incision. The drain is placed posterior to the brachial plexus with the tip into the posterior pleural space. The scalene fat pad is restored to its anatomical position overlying the brachial plexus. Several tacking sutures can be placed to SCM and the periclavicular subcutaneous fascia to hold the fat pad in place. The platysma layer is reapproximated with interrupted sutures, and the skin is closed with subcuticular absorbable stitch.

POSTOPERATIVE MANAGEMENT

The pleural blake drain should be kept to continuous bulb suction, until its removal. An upright chest radiographic examination is performed in the recovery room and each day after the surgery while the drain is in place. Immediate postoperative pain management is accomplished with oral and IV opiates until adequate control can be achieved by oral medications Afterwards, pain management is usually accomplished with a combination of oral narcotics, muscle relaxants, and a nonsteroidal anti-inflammatory agent. These are usually prescribed upon hospital discharge as well. The pleural drain is left in place usually for 2–3 days depending on output and coloration. Ideally, the drain is pulled after the patient is tolerating regular diet with no evidence of lymphatic leak and output is less than 100 cc/24 hr. Patients with neurogenic TOS are usually discharged after 3–4 hospital day stay. Patient with venous TOS are started on 500 units/hr heparin on post-operative day one. If they are tolerating the heparin drip with no evidence of bleeding, then on postoperative day 2 it is advanced to full systemic heparinization and eventually discharged with oral anticoagulation. Physical therapy is resumed the day after surgery and continued upon hospital discharge. It is usually continued after discharge for as long as necessary to allow for the patient to return to optimal level of function.

REFERENCES

1. Sanders RJ. *Thoracic Outlet Syndrome: A Common Sequelae of Neck Injuries*. Philadelphia, PA: Lippincott Williams and Wilkins; 1991.
2. Molina JE. *New Techniques for Thoracic Outlet Syndromes*. New York: Springer; 2012.
3. Illig KA, Thompson RW, Freischlag JA, Donahue DM, Jordan SE, Edgelow PI. *Thoracic Outlet Syndrome*. London: Springer-Verlag; 2013.
4. Thompson RW, Driskill M. Thoracic outlet syndrome: neurogenic. In: Cronenwett JL, Johnston KW, eds. *Rutherford's Vascular Surgery*. 7th ed. Philadelphia, PA: Elsevier; 2010:1878-1898.
5. Sanders RJ, Hammond SL. Management of cervical ribs and anomalous first ribs causing neurogenic thoracic outlet syndrome. *J Vasc Surg*. 2002;36(1):51-56.
6. Emery VB, Rastogi R, Driskill MR, Thompson RW. Diagnosis of neurogenic thoracic outlet syndrome. In: Eskandari MK, Morasch MD, Pearce WH, Yao JST, eds. *Vascular Surgery: Therapeutic Strategies*. Shelton, CT: People's Medical Publishing House-USA; 2010: 129-148.
7. Hempel GK, Rusher AH Jr, Wheeler CG, Hunt DG, Bukhari HI. Supraclavicular resection of the first rib for thoracic outlet syndrome. *Am J Surg*. 1981;141(2): 213-215.
8. Sanders RJ, Raymer S. The supraclavicular approach to scalenectomy and first rib resection: description of technique. *J Vasc Surg*. 1985;2:751-756.
9. Reilly LM, Stoney RJ. Supraclavicular approach for thoracic outlet decompression. *J Vasc Surg*. 1988;8:329-334.
10. Thompson RW, Petrinec D, Toursarkissian B. Surgical treatment of thoracic outlet compression syndromes. II. Supraclavicular exploration and vascular reconstruction. *Ann Vasc Surg*. 1997;11(4):442-451.
11. Sanders RJ, Hammond SL. Supraclavicular first rib resection and total scalenectomy: technique and results. *Hand Clin*. 2004;20:61-70.
12. Duwayri JW, Thompson RW. Supraclavicular approach for surgical treatment of thoracic outlet syndrome. In: Chaikof EL, Cambria RP, eds. *Atlas of Vascular Surgery and Endovascular Therapy: Anatomy and Technique*. Philadelphia, PA: Elsevier; 2014:172-192.

SELF-ASSESSMENT STUDY QUESTIONS AND ANSWERS

Questions

1. The most frequent form of TOS is:
   A. Arterial
   B. Venous
   C. Neurogenic
   D. Combined arterial/venous
   E. Muscular

2. Symptoms of neurogenic TOS due to brachial plexus compression is caused by all of the following except:
   A. Discoloration
   B. Pain
   C. Paresthesias
   D. Weakness
   E. Tingling

3. Lower plexus (C8 and T1) compression can cause ulnar nerve:
   A. Pain in the lateral aspect of the arm
   B. Paresthesias in the medial aspect of the arm
   C. Pain in the first three fingers
   D. Weakness of the thenar muscles
   E. Hypertrophy of the interosseous muscles

4. Upper extremity symptoms of venous obstruction include all of the following except:
   A. Arm swelling
   B. Hand edema
   C. Cyanosis
   D. Discomfort with exertion
   E. Pallor

5. Arterial TOS is associated with all of the following except:
   A. Claudication
   B. Thrombosis
   C. Embolization
   D. Pulsatile mass
   E. Supraclavicular bruit

6. Neurogenic TOS can be diagnosed by:
   A. Upper extremity adduction
   B. Arm dependency
   C. Elevated arm stress test
   D. Decreased radial pulse
   E. Absent ulnar pulse

7. Characteristics of patients with venous TOS include:
   A. Young (20–40 years)
   B. Ultrasound is helpful in diagnosis
   C. Venography is helpful in treatment
   D. Balloon angioplasty is not useful
   E. All of the above

8. A muscle block is most useful in the diagnosis of:
   A. Neurogenic
   B. Arterial
   C. Venous
   D. Combined arterial/venous
   E. Muscular strain

9. Important anatomic components comprising the thoracic outlet include all of the following except:
   A. First rib
   B. Pectoralis minor muscle
   C. Clavicle
   D. Subclavius muscle
   E. Anterior scalene muscle

10. The supraclavicular surgical approach for treatment of TOS includes all of the following except:
    A. Resection of omohyoid muscle
    B. Ligation of thoracic duct
    C. Transection of anterior scalene muscle
    D. Ligation of long thoracic nerve
    E. Removal of first rib

SELF-ASSESSMENT STUDY QUESTIONS AND ANSWERS

Answers

1. C.
2. A.
3. B.
4. E.
5. D.
6. C.
7. E.
8. A.
9. B.
10. D.

CHAPTER

40 Portal Hypertension

Nizar Hariri and Munier Nazzal

OUTLINE

GENERAL CONSIDERATION AND HISTORY

ANATOMY

DIFFERENTIAL DIAGNOSIS OF PORTAL HYPERTENSION

- Extrahepatic Presinusoidal Obstruction
- Intrahepatic Presinusoidal Obstruction
- Intrahepatic Sinusoidal and Postsinusoidal Obstruction
- Extrahepatic Postsinusoidal Obstruction
- Arteriovenous Fistulas

CLINICAL FINDINGS

- Variceal Formation
- Encephalopathy
- Hepatorenal Syndrome

DIAGNOSIS AND EVALUATION OF PATIENTS WITH PORTAL HYPERTENSION

- Noninvasive Evaluation of Portal Hypertension
  - Duplex Ultrasound Imaging
- Serum Markers
- Angiography, Computerized Tomography Angiography (CTA), and Magnetic Resonance Angiography (MRA)

INVASIVE EVALUATION OF PORTAL HYPERTENSION

- Endoscopic Exam

Liver Biopsy

Treatment of Portal Hypertension and Its Complications

- General Consideration in Treatment
- Treatment of Variceal Bleeding

Pharmacotherapy

Endoscopic Treatment Esophageal Variceal Bleeding

Tamponade Therapy

- Balloon Temponade
- Stent Temponade

Transjugular Intrahepatic Portosystemic Shunt

- Surgical Therapy of Portal Hypertension

Nonselective Shunts

- End-to-Side Portacaval Shunt (ECK Fistula)
- Side-to-Side Portacaval Shunt
  - *Interposition Shunts*
  - *Conventional Spleno-Renal Shunt*

Selective Shunts

Nonshunting Procedures

Liver Transplantation

- Surgery in Patients with Portal Hypertension

GENERAL CONSIDERATION AND HISTORY

The history of portal hypertension is intriguing. It is believed that Leonardo Vinci was the first to describe portal hypertension in the fifteenth century. However, Leonardo thought that the changes in the portal vein that becomes large and tortuous cause the changes in the liver, which he described as "liver dires and liver becomes as a frozen bran in color and consistency."

In 1543, Andreas van Wesel (Vesalio in Latin) demonstrated that the blood comes from the heart and not from the liver. He described with a great deal of accuracy the portal system. He described a case of bleeding hemorrhoids which he attributed to the dilatation of the portal branches. Later on, Glisson of London in the seventeenth century demonstrated the details of the portal circulation.[1] The term cirrhosis was mentioned in 1819 by Renee Laennes of Paris. The word cirrhosis is derived from two Greek words: Skirros (Hard fibrotic) and Kirrhos (yellowish).[2] While most of the work was focusing on liver cirrhosis, Augustine Gilbert in Paris introduced the term "portal hypertension" and he described with some details the enlargement of the natural collaterals between the portal and the venous system including the esophageal veins.[3] The portal pressure was measured for the first time by Thompson in 1937, who directly measured the pressure in the portal vein in an open abdomen.[4]

ANATOMY

Blood flow to the liver is provided through both the portal vein and hepatic artery. The portal vein provides approximately 75% of the 1500 mL of blood entering liver each minute. Despite being largely deoxygenated blood, its high flow provides 50% to 70% of the liver's oxygen. The lack of valves in the portal venous system makes it possible to accommodate high flow at low pressure due to low resistance. Additionally, this allows for the measurement of portal venous pressure at any point along the portal venous system.[5] The common hepatic artery provides about 25% of the blood supply to the liver. The hepatic artery arises from the celiac axis and ascends in the hepatoduodenal ligament, then gives the right gastric, gastroduodenal and proper hepatic artery before it divides into right and left hepatic arterial branches in the liver hilum. There are common variations including a replaced right hepatic artery arising from the superior mesenteric artery in 9.6%, and left hepatic artery originating from the left gastric artery (6.6%). In 2.6%, the common hepatic artery has a variant anatomy originating from the superior mesenteric artery and from the aorta. Other anatomical variations include the right hepatic artery arising from the celiac artery (1.8%) and aorta (0.5%).[6]

The portal vein is formed at the level of the second lumber vertebra behind the pancreas. The length of the vein is about 6 to 9 cm reaching the hilum of the liver where it divides into the right and left portal main branches. The left gastric vein joins the portal vein just above the pancreas margin entering at the anteromedial aspect. In about 25% of the cases it joins the splenic vein. Other smaller branches join the portal vein and should be looked for during surgery to avoid bleeding.

At the liver hilum, the portal vein bifurcates to the left portal vein (LPV) and the right portal vein (RPV) that splits to right anterior sectoral (RAS) and right posterior sectoral (RPS) (Figure 40-1).

In the hepatoduodenal ligament, the portal vein lies dorsal and medial to the common bile duct with lymph nodes at the lateral part of the portal vein from the duodenum to the base of the liver.

The venous blood flow out of the liver is made up of three main veins: right, middle, and left hepatic veins. The right hepatic vein drains directly into the inferior vena cava, while the middle and left hepatic veins join outside the liver into a common trunk for draining into the inferior vena cava. Both the hepatic and portal veins do not have valves. Knowledge of these veins is important for procedures, and the relationship to the portal vein branches is essential for procedures such as the transjugular intrahepatic portosystemic shunts (TIPS).[7]

As mentioned above, the total hepatic blood flow is about 1500 mL/minute. This constitutes about 25% of the cardiac output, although the liver accounts only for 2.5% of the body weight. About two-thirds to three-fourths of the blood flow to the liver enters through the portal vein, while the remaining blood enters through the hepatic artery. The blood flow to

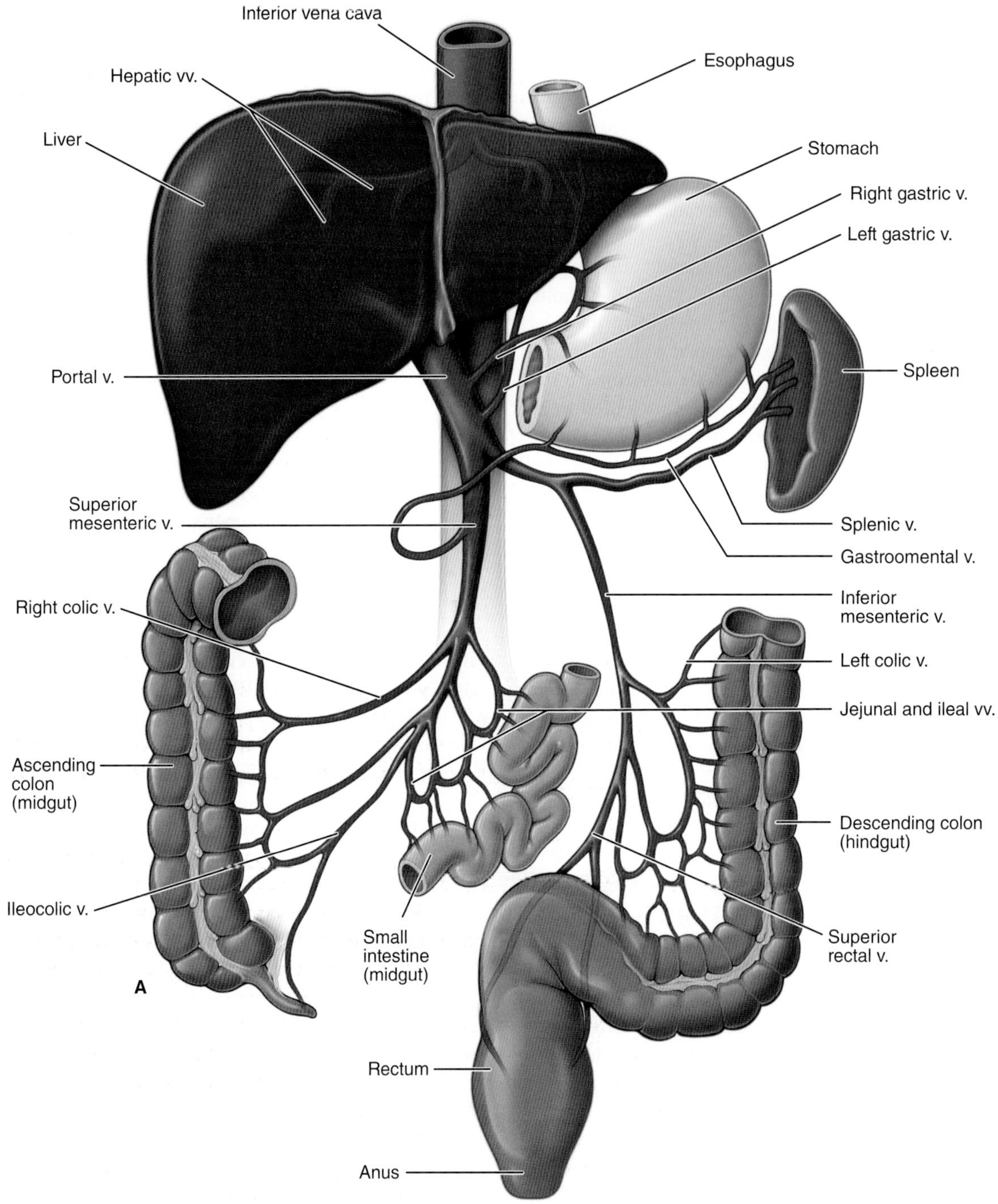

FIGURE 40-1 **Blood flow to the liver.** (Reproduced with permission from Morton D, Foreman KB, Albertine KH. *The Big Picture: Gross Anatomy*. New York, NY: McGraw Hill; 2019.)

the liver through the portal vein is constant while the hepatic artery changes depending on multiple stimuli. Sudden occlusion in the portal vein results in immediate increase in hepatic artery blood flow by 60%, then goes down to baseline, while sudden occlusion of the hepatic artery does not increase blood flow in the portal vein leading to reduction in both portal total blood flow and pressure. The liver derives half of its oxygen supply from portal vein and the other half comes from the hepatic artery.[7]

DIFFERENTIAL DIAGNOSIS OF PORTAL HYPERTENSION

Portal hypertension occurs when there is an abnormal increase in the pressure in the portal vein carrying blood from the visceral organs to the liver. Based on Ohm's Law, change in the pressure equals to the flow times the resistance, ($P = Q \times R$). Therefore, the pressure in the portal vein can be increased by increasing the portal flow, increasing the resistance to the flow in the portal system, or both. Normal portal pressure is between 5 and 10 mmHg.[1] Portal hypertension occurs when portal pressure is elevated above 15 mmHg, usually it averages 20 mmHg and can reach much higher to 50 to 60 mmHg.[7] Additionally, portal hypertension results when the pressure gradient between the portal vein and hepatic veins (hepatic venous pressure gradient, HVPG) is greater than 5 mmHg. However, clinically significant portal hypertension is present when the gradient is more than 10 mmHg.[2]

Portal hypertension can be caused by increase in portal venous flow like in splenomegaly cases associated with myeloid metaplasia. As a result of increased portal flow resistance, hyperdynamic systemic circulation and splanchnic hyperemia occurs (this is the major contributor to the maintenance of flow in the portal systemic collaterals) that contribute to increase in portal blood flow, thus adding to increased portal pressure.[3] The liver can accommodate significant increase in blood flow because of its reserve capacity, so blood flow alone cannot explain the presence of portal hypertension. In cases of arterial-portal fistula, congenital or traumatic in nature, it takes a long time for portal hypertension to develop because of the sinusoidal capability of accommodating such increase in blood flow. If such increase in blood flow persists, sinusoidal sclerosis occurs leading to increase in the liver resistance which will eventually contribute to portal hypertension. So, practically all clinically significant portal hypertension cases are secondary to increased resistance whether directly or indirectly. Because of the increase in the resistance in the liver, a reactionary decrease in the splanchnic vascular resistance secondary to vasodilators such as nitric oxide leading to angiogenesis in the mesentery, which in turn causes increase in the blood flow, thus leading to further increase in the portal hypertension. Portal vein blood flow can fluctuate with blood transfusion or infusion of colloids, which results in an increase in blood volume and portal flow that in turn exaggerates portal hypertension (Figure 40-2). Portal hypertension can be associated with chronic congestive enlargement of the spleen that might be associated hypersplenism with red blood cells, destruction, a condition known as Banit's syndrome. In such cases, splenic embolization or splenectomy will correct the cause of portal hypertension.

As resistance increase in the liver, blood flow in the portal vein becomes slower and less with the increase in portal pressure and higher resistance in the liver. The higher the resistance in the liver, the slower the flow in the portal vein, ranging from 0 to 700 mL/minute. Normally, the direction of blood flow in the portal vein is toward the liver, described as hepatopedal, but increased liver resistance can result in reversal in the direction of flow, described as hepatofugal. Slow blood flow in the portal vein might contribute to portal vein thrombosis which occurs in 16% of patients with advanced liver disease. Portal vein thrombosis further complicates management of portal hypertension by making shunt creation difficult or not possible. Furthermore, once the pressure in the portal vein reaches a high level (30 mmHg), the high resistance diverts blood to collateral circulation. The elevated pressure in the portal venous system will stimulate the development of portosystemic collaterals (Figure 40-3). The most important pathological routes are networks through the coronary and short gastric veins to the azygos vein due to the development of gastroesophageal varicosities. Other sites include recanalization of the umbilical vein (portal vein to left portal vein to umbilical vein to epigastric

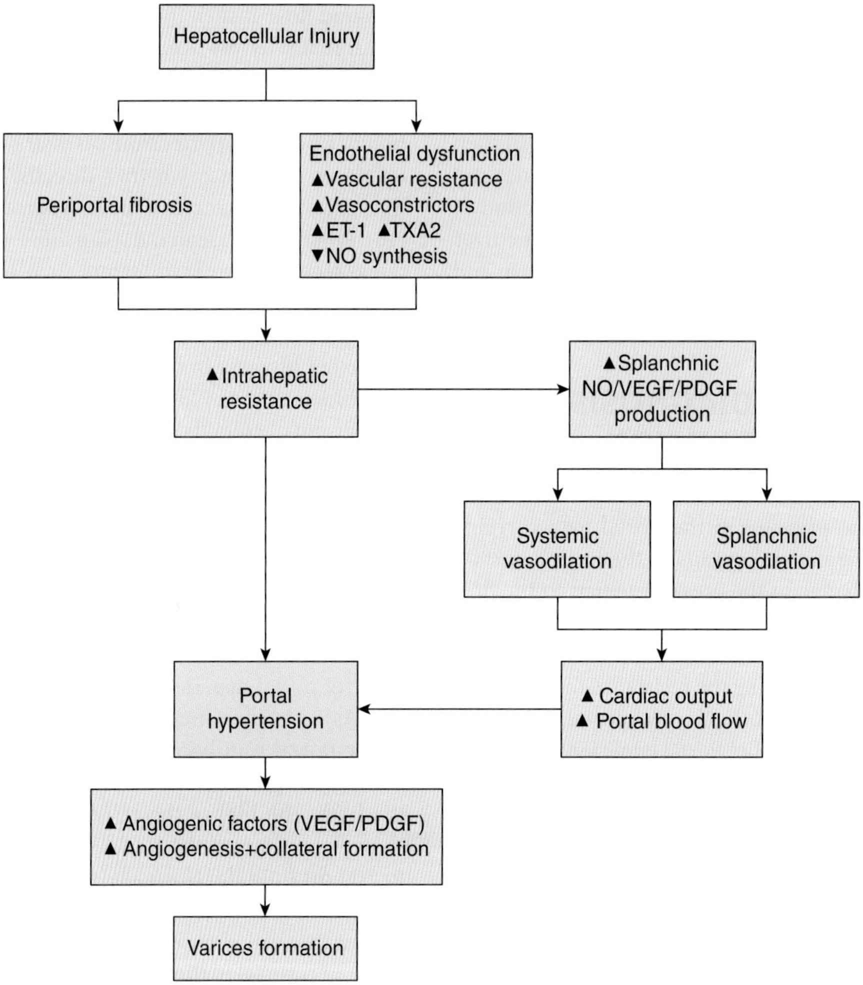

FIGURE 40-2 Pathogenesis of portal hypertension.

veins to caput medusae). Other collaterals include portal vein to superior mesenteric vein and inferior mesenteric vein to retroperitoneal venous collaterals to hemorrhoidal veins to Hemorrhoids.

Sinistral or left-sided portal hypertension refers to portal hypertension secondary to isolated splenic vein thrombosis. This results in gastrosplenic venous hypertension with normal superior mesenteric and portal vein pressures. Left gastroepiploic vein becomes major collateral and only gastric, not esophageal, varicosities develop. Thrombosis of splenic vein with normal flow in the splenic artery causes an increase in the short gastric vein pressure which can cause gastric varices with bleeding causing higher mortality than gastroesophageal variceal bleeding. The traditional treatment of this condition is splenectomy or interruption of the short gastric veins without splenectomy. Splenic artery embolization has been suggested as another treatment method.[8]

Pancreatitis is one of the common causes of splenic vein thrombosis occurring in 14% of patients with risk of GI bleeding of about 12%.[9]

Elevated portal pressure can result from increased hepatic resistance such in cases of fibrosis of the liver and due to active vasoconstriction by norepinephrine, endothelin, and other vasoconstrictors. Conditions

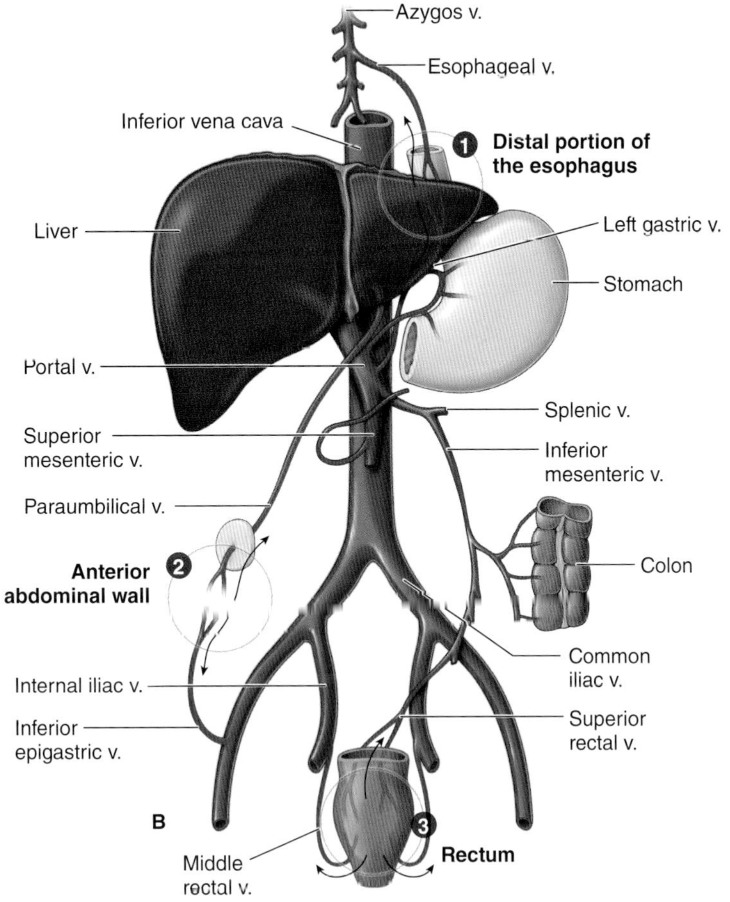

FIGURE 40-3 Collateral blood flow in patients with high portal pressure. (Reproduced with permission from Morton D, Foreman KB, Albertine KH. *The Big Picture: Gross Anatomy*. New York, NY: McGraw Hill; 2019.)

that are associated with increased resistance to flow can be divided into three types based on the area of increased resistance: Prehepatic (portal vein obstruction), hepatic such as in cirrhosis and post hepatic like in Budd-Chiari syndrome (hepatic vein thrombosis), and cardiac causes. These constitute most of the portal hypertension causes (Table 40-1). Based on the location of obstruction, portal hypertension is classified into presinusoidal, sinusoidal, and postsinusoidal. Furthermore, postsinusoidal and presinusoidal conditions are subclassified to intrahepatic and extrahepatic. Increased resistance to flow can occur in cases of sclerosis, fibrosis, or centrilobular swelling in the absence of real fibrosis such as in cases of alcoholic hepatitis and fatty liver. In the absence of real fibrosis, these changes can be transient and might become normal with treatment such as in cases of alcoholic hepatitis and fatty liver.

EXTRAHEPATIC PRESINUSOIDAL OBSTRUCTION

This cause of portal hypertension is less common than other causes. It can occur in children due to infection source like in omphalitis or appendicitis and in adults because of low flow in the portal system secondary to high-resistance hepatic circulation from cirrhosis.

TABLE 40-1 Causes of Portal Hypertension

Increased Resistance to Flow	Increased Portal Blood Flow
Prehepatic (portal vein obstruction)	**Arterial-portal venous fistula**
Congenital atresia/stenosis	
Portal vein thrombosis	
Splenic vein thrombosis	
Extrinsic compression	
Hepatic	**Increased Splenic flow**
Cirrhosis (Portal: alcoholic, nutritional; postnecrotic; biliary; Wilson's disease; hemochromatosis)	Banti syndrome
	Splenomegaly (tropical, myeloid metaplasia)
Acute alcoholic liver disease	
Chronic active hepatitis	
Congenital hepatic fibrosis	
Idiopathic portal hypertension (hepatoportal sclerosis)	
Schistosomiasis	
Sarcoidoisis	
Posthepatic	
Budd-Chiari syndrome	
Veno-occlusive disease	
Cardiac disease (constrictive pericarditis, valvular heart disease, right heart failure)	

Reproduced with permission from Doherty G. *Current Diagnosis and Treatment: Surgery*, 15th ed. New York, NY: McGraw Hill, 2020.

INTRAHEPATIC PRESINUSOIDAL OBSTRUCTION

Portal hypertension can occur due to fibrosis and compression of the portal venules, with subsequent restriction of portal blood flow. Examples include Wilson disease, congenital hepatic fibrosis, sarcoidosis, primary biliary sclerosis with schistosomiasis being the most common in developing countries in which cases the deposition of parasite ova in portal venules can lead to inflammatory reaction, fibrosis, and cirrhosis. In such patients, chronic hepatitis might develop leading to increased resistance in the liver. In these cases, hepatic function is usually preserved in the early stages of the disease. Hemodynamic changes are similar to extrahepatic portal vein obstruction: low hepatic wedge pressure and elevated portal venous pressure.

INTRAHEPATIC SINUSOIDAL AND POSTSINUSOIDAL OBSTRUCTION

Alcoholic hepatitis is the most common cause and is the 10th most common cause of death in the United States of America. Two mechanisms account for the portal hypertension in these patients. The first is due to mechanical obstruction secondary to cirrhosis in damaged liver. The second element is an increase in the splanchnic perfusion, and the genesis of multiple arteriovenous shunts. One-third of the portal blood flow may bypass functional hepatocytes.[3] This will cause high cardiac output and diminished systemic resistance.[4]

The resulting hemodynamic change is consistent with elevated hepatic wedge pressure along with elevated portal vein pressure. Patients have poor hepatic reserve. Selection and timing of the interventions are important aspects in the management of such cases.

EXTRAHEPATIC POSTSINUSOIDAL OBSTRUCTION

Hepatic vein thrombosis results in obstruction to blood flow out of the liver. It results in hepatomegaly and ascites. Thrombosis of the hepatic veins may result from membranous webs, trauma, pregnancy, oral contraceptive pills, and Budd-Chiari syndrome that will cause esophageal varicose, hepatic failure jaundice, massive ascites, and death.[10] Other clinical conditions such as inferior vena cava obstruction, tumors, right sided hear failure can cause similar clinical picture.

ARTERIOVENOUS FISTULAS

Arteriovenous fistulas (AV fistulas) can result from trauma, surgical procedures, or splenic fistula due to splenic artery aneurysms. Formation of fistulas increases blood flow in the portal circulation which can lead to fibrosis and obstruction in the presinusoidal spaces which exacerbates the portal hypertension.[2]

CLINICAL FINDINGS

Patients with chronic liver disease might give history of alcohol ingestions, viral hepatitis, and other hepatic toxic substance. The longer the duration of liver disease, the higher the chance patients will develop portal hypertension.

Signs of portal hypertension include esophageal varices, ascites, splenomegaly, and abdominal wall venous collaterals. Signs such as spider angiomas, palmar erythema, and encephalopathy reflect the presence of chronic liver disease but do not reflect the presence of portal hypertension. Bleeding might be the only sign of portal hypertension.

Bleeding might become complicated by alteration in the mental status, tachycardia, and hypotension, but none of those is pathognomonic of the presence of esophageal varices. Bleeding in patients with esophageal varices and signs of liver disease does not mean that the source of bleeding is from the varices. Many such patients develop complications related to alcoholic consumption such as gastritis and upper gastrointestinal ulcers that can cause bleeding. The presence of splenomegaly and ascites are considered the most specific signs for portal hypertension. The presence of hepatosplenomegaly and massive ascites should raise the suspicion of hepatic vein thrombosis.

VARICEAL FORMATION

In order for the portosystemic collaterals to form, a minimum gradient of 10 to 15 mmHg between the higher portal venous pressure and the lower systemic venous pressure is needed. The vascular resistance in the collateral system increases secondary to increase in flow through the collaterals. The pressure in the collaterals reaches a higher level than the normal portal pressure. This explains why those collaterals still do not normalize the elevated portal venous pressure. The left gastric vein arising from the portal vein and the short gastric veins arising from the splenic vein are the vessels most often affected.

Esophageal varices form after left gastric vein becomes dilated and act as a channel to provide drainage through the azygos vein back to the heart.[11] Those varices are encountered in roughly 50% of patients with cirrhosis at the time of diagnosis but reach to 90% with long-term follow-up. The larger the varices are, the higher the chance bleeding will occur. Over a 2-year period, rupture and bleeding occur in 7% of patients with small <5-mm varices and 30% with larger varices.[12]

Mortality after the first variceal bleed reaches 35%, while rebleeding in the first-year results in 60% mortality. Any additional bleed carries a mortality of 20%.[1,13]

An increase in pressure within the varices to 10 mmHg carries a high risk of bleeding which becomes higher when pressure increases above 12 mmHg. Therapy goal is to keep variceal pressure below 12 mmHg.[11] In addition to pressure, other factors that predict risk of bleeding are Child class of the patient and the presence of erosions on the varices (red-dot signs).[14] Once controlled, the greatest risk of rebleeding is highest within few days after first bleed. The risk reduces rapidly between that point and 6 weeks. Subsequently, the risk of rebleeding returns to the prebleeding rate.[5]

ENCEPHALOPATHY

Encephalopathy occurs in 30% to 40% of patients with decompensated liver disease and is associated with higher mortality.[15] It occurs due to shunting of blood from the dysfunctional hepatocytes in addition to increase in the ammonia and glutamine (derived from ammonia) resulting in increase in false neurotransmitters. The stages of encephalopathy start with mild personality alteration and occasionally with asterixis (stage 1), then drowsiness and mild confusion (Stage 2), obtundation (Stage 3), and lastly coma (Stage 4).[16]

Treatment of encephalopathy is achieved by reduction of ammonia. Lactulose and neomycin reduce ammonia uptake from the gut by altering the intestinal pH, reducing the number of intestinal bacteria, and reducing intestinal transit of protein. Other agents such as levodopa have been used, with mixed results, in improving encephalopathy.[17]

HEPATORENAL SYNDROME

A diagnosis of exclusion. It is believed to occur due to decreased renal perfusion due to ascites and cirrhosis. Clinically, it presents with oliguria, hyponatremia, and low urinary sodium output. It can occur rapidly (deterioration of renal function within 2 weeks) or takes a more chronic course. Rapid deterioration is associated with poor prognosis; 10% of the patient survive hospitalization.[18]

DIAGNOSIS AND EVALUATION OF PATIENTS WITH PORTAL HYPERTENSION

In addition to the presence of signs of chronic liver disease and esophageal varices, blood and chemical tests can help diagnose acute and chronic liver disease.

Both the presence of liver disease and degree of hepatic dysfunction can be evaluated by blood chemistry. Acute liver dysfunction evaluated by alanine aminotransferase (ALT), aspartate aminotransferase (AST), lactic dehydrogenase (LDH), and alkaline phosphate (ALK). Chronic hepatic dysfunction evaluated by prothrombin time and serum albumin. Both correlate with management outcome,[19] but ammonia levels do not correlate well with neurological abnormalities.[12] Decrease in plasma testosterone level has been reported to occur in 90% of men with cirrhosis. Low levels correlate with increased mortality.[20] Hematological evaluation reveals the presence of anemia and hypersplenism. Although splenomegaly is present in almost all portal hypertensive patients, hypersplenism may not develop until later in the course of the disease. The size of the spleen does not correlate with either the degree of hypersplenism or severity of portal hypertension.[21] Hypersplenism is defined by the degree of splenic sequestration, destruction of platelets, and white blood cells. Platelet count less than 50,000/mm^3 and WBC less than 2000/mm^3 support this diagnosis.

Several tests have been used to evaluate hepatic function prior to surgery. The Child-Pugh scoring classification was originally used to assess mortality related to portosystem shunts. This classification depends on the presence of ascites, encephalopathy, serum albumin, serum bilirubin, and prothrombin time (Table 40-2).

Since 2002, liver transplant programs in the United states have used the model for end-stage liver disease (MELD) scoring system to assess the severity of liver disease and to help allocate cadaveric livers for transplant candidates. MELD score is based on serum bilirubin, international normalized ratio (INR), serum creatinine, and dialysis. Later, blood sodium was added to the score (MELDS). MELDs scores may be between 4 and 60. Three months

TABLE 40-2 Child-Pugh Classification in Patients with Chronic Liver Disease

	1 point	2 points	3 points
Ascites	Absent	Slight to moderate	Tense, Refractory
Encephalopathy	None	Grade I–II	Grade III–IV
Serum albumin (g/dL)	>3.5	3.0–3.5	<3.0
Serum Bilirubin (mg/dL)	<2.0	2.0–3.0	>3.0
INR	<1.7	1.7–2.3	>2.3
Child-Pugh Classification	**Score:**		
A (low risk)	**5–6**		
B (moderate)	**7–9**		
C (high risk)	**10–15**		

mortality correlates with MELDS score and varies between almost 3% for MELDs score of 9 and 80% for MELDS score of 40 and above.[22] Both the Child-Pugh classification system and the MELDS scoring systems were originally used in conjunction with predicting mortality in liver failure patients, but latcly are used to predict mortality in patients before liver resection.

NONINVASIVE EVALUATION OF PORTAL HYPERTENSION

Although physical examination can predict the presence of chronic liver disease, it cannot predict the presence of portal hypertension. The two most significant findings are abdominal wall collateral circulation and spider nevi. However, their absence does exclude the presence of portal hypertension. If suspected, portal hypertension diagnosis can be confirmed by a number of tests but measuring the portal venous pressure directly or indirectly remains to the be the final confirmatory test for portal hypertension. Short of direct portal vein pressure measurement, the best method to evaluate the portal pressure, is by measuring hepatic venous pressure gradient (HVPG) which requires invasively catheterizing the hepatic vein and measuring both the hepatic vein pressure and the hepatic wedge venous pressure. The presence of esophageal varices by endoscopy confirms the presence of portal hypertension but cannot accurately predict the severity of the portal hypertension.

Duplex Ultrasound Imaging

Duplex ultrasonography (DU) is the first line for diagnosis and follow-up on patients with portal hypertension. It is noninvasive, low-cost, and can be repeated frequently as needed. Color flow imaging and duplex ultrasound is a great addition to evaluate portal hypertension patients. DU can be used to evaluate the patency of the portal vein as well as the direction of flow. It can be used postshunt placement to evaluate for shunt patency, and direction of flow in addition to the presence of ascites. Presence of collateral circulation and reversal of blood flow in the portal vein is 100% specific for clinically significant portal hypertension. Patients with compensated cirrhosis, specificity drops to about 80% while the sensitivity is only 40% to 70%. The absence of any ultrasound findings does not rule out portal hypertension.[23]

SERUM MARKERS

Platelet count measurement is the most common laboratory finding in portal hypertension. The lower the platelet count, the higher is the correlation with increased hepatic vein–portal vein pressure gradient which indirectly correlates with the presence of esophageal varices. The higher the platelet count, more than 150,000, the higher the chance of esophageal varices. The predictability of platelet count is improved when it is combined with other noninvasive tests. Noninvasive tests in general, including platelet count, are not accurate in patients with compensated cirrhosis for the presence of portal hypertension.[24,25]

Another serum marker that is not frequently used and can predict portal hypertension is the aspartate aminotransferase/platelet ratio index (APRI). It is a noninvasive test used in the diagnosis of fibrosis/cirrhosis in patients with hepatitis C. An APRI score of >1.09 correlated with predicting of HVPG > 12 with 68% diagnostic accuracy with a sensitivity of 66%, specificity of 73%, positive predicative value of 85%, and negative predicative value of 47%.[26]

Other noninvasive tests used include FibroTest which is calculated based on the results of six-parameter blood test. It is used to predict fibrosis, combining α2-macroglobulin, haptoglobin, gamma-glutamyl transferase (GGT), total bilirubin, alanine transaminase, and apolipoprotein A1. FibroTest is independent of ethnic background, gender, viral load, transaminases, or other comorbidities. Another test is platelet count to spleen diameter (PC/SD) ratio were suggested but did not add to accuracy of other tests

Using ultrasound elastography, liver stiffness, and spleen stiffness were evaluated for prediction of clinically significant portal hypertension. Both showed promising results but cannot be used clinically to plan management.[26]

Magnetic resonance elastography (MRE) has been recently used to evaluate both liver stiffness and spleen stiffness. Compared to ultrasound, MRE was proven to be more accurate in liver fibrosis in nonalcoholic fatty liver disease.[27] Their study was based on a literature review and included nine studies reporting about 232 patients. All patients had nonalcoholic fatty liver disease with correlation between MRE and liver biopsy. Based on their pooled analysis, the authors concluded that MRE has high diagnostic accuracy for detection of fibrosis in this group of patients independent of BMI and the degree of inflammation.

Although none of the noninvasive tests each on its own can predict clinically significant portal hypertension, the combination of such tests might improve the accuracy. Integrating liver stiffness (LS), spleen diameter and platelet count into a single ratio (LS X spleen diameter/platelet count) can provide better results than individual tests.[28]

ANGIOGRAPHY, COMPUTERIZED TOMOGRAPHY ANGIOGRAPHY (CTA), AND MAGNETIC RESONANCE ANGIOGRAPHY (MRA)

Angiography used to play a significant role in the diagnosis and management of portal hypertension. It was used to evaluate the anatomy and the severity of portal hypertension. The angiogram can be performed by selecting the superior mesenteric artery and the celiac artery and wait for the venous phase. It is important to evaluate the anatomy of the portal system and the proximity to the systemic venous system to decide on surgical shunts feasibility. Additionally, it is important to measure the hepatic venous wedge pressure, evaluate the anatomy which can demonstrate a coarse mottled parenchymal pattern in cirrhotic patients, and evaluate the direction of flow.[1] Currently, both CTA and MRA are used and replaced the diagnostic value of angiogram. They can also evaluate the liver parenchyma, nodularity of the liver tissue and identify thrombosis in the systemic and portal venous systems.

INVASIVE EVALUATION OF PORTAL HYPERTENSION

ENDOSCOPIC EXAM

Endoscopy should be performed whether the patient is bleeding or not. It helps identify the location of the varices as well as the size. In addition, it can be therapeutic in both acute and chronic bleeding conditions and is used to guide treatment. Every patient with history of portal hypertension should have endoscopy exam to identify presence of varices and presence of other associated conditions such as gastritis and peptic ulcer disease that are frequently encountered with portal hypertension. Part of the evaluation should include the gastric mucosa to evaluate for the presence of gastric varices.[29]

Endoscopy plays the primary role in evaluation and management of patient with portal hypertension. Changes within the gastrointestinal tract secondary to portal hypertension involve the entire gastrointestinal tract. Varices are present in about 50% of patients with cirrhosis, bleeding occurs in about 5% to 15% of patients depending on the size of the varices. In a study published in 1988, 321 patients with liver cirrhosis were prospectively followed for a period of 1 to 38 months. During this period, 26.5% of patients bled. Factors predicting bleeding included patients with worse Child-Pugh score, increased variceal size and the presence of red wale markings ("longitudinal dilated streaks resembling whip marks") on the varices. The authors devised a score index to predict bleeding within 1 year that helped them identify patients for prophylactic treatment.[30] In an attempt to rationalize the use of endoscopy as a diagnostic method for portal hypertension, the Baveno VI consensus reporting stated that in patients with liver stiffness transient elastography (TE) less than 10 kPa in the absence of other known clinical signs rules out compensated advanced chronic liver disease (cACLD) . These patients can be followed without endoscopy while those with TE more than 15 kPa highly suggestive of cACLD. The group of patients with TE between 10 and 15 kPa are suggestive of cACLD but needs more confirmatory tests. Because of false positive results associated with TE, measurement of TE should be performed on two occasions in different days in fasting conditions. In case of cACLD suspicion, methods to confirm diagnosis include liver biopsy, upper GI endoscopy showing varices, collagen proportionate area (CPA) measurement on histology, and hepatic venous pressure gradient (HVPG) measurement with a value of >5 mmHg that indicates sinusoidal hypertension. Clinically significant portal hypertension (CSPH) can be diagnosed if HVPG is 10 mmHg or more (gold standard method). Other methods to diagnose CSPH include imaging showing collateral circulation and TE > 20–25 kPa in at least two occasions. Patients with TE less than 20 kPa and platelet count more than 150,000 have low risk of having varices and thus can be followed without endoscopy with yearly measurements of TE and platelet counts. If either criterion changes, then patient can undergo screening endoscopy. Patients with compensated liver disease and no varices at screening endoscopy but ongoing liver injury such as alcohol consumption surveillance endoscopy to be performed at 2 years. Those with small varices and ongoing liver injury can be followed by yearly endoscopy. While compensated patients with no varices at screening and corrected cause of liver injury, endoscopic screening can be repeated at 3-year interval and at 2-year period if small varices found at screening endoscopy (Figure 40-4).[31]

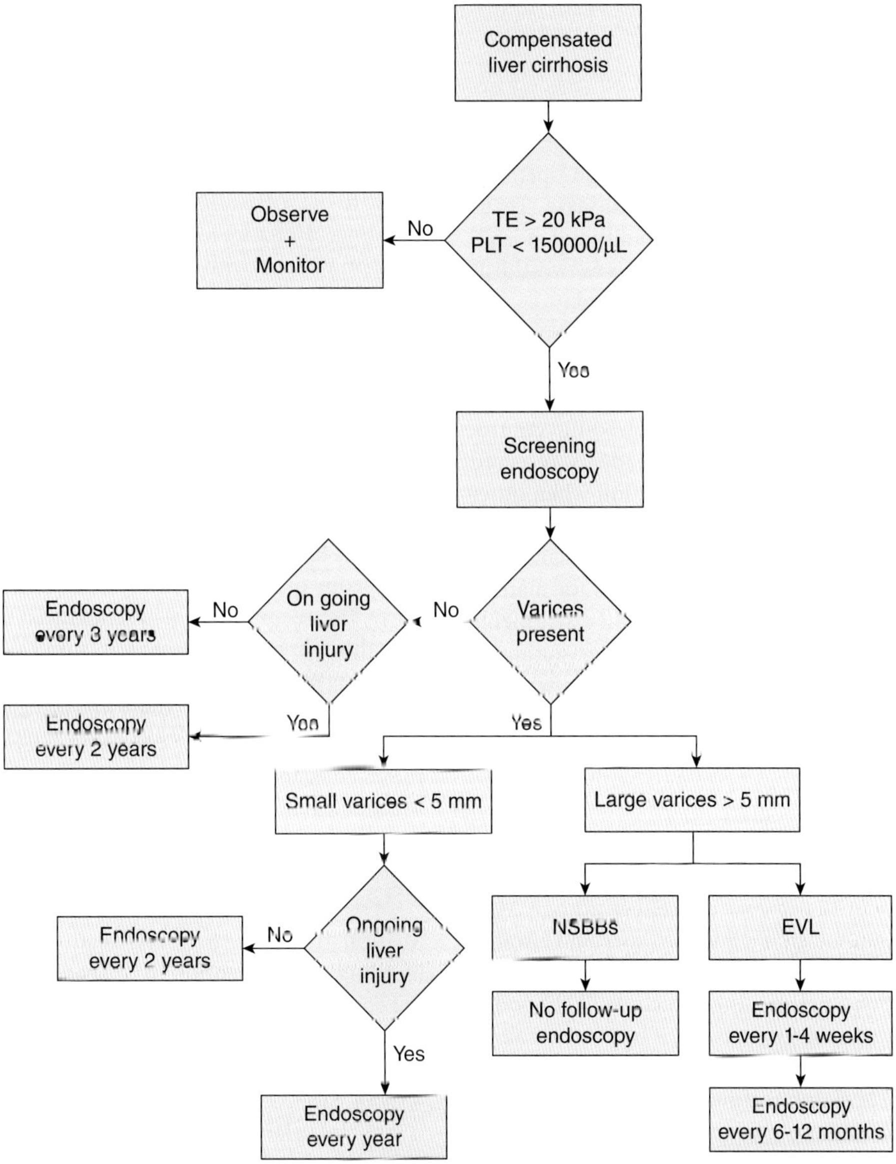

FIGURE 40-4 Endoscopy rationalization in patients with portal hypertension and esophageal varices.

LIVER BIOPSY

Liver biopsy is sometimes indicated to identify the reason for liver failure. It is also important in acute hepatitis setting for being the cause of hemorrhage to give the liver some time to heal before proceeding with any surgical intervention. Liver biopsy is essential to identify reversible causes for liver failure.

TREATMENT OF PORTAL HYPERTENSION AND ITS COMPLICATIONS

General Consideration in Treatment

Portal hypertension patients are often high-operative risk because of decompensated liver disease. Treatments associated with minimal morbidity and mortality should be considered for prophylaxis as two-thirds of the patients with varices will never bleed.

In patients with acute bleeding, nonoperative treatment is preferred. Endoscopic treatment with ligation or sclerosis has become the mainstem of nonoperative treatment with bleeding control achieved in 85%. Balloon tamponade is reserved for severe bleeding with exsanguination when other nonoperative treatments are not successful. TIPS is another management option that will be discussed in detail. It replaced open operative shunts for managing acute variceal bleeding when all other treatments fail. As a result, emergency surgical intervention in most centers is reserved for select patients who are not TIPS candidate.

Randomized studies also showed that somatostatin and long-acting octreotide with adjunct to endoscopic therapy is more effective in controlling bleeding than octreotide alone. Vasopressin can be used to diminish splanchnic blood flow. However, because of the adverse side effect nitroglycerin should be administered simultaneously and titrated to achieve blood pressure control.[5]

Prevention of rebleeding, which its likelihood is around 70% after the first episode, is by pharmacology treatment, chronic endoscopic treatment, TIPS, shunt operations, nonshunt treatment, and liver transplant.

Initial treatment consists of pharmacotherapy or chronic endoscopic treatment with portal decompression by means of TIPSS or operative shunts reserved for failure of first-line treatment. Hepatic transplant for end-stage liver disease patient.[5]

Pharmacotherapy treatment: nonselective beta-adrenergic blockade has shown significant decrease in the rebleeding rate and decrease mortality by a meta-analysis of controlled studies.[32] A combination therapy of beta-blocker and long-acting nitrate (e.g., isosorbide 5-mononitrate) has been shown to be more effective than variceal ligation.[33]

Treatment of Variceal Bleeding

Bleeding remains the most common form of complication in patients of portal hypertension contributing to about one-third of deaths in patient with cirrhosis. Close to half of deaths are secondary to uncontrolled bleeding. Hepatic reserves determine the risk of death in patients with cirrhosis and esophageal bleeding with higher complications and death in patients with Child class C cirrhosis. The risk of rebleeding is highest after the initial bleeding and gradually goes back to baseline by 6 weeks. Because the likelihood of a repeat bleeding is as high as 70%, the management goal should be directed to prevent rebleeding. To achieve this goal, there are three lines of treatment that can be used individually or in combination. The first line of treatment is pharmacotherapy with endoscopy that might need to be repeated more than once. The second line of treatment is TIPSS shunt. The third line of treatment is surgical procedures including shunt procedures (both selective and nonselective) and then finally liver transplant. Choosing the intervention line of treatments depends on the presence of the proper expertise and the urgency of the medical management (Figure 40-5).

PHARMACOTHERAPY

Medical treatment involves treating active variceal bleeding and prevention of rebleeding after a bleeding episode, in addition to primary prevention of the bleeding.

Bleeding usually stops spontaneously in around 40% of cases. The mechanism of bleeding cessation is due to splanchnic vasoconstriction from hypovolemia.[34] Medical therapy includes a number of medications such as vasoactive drugs to lower portal

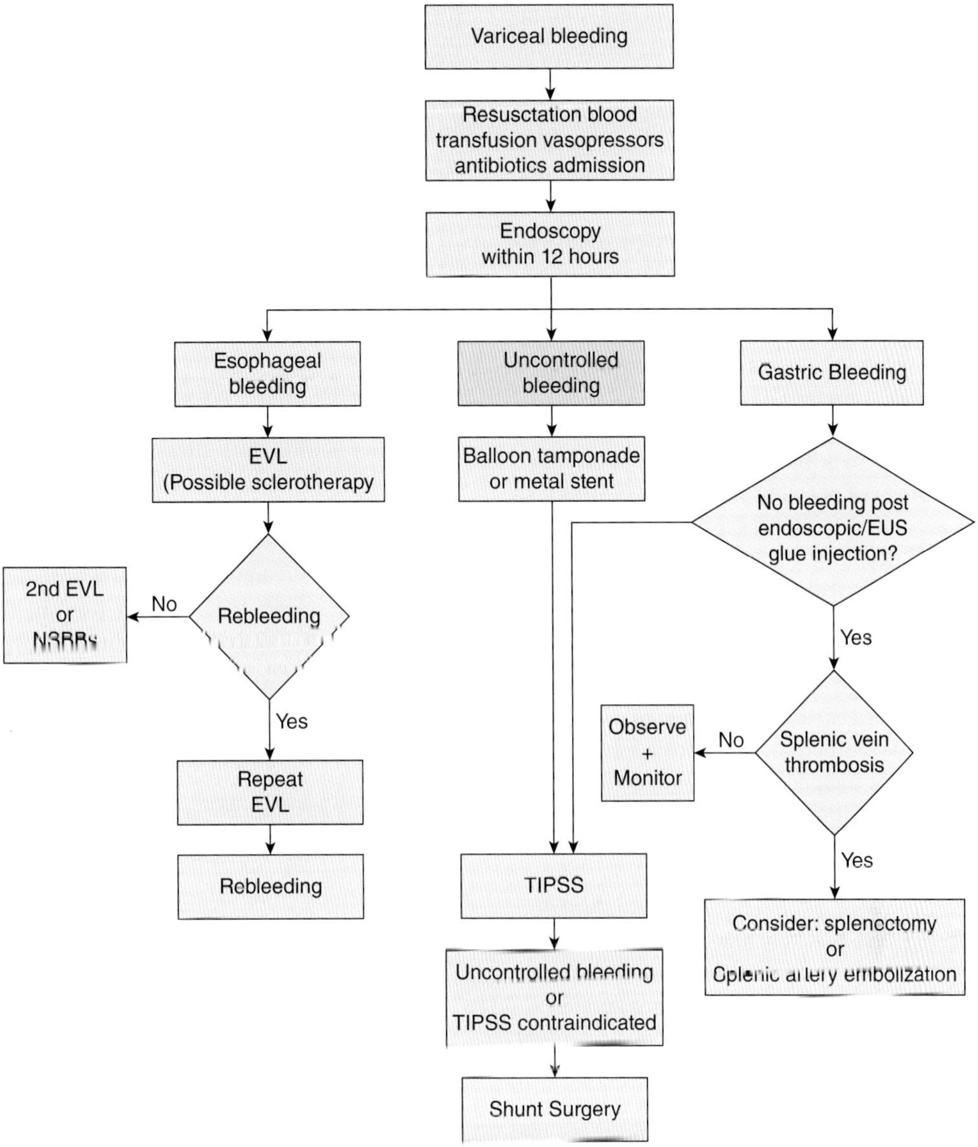

FIGURE 40-5 Management of patients with variceal bleeding.

pressure. They should start even before endoscopy and maintained for up to 5 days. Vasoactive drugs used include Terlipressin, somatostatin, and octreotide. Vasopressin used with nitroglycerine to reduce cardiac side effects and associated angina. Vasocactive drugs act by decreasing splanchnic blood flow that helps to stop the bleeding episodes in 80% of the cases.[34] Vasopressin was reported to decrease mortality, but it can affect cardiac perfusion for which adding sublingual nitroglycerin may help. Octreotide dose is a bolus of 50 μg and then a drip at the same rate 50 μg/h.[35]

Bacterial infection is not uncommon in cirrhotic patients. Up to 20% of cirrhosis patients have bacterial infection on admission and additional 50% develop infection during hospitalization. Infections that are common in cirrhotic patients include spontaneous bacterial peritonitis, spontaneous bacteremia, urinary tract infection and pneumonia. The most common bacterial infection is gram negative species. Both rebleeding rates and mortality are increased in patients with bacterial infections making antibiotic therapy mandatory in patients with variceal bleeding. In a meta-analysis, antibiotics therapy improved survival by an average of 9.1%.[36] Choice of antibiotics depends on local resistance patterns, but third-generation cephalosporins with gram negative coverage are favored. Ceftriaxone 1 g every 24 hours for a period of 7 days is preferred over the previously recommended fluroquinolones.[37]

Nonselective beta blockers (NSBBs) have been used in treatment of portal hypertension. NSBBs, use has been expanded from prevention of bleeding to prevention of decompensation of compensated cirrhosis.[38] In patients with high-risk varices and compensated cirrhosis, NSBB and endoscopic ligation are equally effective in the prevention of first bleed in patients with high-risk varices (medium to large varices, small varices with red wale marks, or in patients with decompensated cirrhosis Child-Pugh B/C).[39] NCBB use include propranolol, nadolol, and carvedilol. Patient should be monitored for low blood pressure and maintain systemic pressure higher than 90 mmHg.

In case of prevention after bleeding a combination of nonselective beta blockers like propranolol or carvidalol and endoscopic treatment with endoscopic band ligation or sclerotherapy will decrease rebleeding risk to less than 50%.[12] For *Primary prevention before any bleeding episode* also nonselective beta blockers and endoscopic band ligation or sclerotherapy repeated every 6 months that can decrease the risk of bleeding in 80% of patients.[39] This can also be offered to patients who are not candidates for TIPSS.

Patients who are treated by nonselective beta blockers showed lower incidence of rebleeding and a trend toward lower mortality.[40] In addition, NSBBs reduce the risk of portal hypertension complication such as ascites and encephalopathy but do not prevent development of varices or the progression of small varices to larger varices.[41] Adding long-acting nitrate reported to be more effective than beta blockers alone and variceal ligation.[42]

ENDOSCOPIC TREATMENT ESOPHAGEAL VARICEAL BLEEDING

In addition to being diagnostic, endoscopy is the first line of interventional management to control bleeding. Because of the poor results of shunting interest in endoscopic therapy was resurrected. In experienced hands, 80% to 90% of the esophageal varices are controlled by endoscopic treatment. Both band ligation and sclerotherapy can be used to control bleeding endoscopically. Generally, band ligation is more effective in controlling bleeding and has less complications and is considered the modality of choice in endoscopic therapy of variceal bleeding. The earlier endoscopic therapy is applied (within 12 hours), the better the results of intervention.

Endoscopic injection sclerotherapy is achieved by using sclerosants such as sodium morrhuate, ethanolamine, alcohol, and sodium tetradecyl sulphate. Other materials have been used in the past. The mechanism of action is to induce tissue necrosis and fibrosis in the area of the varices that will result in obliteration of such varices. It can be achieved with or without balloon compression. Complications of injection sclerotherapy include pain, ulcerations, and in some cases esophageal stricture which is rarely severe. Additionally, it has a relatively high rebleeding from 54% to 82%. Surveillance is required after the initial injection at intervals of 6 months to evaluate for the presence of recurrent varices.[43] Studies in 1980s showed endoscopic sclerotherapy was better than surgery in preventing esophageal bleeding but had higher incidence of recurrence rate, erosions, and ulcerations.[13,44] Because of that banding was introduced by Stiengmann and Goff from Colorado in 1989 being duplicated from hemorrhoidal disease with better results than sclerotherapy. This was modified by Saeed from the Veteran Affairs Hospital in Huston Texas who developed a device that can fire six bands without reloading each time which was the problem in the method described by Steingmann-Goff device.[14,15,45,46] Obliteration of the esophageal varices using this method is achieved by mechanical strangulation using rubber bands which has been the practice for a long time in hemorrhoid therapy. Ligated varices fall off few days after the procedure. Although ligation can be associated with ulcer formation, they are shallower than those encountered with sclerotherapy. Complications of ligation include esophageal laceration, perforation, transient dysphagia, esophageal stricture, retrosternal pain, bleeding, bacteremia, and transient exacerbation of portal hypertensive gastropathy.[47]

Comparison between sclerotherapy and ligation of esophageal varices generally shows ligation to have fewer treatment sessions, similar rate of variceal obliteration, fewer complications, rarely impaired esophageal motility, fewer rebleeding rates, higher recurrence, and possibly better survival.[48]

Other endoscopic interventions include clipping and tissue adhesives, the number of studies using both procedures are small, and difficult to compare with both sclerotherapy and ligation.

Compared to injection sclerotherapy, rebleeding, number of sessions, complications are lower after variceal ligation.[49] Based on the meta-analysis of 17 trials, it is recommended that patients with variceal bleeding be treated with a combination of beta blockers and endoscopic ligation as the first line of treatment. The combination reduced rebleeding rates at 1 and 2 years with lower mortality at 24 months.

After successful endoscopic therapy, patients still have a 50% chance of rebleeding which is highest in the first year, which decreases by about 15% each year. Early relapse occurs in about 20% within the first 24 hours.[50]

Chronic endoscopic therapy can be applied to reduce need for other interventions but should not be the only treatment in patients who live far away from medical centers, and those who are noncompliant. Endoscopic therapy fails in about one-third of patients due to the inability to control bleeding, multiple episodes of bleeding, and gastric varices bleeding. Patients with hypertensive gastropathy should be treated by other modalities such as TIPS, selective and nonselective shunt procedures as well as liver transplant.

TAMPONADE THERAPY

Balloon Temponade

In patients with esophageal varices that cannot be controlled by endoscopic treatment, temporary hemostatic measure using balloon or stents. Sengstaken-Blakemore (SB) tube is inserted through the nose or mouth. Initially, the gastric balloon is inflated using air, then confirmed to be in the stomach by X-ray followed by esophageal balloon inflation to control bleeding by tamponading the bleeding varices. Balloon tamponading reported to control bleeding in up to 80% of cases but is associated by a high rate of complications including esophageal ulceration, aspiration, and potentially esophageal perforation. Rebleeding occurs in 50% of cases after balloon deflation. SB should not be inflated for more than 24 hours to avoid complications.[51,52]

Stent Temponade

Self-expanding covered stents were reported to be a better choice as a bridging therapy in patients with uncontrolled esophageal bleeding. Stents have been used successfully in 80% to 96% to control esophageal bleeding. Stents can be left in place for up to 14 days with lower complications rates and transfusion requirements. Stent migration reported in 20%, and rebleeding in 16%. Mortality rates were comparable between balloon and stent tamponade. In a meta-analysis of five studies, technical success was reported in 96.7% and hemostasis achieved in 93.9% of cases. Rebleeding was achieved in 13.2% with a mortality of 34.5%.[53]

TRANSJUGULAR INTRAHEPATIC PORTOSYSTEMIC SHUNT

Transjugular intrahepatic portosystemic shunt (TIPS) was introduced by Joseph Rosch who was recruited by Dotter in Oregon as a fellow. He later became the Chief of Vascular and Radiology Interventions in Oregon and created the Dotter Institute with first successful TIPSS procedure done in 1988 in Germany. Subsequent experience showed improved bleeding, similar mortality but higher encephalopathy and higher failure that required multiple interventions, and higher cost compared to injections sclerotherapy.[12,54] Creating a shunt between the portal vein and the hepatic vein through a hepatic channel using the internal jugular vein approach is called TIPS (Figure 40-6). Traditional indications of TIPS include ascites refractory to medical therapy, esophageal bleeding not controlled by medical management, hepatic hydrothorax, and Budd-Chiari syndrome. Other nontraditional indications include early

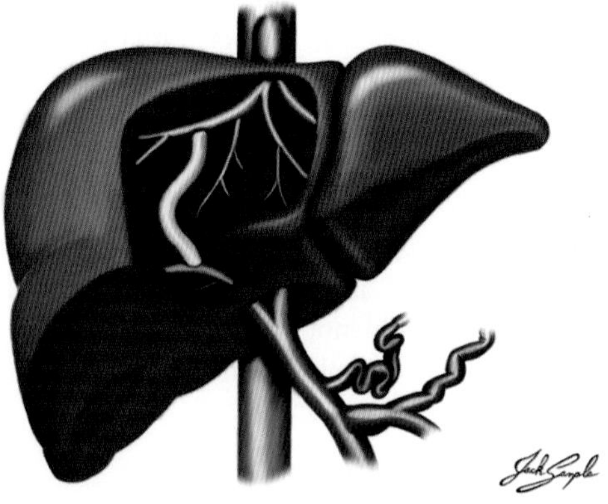

FIGURE 40-6 Transjugular transhepatic portosystemic shunt (TIPSS). (Reproduced with permission from Dr. Jack Sample.)

management of ascites, before nonhepatic abdominal surgery, recanalization of portal vein thrombosis, treatment of hepatopulmonary syndrome, and hepatorenal syndromes.[55]

Patients should be evaluated before placing TIPS by a hepatologist to determine the impact of the shunt on further treatment including liver transplantation. TIPS used to be taken as a temporary control of symptoms until transplant is available; in other words, a short-term solution but it can be a permanent solution in patient who are not expected to live a long time to avoid surgery and reduce bleeding. TIPS is in effect a side-to-side shunt, thus considered a good treatment to control ascites. MELDS score should be calculated before the shunt is placed which help determine survival after shunt placement. Patients with MELDS score more than 19 have decreased survival after TIPS. In such patients, if TIPS is necessary, it should be considered in conjunction with liver transplantation. Patients should be evaluated pre-TIPS by CT scan or MRI to determine the anatomy of the liver and the portal system. In case of compromised renal function, Doppler imaging can be used. Cardiac function should be evaluated by echocardiogram before TIPSS or during the procedure by right heart catheterization as significant congestive heart failure is an absolute contraindication to TIPS. If CHF is due to poor cardiac muscle function or severe pulmonary hypertension, the heart can decompensate after TIPSS procedure due to shifting of the blood to the systemic circulation. In case of fluid overload, CHF can be treated by diuresis before TIPSS. In patients with bacteremia or infection, TIPSS can be seeded by bacteria leading to TIPSSitis. Large or multiple cysts of the liver are considered as contraindication to TIPSS so as patients with biliary obstruction. Refractory hepatic encephalopathy, MELD >19, volume overload or significant valvular heart disease, centrally located liver mass are considered relative contraindication to TIPS. Patients with hepatic encephalopathy are at a higher risk of developing severe encephalopathy. About one-third of patients develop transient encephalopathy after TIPS, but 5% develop severe encephalopathy that require occlusion of the TIPS. Postprocedure, TIPS patients require follow-up by shunt ultrasound surveillance every 6 months. If any sign of stenosis or patient develop ascites, revision of the shunt is required.[55] Before 2001, all TIPS were performed using bare metal stents that were complicated by high rate of restenosis and failure until the covered stent was introduced to the TIPS procedure. Polytetraflurothylene-covered stents are associated with lower failure rates and less restenosis with higher survival. Further improvement was introduced in 2017 using the controlled expansion stents, Viatorr (W. L. Gore & Associates, Flagstaff, Ariz) that can be dilated to a fixed diameter of 8 mm and then dilated further to larger diameter at a later stage. Controlled expansion stents have lower readmissions due to ascites. The incidence of encephalopathy is lower when dilated to 8 mm instead of 10 mm.[56]

Because TIPS can be a time-consuming procedure with high radiation exposure, the ultrasound directed shunts were introduced. This is achieved by intravascular ultrasound which is believed to improve success rate, reduce contrast, time, and the amount of radiation.[57] Compared to endoscopic therapy, TIPSS has lower rebleeding rates (47% vs 19%) at the expense of higher encephalopathy after TIPSS (34%).

Surgical Therapy of Portal Hypertension

It was not until the first half of the twentieth century when management of complications of esophageal bleeding was described by Westfal, then Rowntree, and finally by Sengstaken and Blakemore.[6–8,58–60]

Splenectomy was one of the earliest procedures performed to reduce the portal flow. In 1903, the first successful shunt procedure was done by Vidal who performed a portacaval shunt in a patient who survived 4 months without bleeding.[61] Procedures were done on a low scale because of the results. G. Child collected 500 procedures done worldwide mostly coming from Allan Whipple splenic clinic in New York.[10,62] Then more cases were done between Whipple and Blalock at John Hopkins in Baltimore who was doing the portacaval shunt with everting mattress sutures with success that lead to the more enthusiasm on the shunt procedures.[11,63] After that more cases were done with better understanding of the clinical condition and the complication of shunting. Four prospective randomized studies showed no difference in mortality between medical therapy and surgical therapy with death secondary to liver failure after surgery and variceal bleeding after medical therapy.[12,54] Later other shunts described as more selective were introduced but failed to show superiority when it comes to liver failure compared to nonselective shunts with more complications related to thrombosis of the shunts even when using internal jugular vein as conduit for the shunt.[3,64] After that nonshunt procedures were evaluated with contradicting results such as the Sugiura operation with disconnection systemic and portal circulation that was done in Japan with success that was not reproduced in the Western world, possibly secondary to the differing etiology in liver cirrhosis between both experiences.[12,54] In spite of the multiple surgical procedures described for the treatment of portal hypertension and bleeding varices, none of them is considered to be the ideal procedure for all types of portal hypertension. Factors determining procedure choice include indication of intervention, potential complications such as encephalopathy, rebleeding, and hepatic failure. Shunt procedure basically works by shunting blood from the high-pressure portal system to the lower-pressure systemic veins. In effect part or all of the portal blood that contains hormones, nutrients, and cerebral toxins bypass the liver which contributes to the encephalopathy and accelerated liver failure associate with these shunting procedures. Depending on the proportion of the portal blood shunted, these shunts are classified into selective and nonselective. The selective shunts, in addition to decompressing the portal system, preserve part of the portal blood flow to the liver. They are expected to reduce the complications of nonselective shunting that deprive the liver from portal circulation.

Generally, surgical procedure in patients with portal hypertension can be divided into shunt and nonshunt procedures (Figure 40-7). While the shunt procedures are divided into selective and nonselective. Shunts are the most effective form of treatment to reduce bleeding in patients with portal hypertension. Nonshunt procedures such as esophagogastric devascularization and splenectomy. In a systemic review of Medline and Cochrane library databases comparing the effectiveness of surgical procedures in preventing bleeding and complications, the authors found that there was a higher rate of rebleeding (reported in 10 randomized trials of the review) in patients who underwent devascularization compared to shunting or combined shunting and devascularization with no difference between selective and nonselective shunting. On the other hand, encephalopathy (reported in 11 randomized trials of the review) was higher in shunting patients compared to devascularization patients with no difference between selective and nonselective shunts. As for ascites (reported in three randomized trials of the review), there was no difference between the devascularization and shunt groups. Late mortality after 10 years (reported in seven randomized trials) were the same between both groups, nor was there a different between selective and nonselective shunts.[65] Four prospective randomized studies showed no difference in mortality between medical therapy and surgical therapy with death secondary to liver failure after surgery and variceal bleeding after medical therapy.[12,54] Later other shunts, described as more selective, were introduced but failed to show superiority when it comes to liver failure compared to nonselective shunts with more complications related to thrombosis of the shunts even when using internal jugular vein as conduit for the shunt.[3,64] After that, nonshunt procedures were evaluated with contradicting results such as the Sugiura operation by disconnection of systemic and portal circulation. It was done in Japan with success that was not reproduced in the western world possibly secondary to the differing etiology in liver cirrhosis between both experiences.[12,54]

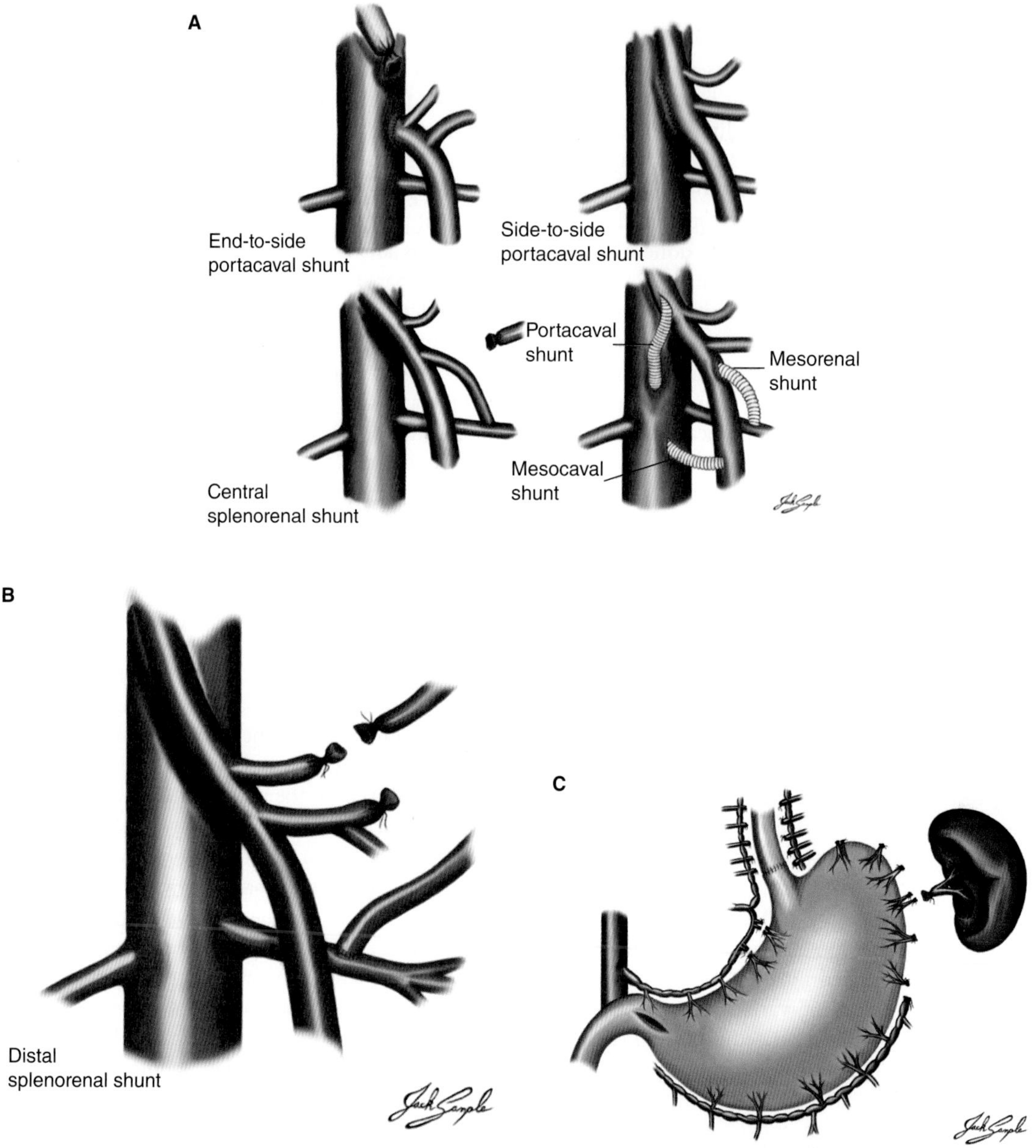

FIGURE 40-7 Shunts procedures for portal hypertension. (**A**) Nonselective shunts (end-to-side portacaval shunt, side-to-side portacaval shunt, interposition shunts (portacaval, mesocaval, mesorenal) and central splenorenal shunt. (**B**) Distal splenorenal shunt (Warren). (**C**) Sugiura devascularization procedure. (Reproduced with permission from Dr. Jack Sample.)

NONSELECTIVE SHUNTS

These shunts work by diverting all the portal blood flow away from the liver into the systemic venous circulation. They are used only when it is not possible to do a TIPSS procedure or failed TIPSS procedure. The nonselective shunts include the following.

End-to-Side Portacaval Shunt (ECK Fistula)

The end-to-side portacaval shunt is the only shunt that diverts all the portal blood to the system venous circulation by connecting the distal end of portal vein into the side of inferior vena cava, while the proximal end of the portal vein is suture closed. As expected, the main complication of the shunt is hepatic encephalopathy and accelerated liver failure due to complete diversion of portal blood away from the liver. Although the shunt was compared in randomized studies to medical therapy, those studies were based mostly on the cross over from failed medical therapy to shunting. In addition, alcoholic cirrhosis was overrepresented in those studies compared to other causes of portal hypertension. While medically treated patients suffered from rebleeding in about 70% of patients, 20% to 40% of shunted patients suffered from severe hepatic encephalopathy.[66]

Other nonselective shunts maintain the continuity of the portal vein but fully divert portal blood away from the liver. These shunts decompress both the intestine and the liver sinusoids, thus are used in patients with uncontrolled ascites in addition to patient with variceal bleeding. They have the same complications as end-to-side porta caval shunts such as hepatic encephalopathy and acceleration of liver failure.

Side-to-Side Portacaval Shunt

Interposition Shunts Shunts between different parts of the portal venous system and the systemic venous circulation can be achieved using interposition grafts. A number of such procedures have been described including portacaval (between the portal vein and the inferior vena cava) interposition graft, mesorenal (superior mesenteric vein to renal vein) interposition graft, and mesocaval (superior mesenteric vein to inferior vena cava) interposition graft. Like all other interposition grafts, thrombosis of the graft is the main complication of such procedures. Unlike conventional splenorenal shunts, the interposition grafts do not dilate with time and are not expected to fully divert the blood from the liver. They will allow decompression of the liver sinusoids which contributes to controlling ascites.

Conventional Spleno-Renal Shunt As the name indicates, this shunt consists of anastomosing the proximal part of the splenic vein to the renal vein. Additionally, splenectomy is performed. The main complication of this shunt is the thrombosis of the splenic vein which is relatively small in size and can be complicated by kinking of the vein. Hepatic encephalopathy is less common with this type of shunt because of the size of the shunt and the subsequent thrombosis that occurs in many patients leading to resumption of full hepatic blood flow. In those patients who shunt stay patent, the vein dilates with time leading to full diversion of blood flow from the liver. Splenectomy, as part of this procedure, might improve thrombocytopenia and leukopenia that occurs in patients with portal hypertension, although such findings are not that common or of clinical significance.

SELECTIVE SHUNTS

The complications related to nonselective shunts lead to attempts to avoid or minimize complications related to completely diverting portal blood away from the liver. In 1967, the distal splenorenal shunt (Warren) was introduced. It provides selective decompression through the short gastric vessels to the spleen, then to the splenic vein into left renal vein through an anastomosis between the splenic vein and the left renal vein. Interruption of the gastroepiploic vein, coronary vein and the umbilicus vein in addition to any other large collaterals will result in maintaining blood flow to the liver through the superior mesenteric vein to the portal vein.[67]

Because of the high flow to the liver and the interruption of many lymphatics and during the procedure, warren shunt might worsen ascites. Because of that, this procedure is contraindicated in patients with intractable ascites. Patients with splenectomy cannot be candidates for such procedure since the spleen the conduit for blood flows from short gastric veins to the splenic vein. Like the conventional splenorenal shunt, a small splenic vein or kinking of the vein can result in showed thrombosis, because of that small splenic vein, less than 7 mm, is considered a contraindication to this procedure. Collateralization of the high-pressure portal flow might result in decompression into the low-pressure shunt; thus, blood flow to the portal vein might be lost in about 50% of the population by the end of the first year. Incomplete separation between the mesenteric and the gastrosplenic venous circulations might contribute to the increased collateralization and loss of selectivity of the shunt. The procedure is technically demanding but certainly within the scope of vascular surgeons. The effectiveness of the distal splenorenal shunts in prevention of hepatic encephalopathy and preservation of the hepatic function is controversial based on the results of a number of controlled studies comparing distal splenorenal shunt and nonselective shunts. However, its effectiveness and preventing rebleeding is comparable to nonselective shunts. Additionally, the role of distal splenorenal shunt and nonalcoholic cirrhotic patients is not consistent in the literature. Distal splenorenal shunt was found to be more effective in preventing rebleeding when compared to chronic endoscopic therapy with similar incidence of hepatic encephalopathy between both types of therapy.

Partial shunting between the portal and the systemic venous systems can be achieved by performing a small vein to vein anastomosis or by using small shunts, 8 to 10 mm as interposition grafts. They effectively decompress the esophageal varices but at the same time preserve the hepatic portal perfusion at the expense of maintaining a degree of portal hypertension. The vein-to-vein anastomosis might dilate with time leading to loss of selectivity in shunting, while the small prosthetic grafts might thrombose with time leading to worsening of portal hypertension and rebleeding.

NONSHUNTING PROCEDURES

Nonshunting procedures include splenectomy and devascularization. Nonshunting procedure maintains portal circulation and portal perfusion to the liver with low incidence of postoperative encephalopathy, liver failure, and longer survival.[68] Sugiura procedure (Figure 40-7C) is a nonshunting procedure for esophagogastric bleeding that was first described in 1973[69] with later modification.[70] In this procedure splenectomy, gastric and esophageal devascularization with esophageal transection using a mechanical stapler via a short gastrotomy. In some cases, highly selective vagotomy is added to the procedure (Figure 40-7C). The Sugiura procedure was originally based on dividing the esophageal and gastric venous plexus from the portal collaterals with preservation of the esophageal collateral system azygous system. A radical devascularization from the left gastric vein to the pulmonary vein could be achieved by a two-step procedure starting with a thoracotomy, then few weeks later by a laparotomy. The complexity of the original procedure and the lack of reproducibility of the Sugiura results lead to modification of the procedure. A one-step transabdominal procedure was described with initial splenectomy followed by devascularization of the upper two-thirds of the lesser curvature and major gastric curvature including the distal 4 to 6 cm of the esophagus via diaphragmatic hiatus. After that an end-to-end anastomosis using stapling device inserted via a small incision in the stomach through the esophagogastric junction to about 6 cm from the junction. Adding the transection part reduces rebleeding but increases stenosis at the junction. Because of the vagotomy part of the procedure, a pyloroplasty drainage procedure is needed. In a review of 22 studies until 2001 with a total patients more than 5000, the incidence of stenosis was 17%, rebleeding 14%, leak 9%, encephalopathy 4% with higher complication in Child class B and C and emergency procedures.[71]

LIVER TRANSPLANTATION

Liver transplantation remains the only therapy to address portal hypertension and cirrhosis; at the same time, liver transplantation is to be considered in patients with end-stage hepatic failure irrespective of the presence of variceal bleeding. It is not a treatment for variceal bleeding. It provides decompression of the portal system and relieves hepatic dysfunction that contributed to portal hypertension. Patients with preserved liver functions but complain of bleeding from esophageal varices such as in patients with schistosomiasis are not considered candidates for liver transplantation. Additionally, patients who are noncompliant with therapy or alcohol consumption are not good candidates for liver transplantation. Patient with early cirrhosis and compensated hepatic function on the reserve such as Child class A and B+ are not considered candidates for liver transplantation. While those patients with advanced liver disease, Child class B and C should be initially treated with pharmacotherapy and TIPS shunts while being evaluated for liver transplantation.

Surgery in Patients with Portal Hypertension

Generally, the risks of surgery in patients with portal hypertension are higher for the same procedure than those without portal hypertension especially those related to fibrosis and cirrhosis of the liver. Because of the presence of hepatic dysfunction metabolism by cytochrome P450 enzymes, biliary excretion, and decrease in plasma binding approach, the metabolism of a number of medications is altered leading to prolong duration of action including anesthesia medications. Opioids such as morphine and oxycodone in addition to certain benzodiazepines such as diazepam and midazolam can cause depressed central nervous system function in patients with hepatic dysfunction. Fentanyl, oxazepam, and temazepam seem not to be much affected in patients with liver cirrhosis. Certain medications such as neuromuscular blocking agents and volatile anesthesia agents reduce blood flow to the liver by up to 36% during the first 30 minutes of the procedure but improves later. Because of that, certain medications such as halothane and enflurane can cause severe hepatitis. While other agents such as isoflurane, sevoflurane, and desflurane have minimal effect and thus preferred as anesthesia agents. Propofol is a safe agent in spite of being metabolized in the liver. Regional anesthesia using spinal or epidural can be complicated by bleeding in patients with liver cirrhosis. Reduction in blood flow to the liver can result from traction on the abdominal viscera, pneumoperitoneum, or positive pressure ventilation which can worsen hepatitis by decreasing blood flow. All those changes in liver function are transient with minimal clinical consequences.[72]

Patients with acute liver failure, acute viral hepatitis, acute alcoholic hepatitis, fulminant liver failure are at increased risk of complications and mortality after elective surgery. In most cases of acute hepatitis, the condition is transient, it is recommended that elective surgery should be be postponed for at least 3 months.[73]

Prediction of mortality and complications in patients with liver cirrhosis and portal hypertension can be based on a number of criteria such as presence of encephalopathy, bilirubin level, albumin level, and international normalized ratio. These represent the basis for Child-Turcotte-Pugh classification which divided risk into three groups: A, B, and C, with C being the worst mortality after elective surgery.[74,75] Another scoring system that is being used for prediction of postoperative mortality is MELD score, which is based on serum bilirubin, INR, creatinine, and sodium that was added later.[76] A 3-month mortality with MELD score of more 40 is 71.3% compared to 1.9% in patients with MELD score of less than 9.

Generally, patients with portal hypertension have higher mortality and complications after nonhepatic surgical procedures compared to those without portal hypertension. Even patients with low MELD score (less than 15) suffered twice mortality rates compared to those with normal liver functions.[77] Patients with liver cirrhosis who are Child class A or MELD score less than 8 can undergo elective surgery, while those with Child class B or MELD score 12 to 15 should proceed with elective surgery with monitoring or choose an alternative treatment to surgery. Patients with a Child score C or MELD score more than 15 should be considered for a liver transplant evaluation or alternatives to surgery, if possible. During surgery, all measures should be taken to avoid hypotension in order to minimize worsening of liver failure.

Emergency procedures carry higher mortality in patients with portal hypertension (19%–57%) compared to elective procedures mortality (6%–18%).[78]

Preoperative ascites is a predictor of complications and mortality in patients with portal hypertension undergoing other surgical procedures. Increased complications might be attributed to the increased severity of portal hypertension. The presence of ascites increases wound complications such as dehiscence, infection, and fluid leakage. To decrease complications, a number of methods have been proposed to control ascites including repeated tapping and draining tubes such as drains. Both methods are associated with increase infection. Peritoneovenous shunting is another method of controlling ascites but is rarely used. TIPSS is the preferred method to control ascites around abdominal surgery. Its procedure was found to have less complications compared to peritoneovenous shunts with improved transplant-free survival after TIPS procedure. The timing between the TIPSS procedure and abdominal surgery is not well-defined.[78]

Postoperatively, certain measures should be taken to avoid complications of liver disease. These include parenteral nutrition, fluid maintenance using albumin, drain removal within 5 to 7 days to minimize chances of infection, diuresis in some cases (reported to worsen kidney function), avoid narcotics, benzodiazepines, and electrolyte imbalance.

REFERENCES

1. Gupta TK, Chen L, Groszmann RJ. Pathophysiology of portal hypertension. *Clin Liver Dis.* 1997;1(1):1-12.
2. Moore WS. *Moore's Vascular and Endovascular Surgery: A comprehensive Review.* 9th ed. Philadelphia, PA: Elsevier, 2018.
3. Shaldon S, Chianduss L, Guevara L. The estimation of hepatic blood flow and intrahepatic shunted blood flow by colloid, heat denatured serum albumin labeled with I^{131}. *J Clin Invest.* 1961;40:1346-1354.
4. Gordon M, DelGuerco L. Late effects of portal systemic shunting procedures on cardiorespiratory dynamics in man. *Ann Surg.* 1972;176:672-679.
5. Townsend C, Beauchamp E, Evers B, Mattox K. *Sabiston Textbook of Surgery.* 19th ed. St Louis, Jason Sicklick, Michael D'Angelica, Yuman Fong MO: Publisher; 2012.
6. Farghadani M, Momeni M, Mhadavi MM. Anatomical variations of celiac axis, superior mesenteric artery, and hepatic artery: evaluation with multidetector computed tomography angiography. *J Res Med Sci.* 2016;21: 129-133.
7. Turcotte S, Jarngin W. Liver and portal venous system. In: Doherty G, ed. *Current Diagnosis and Treatment, Surgery.* 14th ed. New York: McGraw Hill; 2015.
8. Kim HJ, Park E, Hur Y, et al. Splenic Artery Embolization for the Treatment of Gastric Variceal Bleeding Secondary to Splenic Vein Thrombosis Complicated by Necrotizing Pancreatitis: Report of a Case; Case reports in medicine, 2016, www.hindawi .com/journals/crim/2016/1585926/.
9. Butler JR, Eckert GJ, Zyromski NJ, Leonardi MJ, Lillemoe KD, Howard TJ. Natural history of pancreatitis-induced splenic vein thrombosis: a systematic review and meta-analysis of its incidence and rate of gastrointestinal bleeding. *HPB.* 2011;13(12):839-845.
10. Langer B, Stone R, Colapinto R. Clinical spectrum of the Budd-Chairi syndrome and its surgical management. *Ann J Surg.* 1975;129:137-145.
11. Berzigotti A, Escorsell A, Bosch J. Pathophysiology in varecial bleeding in cirrhosis. *Ann Gastroen.* 2016; 14(3):314-325.
12. Bloom S, Kemp W, Lubel J. Portal hypertension: pathophysiology, diagnosis and management. *Intern Med J.* 2015;45:16-26.
13. Nobuyuki T, Yoshitaka T, Tsutsumi M. Management of gastroesohpeal varices in cirrhotic pateints: current status and future directions. *Ann Hepatol.* 2016; 15(3):314-325.
14. Lebrec D, DeFleury P, Rueff B, et al. Portal hypertension, size of esophegeal varices and risk of gastroentistenal bleeding in alcoholic cirrhosis. *Gastroenterology.* 1980;79:1139-1144.
15. Ferro JM, Viana P, Santos P. management of neurologic manifestations in patients with liver disease. *Curr Treat Options Neurol.* 2016;18(8):37.
16. Schenker S, Breen K, Hoyumpa A. Hepatic encephalopathy: current status. *Gastroenterology.* 1974;66:121-151.
17. Fischer JE, Funovics FJ, Falcao HA, Wesdorp RI. L-Dopa in hepatic coma. *Ann Surg.* 1976;183:386-391.
18. Wadei HM, Mai MI, Alisan N, Gonwa TA. Hepatorenal syndrome: patholophysiology and management. *Clinc J Ann Soc Nephrol.* 2006;1:1066-1079.
19. Cello J, Deveney K, Trunkey D. Factors influencing survival after therapeutic shunts. *Ann J Surg.* 1977;134: 146-152.
20. Siniclair M, Grossman M, Gow P, Angus PW. Testosterone in men with advanced liver disease. Abnormalites and implications. *J Gastroenterol Hepatol.* 2015;30:244-251.
21. Rikkers L. Operations for management of esophegeal variceal hemorrahge. *West J Med.* 1982;136:107-121.
22. Organ procurement and transplantation Network/ Scientific Registry of Transplant Recipients annual report. 2007.
23. Berzigotti A, Seijo S, Reverter E, Bosch J. Assessing portal hypertension in liver diseases. *Expert Rev Gastroenterol Hepatol.* 2013;7(02):141-155.

24. Sanyal AJ, Fontana RJ, Di Bisceglie AM, et al.The prevalence and risk factors associated with esophageal varices in subjects with hepatitis C and advanced fibrosis. *Gastrointest Endosc.* 2006;64(06):855-864.
25. Qamar AA, Grace ND, Groszmann RJ, et al. Platelet count is not a predictor of the presence or development of gastroesophageal varices cirrhosis. *Hepatology.* 2008;47(01):153-159.
26. Varma V, Sarin SK, Sharma P, Kumar A. Correlation of aspartate aminotransferase/platelet ratio index with hepatic venous pressure gradient in cirrhosis. *United European Gastroenterol J.* 2014;2(03):226-231.
27. Singh S, Venkatesh S K, Loomba R, et al. Magnetic resonance elastography for staging liver fibrosis in non-alcoholic fatty liver disease: a diagnostic accuracy systematic review and individual participant data pooled analysis. *Eur Radiol.* 2016;26(05):1431-1440.
28. Bohte AE, de Niet A, Jansen L, et al. Non-invasive evaluation of liver fibrosis: a comparison of ultrasound-based transient elastography and MR elastography in patients with viral hepatitis B and C. *Eur Radiol.* 2014;24:638-648.
29. De la Pena J, Brullet E, Sanchez-Hernandez E, et al. Variceal ligation plus Nadolol compared with ligation for prophylaxis of variceal rebleeding: A multicenter trial. *Hepatology.* 2005;41:572-578.
30. North Italian Endoscopic Club for the Study and Treatment of Esophageal Varices. Prediction of the first variceal hemorrhage in patients with cirrhosis of the liver and esophageal varices. A prospective multicenter study. *N Engl J Med.* 1988;319:983-989.
31. De Franchis R, Bravo VI Faculty. Expanding consensus in portal hypertension: report of the bravo VI consensus workshop: stratifiying risk and individualizing care for portal hypertension. *J Hepatol.* 2015;63:743-752.
32. Bernanrd B, Lebrec D, Mathurin P, et al. Beta-Adrenergic antagonist in the prevention of gastrointestinal rebleeding in pateints with cirrhosis: a meta-analysis. *Hepatology.* 1997;25:63-70.
33. Villanueva C, Minana J, Ortiz J, et al. Endoscopic ligation compared with combined treatment with nadolol and isosorbide mononitrate to prevent recurrent variceal bleeding. *N Engl J Med.* 2001;345:647-655.
34. Chen YL, Ghali P. Prevention and management of gastroesophageal varicose in cirrhosis patients. *Int Hepatol.* 2012:750150.
35. Chandler J. Vasopressin and splanchnic shunting. *Ann Surg.* 1982;195:543-553.
36. Bernard B, Grange JD, Khac EN, et al. Antibiotic prophylaxis for the prevention of bacterial infections in cirrhotic patients with gastrointestinal bleeding: ameta-analysis. *Hepatology.* 1999;29(6):1655-1661.
37. Boregowda U, Umapathy C, Halim N, et al. Update on the management of gastrointestinal varices. *W J Gatrointest Pharmacol Ther.* 2019;10(1):1-21.
38. Rodrigues S, Mendoza YP, Bosch J. Beta-blockers in cirrhosis: evidence-based indications and limitations. *JHEP Rep.* 2019;2(1):100063.
39. Svoboda P, Kantorova I, Kozumplik L, Marsova JA. Prospective randomized controlled trial of sclerotherapy vs ligation in the treatment of high-risk esophageal varices. *Surg Endosc.* 1999;13(6):580-584.
40. Bernard B, Lebrec D, Mathurin P, et al. Beta-adrenergic antagonists in the prevention of gastrointestinal rebleeding in patients with cirrhosis: a meta-analysis. *Hepatology.* 1997;25:63-70.
41. Abraldes JG, Tarantino I, Turnes J, Garcia-Pagan JC, Rodés J, Bosch J. Hemodynamic response to pharmacological treatment of portal hypertension and long-term prognosis of cirrhosis. *Hepatology.* 2003;37:902-908.
42. Villanueva C, Minana J, Ortiz J, et al. Endoscopic ligation compared with combined treatment with nadolol and isosorbide mononitrate to prevent recurrent variceal bleeding. *N Engl J Med.* 2001;345:647-655.
43. Lo G-H. The role of endoscopy and secondary prophylaxis of esophageal varices. *Clin Liver Dis.* 2010; 14:307-323.
44. Dzeletovic D, Baron TH. History of portal hypertension and endoscopic treatment of esophageal varices. *Gastrointest Endosc.* 2012;75:1244-1249.
45. Stiegmann GV, Goff JS, Sun JH, et al. Endoscopic variceal ligation: an alternative to sclerotherapy. *Gastrointest Endosc.* 1989;35:431-434.
46. Saeed ZA, Stiegmann GV, Ramirez FC, et al. Endoscopic variceal ligation is superior to ligation and sclerotherapy for esophageal varices: a multicenter prospective randomized trial. *Hepatology.* 1997;25:71-74.
47. Bolognesi M, Balducci G, Garcia Tsao, et al. Complications in the medical treatment of portal hypertension. In: de Franchis R, ed. *Portal Hypertension III. Proceedings of the third Baveno international consensus workshop on definitions, methodology and therapeutic strategies.* Oxford (UK): Blackwell Science; 2001:180-201.
48. Lo G-H. The role of endoscopy and secondary prophylaxis of esophageal varices. *Clin Liver Dis.* 2010; 14:307-323.
49. Funakoshi N, Segalas Largey F, Duny Y, et al. Benefit of combination beta-blocker and endoscopic treatment to prevent variceal rebleeding: a meta-analysis. *World J Gastroenterol.* 2010;16:5982-5992.

50. van Buuren HR, Rasch MC, Batenburg PL, et al. Endoscopic sclerotherapy compared with no specific treatment for the primary prevention of bleeding from esophageal varices. A randomized controlled multicentre trial. *BMC Gastroenterol.* 2003;3:22.
51. Panés J, Terés J, Bosch J, Rodés J. Efficacy of balloon tamponade in treatment of bleeding gastric and esophageal varices. Results in 151 consecutive episodes. *Dig Dis Sci.* 1988;33:454-459.
52. Terés J, Cecilia A, Bordas JM, Rimola A, Bru C, Rodés J. Esophageal tamponade for bleeding varices. Controlled trial between the sengstaken-blakemore tube and the linton-nachlas tube. *Gastroenterology.* 1978;75: 566-569.
53. Shao XD, Qi XS, Guo XZ. Esophageal stent for refractory variceal bleeding: a systemic review and meta-analysis. *Biomed Res Int.* 2016;2016:4054513.
54. Wright AS, Rikkers LF. Current management of portal hypertension. *J Gastrointest Surg.* 2005;9:992-1005.
55. Boike J, Flamm S. Transjugular intrahepatic portosystemic shunts, advances and new uses in patients with chronic liver disease. *Clin Liver Dis.* 2020;24:373-388.
56. Wang Q, He C, Yin Z, et al. Small-diameter covered stents do not affect efficacy but reduce hepatic encephalopathy in transjugular intrahepatic portosystemic shunt for the prevention of variceal rebleeding in cirrhosis. *J Hepatol.* 2017;66(1):S47-S48.
57. Petersen B. Intravascular ultrasound guided direct intrahepatic portacavalshunt:description of technique and technical refinements. *J Vasc Interv Radiol.* 2003; 14(1):21-32.
58. Westfal K. Uber eine Kompressotbehandlung der Blutungen aus Oesophagus varizen. *Deutch Med Wch.* 1930;56:1135-1139.
59. Rowntree LG, Zimmermann EF, Todd MH, et al. Intraoesophageal venous tamponage: its use in a case of variceal haemorrhage from the esophagus. *JAMA.* 1947;135:630-632.
60. Sengstaken RW, Blakemore AH. Balloon tamponage for the control of hemorrhage from esophageal varices. *Ann Surg.* 1950;131:781-788.
61. Vidal ME. Traitment chirurgical des ascites. *Press Med.* 1903;2:747.
62. Child G. Portal hypertension. *N Engl J Med.* 1955;252: 837-47.
63. Sandblom P. The history of portal hypertension. *Proc Roy Soc Med.* 1993;86:544-547.
64. Balducci G, Sterpetti AV, Ventura M. A short history of portal hypertension and of its management. *J Gastr Hepatol.* 2016;31(3):541-545.
65. Yin L, Liu H, Zhang Y, Rong W. The surgical treatment for portal hypertension: a systematic review and meta-analysis. *ISRN Gastroenterol.* 2013;2013:464053.
66. Boyer TD. Portal hypertension and its complications: bleeding esophageal varices, ascites, and spontaneous bacterial peritonitis. In: Zakim D, Boyer TD, eds. *Hepatology: A Textbook of Liver Disease.* Philadelphia, PA: WB Saunders; 1982:464-499.
67. Salam AA. Distal splenorenal shunts: hemodynamics of total versus selective shunting. In: Baker RJ, Fischer JE, eds. *Mastery of Surgery.* 4th ed. Philadelphia, PA: Lippincott Williams & Wilkins; 2001:1357-1366.
68. Ma YG, Li XS, Zhao J, Chen H, Wu MC. Modified sugiura procedure for the management of 160 cirrhotic patients with portal hypertension. *Hepatobiliary Pancrteat Dis Int.* 2004;3:399-401.
69. Sugiura M, Futgawa S. A new technique for treating esophageal varices. *J Thorac Cardiovasc Surg.* 1973;66: 677-685.
70. Ginsberg RJ, Waters PF, Zeldin RA, et al. A modified Sugiura procedure. *Ann Thorac Surg.* 1982;34:258-264.
71. Selzner M, Tuttle-Newhall JE, Dahm F, Suhocki P, Clavien P-A. Current indication of modified Sugiura procedure in the management of variceal bleeding. *J Am Coll Surg.* 2001;193:166-173.
72. Im GY, Lubezky N, Facciuto ME, Schiano TD. Surgery in patients with portal hypertension a preoperative checklist and strategies for attenuating risk. *Clin Liver Dis.* 2014;18:477-505.
73. Mikkelsen WP, Kern WH. The influence of acute hyaline necrosis on survival after emergency and elective portacaval shunt. *Major Probl Clin Surg.* 1974;14: 233-242.
74. Child CG, Turcotte JG. Surgery and portal hypertension. *Major Probl Clin Surg.* 1964;1:1-85.
75. Pugh RN, Murray-Lyon IM, Dawson JL, et al. Transection of the esophagus for bleeding esophageal varices. *Br J Surg.* 1973;60(8):646-649.
76. Wiesner R, Edwards E, Freeman R, et al. Model for end-stage liver disease (MELD) and allocation of donor livers. *Gastroenterology.* 2003;124(1):91-96.
77. Kadry Z, Schaefer EW, Shah RA, et al. Portal hypertension: an underestimated entity? *Ann Surg.* 2016;263(5): 986-991.
78. Wong M, Busuttil R. Surgery in patients with portal hypertension. *Clin Liver Dis.* 2019;23(4):755-780.

SELF-ASSESSMENT STUDY QUESTIONS AND ANSWERS

Questions

1. Which one of the following statements is correct?
   A. The portal vein provides 50% of the blood flow to the liver each minute and 80% of the oxygen.
   B. The portal vein provides approximately 75% of the blood flow to the liver each minute and up to 70% of oxygen.
   C. The portal vein provides approximately 90% of the blood flow to the liver each minute and up to 70% of oxygen.
   D. The portal vein provides approximately 75% of the blood flow to the liver and 25% oxygen.
2. In the pathophysiology of portal hypertension, the following is true:
   A. Increased portal blood flow explains most of the conditions of portal hypertension.
   B. Increased liver resistance is the only mechanism to explain portal hypertension.
   C. Increased blood flow to the liver contributes to sinusoidal sclerosis, which leads to an increase in liver resistance that causes portal hypertension.
   D. All causes of portal hypertension are related to increased liver resistance to portal flow by necrosis of hepatocytes.
3. In patients with portal hypertension increased resistance to flow can lead to:
   A. Reversal of blood flow in the portal vein, hepatopodal flow.
   B. Reversal of blood flow in the portal vein, hepatofugal blood flow.
   C. Blood flow in the portal vein does not get affected by portal hypertension.
   D. Blood flow in the portal vein increases portal hypertension.
4. The model for end-stage liver disease (MELD) scoring system is used to:
   A. Assess the severity of liver disease
   B. Help allocate cadaveric livers for transplant candidates
   C. Predict mortality and prognosis in surgical procedures in patients with liver disease
   D. Predict risk for bleeding from esophageal varices
5. Serum markers used in noninvasive diagnosis of portal hypertension include all of the following except:
   A. Platelet count
   B. Aspartate a minor transferase/platelet ratio index (APRI)
   C. FibroTest which is an ultrasound exam used to predict fibrosis
   D. Haptoglobin, gamma-glutamyl transferase, total bilirubin, alanine transaminase, and apolipoprotein A1.
6. Use of endoscopy can be rationalized in patients with portal hypertension based on the following except:
   A. Liver stiffness transient elastography
   B. Imaging to identity collateral flow
   C. Platelet count.
   D. Hemoglobin level
7. In patients with acute esophageal variceal bleeding, studies showed that:
   A. Endoscopic treatment with ligation or sclerosis can control bleeding in up to 50% of the cases.
   B. Somatostatin and long acting octreotide alone can control bleeding in up to 85% of the cases.
   C. Hepatic reserve determined the risk of death in patients with cirrhosis and esophageal bleeding.
   D. TIPSS is the best method to control acute esophageal variceal bleeding.

SELF-ASSESSMENT STUDY QUESTIONS AND ANSWERS

8. Comparison between sclerotherapy and ligation of esophageal varices shows:
  A. Sclerotherapy and ligation have similar rates of variceal obliteration and number of treatment sessions.
  B. Ligation has fewer complications, less esophageal motility impairment, and fewer rebleeding rates
  C. Better survival with sclerotherapy compared to ligation.
  D. Rebleeding is higher with ligation but survival is better.

9. The following is true about TIPSS shunt:
  A. Indications include bleeding in patients with heart failure.
  B. It is considered a side-to-side shunt.
  C. It is contraindicated in patients with massive ascites.
  D. Liver tumors are considered a contraindication for the shunt.

10. Shunt procedures for portal hypertension include the following except:
  A. End-to-side portacaval shunt is one of the nonselective shunts.
  B. Interposition shunts can be done using artificial grafts or veins.
  C. Sugiura procedure is a selective shunt that reduces the incidence of hepatic encephalopathy.
  D. Warren shunt refers to distal splenorenal shunt which is one of the selective shunts.

SELF-ASSESSMENT STUDY QUESTIONS AND ANSWERS

Answers

1. B.
2. C.
3. B.
4. D.
5. C.
6. D.
7. C.
8. B.
9. B.
10. C.

CHAPTER

41 Hemodialysis Access

Amin Mohamed Ahmed and Ayman Ahmed

OUTLINE

HISTORY AND GENERAL CONSIDERATIONS OF DIALYSIS THERAPY

PREOPERATIVE WORKUP OF PATIENTS

OVERVIEW OF COMMON PERMANENT DIALYSIS ACCESS APPROACHES

- **Autogenous Access**
  - Forearm Access
  - Upper Arm Access
- **Prosthetic Access**
  - Forearm Access
  - Upper Arm Access

PROCEDURE DETAILS

- **Autogenous Venous Constructs**
  - Direct Venous Anastomosis
  - Transposition Venous Anastomosis
  - Postoperative Follow-up
- **Prosthetic Arm Access**
  - Technique of Graft-based Dialysis Access Creation

OVERVIEW OF COMPLEX PERMANENT DIALYSIS ACCESS APPROACHES

- **Complex Autogenous Tissue Dialysis Access Creation**
  - Description of Vein Transposition Procedures
    - *Great saphenous vein transposition*
    - *Brachial vein transposition*
    - *Femoral vein transposition*
  - Description of Vein Translocation Procedures
- **Complex Prosthetic Dialysis Access Creation**
  - Looped Axillary Artery to Axillary Vein Graft
  - Necklace Graft
  - Brachial Artery to Jugular Vein Graft
  - Hemodialysis Reliable Outflow Vascular Access Device (HeRO Device)
  - Lower Extremities Prosthetic Dialysis Access

POSTOPERATIVE COMPLICATIONS

- **Steal Syndrome**
- **Banding**
  - Minimally Invasive Limited Ligation Endoluminal Assisted Revision (MILLER)
  - Distal Revascularization and Interval Ligation (DRIL)
  - Revision Using Distal Inflow (RUDI)
  - Proximal Arteriovenous Anastomosis (PAVA) Creation Procedure
  - Conclusion
- **Bleeding and Hematoma**
- **Aneurysm and Pseudoaneurysm**
- **Infection**
- **Neuropathy**
- **Venous Hypertension**
- **Cardiopulmonary Complications**
- **Graft Thrombosis and Failure**
  - Open Thrombectomy
  - Endovascular Thrombectomy
  - Hybrid Approach

FOLLOW-UP MONITORING OF ESTABLISHED DIALYSIS ACCESS

- **Physical Exam**

Inspection
Palpation
Auscultation
Imaging Studies
LONG-TERM OUTCOMES OF DIALYSIS ACCESS
INDEWELLING DIALYSIS CATHETERS
Technique for Insertion of Temporary Dialysis Access
Short-term Catheters
Long-term Catheters
Complex Long-term Indwelling Catheters
Complication of Catheter Insertion
Pneumothorax
Hemothorax
Air Embolism
Myocardial Rupture and Arrythmias
Central Stenosis
Thoracic Duct Injuries
Arterial Injury
Catheter-related Infections

HISTORY AND GENERAL CONSIDERATIONS OF DIALYSIS THERAPY

End-stage renal disease (ESRD) incidence and prevalence have been steadily increasing since 1980. Reports published by the United States Renal Data System (USRDS) demonstrate that after a plateau in numbers in 2011, the prevalence started increasing again in 2012. This increase has resulted in a total of 746,557 cases at the end of 2017, a significant increase from 56,402 cases recorded in 1980. This is in part due to the increased number of new patients diagnosed with ESRD. This has reached 124,500 new patients in 2017. The increased survival and longevity of life for patients with ESRD accounts for the steady increase in the prevalence of the disease. The modes of treatments for patients include hemodialysis, peritoneal dialysis and kidney transplant. Hemodialysis with approximately two-thirds of patients (67.2%) is the most common method to undergo renal replacement therapy. Naturally, the increased burden of chronic kidney disease (CKD) and ESRD and associated comorbid conditions result in increased Medicare expenditure. A total of $120 billion were spent in 2017 on patients with CKD and ESRD. With recently observed increased prevalence of obesity, diabetes, and survival of patients, it is expected that the impact of CKD and ESRD will only continue to rise.[1]

The development of hemodialysis access has been facilitated with Nobel prize winning work of Alexis Carrel on vascular anastomosis.[2] The first report of hemodialysis in humans dates to 1924, when Georg Haas obtained blood from the radial artery and returned into the cephalic vein using glass canulae. He later placed a cannula from the radial artery to an adjacent vein. However, the first successful hemodialysis attempt was in 1945. Femoral vessels were punctured both to withdraw and reinfuse blood. In 1949, significant progress in hemodialysis was made by Allwall by placing Teflon shunt to function as an arteriovenous fistula. The first patient survived for 11 years after shunt placement. In 1966, Cimino and Brescia are credited with being able to report construction of native arteriovenous fistula by connecting the radial artery to cephalic vein at the wrist. They achieved an impressive 12 out of 14 functioning fistulae with no complications.[3] Since the successful proof of principle, multiple techniques were trialed including saphenous venous transposition to forearm, and femoral artery to femoral vein silastic tube fistulae among other techniques. The inability to find suitable native vein led to the expansion and use of bovine, PTFE and Dacron grafts.

Temporary dialysis catheter became common in the 1980s and 1990s. The preferred route of access was the subclavian vein. This ran out of favor as 50% with indwelling venous catheters placed in that location developed some degree of venous stenosis, which jeopardizes future arteriovenous fistula or graft creation in the ipsilateral arm. The internal jugular vein became the preferred access site to minimize the consequence of venous stenosis. These indwelling catheters are associated with venous stenosis, infective endocarditis, and infections among other complications related to placement. With increased complications rate there was an increase in cost of patient care. The increased risk of sepsis and mortality with the use of temporary catheters can be reduced by early creation of fistulae.[4] The Fistula First Breakthrough initiative was born as a result of collaboration between many medical societies including Centers of Medicare and Medicaid Services (CMS).[5] The Fistula First Breakthrough goal is to increase the use of Arteriovenous fistula in more than 66% of patients on hemodialysis. In order to achieve that it requires collaboration between nephrologist, vascular surgeons, social workers, and multiple team members. Early referral is the cornerstone to reach this goal as dialysis access creation needs some time to heal and mature before it can be used. Patients anticipated to undergo dialysis soon are referred for evaluation and discussion of options for establishing access. Optimizing medical care of patients is of paramount importance to the subsequent placement of dialysis access.

PREOPERATIVE WORKUP OF PATIENTS

Patients with chronic kidney disease often suffer from other comorbid conditions. Collaboration with other health care providers is essential to optimize these conditions. Comprehensive evaluation of patients must be carried out.

A detailed history should be obtained from patients. Particular emphasis on history of upper extremity trauma, previous indwelling catheter, and device placements (e.g., pacemaker, ICD), as well as details on previous attempts of establishing dialysis access. The dominant extremity is identified, as well as the functional status and expectations of patients. Detailed history of other comorbid conditions and their interplay with dialysis access formation is evaluated. Patients are counselled that diabetes mellitus, peripheral vascular disease, and current medication are known to impact the success rate and longevity of dialysis access.

General physical examination is done with evaluation of the cardiopulmonary symptoms, examination of extremities for previous surgical scars, and prominent collateral veins. This physical examination must include a detailed assessment of the arterial and venous systems. Arterial pulses are evaluated for strength, symmetry, and any evidence of atherosclerosis. The Allen test is done to determine the integrity of the palm arch specially before creating distal arteriovenous fistula involving the radial or ulnar artery. The hand is made into a fist, the radial and ulnar artery are compressed, one artery is released, and the hand is relaxed and monitored for perfusion. This is repeated with release of the other artery. Any abnormality of the arterial or venous system detected on physical exam should be evaluated thoroughly with ultrasound (US), pulse volume recordings, angiography, and venography. If a correctable pathology is found, it is corrected prior to establishing dialysis access. Peripheral IV access and blood draws are discouraged and minimized to preserve the superficial veins. Native vein sizes are evaluated with vein mapping preoperatively. Adequate veins for autologous arteriovenous fistula have a diameter of 2 to 3 mm.[6–8] Confirmation of these measurements and distensibility of veins is often done by the duplex US in the operating room.

OVERVIEW OF COMMON PERMANENT DIALYSIS ACCESS APPROACHES

There are different configurations for constructing dialysis access. The goal of these procedure is to establish a conduit that is accessible and can maintain adequate flows to perform dialysis. The preoperative planning is of utmost importance for successful creation of those conduits. Many factors interplay;

however, the principles of location and technique should be widely applied. These principles include the following:

1. Upper extremity is preferred to lower extremity due to high risk of infection with lower extremity access.
2. The nondominant arm is considered first. However, if the nondominant arm does not have adequate veins, there should be no hesitation in considering the dominant arm to create autogenous AV fistula
3. Dialysis access should be placed as far distally on the extremity as possible. This perseveres the proximal sites for future and salvage use.
4. Autogenous AV access is preferred to graft, as autogenous AV access has better long-term patency and reduced risk of complication.

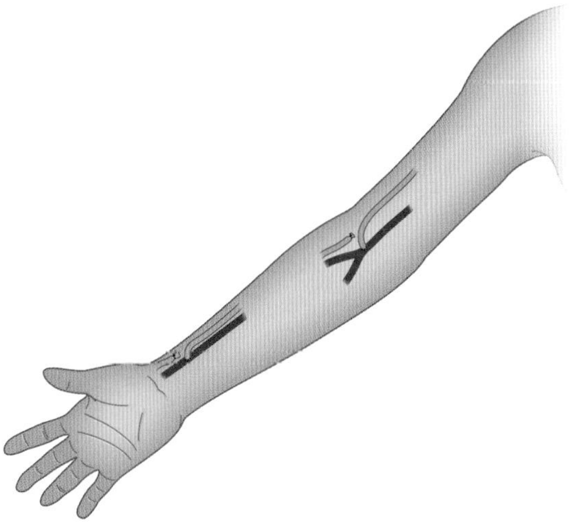

FIGURE 41-1 **Autogenous radiocephalic and brachiocephalic fistula.**

AUTOGENOUS ACCESS

Forearm Access

This is the preferred initial site for constructing dialysis access. The arterial inflow can be from radial, ulnar, or brachial artery. The cephalic vein is used for outflow. The exact location of the fistula is largely determined by the cephalic vein diameter at different levels. Adhering to the principles mentioned earlier, the most distal location is preferred for initial placement. Initial consideration is anastomosing the cephalic vein to radial artery at the anatomic snuff box. This is followed by radiocephalic fistula at the wrist. The radial artery lies in close proximity to cephalic vein and requires minimal mobilization and dissection. Cephalic vein transposition fistula can be done as well. The basilic vein can be used if the cephalic vein is inadequate. If radial artery is not suitable for use, the ulnar and brachial arteries can be used instead (Figure 41-1).

Upper Arm Access

Similar to forearm, the cephalic vein is preferred for use due to anatomic considerations. Again, dialysis access is placed as further distal in the arm as possible. Brachiocephalic fistula is used. If the vein is too far, or there is excess adipose tissue, cephalic vein transposition can be performed to facilitate direct autogenous arteriovenous construction. If cephalic vein is felt to be inadequate to provide outflow, the basilic vein can be used instead. This will invariably require venous transposition due to its deep and distant location in the arm, which can be done as a single stage or two separate stages as mentioned later in this chapter (Figure 41-2).

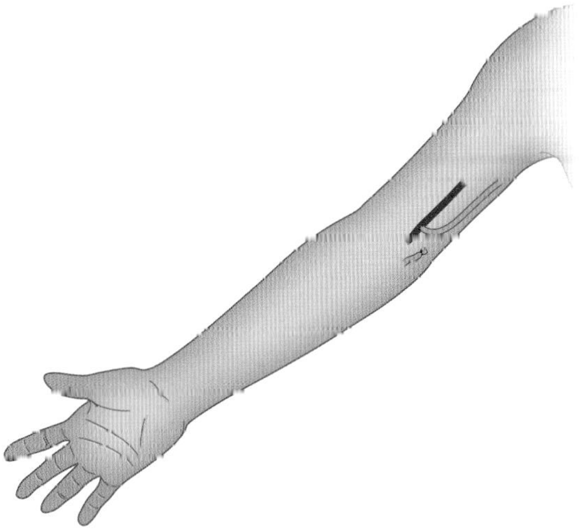

FIGURE 41-2 **Autogenous brachiobasilic fistula.**

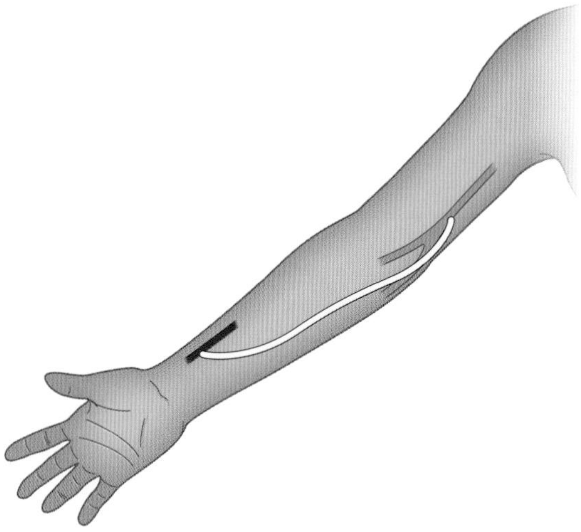

FIGURE 41-3 **Straight forearm AV graft.**

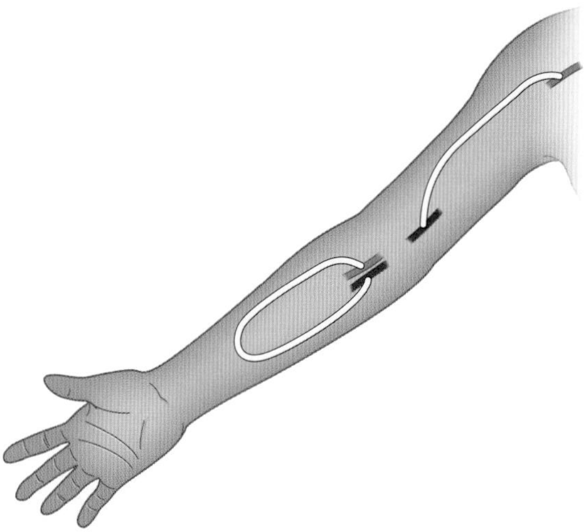

FIGURE 41-4 **Looped forearm graft and straight upper arm graft.**

PROSTHETIC ACCESS

Forearm Access

The use of prosthetic devices is indicated when there are no suitable veins for autogenous access. Arterial inflow can be from radial and brachial arteries. Straight graft connecting the distal radial artery to the ante-cubital forearm cephalic vein is considered first. If it is not feasible, a looped proximal radial or brachial artery to ante-cubital vein is an alternative technique (Figure 41-3).

Upper Arm Access

Prosthetic grafts are reserved for use in the absence of a usable autogenous vein. Brachial artery is used as the inflow. The outflow of the graft can be brachial or axillary vein (Figure 41-4).

PROCEDURE DETAILS

Surgery for dialysis access is performed as an outpatient procedure. It can be done under local anesthesia or regional block, which can be done in designated procedure room prior to moving the patient to the operating room. Occasionally, general anesthesia is utilized. If the side is determined preoperatively, it should be marked in preop area. In situations where the side is yet to be determined, US of the upper extremities is done after induction of anesthesia. This helps as veins often distend after administration of anesthetic which helps determine suitability for use. Once that is complete, the patient is positioned in the supine position. The operative upper extremity is extended and placed on an arm board. The upper extremity is prepped all the way to the axilla.

AUTOGENOUS VENOUS CONSTRUCTS

Direct Venous Anastomosis

1. A longitudinal incision is made along the vein. The vein is dissected free from surrounding tissues and tributaries are ligated.
2. The distal end of the vein is ligated and divided. It is flushed with heparinized saline. This helps confirm that it will distend and aids with identification of branches.
3. Systemic heparin is given, after it is allowed to circulate, the artery is controlled using vessel loupes or clamps.
4. Arteriotomy is made using an 11 blade, it is extended using Potts scissors.
5. End-to-side anastomosis is completed using running 5-0 or 6-0 monofilament nonabsorbable suture.

6. The vessels are allowed to back bleed and flushed with heparinized saline prior to completion of the anastomotic suture line.
7. Hemostasis is obtained and the wound is closed in layers.

Transposition Venous Anastomosis

This can be done in a one or two-step approach. In the one-step approach, the vein is dissected and mobilized close to the skin surface. Tributaries are ligated. The remainder of the steps are identical to the aforementioned technique. The two-steps approach entailed creating the arteriovenous anastomosis without dissecting and mobilization of the vein. The access is allowed to mature for 4 to 6 weeks. If the access matures, the second stage is performed. During this portion, the vein is dissected, mobilized, and placed in a more superficial location to make access easier.

There are benefits and risks with each approach. The one-step approach eliminated the risk of a second anesthetic exposure. It is also more convenient from a scheduling standpoint both for patients and providers. However, the drawback is that failure of maturation of the access renders patient hesitant about another operation since they have already undergone an extensive procedure. The two-stage approach invites the possibility of complications from a second anesthetic exposure. It is also more difficult to schedule and accommodate both patients and providers' schedules. On the other hand, it may have better maturation rate as the vein is allowed to mature in a native tissue plain before superficialization.

Postoperative Follow-up

The autogenous venous access is evaluated for maturation at 4 to 6 weeks after placement. Duplex US is used to measure flows within the fistula and ensure adequate diameter and location. One of the common rules used to assess dialysis access maturation is the rule of 6s. Mature autogenous venous access showed to be at least 6 mm wide, not more than 6 mm deep to the skin and must maintain a minimum flow of 600 mL/min. On clinical exam, mature dialysis access should be easily palpable with good thrill. Dialysis access failure may require additional procedures to help with maturation (e.g., arterial and venous angioplasties/stenting, venous side branches identification and ligation, vein mobilization and superficialization, balloon-assisted maturation).

PROSTHETIC ARM ACCESS

There are multiple grafts that were engineered to be used for dialysis access. There is no clear evidence that one graft is superior to others. As a result, the choice of graft to be used is according to the surgeon's preference in conjunction with consideration of the circumstances. Most grafts are accessed for dialysis within 2 to 3 weeks of implantation. Generally speaking, once the skin incision heals, the graft can be used for dialysis. Some grafts allow earlier use for dialysis, the Acuseal graft can be used within 24 hours of surgery. The patency and complications of Acuseal grafts are comparable to ePTFE grafts.[9] Having an established dialysis access can facilitate and expedite removal of indwelling dialysis central venous lines.

Technique of Graft-based Dialysis Access Creation

1. This will often require more than one incision, depending on the location of artery and vein and tunneling route.
2. The artery and vein are dissected in situ, there is no need to ligate the tributaries of the vein.
3. The graft is tunneled between the two incisions using a tunneling device, looped configuration may require a third incision at the apex of the loop. Systemic heparin is given.
4. Arteriotomy is made using an 11 blade, it is extended using Potts scissors to 5 to 6 mm. The end-to-side anastomosis is created using 5-0 or 6-0 monofilament nonabsorbable suture in a running continuous fashion.
5. The graft is flushed with heparinized saline and graft to vein anastomosis is created using 5-0 or 6-0 monofilament nonabsorbable suture in an end-to-side fashion.
6. Hemostasis is obtained and the wound is closed in layers.

OVERVIEW OF COMPLEX PERMANENT DIALYSIS ACCESS APPROACHES

There is a steady increase in the number of patients with no options for conventional dialysis access creation. This increase is a result of the increased survival of patients with chronic kidney disease and better management of medical comorbidities. These patients have typically exhausted their upper extremity options for dialysis access either via previous access surgery or device placement. This unique dilemma requires extensive evaluation and planning to resolve. Figure 41-5 shows a suggested flow chart for decision-making in hemodialysis access creation.

Evaluation of patients for complex dialysis access starts with history and physical examination. Inquiry into previous AV access is made and examination of surgical scars and upper extremities is performed. One must ensure depletion of all upper extremity access options. This evaluation must include duplex US, angiography, and venography. Occasionally, a

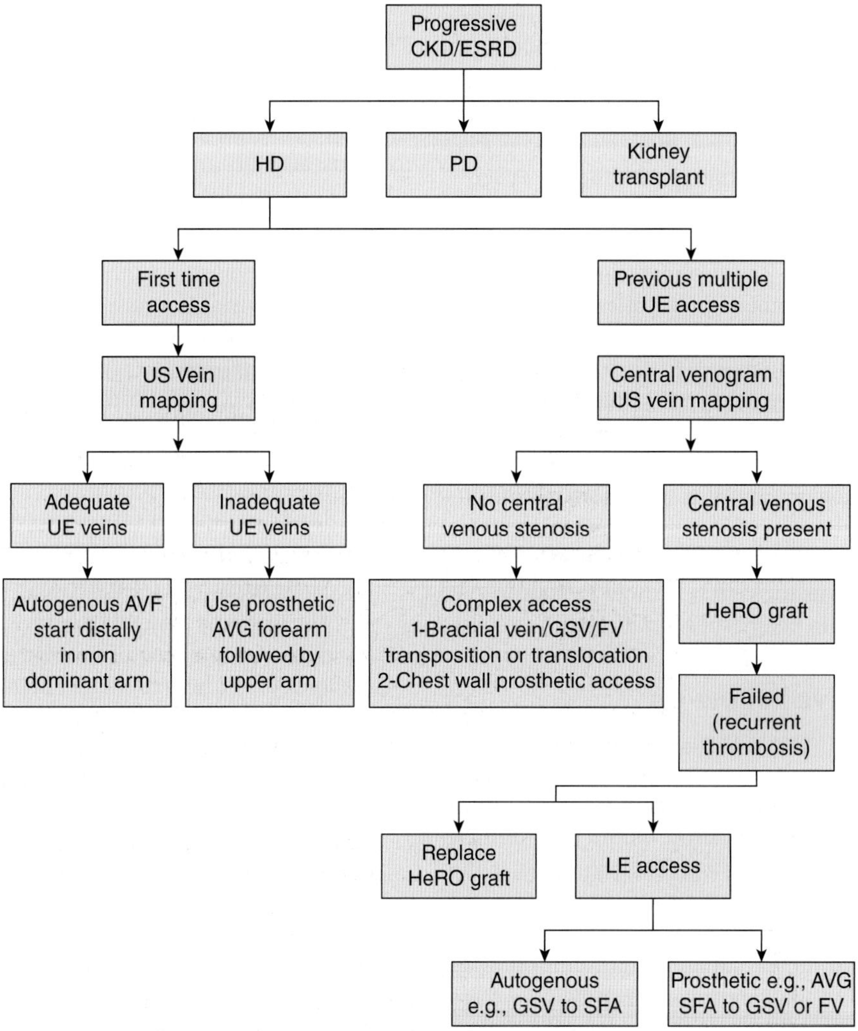

FIGURE 41-5 Flow chart for decision-making in hemodialysis access creation.

correctable lesion is identified and corrected, and this allows conventional dialysis access construction.

Once a patient is deemed a candidate for complex dialysis access procedure, detailed assessment of their arterial and venous system, medical comorbidities, body habitus, and functional evaluation is carried out. Unlike conventional dialysis access, there are no guidelines for choice of access constructed. Extensive data is not available on the patency and complication of such access procedures.

COMPLEX AUTOGENOUS TISSUE DIALYSIS ACCESS CREATION

These entail various procedure. The fundamental concept of which is the use of native veins as conduits for dialysis access. This involves both vein transposition and vein translocation procedures. Vein transposition includes mobilization of a great saphenous, brachial, or femoral vein and anastomosing them to nearby arteries. Vein translocation is the harvest of a vein and utilizing it to construct arteriovenous anastomosis at a different anatomic region.

Description of Vein Transposition Procedures

Vein transposition procedure starts of by dissecting the vein and ligating the tributaries to give it further mobility. For the great saphenous vein this can be done through skip incisions or endoscopically to minimize wound complications. The brachial veins are often paired and multiple. The largest of these veins is used to create a fistula.

Great saphenous vein transposition The great saphenous must be 3 mm in diameter to be considered for this procedure. The vein is harvested, and tributaries are ligated. Adequate length of vein is mobilized. The vein is transected and tunneled in a looped subcutaneous tunnel and anastomosed to the superficial femoral artery (Figure 41-6).

Brachial vein transposition This can be done in a one or two-step fashion similar to basilic vein-based access procedure. The brachial artery and vein are exposed in the antecubital area. The largest brachial vein is anastomosed to the brachial artery. In the one-step fashion, the vein is mobilized and placed in a subcutaneous location. In the two-step technique, the access is allowed to mature prior to placing in a subcutaneous location.

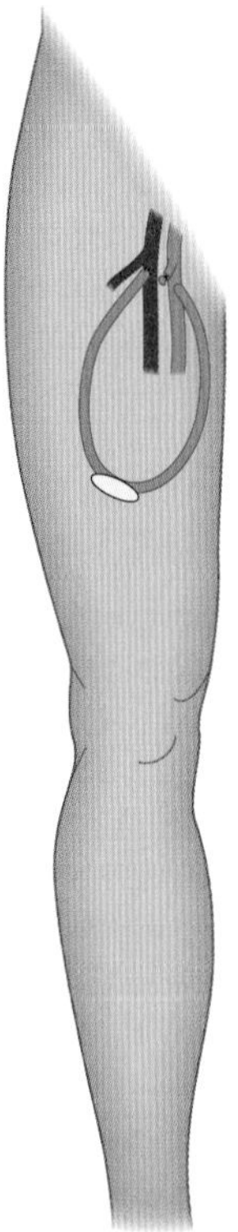

FIGURE 41-6 GSV transposition and thigh femoral artery to femoral vein AV fistula.

Femoral vein transposition The femoral vein is dissected down to the knee to obtain adequate length. The deep femoral veins are preserved. The vein is tunneled in a subcutaneous tunnel and anastomosed to the superficial femoral artery in the distal thigh. Occasionally, the vein does not have adequate length for tunneling. Creating a composite graft by anastomosing PTFE to provide additional length has been described.

Description of Vein Translocation Procedures

The saphenous vein and femoral veins are used for translocation procedure. Patients must have patent central veins to allow the use of the upper extremity for constructing a translocated vein-based access.

The saphenous vein and femoral veins are harvested down to the knees. Tributaries are ligated. Both veins have valves and must be reversed for use as a dialysis conduit. The harvested vein is used to create a brachial artery to axillary vein dialysis access.

COMPLEX PROSTHETIC DIALYSIS ACCESS CREATION

This is often easier than vein translocation and transposition procedure as they require limited dissection. Prosthetic graft use has been described in the chest and lower extremities.

There are three commonly described upper chest prosthetic dialysis access. Looped axillary artery to axillary vein, necklace, and brachial artery to jugular vein grafts. This is preferred to lower extremity access in obese patient due to the lower risk of infection. Venography to exclude or treat central venous stenosis must be done prior to constructing dialysis access.

Looped Axillary Artery to Axillary Vein Graft

The axillary artery and vein are dissected in infraclavicular location. Looped PTFE graft is anastomosed in an end-to-side fashion to the ipsilateral axillary artery and axillary vein. An incision at the apex of the loop is often needed to tunnel the graft. The final configuration is arranged so that the arterial anastomosis is perpendicular, and the venous anastomoses is in the same line as the axillary vein (Figure 41-7).

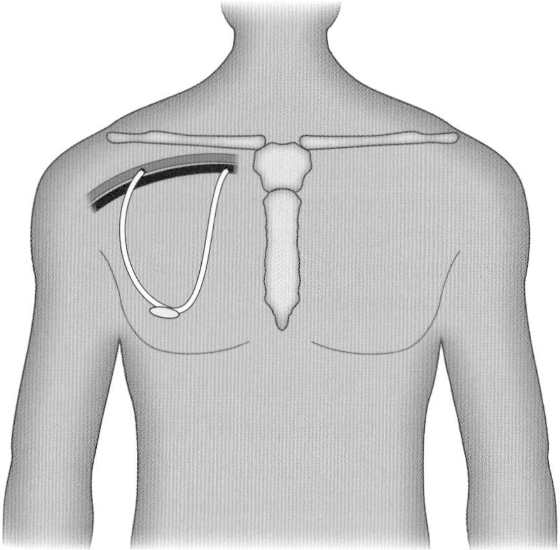

FIGURE 41-7 Looped axillary artery to ipsilateral axillary vein graft.

Necklace Graft

This configuration connects the axillary artery on one side to the axillary vein on the contralateral side using PTFE graft. This makes percutaneous interventions more difficult as the graft lies in a straight orientation (Figure 41-8).

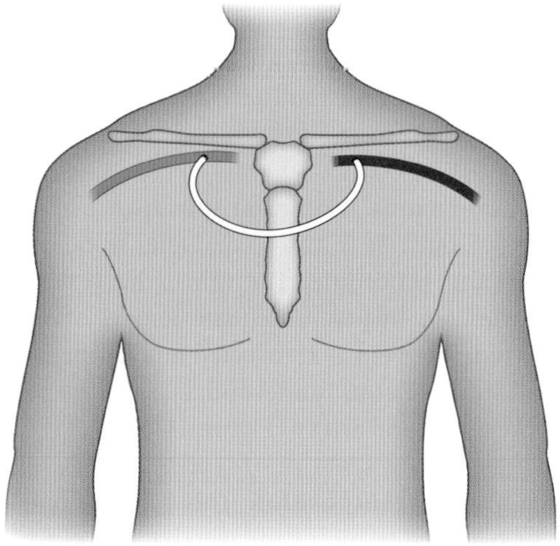

FIGURE 41-8 Necklace axillary artery to axillary vein graft.

Brachial Artery to Jugular Vein Graft

PTFE graft is used to connect the brachial artery to the ipsilateral jugular vein in a looped configuration.

Hemodialysis Reliable Outflow Vascular Access Device (HeRO Device)

This is usually the last effort prior to moving to a lower extremity dialysis access creation. The HeRO device is made up of two components: the arterial component is synthesized of prosthetic graft and is anastomosed to the brachial artery; the venous

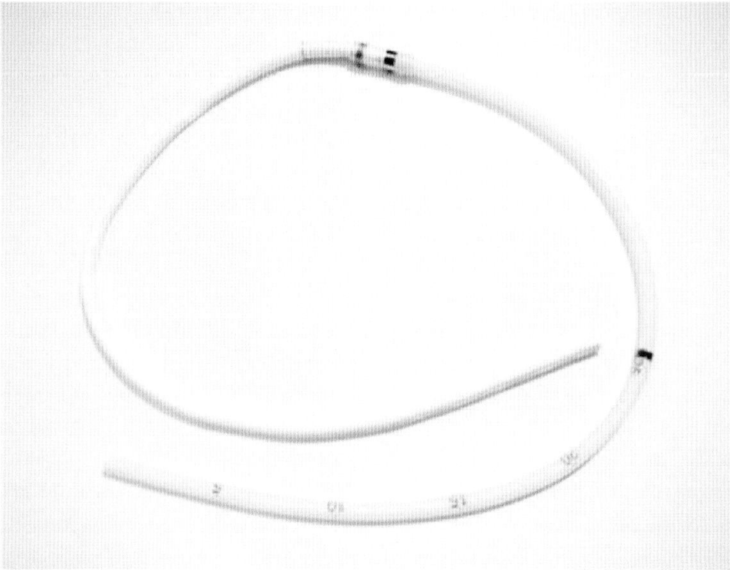

FIGURE 41-9 HeRO graft.

component is a tunneled catheter that ends at the right atrium. The two components are connected in the deltopectoral grove. There is a high risk of steal syndrome and cardiac complication with the use of HeRO device. It should not be used in patients with small brachial arteries and in patients with heart failure (Figure 41-9).

Lower Extremities Prosthetic Dialysis Access

These entail multiple configuration. The fundamental principle is connecting the superficial femoral artery to the femoral or great saphenous vein using PTFE grafts. This can be straight from the distal superficial femoral artery to the femoral vein. It can also be looped from the proximal superficial femoral artery to the femoral vein. The graft is tunneled in a subcutaneous location to allow easy access into the graft (Figure 41-10).

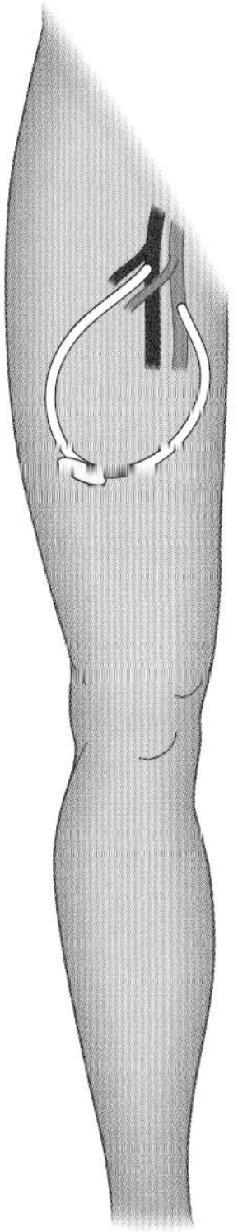

FIGURE 41-10 Looped femoral artery to femoral vein graft.

POSTOPERATIVE COMPLICATIONS

A wide range of postoperative complications can occur. Providers who are responsible for caring for patients with hemodialysis must be familiar with these complications. Early detection and intervention are essential for maintenance and salvation of dialysis access.

STEAL SYNDROME

Steal syndrome is defined as access-related hand ischemia. It is a consequence of preferential blood flow through the low-resistance venous anastomosis. Reversal of flow in the artery distal to the arteriovenous anastomosis is often observed, but it is not diagnostic. Many ESRD patients suffer from peripheral arterial disease and increased resistance in arterial segments, this further increases the gap in resistance between the two vascular beds.

They are four stages of steal syndrome. Stage I is asymptomatic and retrograde inflow of blood into the access during diastole is observed. It's a frequent finding in arteriovenous fistula and graft. It does not require an intervention. In stage II, patient will experience pain only during exercise or dialysis. Often intervention is not required; however, close monitoring is needed to early detect deterioration to stage III. In stage III, patient will develop rest pain and in stage IV, patient will have tissue necrosis. Stage III, IV, and sometimes stage II require surgical intervention to correct the steal syndrome or sacrifice the dialysis access.

One unique presentation of steal is ischemic monomelic neuropathy (IMN), it is believed to result from impaired flow in the vasa nervosum resulting in severe sensorimotor dysfunction of the ulnar, radial, and median nerves without obvious tissue loss. Symptoms manifest itself usually immediately after access creation. The presence of palpable pulse helps to distinguish it from steal syndrome. It is more common in diabetics and brachial artery-based access. If the ischemia is not reversed immediately (usually by sacrificing the newly created access), irreversible neural damage and permanent extremity impairment can occur.

Diagnosis of steal syndrome starts with history and physical examination. Examination of distal pulses with palpation and doppler techniques is carried out. Demonstration of augmentation of arterial flow with compression of the dialysis access, and improvement of patient symptoms are diagnostic in many situations. Pulse oximetry applied to the digits and monitoring the oxygen saturation wave form is another useful technique. In critical ischemia as in stage III or stage IV, transcutaneous oxygen partial pressure ($tcpO_2$) is lower than 30 mmHg, while digital arterial pressures are below 50 mmHg and digital brachial pressure index is below 0.6. With compression, these numbers significantly improve. These objective tests can help in the diagnosis process.

The decision to treat steal syndrome is dependent on the severity of symptoms, as mentioned before. Mild symptoms can be observed and managed expectantly. Tissue loss and severe symptoms require immediate recognition and intervention. Treatment options include banding, distal revascularization and interval ligation (DRIL), revision using distal inflow (RUDI), and proximalization arteriovenous anastomosis (PAVA).

BANDING

To be used in high flow associated steal and it is narrowing of the venous outflow to increase the resistance in outflow bed. Our preferred technique is placing a monofilament permanent suture around the vein. Coronary artery dilators are used to help with vein sizing.

Minimally Invasive Limited Ligation Endoluminal Assisted Revision (MILLER)

Recently described minimally invasive technique for fistula banding by a group of US interventional nephrologist is done in the radiology suite or the outpatient office. The vein or the graft is exposed close to the arterial anastomosis and banding is performed by tying a nonabsorbable suture around the access over an inflated 4- or 5-mm balloon under fluoroscopic or US guidance. Pre- and postbanding flow are obtained through US. Reduction in flow after banding provides an objective measurement regarding the adequacy of the performed banding.

Distal Revascularization and Interval Ligation (DRIL)

It involves two components, the first one is ligating the artery distal to the arteriovenous anastomosis. The second component is an arterial bypass that is created from an area proximal to the arteriovenous anastomosis to an area distal to the ligated vessel using great saphenous vein, if available. There should be at least 6 cm or more distance between the proximal bypass anastomosis and the access anastomosis to prevent retrograde diastolic flow in the graft. The first component can be sufficient for treatment of steal in distal radiocephalic fistula (DRAL; Distal radial artery ligation) as long as the ulnar artery and the palmar arch are patent. The DRIL procedure has been shown to result in immediate relief of steal symptoms in the majority of patients with excellent long-term patency for both the fistula and arterial bypass.

Revision Using Distal Inflow (RUDI)

RUDI is another technique that is similar to banding useful in high-flow–associated steal syndrome. It comprises two steps, the first is ligation of the conduit at the first part of the vein and migrating the arterial anastomosis to a more distal location in the arterial tree. Moving the arterial anastomosis to the forearm radial or ulnar artery can effectively reduce access flow by more than 50%. This will often require the use of venous or prosthetic grafts. RUDI should only be used if the forearm artery not used for distal inflow is patent; otherwise there will be a high risk of persisting steal.

Proximal Arteriovenous Anastomosis (PAVA) Creation Procedure

Another technique is to move the arteriovenous anastomosis more proximally. The original arteriovenous anastomosis is ligated, and an interposition graft is used to connect the access vein or graft with inflow artery more proximally so more proximal arterial collaterals can contribute to peripheral blood supply. Although PAVA has been widely used, systemic studies have rarely been published. In a prospective series by Zanow et al., 30 patients underwent PAVA, and complete relief of symptoms was reported in 84% of the patients with excellent access patency rates.[10] PAVA is an alternative to DRIL in normal flow–associated steal syndrome, especially in patients without suitable bypass vein and in patients with graft access. PAVA doesn't need vein harvest as PTFE graft can be used for proximal inflow of the access. When the central anastomosis of the interposition graft in PAVA is created on the central brachial or axillary artery and when the graft used for feeding the access has a diameter of 5 or 6 mm, PAVA enhances access flow. Therefore, in low-flow–associated steal syndrome, PAVA could be the best if not the only option to preserve both the access and the extremity.

Conclusion

Banding, MILLER, and RUDI are indicated in high-flow–associated steal syndrome. DRIL is very effective in high- and normal-flow–associated steal syndrome but is a time-consuming procedure and requires ligating the native artery. PAVA can be equally effective to DRIL while it is less invasive. Moreover, PAVA is the only option in low-flow–associated steal syndrome to optimize both access and peripheral circulation flow; however, careful assessment and treatment of arterial stenosis is needed before considering PAVA or related procedures.

BLEEDING AND HEMATOMA

Patients with ESRD have coagulopathy due to multiple factors. Uremia affects platelet functions regardless of count. The chronic anemia associated with CKD affects the dynamics of blood flow, in normal subjects with laminar flow red blood cells occupy the center and platelet are in the periphery in proximity to vessel wall, anemia also results in an increase in nitric oxide, which is a known platelet inhibitor. In addition, patients with CKD have impaired clearance of medications which can cause coagulopathy.

Minor bleeding complications like a small postoperative hematoma can be managed expectantly. If the hematoma is causing flow limiting compression of the outflow vein, it may require evacuation. Major postoperative bleeding requires a trip back to the operating room to control surgical bleeding. Protamine can be given to reverse the effect of heparin. Platelet transfusion is considered on individual bases. Transfused platelets lose their function after a few hours due to uremia.

Patients with ESRD are at an increased bleeding risk with procedures and surgeries. Coordination of dialysis and timing of procedure is optimal to minimize the effect of uremia. Ideally patients should be dialyzed the day before surgery.

ANEURYSM AND PSEUDOANEURYSM

Aneurysmal degeneration of fistula occurs most commonly at puncture site. Repeated puncture at the same location increases the risk of aneurysm development. Pseudoaneurysms can affect both autogenous and prosthetic dialysis access. It is more common with grafts.

Aneurysms present an increase in the size of the fistula. This can cause skin changes ranging from erythema and ulceration of the skin, and potential fistula rupture and catastrophic hemorrhage. The risk of rupture is related to the diameter of the fistula. It is also increased in the setting of infection.

Pseudoaneurysms do not have all three layers of blood vessels. Their lining is made of adventitia or adventitia and media. These are more common with grafts. They result from repeated puncture at the same location and inappropriate compression of the access after needle removal.

INFECTION

Infections are a serious cause of morbidity and mortality in patients with CKD and ESRD. The majority of the infection burden is secondary to temporary catheters use for dialysis.[11] Native arteriovenous fistula has lower risk of infection when compared to prosthetic graft. Graft infection originates as a localized infection or can result from systemic bacteremia. The presentation of infected dialysis access can be obvious when it presents with fevers, erythema, tenderness, swelling, and warmth over the fistula. It can be subtle and present with low-grade fever, draining sinus, and minor systemic signs of infections. Poor patient hygiene, diabetes, immunosuppression, and other comorbidities contribute to the risk of infection. Femoral location is associated with increased risk of infection when compared with upper extremity locations.

Patients suspected of having infected dialysis access should be investigated by obtaining blood cultures, CBC, ESR, and CRP levels. Imaging studies are not necessary. However, if there is uncertainty about the diagnosis, then a tagged white blood scan can help with the localization of infection. Empiric antibiotics are started immediately. Staphylococcus aureus is covered as it is the most common organism causing graft infection. Combination antibiotics is often used to cover both coagulase positive and negative species. The failure of medical treatment in clearing infection is high. Therefore, we recommend excision of the infected segments of the prosthetic graft and creating new dialysis access in new location or through a different tunnel.

NEUROPATHY

Peripheral neuropathy is commonly seen in patients with ESRD. Diabetes is a common comorbidity affecting patients with CKD. It is typically symmetrically distributed in gloves and stocking distribution. It presents as numbness, paresthesia, and neuropathic pain. Uremia in itself is associated with neuropathy manifesting as loss of fine sensory functions and tendon reflexes. It typically improves with commencement of dialysis and transplant. In addition, patients with ESRD continue to experience compression neuropathies. This includes carpal tunnel syndrome and compression by aneurysms and hematomas.

Ischemic monomelic neuropathy is a unique diagnosis which was mentioned earlier in this chapter.

VENOUS HYPERTENSION

The increased flow through the central vein is a direct consequence of arteriovenous anastomosis. This increased flow is well tolerated by many patients. Occasionally, it causes significant venous hypertension in patients with stenosis of central veins. The most common etiology for central venous stenosis is indwelling venous catheters placements, and indwelling devices. It is more common with subclavian-based access. Therefore, the recommended initial location of temporary dialysis catheter placements is through the internal jugular vein. In fact, venography is recommended prior to the placement of dialysis access in patients with previous subclavian vein lines. The second most common cause is neointimal hyperplasia affecting the central veins.

Venous hypertension presents itself in many different ways. It is occasionally asymptomatic in patients with well-established collateral veins. It is usually first noticed with increased and prolonged bleeding after needle removal at the end of a dialysis session. On physical examination, there is an increased superficial venous collaterals and persistent edema of the extremity is also a feature of venous hypertension. On palpation, there is an increased pulsatile impulse on the dialysis access.

Duplex US is the initial diagnostic test. However, it is limited by poor visualization of more central veins. Venography is the next step in evaluating patients with suspected venous hypertension. Balloon angioplasty improves the pressure gradient and can increase the patency of the dialysis access. Stenting is occasionally used across these lesions. While it improves the immediate success rate, it does not increase long-term patency.

Surgery is rarely used to treat venous hypertension. Venous bypasses and reconstructions of veins are surgical options. Ligation of the dialysis access is the last resort solution. It is used when other modalities fail. It is discouraged as it results in the loss of the dialysis access.

CARDIOPULMONARY COMPLICATIONS

In the first few weeks after establishing dialysis access, there is an increase in cardiac output to compensate for the increased demand of flow through the low-resistance arteriovenous anastomosis. Patients with preexisting cardiac dysfunction can develop high output heart failure. This is managed by banding of the access and other flow restrictive procedures.

Coronary steal syndrome is a unique complication in patients with dialysis access in the ipsilateral extremity as an internal mammary artery graft. Patients with proximal subclavian artery stenosis are at an increased risk for this condition. The decreased resistance through the dialysis access can cause decreased or reversal of flow through the internal mammary artery (IMA). Patients with preexisting IMA coronary graft should be investigated by CTA to ensure the patency of the proximal subclavian artery. Some have even recommended avoiding establishing dialysis access on the same side as the IMA grafts.[12]

GRAFT THROMBOSIS AND FAILURE

Predicting which graft will thrombose and fail is difficult. Although there are predictors of graft dysfunction, the rate of progression is variable. Decreased flow through the dialysis access warrants investigation with duplex US and angiographic studies. Anatomic abnormalities are corrected, including flow limiting central venous stenosis and arterial inflow anomalies. Graft thrombosis presents as loss of thrill overlying the dialysis access and absence of flow through the conduit. Graft failure is the inability of the access to maintain adequate flows for dialysis. It is usually identified at dialysis centers by dialysis nurses.

Loss of dialysis access requires immediate attention. Patients' electrolytes and serum studies are checked and their need for emergent dialysis is identified. If patients need emergent dialysis, temporary dialysis catheters are placed until salvage of failing graft or establishing new access. This invites a host of complications associated with indwelling catheters, including infection, central venous stenosis, and procedural complications.

The most common cause of decline of graft function is neointimal hyperplasia. It commonly develops at the venous anastomosis. This is corrected by balloon angioplasty of the area. Long inflation times (2–3 minutes) and high-pressure balloons are used. Any "waisting" is corrected using angioplasty. Improved diameter of lesion indicates technical success. Pressure measurements can be done as well to confirm a change in hemodynamics. Occasionally, surgical revision of the venous anastomosis is required to correct this issue.

Graft thrombosis is formation of clots and absence or near absence of flow in a dialysis access. US demonstrates no flow or minimal flow in the graft. The key principle used to prevent this complication is early recognition of decline in graft function and correction of these abnormalities. Multiple interventions were considered and used as adjuncts to maintain graft patency. However, no conclusive evidence is available. Blood thinners were widely investigated, and it was found that they increase the bleeding events with no improvements in graft patency.

Graft thrombosis is treated by removal of clots from the graft. This can be done in an open or endovascular or hybrid approach.

Open Thrombectomy

This can be done under local anesthesia—an incision is made overlying the graft in a location proximal to the area of thrombosis. The fistula is dissected and controlled with vessel loops. A horizontal incision is made in the graft. Fogarty embolectomy catheters are passed in antegrade and retrograde directions and clots are retrieved. The fistula is allowed to back bleed and forward bleed. The graft is closed using permanent 5-0 or 6-0 monofilament suture in an interrupted fashion. The skin is closed in layers.

Prosthetic grafts have higher success rate of open mechanical thrombectomy. They also have high success rates with repeated thrombectomy. This can be explained by the fact that their inner lining is not composed of vascular endothelium. Vascular endothelium is prone to further neointimal hyperplasia and to damage from thrombectomy balloons.

Endovascular Thrombectomy

The development of endovascular thrombectomy technique is a continuation of the development of minimally invasive techniques in the treatment of patients with vascular disease. This is performed in the cath lab or the hybrid operating room. After establishing access and placement of an antegrade sheath in the dialysis access toward the venous outflow, mechanical thrombectomy devices are used to fragment the clots. Some of these clots are suctioned, and the majority passes into the central veins and into the pulmonary artery. These emboli have minimal to no consequence on the pulmonary circulation. After the mechanical thrombectomy, a retrograde sheath is placed toward the arterial inflow and either regular or over the wire size 3F Fogarty catheter is used to remove the arterial plug. Completion angiogram is necessary to reveal the underlying etiology behind the fistula/graft thrombosis and to be treated accordingly. Caution should be exercised in patients with aneurysmal degeneration of their fistula or large burden of clot that extends into their central venous system (can be assessed by pull back central venogram at the beginning of the procedure), as these patients may benefit from thrombolysis to minimize the risk of massive pulmonary embolism. The benefits of the endovascular technique is limiting the incision area and allowance of radiographic evaluation of other abnormalities.

Hybrid Approach

The hybrid approach is a combination of the open and endovascular techniques. It allows further investigation of the cause of graft thrombosis.

FOLLOW-UP MONITORING OF ESTABLISHED DIALYSIS ACCESS

After initial successful maturation and function dialysis access, it should be monitored regularly. Some aggressive recommendations suggest that it should be done monthly. Dialysis centers can identify situations where there is malfunction dialysis access. High venous pressure and poor flows are detected by dialysis machines. Physical exam is extremely useful and both sensitive and specific of detection of abnormalities of autogenous dialysis access dysfunction.[13,14] Arteriovenous grafts do not allow the same degree of reliability. Duplex US and fistulogram are used to recognize and identify the cause of suboptimal dialysis access.

PHYSICAL EXAM

The physical examination of dialysis access follows the principle of general physical exam. It starts with inspection followed by palpation then auscultation.

INSPECTION

The skin overlying the fistula/graft is evaluated for breakdown or infection. Aneurysmal enlargement of fistula can be seen occasionally. Venous stenosis is suggested by prominent collateral veins as well as prolonged bleeding after dialysis needle removal. The arm with the fistula is lifted above the heart level and monitored for flattening of the fistula. The fistula should decompress spontaneously, if it does not, this suggests venous stenosis.

PALPATION

Palpation of the fistula is done using the palm of the hand. It is done along the entire length of the arteriovenous fistula/graft. A normal fistula/graft should have systolic and diastolic flow with no pulsatility. Pulsatile impulse indicates venous stenosis. Diminished flow suggests inflow stenosis. An absent thrill and pulse are features of thrombosed access.

AUSCULTATION

Normal grafts have bruits on auscultation. These have the same characteristics of normal thrills, with both systolic and diastolic flows. Venous stenosis increases the systolic component of the auscultated sounds.

IMAGING STUDIES

Duplex US is used to measure the flow in AV fistulas and grafts. Evidence of access abnormality includes flow that is less than 600 mL/min or decreased by one quarter (25%) in 4 months. Abnormalities detected on US warrant fistulogram and possible intervention to correct these abnormalities. Duplex can also identify poor inflow from arterial disease and fistula steal syndrome. US also identifies structural abnormalities such as hematoma, pseudoaneurysm, aneurysm, and presistent side branches.

LONG-TERM OUTCOMES OF DIALYSIS ACCESS

Agreed upon standardized terms were described to standardize reporting of dialysis access surgery outcomes. Primary Patency is the time interval from placement of dialysis access to any intervention that aims at maintaining or reestablish access before it completely fails.[15] Assisted primary patency is the interval from placement of dialysis access till access thrombosis. This may include procedures dedicated to maintain patency and function of the access. Secondary patency is the interval from access placement till access abandonment. This includes all interventions intended to restore function to thrombosed access.

Autogenous AV access has better primary and secondary patency rates when compared with prosthetic AV access. The 6-month primary patency rate for autogenous dialysis access is 72% (95% confidence interval [CI], 70%–74%). The 6-month primary patency rate for prosthetic access is 58% (95% CI, 56%–61%). The superiority of autogenous AV access continued to be demonstrated at 18 months with primary patency of 51% (95% CI, 48%–53%), compared to 33% (95% CI, 31%–36%) for prosthetic access.

Autogenous AV access also has better short- and long-term secondary patency rates. Autogenous accesses have a secondary patency rate of 86% (95% CI, 84%–88%) at 6 months, the corresponding patency of prosthetic access is 76% (95% CI, 73%–79%). The secondary patency of autogenous access is 77% (95% CI, 74%–79%) at 18 months, and secondary patency rate for prosthetic accesses is 55% (95% CI, 51%–59%).[16] It is worth mentioning that autogenous AV access has a considerable primary failure rate (15%).[17]

INDEWELLING DIALYSIS CATHETERS

All discussions involving dialysis access must include dialysis catheters. In the year 2017, 80% of patients starting hemodialysis in the US were achieving that through central venous catheter.[1] This proportion is similar to previous reports despite initiatives like fistula first and multiple societal efforts. Hispanic ethnicity, age <45 years, congestive heart failure, or other cardiac diseases are risk factors.

There are many designs of indwelling dialysis catheters. There are different configurations of catheters' tip. No conclusive evidence of superiority of any design over the other. The goal of these catheters is to achieve adequate flow approximately 300 mL/min to maintain hemodialysis with minimal recirculation. The catheters have two lumens. One lumen is the inflow from the dialysis machine to the patient "venous lumen". The second one is the outflow from the patient to the dialysis machine "arterial lumen". The physical separation of the two lumens aims to prevent recirculation. Recirculation is the phenomenon of dialyzed blood reentering the catheter lumen without entering the systemic circulation. This causes inadequate clearance of solutes and ineffective dialysis. The preferred location for placement is the right internal jugular vein. Catheters placed in the right internal jugular vein have the best patency rate. Femoral vein catheters are associated with increased risk for infection. Subclavian-based access is discouraged due to the associated risk of central venous stenosis.

The evaluation of patients for placing temporary dialysis catheter includes a detailed history and physical exam, and Duplex US of the accessible central venous system. Any difficulty with placement should warrant aborting the procedure and further investigation by venography. Venography can be conventional using fluoroscopy, magnetic resonance venography, or computed-tomography venography.

The types of catheters can be categorized into short-term use catheters and long-term use catheters.

Short-term use catheters are used in inpatients and for 1 to 2 weeks. It is commonly placed for patients that need immediate dialysis with expected return of renal function. These catheters are not cuffed and are not tunneled. Long-term use catheters are used to maintain dialysis in patients awaiting placement, maturation, or salvation of established dialysis access. Occasionally, they are used for long term in patients who exhausted the options for fistula creation or those with significant comorbidities that precludes surgical creation of fistula. These long-term use catheters are characterized by tunneling and the presence of a cuff that fixes it in place and prevents ascending infection along the catheter.

TECHNIQUE FOR INSERTION OF TEMPORARY DIALYSIS ACCESS

Short-term Catheters

These catheters can be placed at the bedside or in the cath lab. US evaluation of the vein for compressibility and patency is done. The area of insertion is prepped and draped. Sterile precautions are carried out. Local anesthesia is injected into the insertion site. Under US guidance and using a Seldinger technique, temporary dialysis catheter is inserted. Postplacement chest x-ray confirms the location of the tip and evaluates for procedure-related complications.

Long-term Catheters

These catheters are placed in the cath lab with the aid of fluoroscopy. The vein is evaluated by US and confirmed to be compressible and patent. The area of insertion is prepped and draped. This includes the neck and upper chest on the same side. Local anesthesia is used at the insertion sites including chest wall. Using large bore needle under US, the vein is accessed. The guidewire is introduced into the vessels. Fluoroscopy confirms good position of the wire. A skin incision is made adjacent to the wire. The catheter is tunneled from the anterior upper chest to the neck incision around the wire. The peel away sheath is introduced over the wire. The wire and dilator are removed. The catheter is passed through the sheath as the sheath is being peeled off. X-ray confirms proper position of the catheter tip. It is secured at the chest wall and the neck incision is closed. As these catheters have a predetermined length, appropriate catheter length should be selected based on the access site (e.g., right internal jugular, left internal jugular, or femoral vein) (Figure 41-11).

COMPLEX LONG-TERM INDWELLING CATHETERS

These are rarely utilized and used as last resort in patients with no alternatives for creating dialysis access with thrombosed central veins. The thrombosed central veins preclude internal jugular vein use for catheter insertion. This situation is rarely encountered and there is limited long-term data on this approach. These catheters can be placed directly into the superior vena cava. This is placed transthoracically using radiological guidance. Alternatively, the superior vena cava is recanalized from the inferior vena cava. The inferior vena cava is another site that can be used for placement of long-term

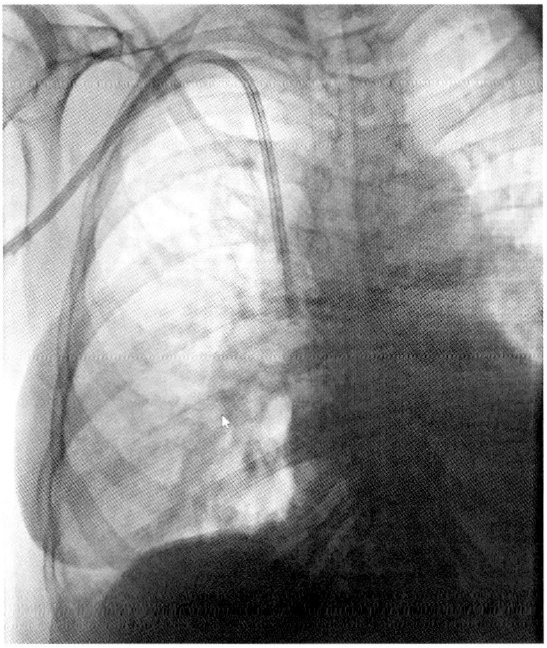

FIGURE 41-11 Tunneled dialysis catheter in appropriate location.

dialysis catheters. This can be placed transhepatically or through the back.

These unusual locations for long-term catheter placement are often reported to have a significant complication burden and requiring frequent interventions.

COMPLICATION OF CATHETER INSERTION

Pneumothorax

Pneumothorax is the collection of air in the pleural space. It is a result of pleural puncture during line placement. This condition is less frequent now with routine use of US guidance. A small pneumothorax in an asymptomatic patient can be observed and managed expectantly. Large pneumothorax requires treatment with insertion of tube thoracostomy. Tension pneumothorax requires immediate needle decompression followed by tube thoracostomy insertion. Pneumothorax can also present in a delayed fashion. This is believed to be due to the small puncture of the pleural space and slow accumulation of air.

Hemothorax

Hemothorax is collection of blood in the pleural space. It occurs with an injury to a vessel. It usually occurs with back wall puncture, concomitant with pleural puncture. It can happen at any step of insertion of lines. Any resistance of advancement of wire, dilator, or catheter should lead the proceduralist to stop and evaluate the causes for resistance. It is treated with tube thoracostomy to prevent adhesions in the pleural cavity and superinfection of the pooling blood. The injured vessel most commonly stops bleeding spontaneously with no need for intervention. Rarely endovascular or open intervention is required to achieve hemostasis.

Air Embolism

Air embolism is the passage of air into the central veins and into the pulmonary artery. It can cause cardiac arrest. It commonly occurs during the insertion or removal of the catheter. During insertion, having the needle open to air may allow air to suck into the vessel. Placing the patient in Trendelenburg position during insertion can decrease the risk of air embolism. During removal of the line, pressure must be held at the insertion site to prevent air from entry into the circulation. If the condition develops, the patient is positioned in the left lateral decubitus position to allow the air bubble to migrate to the right ventricle. The catheter is advanced, and air is suctioned out.

Myocardial Rupture and Arrythmias

This is a rare complication of indwelling line placement. It can occur due to wire, dilator, or catheter injury to cardiac walls. It is more common in pediatric population. It causes pericardial effusion and possible tamponade. It is treated by pericardiocentesis. The bleeding resolves spontaneously and drainage of the pericardium is effective treatment. Rarely, ongoing bleeding requires median sternotomy and formal cardiac repair.

Cardiac arrythmias occur as a consequence of irritation of the myocardium by the wire. Observing the markers of depth on the wire during advancement ensures that the wire is not progressing too far into the heart and ideally is to advance the wire into the IVC rather than into the ventricle. Proper position of the catheter tip is important in preventing this complication. The optimal location of the dialysis catheter tip on standard chest radiograph is proximal to the cardiac shadow and overlying the right mainstem bronchus impression.

Central Stenosis

The presence of catheters in central vein induces thrombosis and neointimal hyperplasia. It is more common with subclavian vein cannulation than with other sites. The higher rate with subclavian location suggests a mechanical contribution from the clavicle and first rib to vein damage. The thrombi associated with indwelling lines are frequently inconsequential and rarely result in pulmonary embolism.

Thoracic Duct Injuries

This is a unique complication of left-sided catheter placement. The thoracic duct is injured at its insertion at the left subclavian vein and left internal jugular vein confluence. This can result in a chylothorax, which is diagnosed by high fat content of the pleural fluid. The leakage stops spontaneously most of the time.

Arterial Injury

Arterial sticks and insertion of catheters should be a rare occurrence with the use of US during line insertion. It commonly occurs in emergent situations, in hypotensive and hypoxic patients. If the artery was not dilated, holding pressure is sufficient treatment and catheter insertion can be reattempted. If the catheter was already placed in the carotid artery, formal exploration and repair of the artery is performed in the operating room. Subclavian artery misplacement of catheter is more difficult to manage conservatively. The clavicle prevents applying direct pressure on the artery. It is often treated by removal of the catheter in the angio suite with stenting of the area of arterial puncture.

Catheter-related Infections

It usually presents as localized infection at the insertion site of the catheter. It can also present as disseminated blood stream infection or infection of the subcutaneous tunnel. It is most commonly caused by *Staphylococcus Aureus*. Localized infection is treated with antibiotics. More diffuse infection occasionally requires complete removal of the catheter with insertion at a different site or exchange of the catheter over a wire. Removal of the catheter and "line holiday" is the preferred modality of treatment, however that can be limited by patient's condition.

REFRENCES

1. United States Renal Data System. 2019 USRDS annual data report: Epidemiology of kidney disease in the United States. National Institute of Diabetes and Digestive and Kidney Diseases (NIDDK).
2. Konner K. History of vascular access for haemodialysis. *Nephrol Dial Transplant*. 2005;20(12):2629-2635.
3. Brescia MJ, Cimino JE, Appel K, Hurwich BJ. Chronic hemodialysis using venipuncture and a surgically created arteriovenous fistula. *N Engl J Med*. 1966;275(20):1089-1092.
4. Oliver MJ, Rothwell DM, Fung K, Hux JE, Lok CE. Late creation of vascular access for hemodialysis and increased risk of sepsis. *J Am Soc Nephrol*. 2004;15(7):1936-1942.
5. Lok CE. Fistula first initiative: advantages and pitfalls. *Clin J Am Soc Nephrol*. 2007;2(5):1043-1053.
6. Silva MB Jr, Hobson RW II, Pappas PJ, et al. A strategy for increasing use of autogenous hemodialysis access procedures: impact of preoperative noninvasive evaluation. *J Vasc Surg*. 1998;27(2):302-308.
7. Mendes RR, Farber MA, Marston WA, Dinwiddie LC, Keagy BA, Burnham SJ. Prediction of wrist arteriovenous fistula maturation with preoperative vein mapping with ultrasonography. *J Vasc Surg*. 2002;36(3):460-463.
8. Huber TS, Ozaki CK, Flynn TC, et al. Prospective validation of an algorithm to maximize native arteriovenous fistulae for chronic hemodialysis access. *J Vasc Surg*. 2002;36(3):452-459.
9. Glickman MH, Burgess J, Cull D, Roy-Chaudhury P, Schanzer H. Prospective multicenter study with a 1-year analysis of a new vascular graft used for early cannulation in patients undergoing hemodialysis. *J Vasc Surg*. 2015;62(2):434-441.
10. Zanow J, Kruger U, Scholz H. Proximalization of the arterial inflow: a new technique to treat access-related ischemia. *J Vasc Surg*. 2006;43(6):1216-1221.
11. Nassar GM, Ayus JC. Infectious complications of the hemodialysis access. *Kidney Int*. 2001;60(1):1-13.

12. Cuthbert GA, Kirmani BH, Muir AD. Should dialysis-dependent patients with upper limb arterio-venous fistulae undergoing coronary artery bypass grafting avoid having ipsilateral in situ mammary artery grafts? *Interact Cardiovasc Thorac Surg.* 2014;18(5):655-660.
13. Asif A, Leon C, Orozco-Vargas LC, et al. Accuracy of physical examination in the detection of arterio-venous fistula stenosis. *Clin J Am Soc Nephrol.* 2007; 2(6):1191-1194.
14. Salman L, Beathard G. Interventional nephrology: physical examination as a tool for surveillance for the hemodialysis arteriovenous access. *Clin J Am Soc Nephrol.* 2013;8(7):1220-1227.
15. Sidawy AN, Gray R, Besarab A, et al. Recommended standards for reports dealing with arteriovenous hemodialysis accesses. *J Vasc Surg.* 2002;35(3):603-610.
16. Huber TS, Carter JW, Carter RL, Seeger JM. Patency of autogenous and polytetrafluoroethylene upper extremity arteriovenous hemodialysis accesses: a systematic review. *J Vasc Surg.* 2003;38(5):1005-1011.
17. Rooijens P, Tordoir J, Stijnen T, Burgmans J, Yo T. Radiocephalic wrist arteriovenous fistula for hemodialysis: meta-analysis indicates a high primary failure rate. *Eur J Vasc Endovasc Surg.* 2004;28(6):583-589.

SELF-ASSESSMENT STUDY QUESTIONS AND ANSWERS

Questions

1. Goal of Fistula First Breakthrough initiative is:
   A. To increase the use of AVF in > 66% of patients on hemodialysis.
   B. It requires collaboration between nephrologists, vascular surgeons, social workers, and multiple team members.
   C. Early referral is the cornerstone to reach this goal as dialysis access creation needs some time to heal and mature before it can be used.
   D. All of the above.

2. The following is correct about Allen's test:
   A. A tourniquet is routinely placed in the upper arm to perform Allen's test.
   B. It is done to determine the integrity of plantar arch before thigh AVF/AVG.
   C. It is done to determine the integrity of palm arch before creating distal forearm AVF involving the radial or ulnar artery.
   D. It is done using duplex ultrasound.

3. Which of the following is considered when creating a hemodialysis access?
   A. Lower extremity is preferred to upper extremity due to lower risk of infection.
   B. Dialysis access should be placed as far distally on the extremity as possible to preserve the proximal sites for future use.
   C. Dominant arm is considered first.
   D. AVG has better long-term patency and reduced risk of infection.

4. One of the common rules to assess AVF maturation is the rule of 6s, what does it entitle?
   A. flow > 600 mL/min
   B. fistula diameter < 6 mm
   C. depth from the skin surface > 6 mm
   D. to be used 6 weeks after creation

5. In stage III steal syndrome, the patient will experience:
   A. Asymptomatic with retrograde flow of blood into the access during diastole is observed.
   B. Patient will experience pain only during exercise or dialysis. Often intervention is not required, but close monitoring is needed.
   C. Rest pain.
   D. Tissue loss.

6. The following is/are correct regarding ischemic monomelic neuropathy (IMN):
   A. Absence of distal pulses is diagnostic for IMN.
   B. If the ischemia is not reversed immediately, irreversible neural damage can occur.
   C. It is believed to result from impaired flow in the vasa vasorum.
   D. Both B and C are correct.

7. Why ESRD patients are more prone to bleeding complications?
   A. ESRD patients tend to have low platelet count that affects their ability to form clots.
   B. The chronic anemia associated with CKD affects the dynamics of blood flow.
   C. Anemia associated with ESRD is also known to decrease nitric oxide, which is a known platelet stimulator.
   D. ESRD patients are more prone to bleeding complications only if they are receiving anticoagulation, given the impaired clearance of medication.

SELF-ASSESSMENT STUDY QUESTIONS AND ANSWERS

8. What are the long-term outcomes of autologous AV access Vs prosthetic access?
   A. Autologous AV access has better primary patency that approaches 51% at 18 months.
   B. Autologous AV access has better secondary patency approaching 77% at 18 months.
   C. Prosthetic AV access has better secondary patency rate approaching 77% at 18 months.
   D. Both A and B are correct.

9. What is the purpose of the physical separation of the two lumens in indwelling dialysis catheter?
   A. To minimize risk of clotting of the dialysis circuit
   B. To provide adequate flow to the dialysis machine
   C. To prevent recirculation
   D. To avoid high venous pressure

10. The following is/are true in treating dialysis catheter-related infection:
   A. Localized infection can be treated with antibiotics.
   B. Most commonly caused by staphylococcus Aureus.
   C. More diffuse infection occasionally requires complete removal of the catheter with line holiday and new catheter insertion at a different site.
   D. All of the above are correct.

SELF-ASSESSMENT STUDY QUESTIONS AND ANSWERS

Answers

1. D.
2. C.
3. B.
4. A.
5. C.
6. D.
7. B.
8. D.
9. C.
10. D.

CHAPTER

42 Peripheral Vascular Trauma

Sarah Hill and Mallory Williams

OUTLINE

MANAGEMENT OF PERIPHERAL VASCULAR INJURY
- **Introduction**
- **Epidemiology**
- **Preoperative Trauma Management**
  - Airway and Breathing Management
  - Circulation Management
  - Extremity Tourniquet Management
  - Disability Management
- **Diagnoses**
- **Type of Vessel Injuries**
- **Operative Management**
  - Operative Exposure and Vascular Control
  - Arterial Repair
  - Venous Repair
  - Specific Injuries
    - *Brachial Vessel Injuries*
    - *Ulnar and Radial Artery Injuries*
    - *Common Femoral Vascular Injuries*
    - *Superficial Femoral Vessels*
    - *Popliteal Injuries*
  - Medial Exposure of the Popliteal Vessels
    - *Supragenicular Exposure*
    - *Infragenicular Exposure*
    - *Lateral Exposure of the Popliteal Vessels*
    - *Tibial Injuries*
- **Postoperative Complications**
  - Early Complications
    - *Postoperative Hemorrhage*
    - *Thrombosis and Limb Ischemia*
    - *Compartment Syndrome*
    - *Surgical Site Infection*
  - Late Complications
    - *Pseudoaneurysms*
    - *Venous Insufficiency*
    - *Neurological Complications*
- **Special Scenarios**
  - The Mangled Extremity
  - Vascular Damage Control Approach
  - Stenting
  - Injuries with Poor Functional Outcomes
  - Postoperative Management

MANAGEMENT OF PERIPHERAL VASCULAR INJURY

INTRODUCTION

Injury to the major named arteries and veins of the upper and lower extremity while infrequent still poses significant challenges for both civilian and military trauma teams. There are major differences in military and civilian mechanisms which present as different magnitudes of tissue destruction and therefore vascular injury. Effective management of peripheral vascular trauma is essential to preservation of both life and limb in trauma patients. This chapter will detail an evidence-based approach to the diagnosis, preoperative trauma management, operative management, and postoperative management of common patterns of peripheral vascular trauma.

EPIDEMIOLOGY

Peripheral vascular injuries account for approximately 2% to 3% of injuries in the National Trauma Data Base over the last decade. Vascular injuries are associated with approximately 7% of penetrating injuries.[1] Arterial injuries were associated with 43% concomitant bone fractures, and venous injuries occurred in 20% of patients studied.[2] Vascular injuries are associated with less than 0.5% of all limb fractures.[3] Extremity injuries compose 50% to 60% of United States Armed Forces casualties in Iraq and Afghanistan and 12% of this cohort have combat-related vascular injuries.[4] In the modern era, war injuries of the lower extremity occur primarily from improvised explosive devices and therefore tissue devitalization in conjunction with vessel trauma occurs.

PREOPERATIVE TRAUMA MANAGEMENT

Airway and Breathing Management

The initial evaluation of a patient presenting following traumatic peripheral vascular injury is guided by advanced trauma life support (ATLS) guidelines. The emergency medical technician's prehospital description of mechanism of injury, scene of events, and clinical course in route to the trauma center may all lend important details relevant to determining the patient's pattern of injury. Establishing that the patient has a patent airway and appropriate oxygenation and ventilation is the critical first priority for all trauma patients. For patients who have obvious physiologic signs of being in hypovolemic shock, orotracheal intubation and activation of the massive transfusion protocol are essential first steps.

Circulation Management

The circulation evaluation during the primary survey of ATLS is critical to understand and execute efficiently. It begins with the establishment of large bore intravenous catheters for patients in hypovolemic shock. If establishment of upper extremity catheters are not technically possible, the trauma team should quickly move to preferably establish 8 French line placement in an uninjured lower extremity. Similarly, peripheral intravenous lines should not be established in injured upper extremities. Intraosseous catheters should also not be placed in injured extremities. It is important to note that standard polyurethane or silicone central lines are 7 French and from 15 to 30 cm long and thus are not appropriate for trauma resuscitation. With the establishment of intravenous access, trauma laboratory studies should be obtained. These include a complete blood count, basic metabolic panel, serum lactate, type and crossmatch, and activated prothrombin and prothrombin time. The most important study to prioritize is the type and crossmatch. For patients with obvious sources of active hemorrhage, a hemostatic resuscitation should be initiated. A hemostatic resuscitation is defined by minimal crystalloid with a low ratio of blood to plasma and platelet transfusion regimen. Concomitant with hemostatic resuscitation and massive transfusion these patients will receive tranexamic acid at a dose of 1 g over 10 minutes if their injury was within hours of arrival to the trauma center.

Assessment of the peripheral pulses should be performed. Immediate recognition of hard signs of vascular trauma is important as they are 92% to 95% sensitive for an injury. These are delineated in Table 42-1 and include the presence of pulsatile bleeding, expanding hematoma, pulsatile hematoma, bruit or thrill, and ischemia. Signs of ischemia may

TABLE 42-1 Signs of Vascular Trauma

Hard Signs	Soft Signs
Pulsatile bleeding	Proximity of injury to a named vessel
Absent pulses	Diminished pulses
Acute ischemia	ABI <0.9
Expanding or pulsatile hematoma	Large hematoma
Bruit or thrill	Associated nerve injury

be generally recalled using the six P's: pain, pallor, paresthesia, poikilothermia, paralysis, and pulselessness. In comparison, soft signs of vascular injury include a reported history of hemorrhage, presence of a nonexpanding nonpulsatile hematoma, present but diminished pulses, and injury in proximity to a named blood vessel. The majority of vascular injuries, especially those involving the extremities, may be diagnosed during a physical exam, coupled with the utilization of ankle-brachial or wrist-brachial indices. It is our protocol at our Level I trauma center to perform and document arterial brachial indices (ABIs) for patients with extremity trauma on both the unaffected and injured extremity. For patients with an ABI of less than 0.9, this examination is 87% sensitive and 97% specific for arterial injury. These patients will go on to receive computed tomography angiography of the lower extremity for a more specific diagnosis of peripheral vascular injury. Patients with hard signs of vascular injury secondary to trauma should proceed to the operating room for exploration.

Extremity Tourniquet Management

Management of tourniquets becomes very important in peripheral vascular trauma. For patients exsanguinating from an extremity, direct pressure should be applied over the wound to stop active hemorrhage. Trauma team members should then place a tourniquet directly above the wound and turn the windlass until active hemorrhage has stopped. If the patient continues to hemorrhage with one tourniquet in place, an additional tourniquet should be placed above the first tourniquet in the same manner. Upon hemorrhage cessation, the tourniquet placement times should be documented and the primary survey should be completed. The massive transfusion protocol should be initiated as well, and the patient should then be operatively managed. For more complicated junctional hemorrhage in the trauma bay, we have had more success with continued direct pressure and moving the patient to the operating room for both supra inguinal ligament and infra inguinal ligament vessel control. We also utilize direct pressure for axillary hemorrhage in the trauma bay.

Placement of tourniquets is a lifesaving intervention for peripheral vascular trauma. The caveat is that tourniquets must be placed before the patient develops shock. Those tourniquets placed before shock were associated in prospective combat data as being associated with 90% survival. For tourniquets that are already in place at the time of trauma evaluation, we routinely unwind the windlass by half rotations while directly observing the wound. This is important so as to be able to quickly reapply the requisite pressure for hemorrhage control if needed. We do not remove the tourniquet initially when evaluating the wound. It is also important to note that in many contemporary instances, the tourniquet has been placed for venous injury that can be controlled with lower pressure dressings without eliminating perfusion to the limb. This prevents further unnecessary ischemia time and development of limb ischemia.

Disability Management

There are four important constituents of the extremity that should be focused on during trauma management: the bones, muscles and tendons, nerves, and the vasculature. As mentioned previously, with arterial injuries there is a high incidence of concomitant bone fractures. Comminuted fractures of the bone can compromise arterial blood supply and the corresponding pulse examination. Bones should be splinted with a neurovascular examination following this procedure. Assessment of motor and sensory should be performed and documented. When there are both fractures and vascular injuries, restoration of blood supply to the limb and cessation of hemorrhage should be the priority. If ever faced with the unfortunate choice of life or limb, the surgeon's actions should always be interpretable as first preserving the patient's life.

DIAGNOSES

High-resolution multidetector computed tomography angiography is the gold standard for diagnosis.[5,6] This study remains the most frequently utilized study for diagnosing specific peripheral vascular injuries in trauma centers. Computed tomography angiography (CTA) is relatively quick, noninvasive, and specific for vascular injuries. Furthermore, other studies can be obtained simultaneously. However, consideration must be given to risks including but not limited to contrast-induced injury and radiation exposure. Two prospective studies have demonstrated 100%

sensitivity and specificity for the identification of peripheral vascular injuries.[7] For those patients who are hemodynamically stable and demonstrate physical examination pulse deficits or an ABI of <0.9, CTA of the extremity should be test of choice. The CT angiographic signs of arterial injuries in the extremities are active extravasation of contrast material, pseudoaneurysm formation, abrupt narrowing of an artery, loss of opacification of a segment of artery, and arteriovenous fistula formation.

Other imaging modalities are often useful when localizing a vascular lesion with a variety of diagnostic and/or therapeutic considerations. Duplex ultrasonography (DUS) may be utilized at the bedside or in the operating room and is highly accurate in the setting of a trained technician or operator. The utilization of DUS could preclude unnecessary angiography or CTA in certain patients.

The role of postoperative on table angiography postrepair in patients is well established. The goals of this procedure are to establish direct radiographic evidence of patency of the repair. Many hybrid operating rooms are now available but they are usually separate from the main trauma room. Tabletop angiograms should begin with establishing the patient's allergies with the nurse. Next, it is necessary to know that the operating room table is capable of having appropriate x-ray plate placement beneath the area of interest and that there is fluoroscopic capability. Surgeons should be protected by lead draping including thyroid shields before beginning the procedure. The proximal artery is often already exposed and clamped and/or controlled with a Potts tie with a vessel loop during the repair. The vessel should be accessed with the appropriate size catheter to inject contrast (see Table 42-2). We utilize Visipaque 320 contrast dye diluted with 100 mL of saline in a 30-mL bottle. Handheld injection is sufficient for infrainguinal studies. Injection rates and volumes can be found in Table 42-2. Postoperative Doppler studies are also performed with palpation of pulses.

TABLE 42-2 Contrast Injection Rate and Injection Volume

Location	Catheter	Injection Rate (mL/s)	Injection Volume
Aortoiliac	5 Fr	14–16	15–25
CFA–SFA–Pop	4–5 Fr	5–7	16–20
Run: CFA–Pop	4–5 Fr	4	9–12
SFA	4–5 Fr	4–5	8–10
Run: Below knee	4 Fr	3–4	10–12
Below knee	4 Fr	3–4	5–7
Below the ankle	4 Fr	3–4	5–7

TYPE OF VESSEL INJURIES

The five types of vessel injury can be found in Table 42-3.[8,9] Two of these injury types present with hard signs of vascular trauma and should be immediately taken to the operative room except in very rare cases (i.e., multisystem trauma – pelvic fracture). The guiding principle in trauma of life over limb should always be followed. All five injury types have decreased pulse and may occur due to either penetrating trauma or boney fractures (Table 42-4). The American Association for the Surgery of Trauma Organ Injury Scale has graded peripheral vascular trauma (Table 42-5).[10]

TABLE 42-3 Types of Vessel Injury

Vessel Injury Type	Radiographic Findings	Physical Findings
Intimal injuries	Subintimal hematomas, flaps, disruptions	Decreased pulse & ABI
Total vascular wall defects	Pseudoaneurysm	Bleeding and hematomas with decreased pulse & ABI
Total vessel disruption	Vessel occlusion	Bleeding and absent pulse
Arteriovenous fistula	Acquired arterial–venous connection	Palpable thrill and decreased pulse
Spasm	Partial vessel occlusion	Decreased pulse

TABLE 42-4 Patterns of Associated Musculoskeletal and Other Structures with Specific Vessel Injury

Vessel	Musculoskeletal	Other
Carotid artery	Cervical spine	Vertebral vein
	Mandible, Le Fort II/III facial fracture	Carotid artery
	Skull base	Trachea, esophagus
Vertebral artery	Cervical spine (vertebral foramina)	Jugular vein
	Skull base	Carotid artery
Subclavian artery or vein	Clavicle	Thoracic duct (left)
	Sternum, manubrium	Brachial plexus, recurrent laryngeal nerve
Axillary artery or vein	Shoulder, proximal humerus	Brachial plexus, axillary nerve
Brachial artery	Midhumerus	Ulnar nerve
	Biceps, triceps	Median nerve
Radial or ulnar artery	Elbow fracture or dislocation	Distal radial nerve (sensation only)
	Radius, ulna, wrist	Ulnar nerve
	Forearm and hand flexor tendons	
Thoracic great vessels	Sternum, manubrium	Innominate vein, recurrent laryngeal nerve
Descending aorta	Thoracic spine	Esophagus
	Posterior rib fracture or dislocation	Lung
	Diaphragm	Left subclavian vein (blunt)
Abdominal aorta or vena cava	Thoracic or lumbar spine	Zone 1 retroperitoneal hematoma
Suprarenal	T12-L2 (with or without spinal cord injury)	Stomach, transverse colon, pancreas
Infrarenal	L2-sacral fractures	Duodenum, small bowel
Portal vein or superior mesenteric vein	Lumbar spine fracture or ligament injury	Zone 4 retroperitoneal hematoma
	Rib fractures	Duodenum (second or third portion), head of pancreas
		Portal triad (hepatic artery, common bile duct)
Renal artery or vein	Lumbar spine	Zone 2 retroperitoneal hematoma
	Posterior rib fracture or dislocation	Kidney, proximal ureter, adrenal or gonadal vessels
Iliac vessels	Pelvic fracture	Zone 3 retroperitoneal hematoma
	Sacral fracture	Cecum (right), sigmoid colon (left)
	Sacroiliac joint disruption	Bladder, ureters

(Continued)

TABLE 42-4 Patterns of Associated Musculoskeletal and Other Structures with Specific Vessel Injury—Continued

Vessel	Musculoskeletal	Other
Femoral artery or vein	Pelvic fracture	Femoral nerve, sciatic nerve (rare)
	Acetabulum	Inguinal ligament
	Proximal to mid-femur	Spermatic cord
Popliteal artery or vein	Dislocated or "floating" knee	Tibial nerve
	Distal femur, proximal tibia	Calf compartment syndrome
Tibioperoneal vessels	Tibia, fibula	Tibial nerve, peroneal nerve (footdrop)
	Ankle fracture or dislocation	Calf compartment syndrome

TABLE 42-5 Peripheral Vascular Organ Injury Scale

Grade*	Description of Injury	ICD-9	AIS-90
I	Digital artery/vein	903.5	1–3
	Palmar artery/vein	903.4	1–3
	Deep palmar artery/vein	904.6	1–3
	Dorsalla pedia artery	904.7	1–3
	Plantar artery/vein	904.5	1–3
	Non-named arterial/venous branches	903.8/904.7	1–3
II	Basilic/cephalic vein	903.8	1–3
	Saphenous vein	904.3	1–3
	Radial artery	903.2	1–3
	Ulnar artery	903.3	1–3
III	Axillary vein	903.02	2–3
	Superficial/deep femoral vein	903.02	2–3
	Popliteal vein	904.42	2–3
	Brachial artery	903.1	2–3
	Anterior tibial artery	904.51/904.52	1–3
	Posterior tibial artery	904.53/904.54	1–3
	Peroneal artery	904.7	1–3
	Tibioperoneal trunk	904.7	2–3

TABLE 42-5 Peripheral Vascular Organ Injury Scale—Continued

Grade*	Description of Injury	ICD-9	AIS-90
IV	Superficial/deep femoral artery	904.1/904.7	3–4
	Popliteal artery	904.41	2–3
V	Axillary artery	903.01	2–3
	Common femoral artery	904.0	3–4

*Increase one grade for multiple grade III or IV injuries involving >50% vessel circumference. Decrease one grade for < 25% vessel circumference disruption for grades IV or V.

Reproduced with permission from Moore EE, Malangoni MA, Cogbill TH, et al. Organ injury scaling VII: cervical vascular, peripheral vascular, adrenal, penis, testis, and scrotum. *J Trauma.* 1996;41(3):523–524.

OPERATIVE MANAGEMENT

The goals of operative management of peripheral vascular trauma are hemorrhage control and timely restoration of limb perfusion. Patients who present without a pulse should be taken directly to the operating room. When other life-threatening injuries are not being prioritized, limb preservation mandates timely evaluation and intervention. Further, patients with an ABI of less than 0.9 in the injured extremity found to have arterial injuries with computed tomography should be immediately operatively managed. An algorithm for management of peripheral vascular trauma can be found in Figure 42-1.

Operative Exposure and Vascular Control

The two essential components of operative management of peripheral vascular trauma are operative exposure and obtaining both proximal and distal vascular control. Operative exposure begins with patient positioning and understanding precise incision location and anatomy. The incision length and location are planned in order to give the surgeon easy access to the proximal vessel above the injury for clamping or placing a vessel loop in a Potts tie configuration. At times, this will mean entering into the adjacent proximal cavity such as the abdomen or retroperitoneum to obtain vascular control.

If a tourniquet is in place, the tourniquet is removed and precise manual pressure is substituted with a hand gloved sterilely while the patient is prepped. A sterile tourniquet is then applied and a decision is made regarding heparinization of the patient with 5000 units as an intravenous bolus of heparin. Most times, this can be done safely as there is an isolated gunshot or stab wound. In a setting in which the patient has multiple wounds or there is uncertainty whether the injury is isolated, the patient is not heparinized. Junctional tourniquets may be rarely encountered in civilian practice, but they mandate entry into the proximal cavity for control of the large inflow vessels. This is true whether they are applied at the axillary or groin region. In this very unique event, sterility is prioritized after hemorrhage control. These tourniquets should not be taken down until the surgeon is ready to achieve proximal control (manual compression may be far less precise).

Vasculature control may be achieved via external compression or luminal occlusion. External compression methods include manual, sponge stick, forcep, vascular clamps, or silastic vessel loops in a Potts tie configuration. Luminal occlusion methods include Fogarty balloon catheters on a three-way stopcock and resuscitative endovascular balloon occlusion of the aorta (REBOA). While utilization of a Foley has been asserted as useful, we have found it unhelpful in both vessels and chambers. Silastic vessel loops are applied by a double pass around the vessel and then retracting until flow ceases. Table 42-6 illustrates anatomical locations of proximal and distal control and repairs for peripheral vascular trauma.

Arterial Repair

The steps in repairing vascular trauma are stepwise: diagnose the injury, expose the injury, control

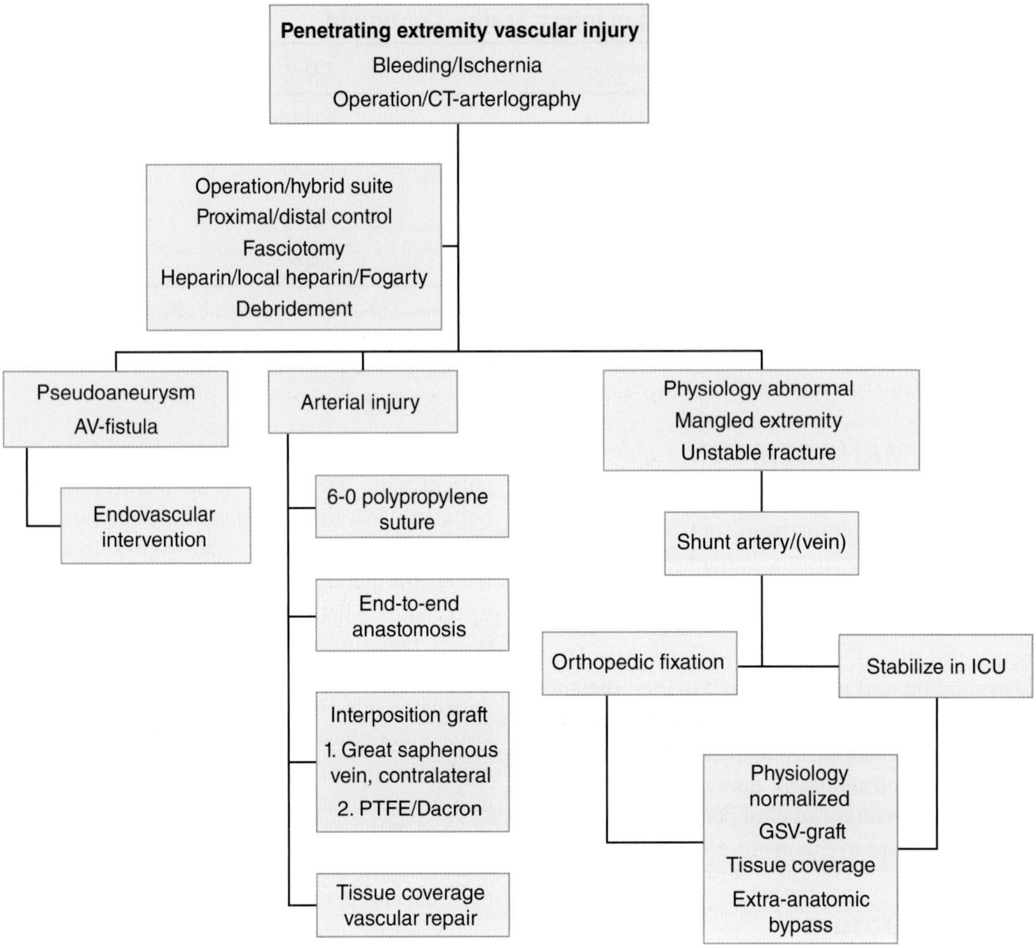

FIGURE 42-1 Management of penetrating peripheral vascular injury.

the bleeding vessels, explore the injured region and define the vessel injury, and repair the injury. During the exposure of the injured artery, the surgeon must be aware that the vessel may retract significantly in the muscle compartment if it is fully severed. This can be protective and assist in controlling hemorrhage. Exploration proximal to the injury may be needed in the appropriate plane to locate the injured proximal segment of vessel. Once the region of injury has been explored and the arterial injury has been well defined, the arterial vessel edges should be sharply debrided to normal appearing adventitia, media, and intima. Debridement is classically described first followed by passage of a Fogarty balloon catheter proximally and distally to remove potential thrombus. If possible, pass the Fogarty balloon catheter before debridement of the vessel edges to limit the handling of the intact vessel wall before suture repair. This minimizes iatrogenic damage to the vessel prior to repair. An olive-tipped syringe with heparinized saline is utilized to carefully flush both proximally and medially. Finally, an assessment of whether a tension-free arterial repair with adequate diameter can be performed should be made. Excessive tension will result in thrombosis and limb ischemia.

Primary repairs may be performed on partial short transverse lacerations from knife wounds of the arterial wall without overly constricting the

TABLE 42-6 Anatomical Location of Proximal and Distal Control for Peripheral Vascular Trauma

Peripheral Vascular Injury	Proximal Control	Incision	Repair
Common femoral artery (groin wound)	Abdomen Retroperitoneum—more time to obtain Proximal CFA just below inguinal ligament	Abdomen—lower midline Iguinal incision—vertical or horizontal	Tension-free primary repair and/or with vein patch Vein interposition Graft interposition
Superficial femoral artery (mid-thigh wound)	Above injury on SFA	Proximal to hematoma or wound and then extend distally once proximal control is obtained.	Tension-free primary repair and/or vein patch Vein interposition Graft Interposition
Popliteal artery (behind the knee wound)	Proximal popliteal or SFA	Medial thigh just proximal to the knee	Tension-free primary repair Ligation with bypass graft
Brachial artery	Axillary artery Proximal brachial artery	Medial arm to ipsilateral infraclavicular region Medial arm (bicipital groove) to antecubital fossa	Tension-free primary repair or interposition graft
Radial & ulnar artery	Proximal artery	Anterior wrist over artery	Tension-free primary repair

diameter of the vessel and impeding arterial flow. These lacerations should be extended in order to adequately examine the intima. The injury can then be primarily repaired with a permanent suture. An interrupted technique but a running suture is equally effective. Longitudinal lacerations of the vessel cannot be repaired without compromising the diameter of the artery. These injuries should be extended so as to evaluate the intima and debride when needed. Closure with a vein patch is preferred but polytetrafluoroethylene (PTFE) patch is acceptable in the common and superficial femoral artery.

In the setting of complete transection of the artery surgical dogma has proclaimed a "2-cm Rule" for the length of brachial artery and superficial femoral artery that can be resected and still accommodate a primary anastomosis. Tension should be assessed before performance of any arterial anastomosis. Mobilization of proximal and distal segments of the injured artery must yield adjacent ends without tension with the extremity fully extended at the joint. If this cannot be achieved, an interposition graft should be utilized. Autologous greater saphenous vein harvested from the contralateral uninjured extremity is the graft of choice. Autologous greater saphenous vein is preferred due to tissue properties such as elasticity, less thrombogenicity, and similar diameter of major arteries in both the arms and legs. However, in some instances both extremities are injured. PTFE can be used for the brachial artery, common femoral artery (CFA), and superficial femoral artery (SFA) in these instances. Patency rates using PTFE are improved over previous historical experiences with synthetic grafts and infection rates are low even in marginal wounds. PTFE and vein interposition grafts have equal patency rates above the popliteal artery. PTFE grafts are inferior to vein at the level of the below knee popliteal artery and distally. PTFE graft for traversing joints and smaller than 6-mm in diameter should not be utilized. Both synthetic interposition grafts and veins must have adequate tissue coverage to prevent graft complications. All arterial repairs should be evaluated intraoperatively both with pulse examination and Doppler or Duplex ultrasound studies. Intraoperative angiography can also be performed.

Single arterial vessel injuries in the distal upper and lower extremity may be ligated and not repaired or reconstructed. At the time of exploration for hemorrhage control robust back bleeding from the distal segment of the vessel can be reassuring of the surgeon's ability to ligate the vessel. As always, assessment of the distal pulses with Doppler studies should be done as well as arteriography if needed.

Venous Repair

While most minor venous injuries are ligated and this operative decision is well tolerated over long term, a discussion of venous repair is both important and informative to any complete academic considerations of peripheral vascular trauma. Although ligation is performed in patients who are undergoing only vascular damage control, primarily repair of major veins with a running Prolene suture or autologous vein patch angioplasty is recommended. A major complication of venous trauma is thrombosis. Therefore, the goal of this procedure is to maintain the vessel diameter. The principles behind venous repair are similar to arterial repair. Small partial transections may be primarily repaired. More extensive circumferential transections may require interposition of saphenous vein panel graft. This is particularly true when longitudinal vessel injuries are encountered. In general, the great saphenous vein is harvested and then the vein is opened longitudinally with Potts scissors. This vein is wrapped around a tubular structure (i.e., thoracostomy tube) and sewn in a spiral fashion. The interposition vein graft is then sewn in an end-to-end fashion with the injured vessel. All venous repairs should be surveilled in the postoperative period with physical examination, Doppler evaluation, and duplex studies, acknowledging the increased risk of deep venous thrombosis.

Ligation of the named deep veins in the lower extremity will lead to high pressures in the venous system in the lower leg and these patients may go on to develop compartment syndrome and require four-compartment fasciotomy. Therefore, if ligation is performed, extremity compression and elevation should be prioritized postoperatively, and a thorough neurovascular assessment should be performed at least as frequently as each shift.

Specific Injuries

Brachial Vessel Injuries Injuries to the brachial artery of the upper extremity most commonly occur from penetrating trauma. While fracture caused by blunt trauma can also injure the artery, this is a much less common mechanism. The most common fracture associated with the brachial artery injury is the supracondylar humerus fracture. This is a fracture of the humerus at its narrowest point above the elbow. This fracture is caused by a fall on an outstretched elbow and is the most common upper arm fracture in children. Brachial artery injuries that are actively bleeding are well controlled by a tourniquet. The diagnosis of an arterial injury should be suspected, taking care to examine both along the course of the artery and over the radial and ulnar branches. Doppler studies can also be performed. Formal angiography is usually not required.

Exposure of the injured segment of the artery is made via an incision over the medial aspect of the arm overlying the pulse in the bicipital groove. For proximal artery injuries, this incision may need to be extended onto the chest in the infraclavicular region for proximal control of the axillary artery. Distal artery injuries may require that the incision is carried across the antecubital fossa in an "S" type shape. We use vessel loops in a Potts tie configuration for partial transections. For complete transections, Bulldog vascular clamps are used to obtain control. Intravenous bolus heparinization with 5000 units is well tolerated in isolated injuries. As mentioned in the arterial repair section, debridement and passing of a Fogarty balloon catheter both proximally and distally is performed. The proximal and distal segments are then flushed with heparinized saline. An assessment is made for a tension-free repair versus interposition graft. Before tying down the last stitch, the proximal clamp should be removed so as to flush all air out of the lumen. Doppler studies and pulse evaluations should be performed after repair. Postoperative angiography can also be performed.

There is no role for brachial vein repairs although this can be attempted. Saphenous vein grafts should be the first-line conduit when interposition grafts are needed. PTFE should be used rarely as a second-line graft in the upper extremity. It is also important to note that brachial artery injuries are associated with median nerve injury. These nerve repairs should be performed by experienced surgeons in a delayed fashion if needed.

Ulnar and Radial Artery Injuries Whenever there is only one injured forearm artery, it may be ligated. In the setting of no other injuries these vessels can also be repaired. The ulnar artery is the larger artery and is the dominant blood supply to the hand in 60% of patients. The ulnar artery is the major blood supply to the palmar surface of the hand and the radial artery is the major blood supply to the dorsum. Both arteries contribute to the superficial and deep palmar arches. In a little less than a third of patients the palmar arches are incomplete.

An Allen's test can be performed quickly to evaluate blood flow to the hand. The modified Allen's test is performed by digitally compressing both the radial and ulnar arteries at the level of the wrist causing blanching of the palm. Upon release of compression of either artery, the palm should become flushed within 6 seconds. This is considered a positive test. The modified Allen's test has a sensitivity of 55% and specificity of 92% for a diagnostic accuracy of 79%. The palm can be evaluated after compressing the artery without injury for capillary refill within 6 seconds.

Common Femoral Vascular Injuries

Exposing the Femoral Vessels The patient should be placed in the supine position and the field should be prepped from the level of the umbilicus to the knee. The contralateral leg should also be prepped in the case that a saphenous graft conduit is required. A vertical incision is made either directly over the hematoma and extended above the groin crease or if there is no hematoma then a vertical incision is made at the point 2/3 of the way between the anterior superior iliac spine and the pubic tubercle. Dissection is carried down through the subcutaneous tissue to the femoral sheath. This can be guided by palpation of the pulse if the injury type allows for continued arterial pulse. In patients who are actively bleeding, the aim of the surgeon is proximal and distal control. Therefore, approaching the vessel both proximally and then distally should be the preferred strategy for these patients. The option of achieving proximal control of the external iliac artery in the retroperitoneum of the abdomen first and then approaching the groin is also performed in some cases. Upon entering the femoral sheath, the femoral vein is medial to the artery. The femoral artery must be controlled proximally, distally, and at the profunda.

Similar to brachial injuries, penetrating trauma is the most common mechanism for common femoral vascular injuries, and hemorrhage is the major presenting sign. Combined arterial and venous injuries occur commonly and diagnosis can be made via physical exam and review of the injury pattern. Massive transfusion protocols are critical elements to the preoperative management of these injuries. Most patients will have also been injured within 3 hours and be eligible to receive tranexamic acid. Tourniquets may be effective but proximal injuries may prevent them from being applicable except in the case of junctional tourniquets. In this scenario, incisions superior to the inguinal ligament are required to obtain proximal control of the external iliac artery. This vessel can be controlled with either a silastic vessel loops in a Potts tie configuration or a Satinsky vascular clamp. A vertical incision over the common femoral vessels provides exposure. For control of the common femoral artery a Satinsky clamp is used. The steps of the repair follow the same principles as described, with repair utilizing 5-0 Prolene suture. Extensive injuries to the profunda femoral or deep branch should be ligated. When injured, the common femoral vein should be repaired if possible.

Superficial Femoral Vessels Injuries to the superficial femoral vessels are diagnosed by presentation, pulse examination, and Doppler studies. The incision is made on the anterior medial thigh, and the sartorius muscle is retracted anteriorly to expose the superficial femoral vessels. Many times, continuing hemorrhage will lead the surgeon to the injury. Proximal and distal control can be obtained with silastic vessel loops. Principles of arterial repair are the same as outlined above. Most of these injuries will require an interposition graft. The superficial femoral vein should be repaired if possible but also can be ligated.

Popliteal Injuries The popliteal artery is a continuation of the superficial femoral artery as it enters into the hiatus of the adductor magnus muscle posterior to the knee. It is this particular anatomy that becomes critical when blunt forces cause posterior displacement of the tibial bone. The popliteal artery gives rise to the anterior and posterior tibial artery and is accompanied by two popliteal veins that are usually never completely transected. Popliteal artery injuries are more commonly caused by blunt trauma. Specifically, posterior dislocation of the knee is associated with a 20% to 30% rate of popliteal artery occlusion. This injury is caused due to the anatomy of the popliteal artery as it relates to the adductor and gastrocnemius muscles as it traverses the knee joint. The posterior aspect of the tibial plateau, when dislocated, stretches the popliteal artery and subsequently causes injury. Patients with posterior knee dislocation should always be screened with CT angiography for popliteal artery injury. This screening should be performed even if ABIs are normal and pulses are intact. Gunshot wounds are also an important mechanism of injury to the popliteal vessels. Of note, in the setting of popliteal vessel injury, thrombosis is more common than hemorrhage.

Medial Exposure of the Popliteal Vessels

Supragenicular Exposure Management of popliteal vessel injuries are conducted by the algorithm already outlined. After diagnosis of the injury, exposure of the suprageniculate and infrageniculate popliteal vessels are achieved by an incision on the medial thigh. The patient should be positioned supine with the leg rotated laterally and flexed with a bump placed beneath the knee joint of the extremity. A 12-cm incision ending at approximately the level of the superior edge of the medial patella should be performed between the vastus medialis and sartorius muscles. The greater saphenous vein is encountered in a more posteromedial position. The popliteal fossa is entered above the sartorius muscle after the fascia is incised. The popliteal artery can be palpated against the femur bone. The popliteal veins are usually located in a posterolateral position to the artery. Proximal and distal control can be achieved with silastic vessel loops.

Infragenicular Exposure The patient should be positioned in a supine position with the leg rotated laterally and flexed with a bump placed beneath the knee joint of the extremity. Make a longitudinal incision from below the edge of the tibia along the course of the great saphenous vein. This incision is carried through subcutaneous tissue and fascia into the deep posterior compartment. The below-knee popliteal vessels are located deeply and are partially covered by the origin of the soleus muscle. Removal of the soleus origin medially facilitates exposure of the tibioperoneal trunk and origin of the anterior tibial artery. This exposure is rarely necessary for exposure of the popliteal artery itself. Proximal and distal control of the vessels can be achieved with silastic vessel loops.

Lateral Exposure of the Popliteal Vessels

Supragenicular Exposure The patient should be placed in the supine position. The leg should be rotated medially, with flexed knee, and a bump should be placed underneath the knee joint. A 12-cm incision is made between the vastus lateralis and the biceps femoris muscles. The incision is carried through the subcutaneous tissue and fascia. A generous incision on the fascia lata is performed. When a bypass is required, a cruciate incision is made to prevent bypass graft impingement by the dense fascia lata fibers. A Beckman retractor is placed and the popliteal space is entered. The sciatic nerve, then popliteal vein will be encountered first. To expose the popliteal artery, gently retract the sciatic nerve posteriorly and then mobilize and retract the popliteal vein.

Infragenicular Exposure The lateral approach is rarely performed in trauma. While this approach may be particularly useful to avoid scarring from a previous medial approach, it is easiest to expose the popliteal vessels using the approach with which the surgeon is most familiar. Place the incision posterior to the head of the fibula and extend along the course of the fibula and directly on top of it. Note the location of the common peroneal nerve, which courses from posterior to anterior around the neck of the proximal fibula just below its head, before it branches into the superficial and deep peroneal nerves. Circumferentially elevate the periosteum of the fibula and excise the exposed segment of the fibula with a saw. The popliteal vessels and branches are found directly beneath the fibular periosteum, with the artery usually located anterior to the posterior tibial nerve and the popliteal vein. Extending the dissection distally allows exposure and control of the distal popliteal artery as well as the origins of the anterior tibial and the tibioperoneal trunk.

Popliteal artery injuries are rarely managed by primary repair. Saphenous vein interposition grafts are the preferred method of reconstruction. PTFE should never be considered unless there are no upper or lower extremity conduits for reconstruction. Restoration of perfusion to the distal limb is the priority. Although vascular reconstruction should be performed first in most cases, vascular shunts may be used initially if the orthopedic repair is being performed first. This shunt must be monitored for patency. While four-compartment fasciotomy of the lower extremity is usually performed prior to completion of the initial surgery, when there are both arterial and venous injuries four-compartment fasciotomy is required. A National Trauma Data Bank Study demonstrated a 2% mortality and an amputation rate of 19% with an increasing trend toward endovascular management for these injuries.[11]

In the above sections on popliteal vessel exposure, it cannot be overemphasized that principles of vascular reconstruction are appropriate inflow and outflow, in-line graft positioning, and appropriate tissue coverage of the interposition graft.

Tibial Injuries Individual tibial vessel injuries can be ligated if there is sufficient flow through the remaining intact vessels. Intraoperative arteriography is helpful in making this determination. When there are multiple injuries to the tibial vessels, reconstruction should be done with a saphenous vein interposition graft to the distal tibial artery where tissue coverage can occur easily.

POSTOPERATIVE COMPLICATIONS

Early Complications

The major early postoperative complications in peripheral vascular trauma are postoperative hemorrhage, thrombosis and limb ischemia, compartment syndrome, and surgical site infection.

Postoperative Hemorrhage It is rare that continued hemorrhage in the postoperative period occurs but occasionally there are acceptable reasons for this occurrence. Hemorrhage control should be the objective of the index operation as this is consistent with prioritizing life over limb. However, use of systemic anticoagulation as adjuvant therapy to arterial repairs while not usually necessary may cause hemorrhage at wound sites that were not bleeding at the time of closure. Also, infrequently, with the restoration of both circulating volume and mean arterial pressure, bleeding not seen at the time of the exploration and repair may occur. Finally, anastomotic dehiscence may occur in open wounds when vessel repairs and grafts do not have appropriate tissue coverage or additional negative pressure wound therapy devices are applied to the wound (even at low pressures). This manifests as graft erosion and resultant hemorrhage. Obscuration of the wound with such devices can conceal bleeding. Mortality in such a case is devastating and preventable. Classically, we have not described these events in textbooks although they have been discussed in trauma peer reviews extensively.

Thrombosis and Limb Ischemia For all patients who undergo vascular repairs or reconstruction the postoperative period must include surveillance of limb perfusion. The practice of patient handoffs lends itself to either missed surveillance or misinterpreted vascular examinations. These patients should ideally have handoff of their care at the bedside with a shared assessment of the pulses. Further, vein ligations place patients at higher risk for deep venous thrombosis. Duplex ultrasound should be utilized to screen these patients weekly for DVT. For patients with arterial repairs or reconstructions, vascular checks should be performed at a minimum of every hour for high-risk anastomoses. Doppler studies should be performed and documented. Pulse checks can be variable dependent upon experience of the examiner and on patient body habitus. Changes in pulses and Doppler studies not consistent with hemodynamics should result in returning the patient to the operating room for exploration of the vascular repair. Initiation of systemic anticoagulation alone is an inappropriate response to an acute change in pulse examination, especially as the most common etiology of early repair failure is technical error.

Compartment Syndrome Due to the strong association between extremity vascular injury and ischemia-reperfusion injury, compartment syndrome should always be considered. In addition to physical examination, compartment pressures may be directly measured using a Stryker needle. Delta pressure, the difference between diastolic pressure and compartment pressure, less than 30 mmHg is highly concerning for compartment syndrome. Treatment is decompressive fasciotomy, taking care to open all compartments.

Compartment syndrome of the thigh is typically caused by high-energy trauma resulting in femur fracture, but can also be the result of a large hematoma, especially in an anticoagulated patient. The thigh contains three muscular components: the anterior quadriceps, posterior hamstrings, and medial adductors. Decompression may be obtained first via a 20-cm lateral incision between the anterior and posterior compartments. The anterior compartment is the first to be encountered, and sharp incision of the fascia is used to release it. Dissection to the lateral intermuscular septum is obtained by bluntly retracting the vastus lateralis and either ligating or cauterizing the crossing branches of the deep femoral artery (profunda femoris). An incision through the intermuscular septum allows inspection and release of the posterior compartment. If the medial compartment remains tense upon palpation, a medial incision may be made; however, if the medial compartment is sufficiently relaxed following lateral decompression of the anterior and posterior compartments, further decompression is not often necessary. Medial decompression is accomplished via a medial incision from proximal- to mid-thigh followed by sharp incision of the fascia of the medial compartment.

Four-compartment fasciotomy of the lower leg is performed via medial and lateral incisions; the medial incision provides access to the deep and superficial posterior muscle compartments and the lateral incision provides access to the anterior and lateral compartments. Care should be taken to avoid the superficial peroneal nerve when performing the lateral incision, which courses over the fibular head.

Compartment syndrome of the upper arm is addressed using 15-cm anterior and posterior incisions, facilitating release of both biceps and brachialis release through the anterior incision and triceps release through the posterior incision. Compartment syndrome of the forearm is often sustained following crush or high-energy injuries. Decompression requires release of each individual component of the anterior and posterior compartments as well as the mobile wad of three, consisting of the extensor carpi radialis longus, extensor carpi radialis brevis, and brachioradialis. This is accomplished via a single longitudinal volar incision from the antecubital fossa to the crease of the wrist and either one or two longitudinal dorsal incisions. All muscles of the forearm must be meticulously inspected and debrided or decompressed as needed, as isolated compartment syndrome has been described.

In the setting of delayed diagnosis of compartment syndrome, often a result of prioritizing lifesaving efforts over limb-saving endeavors, fasciotomy and debridement should not be undertaken if it is felt that compartment syndrome has been ongoing for greater than 48 hours. This is due to the increased risk of infection among these patients, with little to no improvement in symptoms or limb function. Instead, these patients should be managed with supportive care, largely consisting of hydration to prevent kidney injury due to rhabdomyolysis as well as splinting of any muscle contractures.

Surgical Site Infection Wound infection at the site of a vascular repair is a potential devastating event. Extension of the infection to the repair or graft may cause failure or the reconstruction. Furthermore, opening the wound may expose the repair to infection, again leading to failure of the reconstruction. Thus, layered closure of the wounds to appropriately cover the repair is essential. In complicated wounds, a muscle flap may be required. The sartorius muscle is a convenient choice for the SFA. Open wounds can cause desiccation of the vessel repair and lead to hemorrhage. Infected wounds should be debrided and re-closed with tissue additional coverage over the vessel if possible.

Late Complications

Late complications of peripheral vascular trauma include anastomotic complications, venous insufficiency, and neurological complications.

Pseudoaneurysms Following penetrating trauma to the lower extremity, pseudoaneurysms can occur months or years after the initial injury. Most pseudodaneuryms are a result of penetrating trauma. Clinical signs of pseudoaneurysms include pulsatile mass, murmur over its localized region, palpable thrill, pain, and extremity edema. Pseudoaneurysms cause pain by compressing the adjacent structures, can contain thrombus, and can cause regional ischemia due to distal embolism. The most common presenting symptom is pain followed by a pulsatile mass. Open surgery is generally used for major axial vessels and smaller arteries may be managed with an endovascular approach.

Venous Insufficiency The early sequel of ligation or complex venous repair is limb edema. Phlegmasia syndromes are rare. The challenge in the literature with describing chronic venous insufficiency is the lack of long-term follow-up in this patient population.

Neurological Complications While immediate neurological complications of causalgia are more common in peripheral vascular trauma, delayed pain syndromes do occur, particularly with gunshot wounds in the extremity. These pain syndromes once thought to be infrequent are now more commonly acknowledged and treated with multimodal pain management and physical therapy. Upper extremity gunshot wounds are associated with neurological abnormalities such as palsies. Rates of such palsies range from 15% to 63% in the literature. These palsies are not related to injury to the vasculature or retained fragments. Early exploration has found nerve laceration, delayed exploration of these injuries can result in increased morbidity. The peroneal nerve was the most injured peripheral nerve of the lower extremity in a review of 60,422 leg injuries from the Trauma Register DGU between 2002 and 2015. The overall peripheral nerve injury rate was 1.8% in this large Central European Trauma Registry, and car and motorbike incidents were the leading causes of these injuries.[12] The same authors reviewed this trauma registry and found 49,382 upper extremity injuries with 3.3% peripheral nerve injuries.[12] Brachial plexopathies were very common from blunt trauma. Coexistent humerus and ulnar fractures as well as vascular lacerations were associated with peripheral nerve injury.

SPECIAL SCENARIOS

The Mangled Extremity

Mangled extremities are arms or legs that have three of four components (soft tissue, bone, vessel, and nerve) injured. These injuries result from high energy mechanisms. While salvage rates for this injury have improved significantly, in some cases, amputation results in superior clinical outcomes.[12] The acute management of insensate nonfunctional limbs historically has been controversial. For this reason, accurate assessment of the injury is performed. The Mangled Extremity Severity Scoring System is one of several well validated scoring systems for evaluation (see Table 42-7). Patients with scores equal to or exceeding 7 are recommended to undergo amputation and fitting for prosthesis.[13–15]

Vascular Damage Control Approach

Damage control principles govern our modern trauma approach. These principles are aimed at rapid control of hemorrhage and then a staged approach to avoid the lethal triad of acidosis, hypothermia, and coagulopathy. Prolonged vascular repairs in the setting of deranged physiology prioritize limb salvage over life and should not occur. Shunt placement or the difficult but necessary operative decision of ligation with the expectation of amputation in an effort to preserve the life of the patient is the right surgical decision. This decision usually occurs in the setting of concomitant severe thoracoabdominal injuries. Other rationale for early amputation includes mangled extremities with extensive soft tissue and skeletal injuries in the setting of a vascular injury and loss of sensation in the limb. Operative consultation often helps to document injury pattern and develop consensus around amputation decisions.

In the setting of isolated extremity injuries, ligation of major injuries should only occur if adequate

TABLE 42-7 Mangled Extremity Severity Scoring System

Criterion	Score
Skeletal/Soft Tissue Injury	
Low energy	1
Medium energy	2
High energy	3
Very high energy	4
Limb Ischemia	
Pulse reduced or absent (but normal perfusion)	1*
Pulseless, diminished capillary refill	2*
Cool, paralyzed, insensate, numb	3*
Shock	
SBP always >90 mmHg	0
SBP transiently <90 mmHg	1
SBP persistently <90 mmHg	2
Age	
<30 years	0
30–50 years	1
>50 years	2

*Double value if duration of ischemia exceeds 6 hours.

collateral flow. This should be assessed by palpation and Doppler studies. The radial or ulnar artery in the upper extremity usually can be ligated and similarly the anterior tibial or posterior tibial artery may be ligated in the lower extremity. However, ligation of the brachial, external iliac, superficial femoral, or popliteal arteries will likely result in limb threatening ischemia. These injuries should be stented.

Stenting

Vascular stenting is a critical strategy in the damage control approach to extremity vascular trauma. Placement of a 10 or 12 French stent in the injured proximal and distal segments of the artery allow for continued perfusion for stabilization of fractures or return to the intensive care unit for resuscitation and establishment of coagulo-competence. When commercially available vascular stents are not available, then sterile intravenous tubing, pediatric endotracheal tubes, or endotracheal suction tubing are all alternatives if appropriately sized.

After diagnosis, adequate proximal and distal control of the injured vessel should be established. Clearance of luminal thrombus is performed with a Fogarty catheter. Regional heparinized saline is injected with an olive-tipped syringe. In the setting of multicavity injury pattern, I do not perform systemic heparinization. The shunt should be carefully placed in the proximal and distal segment of the injured vessel. Care should be taken not to dissect the intima. A 2-0 silk is utilized to stabilize the shunt in location. A tie should be done both proximal and distally and around the center of the shunt. Shunting of the proximal veins should also be done to maintain the option for repair. Definitive vessel repairs should only be done when acidosis, hypothermia, and coagulopathy has been reversed. When it is the decision of the surgeon to perform ligation in a damage-control manner, then fasciotomy should also be performed.

Injuries with Poor Functional Outcomes

There are combined vascular and skeletal injuries that have very poor functional outcomes. Posterior knee dislocation with popliteal artery and vein and scapulothoracic dislocation injury with axillary artery injury. Both of these injuries are associated with both a delay in the vascular repair and association with early thrombosis, which puts the patient at risk for limb loss.

Postoperative Management

Systemic heparinization should be used whenever possible following repair of a peripheral vascular injury. Patients who have sustained traumatic brain injury (TBI), extensive torso trauma, or multiple injuries are not candidates for systemic heparin. Systemic heparin should also be avoided in the setting of existing coagulopathy, massive hemorrhage, hypothermia, and/or hypotension. Nevertheless, local heparinization may prevent thrombotic complications at the site of vascular injury and repair.

REFERENCES

1. Frykberg ER, Dennis JW, Bishop K, Laneve L, Alexander RH. The reliability of physical examination in the evaluation of penetrating extremity trauma for vascular injury: results at one year. *J Trauma.* 1991;31(4):502-511.
2. Franz RW, Shah KJ, Halaharvi D, Franz ET, Hartman JF, Wright ML. A 5-year review of management of lower extremity arterial injuries at an urban level I trauma center. *J Vasc Surg.* 2011;53(6):1604-1610.
3. Schlickewei W, Kuner EH, Mullaji AB, Götze B. Upper and lower limb fractures with concomitant arterial injury. *J Bone Joint Surg Br.* 1992;74(2):181-188.
4. Patel JA, White JM, White PW, Rich NM, Rasmussen TE. A contemporary, 7-year analysis of vascular injury from the war in Afghanistan. *J Vasc Surg.* 2018;68(6):1872-1879.
5. Inaba K, Potzman J, Munera F, et al. Multi-slice CT angiography for arterial evaluation in the injured lower extremity. *J Trauma.* 2006;60:502-506.
6. Inaba K, Branco BC, Reddy S, et al. Prospective evaluation of multidetector computed tomography for extremity vascular trauma. *J Trauma.* 2011;70(4):808-815.
7. Seamon MJ, Smoger D, Torres DM, et al. A prospective validation of a current practice: the detection of extremity vascular injury with CT angiography. *J Trauma.* 2009;67(2):238-243; discussion 243-244.
8. Feliciano DV. Evaluation and treatment of vascular injuries. In: Browner BD, Jupiter JB, Levine AM, Trafton PG, Krettek C, eds. *Skeletal Trauma: Basic Science, Management and Reconstruction.* Philadelphia, PA: Saunders Elsevier; 2009:323-340.
9. Wahlgren CM, Riddez L. Penetrating vascular trauma of the upper and lower limbs. *Curr Trauma Rep.* 2016; 2:11-20.
10. Moore E, Malangoni M, Cogbill T, et al. Organ injury scaling VII: cervical, peripheral vascular, adrenal, penis, testis, and scrotum. *J Trauma.* 1996;41:523-524.
11. Tan T-W, Armstrong FD, Zhang WW. Review of surgical treatment of popliteal artery injury: outcomes of open vs endovascular repair. *Vasc Dis Manag.* 2016; 13(8):176-182.
12. Huckhagel T, Nüchtern J, Regelsberger J, Gelderblom M, Lefering R, the TraumaRegister DGU®. Nerve trauma of the lower extremity: evaluation of 60,422 leg injured patients from the TraumaRegister DGU® between 2002 and 2015. *Scand J Trauma Resusc Emerg Med.* 2018;26:40.
13. Rush RM Jr, Kjorstad R, Starnes BW, Arrington E, Devine JD, Andersen CA. Application of the mangled extremity severity score in a combat setting. *Mil Med.* 2007;172:777-781.
14. Behdad S, Rafiei MH, Taheri H, et al. Evaluation of mangled extremity severity score (MESS) as a predictor of lower limb amputation in children with trauma. *Eur J of Pediatr Surg.* 2012;22(6):465-469.
15. Robertson PA. Prediction of amputation after severe lower limb trauma. *J Bone Joint Surg Br.* 1991;73(5): 816-818.

SELF-ASSESSMENT STUDY QUESTIONS AND ANSWERS

Questions

1. Patients with penetrating trauma to the extremity should receive what initial screening physical examination?
   A. Duplex ultrasound
   B. CT Angiography
   C. ABIs on both the injured and noninjured extremity
   D. ABIs on the injured extremity only
   E. None of the above

2. A patient with a gunshot wound to the leg and pulselessness should undergo what management?
   A. ABIs on both the injured and noninjured extremity
   B. ABIs on just the injured extremity
   C. CT angiography
   D. Operative exploration of the extremity
   E. None of the above

3. A patient with a stab wound to the right antecubital fossa who has pulsatile bleeding at the site of injury is taken to the operating room for exploration. A tension-free primary repair is performed 5 hours postinjury and distal pulses return. What additional procedure should be performed?
   A. Volar fasciotomy
   B. Additional heparinization
   C. Postoperative CT angiogram
   D. Negative pressure wound therapy for incision
   E. None of the above

4. A tourniquet is applied in the field to a patient with a stab wound to the left upper extremity. The windlass is released and no bleeding is seen at the site of the injury. How should the tourniquet be managed going forward in the patient's care?
   A. The tourniquet should be removed.
   B. The tourniquet should be reapplied with less turns of the windlass (looser).
   C. The tourniquet should be reapplied with more turns of the windlass (tighter).
   D. The tourniquet should be kept down but remain around the extremity for reapplication if the patient bleeds.
   E. None of the above is correct.

5. A 45-year-old male suffers a right midshaft femur fracture with an ABI of 0.65 for the injured limb. CTA of the leg demonstrates a cut off of the superficial femoral artery. The first priority for the vascular trauma management of this patient is?
   A. ORIF of the right femur
   B. Reestablishment of blood flow in the extremity
   C. Establishment of a massive transfusion protocol
   D. Repeating the ABIs
   E. None of the above

6. Early graft occlusion after arterial repair requires?
   A. Heparinization to a higher PTT
   B. TPA
   C. CT Angiogram
   D. Re-exploration of the graft to evaluate for technical error
   E. None of the above

SELF-ASSESSMENT STUDY QUESTIONS AND ANSWERS

7. When exploring a femoral artery injury in the lower extremity the incision should be made in what relation to the hematoma?
A. Superior to the hematoma
B. Inferior to the hematoma
C. Medial to the hematoma
D. Directly above the hematoma and extended to above the groin crease
E. None of the above

8. When a major vein has been ligated in the lower extremity the management postoperatively should include which of the following?
A. Leg elevation
B. DVT prophylaxis as soon as clinically possible
C. Compression
D. All of the above
E. None of the above

9. Supragenicular exposure of the popliteal artery is performed by dissecting between what muscles?
A. Vastus medius and sartorius muscles
B. Vastus medius and vastus lateralis
C. Vastus medius and adductor longus
D. None of the above

10. A 23-year-old male is postoperative day 1 from a reverse saphenous vein graft for a superficial femoral artery injury. He had palpable pulses upon leaving the operating room and now is found to have no pulse in the injured extremity. The next step in management is
A. CTA of the injured extremity to evaluate the graft
B. Heparinization
C. Warm the extremity and evaluate Doppler signals
D. Re-exploration of the saphenous vein graft
E. None of the above

SELF-ASSESSMENT STUDY QUESTIONS AND ANSWERS

Answers

1. C.
2. D.
3. A.
4. D.
5. B.
6. D.
7. D.
8. D.
9. A.
10. D.

CHAPTER

43 Neck Vascular Trauma

Ahmad Zeineddin and Mallory Williams

OUTLINE

- INTRODUCTION
- CLINICAL ANATOMY
- PENETRATING CERVICAL VASCULAR INJURIES
- MANAGEMENT OF SPECIFIC INJURIES
- CAROTID ARTERY INJURY
- INTERNAL JUGULAR VEIN INJURY
- VERTEBRAL ARTERY
- SUBCLAVIAN VESSELS
- THYROIDAL VESSEL INJURIES
- BLUNT CEREBROVASCULAR INJURIES (BCVI)
- OPERATIVE APPROACH TO VASCULAR INJURIES IN THE NECK

INTRODUCTION

Vascular injury may be present in up to 3% to 20% of cases of blunt and penetrating craniocervical injury.[1] There are three major mechanisms of vascular trauma in the neck, penetrating, blunt, and strangulating. Blunt carotid and vertebral injuries (BCVI) are infrequent and are 1% to 3% of all injuries, but the mortality is much higher than penetrating neck injuries. BCVI has a mortality of 23% to 28%, and over 50% of survivors have permanent neurologic sequelae.[2] Penetrating neck injuries comprise 1% of trauma registry cases but likely much less than 0.5% of all adult trauma; however, mortality is as high as 10%. The most common injuries are aerodigestive tract injuries (10%), but internal jugular (IJ) vein (9%) and carotid artery (6.6%) trauma is also frequent. Management of penetrating vascular trauma in the region of the neck requires a detailed understanding of both anatomy and surgical treatment options which we review in this chapter.

CLINICAL ANATOMY

Historically, penetrating injuries to the neck are divided into three zones dictating management (Figure 43-1)[3,4]:

- Zone I, originally located below the clavicles,[3] later revised as below the cricoid membrane,[4] includes the innominate vessels, the origin of the common carotid (CC) artery, the subclavian vessels and the vertebral artery, the brachial plexus, the trachea, the esophagus, the apex of the lung, and the thoracic duct and injuries are generally managed as thoracic injuries.
- Zone II, between the cricoid cartilage and the angle of the mandible, includes the carotid and vertebral arteries, the IJ veins, trachea, and the esophagus. Management of these injuries has been most controversial and has evolved over the decades as will be discussed later.
- Zone III, extending from the angle of the mandible to the base of the skull, includes the

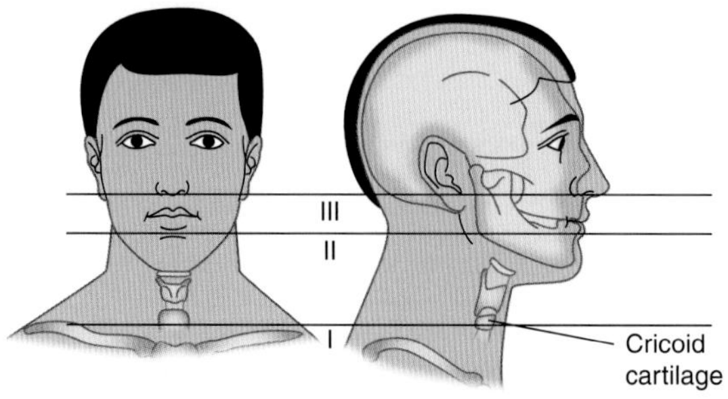

FIGURE 43-1 **Saletta zones of the neck.**

distal carotid and vertebral arteries and the pharynx, and injuries to this zone are most difficult to access and are mostly managed with endovascular techniques.

The right carotid arises from the brachiocephalic trunk, roughly at the sternoclavicular joint, while the left carotid arises from the arch of the aorta. Each CC then travels cephalad lateral to the trachea and esophagus within the carotid sheath and along the IJ veins and vagus nerves. The CC bifurcates around the superior border of the thyroid cartilage at the level of C4, giving rise to the internal carotid (IC), which continues cephalad within the carotid sheath and enters the skull, and the external carotid (EC), which exits the carotid sheath and supplies the thyroid, larynx, pharynx, face, and scalp. The IJ veins begin their course at the base of the skull at the jugular foramen and travel inferiorly in the carotid sheath lateral to the IC then the CC to join the subclavian vein at the root of the neck. The vagus nerve lies between the two vessels and posteriorly.

The other pair of major cervical arteries are the vertebral arteries. The vertebral artery arises from the subclavian artery medial to the anterior scalene muscle and travels cephalad within the transverse foramen of the cervical vertebrae starting at C6 and enters the skull through the foramen magnum to converge in the basilar artery.

PENETRATING CERVICAL VASCULAR INJURIES

Penetrating neck injuries make up 1% of trauma presentations in the United States, with a mortality rate ranging between 3% and 6%. The IJ vein is most commonly injured. Arterial injuries make up 25% of penetrating neck injuries, with the carotid injured in 80% and the vertebral in 43% of those.[5] Arterial injuries are the major cause of mortality from penetrating neck injuries and can be as high as 50% of those injured,[6] with 80% of that being attributed to ischemic stroke and the remainder to exsanguination.[7]

As with other traumatic injuries, hemodynamically unstable patients unresponsive to resuscitation belong in the operating room for emergent exploration. Similarly, patients presenting with hard signs of vascular injury (see Table 43-1) require immediate exploration and control of hemorrhage. Hemodynamically stable patients or patients with soft signs of vascular injury can undergo further diagnostic evaluation to determine the extent of injury and the need for and planning any operative intervention.

Penetrating injuries to Zone II were historically managed with mandatory operative exploration in the mid-twentieth century. In the past 2 to 3 decades, however, there has been a shift in the management toward a more selective approach for hemodynamically stable patients. Mandatory exploration resulted in a negative exploration rate of 53% to 69%.[8–12] However, around 15% had positive explorations with negative clinical examinations.[9] With the advancements in diagnostic modalities, selective management has been increasingly practiced. Arteriography and laryngoscopy/bronchoscopy reached 100% accuracy while esophagogram reached 90% accuracy.[13] Moreover, a nonzonal approach has been suggested,

TABLE 43-1 **Hard and Soft Signs of Vascular Injury in the Neck**

Hard Signs	Soft Signs
Absent pulse	Decreased pulse
Pulsatile bleeding	Minor bleeding/history of active hemorrhage
Expanding hematoma	Nonexpanding hematoma
Audible bruit or palpable thrill	Associated nerve injury
Neurological signs of ischemia	Injury in proximity to major vessel

where unstable patients undergo emergent operative exploration, and stable patients undergo appropriate diagnostic studies to include a multidetector helical computed tomography with angiography, regardless of the traditional zone of injury.[5,14,15]

MANAGEMENT OF SPECIFIC INJURIES

Initial management of neck injuries is guided by the Advanced Trauma Life Support Protocol. This is essential to understand because aerodigestive injuries are both leading causes of death in the acute and delayed setting. Establishing a definitive airway that protects the patient from hypoxia and death both from external and internal airway obstruction must be the priority. The airway must be recognized as a potential location for the drainage of arterial or venous hemorrhage. Early intubation allows for a screening evaluation of the airway in the setting of penetrating neck trauma and protection from hemorrhage into the trachea. A copious amount of blood during intubation is not consistent with isolated airway injury. If possible, safe passage of an endotracheal tube with suctioning should be the course of action.

Zone I injuries may cause pneumothorax and require thoracostomy tube placement. If a thoracostomy tube is not placed before induction of general anesthesia and institution of positive pressure ventilation, a tension pneumothorax may develop. Patients who are hemodynamically unstable with hard or soft signs of hemorrhage should have prompt vascular access established in the upper extremities and a Massive Transfusion Protocol activated, which includes tranexamic acid if the injury occurred within 3 hours. In Zone I injuries on a particular side of the patient, where there is a concern for a great vessel venous injury, intravenous administration may be infused through the contralateral extremity.

An accurate neurological examination should be achieved when possible. This is very important when undergoing operative decision-making of whether to repair or ligate the carotid artery. Patients with fixed neurological deficits should not be revascularized. Therefore, patients with these neurological deficits may undergo carotid artery ligation. The preference is to repair the carotid artery and this is achievable frequently. Historically, 30% neurological deficit rate was reported when carotid artery injuries were ligated during World War I.

Historically, mandatory exploration, selective exploration, and observation are the three different approaches to the management of penetrating neck injuries. For hemodynamically stable patients, either selective management or observation should be chosen. Mandatory exploration has been shown to have a very high negative exploration rate, cause significant morbidity, and miss injuries. While initially, mandatory exploration was chosen to avoid missing aerodigestive and vascular injuries, selective or observation management was demonstrated to be a superior approach in hemodynamically stable patients. Demetriades et al., demonstrated that the lack of hard signs of vascular and aerodigestive trauma findings had a 100% negative predictive value and are extremely reliable in excluding these wounds from the clinical picture.[16]

CAROTID ARTERY INJURY

The management of carotid artery injuries is based on the anatomical zone of the injury in the anterior neck. Zone II injuries are approached through an incision along the anterior border of the sternocleidomastoid muscle. The head should be rotated away from the injury. Exposure of the carotid artery is technically achieved in the same manner as when performing carotid endarterectomy. Dissection is carried out down to the carotid sheath and the facial vein is divided, and IJ vein is retracted laterally for exposure of the vessel. Primary repair of the artery should be done with an interrupted 6-0 Prolene suture. When primary repair is not possible, vein patch angioplasty should be done using the adjacent facial vein when conducive, Gortex graft, or Bovine pericardium. A continuous 6-0 Prolene suture may be utilized when performing a patch angioplasty. For injuries of the IC vessel that are closer to the skull base, subluxation of the temporomandibular joint, division of the posterior belly of the digastric muscle, and division of the styloid process, stylomandibular, and stylohyoid ligaments may be necessary to gain access to the vessel. The preferred incision for this exposure is a curvilinear incision starting at the mid-anterior sternocleidomastoid border and extending to the posterior auricular region to beyond the mastoid.

The role of endovascular stenting in the setting of penetrating neck injuries is evolving and there are successful reported cases throughout the literature.

INTERNAL JUGULAR VEIN INJURY

Lacerations to the IJ vein should be repaired with lateral venography with a 6-0 Prolene. When the venous repair results within 50% constriction of lumen then ligation is a reasonable operative decision. Some IJ vein injuries extend downward into the thoracic inlet. These injuries require extending the anterior border sternocleidomastoid incision into a median sternotomy. Similarly, the incision can be extended laterally for exposure of the subclavian vessels. The data suggest that the IJ vein is injured more in penetrating trauma than in blunt mechanisms.

VERTEBRAL ARTERY

Vertebral artery injuries secondary to penetrating trauma are extremely rare (<1%). The largest National Trauma Data Bank study includes 476 injuries, only 6% were operatively managed. The most common mechanism for operative management was stab wounds and vertebral artery injuries were associated with injury to the external or IJ vein. Angioembolization was performed in 8%. Eighty-six percent of patients were managed nonoperatively. The stroke rate in this series was 3% and most correlated with concomitant carotid artery injury. The mortality rate for the series was 19% and 28% in patients managed operatively. Vertebral artery injuries should be ligated. The subclavian vein is anterior to the artery and therefore retraction of this vein may be necessary to appropriately visualize the vertebral artery. Vertebral artery dominance in the population is left 45%, right 30%, and codominant 25%. Attempts at preservation of the dominant vertebral artery should be made if known. The benefits of this operative decision-making are unknown.

SUBCLAVIAN VESSELS

Subclavian vessels may be injured in Zone I neck trauma. Patients with penetrating Zone I neck injuries that are hemorrhaging should undergo a thoracotomy incision. A median sternotomy with cervical extension is performed for right subclavian vessels and a high (above the nipple) anterior lateral thoracotomy combined with a supraclavicular incision for left subclavian vessels. These injuries can be repaired through horizontal supraclavicular and/or infraclavicular incisions or high anterolateral thoracotomy or median sternotomy. Subclavian vessel injuries can be repaired with anterior or lateral arteriorrhaphy or interposition grafts.

THYROIDAL VESSEL INJURIES

The superior and inferior thyroid artery and vein originate from the EC artery and the thyrocervical trunk, respectively. These vessels can bleed significantly if they are not effectively controlled at the time of the exploration. Ligation of these vessels with a 2-0 free silk tie should be done. Care should be taken when ligating the superior thyroidal artery at the superior pole of the thyroid to avoid injury to the external branch of the superior laryngeal nerve. Injury to the gland can often be controlled with 2-0 silk sutures through the parenchyma.

BLUNT CEREBROVASCULAR INJURIES (BCVI)

BCVI has been recognized to have a much higher prevalence in trauma patients than previously thought. Previous estimates of a rate of 1 in every 1,000 patients were based on patients diagnosed after developing neurological sequelae of these injuries, which carry morbidity of 80% and mortality of up to 40%.[17–19] The screening of asymptomatic patients found the rate of those injuries to be at least 10 times higher at 1%, or even higher in more severely injured patients.[2] This has led to a big controversy on the breadth of screening for BCVI in our trauma population.

Current guidelines recommend screening any trauma patient with unexplained neurological symptoms, blunt trauma patients with epistaxis from arterial

TABLE 43-2 Treatment for CTA-Detected BCVI

Grade of Injury	Treatment
I—intimal irregularity with <25% narrowing	Aspirin or Heparin
II—dissection or intramural hematoma with >25% narrowing	Aspirin or Heparin (no bolus), can be bridged to Warfarin (goal INR 2–3)
III—pseudoaneurysm	Usually require intervention; surgery or endovascular
IV—Occlusion	Stenting to restore flow in early neurologic deficits should be considered
V—Transection/extravasation	

source, and asymptomatic patients at high risk for BCVI, which includes: GCS≤8; petrous bone fracture; diffuse axonal injury; cervical spine fracture particularly those with a fracture of C1 to C3 and those with a fracture through the foramen transversarium; cervical spine fracture with subluxation or rotational component; and Lefort II or III facial fractures.[17] In addition, the Denver screening criteria include patients with basilar skull fracture, Lefort II/III, cervical hematoma, cervical bruit, and hanging/anoxia.[20–23]

The gold standard diagnostic modality is a four-vessel cerebral angiography. However, the less invasive computed tomography angiography (CTA) performed in a multislice (8+), multidetector scanner provides similar accuracy and can be used to guide therapy (Table 43-2).[17,23–26]

Follow-up imaging at 7 days is recommended to confirm the diagnosis of BCVI.[17,23] Continue antithrombic treatment with LMWH or antiplatelet therapy followed by repeat imaging at 3 months to guide continuation or discontinuation of antithrombic treatment.[23]

OPERATIVE APPROACH TO VASCULAR INJURIES IN THE NECK

Zone I injuries are managed based on the hemodynamics of the patient and the likely injury. Highly unstable patients with injuries to the great vessels in the superior mediastinum are managed with a high ipsilateral anterolateral thoracotomy and hemorrhage control with packing or direct clamping. A slightly unstable patient would require a sternotomy with cervical or supraclavicular extension depending on the site of the injury. A more tailored incision and operative plan can be made in stable patients who can undergo CTA.[20]

The goals of operative intervention in Zone II injuries are hemorrhage control and rapid reversal of brain ischemia and neurological deficits. The incision will depend on the site and zone of injury to achieve adequate exposure for proximal and distal control. It is acceptable to ligate a unilateral IJ injury. However, bilateral IJ injuries require repair of at least one of the veins to avoid the high morbidity and mortality associated with bilateral ligation of the IJVs.[27,28] Similarly, unilateral EC ligation is well tolerated. However, bilateral EC ligation is rare and may result in cerebral ischemia.[29]

Common and IC injuries require repair, as ligation performed historically resulted in a 30% stroke rate and 45% rate of procedural mortality.[30,31] Repair options include primary arteriorrhaphy for minimal lateral injuries, a patch angioplasty, or a segmental resection and insertion of interposition graft. Field contamination may direct the choice of patch or graft, saphenous vein, or polytetrafluoroethylene (PTFE).[20,32–34] Other surgical options for reconstruction include the use of the proximal EC as an interposition graft after ligation of the distal part.[20,31] The superficial femoral artery has also been used as a graft to reconstruct the CC, followed by a PTFE interposition graft to replace the SFA.[31,35] Systemic anticoagulation is indicated when appropriate in light of concomitant injuries and when an interposition graft is needed. An intraluminal shunt is indicated when inadequate backflow is noted, or extensive repair at the base of the skull is expected.[20]

Vertebral artery injuries are managed endovascularly.[36] When encountered during exploration, hemorrhage control can be obtained with packing or the use of bone wax. This is followed by postoperative imaging and endovascular intervention as needed. Due to the risk of antegrade thrombosis after this injury, systemic anticoagulation is indicated.[20]

Rare Zone III carotid injuries can be temporized with balloon tamponade using a Foley catheter. If unsuccessful, a proximal oblique incision to expose the IC is needed, followed by passage of a Fogarty balloon catheter, and a plan for definitive endovascular intervention.[20]

REFERENCES

1. Ssenyonga PK, Le Feuvre D, Taylor A. Head and neck neurovascular trauma: clinical and angiographic correlation. *Interv Neuroradiol.* 2015;21(1):108-113.
2. Biffl WL, Moore EE, Ryu RK, et al. The unrecognized epidemic of blunt carotid arterial injuries: early diagnosis improves neurologic outcome. *Ann Surg.* 1998;228(4):462-470.
3. Monson DO, Saletta JD, Freeark RJ. Carotid vertebral trauma. *J Trauma.* 1969;9(12):987-999.
4. Roon A, Christensen N. Evaluation and treatment of penetrating cervical injuries. *J Trauma.* 1979;19(6):391-397.
5. Nowicki JL, Stew B, Ooi E. Penetrating neck injuries: a guide to evaluation and managementx. *Ann R Coll Surg Engl.* 2018;100(1):6-11.
6. Bladergroen M, Brockman R, Luna G, Kohler T, Johansen K. A twelve-year survey of cervicothoracic vascular injuries. *Am J Surg.* 1989;157(5):483-486.
7. Brywczynski JJ, Barrett TW, Lyon JA, Cotton BA. Management of penetrating neck injury in the emergency department: a structured literature review. *Emerg Med J.* 2008;25(11):711-715.
8. Tisherman SA, Bokhari F, Collier B, et al. Clinical practice guideline: penetrating zone II neck trauma. *J Trauma.* 2008;64(5):1392-1405.
9. Elerding SC, Manart FD, Moore EE. A reappraisal of penetrating neck injury management. *J Trauma.* 1980;20(8):695-697.
10. Bishara RA, Pasch AR, Douglas DD, Schuler JJ, Lim LT, Flanigan DP. The necessity of mandatory exploration of penetrating zone II neck injuries. *Surgery.* 1986;100(4):655-660.
11. Sheely CHII, Mattox KL, Reul GJJ, Beall ACJ, DeBakey ME. Current concepts in the management of penetrating neck trauma. *J Trauma.* 1975;15(10):895-900.
12. Ayuyao AM, Kaledzi YL, Parsa MH, Freeman HP. Penetrating neck wounds. Mandatory versus selective exploration. *Ann Surg.* 1985;202(5):563-567.
13. Meyer JP, Barrett JA, Schuler JJ, Flanigan DP. Mandatory vs selective exploration for penetrating neck trauma: a prospective assessment. *Arch Surg.* 1987;122(5):592-597.
14. Shiroff AM, Gale SC, Martin ND, et al. Penetrating neck trauma: a review of management strategies and discussion of the "No Zone" approach. *Am Surg.* 2013;79(1):23-29.
15. Osborn TM, Bell RB, Qaisi W, Long WB. Computed tomographic angiography as an aid to clinical decision-making in the selective management of penetrating injuries to the neck: a reduction in the need for operative exploration. *J Trauma.* 2008;64(6):1466-1471.
16. Demetriades D, Theodorou D, Cornwall E, et al. Evaluation of penetrating injuries of the neck: prospective study of 223 patients. *World J Surg.* 1997;21(1):41-48.
17. Bromberg WJ, Collier BC, Diebel LN, et al. Blunt cerebrovascular injury practice management guidelines: the Eastern Association for the Surgery of Trauma. *J Trauma.* 2010;68(2):471-477.
18. Cogbill TH, Moore EE, Meissner M, et al. The spectrum of blunt injury to the carotid artery: a multicenter perspective. *J Trauma.* 1994;37(3):473-479.
19. Davis JW, Holbrook TL, Hoyt DB, Mackersie RC, Field TO, Shackford SR. Blunt carotid artery dissection: incidence, associated injuries, screening and treatment. *J Trauma.* 1990;30(12):1514-1517.
20. Sperry JL, Guardiani E, Snow G, Meenan K, Feliciano DV. Neck and larynx. In: Feliciano DV, Mattox KL, Moore EE, eds. *Trauma.* 9th ed. McGraw Hill; 2020. http://accesssurgery.mhmedical.com/content.aspx?aid=1175133391
21. Geddes AE, Burlew CC, Wagenaar AE, et al. Expanded screening criteria for blunt cerebrovascular injury: a bigger impact than anticipated. *Am J Surg.* 2016;212(6):1167-1174.
22. Burlew CC, Biffl WL, Moore EE. Blunt cerebrovascular injuries in children: broadened screening guidelines are warranted. *J Trauma Acute Care Surg.* 2012;72(4):1120-1121.
23. Brommeland T, Helseth E, Aarhus M, et al. Best practice guidelines for blunt cerebrovascular injury (BCVI). *Scand J Trauma Resusc Emerg Med.* 2018;26(1):1-10.
24. Berne JD, Reuland KS, Villarreal DH, McGovern TM, Rowe SA, Norwood SH. Sixteen-slice multi-detector computed tomographic angiography improves the accuracy of screening for blunt cerebrovascular injury. *J Trauma.* 2006;60(6):1204-1210.
25. Eastman AL, Chason DP, Perez CL, McAnulty AL, Minei JP. Computed tomographic angiography for the diagnosis of blunt cervical vascular injury: is it ready for primetime? *J Trauma.* 2006;60(5):925-929; discussion 929.

26. Biffl WL, Egglin T, Benedetto B, Gibbs F, Cioffi WG. Sixteen-slice computed tomographic angiography is a reliable noninvasive screening test for clinically significant blunt cerebrovascular injuries. *J Trauma*. 2006; 60(4):742-745.
27. Inaba K, Munera F, McKenney MG, et al. The nonoperative management of penetrating internal jugular vein injury. *J Vasc Surg*. 2006;43(1):77-80.
28. McGovern PJ, Swan KG. Management of bilateral internal jugular venous injuries. *Injury*. 1985;16(4):259-260.
29. Nasr MM. Bilateral external carotid artery ligation: a life saving procedure in severe maxillofacial trauma. *Int J Surg Case Rep*. 2015;8:81-83.
30. Lawrence KB, Shefts LM, McDaniel JR. Wounds of common carotid arteries; report of 17 cases from World War II. *Am J Surg*. 1948;76(1):29-37.
31. Karaolanis G, Maltezos K, Bakoyiannis C, Georgopoulos S. Contemporary strategies in the management of civilian neck zone II vascular trauma. *Front Surg*. 2017; 4(September):1-10.
32. Brown MF, Graham JM, Feliciano DV, Mattox KL, Beall AC, DeBakey ME. Carotid artery injuries. *Am J Surg*. 1982;144(6):748-753.
33. Feliciano DV. A new look at penetrating carotid artery injuries. *Adv Trauma Crit Care*. 1994:319-345.
34. Feliciano DV. Management of penetrating injuries to carotid artery. *World J Surg*. 2001;25(8):1028-1035.
35. Jacobs JR, Arden RL, Marks SC, Kline R, Berguer R. Carotid artery reconstruction using superficial femoral arterial grafts. *Laryngoscope*. 1994;104(6 Pt 1):689-693.
36. Albuquerque FC, Javedan SP, McDougall CG. Endovascular management of penetrating vertebral artery injuries. *J Trauma*. 2002;53(3):574-580.

SELF-ASSESSMENT STUDY QUESTIONS AND ANSWERS

Questions

1. The borders of Zone II of the neck are?
   A. The cricoid cartilage and sternoclavicular joint
   B. The first rib and the angle of the mandible
   C. The cricoid cartilage and the angle of the mandible
   D. None of the above
   E. All of the above

2. The appropriate incision location for penetrating trauma to Zone II of the neck with a unilateral hematoma is?
   A. Anterior border of the sternocleidomastoid muscle
   B. Transverse incision at the level of the cricoid cartilage
   C. An incision directly over the hematoma extended vertically both superior and inferior
   D. None of the above
   E. All of the above

3. Penetrating trauma to the jugular vein should be definitively managed how?
   A. Attempted primary repair but ligation if primary repair is not possible
   B. Ligation without any other considerations
   C. Packing
   D. None of the above
   E. All of the above

4. Selective management of Zone II injuries requires?
   A. Physical examination to detect injuries
   B. Screening CTA to evaluate injuries
   C. Operative exploration for all patients
   D. None of the above
   E. All of the above

5. Blunt carotid and vertebral injuries are rare but should be screened for in what circumstances?
   A. Patients with GCS < 8
   B. Patients with injuries to C1-C3
   C. Patients with petrous bone fracture
   D. Patients with Lefort II or III injuries
   E. All of the above

6. Zone I injuries may be associated with what other injury?
   A. Pneumothorax
   B. Rib fracture
   C. Anterior scalene muscle injury
   D. None of the above
   E. All of the above

7. A 35-year-old male who fell from a two-story window presents unconscious with only evidence of a C3 fracture. What further initial management should the patient receive?
   A. CTA of the neck vessels
   B. MRI of the spine
   C. CT of the pelvis
   D. EEG
   E. All of the above

SELF-ASSESSMENT STUDY QUESTIONS AND ANSWERS

8. Operative exposure of the carotid artery involves which maneuvers?
A. Incision at the anterior border of the sternocleidomastoid muscle, division of the facial artery, and retraction of the internal jugular vein
B. Incision at the anterior border of the sternocleidomastoid muscle, division of the facial vein, and retraction of the internal jugular vein
C. Incision at the anterior border of the sternocleidomastoid muscle, division of the SCM muscle
D. None of the above
E. All of the above

9. Repair options for the carotid artery include?
A. Saphenous vein or PTFE patch
B. Superficial femoral artery interposition graft with PTFE interposition for SFA repair
C. PTFE interposition graft
D. Proximal external carotid interposition graft
E. All of the above

10. When should a shunt be used while repairing the carotid artery?
A. Inadequate backflow
B. Expected lengthy repair
C. Prolonged repair of the carotid artery at the base of the skull
D. None of the above
E. All of the above

SELF-ASSESSMENT STUDY QUESTIONS AND ANSWERS

Answers

1. A.
2. A.
3. A.
4. B.
5. E.
6. E.
7. A.
8. B.
9. E.
10. E.

CHAPTER

44 Central Vascular Trauma

Mallory Williams and Mohamed F. Osman

OUTLINE

EPIDEMIOLOGY

BLUNT TRAUMA

DIAGNOSIS

- **Physical Examination**
- **Computed Tomography of the Abdomen**
- **Focused Assessment with Sonography in Trauma**
- **Exploratory Laparotomy**

GENERAL PRINCIPLES OF MANAGEMENT OF ABDOMINAL VASCULAR TRAUMA

- **Damage Control Principles**
- **Operative Management**
  - Aortic Control
    - *Supraceliac aortic control*
    - *Thoracic aortic control*
    - *Resuscitative endovascular balloon occlusion of aorta (REBOA)*
    - *Accessing the femoral artery*
  - Aortic Zones
    - *Placement of the balloon catheter*
  - Evidence for REBOA

MANAGEMENT OF PENETRATING ABDOMINAL VASCULAR INJURIES

- **Zone I Vascular Injuries (Central Abdominal Hematoma)**
  - Suprarenal Aortic Control
  - Supramesocolic Vascular Injuries/Suprarenal Aortic Injuries
  - Celiac Axis Injuries
  - Superior Mesenteric Artery Injuries
  - Superior Mesenteric Vein Injuries
  - Proximal Renal Artery Injuries
  - Inframesocolic Vascular Injuries
  - Infrarenal Aortic Injuries

MANAGEMENT OF BLUNT TRAUMATIC ABDOMINAL VASCULAR INJURY

- **Zone II Abdominal Vascular Injuries**

ENDOVASCULAR MANAGEMENT OF RENAL TRAUMA

- **Penetrating Injuries**

ZONE III ABDOMINAL VASCULAR INJURIES

- **Iliac Artery**
- **Iliac Vein**

EPIDEMIOLOGY

Abdominal vascular injuries are mostly represented in major urban civilian trauma centers. This is quite different when compared to abdominal vascular injuries seen in the war, which range from 2% to 3% from World War II to the Iraqi War.[1–3] Currently, blunt mechanisms are responsible for approximately 5% of these injuries while penetrating trauma accounts for 10%.[4] In the classical trauma literature, gunshot wounds are responsible for up to 25% of abdominal vascular injuries.[5] In a more recent 10-year review, 78% of patients experiencing abdominal vascular trauma had gunshot wounds and 42% of these patients had injuries to multiple abdominal vessels.[6] In all cases, prolonged shock from uncontrolled hemorrhage is associated with mortality.

BLUNT TRAUMA

The typical mechanism associated with abdominal vascular injuries is not blunt force trauma but rather penetrating trauma. However, when blunt force trauma is the cause of abdominal vascular injuries, it results from an acceleration–deceleration pattern that produces an avulsion of branches of major vessels causing hemorrhage. The other pattern is a blunt force that produces thrombosis which typically occurs after tearing of the intimal layer of arterial wall and can be seen after renal vascular trauma. Finally, cases where there are full thickness tears to the vascular wall lead to massive hemorrhage and/or pseudoaneurysms can occur. Massive hemorrhage can result from blunt force trauma and renal vein, mesenteric vessel, or aortic disruption. Frequently, seat belt injuries present with an exquisitely tender abdominal examination and ecchymoses over the distribution of the seat belt across the abdomen. These patients with pseudoaneurysms classically are seen with blunt hepatic trauma and can present with hematemesis after high-grade liver injury. These patients require hepatic angiography and coil embolization of the pseudoaneurysm of the hepatic artery. Interventional radiology techniques for the control of hepatic hemorrhage are discussed below.

DIAGNOSIS

PHYSICAL EXAMINATION

Physical examination must always be our initial approach to a trauma patient. Fifty percent of patients who arrive at the trauma center in shock (SBP < 80 mmHg) will have major vascular injuries.[7] Patients in shock will have cool skin and may have altered consciousness. Furthermore, pulse rate and character are valuable in determining the likelihood of hemorrhage from abdominal vascular trauma. Patients who are not on heart rate control medications and who manifest high pulse rates (heart rate $>$ 100) with thready characteristics should be suspected of having an ongoing hemorrhage. A distal pulse is absent in 90% of patients who have a major arterial injury.[8] Understanding the events of the scene are very helpful because the context of certain traumas will lead to greater suspicions of abdominal vascular injury (i.e., high-speed collision vs ground-level fall). Abdominal tenderness and abdominal wall hematoma at physical examination are also findings highly suspicious for intra-abdominal vascular injury. The central dictum is to locate the blood loss in a body cavity. Therefore, abdominal distention in the setting of shock should always be considered findings associated with abdominal vascular trauma. One specific physical examination finding is the seat belt sign or abdominal wall contusion extending across the abdomen in the distribution of the restraining device. Approximately, 30% of patients presenting with a classic seat belt–related abdominal wall bruises at physical examination have associated significant intra-abdominal injury.[9]

COMPUTED TOMOGRAPHY OF THE ABDOMEN

Computed tomography is the imaging study of choice for the evaluation of hemodynamically stable patients with abdominal trauma. The efficiency of this study has led many traumatologists to widen the traditional selection criteria based on hemodynamic stability. The so-called "quasi" stable patient is currently often taken to the CT scanner because of the overall speed and value of the information. This is not appropriate for hospital facilities without the capabilities for definitive surgical management. Such imaging studies are often interpreted by surgeons for the presence or absence of gross blood in the peritoneal cavity and organ injury. The structural setup of the trauma center in relation to the distance of the CT scanner from the trauma resuscitation bay and the operating room become determining elements of whether this type of clinical decision-making is deployed. But it must be acknowledged that the overall efficiency of gaining a tremendous amount of clinical information has been greatly increased. For patients with blunt mechanisms to the body, CT scanning has an accuracy of 98.3%.[10] For hemodynamically stable patients with penetrating trauma, CT scanning has also been shown to be useful. The use of mandatory exploratory laparotomy for stab wounds of the anterior abdominal wall resulted in 30% to 50% nontherapeutic operations.[10–14] Triple-contrast CT has an excellent sensitivity ranging from 89% to 100% for excluding injury requiring trauma laparotomy.[15,16] Nontherapeutic laparotomy rates with triple-contrast CT are now as low as 3%.[17] CT scanning that demonstrates no intra-abdominal injuries has also been shown to be cost-effective by facilitating definitive triage and early discharge.[18]

FOCUSED ASSESSMENT WITH SONOGRAPHY IN TRAUMA

Focused assessment with sonography in trauma (FAST) when performed serially has demonstrated 85% sensitivity for hemoperitoneum necessitating laparotomy.[19] Surgeon performing sonography in trauma patients was most accurate for hypotensive patients with blunt abdominal trauma with a sensitivity and specificity of 100%.[20] While across all trauma patients computed tomography is a more accurate study for hemoperitoneum, it is the hemodynamically unstable patient who will not receive this imaging modality. Therefore, those patients with hypotension who are not rapid responders to fluid resuscitation require rapid exploratory laparotomy. FAST examinations provide both accurate and efficient diagnoses of abdominal hemorrhage. FAST should be the initial imaging examination for all patients suspected of having trauma.

EXPLORATORY LAPAROTOMY

Although rarely discussed in major trauma textbooks, exploratory laparotomy for diagnosis of abdominal vascular injuries does and should occur. There are several scenarios of trauma patients experiencing hemodynamic lability or falling serum hemoglobin levels after admission, which lead to exploratory laparotomy in the setting of poorly defined abdominal injuries. Hemodynamically stable patients experiencing thoracoabdominal trauma may go for a diagnostic laparoscopy to evaluate the left diaphragmatic leaflet because of the poor sensitivity of CT scanning for detection of these injuries. Episodes of hypotension in the CT scan suite or in the route to the operating room often cause surgeons to perform exploratory laparotomies instead of the initially intended procedure. The algorithm for the management of pelvic fractures in patients with hypotension includes exploratory laparotomy. One component of this procedure is to effectuate preperitoneal packing for hemorrhage control and the other is to perform exploration of the abdominal cavity to diagnose or rule out associated injuries secondary to the significant force involved in the trauma. Furthermore, although rare, the patient with the so-called "soft" blood pressure, who is a transient responder in the setting of low-grade solid organ injuries and no definitive major vessel injury on imaging, may eventually undergo abdominal exploration for intermittent hypotension not explained by current injuries. And finally, the rarest clinical scenario that I have witnessed is the patient with delayed cardiac tamponade secondary to a thoracoabdominal stab wound where blood evacuated the pericardial space initially through the pericardial defect and therefore masked the hemodynamic consequences of the injury. When the evacuation of blood from the pericardial space ceased, then the patient became hypotensive. During this period, he was placed on the operating room table for diagnostic laparoscopy. He went on to receive a diagnostic laparotomy simultaneously with a left lateral thoracotomy.

GENERAL PRINCIPLES OF MANAGEMENT OF ABDOMINAL VASCULAR TRAUMA

DAMAGE CONTROL PRINCIPLES

Abdominal vascular trauma that leads to massive hemorrhage requires implementation of damage control protocols. Damage control surgery (DCS) is divided into three phases: (1) abbreviated laparotomy (2) intensive care unit, and (3) definitive surgery. DCS principles shorten the time that patients spend in their initial operative exploration to avoid the development of the vicious triad of hypothermia, coagulopathy, and acidosis. The goals of the abbreviated laparotomy are for the early control of hemorrhage and gastrointestinal and genitourinary contamination followed by a staged approach to definitive surgery. Massive transfusion protocols that include both blood components and the antifibrinolytic, tranexamic acid, should be employed early in the management of these patients. Duchesne demonstrated that when DCS principles were combined with damage control resuscitation or limited crystalloid infusion until hemorrhage control was performed together with balanced ratio blood component transfusion, superior clinical outcomes were achieved.[21] When DCS coordinated surgical intensive care is a critical aspect of the damage control paradigm and it allows for the rapid correction of acidosis and hypothermia, both improving overall mortality and making possible the return to the operating room for definitive surgery. Goals that should be achieved during the ICU phase of care are a core body temperature above 35°C, a serum pH between 7.30 and 7.45, base deficit greater than −5, correction of platelet levels to above 50,000, and a pro time of < 12 seconds (see Table 44-1). These patients have open abdominal cavities and therefore an additional element of the ICU phase must be an improvement of overall abdominal wall compliance through mobilization of fluid from the third space by active diuresis if the patient can tolerate this without producing hypotension. Diuresis may also decrease bowel wall edema and facilitate abdominal wall closure without advanced reconstructive techniques.

OPERATIVE MANAGEMENT

Patients are prepped in the trauma operating room from the chin to mid-thighs with either a povidone-iodine solution or chlorhexidine gluconate solution. A nasogastric or oral gastric tube and Foley catheter are inserted. Intravenous access should be obtained with large bore peripheral catheters in the upper extremities. When this is not possible due to shock or fractured extremities, 8 French cordis should be placed in the femoral vein preferably. When there is thoracoabdominal penetrating trauma mechanism and hypotension, intravenous access should be obtained above and below the diaphragm. The blood bank should be notified by the circulating nurse of the operating room number and location for the delivery of blood products. Surgical time-outs are effective elective surgery protocols that are generally not applicable in trauma cases. These patients should receive preoperative antibiotics if possible and an incision should be made as soon as it can be performed.

The incision made is from the patient's sternum to the pubic symphysis. Preparation is made to pack off all four quadrants of the abdomen with laparotomy sponges upon entering the peritoneal cavity. Attention to where hemorrhage or hematoma is allowed for an understanding of what abdominal vascular structures may be injured. This is conceptualized using the Abdominal Zone System (see Figure 44-1). Zone I is the central area of the abdomen where the aorta and vena cava are located in the retroperitoneal plane as well as the origins of the renal arteries and veins as well as the superior and inferior mesenteric vessels. Zone II is the lateral retroperitoneal aspects of the abdominal cavity, which include the middle and distal right and left renal arteries and

TABLE 44-1 Zone I Hematomas, Potential Vascular Injuries, Aortic Control Maneuvers

Region of Zone I Hematoma	Potential Vascular Injuries	Aortic Control Maneuver
Supramesocolic	Suprarenal abdominal aorta	Split lesser omentum and hiatus
	Proximal superior mesenteric artery	Left medial visceral rotation
	celiac axis	Above and REBOA
	Proximal renal artery	
Inframesocolic	Infrarenal abdominal aorta	Upward retraction of the transverse mesentery and evisceration of the small bowel to the right Retroperitoneum is opened to left renal vein Clamp inferior to left renal vein
	Inferior vena cava	
		Right medial visceral rotation

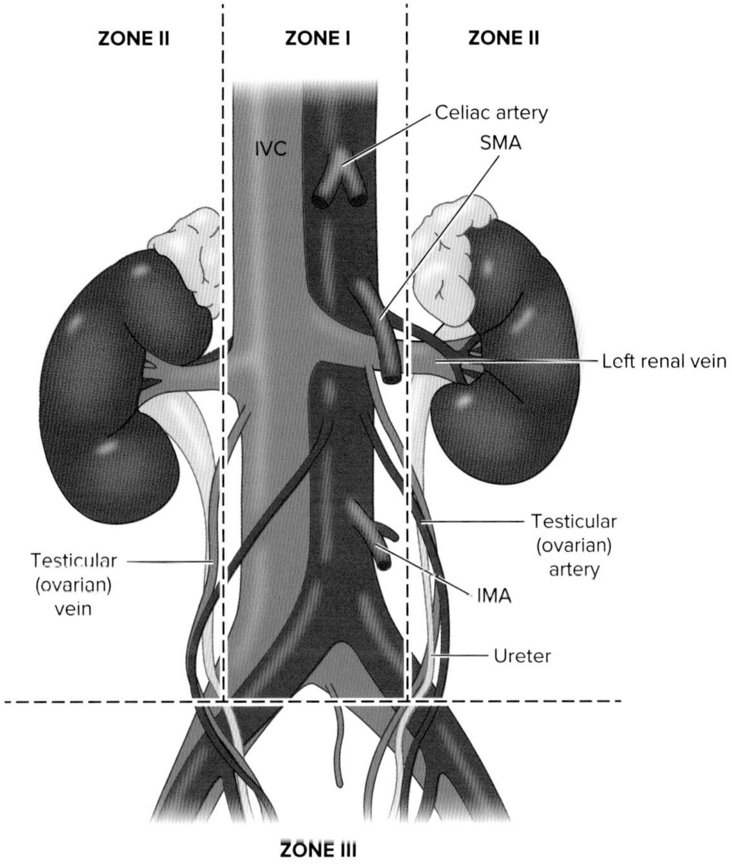

FIGURE 44-1 **Zones of abdominal vascular injury.**

veins. Zone III includes the right and left iliac arteries and veins. In this chapter, we discuss the porta hepatis as a unique subsection of the abdomen. However, traditionally superior mesenteric vein (SMV)–portal vein injuries are included in Zone I vascular injury discussions. After careful packing of all four quadrants of the abdomen, a coordinated approach with the anesthesiologist should be utilized to resuscitate the patient in order to restore the circulating volume. It may be necessary to have an additional member of the anesthesia team to join this effort for maximal effectiveness. Blood products should be administered through a rapid transfuser with a heated line. Intravenous antibiotics should be readministered during the operating serial, arterial blood gases will be necessary to inform the surgical team of the patient's physiology. Base deficits that continue to exceed 6 mmol/L should prompt implementation of damage control surgery strategies.

Aortic Control

Supraceliac aortic control If intra-abdominal packing and infusion of blood components are ineffective in elevating the mean arterial pressure, supraceliac control of the abdominal aorta should be achieved through rightward retraction of the left lateral segment of the liver and dissection through the gastro hepatic ligament followed by lateral retraction of the esophagus and stomach. At this point, a sponge stick or the more reliable compression of the aorta against the spine can be achieved with hand compression. If an aortic clamp is to be applied, the right crus of the diaphragm is transected with Metzenbaum scissors for appropriate exposure of the vessel.

Thoracic aortic control In scenarios where the proximal abdominal aorta is injured and supraceliac control is not possible, then a left anterior lateral thoracotomy can be performed. An incision with a number 10 blade should be carried out from the sternum to the posterior axillary line above the fifth rib. The intercostal muscles should be incised and the rib retractor should be inserted. The inferior pulmonary ligament lung should be retracted upward and the aorta can be cross-clamped with a straight Satinsky or side biting clamp at the level of the diaphragm after blunt dissection of the vessel.

Resuscitative endovascular balloon occlusion of aorta (REBOA) REBOA is hemorrhage control via aortic endoluminal placement of a balloon catheter (Figure 44-2). These advanced techniques are for nonresponders to resuscitation which typically are patients with abdominal vascular injuries experiencing noncompressible rapid exsanguination. Experienced trauma surgeons have always intuitively known that the time and maneuvers necessary to expose and control the abdominal vascular injury both caused additional hemorrhage and stress. Technical ability in trauma surgery was often defined in terms of navigating these challenging clinical scenarios in order to preserve the life of these patients. As a traumatologist who also serves as a combat surgeon, I recognize the tremendous importance of innovating hemorrhage control procedures. REBOA provides a sensible strategy for controlling excess hemorrhage from abdominal vascular injuries that can be implemented in austere environments such as those where forward resuscitative surgical teams and other specialized surgical teams operate. Discussion of important details of this procedure are presented in this chapter; however, a more complete examination of this technique is reviewed in Chapter 46.

Accessing the femoral artery REBOA is performed through a direct cut down to the femoral artery or

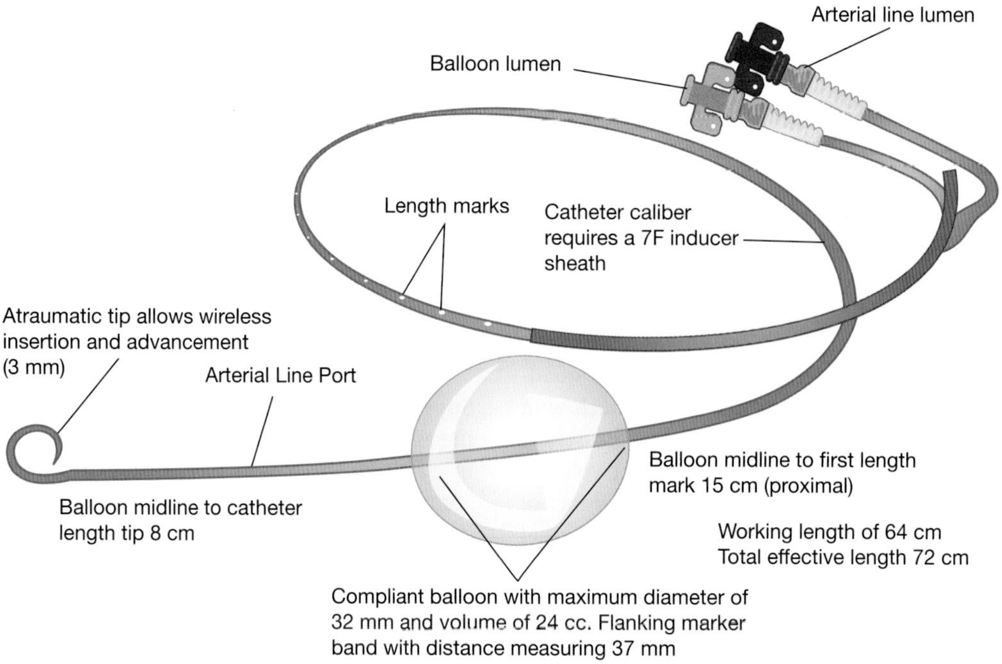

FIGURE 44-2 REBOA catheter.

percutaneous Seldinger technique. It cannot be overstated how important gaining initial access to the common femoral artery is. The cut-down is performed after palpation of the femoral artery pulse which is most commonly located at the halfway point between the anterior superior crest of the iliac bone and the pubic tubercle. The femoral artery lies anterior and lateral to the femoral vein. A single anterior wall puncture should be performed whether using a cut-down or Seldinger procedure for access of the vessel. There is an association between low puncture sites and both pseudoaneurysms and arteriovenous fistulas as well as a high risk of retroperitoneal bleeding with high puncture sites.[22] The femoral pulse is over the CFA in approximately 93% of limbs, and the CFA is over the medial aspect of the femoral head in 78% of limbs.[22] So the most reliable landmark for both the incision for cut down and the arterial puncture is the maximal arterial pulse. For patients with weak or absent pulses due to hemorrhage, the most reliable landmark in individuals of average body build is 2 finger breadths (2.5 cm) lateral to the pubic tubercle below the inguinal ligament. In the American Association for the Surgery of Trauma AORTA Registry, up to 50% of patients required cut downs for accessing the common femoral artery for REBOA.[23] Both fluoroscopic and ultrasound-guided arterial puncture can be utilized as well. The incidence of pseudoaneurysm formation can be significantly reduced to 2.6% with the use of ultrasound guidance mainly by avoiding inadvertent puncture of the external iliac artery and superficial and deep femoral artery.[24] In a prospective evaluation of ultrasound-guided CFA puncture, it was found that the ultrasound-guided technique reduced the time to puncture and the number of attempts in obese patients and patients with weak or absent pulses.[24]

Aortic Zones

There are three aortic zones for placement of the occluding balloon catheter. Zone I is in the descending aorta distal to the subclavian artery to above the celiac artery. Zone II is defined as between the celiac artery and the renal arteries. Balloon occlusion should not occur in this zone. Zone III is the aortic and vena cava bifurcations. Measurements for placement of the catheter in the different zones must be performed. For Zone I placement, measurement is done from the sternal notch to the access site of the common femoral artery. For Zone III placement, the measurement is from the xiphisternal process to the access site of the common femoral artery. There are both fluoroscopically guided balloon catheters and those that do not require image guidance for placement.

Placement of the balloon catheter The major initial step in the placement of the balloon catheter is the establishment of access to the common femoral artery. First-generation balloon catheters required 7 French access catheter. The catheter is then preflushed before placement. After placement of the catheter, the balloon is inflated to occlude or partially occlude the aorta. For patients receiving total occlusion, the contralateral pulse of the common femoral artery should be absent. Attention to stabilization of the balloon catheter in its final position is essential to prevent the known complication of balloon migration. Limits of timing of a balloon catheter occluding either Zones I or II have not been well established. Current expert opinion is evolving around a Zone I occlusion time of 30 minutes as optimal.

Complications:

- Balloon migration
- Arterial puncture complications
- Distal embolization
- Amputation

Evidence for REBOA

The initial clinical series by Brenner et al., described six patients with a mean systolic pressure of 50 mmHg and a base deficit of 13 mmol/L.[25] Insertion of the catheter with three placements in Zones I and III, placements in Zone III resulted in a mean increase in systolic blood pressure by 55 mmHg.[25] There are several large series that support the use of endovascular balloon occlusion in exsanguinating noncompressible hemorrhage.[26–29] Even with more innovative smaller introducers (7 Fr) and partial occlusion techniques, the issue however remains controversial. An American national study demonstrated no improvement in overall survival.[30] It remains to be seen whether this is an intervention that can be successfully deployed to prehospital trauma personnel in America. Limited success has been already demonstrated in London.[31] What can be clearly stated is that the feasibility of deploying a resuscitative balloon for aortic occlusion has been demonstrated and mean arterial pressures are significantly elevated.

MANAGEMENT OF PENETRATING ABDOMINAL VASCULAR INJURIES

In the contemporary literature, a multicenter review of trauma laparotomies in patients with an average Injury Severity Score of 19 revealed a mortality rate of 21% with 60% of these deaths being due to hemorrhage.[32] Therefore, approximately one in five trauma patients receiving laparotomy at reputable American College of Surgeons' verified trauma centers for severe injuries result in death with the majority being due to hemorrhage.

ZONE I VASCULAR INJURIES (CENTRAL ABDOMINAL HEMATOMA)

Suprarenal Aortic Control

All Zone I vascular injuries resulting from penetrating trauma should be explored. Zone I is divided by the transverse mesocolon into the supramesocolic region and the inframesocolic region. Abdominal exploration with the identification of a hematoma in either of these regions suggests vascular structures that have been injured (see Table 44-1). Supramesocolic hematomas suggest injury to the suprarenal aorta, proximal superior mesenteric artery (SMA), and proximal renal artery. In these clinical scenarios, control of the aorta as it enters the abdomen at the diaphragm is important. We have already discussed several methods of obtaining aortic control at the diaphragm. Another critical maneuver for achieving aortic control is a left visceral medial rotation that includes mobilization of the descending colon, left kidney and spleen, tail of the pancreas, and fundus of the stomach to the midline. When performed appropriately, the left lateral portion of the aorta from the aortic hiatus to the bifurcation is exposed for control of its branches. Care must be taken not to damage the spleen, tail of the pancreas, and kidney, and its vasculature during this mobilization. When possible, do not mobilize the kidney with this maneuver. Exposing the distal thoracic aorta by transecting the left diaphragmatic crus is helpful for clamp placement. Transection of the crus is usually best performed at about the 2 o'clock position. The left visceral medialization requires more time than controlling the suprarenal aorta through the lesser omentum with digital dissection of the hiatal muscle fibers. However, a surgeon's experience with each of these techniques ultimately determines the time to completion of aortic control with these maneuvers. It is quick to obtain a sponge stick on the suprarenal aorta at the hiatus after a longitudinal transection of the lesser omentum and leftward retraction of the esophagus and stomach. At this time, a left medial visceral rotation maneuver can be performed for exposure of aortic branches.

Active hemorrhage from the supraceliac aorta may require division of the celiac axis to accommodate repair of the aorta. This leads to gallbladder necrosis and therefore mandates a cholecystectomy likely at a later operation where definitive management is being performed within the damage control paradigm.

Supramesocolic Vascular Injuries/ Suprarenal Aortic Injuries

Survival after injury to the suprarenal aorta is low (<40%) and highly dependent on the experience of the team caring for these patients. Small penetrating lacerations to the suprarenal aorta should be repaired with lateral arteriorrhaphy with 3-0 polypropylene suture. Small adjacent injuries can be connected and repaired as one with polypropylene suture in a transverse manner so as not to narrow the vessel. Patch angioplasty should be performed when there are larger defects in the aortic wall where attempts at repair will only narrow the vessel or produce tension on the suture line.

Polytetrafluoroethylene (PTFE) is recommended for patch angioplasty. In the setting of contamination secondary to hollow viscus injury, spillage from the injured intestine is controlled and the bowel is packed out of the field. The trauma surgeon and operative team should change gloves and utilize new instruments to perform the aortic repair. Synthetic material is used for either patch angioplasty or interposition grafts. A logical separation of the repair of the aorta and the hollow viscus injury must be executed. When an interposition graft is required, proximal and distal control should be obtained as an assessment for the feasibility of safe anticoagulation. At the completion of sewing the graft, the distal clamp is released and the proximal clamp is released slowly and in coordination with the anesthesiologist administering fluid to avoid hypotension. The retroperitoneum should be irrigated and closed when possible. Aortic segmentectomy followed by end-to-end anastomosis is technically risky. The overall mobility of the aorta in this region is low and an anastomosis with tension is likely to fail.

Cross-clamping of the supraceliac aorta can result in severe lower extremity ischemia. Lower extremity compartment pressures below the knees bilaterally should be measured, and if they exceed 30 to 35 mmHg, four-compartment fasciotomies of each extremity should be performed. Baseline pulse examinations should be documented. In patients receiving damage control surgery, this procedure should be able to be performed either quickly with a double team approach in the operating room or in the trauma intensive care unit while concomitant warming and resuscitation are taking place. Consistent with the bloody triad of acidosis, hypothermia and coagulopathy fasciotomy sites can be the source of significant blood loss and therefore fasciotomies may be delayed with serial lower extremity pressure monitoring until compartment pressures are closer to 35 mmHg and there has been time to resolve coagulopathy.

Celiac Axis Injuries

This is a very rare injury pattern. Asensio documents a series of 13 patients with a 62% mortality. Complex repair should not be attempted as all survivors received ligations of the celiac axis and chole cystectomy. Injuries requiring simple repairs may be attempted. The left gastric artery and proximal splenic arteries should be ligated. The diameters of their lumens make viable repair with lateral arteriorrhaphy infrequent. The common hepatic artery lumen has a wider diameter and may be repaired with lateral arteriorrhaphy, end-to-end anastomosis, saphenous vein, or prosthetic interposition graft. The hepatic artery may be ligated proximal to the gastroduodenal artery.

Superior Mesenteric Artery Injuries

These injuries carry high mortality of 43%. The SMA is divided into what is called Fullen Zones and management of injuries to this artery is based on the Fullen Zone of injury (see Figure 44-3). Fullen Zone I injuries to the SMA are managed by either division of

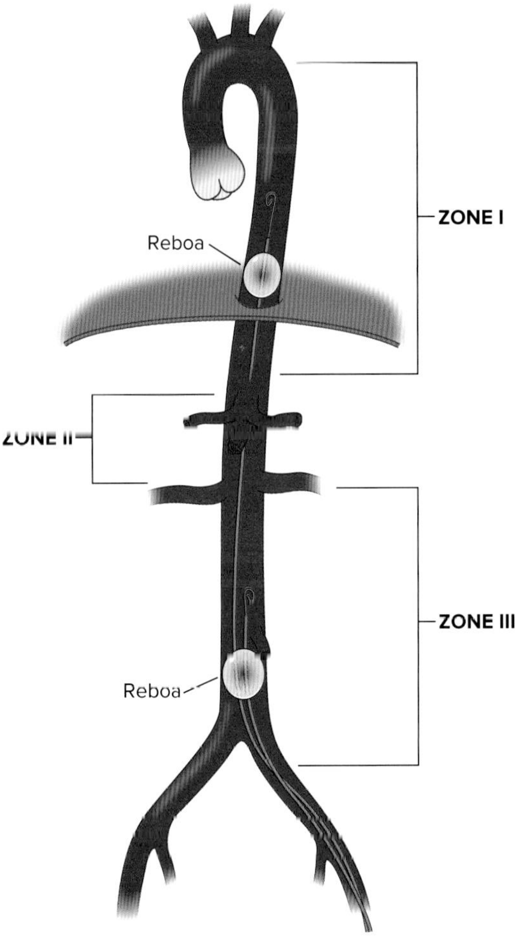

FIGURE 44-3 **Zones of REBOA placement.**

the pancreas to access the artery at its origin and then achieve proximal and distal control or via left medial visceral rotation and clamping of the origin of the SMA. When exposing the SMA with left medial visceral rotation, the left kidney need not be mobilized thus sparing it and its vasculature the risk of injury. Fullen Zone II of the SMA is between the inferior edge of the pancreas and the base of the transverse mesocolon. Injury to the SMA in Fullen Zones I and II threaten intestinal viability, particularly the cecal and ascending colon. For patients who are being managed with damage control strategies, a vascular shunt should be placed in surgically debrided ends of the injured vessel and definitive repair should be delayed until the patient is resuscitated and more physiologically normal. When replacement of the proximal SMA is required, it is preferred to place the saphenous vein or prosthetic graft on the infrarenal aorta away from the pancreas and other upper abdominal injuries. These grafts should be fashioned to be positioned through the posterior aspect of the mesentery to the remaining SMA in an end-to-side fashion. Fullen Zones III and IV SMA segments should be repaired but due to distal small luminal diameter, they are sometimes ligated. When ligation occurs or failure of repairs distal ilium and right colon may require resection.

Superior Mesenteric Vein Injuries

These injuries are very survivable when they are identified and managed appropriately with ligation or repair. The SMV lies to the right of the SMA. While the dictum of being able to ligate all veins is true. This should not be the first choice when this vessel is injured. Injury to the SMV as its junction with the splenic vein is challenging to control due to the amount of hemorrhage and the adjacent structures obstructing the surgeon's ability to gain proximal and distal control of the vein. Similar to the management of Fullen Zone I SMA injuries, the pancreas may need to be divided between two clamps to gain the needed access to the proximal vessel. The more common injury pattern is a laceration or injury inferior to the pancreas. These injuries can be repaired with 5-0 polypropylene sutures. Posterior injuries to the SMV are more difficult because of branches entering the vein. When near transection has occurred, ligation with reanastomosis in an end-to-end fashion can be achieved. When ligation is the management for injury to the SMV, it is very important to fluid resuscitate these patients over the next 3 days due to the peripheral hypovolemia that occurs as a result of splanchnic hypervolemia.

Proximal Renal Artery Injuries

Left medical visceral rotation exposes the left lateral aorta and the left renal artery. The right renal artery may be most reliably exposed with a right medial visceral rotation. The right renal artery can also be located through the base of the mesocolon beneath the left renal vein and between the infrarenal abdominal aorta and vena cava. These injuries should be exposed and repaired after proximal and distal control has been obtained.

Inframesocolic Vascular Injuries

Vessels in Zone I inframesocolic region are the infrarenal abdominal aorta and the inferior vena cava. Central hematoma occurring in the inframesocolic region results from one of these vessels. Hematoma or hemorrhage that is coming through the right colonic mesentery or to the right of the midline is consistent with injury to the inferior vena cava or liver. The injury is most commonly found beneath the tallest aspect of the hematoma. When efforts to gain control are challenging, finger dissection through the hematoma to compress the injury in the vessel can be very effective. The complications of this maneuver, namely excess hemorrhage from clot disruption, are illustrative of the discussion in the REBOA section regarding avoiding the additional hemorrhage and stress of gaining operative control of the injured vessel through endoluminal approaches for occlusion. Open operative approaches to achieve control of the infrarenal abdominal aorta are performed with cephalad retraction of the transverse mesocolon and rightward evisceration of the small bowel. The retroperitoneum is then opened in the midline and the infrarenal aorta is exposed to the left renal vein and a vascular clamp is applied inferior to the left renal vein. The alternative method is a right medial visceral rotation that is very familiar to trauma surgeons. The peritoneal reflection of the right colon is taken down and the colon is mobilized to the right (the kidney can stay in its fossa). A Kocher procedure is then performed and the duodenum is mobilized medially off of the anterior vena cava. This exposes the infrahepatic vena cava. Whenever a clamp is placed on the vena cava, blood flow to the heart is severely decreased and therefore considerations should be given to concomitant clamping of the infrarenal aorta to avoid hypotension.

Infrarenal Aortic Injuries

The infrarenal aorta is exposed similarly as described above. Proximal control can be achieved with a vascular clamp just inferior to the left renal vein. Distal control with a vascular clamp should be performed inferior to the injury zone. Primary repair of injuries can be achieved with 3-0 Prolene suture or interposition graft or patch angioplasty in noncontaminated fields. When infrarenal aortic ligation is necessary, extraanatomic bypass is required for revascularization of the lower extremities. This is usually done in a delayed fashion for patients undergoing damage control management.

MANAGEMENT OF BLUNT TRAUMATIC ABDOMINAL VASCULAR INJURY

ZONE II ABDOMINAL VASCULAR INJURIES

Blunt force trauma that increases abdominal pressure and causes trauma to the renal vessels or kidneys occasionally requires surgery. Blunt renal trauma in the adult population was caused primarily by motor vehicle accidents (MVAs) (63%), followed by falls (43%), sports (11%), and pedestrian accidents (4%), while blunt trauma in the pediatric population was caused by more falls (27%) and pedestrian accidents (13%) and fewer MVAs (30%).[33] The major elements that cause renal trauma are deceleration and acceleration forces. Deceleration forces on the renal attachments (Gerota facia in the retroperitoneum, and the renal pedicle and ureteropelvic junction) cause rupture or thrombosis. Acceleration forces push the kidney against its surrounding boney structures such as the ribs and spine, and cause parenchymal and vascular injuries.[34] Contrast-enhanced computed tomography of the abdomen is the diagnostic study of choice for hemodynamically stable patients. Postcontrast phases identify vascular and parenchymal damage including the presence of active extravasation of contrast. Delayed phase can visualize the collecting system and ureteric injury. For Zone II injuries, the most important decision for intervention seen on CT scan will be whether renal revascularization within a 5-hour window after trauma is achievable.

Indications for operative exploration and renal intervention are hemodynamic instability and unresponsiveness to aggressive resuscitation due to renal hemorrhage, grade 5 vascular injuries, and an expanding or pulsatile perirenal hematoma found during laparotomy performed for associated injuries. Expanding hematomas should be explored in Zone II. Nonexpanding hematomas caused by blunt trauma should not. Angiographic failure at embolization or renal artery thrombosis is a relative indication for surgery.

ENDOVASCULAR MANAGEMENT OF RENAL TRAUMA

Endovascular therapy for blunt abdominal vascular trauma has been best applied to the kidneys. Embolization of bleeding arteries with preservation of normal renal function has been well described.[35-37] This management should be applied to hemodynamically normal patients.

PENETRATING INJURIES

Hemodynamically unstable patients with penetrating injuries to Zone II require exploration. Hematomas in this region, whether expanding or not, should be explored to rule out and repair not just vascular injuries but also renal pelvic trauma. Persistent attempts to repair renal vascular structures should be avoided as they may lead to excess bleeding. Whether a functional contralateral kidney is present or not, hemorrhage control must be achieved to prevent mortality. In the setting of patients in hemorrhagic shock, renal preservation should not come before hemorrhage control. Mobilization of the kidney from Gerota's fascia into the midline positions the renal vascular structures perpendicular to the midline aorta and vena cava allowing for clamping. Complex repairs are usually not required. If ligation of the right venal vein is necessary, nephrectomy should be performed at the initial or take-back operation. While left renal vein repair is preferred, the medial left renal vein can be ligated as long as the adrenal and gonadal veins are intact. Renal artery repairs can be done primarily or interposition grafts using PTFE or saphenous vein. It must again be said that in the setting of hemodynamic instability, nephrectomy is likely the best surgical management.

ZONE III ABDOMINAL VASCULAR INJURIES

The iliac artery and vein are located in the pelvic retroperitoneal region. The gonadal vessels also cross these structures in the pelvis. The majority of these injuries are due to penetrating trauma. However, blunt trauma to the pelvis can result in an open book fracture that displaces the boney pelvis into the venous plexus. All retroperitoneal hematomas caused by penetrating mechanisms should be explored. The focus should be on the identification and cessation of hemorrhage after obtaining proximal and distal control of the vessels. An evaluation of the ureter on the ipsilateral side of the hematoma should also be a priority after hemorrhage control has been achieved. Retroperitoneal hematomas caused by blunt mechanisms should be explored only if they are expanding or if ipsilateral femoral pulse is absent. The maneuvers to be considered for control of hemorrhage in this anatomical region are primary vascular repairs with 5-0 Prolene suture, interposition grafts with PTFE, and saphenous vein patch angioplasties. Preperitoneal packing for venous bleeding secondary to pelvic fractures leading to hemodynamic stability is also an essential trauma maneuver in damage control surgery.

ILIAC ARTERY

Iliac vessel injuries have an incidence just over 10% of all cardiovascular injuries with mortality of just under 50%.[38,39] These vessels are exposed by mobilization of the small intestines to the right upper quadrant and entering the retroperitoneum over the aortic bifurcation. Active bleeding will be encountered beneath the highest point of the hematoma. Injuries to the common iliac artery (CIA) or external iliac artery (EIA) should be preferably repaired primarily or interposition grafts should be performed. If the patient is hemodynamically unstable, temporarily shunting these vessels and employing a damage control strategy on either of these vessels is ligated which will lead to a high above-knee amputation. However, the internal iliac artery can be ligated without such consequences. Stable patients may receive complex arterial reconstruction and repairs. Unstable patients should be temporarily shunted with a similarly sized tubular structure secured at both ends of the arteriotomy. Pelvic infection may also be a reason to delay end-to-end anastomosis in favor of revascularization from contralateral limb (i.e., femoral–femoral bypass). Another option would be temporary shunting to allow time for reduction of bioburden followed by delayed end-to-end anastomosis. This would depend on overall contamination levels. Endovascular approaches to iliac artery injuries have been described. Both covered stents to control iliac artery injury as well as initial balloon temporary occlusion before operative repair of injuries have been demonstrated.

ILIAC VEIN

Iliac vein injuries are associated with iliac artery injuries. Exposure of the iliac veins is performed as described for Zone III arterial injuries. Right common iliac vein injuries are challenging to expose due to their posterior position to the bifurcation of the aorta. Historically, temporary transection of the right CIA with mobilization of the vessel to the left is an approach described for exposing the right common iliac vein. This is seldom performed now. Smaller venous injuries are repaired primarily with 5-0 Prolene suture. Larger venous injuries should be repaired with interposition grafts or contralateral saphenous vein patch angioplasty. A study demonstrates that patency rates for complex venous reconstructions are 73% at 30 days.[40] If necessary, iliac vein injuries can be ligated with minimal complications. All postoperative repairs should be placed on anticoagulation to prevent thrombosis.

REFERENCES

1. Barr J, Cherry KJ, Rich NM. Vascular surgery in World War II: the shift to repairing arteries. *Ann Surg*. 2016;263(3):615-620.
2. DeBakey ME, Simeone FA. Battle injuries of the arteries in World War II: an analysis of 2,471 cases. *Ann Surg*. 1946;123:534-579.
3. Beekley AC, Blackbourne LH, Sebesta JA, et al. Selective nonoperative management of penetrating torso injury from combat fragmentation wounds. *J Trauma*. 2008;64(2 Suppl):S108-S116; discussion S116-7.
4. Cox EF. Blunt abdominal trauma. A 5-year analysis of 870 patients requiring celiotomy. *Ann Surg*. 1984; 199(4):467-474.
5. Feliciano DV, Burch JM, Spjut-Patrinely V, Mattox KL, Jordan GL Jr. Abdominal gunshot wounds. An urban trauma center's experience with 300 consecutive patients. *Ann Surg*. 1988;208(3):362-370.
6. Davis TP, Feliciano DV, Rozycki GS, et al. Results with abdominal vascular trauma in the modern era. *Am Surg*. 2001;67(6):565-570; discussion 570-571.
7. Drapanas T, Hewitt RL, Weichert RF 3rd, Smith AD. Civilian vascular injuries: a critical appraisal of three decades of management. *Ann Surg*. 1970;172(3):351-360.
8. Rose SC, Moore EE. Trauma angiography: the use of clinical findings to improve patient selection and case preparation. *J Trauma*. 1988;28(2):240-245.
9. Hayes CW, Conway WF, Walsh JW, Coppage L, Gervin AS. Seat belt injuries: radiologic findings and clinical correlation. *Radiographics*. 1991;11(1):23-36.
10. Peitzman AB, Makaroun MS, Slasky BS, Ritter P. Prospective study of computed tomography in initial management of blunt abdominal trauma. *J Trauma*. 1986;26(7):585-592.
11. Demetriades D, Rabinowitz B. Indications for operation in abdominal stab wounds: a prospective study of 651 patients. *Ann Surg*. 1987;205(2):129-132.
12. Chiu WC, Shanmuganathan K, Mirvis SE, Scalea TM. Determining the need for laparotomy in penetrating torso trauma: a prospective study using triple-contrast enhanced abdominopelvic computed tomography. *J Trauma* 2001;51(5):860-868; discussion 868-869.
13. Goodman CS, Hur JY, Adajar MA, Coulam CH. How well does CT predict the need for laparotomy in hemodynamically stable patients with penetrating abdominal injury? A review and meta-analysis. *AJR Am J Roentgenol*. 2009;193(2):432-437.
14. Jansen JO, Inaba K, Resnick S, et al. Selective nonoperative management of abdominal gunshot wounds: survey of practise. *Injury*. 2013;44(5):639-644.
15. Hauser CJ, Huprich JE, Bosco P, Gibbons L, Mansour AY, Weiss AR. Triple-contrast computed tomography in the evaluation of penetrating posterior abdominal injuries. *Arch Surg*. 1987;122(10):1112-1115.
16. de Vries CS, Africa M, Gebremariam FA, van Rensburg JJ, Otto SF, Potgieter HF. The imaging of stab injuries. *Acta Radiol*. 2010;51(1):92-106.
17. Shanmuganathan K, Mirvis SE, Chiu WC, Killeen KL, Hogan GJ, Scalea TM. Penetrating torso trauma: triple-contrast helical CT in peritoneal violation and organ injury—a prospective study in 200 patients. *Radiology*. 2004;231(3):775-784.
18. Phillips T, Sclafani SJ, Goldstein A, Scalea T, Panetta T, Shaftan G. Use of the contrast-enhanced CT enema in the management of penetrating trauma to the flank and back. *J Trauma*. 1986;26(7):593-601.
19. Lee BC, Ormsby EL, McGahanJP, Melendres GM, Richards JR. The utility of sonography for the triage of blunt abdominal trauma patients to exploratory laparotomy. *AJR Am J Roentgenol*. 2007;188:415-421.
20. Rozyki G. Surgery performed ultrasound in the assessment of truncal injuries. *Ann Surg*. 1998;288:557-567.
21. Duchesne JC, Kimonis K, Marr AB, et al. Damage control resuscitation in combination with damage control laparotomy: a survival advantage. *J Trauma*. 2010;69(1); 46-52.
22. Gabriel M, Pawlaczyk K, Waliszewski K, Krasiński Z, Majewski W. Location of femoral artery puncture site and the risk of postcatheterization pseudoaneurysm formation. *Int J Cardiol*. 2007;120:167-171.
23. DuBose JJ, Scalea TM, Brenner M, et al. The AAST prospective aortic occlusion for resuscitation in trauma and acute care surgery (AORTA) registry: data on contemporary utilization and outcomes of aortic occlusion and resuscitative balloon occlusion of the aorta (REBOA). *J Trauma Acute Care Surg*. 2016;81(3):409-419.
24. Dudeck O, Teichgraeber U, Podrabsky P, et al. A randomized trial assessing the value of ultrasound guided puncture of the femoral artery for interventional investigations. *Int J Cardiovasc Imaging*. 2004;20:363-368.
25. Brenner ML, Moore LJ, DuBose JJ, et al. A clinical series of resuscitative endovascular balloon occlusion

of the aorta for hemorrhage control and resuscitation. *J Trauma Acute Care Surg*. 2013;75(3):506-511.
26. Pieper A, Thony F, Brun J, et al. Resuscitative endovascular balloon occlusion of the aorta for pelvic blunt trauma and life-threatening hemorrhage: a 20-year experience in a level I trauma center. *J Trauma Acute Care Surg*. 2018;84(3):449-453.
27. Darrabie MD, Croft CA, Brakenridge SC, et al. Resuscitative endovascular balloon occlusion of the aorta: implementation and preliminary results at an academic level I trauma center. *J Am Coll Surg*. 2018; 227(1):127-133.
28. Brenner M, Inaba K, Aiolfi A, et al. Resuscitative endovascular balloon occlusion of the aorta and resuscitative thoracotomy in select patients with hemorrhagic shock: early results from the American Association for the surgery of trauma's aortic occlusion in resuscitation for trauma and acute care surgery registry. *J Am Coll Surg*. 2018;226(5):730-740.
29. Brenner M, Teeter W, Hoehn M, et al. Use of resuscitative endovascular balloon occlusion of the aorta for proximal aortic control in patients with severe hemorrhage and arrest. *JAMA Surg*. 2018;153(2):130-135.
30. Joseph B, Zeeshan M, Sakran JV, et al. Nationwide analysis of resuscitative endovascular balloon occlusion of the aorta in civilian trauma. *JAMA Surg*. 2019; 154(6):500-508.
31. Lendrum R, Perkins Z, Chana M, et al. Pre-hospital resuscitative endovascular balloon occlusion of the aorta (REBOA) for exsanguinating pelvic haemorrhage. *Resuscitation*. 2019;135:6-13.
32. Harvin JA, Maxim T, Inaba K, et al. Mortality after emergent trauma laparotomy: a multicenter, retrospective study. *J Trauma Acute Care Surg*. 2017;83(3):464-468.
33. Voelzke BB, Leddy L. The epidemiology of renal trauma. *Transl Androl Urol*. 2014;3:143-149.
34. Schmidlin F, Farshad M, Bidaut L, et al. Biomechanical analysis and clinical treatment of blunt renal trauma. *Swiss Surg*. 1998:237-243.
35. Sclafani SJ, Becker JA. Interventional radiology in the treatment of retroperitoneal trauma. *Urol Radiol*. 1985;7(4):219-230.
36. Hagiwara A, Sakaki S, Goto H, et al. The role of interventional radiology in the management of blunt renal injury: a practical protocol. *J Trauma*. 2001;51(3): 526-531.
37. Boufi M, Bordon S, Dona B, et al. Unstable patients with retroperitoneal vascular trauma: an endovascular approach. *Ann Vasc Surg*. 2011;25:352-358.
38. Asensio JA, Petrone P, Roldan G, et al. Analysis of 185 iliac vessel injuries: risk factors and predictors of outcome. *Arch Surg*. 2003;138:1187-1193; discussion 1193-1194.
39. Mattox KL, Feliciano DV, Burch J, et al. Five thousand seven hundred sixty cardiovascular injuries in 4,459 patients. Epidemiologic evolution 1958 to 1987. *Ann Surg*. 1989;209:698-705; discussion 706-707.
40. Pappas PJ, Haser PB, Teehan EP, et al. Outcome of complex venous reconstructions in patients with trauma. *J Vasc Surg*. 1997;25:398-404.

SELF-ASSESSMENT STUDY QUESTIONS AND ANSWERS

Questions

1. Central abdominal hematomas from penetrating trauma should be managed how?
   A. They should be monitored, if not expanding.
   B. They should be operatively explored with medial visceral rotations for vascular control.
   C. They should be operatively explored without vascular control.
   D. They should be packed.
   E. None of the above are correct.

2. Left visceral rotation gives the surgeon access to which vessels?
   A. Abdominal aorta
   B. Superior mesenteric artery
   C. Celiac artery
   D. Splenic artery
   E. All of the above

3. The proximal renal vessels are found in which abdominal vascular zone?
   A. Zone I
   B. Zone II
   C. Zone III
   D. None of the above

4. The principles for the management of hepatic trauma include?
   A. Packing above and beneath the liver
   B. Pringle manouver = control of the hepatoduodenal ligament
   C. Mobilization of the liver
   D. Hepatic resection
   E. All of the above

5. An infrahepatic caval injury should be exposed by which maneuver?
   A. Right medial visceral rotation
   B. Right medial visceral rotation and Kocher maneuver
   C. Right medial visceral rotation and mobilization of the right hepatic lobe away from the diaphragm
   D. None of the above

6. Damage control principles imply?
   A. Control hemorrhage and gastrointestinal and genitourinary spillage and delay complex repairs and abdominal closure until improvement of physiological parameters in the SICU
   B. Achieve definitive repair of all injuries at the initial operation
   C. Achieve definitive repair of all major injuries at the initial operation
   D. None of the above

7. To gain improved access to the supraceliac aorta what is performed?
   A. Transection of the right cruz of the diaphragm
   B. Transection of the left cruz of the diaphragm
   C. Left anterolateral thoracotomy
   D. None of the above

8. What additional procedure should be performed after supraceliac aortic clamping?
   A. Bilateral four-compartment fasciotomies
   B. Left colon resection
   C. Heparinization
   D. Postoperative caval interruption

9. Which is true of iliac vein injuries?
   A. They may be ligated.
   B. Patients should be placed on anticoagulation postoperatively.
   C. They may be difficult to expose if injuries occur in the right iliac vein.
   D. All of the above are correct.

10. Noncompressible hemorrhage in the trunk can be managed with REBOA. Which of the following is true concerning the application of REBOA?
    A. Placement of the balloon should be Zone I of the Aorta.
    B. Complications include balloon migration, distal embolization, and amputation.
    C. Optimal Zone I occlusion times are 30 minutes.
    D. All of the above are correct.

SELF-ASSESSMENT STUDY QUESTIONS AND ANSWERS

Answers

1. B.
2. E.
3. A.
4. E.
5. B.
6. A.
7. B.
8. A.
9. D.
10. D.

CHAPTER

45 Thoracic Vascular Trauma

Mallory Williams and Abraham Lebenthal

OUTLINE

INTRODUCTION

THORACIC CAVITY ANATOMY

BLUNT TRAUMA

MANAGEMENT OF SPECIFIC INJURIES

- Preoperative Management and Decision-making
- Blunt Cardiac Trauma

DESCENDING THORACIC AORTA

- Thoracic Endovascular Aortic Repair (TEVAR)
  - Role of CT Angiography and Intravascular Ultrasound in Diagnosis
  - Endograft Sizing and Deployment
  - Society of Vascular Surgeons Clinical Practice Guidelines for TEVAR in TAI
  - Eastern Association for the Surgery of Trauma Clinical Guidelines for Diagnostic and Management of Blunt Aortic Injuries
  - Screening and Complications

TEVAR VERSUS OPEN MANAGEMENT

NONOPERATIVE MANAGEMENT

PENETRATING TRAUMA

MANAGEMENT OF SPECIFIC INJURIES

- Cardiac Injuries
- Ascending Aorta
- Transverse Aortic Arch
- Innominate Artery

DESCENDING THORACIC AORTA

- Thoracic Vena Cava
- Subclavian Artery
- Subclavian Vein
- Left Carotid Artery
- Pulmonary Artery
- Pulmonary Veins
- Internal Mammary Artery
- Azygous Vein

INTRODUCTION

Trauma to the major vascular structures of the thoracic cavity is caused by either penetrating mechanisms or acceleration–deceleration forces that tear vascular structures that are fixed within the thoracic cavity. Less than 10% of blunt injuries and only 15% to 30% of penetrating injuries in the thoracic cavity will require thoracotomy.[1] Traditionally, of the patients receiving thoracotomy, only 25% will have a thoracic vascular injury.[2] While penetrating injuries may damage any thoracic vascular structure, blunt injuries typically only impact the thoracic aorta, innominate artery, and intercostal vessels. Both blunt and penetrating vascular trauma to the chest can be lethal. However, most thoracic vascular injuries will require only airway management and thoracostomy tube for the drainage of the resulting hemothorax.[1]

THORACIC CAVITY ANATOMY

The thoracic cavity is an articulating musculoskeletal framework that houses the aerodigestive tract, lungs, heart, and great vessels. Because this is a dynamic cavity designed for both active and passive ventilation, the position of the rib cage changes during the respiratory cycle. The greatest thoracic cavity mobility is noted between ribs 7 and 10. Therefore, it should be understood that this is where most fractures occur. The next most common fractures occur at ribs 4 to 6. Hence, these intercostal vessels are the most susceptible to injury and hemorrhage. The muscular covering of the thorax includes the pectoralis major and minor muscles anteriorly, the latissimus dorsi and serratus anterior muscles laterally, and the trapezius, levator scapulae, serratus posterior rhomboid major and minor, latissimus dorsi muscles posteriorly. These muscles provide a protective coat to the rib cage and help to define a very well-protected superior anterior and posterior section of the rib cage versus a less well-protected inferior anterior and lateral sections. This anatomical structure explains why most rib fractures will occur in the lateral or anterolateral section and less in the posterior section. Penetrating trauma occurring between the nipples and the clavicles and sternocostal margin or the "cardiac box" is particularly concerning because of the underlying great vessel and cardiac structures. Blunt trauma that arises from an acceleration–deceleration mechanism can produce the "ripping" force that tears the descending aorta between the ligamentum arteriosum and the left subclavian artery. These are the two major anatomical considerations for the most severe thoracic vascular injuries.

BLUNT TRAUMA

Blunt trauma is the most common source of injury to thoracic vascular structures. Blunt trauma mechanisms causing thoracic vascular injuries are usually fall from heights, motor vehicle or motorcycle collisions, or sky accidents. The innominate artery origin, pulmonary veins, vena cava, and most commonly the descending thoracic aorta are particularly at risk from blunt trauma. The recognized mechanisms of blunt great vessel injury include the following: a) shear forces, b) compressive forces, and c) intraluminal hypertension at the time of the trauma. Shearing forces primarily cause injury due to the relative increased mobility of the thoracic vessel adjacent to the fixed portion of the same vessel. Therefore, the atrial attachments of the pulmonary veins and vena cava as well as the fixation of the descending thoracic aorta at the ligamentum arteriosium and diaphragm make these vessels at risk of injury from significant blunt trauma. The innominate artery can be compressed between the boney structures of the sternum and the vertebrae with anterior blows to the chest.

MANAGEMENT OF SPECIFIC INJURIES

PREOPERATIVE MANAGEMENT AND DECISION-MAKING

Advanced Trauma Life Support principles should guide the management of these patients. For patients who have hemodynamic stability, computed tomographic angiography of the chest should be performed for the diagnosis. At this time, patients without concomitant head injuries should be managed with permissive hypotension of 55 to 60 mmHg. These patients should be taken to the operating room for either thoracic endovascular aortic repair (TEVAR) or thoracotomy. Patients who arrive with hypotension and are nonresponders to resuscitation have a poorer prognosis. After endotracheal intubation, the establishment of wide bore intravenous access, and activation of the massive transfusion protocol, an extended Focused Assessment of Sonography in Trauma examination should be performed along with a chest and pelvis radiograph. FAST examinations that demonstrate blood in the left hemithorax should raise suspicion of injury to the thoracic aorta. Chest radiograph imaging should be evaluated for signs consistent with blunt traumatic aortic injury (see Table 45-1). These patients should proceed to the operating room for left anterior lateral thoracotomy and repair of the thoracic aorta with a clamp and sew technique. The difficulty occurs when there is concomitant abdominal solid organ injury and blood on FAST examination or pelvic fractures. These findings can be associated with thoracic aortic injury and yet obscure the diagnosis. Chest radiographic findings should be carefully reviewed. Sometimes, trauma laparotomy to clear the abdomen of life-threatening hemorrhage still precedes thoracotomy. In the setting of thoracic aortic rupture, valuable time may be lost if two teams are not working simultaneously. Damage control principles should clearly be instituted. When

TABLE 45-1 Chest Radiograph Signs of Blunt Traumatic Aortic Injury

Widening (Bleeding)	Movement of Aerodigestive Tract Structures	Obliteration and Bleeding	Fractures
Mediastinum	Deviation trachea to the right	Aortic knob	1st rib
Paratracheal stripe	Deviation of the esophagus to the right	Aortopulmonary window	2nd Rib
Paraspinal interfaces	Depression of the left main stem bronchus	Apical capping	Scapula
	Elevation of the right main stem bronchus	Left hemothorax	

life-threatening injuries are found in both cavities, overall survival is poor but this should not mirror the overall trauma team effort.

BLUNT CARDIAC TRAUMA

The classic terminology has been "cardiac contusion." The range of what is now termed blunt cardiac injury can range from "bruises" of the myocardium to rupture. This results from mechanical compression of the heart between the sternum and the vertebral column. The range of injuries includes chamber rupture, coronary thrombosis, septal rupture, and chordae tendineae or papillary muscle ruptures. The injury can result in dysrhythmias. Blunt cardiac injury occurs most often to the right ventricle, but for those patients alive on arrival to the hospital, it is the right atrium that is most often ruptured. This injury occurs at the superior vena cava–right atrial junction, inferior vena cava–right atrial junction, and atrial appendage. Blunt injuries causing pericardial and diaphragmatic tears allow for displacement of the heart from its normal mediastinal position. This can produce obstructive shock and replacing the heart into its usual position is required for stabilization. Traumatic disruption of the abdominal aorta is associated with cardiac rupture in 25% of cases.[2]

DESCENDING THORACIC AORTA

Blunt injuries to the descending thoracic aorta have very high mortality. The isthmus (distal to the left subclavian artery) is the most common location for rupture (50%-70% of the cases, followed by the ascending aorta or aortic arch (18%), and the distal thoracic aorta (14%).[2] For those patients who make it to the hospital and are hemodynamically stable, endovascular approaches should be the management choice. When compared to open approaches, endovascular approaches have lower initial mortality and lower complication rates such as paraplegia. Patients who are hemodynamically unstable and nonresponders to resuscitation should be taken emergently to the operating room for thoracotomy and clamp and sew repairs of the aorta.

THORACIC ENDOVASCULAR AORTIC REPAIR (TEVAR)

Role of CT Angiography and Intravascular Ultrasound in Diagnosis

TEVAR has been demonstrated to be an effective approach to blunt traumatic aortic injury. Hybrid operating rooms greatly facilitate this procedure. The abdomen and bilateral groins are prepped. Femoral artery access is obtained on the more suitable side based on CTA imaging. Aortic arch angiography is performed to define the injury. Cerebrovascular anatomy is also evaluated if the left subclavian artery origin is to be covered. In the setting of continued hemodynamic instability, some endovascular surgeons will perform intravascular ultrasound (IVUS). IVUS has been reported to be extremely valuable in diagnosing traumatic aortic injury when CTA and angiography have been equivocal.[3] Specifically, angiography was twice as likely to be equivocal when patients were studied after having equivocal CTA findings (5% for angiography vs 2.5% for IVUS).[3] TAI is classified into four groups (see Table 45-2). Grade I are intimal tears, Grade II are intramural hematomas, Grade III are pseudoaneurysms), and Grade IV are ruptures. Patients with

TABLE 45-2 Grades of Aortic Injury and Management

Grades of Aortic Injury	Injury	Management
Grade I	Intimal tear	Medical
Grade II	Pseudoaneurysm	Repair
Grade III	Intramural hematoma	Repair
Grade IV	Rupture	Repair

Grade I injuries can be managed with medical therapy (anti-impulse control). A repeat CTA study can be performed in 6 weeks. Most Grade I injuries heal with medical therapy. Patients with injuries Grades II to IV require repair. Thoracic endograft devices are required for patients with Grade II to IV injuries.

Endograft Sizing and Deployment

The sizing of these devices is performed based on thin-cut CTA imaging. The average diameter of the thoracic aorta among patients with aortic tears is 19.3 cm. Manufacturers recommend 15% to 20% oversizing of grafts. Compression and infolding are complications with higher degrees of oversizing. There are now FDA-approved devices for the thoracic aorta that can be utilized. Patients who present with small aortas are still challenging. Off-label usage of abdominal endografts has been done. Heparinization should only be done if isolated thoracic vascular injuries are present. After diagnosis, the thoracic endograft is deployed. Certain manufacturer sheaths allow for use of more than one device facilitating the procedure. Covering of the left subclavian artery is sometimes needed to obtain a proximal landing zone or gain better apposition with the lesser curvature of the aortic arch. Over 85% of descending thoracic aortic injuries are within 1 cm of the orifice of the left subclavian artery. Many surgeons will perform selective delayed subclavian artery revascularization. In cases of incomplete apposition of the graft at the proximal landing zone or proximal type I, endoleak selective balloon angioplasty can be performed. Reversal of heparin with protamine should be done. Completion angiography is the final procedure before sheath removal.

Society of Vascular Surgeons Clinical Practice Guidelines for TEVAR in TAI[4]

A review included 7768 patients from 139 studies, and the mortality rate was significantly lower in patients who underwent endovascular repair, followed by open repair and nonoperative management (NOM) (9%, 19%, and 46%, respectively; $P < 0.01$). The majority opinions of the committee suggested the following:

1. Timing of TEVAR in a stable patient. The committee suggested urgent repair (<24 hours) in the absence of other serious concomitant injuries or repair immediately after other injuries have been treated, but at the latest, prior to hospital discharge.
2. Management of minimal aortic injuries. The committee suggested expectant management with serial imaging for Grade I injuries and repair for injuries in Grades II to IV.
3. Type of repair in young patients. Endovascular repair regardless of age, if anatomically suitable.
4. Management of the left subclavian artery. The committee suggested selective revascularization.
5. Systemic heparinization. The committee suggested routine heparinization, but at a lower dose than in elective TEVAR.
6. Spinal drainage. The committee did not suggest routine spinal drainage.
7. Choice of anesthesia. The committee suggested general anesthesia.
8. Femoral access technique. The committee suggested open femoral exposure.

Eastern Association for the Surgery of Trauma Clinical Guidelines for Diagnostic and Management of Blunt Aortic Injuries[5]

Eastern Association for the Surgery of Trauma Clinical Guidelines were published in the year 2000. No Level I recommendations were made by the EAST Clinical Guidelines Committee. However, Level II and III recommendations were written. Level II recommendations are as follows:

1. The possibility of a blunt aortic injury should be considered in all patients who are involved in a motor vehicle collision regardless of the direction of impact.
2. The chest x-ray is a good screening tool for determining the need for further investigation. The most significant chest x-ray findings include (but are not limited to): widened mediastinum, obscured aortic knob, deviation of the left mainstem bronchus or nasogastric tube, and opacification of the aortopulmonary window.
3. Angiography is a very sensitive, specific, and accurate test for the presence of blunt aortic injury. It is the standard by which most other diagnostic tests are compared.
4. Computed tomography of the chest is a useful diagnostic tool for both screening and diagnosis of blunt aortic injury. Spiral or helical CT scanners have an extremely high negative predictive value and may be used alone to rule out blunt aortic injury. When these scanners are used, angiography may be reserved for patients with indeterminate scans.
5. Prompt repair of the blunt aortic injury is preferred. If the patient has more immediately life-threatening injuries that require intervention such as emergent laparotomy or craniotomy, or if the patient is a poor operative candidate due to age or comorbidities, the aortic repair may be delayed. Medical control of blood pressure is advised until surgical repair can be accomplished.

Screening and Complications

CTA is the gold standard for follow-up imaging after TEVAR procedures. CTA acquires high-quality images that can then be postprocessed. Precontrast images are evaluated for the integrity of the metallic components of the stent graft. It is also important to understand aortic calcifications so that they are not confused with endoleaks on contrast images. Contrast-phase images allow for luminal pathology with great accuracy. The position of the stent-grafts is evaluated and aortic branch vessel patency is examined. The ends of endografts are evaluated for type I endoleaks and the stent-graft is examined for type III endoleaks. Delayed imaging is important to assess for slower filling type II endoleaks. Postprocedure imaging protocols for screening can vary but one standard schedule was CTA imaging at 30 days, 60 days, and 6 months.

Complications of TEVAR are endoleaks, graft migration, graft infection, retrograde dissection, and access vessel rupture. These topics are covered in other chapters of this textbook. But graft collapse is particularly common when TEVAR is performed for traumatic aortic injury.

TEVAR VERSUS OPEN MANAGEMENT

Several meta-analyses demonstrate a decreased mortality but similar morbidity (including paraplegia) for patients with blunt thoracic aortic injury undergoing TEVAR versus open repair.[6] It should be pointed out that the incidence of cerebrovascular accidents is reported to be higher with TEVAR.[6] But because of the associated injuries that can and do not occur infrequently (particularly, the least desired concomitant traumatic brain injury), TEVAR is now the preferred option for management of this injury.

NONOPERATIVE MANAGEMENT

NOM of blunt thoracic aortic injury was once not considered an option and then gradually became highly controversial. It is now accepted that in small groups of well-defined patients, NOM can be successfully performed based on the analysis of CT angiography.[6] In fact, data for Grades I and II blunt thoracic aortic injuries mortality and morbidity have not been reported differently for TEVAR and NOM groups.[7] It should be emphasized that these are hemodynamically stable patients with minimal injuries.

PENETRATING TRAUMA

The most common penetrating mechanisms in thoracic vascular injury are gunshot wounds or stab wounds. The majority of these injuries are to the chest wall structures (ribs, muscles, and intercostal vessels), and lungs. The most common vessels to be injured by penetrating trauma mechanisms are the intercostal vessels. Rarely is a thoracotomy required for the circumferential ligation of intercostal vessels around the rib on both sides of the fracture. Thoracostomy tube drainage is usually sufficient for the management of these patients.

MANAGEMENT OF SPECIFIC INJURIES

The management of great vessel injury secondary to penetrating trauma is facilitated by exposing the injury through thoracic incisions (Table 45-3). Some injuries are simply not survivable even though the patient may arrive at the hospital with signs of life.

TABLE 45-3 Thoracic Incisions for Great Vessel Injuries

Great Vessel Injury	Incisions
Uncertain injury (hemodynamically unstable)	Left anterior lateral thoracotomy +/− Transverse sternotomy +/− Right anterolateral thoracotomy (clamshell thoracotomy)
Ascending aorta	Median sternotomy
Transverse aortic arch	Median sternotomy +/− neck distention
Pulmonary artery	Median sternotomy
Innominate artery	Median sternotomy with right cervical extension
Right subclavian artery or vein	Median sternotomy with right cervical extension
Left common carotid artery	Median sternotomy with left cervical extension
Innominate vein	Median sternotomy
Intrathoracic vena cava	Median sternotomy
Descending thoracic aorta	Left posterolateral thoracotomy (4th intercostal space)
Right or left hilar	Ipsilateral posterolateral thoracotomy
Pulmonary vein	Ipsilateral posterolateral thoracotomy

CARDIAC INJURIES

Patients who survive with anterior stab wounds to the chest usually exhibit tamponade physiology and have right ventricular injuries. These injuries should be managed with an Emergency Department anterolateral thoracotomy resulting in a pericardotomy and cardiorrhaphy with a pledgeted 2-0 Prolene suture on an MH needle. Cardiac lacerations near coronary arteries should receive cardiorrhaphy by placement of sutures deep into the coronary vessel. Most cardiac injuries will not require cardiac bypass. Complex injuries that involve the valvular structures or coronary arteries will require cardiac bypass. Coronary artery has a mortality rate that approximates 70%. Suture ligation of the artery is performed with bypass grafting employed for hemodynamically stable patients with proximal left coronary artery injuries. The efficient decision to utilize a left anterolateral approach to release the cardiac tamponade in the repair of these injuries is very consequential.

ASCENDING AORTA

This is usually a fatal injury but if patients make it to the operating room, cardiopulmonary bypass is usually required in addressing this injury. Specifically, if aortic root replacement is required or if there are concomitant anterior and posterior arterial defects, then bypass should be used. Patients who are hemodynamically stable upon arrival to the trauma center have higher survival rate.

TRANSVERSE AORTIC ARCH

Exposure to these injuries is achieved through median sternotomy with extension to the neck to obtain access to the arch and brachiocephalic branches. The innominate vein can be divided to further enhance exposure. Cardiopulmonary bypass is required when approaching transverse aortic injury trauma when there are posterior wall or concomitant pulmonary artery injuries. For simple lacerations, primary repair can be performed with lateral aortorrhaphy with 3-0 or 4-0 polypropylene suture.

INNOMINATE ARTERY

Exposure to the injuries of the innominate artery is achieved through a median sternotomy with a right cervical extension. Division of the innominate vein enhances the exposure of the artery. Lateral arteriorrhaphy with 4-0 polypropylene suture can be a successful technique for some injuries. For experienced surgeons, bypass exclusion procedure can also be used. A graft is placed from the ascending aorta to the distal innominate artery (immediately proximal to the bifurcation of the right subclavian artery and carotid arteries). Proximal and distal controls are obtained, and after the bypass graft is completed, the hematoma can be entered and the proximal innominate artery can be oversewn.

DESCENDING THORACIC AORTA

Injury to the descending thoracic aorta is approached through a posterolateral thoracotomy through the fourth intercostal space. The standard repair is called a clamp and sew technique. Adjunctive approaches include pharmacologic control of hypertension, passive bypass shunts, and cardiopulmonary bypass or atriofemoral bypass. Proximal control is gained at the level of the transverse aortic arch. Umbilical tapes are passed around the arch between the left carotid and subclavian arteries. The left subclavian artery is also encircled by an umbilical tape. If the injury extends to the ascending aorta, then cardiobypass should be available. Vascular clamps should be applied to the proximal aorta, distal aorta, and left subclavian artery. The hematoma is entered and back bleeding from the intercostal arteries is controlled. The proximal and distal ends of the aorta are completely transected and dissected away from the esophagus and an interposition graft is sewed in place with a 3-0 polypropylene suture. The major complication of this repair is paraplegia. This complication is related to perioperative hypotension, ligation of intercostals, and duration of clamp time.

THORACIC VENA CAVA

Median sternotomy is used to approach these injuries. Anterior injuries can be repaired after clamping with a partial occluding clamp. Posterior wall injuries usually require cardiopulmonary bypass. Intracaval shunts are not likely to be successful if not deployed early in the procedure and by experienced surgeons. Thoracic inferior vena cava injuries produce cardiac tamponade. Exposure of the thoracic inferior vena cava is done with the assistance of cardiopulmonary bypass. Repair is achieved inside the cava via the right atrium. Cardiothoracic surgeon assistance is helpful.

SUBCLAVIAN ARTERY

Cervical extension of a median sternotomy exposes the right subclavian artery. Repair of these injuries is performed with later arteriorrhaphy with 4-0 polypropylene suture. Left subclavian artery injuries are repaired through a left anteriolateral thoracotomy at the second or third intercostal space. A separate supraclavicular incision can be used for distal control. The phrenic nerve lies anterior to the anterior scalene muscle and attention to this anatomy should be paid to avoid its injury. Injuries are usually repaired with lateral arteriorrhaphy or interposition graft. Associated lung injuries should be stapled through wedge resection or pulmonary tractotomy. Common pitfalls are attempted repair via the deltopectoral groove without proximal control. Exsanguination can occur. Removal of the proximal clavicle helps to achieve proximal control of the artery.

SUBCLAVIAN VEIN

Exposure of subclavian veins is the same for the arteries. Lateral venorrhaphy with 4-0 polypropylene for repair or suture ligation is the approach to an injury

LEFT CAROTID ARTERY

Similar to the innominate artery, a median sternotomy with left cervical extension exposes the vessel.

Vascular shunts can be used. When transection of the artery at the origin, a bypass graft is the preferred approach over end-to-end anastomosis. Other injuries can be repaired with 5-0 polypropylene.

PULMONARY ARTERY

These are usually lethal injuries both because of the blood loss and the time to exposure. Intrapericardial pulmonary arteries are exposed through median sternotomy. The main and proximal left pulmonary arteries are exposed with minimal dissection. The intrapericardial right pulmonary artery can be found with dissection between the superior vena cava and ascending aorta. Anterior injuries are repaired primarily but posterior injuries are repaired with the assistance of cardiopulmonary bypass. Distal pulmonary artery injuries are exposed through an ipsilateral posterolateral thoracotomy. Major hilar injuries may require pneumonectomy as a life-preserving procedure.

PULMONARY VEINS

Exposure of pulmonary veins is through an ipsilateral posterolateral thoracotomy. When major hemorrhage is encountered, it should be controlled by clamping the hilum of the respective lung. If ligation of the pulmonary vein is performed, the corresponding lobe should be resected. Pulmonary vein injuries are associated with concomitant cardiac, pulmonary artery, aorta, and esophagus injuries.

INTERNAL MAMMARY ARTERY

These injuries can cause large hemothorax or pericardial tamponade. When encountered at the time of thoracotomy, these vessels are ligated. Similarly, when a clamshell thoracotomy is performed, these vessels are injured and should be controlled with suture ligation.

AZYGOUS VEIN

Exposure to this injury is through ipsilateral thoracotomy. These injuries are difficult to evaluate through median sternotomy. This is a potentially fatal injury because of the drainage of this vein into the superior vena cava. These injuries are best managed through suture ligation.

REFERENCES

1. *Advanced Trauma Life Support: Student Course Manual.* Chicago, IL: American College of Surgeons Committee on Trauma; 2018.
2. Wall MJ, Tai P, Mattox KL. Heart and thoracic vascular injuries. In: Feliciano DV, Mattox KL, Moore EE, eds. *Trauma.* McGraw Hill; 2020:485-511.
3. Azizzadeh A, Valdes J, Miller CC, et al. The utility of intravascular ultrasound compared to angiography in the diagnosis of blunt traumatic aortic injury. *J Vasc Surg.* 2011;53:608-614.
4. Lee WA, Matsumura JS, Mitchell RS, et al. Endovascular repair of traumatic thoracic aortic injury: clinical practice guidelines of the Society for Vascular Surgery. *J Vasc Surg.* 2011;53:187-192.
5. Fox N, Schwartz D, Salazar JH, et al. Evaluation and management of blunt traumatic aortic injury: a practice management guideline from the Eastern Association for the surgery of trauma. *J Trauma Acute Care Surg.* 2015;78(1):136-146.
6. Bottet B, Bouchard F, Peillon C, Baste J-M. When and how should we manage thoracic aortic injuries in the modern era? *Interact Cardiovasc Thorac Surg.* 2016;23(6):970-975.
7. Dubose JJ, Azizzadeh A, Estrera AL, Safi HJ. Contemporary management of blunt aortic trauma. *J Cardiovasc Surg (Torino).* 2015;56(5):751-762.

SELF-ASSESSMENT STUDY QUESTIONS AND ANSWERS

Questions

1. The most common thoracic vessels susceptible to injury are
   A. Intercostal vessels beneath ribs 1-3
   B. Intercostal vessels beneath ribs 4-6
   C. Intercostal vessels below rib 10
   D. Intercostal vessels beneath ribs 7-10
   E. None of the above

2. Permissive hypotension for patients with blunt traumatic aortic disruption without head injuries is maintained at what pressure?
   A. Between 50 and 55 mmHg
   B. Between 50 and 60 mmHg
   C. Between 60 and 70 mmHg
   D. Between 45 and 55 mmHg
   E. None of the above

3. Traumatic rupture of the aorta is associated with cardiac rupture in what percentage of patients?
   A. 5%
   B. 10%
   C. 33%
   D. 25%
   E. None of the above

4. The average diameter of the aorta among patients with aortic tears is?
   A. 15 cm
   B. 20 cm
   C. 19 cm
   D. 23 cm
   E. None of the above

5. When should a stable patient with traumatic aortic injury receive TEVAR?
   A. Within 12 hours
   B. Within 24 hours
   C. Within 48 hours
   D. Within 36 hours
   E. None of the above

6. Complications of TEVAR include?
   A. Endoleaks
   B. Graft migration
   C. Graft infection
   D. Retrograde dissection
   E. All of the above

7. Chest radiographic findings of blunt traumatic aortic disruption are
   A. Left hemothorax
   B. Apical capping of the left thorax
   C. Inferior depression of the left mainstem bronchus
   D. Deviation of the NGT to the right
   E. All of the above

8. For an uncertain thoracic vascular injury, the incision performed should be
   A. Median sternotomy
   B. Left anterolateral thoracotomy
   C. Right thoracotomy
   D. Left posterolateral thoracotomy
   E. None of the above

9. The incision performed to expose the right subclavian artery and vein?
   A. Median sternotomy with right extension along the anterior border of SCM
   B. Right anterolateral thoracotomy
   C. Right posterolateral thoracotomy
   D. Median sternotomy
   E. None of the above

10. The initial exposure of a left subclavian artery injury is performed through what incision?
   A. Median sternotomy
   B. Left anterolateral thoracotomy
   C. Left posterolateral thoracotomy
   D. Median sternotomy with extension to the left anterior border of the SCM
   E. None of the above

SELF-ASSESSMENT STUDY QUESTIONS AND ANSWERS

Answers

1. D.
2. B.
3. D.
4. D.
5. B.
6. E.
7. E.
8. B.
9. A.
10. B.

CHAPTER

46 Resuscitative Endovascular Balloon Occlusion of the Aorta for Vascular Trauma

Maaz Zuberi and Mallory Williams

OUTLINE

INTRODUCTION
HISTORICAL PERSPECTIVE OF AORTIC CONTROL FOR TORSO HEAMMORAGE
INDICATIONS
CONTRAINDICATION
PREPERATION AND EQUIPMENT
DEVICES
TECHNIQUE
Accessing the Femoral Artery
Balloon Catheter Selection and Insertion
Balloon Inflation
Operative Definitive Hemostasis
Balloon Deflation
Sheath Removal
COMPLICATIONS AND PITFALLS
CONCLUSION AND OUTCOMES

INTRODUCTION

Uncontrolled hemorrhage remains the leading cause of preventable death in most military and civilian trauma patients that present to the hospital.[1,2] ATLS (advanced trauma life support) dictates immediate control of hemorrhage as one of the most important aspect of management. Direct pressure and tourniquet-based proximal control can suffice to obtain extremity hemostasis, but a significant proportion of patients with torso injuries have noncompressible hemorrhage. Effective operative management for these patients includes aortic occlusion by either resuscitative endovascular balloon occlusion of the aorta (REBOA) and resuscitative thoracotomy with aortic cross clamping.

REBOA is currently a reliable means of obtaining torso hemorrhage control. This gives time for the trauma surgeon to achieve definitive operative hemostasis of torso injuries. REBOA represents a significant expansion of the trauma surgeon's tool kit for hemorrhage control and potential salvage of these patients.

HISTORICAL PERSPECTIVE OF AORTIC CONTROL FOR TORSO HEAMMORAGE

Although the oldest reported successful case of resuscitative thoracotomy dates as far back as 1896 by Luwig Rehn, the first formal report of an immediate ED thoracotomy for a hemodynamically unstable trauma patient was by Beall et al., in 1967.[3,4] The applicability of the technique was further broadened in 1976 when Ledgerwood described pre-laparotomy thoracotomy with aortic clamping for abdominal exsanguination.[5] The left lateral thoracotomy with aortic cross clamping avoided hemodynamic collapse caused by a laparotomy and associated release of tamponade of an abdominal bleed. It also gave access to repair cardiac injuries, release cardiac tamponade, and perform open cardiac massage.

In contrast to the open technique, the minimally invasive endovascular approach to proximal aortic control was first described in the military by CW Hughes in 1954, but was not widely utilized due to the cumbersome nature of early endovascular techniques and lack of appropriate training and equipment.[6] There were civilian attempts made in the pre-endovascular era in the 1980s to expand on the concept, but had poor outcomes.[7] With the advent of the endovascular era in the early 2000s, and increased experience of the vascular surgeons, REBOA became common to control hemorrhage in the setting of a ruptured abdominal aortic aneurysm.[8] This led to a renewed interest in REBOA for trauma hemorrhage control. High-quality translational research with animal models was conducted with promising results including improved hemorrhage control, rapid improvement in systolic blood pressures, reduction in acidosis, and improved outcomes to a thoracotomy. These studies lead to a resurgence in REBOA use by the trauma surgeon in the late 2000s for abdominal injuries with promising results from the AAST (American Association for Surgery of Trauma) AORTA study group. In the review, 85 REBOA patients were compared to 202 resuscitative thoracotomy patients, and survival was higher in the REBOA group (10% vs 3%).[9,10]

INDICATIONS

There is not enough data to describe absolute indications for REBOA; however, all patients with rapid exsanguination of abdominal injuries may be candidates for REBOA. These patients are divided into two categories: (1) those without a palpable pulse with cardiopulmonary arrest and (2) those with a palpable pulse but hypotensive and nonresponders to resuscitation. REBOA is noted to be better applied prior to cardiovascular collapse.

Based on the US department of defense Joint Commission REBOA algorithm (Figure 46-1), in patients with blunt injury without a pulse and CPR < 5minutes and **no cardiac tamponade or large pneumothorax on imaging**, REBOA is strongly considered to improve cerebral and coronary perfusion. Recent studies show improved outcomes in this subset of patients with endovascular versus open approach, likely due to the higher cardiac compression ratio, since CPR does not have to be stopped to place the intra-aortic balloon.[10]

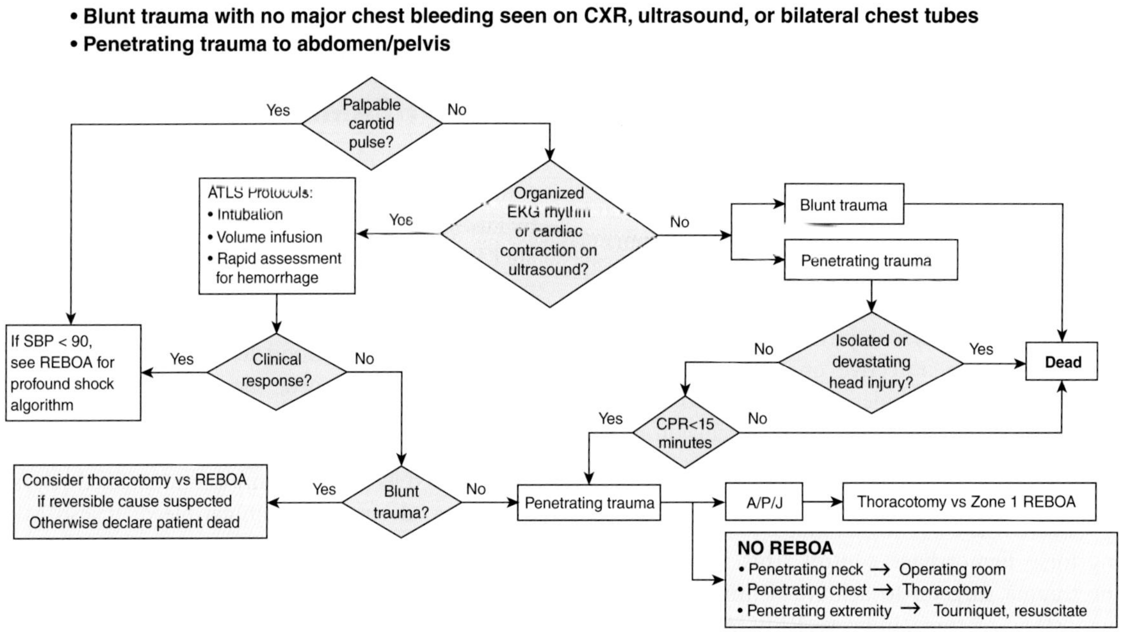

FIGURE 46-1 Resuscitative aortic occlusion decision algorithm in pulseless. (Reproduced with permission from Joint Trauma System: Joint Trauma System Clinical Practice Guidelines (JTS CPG). Resuscitative Endovascular Balloon Occlusion of the Aorta (REBOA) for Hemorrhagic Shock (CPG ID:38); 2017.)

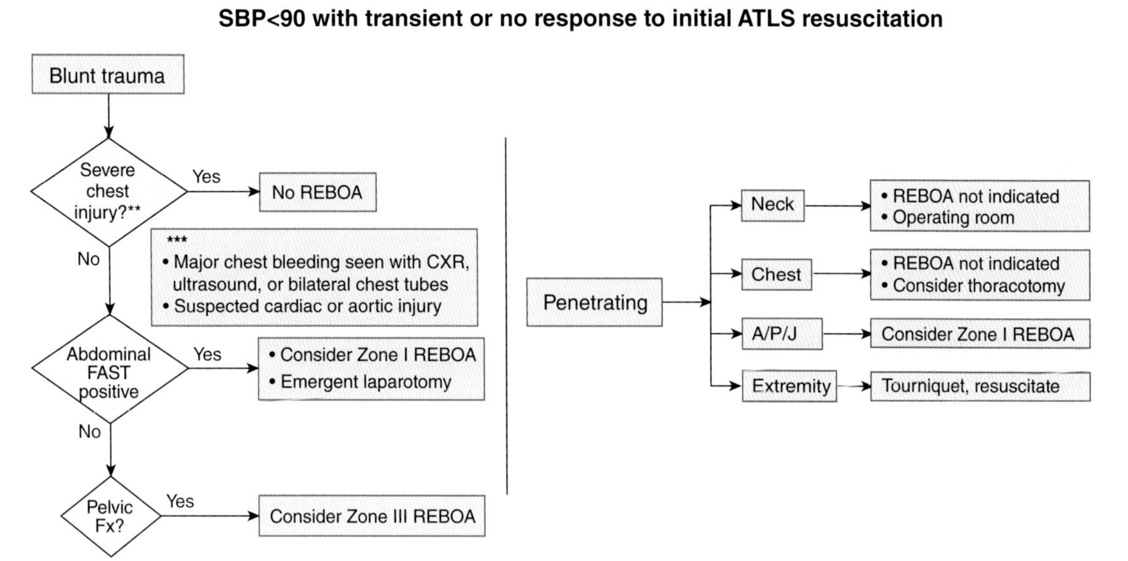

FIGURE 46-2 Resuscitative aortic occlusion decision algorithm in hypotensive patient. (Reproduced with permission from Joint Trauma System: Joint Trauma System Clinical Practice Guidelines (JTS CPG). Resuscitative Endovascular Balloon Occlusion of the Aorta (REBOA) for Hemorrhagic Shock (CPG ID:38); 2017.)

In patients with blunt injury and a palpable pulse, severe TBI, injury below the diaphragm, and refractory hypotension with systolic blood pressure <90 mmHg, after ruling out thoracic injuries, REBOA should be considered (based on a consensus conference using the Delphi method) (Figure 46-2). Early exposure and access to the common femoral artery (CFA) is recommended as this is the most time-consuming part of the REBOA device placement. This maneuver is especially well described in pelvic injuries as a bridge to angiographic or operative pelvic hemorrhage control.[11]

In the setting of penetrating injury, REBOA is only indicated in injuries below the diaphragm.

CONTRAINDICATION

Patients with nonsurvivable injuries, and those with extended periods of CPR (commonly >15 minutes), should not receive REBOA. Patients with thoracic, neck, and extremity injuries should not receive REBOA. In patients with penetrating or blunt thoracic injuries including tamponade or pneumothorax, open ED thoracotomy should be performed as it is both diagnostic and therapeutic. In patients with widened mediastinum and thoracic aorta injury, REBOA is contraindicated as it can worsen the aortic injury. Inability to obtain femoral access, such as in patients with significant peripheral arterial disease or prior groin surgery, remains a relative contraindication.

PREPERATION AND EQUIPMENT

The patients should be supine with an x-ray board under the trauma stretcher at the patients mid torso. If available, the patient should receive prophylactic antibiotics and standard groin prep with chlorhexadine. Preparation to place a REBOA and early access to the CFA should be made prior to hemodynamic collapse.

DEVICES

Currently available endovascular balloon catheters include over-the-wire and free-wire options.

Common example of over-the wire catheter includes the Coda Balloon™ (Cooks medical). These catheters require a larger femoral sheath, a 0.035" platform wire and fluoroscopy to control positioning. In these catheters, the balloon is located at the tip of

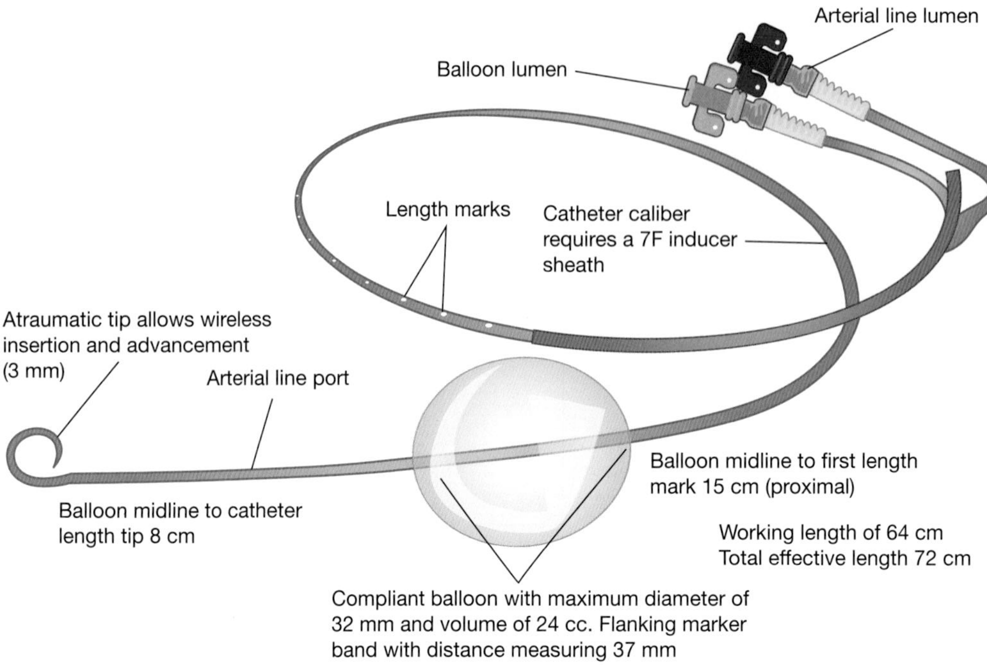

FIGURE 46-3 **A diagram depicting the ER REBOA catheter.**

the catheter and external landmarks used for catheter length for aortic Zone 1 is the xiphoid process, and for Zone 3 is the umbilicus.

In comparison, free-wire low-profile devices that include ER-REBOA™ (Prytime Medical) do not require use of radiography for appropriate positioning (Table 46-1). These devices have a small Nitinol wire inside the catheter hypo-tube design providing enough stiffness for quick positioning without imaging. In these catheters, the balloon is located away from the tip of the catheter and external landmarks used for catheter length for aortic Zone 1 is the sternal notch, and for Zone 3 is the xiphoid process (Figure 46-3).

Recent advances in REBOA catheter design includes an inner lumen that can accommodate a 0.025" wire assembly to facilitate endovascular intervention (P-REBOA PRO™), and catheters with integrated pressure monitoring to regulate intermittent partial pressure regulated aortic occlusion.

TABLE 46-1 Available REBOA Catheters

Catheter Type	Over-the-wire	Free-wire
	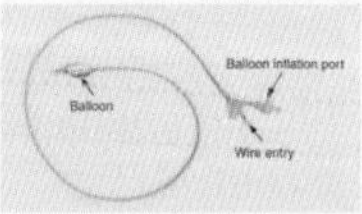	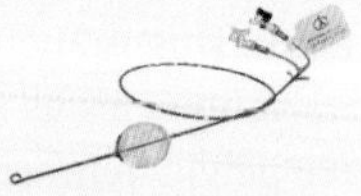
Brand examples	Coda type (Cook medical)	ER-REBOA (Prytime Medical)
Sheath size required	12 Fr	7–8 Fr
Landmark for Zone 1	Xiphoid process	Sternal notch
Land mark for Zone 3	Umbilicus	Xiphoid process
Need for fluoroscopy	Yes	No

TECHNIQUE

There are six fundamental steps to placement of a REBOA device: (1) Arterial access and sheath placement; (2) balloon catheter selection and insertion; (3) balloon inflation; (4) operative definitive hemostasis; (5) balloon deflation; (6) sheath removal.

ACCESSING THE FEMORAL ARTERY

REBOA is performed through a direct cut down to the femoral artery or percutaneous Seldinger technique either with a new percutaneous access with a needle or a wire exchange through an already existing arterial line. This is the most time-consuming and rate-limiting step of the REBOA procedure. It cannot be overstated how important gaining the initial access to the CFA is. Accidental access into the superficial femoral artery greatly increases the risk of ipsilateral leg ischemia and thromboembolic events due to the smaller caliber of the vessel in proportion to the sheath. The cut down is performed using a vertical groin incision after palpation of the CFA pulse, which is most commonly located at the half way point between the anterior superior crest of the iliac bone and the pubic tubercle just below the inguinal canal. The femoral artery lies anterior and lateral to the femoral vein. A single anterior wall puncture should be performed whether using a cut down or Seldinger procedure for access of the vessel. There is an association between low puncture sites and both pseudoaneurysms and arteriovenous fistulas as well as a high risk of retroperitoneal bleeding with high puncture sites.

The femoral pulse is over the CFA in approximately 93% of limbs, and the CFA is over the medial aspect of the femoral head in 78% of limbs.[12] So the most reliable landmark for both the incision for cut down and the arterial puncture is the maximal arterial pulse. For patients with weak or absent pulses due to hemorrhage, the most reliable landmark in individuals of average body build is 2 finger breadths (2.5 cm) lateral to the pubic tubercle below the inguinal ligament. In the American Association for the Surgery of Trauma, AORTA Registry up to 50% of patients required cut downs for accessing the CFA for REBOA. Both fluoroscopic- and ultrasound-guided arterial puncture can be utilized as well. The incidence of pseudoaneurysm formation can be significantly reduced to 2.6% with the use of ultrasound guidance, mainly by avoiding inadvertent puncture of the external iliac artery and superficial and deep femoral artery.[13] In a prospective evaluation of ultrasound-guided CFA puncture, the technique reduced the time to puncture and the number of attempts in patients with high BMI and those with weak or absent pulses.[14]

Once access has been established, an access sheath (longer for over the wire and shorter for wire-free catheters) of 7-14 Fr is advanced over a wire. The size of the sheath should accommodate the balloon without resistance, and during the access one should not push any wires or sheaths if resistance is felt. Next the wire and tapered introducer should be removed and the sheath flushed with 10 cc of heparin (10 units/ml) and 0/9% saline.

BALLOON CATHETER SELECTION AND INSERTION

There are three aortic zones for placement of the occluding balloon catheter. Zone 1 is in the descending aorta just distal to the subclavian artery to above the celiac artery. Zone 2 is defined as between the celiac artery and the renal arteries. Balloon occlusion should not occur in this zone. Zone 3 is the aortic and vena cava bifurcations (Figure 46-1). Measurements for placement of the catheter to the different zones must be performed and is different for the ER-REBOA wire-free catheter and the Coda over-the-wire catheter, based on where the catheters balloon is in relation to the tip of the catheter.

For the ER-REBOA wire-free catheter system for Zone I placement, measurement is done from the sternal notch (or 47 cm) to the access site of the CFA. For Zone 3 placement the measurement is from the xiphisternal process (or 27 cm) to the access site of the CFA. The ER-REBOA is advanced into the sheath taking care to keep the centered P-tip unfurled using the peel away sheath. Fluoroscopy is not required for placement.

For the Coda over-the-wire balloon catheter, since the balloon is located at the tip of the catheter,

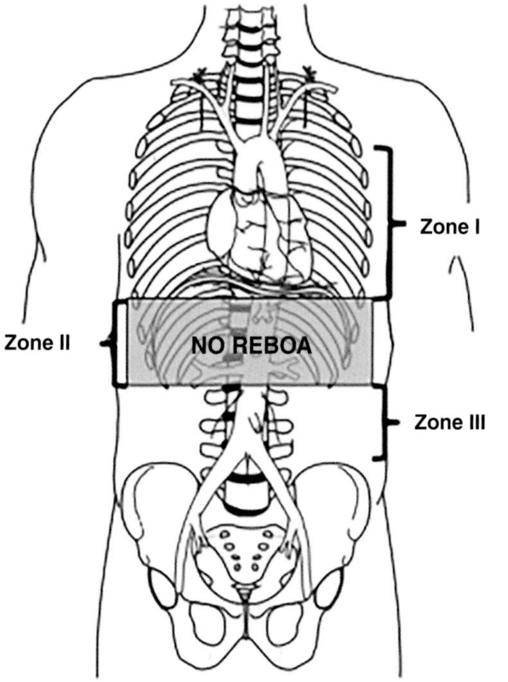

FIGURE 46-4 **Diagram representing the REBOA Zones.** (Reproduced with permission from Joint Trauma System: Joint Trauma System Clinical Practice Guidelines (JTS CPG). Resuscitative Endovascular Balloon Occlusion of the Aorta (REBOA) for Hemorrhagic Shock (CPG ID:38); 2017.)

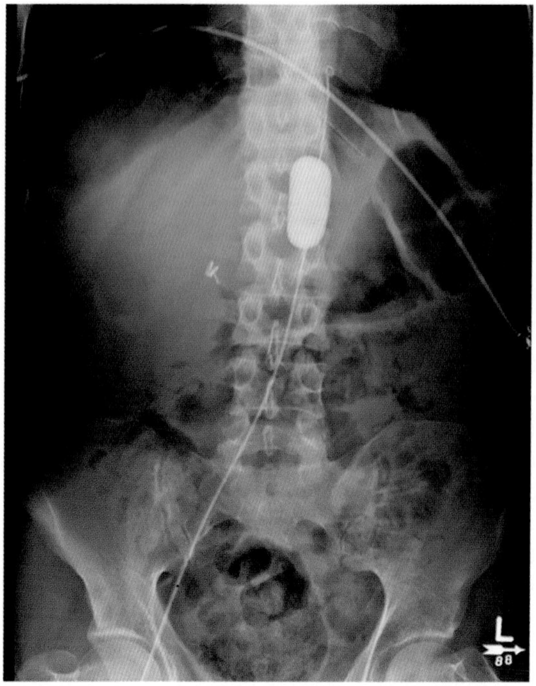

FIGURE 46-5 **X-ray demonstrating the cylindrical contour of the REBOA balloon showing complete aortic occlusion.** (Reproduced with permission from Hörer T, DuBose JJ, Rasmussen TE, et al. *Endovascular Resuscitation and Trauma Management: Bleeding and Haemodynamic Control.* Switzerland: Springer Nature; 2020.)

Zone 1 placement is measured from the xiphoid process, and Zone 3 from the umbilicus to the access site of the CFA. Over a 0.035 assembly, a long working wire of intermediate stiffness is first inserted into the aorta, and exchanged for a stiffer wire (Amplatz or Benson). Fluoroscopy is recommended to ensure that the wire remains in the thoracic aorta. Experimental use of the ultrasound with microbubble contrast and the sub-xiphoid window as an alternative to fluoroscopy is under investigation.[15]

BALLOON INFLATION

After placement of the catheter, the balloon is inflated to occlude or partially occlude the aorta. A 10-20 ml Luer lock syringe should be filled with a dilute mix of saline and contrast. Thick contrast can occlude the port, hence it should always be diluted before injecting into the balloon. The balloon should be inflated slowly to prevent over inflation and rupture. Rough estimation of balloon volume required for total aortic occlusion is 8 mL for Zone I and 3 mL for Zone III.

For over-the-wire catheters, the sheath should be maintained in place to prevent balloon migration during inflation, and the wire should not be removed. Once resistance is felt, a step up is noted in the A line tracing or the balloon adopts the cylindrical shape of the aorta, inflation is complete (Figure 46-5). An x-ray should be performed to document correct placement of the balloon.

For patients receiving total occlusion of the aorta, the contralateral pulse of the CFA should be absent. Left brachial pulse should be palpated and should be present ensuring the balloon is below the left subclavian artery. Attention to stabilization of the balloon catheter in its final position is essential to prevent the known complication of balloon migration. Most surgeons stitch the catheter in place within 5 cm of the access sheath.

OPERATIVE DEFINITIVE HEMOSTASIS

Once the balloon is inflated and the catheter is secured, the inflating syringe should remain attached to the balloon port, and stop cock should be placed in off position. Measures should now be taken for definitive hemorrhage control, either with a laparotomy in setting of peritonitis and abdominal bleed, or angiography and embolization in the setting of pelvic bleeding and pelvic fractures. As the patients, hemodynamics improve with placement of a REBOA device, the trauma team may develop a false sense of safety and become more relaxed in their interventions. It is the job of the trauma surgeon to ensure that the patients gets expeditious definitive control of hemorrhage. Limits of timing of a balloon catheter occluding either Zone I or Zone III has not been well established. Current expert opinion is evolving around a Zone I occlusion time of 30 minutes as optimal and a Zone III at 60 minutes; however, all efforts must be made to reach hemostasis and balloon deflation as soon as possible.

BALLOON DEFLATION

Once hemorrhage has been controlled, the balloon should be deflated. Deflation requires close communication with the anesthesia team because it leads to sudden release of toxins and reduction in afterload. Preferably, the anesthesia team should be prepared to provide aggressive fluid resuscitation. The balloon should be incrementally deflated <1 ml at a time over the course of 5-15 minutes, as sudden deflation can lead acute hemodynamic compromise. Even small reduction in balloon volume leads to significant increase in aortic flow. During a laparotomy, partial deflation of the balloon helps identify new areas of bleeding that can be controlled systematically. Once the balloon has been fully deflated, it is usually left in place till the completion of the laparotomy, in case reinflation is required.

SHEATH REMOVAL

Once the balloon is no longer required, the securing sutures should be cut and catheter should be removed from the sheath. With sheath removal, the common femoral access site needs to be managed. The sheath should be flushed with 100 ml of heparinized saline prior to removal. The sheath should not be removed if the patient is severely coagulopathic. In some centers, it is customary to perform a completion angiogram of the ipsilateral leg to ensure adequate blood flow. The arteriotomy can be closed with a suture in the open cut-down approach after a thorough proximal and distal Fogarty thromboembolectomy, or in a percutaneous approach, it can be closed with a closure device (Angioseal) or managed with direct pressure for 20 minutes. It is imperative to examine the ipsilateral leg and ensure pulses are present after sheath removal and no discrepancy in ABI is evident. Serial neurovascular checks for 12 hours pos REBOA removal are recommended. In some centers, a femoral ultrasound is performed at 72 hours to ensure no thrombus has formed, since the procedure is done without systemic heparin.

COMPLICATIONS AND PITFALLS

Although REBOA has emerged as a useful tool in the trauma surgeon's armamentarium, it is not without its complications and pitfalls. The largest review on REBOA has noted groin complications (i.e., pseudoaneurysms) in 5.6% of patients and lower extremity amputations in 2.1% of patients.[16]

A common operational pitfall includes making the decision to perform REBOA too late, as mortality increases once the patient loses pulses. Early cannulation of the CFA and utilization of a wire-free device in a hypotensive nonresponder, which is the rate-limiting step to the procedure can increase the efficiency of aortic occlusion. Accidental placement of the REBOA catheter in the superior vena cava and inflation of the balloon can lead to acute hemodynamic collapse due to loss of preload. Similarly accidental placement in a branch vessel can lead to damage to the vessel and further bleeding.

Unfamiliarity of the femoral anatomy and its variations with insertion of the REBOA catheter below the femoral artery bifurcation can greatly increase the risk of thromboembolism and ischemic injury to the ipsilateral leg. Some patients may present with unrecognized proximal femoral or iliac artery transection, which prevents access to the side of the injury. In this setting, contralateral access at the site with stronger pulse should be attempted but there should be a low threshold to convert to an ED resuscitative thoracotomy.

In patients where the guidewire or catheter does not pass freely, attempt should be made to access the contralateral groin. You should never push against resistance. Overinflation of the balloon can lead to rupture and intimal injury to the thoracic aorta with dissection. Rupture can be diagnosed with sudden drop in blood pressure, or blood noted in the syringe and balloon port on aspiration. If the patient still requires aortic control, the catheter can be replaced with a new one and balloon occlusion reattempted. Similarly, inappropriate inflation in Zone II can lead to bowel ischemia and renal injury. Failure to adequately secure the catheter can lead to balloon migration and injury to the aorta.

Failure to work with heightened urgency with improvement in vital signs after REBOA placement can lead to prolong inflation of the aortic balloon and subsequent ischemic injury to end organs. Similarly, early deflation of the balloon prior to adequate hemostasis can lead to prolong bleeding and hemodynamic collapse. Removal of arterial sheath while the patient is coagulopathic can lead to major hemorrhage from the access site.

As with all procedures requiring arterial cannulation, REBOA is associated with access site-related complication. Inadvertent cannulation of the superficial femoral artery instead of the CFA increases the risks of all complications. There is a known risk of thromboembolic event, especially in the absence of systemic anticoagulation therapy during the sheath placement. Recent studies have noted a REBOA-related embolism rate of 4.3%.[17] Thrombus can form along the whole assembly from the tip of the catheter to the access site. It is imperative that post REBOA neurovascular checks are performed of the ipsilateral extremity.

Access site dissection can occur as a result of balloon trauma. Angiography should be routinely utilized prior to sheath removal to diagnose this complication early and involve vascular surgery for definitive management.

CONCLUSION AND OUTCOMES

Data on the outcomes of REBOA are limited and contradictory and mostly consist of observational studies from single center retrospective reviews.

Although early results from US studies are promising, the largest study evaluating outcomes for Zone I REBOA comes from the Japanese Trauma Data bank. They reviewed 452 patients with or without REBOA intervention with matched injury severity scores, and found that mortality was significantly increased for those who underwent REBOA compared to those that did not. (Odds ratio 0.3, 95% CI 0.23–0.4).[18] However, it must be noted that the standard use of REBOA in Japan is more aggressive since a majority of emergency room physicians are double boarded in interventional radiology and may have overused REBOA beyond the strict parameters that are utilized in the US. Multiple case series from the US and Japan have shown varying results, for example, in contrast a series of 24 severely injured patients in which REBOA was used shows an actual survival of 29.2% compared to a predicted survival of 12.5%.[19]

When compared to Zone I REBOA, Zone III REBOA use has been studied even less. Two US-based groups have reported case series for utilization of Zone III REBOA for pelvic fractures and noted a survival advantage with REBOA. A two patient-based study showed systolic blood pressure elevation from 80s to 120s after placement of Zone III REBOA in patients with pelvic fractures.[20] Another study showed that the predicted survival of such patients was 39% compared to the actual survival of 46% in a 13 patient-based case series.[21] REBOA is a method for proximal aortic control that while still being actively reviewed has become one of the tools for hemorrhage control both in civilian and military trauma teams.

REFERENCES

1. Teixeira PGR, Inaba K, Hadjizacharia P, et al. Preventable or potentially preventable mortality at a Mature Trauma Center. *J Trauma*. 2007;63(6):1338-1347.
2. Kisat M, Morrison JJ, Hashmi ZG, Efron DT, Rasmussen TE, Haider AH. Epidemiology and outcomes of non-compressible torso hemorrhage. *J Surg Res*. 2013;184(1): 414-421.
3. Beck CS. Wounds of the heart. *Arch Surg*. 1926;13:205.
4. Beall AC, Diethrich EB, Crawford HW, Cooley DA, De Bakey ME. Surgical management of penetrating cardiac injuries. *Am J Surg*. 1966;112:686-692.

5. Ledgerwood AM, Kazmers M, Lucas CE. The role of thoracic aortic occlusion for massive hemoperitoneum. *J Trauma*. 1976;16(8):610-615.
6. Hughes CW. Use of an intra-aortic balloon catheter tamponade for controlling intra-abdominal hemorrhage in man. *Surgery*. 1954;36(1):65-68.
7. Gupta BK, Khaneja SC, Flores L, Eastlick L, Longmore W, Shaftan GW. The role of intra-aortic balloon occlusion in penetrating abdominal trauma. *J Trauma*. 1989; 29(6):861–865.
8. Greenberg RK, Srivastava SD, Ouriel K, et al. An endoluminal method of hemorrhage control and repair of ruptured abdominal aortic aneurysms. *J Endovasc Ther*. 2000;7(1):1–7.
9. Brenner M, Teeter W, Hoehn M, et al. Use of resuscitative endovascular balloon occlusion of the aorta for proximal aortic control in patients with severe hemorrhage and arrest. *JAMA Surg*. 2018;153(2):130–135.
10. Brenner M, Inaba K, Aiolfi A, et al. Resuscitative endovascular balloon occlusion of the aorta and resuscitative thoracotomy in select patients with hemorrhagic shock: early results from the American Association for the Surgery of Trauma's Aortic occlusion in resuscitation for trauma and acute care surgery registry. *J Am Coll Surg*. 2018;226(5):730–740.
11. Joint Trauma System. (2017). *Clinical Practice Guidelines (CPGs). Joint Trauma System*. The Department of Defense Center of Excellence for Trauma. https://jts.amedd.army.mil/index.cfm/PI_CPGs/cpgs
12. Baum PA, Matsumoto AH, Teitelbaum GP, Zuurbier RA, Barth KH. Anatomic relationship between the common femoral artery and vein: CT evaluation and clinical significance. *Radiology*. 1989;173:775–777.
13. Gabriel M, Pawlaczyk K, Waliszewski K, Krasiński Z, Majewski W. Location of femoral artery puncture site and the risk of postcatheterization pseudoaneurysm formation. *Int J Cardiol*. 2007;120:167–171.
14. Dudeck O, Teichgraeber U, Podrabsky P, Haenninen EL, Soerensen R, Ricke J. A randomized trial assessing the value of ultrasound-guided puncture of the femoral artery for interventional investigations. *Int J Cardiovasc Imaging*. 2004;20:363–368.
15. https://pubmed.ncbi.nlm.nih.gov/28215930/ *US guided reboa*
16. DuBose JJ, Scalea TM, Brenner M, et al. The AAST prospective aortic occlusion for resuscitation in trauma and acute care surgery (AORTA) registry: data on contemporary utilization and outcomes of aortic occlusion and resuscitative balloon occlusion of the aorta (REBOA). *J Trauma Acute Care Surg*. 2016;81:409–419.
17. Manzano-Nunez R, Orlas CP, Herrera-Escobar JP, et al. A meta-analysis of the incidence of complications associated with groin access after the use of resuscitative endovascular balloon occlusion of the aorta in trauma patients. *J Trauma Acute Care Surg*. 2018;85:626–634.
18. Norii T, Crandall C, Terasaka Y. Survival of severe blunt trauma patients treated with resuscitative endovascular balloon occlusion of the aorta compared with propensity score-adjusted untreated patients. *J Trauma Acute Care Surg*. 2015;78:721–728.
19. Saito N, Matsumoto H, Yagi T, et al. Evaluation of the safety and feasibility of resuscitative endovascular balloon occlusion of the aorta. *J Trauma Acute Care Surg*. 2015;78:897–903.
20. Martinelli T, Thony F, Decléty P, et al. Intra-aortic balloon occlusion to salvage patients with life threatening hemorrhagic shocks from pelvic fractures. *J Trauma*. 2010;68:942–948.
21. Brenner ML, Moore LJ, DuBose JJ, et al. A clinical series of resuscitative endovascular balloon occlusion of the aorta for hemorrhage control and resuscitation. *J Trauma Acute Care Surg*. 2013;75:506–511.

SELF-ASSESSMENT STUDY QUESTIONS AND ANSWERS

Questions

1. The indications for REBOA are?
   A. No palpable pulse in cardiac arrest with noncompressible hemorrhage
   B. Palpable pulse with noncompressible hemorrhage who are nonresponders to resuscitation
   C. None of the above
   D. All of the above

2. The most time-consuming aspect of this procedure is?
   A. Having equipment ready at the bedside
   B. Accessing the common femoral artery
   C. Placement of the aortic balloon in Zone 1
   D. Passing a guide wire
   E. None of the above

3. What are the external surface markers for Zone 1 and Zone III?
   A. The sternal notch and the umbilicus
   B. The nipple and the umbilicus
   C. The cricoid and the pubic symphysis
   D. The sternal notch and the pubic symphysis
   E. None of the above

4. What is the the most reliable location for the common femoral artery in patients with a weak pulse from hemorrhage?
   A. 3 finger breadths from the pubic tubercle
   B. 2 finger breadths from the pubic tubercle
   C. 1 finger breadth from the pubic tubercle
   D. None of the above

5. Define Zone II of the aorta.
   A. Between the renal arteries and the SMA
   B. Between the renal arteries and the celiac artery
   C. Between the renal arteries and the hepatic artery
   D. None of the above

6. In an average sized individual, what is the distance from the xiphisternal process to the access site in the common femoral artery?
   A. 40 cm
   B. 35 cm
   C. 27 cm
   D. 45 cm
   E. None of the above

7. What is the amount of saline and contrast required to fill the balloon to occlude Zone 1?
   A. 5 cc
   B. 8 cc
   C. 10 cc
   D. 15 cm
   E. None of the above

8. What is the amount of saline and contrast required to fill the ballon to occlude Zone III?
   A. 5 cc
   B. 6 cc
   C. 3 cc
   D. 7 cc
   E. None of the above

9. What is the current recommendation for timing of Zone III occlusion?
   A. 35 minutes
   B. 45 minutes
   C. 25 minutes
   D. 60 minutes
   E. None of the above

10. What is the procedure for deflating the aortic balloon?
   A. 1 cc at a time over 5–15 minutes with resuscitating
   B. 0.5 cc at a time over 5–15 minutes with resuscitation
   C. 2 cc at a time over 5 minutes with resuscitation
   D. 2 cc at a time over 10 minutes with resuscitation
   E. None of the above

SELF-ASSESSMENT STUDY QUESTIONS AND ANSWERS

Answers

1. D.
2. B.
3. A.
4. B.
5. B.
6. C.
7. B.
8. C.
9. D.
10. A.

CHAPTER

47 Compartment Syndrome

Nabil A. Ebraheim and David Yatsonsky, II

OUTLINE

GENERAL CONSIDERATIONS/HISTORY
BASIC ANATOMY
PATHOPHYSIOLOGY/ASSOCIATED MOLECULAR PROBLEMS
CLINICAL FINDINGS
DIFFERENTIAL DIAGNOSIS
DIAGNOSIS
MANAGEMENT OF THE CLINICAL PROBLEM
Endovascular Options
OPEN SURGERY
Fasciotomies
COMPLICATIONS
VOLKMANN'S ISCHEMIC CONTRACTURE
CHRONIC EXERTIONAL COMPARTMENT SYNDROME

GENERAL CONSIDERATIONS/HISTORY

Compartment syndrome (CS) has been identified as a disease state since 1881 by German surgeon Richard Von Volkmann.[1] However, the potential harm of increased intra-compartmental pressure was first observed by Hippocrates in 400 BC. Volkmann noted paralysis and contracture and suggested that it came simultaneously because of an interruption to the blood supply of the affected muscles.[1,2] The first surgeon to reproduce ischemic contracture was Paul Jepson in 1924 while working at the Mayo Foundation.[1] He demonstrated that prompt surgical decompression could prevent these contractures.[1]

Acute compartment syndrome (ACS) is a condition in which increased pressure (from any source) within a closed space comprises the circulation to the tissues contained within this space[2] (Figures 47-1 and 47-2). Without urgent decompression, tissue ischemia, necrosis, and functional impairment will occur.[1,3,4] Almost any injury can cause this syndrome including fractures, soft tissue injury, crush syndrome, burns, decreased compartment size, vigorous exercise, and more (Figures 47-1 and 47-3).[2–4] According to a study by McQueen et al. (2000), which examined 164 patients with CS, 69% had an associated fracture of which approximately half were tibial shaft fractures (Figure 47-3).[2] CS is also frequently secondary to reperfusion following arterial occlusion.[3]

There are numerous risk factors for CS including young age, usually under 35, male gender, tibial fractures, high-energy forearm fractures, bleeding, and diathesis/anticoagulants (Figure 47-4).[3] Alternatively, there are numerous risk factors for misdiagnosing ACS including altered level of consciousness, regional anesthesia, patient-controlled analgesia, children, and associated nerve injuries.[3] Exertional compartment syndrome is divided into two forms: acute exertional compartment syndrome (AECS) and acute on-top-of chronic exertional CS. AECS exists when intracompartmental pressure is elevated to a level and duration such that immediate

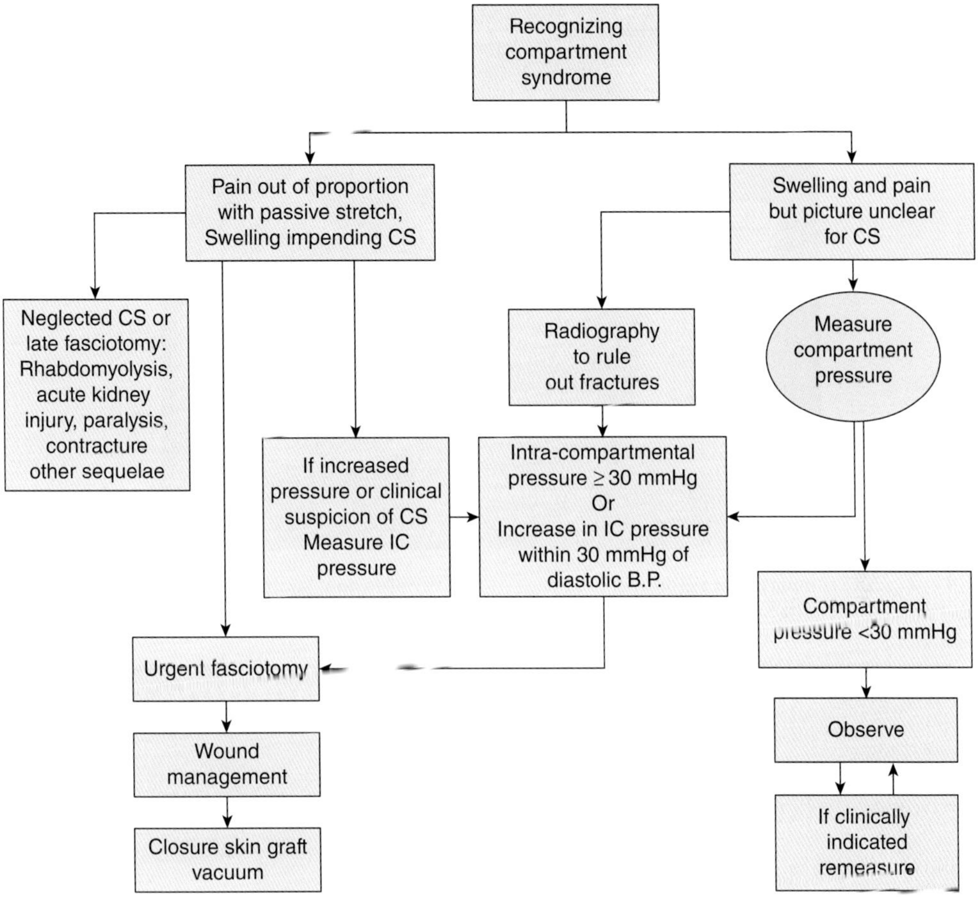

FIGURE 47-1 **Flow chart demonstrating clinical presentation, workup, treatment, neglected compartment syndrome, and various outcomes.**

decompression is necessary to prevent necrosis, which occurs in individuals performing strenuous activity above his or her normal level of training.[3] Acute on-top-of chronic exertional CS exists when a chronic CS proceeds to an acute form which requires decompression. For example, military recruits may be forced to exercise while suffering from a chronic exertional CS and need urgent fasciotomies.

BASIC ANATOMY

CS can involve any myofascial compartment within the body. Compartments most at risk due to fractures include leg, forearm, thigh, hand, foot, gluteal, and shoulder.

Tibial fractures are the most common. The compartments of the lower extremity are particularly susceptible to elevated compartment pressures.[5] Up to 45% of all CS cases involving the lower leg are caused by tibial fractures.[5,6] Clinicians should have a high index of clinical suspicion for CS.[5] There are four quadrants of the lower leg: anterior compartment, lateral compartment, deep posterior compartment, and superficial posterior compartment.[5,6] The anterior compartment tibialis anterior, extensor hallucis longus, extensor digitorum longus, and fibularis tertius.[5] The boundaries of the anterior compartment include deep fascia of the leg, anteriorly, interosseous membrane, the lateral surface of the tibia, medially, and the anterior intermuscular septum, and

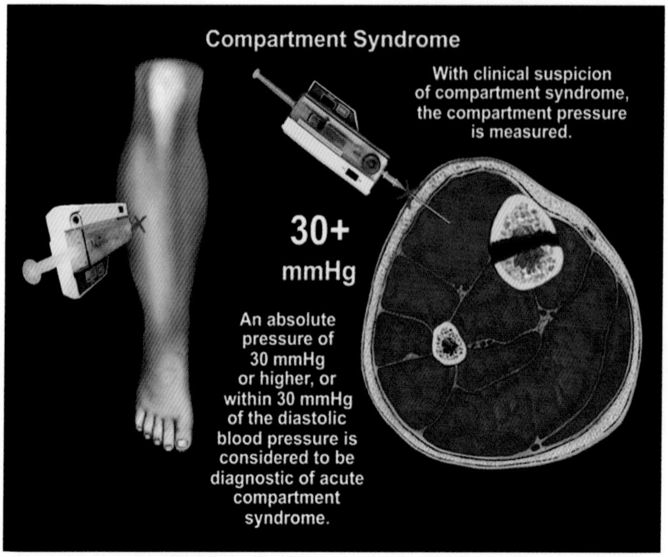

FIGURE 47-2 **Acute compartment syndrome.** This image depicts a swollen right lower extremity being measured with a manometer, following a tibial fracture.

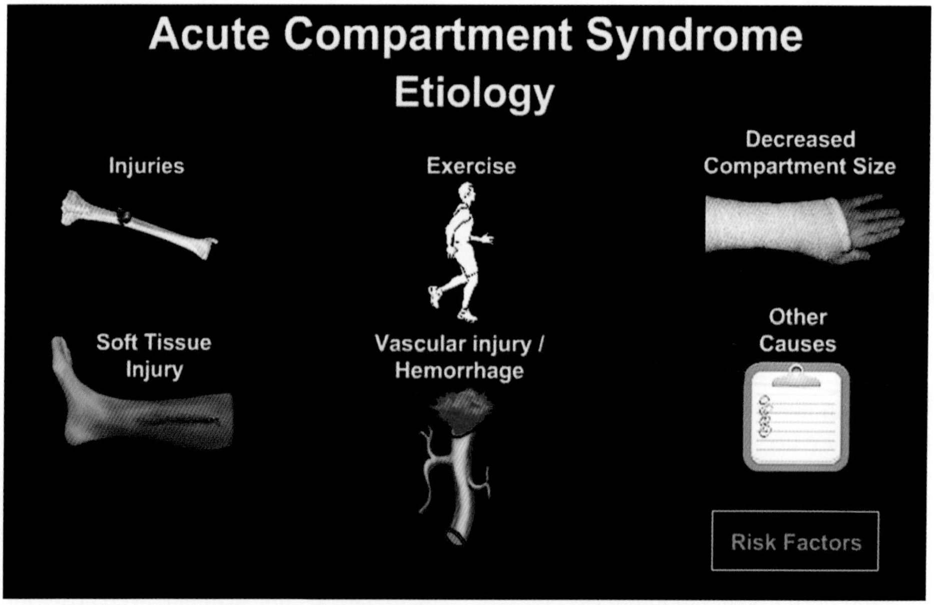

FIGURE 47-3 **Acute compartment syndrome etiology.** This image depicts various causes of acute compartment syndrome including fractures, soft tissue injuries, exercise, vascular injury/hemorrhage, decreased compartment size, and additional causes.

medial surface of fibula, laterally.[5,6] The muscles of the anterior compartment are innervated by the deep peroneal nerve (L4-S) and anterior tibial artery.[5] The lateral compartment also known as the peroneal compartment is composed of the peroneus brevis and peroneus longus.[5,6] The borders of the lateral compartment include the anterior intermuscular septum, anteriorly; the posterior intermuscular septum,

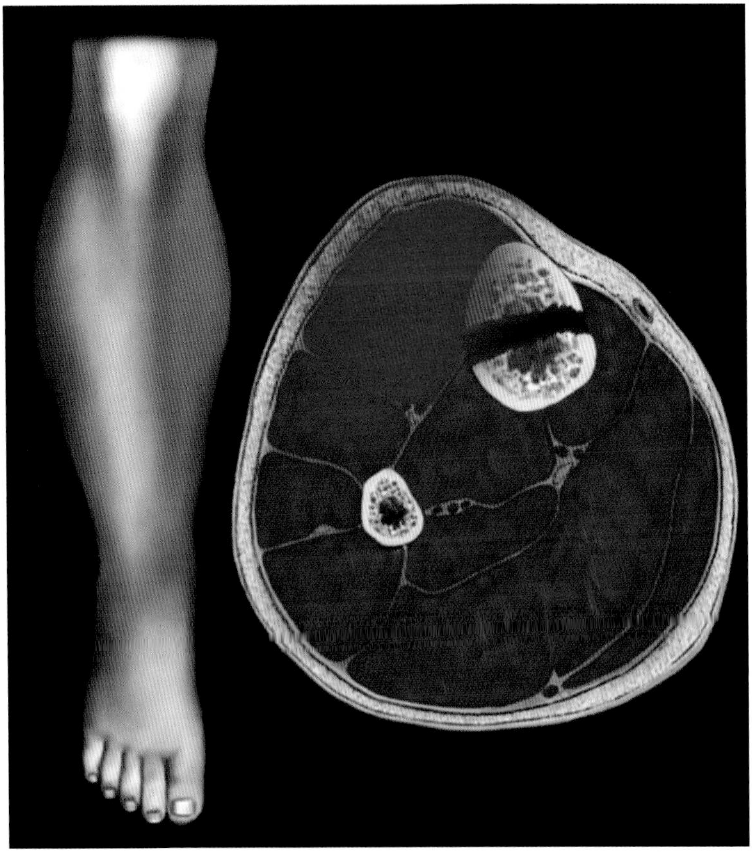

FIGURE 47-4 **This animation depicts a tibial fracture, swelling, and erythema, consistent with a limb afflicted with acute compartment syndrome.**

posteriorly; the fibula, medially; and the deep fascia of the leg, laterally.[5] It is innervated by the superficial peroneal nerve and receives its blood supply from the perforating branches of the anterior tibial artery and peroneal artery.[5] Venous drainage includes drainage into small saphenous veins superficially and fibular veins which drain into the posterior tibial vein.[5] The deep posterior compartment is composed of the tibialis posterior, flexor digitorum longus (FDL), flexor hallucis longus, and the popliteus muscles.[5] This compartment is innervated by the tibial nerve and receives blood supply from branches of the posterior tibial artery and fibular artery.[5] The borders of this compartment include the deep transverse fascia, anteriorly; the transverse intermuscular septum, posteriorly; and the deep fascia of the leg medially and laterally.[5] The superficial posterior compartment of the lower leg is composed of the plantaris and triceps surae; the medial and lateral heads of the gastrocnemius muscle and the soleus muscle.[5] This compartment is innervated by the tibial artery and receives blood supply from branches of the posterior tibial artery and fibular artery.[5] The borders of the posterior compartment include the transverse intermuscular septum, anteriorly, and the deep fascia of the leg medially, laterally, and posteriorly.[5] Most can be treated by dual medial/lateral fasciotomy approach or single lateral approach fasciotomies.[5,6]

The forearm is the next most common place for CS to occur.[6,7] Distal radius fractures are the second most common cause of CS following tibial fractures.[7] Forearm CS is usually caused by fractures.[6–9] The most common fractures causing forearm CS are supracondylar humerus fractures and both-bone radius and ulna fractures.[6–8] Rare etiologies include constrictive bandages, roller injuries, limb compression, arterial catheterization, and nephrotic syndrome.[7,8] In 5% of gunshot wounds to the forearm, patients will develop CS within 24 hours.[10] The forearm contains five compartments: superficial volar, deep volar, Henry's mobile wad, superficial dorsal, and deep dorsal compartments.[7,9] Most cases can be treated by release of the volar compartments. The mobile wad or mobile wad of Henry is also known as the "lateral compartment" or "radial group" is composed of the brachioradialis, extensor carpi radialis brevis, and extensor carpi radialis longus.[7,9] It is innervated by the radial nerve and CS of this compartment leads to decreased sensation along the radial nerve distribution in the hand.[7,9] The superficial volar compartment is composed of flexor carpi ulnaris, flexor digitorum superficialis, flexor carpi radialis, and pronator teres.[6,7,9] The deep volar compartment contains the flexor digitorum profundus and flexor pollicis longus.[6,7,9] The dorsal compartment contains the extensor carpi ulnaris.[6,7,9]

The arm is composed of two compartments: anterior and posterior.[8,12] The anterior compartment is bounded by the humerus posteriorly, the lateral and medial intermuscular septa, and the brachial fascia anteriorly.[8,9,11] The posterior compartment is bounded by the humerus and the lateral and medial intermuscular septa, and posteriorly by the brachial fossa.[8,9,11] The anterior compartment contains the biceps brachii, the brachialis, corachobrachialis, and brachoradialis in the lower one-third, and the posterior compartment contains the triceps brachii and aconeus.[8,9,11] The anterior compartment contains the median nerve, the musculocutaneous nerve, the ulnar nerve in the upper two-thirds and the radial nerve in the lower one-third.[8,9,11] CS in the biceps, triceps, or deltoid regions is usually seen when patients are found down for prolonged periods of time, such as in patients with drug overdoses.[8,9,11]

CS of the hand is often the result of iatrogenic injuries from IV's or A-lines.[8,9,12] Other etiologies include snake bites, crush injuries, burns, trauma, and prolonged pressure.[8,12] The hand is generally considered to have 10 muscle compartments, which include the thenar, hypothenar, adductor pollicis, 4 dorsal interosseous, and 3 volar interosseous compartments.[9,11] Within the dorsal interosseous compartment are the territories of the median and ulnar nerve and the four dorsal interossei.[9,11] The volar interosseous compartment contains the nerve territories of the median and ulnar nerve as well as three volar interossei.[9,11] The thenar compartment contains the territory of the recurrent branch of the median nerve, the superficial branch of the radial nerve, and the following muscles: abductor digiti minimi brevis, flexor pollicis brevis, and opponens pollicis.[8,9,11,12] The hypothenar compartment is innervated by the superficial and deep branches of the ulnar nerve. It contains the abductor digiti minimi, flexor digiti minimi brevis, and opponens digiti minimi.[9,11,12]

CS of the buttocks is quite rare. CS of the buttocks are often secondary to prolonged surgical procedures or drug overdoses.[13,14] If this is not detected early, gluteal CS can lead to severe muscle necrosis, renal failure, sepsis, and possibly death.[4,13,14] The buttocks are divided into four compartments conventionally.[9,13,14] These include the iliopsoas compartment, the anterolateral compartment, the gluteus maximus compartment, and the gluteus medius and minimus compartment.[13,14] The gluteal compartments are generally considered to include the tensor fascia lata, the gluteus medius and minimus compartment, and the gluteus maximus compartment.[9,13,14] The sciatic nerve is the primary motor and sensory nerve. It should be protected during pressure measurements and subsequent fasciotomies.[9,13,14],

The pelvis is highly unlikely location for CS.[15–17] It is primarily a result of anticoagulant medications, hemophilia, severe trauma, rupture of an abdominal aortic aneurysm, percutaneous posterolateral discectomy and decompression, and traumatic iliopsoas hematomas.[15] Iliopsoas compartment includes the psoas major, psoas minor, and iliacus muscles.[9,11] It also contains the many lumbar nerve roots which become the lateral femoral cutaneous nerve and femoral nerve, which splits into many branches below the inguinal ligament.[9,11,15–17]

Thigh CS is an uncommon occurrence; it is most commonly secondary to blunt trauma often accompanying a femoral fracture.[18–20] It is imperative to have a high index of suspicion even in the instance of minor trauma in the instance of hemophilia or anticoagulation therapy.[18–20] Rarer causes include vascular injury, intramedullary nailing, and iliofemoral deep vein thrombosis (DVT).[18,19,20] Thigh compartments include the anterior compartment, medial compartment, and posterior compartment.[9,19] The medial compartment contains the adductor longus, the adductor brevis, the adductor magnus, and the gracilis. It is innervated by the obturator nerve.[9,19] The anterior compartment contains the quadriceps femoris and the sartorius muscles.[9,19] The anterior compartment is innervated by the femoral and saphenous nerve.[9,11,19] The anterior compartment is the most impacted in CS of the thigh.[9,11,19] The posterior compartment of the thigh contains the hamstrings: biceps femoris, semitendinosus, and semimembranosus.[9,11,19] The posterior compartment contains and is innervated by the sciatic nerve: primarily the tibial nerve, while the biceps femoris is innervated by the common fibular nerve.[6,9,11,18,19]

The foot is another unlikely site for CS. There are nine compartments of the foot.[6] Among these are the four general compartments; interossei compartments, adductor hallucis compartment, lateral compartment, and central compartments.[5,6,9] Of note, the deep central compartment of the foot communicates with the deep posterior compartment of the lower leg.[6,20] Therefore, injuries may contribute to CS in both of these compartments.[6,20] The central compartments are composed of the superficial central compartment which contains the FDL and brevis.[9] The medial compartment contains abductor hallucis; flexor hallucis brevis; tendon of flexor hallucis brevis; and medial plantar arteries, veins, and nerves.[5,6,9,20] The interosseous compartment contains the dorsal interossei muscles; plantar interossei muscles; and plantar lateral artery, vein, and nerve.[5,6,9,20] The lateral compartment contains the abductor digiti minimi/quinti; the flexor digiti minimi; opponens digiti minimi; and branches of the lateral plantar artery, vein, and nerve.[5,6,9,20] The central compartment is composed of three levels. The first level contains the adductor hallucis; the second level contains the quadratus plantae, lumbrical muscles, and tendons of the FDL.[5,6,9,20] The third level contains the flexor digitorum brevis. Insults which would merit a high index of clinical suspicion for foot CS include calcaneal fractures, tibial fractures, and crush injuries.[5,6,9,20]

PATHOPHYSIOLOGY/ASSOCIATED MOLECULAR PROBLEMS

Mechanisms including fractures, contusions, bleeding disorders, burns, trauma, postischemic swelling, gunshot wounds, exercises, crush syndrome, decreased compartment size, and a variety of other etiologies may all initiate a sequence of events that produces CS.[4,21,22] The exact pathophysiology is still the topic of debate, but prominent theories hold that obstruction at the small blood vessels occurs.[6,21] In a rabbit study by Matsen et al, increased tissue pressures lead to compromised blood flow and decreased pO_2 muscle tissue.[22] Reduced blood flow leads to ischemia, necrosis, irreversible damage to the afflicted limb, and possible systemic conditions resulting from traumatic rhabdomyolysis, and reperfusion injury.[21,22] Three main theories describe the pathophysiology of CS. The critical closing pressure theory holds that when transmural pressure, which is the difference between intravascular pressure and tissue pressure drops, there is a critical closing pressure in the small vessels, and they become obstructed.[23] A second theory called the arteriovenous (AV) gradient theory iterates that increases in local pressure reduces the local AV pressure gradient thus reducing blood flow. When flow diminishes to less than the metabolic demands of the tissues, not necessarily zero, functional abnormalities result.[23] A third theory, the microvascular occlusion theory holds that capillary occlusion is the main mechanism reducing blood flow in ACS.[6,23]

Resting compartment pressure is usually less than 10 mmHg for adults, ±4 mmHg according to most sources.[3,6] In children, however, the resting compartmental pressures are generally higher.[24] On average, pressures in the four compartments varied between 13.3 mmHg and 16.6 mmHg in the children and between 5.2 mmHg and 9.7 mmHg in adults.[5,6]

The typical sequence of CS is the initiating event, edema-hemorrhage-accumulation, elevated compartment pressures, venous obstruction, and further elevation of compartment pressures.[5,6,22,24] An increase to 30 mmHg within a compartment or to within 30 mmHg of diastolic blood pressure will lead to impending CS.[6,22] Within the first 3–4 hours, the muscular changes are still typically reversible.[6,22] After 6 hours, there are clear variable damage to the tissue compartments.[6,22] After 8 hours following onset of CS, irreversible changes have befallen the muscles.[6,22] Nerve damage is also longitudinal in progression in CS. Within the first 2 hours, there is loss of nerve conduction.[6,22] After 4 hours, neuropraxia develops.[6,22] At this point, the nerve is still in place but can no longer transmit impulses.[6,22] After 8 hours following the onset of CS, total axonotmesis and a secondary scar has occurred, and irreversible damage has occurred to the nerves (Figure 47-1).[6,22] Theories of nerve damage due to ACS vary.[6,22] Viable pathophysiological mechanisms include ischemia, ischemia plus compression, and toxic effects of local acidosis.[6,22,23]

Pathophysiology of acute ischemia is secondary to increased compartmental pressure.[6,22] In untreated CS Volkmann's intrinsic contracture may occur, for instance, in the foot claw toes are a result (Figure 47-1).[25]

CLINICAL FINDINGS

Patients with CS may present in a variety of instances but usually after trauma involving a fracture, soft tissue damage, vascular injury, decreased compartment size, as well as other injuries or insults.[2,3,6] Following these traumatic injuries, patients may acutely or gradually experience increased compartmental pressure and subsequent pain.[2,6] These patients experience significant pain, particularly pain out of proportion to muscle stretch.[2,6] The traditional six P's, which include pain, pallor, paresthesia, pulselessness, poikilothermia, and paresis/paralysis, were used to diagnose CS; however, these symptoms, excluding pain, are misleading.[6,23] These are late presentations of the disease and may not be observed until the CS is fully established and the damage is irreversible (Figure 47-1).[6,23] CS needs to be diagnosed early in the impending stage.[2,3,6] The afflicted compartment is often tense to the examiner.[2,3,6] The symptoms are not always chronological and oftentimes pulseless, paresthesia, paralysis are later findings and associated with more significant ischemia and poorer clinical outcomes.[6,23] Prolonged ischemia, over 6–8 hours are more likely to suffer lasting effects.[6,22,23] Furthermore, patients who experience reperfusion after permanent ischemia has ensured will experience other serious insults such as myoglobinuria, acute kidney injury.[4,6]

Swelling is often heralded as an indicator of CS.[2,4,6] A swollen and tense compartment is a direct manifestation of increased intracompartmental pressure.[2,6,22] Swelling, and palpable tenderness are considered crude indicators and may be difficult to appreciate in deeper compartment manifestations.[2,6,22]

The six P's are not considered diagnostic criteria but are late term sequelae and some will be discussed individually.[6]

Pain out of proportion is often the primary and most reliable sign of impending CS. Escalating pain that is unrelieved by immobilization and requires increasing analgesia should elicit a high index of suspicion. Pain with passive stretch represents another common and relatively early marker of CS.[6] As CS progresses and ischemia, necrosis, and nerve injury manifest, the pain sensation may be lost.[2,6,26]

Paresthesia and sensory deficits are another late manifestation of CS.[2,6] Elevated compartment pressure leads to nerve ischemia which leads to sensory deficits within the distribution of the involved nerves.[2,6] Therefore, anatomical knowledge of the contents of each compartment is necessary in identifying the source of the afflicted compartment clinically. It should be noted that nerve damage may lead to paresthesia and/or dysesthesia independent of CS secondary to initial injury.[2,6]

Pulselessness is a rare presentation of CS.[6] As intracompartmental pressure increases, small vessels become occluded.[6,22,23] As intracompartmental pressure exceeds diastolic pressure, arteriolar and capillary perfusion are blocked and the muscles become ischemic.[6,22,23] Systolic blood pressure, however, is still forcing blood into the arteries of a compartment distally, commonly producing a pulse and capillary refill despite the established CS.[6,22,23] Pulselessness, therefore, is a very late sign indicating that intracompartmental pressure has increased enough to surpass systolic blood pressure and occlude a major artery.[6,22,23] Once pulselessness presents, there is considered to be total ischemia and fully established CS.[6,22,23] Now, tissue damage is likely severe and may necessitate amputation.[6,25,26]

Compartment pressures will be elevated in these patients.[2,3] A resting pressure of less than 10 mmHg is normal for compartment pressure.[6] Of note, there is moderate variability in children versus adults. Children often have pressure variation in the compartments of the lower leg: 13.3 mmHg and 16.6 mmHg, whereas adults are commonly between 5.2 mmHg and 9.7 mmHg.[6,24] When a patient has CS, the afflicted compartment will have an increase in pressure to 30 mmHg or within 30 mmHg of the diastolic blood pressure.[2,6] The diagnosis of CS is not limited to the compartmental pressure however if the patient has symptoms consistent with CS. The test may be falsely negative due to user error. In this case a fasciotomy is still indicated.[5,6,27,28]

According to Ulmer et al. (2002), sensitivity of individual clinical findings is low, but if three or more clinical findings are present simultaneously, the probability of CS increases precipitously.[27]

DIFFERENTIAL DIAGNOSIS

CS can be confused with cellulitis, DVT, emergent necrotizing fasciitis, gas gangrene, peripheral vascular injury, fracture, rhabdomyolysis, nerve entrapment, radiculopathy, fascial defects, nerve injury, arterial injury, and medial tibial stress syndrome (shin splints).[6,9,11] It is imperative to rule out CS if this is a concern of the clinician at time of injury.[2,3,6] Patients with CS will present with pain and may have redness which can be mistaken for DVT, cellulitis, necrotizing fasciitis, vascular injury, and other infectious or traumatic conditions.[6,22]

The various etiology of limb CS can be further classified based on the cause of the insult.

Orthopedic causes of CS are primarily fracture related.[2,3,6] Such causes include tibial shaft, distal radius, and ulnar fractures most commonly.[6] Tibial shaft fractures result in CS ranging from 1% to 29% based on numerous studies including McQueen et al.[29,30] There is not a significant difference in CS in the case of open or closed tibial shaft fractures.[6,29,30]

Vascular causes of CS include arterial and venous injuries.[6,30] Popliteal artery and veins are susceptible, especially with concomitant tibial fractures.[30] Many patients with injury to the popliteal artery and vein will require urgent fasciotomy.[30] Other vascular etiology for CS includes embolectomy, thrombolysis, bypass surgery, via reperfusion injury.[31] In this capacity, revascularization of a compartment following prolonged ischemia leads to tissue swelling and compartmental hypertension. Furthermore, iliofemoral thrombosis, causing phlegmasia cerulea dolens, an advanced precursor to venous gangrene, can lead to CS.[32,33]

Iatrogenic causes are another significant source of CS. Such causes include but are not limited to drugs, anti-shock garments, prolonged surgeries including Lloyd-Davies position, Trendelenburg position with legs apart, which results in necrosis of soft tissue.[12,34,35] Hematologic disorders and mismanagement can also lead to CS. Excess anticoagulation, spontaneous bleeds in hemophiliac patients, and inadvertent injection of pressurized fluids are potential sources for CS.[36]

Soft tissue causes are another potential source of CS. In the absence of a fracture trauma such as crush injury or a direct blow to a muscle compartment may lead to CS.[26,37] These phenomena are much more common in patients with underlying coagulopathies or bleeding disorders.[37] The continued use of injured muscles may further increase ICP and bleeding, thus contributing to CS.[6,37] Burns are an additional source of CS.[38] Drug and alcohol use and their relationship with CS are well-documented as many of these sequelae are associated with prolonged periods of being "down" or incapacitated resulting in ischemia to compressed limb.[14] Intra-arterial injections of barbiturates such as IV diazepam may cause vascular damage.[4,6] In patient populations with drug addictions, this may lead to nontraumatic rhabdomyolysis and subsequent CS.[4,6]

DIAGNOSIS

CS is a clinical diagnosis. All other diagnostic methods are adjuncts. However, there are significant signs, symptoms, and diagnostic indications to be aware of.[3,6] CS can be diagnosed by measuring an intracompartmental pressure greater than 30 mmHg or an increase in compartmental pressure within 30 mmHg of diastolic BP.[2,3,6] However, this does not need to be met if the clinical picture is consistent with CS in which case, urgent fasciotomy is still necessary.[4,6]

Decompression of the involved compartments is indicated if the differential pressure falls to under 30 mmHg. If the differential pressure is over 30 mmHg, relatively high absolute pressures require only observation, but continued monitoring is necessary until the pressure differential is rising steadily and the absolute pressure is falling.[17] In patients with concern for CS, it is imperative to check blood urea nitrogen (BUN), creatinine, electrolytes, creatine kinase, glomerular filtration rate, urine myoglobin, and lactic acid to monitor for myoglobinuria, and possible acute kidney injury.[5,6,23]

CS of the buttock includes paresthesia in the distribution of the sciatic nerve, tenderness over the buttocks, pain with flexion and adduction of the hip, weakness of extension.[13,14] To diagnose CS of the buttocks, the entry point of the manometer would be in the anterosuperior quadrant.[13,14]

When considering pelvic CS, although very rare, it typically presents with flexion and adduction of the hip, pain with passive extension of the hip, paresthesia around the medial aspect of the knee and leg in the distribution of the saphenous nerve (secondary to compressive hematoma), and tenderness along the inguinal ligament.[6,9,17,34] Manometer measurement of the iliopsoas compartment is difficult.[17,38]

MRI or CT scan is appropriate for diagnosis of iliopsoas hematoma.[15,16] If the hematoma/vascular pathology is amenable to coagulable, this should be done immediately, otherwise surgical intervention may be necessary.[15,16]

CS of the thigh varies clinically based on which compartment is affected.[9,11,18,19] Anterior CS presents with tenderness over the anterior compartment; pain with knee in extension; pain with passive flexion of the knee; paresthesia over the medial aspect over knee, leg, and foot; and weakness on knee extension.[18,19] The posterior compartment will present with tenderness along the posterior aspect of the thigh, pain with passive knee extension, weakness on knee flexion, and sciatic nerve may be involved when pressures are great but sensory changes are rare.[9,11,18,19] The medial compartment presents with pain along the medial aspect of the thigh and pain with passive hip abduction.[9,11,18,19]

CS of the leg is possible due to applied traction during reaming in the intramedullary nailing of tibial fractures may transiently raise compartment pressure as high as 180 mmHg.[29,30,39] The lower leg may tolerate the elevation transiently; however, many authors believe pressure monitoring should be completed during nailing.[39,40] Also, pneumatic anti-shock garment are an additional source of possible CS.[39,40]

CS of the foot is a rare and difficult to measure phenomenon.[5,6] Therefore, a high index of clinical suspicion merits an urgent fasciotomy.[5,6] If measured properly, intracompartmental pressures above 40 mmHg or within 30 mmHg are reliable indicators.[5,6]

CS of the hand is measured by inserting the manometer needle at the site of maximally swelling.[6,8,24] In a review of CS of the hand (Oulette et al.) assert that indication of fasciotomy in the hand should be enacted when intracompartmental pressure is 15 mmHg–25 mmHg in the presence of clinical symptoms.[12] In the absence of clinical symptoms ≥30 mmHg or within 30 mmHg of diastolic pressure still necessitate fasciotomy.[8,12]

MANAGEMENT OF THE CLINICAL PROBLEM

The acute and definitive management of CS is urgent fasciotomy.[2,3,6] There is not an adequate medical management for this condition.[2,3,6], Immediate management, however, entails removing offending dressing, casts, or other sources of compression.[4] There are sequelae associated with CS, oftentimes even if it is managed appropriately.[4,22,23] Among the possible complications of CS include persistent pain, paralysis, necrosis, and amputation.[22,23]

There is no medical management for ACS, but great care must be assessed for serum chemistry, myoglobinemia, hypovolemia, urinalysis, and metabolic acidosis.[4,23] To avoid renal failure hydration, serum chemistries, and frequent urinalyses are integral.[4] Chronic pain following CS, however, can be managed by physiotherapy and NSAIDs.[2,3,6,22]

Regarding iliopsoas CS, management varies based on presentation.[15,16] Iliopsoas hematomas are usually treated conservatively.[15,16] However, severe trauma may require surgical intervention.

ENDOVASCULAR OPTIONS

In iliiopsoas hematomas, controlling the bleeding is of paramount importance. In the case of CS, extensive debridement of necrotic tissue may be necessary.[15,16]

OPEN SURGERY

FASCIOTOMIES

CS of the leg is the most common location of CS.[1-3,6], Up to 45% of CS cases of the lower leg are due to tibial fractures.[2,3,29,30] The leg is composed of four compartments: the anterior compartment, the lateral compartment, the superficial posterior compartment, and the deep posterior dompartment.[6,9] Dual medial/lateral fasciotomy approach or single lateral approach fasciotomies can be effective (Figure 47-5A-D).[4,6,8] Anterior and lateral compartments can be released using the anterolateral two incision approach (Figure 47-5).[6,8] This includes a single longitudinal incision beginning at the middle of the leg 2 cm anterior to the fibular shaft.[8] It can instead be placed directly between the tibial crest and fibula. This separates the anterior and lateral compartments and allows access to each.[8] For elective chronic syndromes a smaller 4 cm–5 cm incision may be sufficient.[6,8] However, in an acute traumatic setting a 15 cm incision is used.[6,8] For release of the anterior compartment, the septum is identified, small nicks are made in the fascia of the intermuscular septum halfway between the septum and tibial crest.[6,8] Fascia can then be opened proximally and distally (Figure 47-4).[6,8] Proximally aim for patella and distally aim for the center of the ankle to maintain anterior release.[6,8] Care should be taken to avoid straying too medially and injuring the dorsalis pedis.[8] For lateral compartment fasciotomy, the incision should be made

A

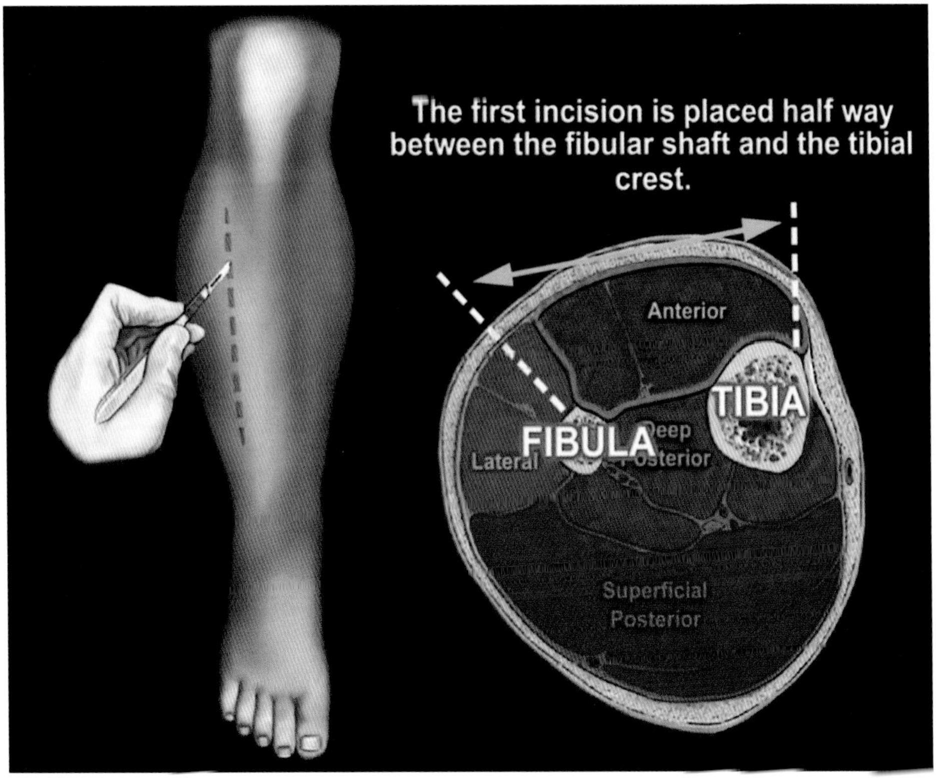

FIGURE 47-5 **A)** This figure demonstrates the first incision in the release of lower extremity compartment syndrome though the lateral compartment. Incision is made halfway between the fibular shaft and tibial crest. **B)** This depicts a lateral incision release of the anterior compartment. Lateral incision releases anterior and lateral compartments. **C)** This image demonstrates the release of the posterior compartments through a medial incision. This incision is made medial to the previous incision, 2cm posterior to the tibial margin. **D)** This animation depicts the medial incision in a lower leg fasciotomy. This incision first releases the superficial posterior compartment, then the deep posterior compartment.

B

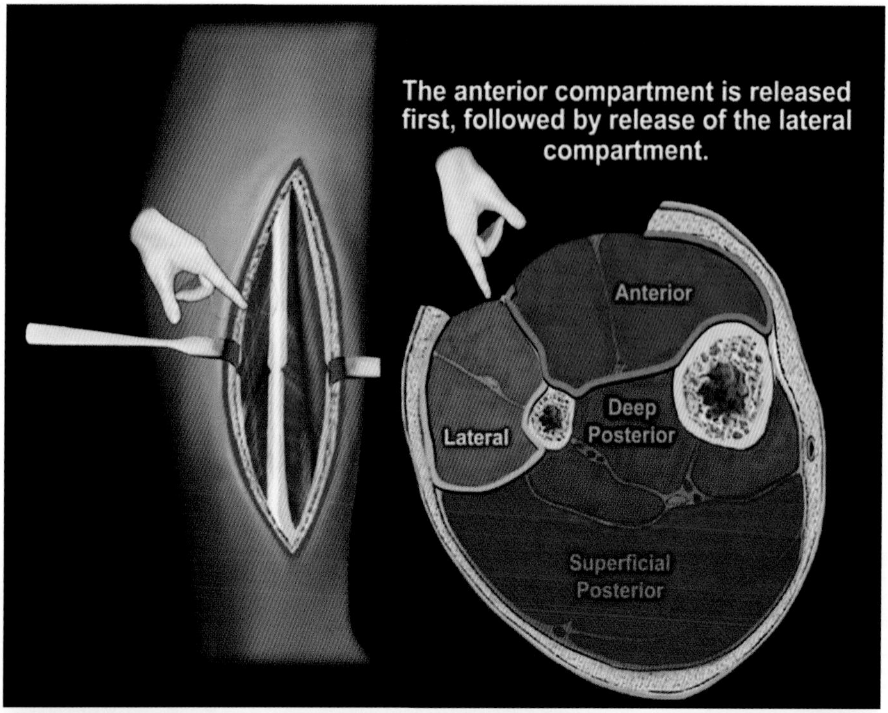
The anterior compartment is released first, followed by release of the lateral compartment.
Anterior
Lateral
Deep Posterior
Superficial Posterior

C

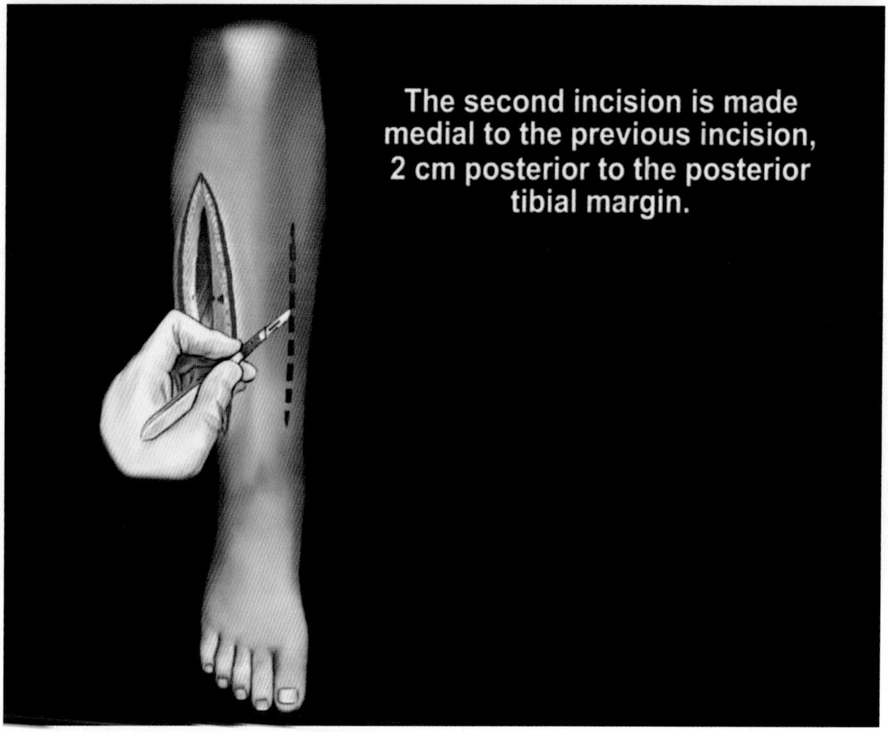
The second incision is made medial to the previous incision, 2 cm posterior to the posterior tibial margin.

FIGURE 47-5 Continued

D

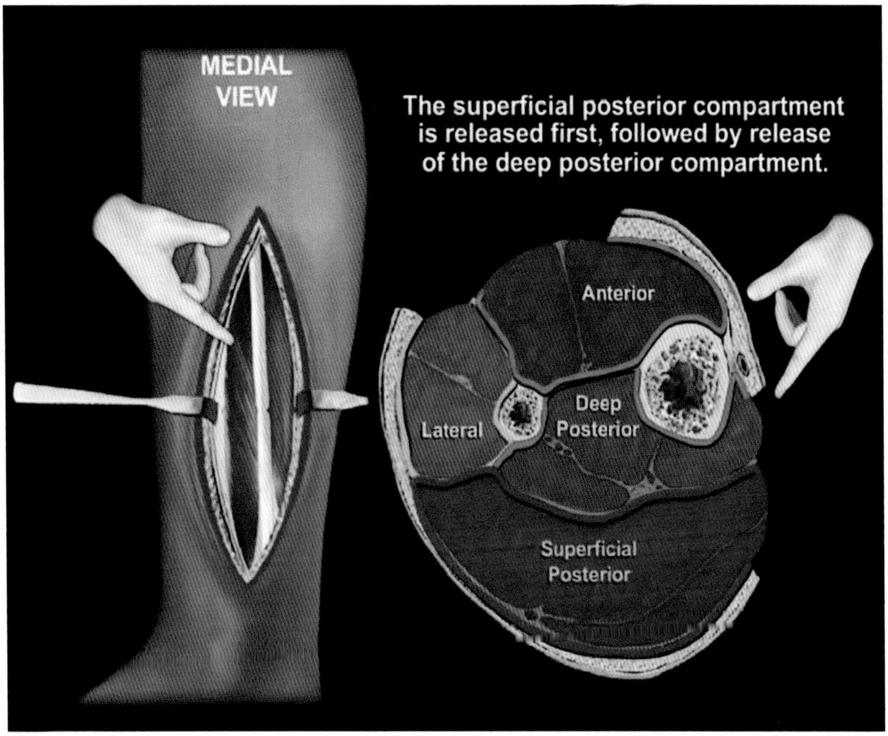
MEDIAL VIEW
The superficial posterior compartment is released first, followed by release of the deep posterior compartment.
Anterior
Lateral
Deep Posterior
Superficial Posterior

FIGURE 47-5 **Continued**

in line with the fibular shaft, distally toward the lateral malleolus, protecting the superficial peroneal nerve.[8] The posteromedial incision, which is a two incision technique, releases the deep and superficial posterior compartments.[8] A single 15 cm longitudinal incision is made in the distal aspect of the leg, 2 cm posterior to the medial palpable edge of the tibia.[6,8] At the fascia, dissection should be completed anteriorly to posterior tibial margin to avoid the saphenous vein and nerve.[8] The superficial compartment can be released while retracting the saphenous vein and nerve.[6,8] The deep posterior compartment includes the soleus which takes origin from the proximal one-third of the tibia and fibula and covers the proximal portion of the deep posterior compartment to release this compartment; the soleal bridge should be detached and retracted posteriorly to expose the fascia covering the FDL and tibialis posterior.[6,8] Releasing the fascia over the FDL is necessary to release the posterior compartment, with the fascia under the belly of the soleus being released both distally and proximally.[6,8]

CS of the arm is rare as there are fewer broad tendons and ligaments in the arm.[1,8] The brachial fascia often yields more than that of the lower extremity.[1,6,8] Causes of the arm include trauma burns, fracture of the neck of the humerus, muscle avulsion, prolonged tourniquet use, steroids in athletes, severe bleeds secondary to thrombolytic therapy, and prolonged pressure on the arm during unconsciousness as a result of alcohol or drug use.[1,6,8] For an anterior compartment fasciotomy, an anterolateral incision can be used to evacuate the anterior compartment of the upper arm.[6,8] A longitudinal cut would be made from the anterior compartment of the groove to the elbow flexion crease, releasing the pressure on the biceps brachii, brachialis, and coracobrachialis muscles.[7,8] For a posterior compartment fasciotomy, a longitudinal midline longitudinal incision needs to be made over the posterior compartment releasing pressure on the triceps brachii and anconeus muscles.[7,8]

Forearm compartments are usually caused by fractures, most commonly supracondylar humerus fractures and both-bone radius and ulna fractures.[7,8] Rarer etiologies include constrictive bandages, roller injuries, limb compression, arterial catheterization, and nephrotic syndrome.[7,8] In patients with low-velocity gunshot wounds to the forearm, 5% to 10% will develop within 24 hours.[10] The five compartments of the forearm include the superficial volar compartment, deep volar compartment, Henry's mobile wad, and superficial dorsal, and deep dorsal compartments.[8] Usually, release of the volar compartment will treat forearm CS (Figure 47-6A,B).[8,9,11] The two approaches for forearm fasciotomies include the volar and dorsal approach (Figure 47-6).[8,9,11] The volar approach includes a deep curvilinear incision, following Henry's approach.[8,9,11] The superficial fascia is released then the flexor carpi radialis and palmaris longus, retracted to the ulnar side. The deep volar compartment is then released (Figure 47-6). If indicated, the carpal tunnel may also be released.[8,41,42] The dorsal approach starts 10 cm distally to the lateral epicondyle of the humerus.[8,41,42] A deep longitudinal incision is made down the dorsal forearm between the extensor digiti minimi and the extensor carpi ulnaris.[8,41,42] From this approach, the superficial dorsal and mobile wad compartments as well as the deep dorsal compartments can be released. It is imperative to avoid the posterior interosseous nerve.[8,41,42]

It is generally considered that the hand is composed of 10 muscle compartments: 1 thenar, 1 hypothenar, 1 adductor pollicis, 4 dorsal interosseus, and 3 volar interosseous compartments (Figure 47-9).[8,11,12] CSs of the hand are often a result of iatrogenic injuries from IV's or arterial lines, but can be a result of crush injuries, burns, trauma, and snake bites.[8,12] The fasciotomies are two dorsal incisions of the hand in line with the second and fourth metacarpals.[8,12] These two incisions are usually sufficient to release all compartments.[12] Occasionally, the dorsal incisions are not enough to release pressure.[12] Additional incisions and/or a carpal tunnel release may be necessary.[8,12] In the

A

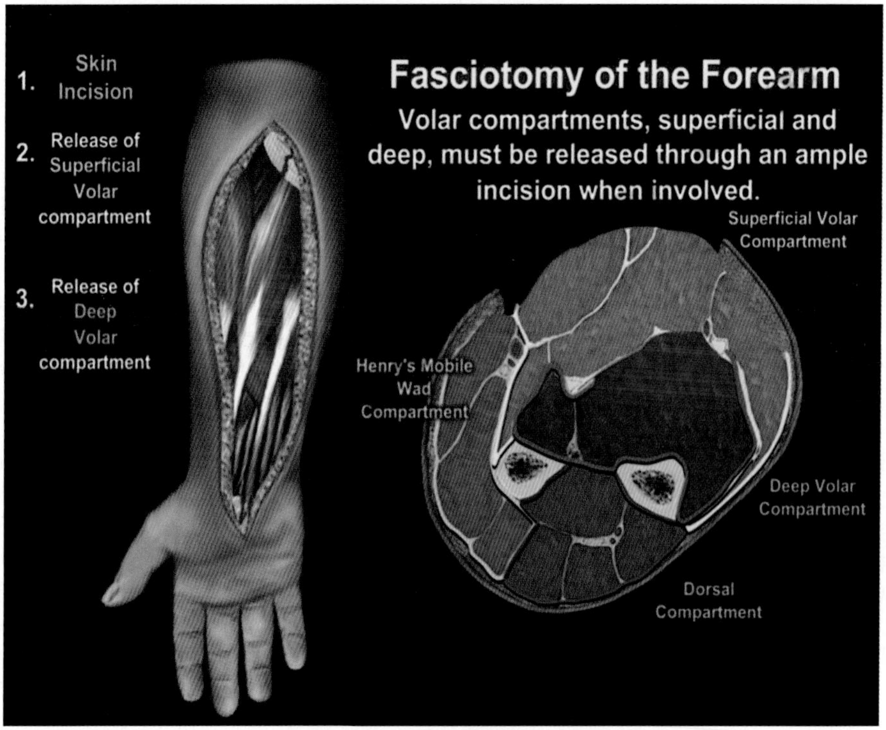

FIGURE 47-6 **A)** This image depicts a forearm depicting a volar fasciotomy. The volar compartments can be released through this approach. An ample incision is necessary to release the superficial and deep compartments. **B)** This image depicts a dorsal release of the forearm after compartment syndrome. The dorsal compartment can be released using this method.

B

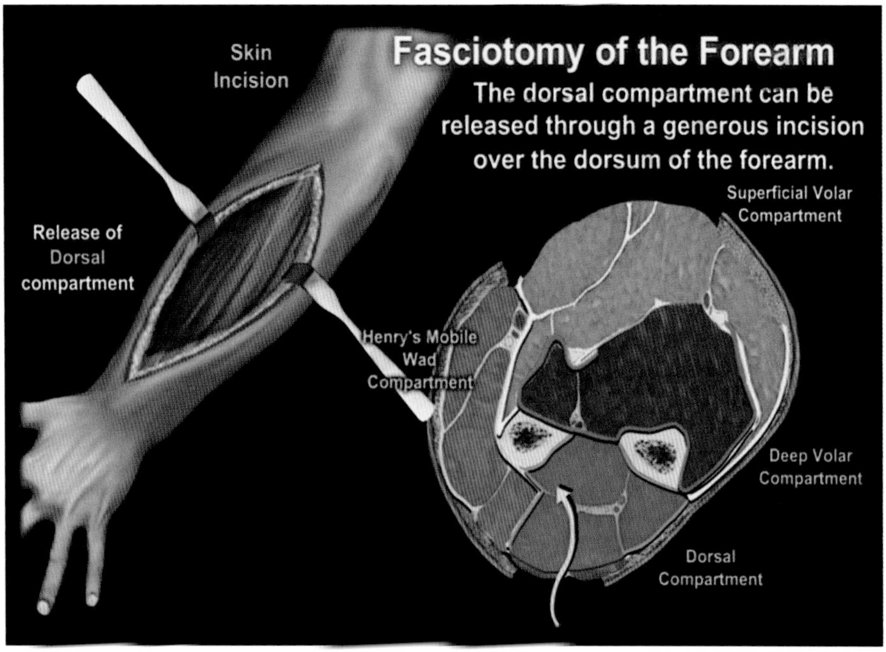

FIGURE 47-6 Continued

event of a severe trauma or a snakebite, a finger fasciotomy may be necessary.[8,12] In this case, an incision must be made where the flexor crease ends.[8,12] A dissection is made across the digit superficially to the flexor tendon sheath.[8,12] The neurovascular bundles are retracted volarly and dissection is completed across the digit.[8,12]

The buttocks are composed of four compartments: the anterolateral compartment, the iliopsoas compartment, the gluteus medius and gluteus minimus compartment, and the gluteus maximus compartment.[9,11,13,14] The fasciotomy for gluteal CS is performed by dissecting through the tensor fascia lata.[13,14] The gluteus medius is decomposed by epimysiotomy.[13,14] Note: for patients with sciatic or peroneal nerve palsy, the sciatica nerve must be inspected intraoperatively to exclude direct damage to the nerve.[13,14]

Iliopsoas CS requires a fasciotomy using the anterolateral pelvic approach.[15,16]

CS of the thigh is most commonly in the anterior compartment.[6,8,9] Release of the anterior compartment of the thigh is made through a lateral incision.[6,8,9] The lateral incision follows a line from distal to the intertrochanteric line as needed (Figure 47-7).[26] Release of the tensor fascia lata is indicated. Release of the medial compartment of the thigh is accomplished by a medial incision beginning from the iliac crest extending to the medial epicondyle of the femur.[6,19,43]

For shoulder fasciotomies, the saber-type incision is made through the skin over the deltoid compartment.[44] Deltopectoral approach may also be taken releasing subacromial space.[44] And the skin is pulled back with retractors. Blunt scissors are used to cut through the fascia over the deltoid compartment.[8,9,44]

CS of the foot is a rare presentation.[25] Crush injuries are the most common cause of CS of the foot.[25] Emergent fasciotomies of all compartments include dual dorsal incisions, which is considered the gold standard.[6,25,45] The first incision is a dorsal medial incision made medial to the second metatarsal, which releases the 3rd and 4th interosseous, lateral, superficial, and middle central compartments.[6,45] The dorsal fascia of each interosseous compartment incision is longitudinal.[6,45] A medial incision may be necessary for decompression of the calcaneal compartment.[6,45] Alternatively, a single medial incision may be employed.[6,25] This requires one medial incision to release all nine compartments and is considered technically challenging.[6,25,45]

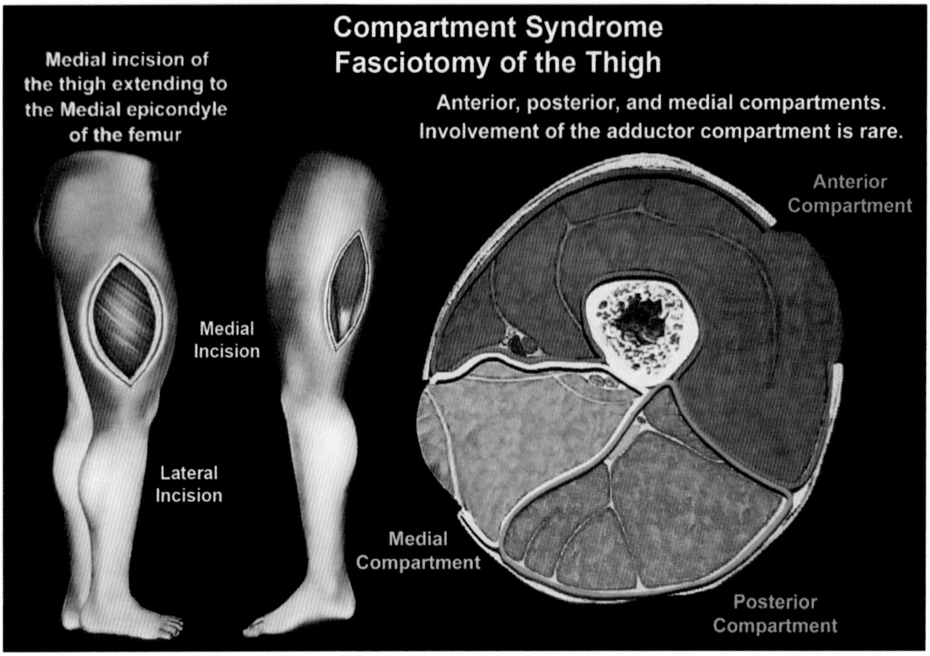

FIGURE 47-7 This image demonstrates a thigh fasciotomy. Both medial and lateral incisions are demonstrated. The medial compartment is released by the medial incision. The anterior compartment is released by the lateral incision.

COMPLICATIONS

Complications of CS include a variety of sequelae including Volkmann's ischemic contracture, chronic exertional CS, acute kidney injury, and subsequent neurovascular compromise.[2,3,6,23] Untreated CS may also lead to muscle necrosis requiring limb amputation.[23] Each is treated on a case-by-case basis.[6] Additionally, fasciotomies are the only definitive treatment for ACS.[2] However, fasciotomies are also associated with a variety of complications including prolonged hospitalization, infection, osteomyelitis, delayed bone healing, need for secondary surgeries, chronic venous insufficiency, weakness, cosmetic problems, and subsequent changes.[2,3,6,23]

VOLKMANN'S ISCHEMIC CONTRACTURE

Volkmann's contracture is a late complication of untreated ischemic injuries including CS, crush injuries, fractures, and vascular injuries.[25,46,47] Rarely, it can be caused by bleeding disorders, excessive exercise, and injection of certain medications.[25,46,47] The ischemia causes muscle and nerve necrosis in the afflicted compartment.[25,46,47] Necrotic tissue eventually scars and is replaced by fibrous tissue through fibroblastic proliferation.[25,46,47] This results in contracture and nerve palsy (Figure 47-7).[25,46,47] Without release, the limb involved will become deformed, dysfunctional, and insensate.[25,46,47] These changes may occur as late as 3–4 months following onset of ischemia. This may necessitate amputation.[25,46,47]

When Volkmann's contracture involves the forearm, it typically results in claw hand. Patient will have elbow flexion, wrist flexion, forearm pronation, thumb flexion and abduction, metacarpophalangeal (MP) extension, and interphalangeal (IP) flexion.[25,47] In the lower limb, Volkmann's ischemic contracture will result in several manifestations based on afflicted compartment (Figure 47-8A,B).[25,46] The deep posterior compartment results in dorsiflexion of talus, heel varus, clawing of toes, fixed cavus forefoot adduction, and equinus. In the anterior compartment, it results

A

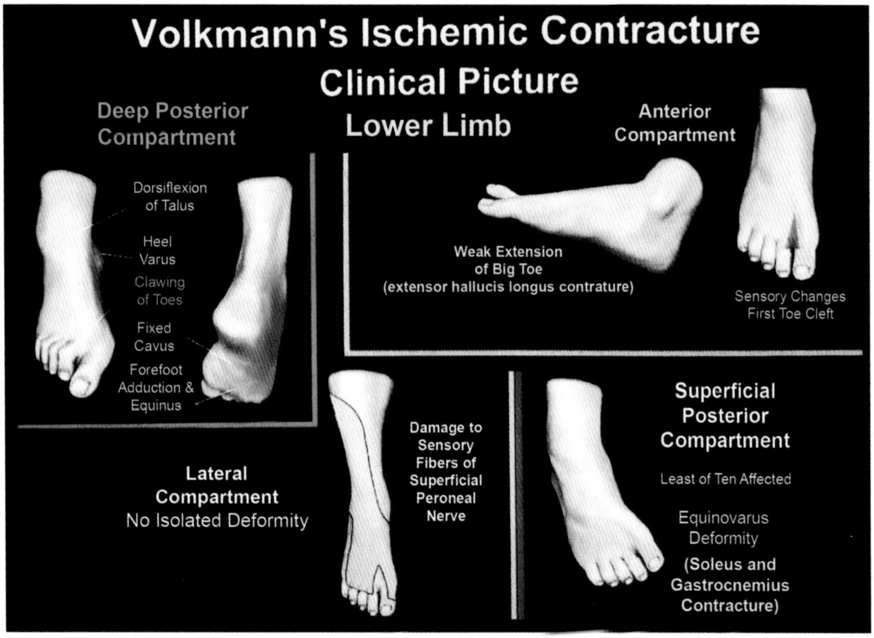

B

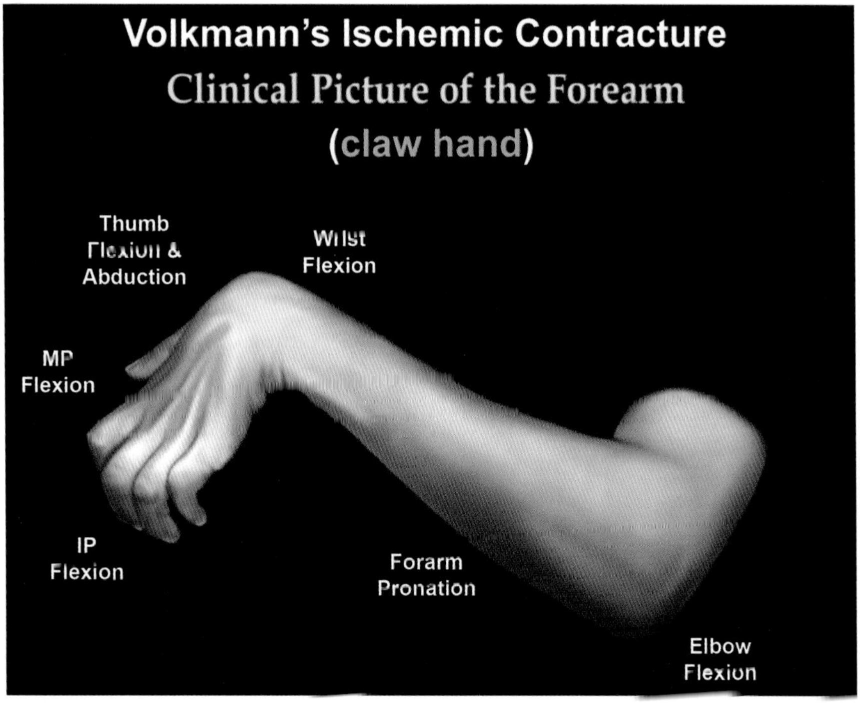

FIGURE 47-8 **A)** This image demonstrates Volkmann's Ischemic Contracture of the foot. It depicts effects of deep posterior compartment, lateral compartment, anterior compartment, and superficial posterior compartment involvement. **B)** This image demonstrates Volkmann's Ischemic Contracture (claw hand) of the upper extremity. This includes thumb flexion and abduction, wrist flexion, MP flexion, IP flexion, forearm pronation, and elbow flexion.

in weak extension of great toe through hallucis longus contracture and sensory changes in the webspace of great toe and second toe.[9,11,46] The lateral compartment results in sensory changes in the distribution of the superficial peroneal nerve.[9,11,46] The superficial posterior compartment, which is least often affected, results in equinovarus deformity consistent of gastrocnemius contracture.[25,46]

CHRONIC EXERTIONAL COMPARTMENT SYNDROME

Chronic exertional compartment syndrome (CECS) is an exercise-induced neuromuscular condition which occurs when a compartment cannot accommodate the increase in muscle volume during exercise.[48–50]

At the afflicted compartments, the symptoms include pain, tenderness, swelling, and possibly paresthesia (Figure 47-9).[48,49] Symptoms frequently become predictable after a certain amount of exertion.[48,49] In 80% to 95% of the cases, CECS affects the lower extremity although it has been reported in forearm, hand, thigh, and foot compartments.[48] In these patients, resting compartment pressure is frequently greater than 15 mmHg.[48] This typically presents as pain, swelling, claudication, and possibly paresthesia.[48] It is often bilateral in 80% to 95% of patients most commonly affecting the anterior leg compartment 40% to 60%, the deep posterior compartment 32% to 60%, and the lateral compartments in 12% to 35% of patients.[48] Fascial herniations may be evident in 40% to 60% of patients.[49]

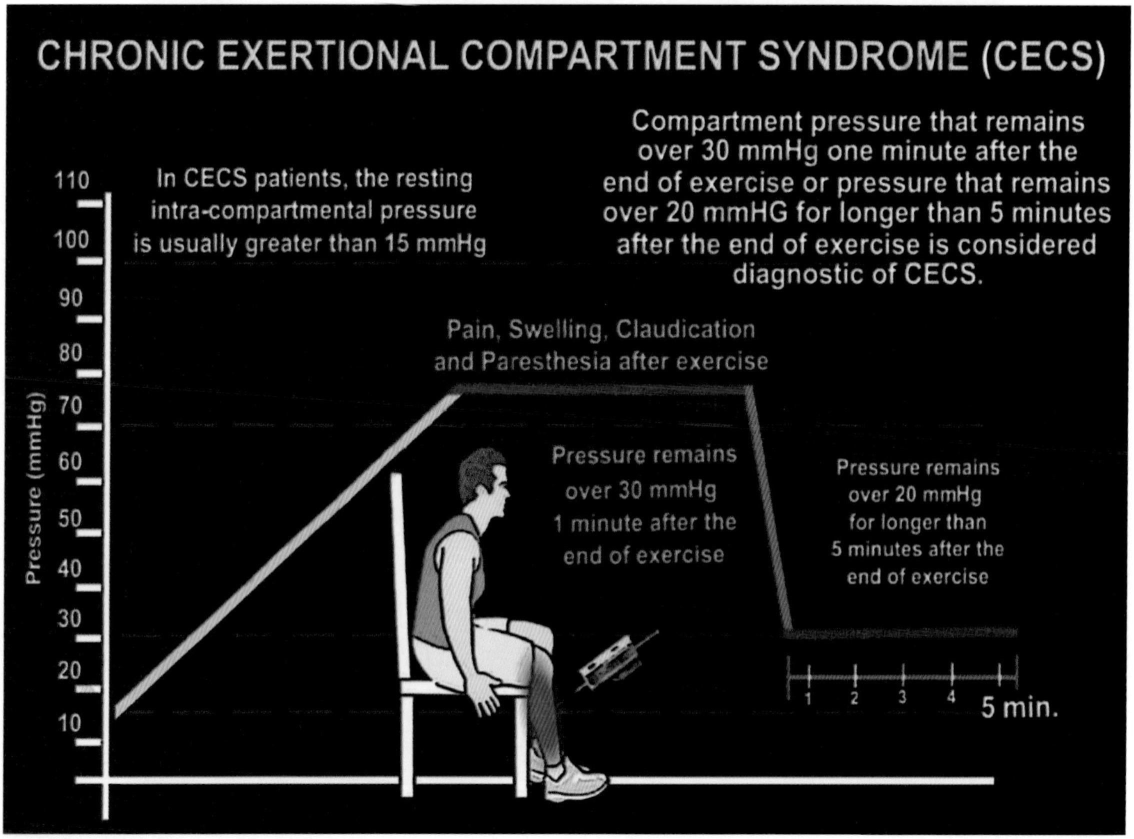

FIGURE 47-9 This animation demonstrates chronic exertional compartment syndrome (CECS). It depicts the symptoms and pathophysiology after exercise and sustained elevated compartmental pressure following exercise.

CECS in the presence of clinical findings is diagnosed with one or more of the following: (a) a pre-exercise pressure greater than or equal to 15 mmHg; (b) a 1-minute postexercise pressure of greater than or equal to 30 mmHg; or (c) a 5-minute postexercise pressure of greater than or equal to 20 mmHg.[50]

REFERENCES

1. Gourgiotis S, Villias C, Germanos S, Foukas A, Ridolfini MP. Acute limb compartment syndrome: a review. *J Surg Educ*. 2007;64(3):178-186.
2. McQueen MM. (v) Acute compartment syndrome in tibial fractures. *Curr Orthop*. 1999;13(2):113-119.
3. McQueen MM, Gaston P, Court-Brown CM. Acute compartment syndrome: who is at risk? *J Bone Joint Surg Br*. 2000;82(2):200-203.
4. Donaldson J, Haddad B, Khan WS. The pathophysiology, diagnosis and current management of acute compartment syndrome. *Open Orthop J*. 2014;8:185-193
5. Frink M, Hildebrand F, Krettek C, Brand J, Hankemeier S. Compartment syndrome of the lower leg and foot. *Clin Orthop Relat Res*. 2010;468(4):940-950.
6. Rockwood CA, Green DP. *Rockwood and Green's Fractures in Adults*. Vol. 1. Philadelphia, PA: Lippincott Williams & Wilkins; 2010.
7. Kannam S, Cardwell AB. The forearm: anatomy of muscle compartments and nerves. *Am J Roentgenol*. 2000; 174(1):151-159.
8. Seiler JG 3rd, Casey PJ, Binford SH. Compartment syndromes of the upper extremity. *J South Orthop Assoc*. 2000;9(4):233-247.
9. Moore KL, Agur AMR, Dalley AF II *Essential Clinical Anatomy*. 2nd ed. Philadelphia, PA: Lippincott Williams & Wilkins; 2002.
10. Moed BR, Fakhouri AJ. Compartment syndrome after low-velocity gunshot wounds to the forearm. *J Orthop Trauma*. 1991;5(2):134-137.
11. Wheeless CR, Nunely JA, Urbaniak J. *Wheeless' Textbook of Orthopaedics*. Brooklandville, MD: Data Trace Internet Publishing; 2009.
12. Ouellette EA, Kelly R. Compartment syndromes of the hand. *J Bone Joint Surg*. 1996;78(10): 1515-1522.
13. Bleicher RJ, Sherman HF, Latenser BA. Bilateral gluteal compartment Syndrome. *J Trauma*. 1997;42(1): 118-122.
14. Kumar V, Saeed K, Panagopoulos A, Parker PJ. Gluteal compartment syndrome following joint arthroplasty under epidural anesthesia. *J Orthop Surg (Hong Kong)*. 2007;15(1):113-117.
15. Heim M, Horoszowski H, Seligsohn U, Martinowitz U, Strauss S. Iliopsoas hematoma: its detection, and treatment with special reference to hemophilia. *Arch Orthop Trauma Surg*. 1982;99:195-197.
16. Robinson DE, Ball KE, Webb PJ. Iliopsoas hematoma with femoral neuropathy presenting a diagnostic dilemma after spinal decompression. *Spine*. 2001; 26(6):135-138.
17. Smith WR, Ziran BH, Morgan SJ. *Fractures of the Pelvis and Acetabulum*. Miami, FL: Information Healthcare USA, Inc.; 2007.
18. Heidepriem RW, Frey SE, Robinson D, Tapscott WJ, Spence RK. Thigh compartment syndromes: diagnosis and surgical treatment. *Vascular*. 2004;12(4):271-272.
19. Ojike NI, Roberts CS, Giannoudis PV. Compartment syndrome of the thigh: a systematic review. *Injury*. 2010;41(2):133-136.
20. Hansen ST. *Functional Reconstruction of the Foot and Ankle*. Philadelphia, PA: Lippincott Williams & Wilkins; 2000.
21. Heppenstall RB, Sapega AA, Scott R, et al. The compartment syndrome. An experimental and clinical study of muscular energy metabolism using phosphorus nuclear magnetic resonance spectroscopy. *Clin Orthop Relat Res*. 1988;(226):138-155.
22. Matsen FA, King RV, Krugmire RB Jr, et al. Physiological effects of increased tissue pressure. *Int Orthop*. 1979; 3(3):237-244.
23. Mauffrey C, Hak DJ, Martin MP III, eds. *Compartment Syndrome: A Guide to Diagnosis and Management*. Cham (CH): Springer; 2019.
24. Stuadt JM, Smeulders MJC, van der Horst CMAM. Normal compartment pressures of the lower leg in children. *J Bone Joint Surg Br*. 2008;90(2):215-219.
25. Mubarak SJ, Hargens AR. *Compartment Syndrome and Volkmanns Contracture*. Philadelphia, PA: W.B. Saunders Company; 1981.
26. Mubarak SJ, Pedowitz RA, Hargens AR. Compartment syndromes. *Curr Orthop*. 1989;3(1):36-40.
27. Ulmer T. The clinical diagnosis of compartment syndrome of the lower leg. *J Orthop Trauma*. 2002;16:572-577.
28. Matsen FA III. Compartmental syndromes: an unified concept. *Clin Orthop Relat Res*. 1975;113:8-14.
29. McQueen MM, Christie J, Court-Brown CM. Acute compartment syndrome in tibial diaphyseal fractures. *J Bone Joint Surg Br*. 1996;78(1):95-98.
30. McQueen MM, Court-Brown CM. Compartment monitoring in tibial fractures: the pressure threshold for decompression. *J Bone Joint Surg Br*. 1996;78(1):99-104.
31. Shah DM, Bock DE, Darling RC III, Chang BB, Kupinski AM, Leather RP. Beneficial effects of hypertonic

mannitol in acute ischemia—reperfusion injuries in humans. *Cardiovasc Surg*. 1996;4(1):97-100.

32. Weinmann EE, Salzman EW. Deep-vein thrombosis. *N Engl J Med*. 1994;331(24):1630-1641.
33. Wood KE, Reedy JS, Pozniak MA, Coursin DB. Phlegmasia cerulea dolens with compartment syndrome: a complication of femoral vein catheterization. *Crit Care Med*. 2000;28(5):1626-1630.
34. Aprahamian C, Gessert G, Bandyk DF, Sell L, Stiehl J, Olson DW. MAST-associated compartment syndrome (MACS): a review. *J Trauma*. 1989;29(5):549-555.
35. Chase J, Harford F, Pinzur MS, Zussman M. Intraoperative lower extremity compartment pressures in lithotomy-positioned patients. *Dis Colon Rectum*. 2000; 43(5):678-680.
36. Perez RO, Pecora RA, Giannini CG, Nahas SC, Habr-Gama A. Lower limb compartment syndrome associated with Lloyd-Davies/lithotomy position in colorectal surgery. *Hepato-gastroenterology*. 2004;51(55):100.
37. Rööser B, Bengtson S, Hägglund G. Acute compartment syndrome from anterior thigh muscle contusion: a report of eight cases. *J Orthop Trauma*. 1991; 5(1):57-59.
38. Perron AD, Brady WJ, Keats TE. Orthopedic pitfalls in the ED: acute compartment syndrome. *Am J Emerg Med*. 2001;19(5):413-416.
39. Blick SS. Brumback RJ, Poka A, Burgess AR, Ebraheim NA. Compartment syndrome in in open tibial fractures. *J Bone Joint Surg Am*. 1986;68(9):1348-1353.
40. Vahedi MH, Ayuyao A, Parsa MH, Freeman HP. Pneumatic antishock garment-associated compartment syndrome in uninjured lower extremities. *J Trauma*. 1998;38(4):616-618.
41. Hobson RW, Wilson SE, Veith FJ. *Vascular Surgery*. 2nd ed. New York, NY: McGraw Hill, Inc.; 1994.
42. Gelberman RH, Garfin SR, Hergenroeder PT, Mubarak SJ, Menon J. Compartment syndromes of the forearm: diagnosis and treatment. *Clin Orthop Relat Res*. 1981;161:252-261.
43. Boland MR, Heck C. Acute exercise-induced bilateral thigh compartment syndrome. *Orthopedics*. 2009;32(3): 218.
44. Cagle PJ, Shukla DR, Parsons BO. Deltoid compartment syndrome following shoulder arthroscopy: a case report. *Clin Arch Bone Joint Dis*. 2018;1(004).
45. Browner BD, Jupiter JB, Levine AM, Trafton PG. *Skeletal Trauma*. 3rd ed. Amsterdam: Elsevier; 2003.
46. Bottme MJ, Santi MD, Prestianni CA, Abrams RA. Ischemic contracture of the foot and ankle: principles of management and prevention. *Orthopedics*. 1996;19(3): 235-244.
47. Eaton RG, Green WT. Volkmann's ischemia. A volar compartment syndrome of the forearm. *Clin Orthop*. 1975;113:58-64.
48. Mazerolle SM, McDermott B, Silverberg E. Bilateral exertional compartment syndrome. *Athl Ther Today*. 2008;13(3):20-23.
49. Bong MR, Polatsch DB, Jazrawi LM, Rokito AS. Chronic exertional compartment syndrome: diagnosis and management. *Bull Hosp JT Dis*. 2005;62:77-84.
50. Pedowitz RA, Hargens AR, Mubarak SJ, Gershuni DH. Modified criteria for the objective diagnosis of chronic compartment syndrome of the leg. *Am J Sports Med*. 1990;18(1):35-40.

SELF-ASSESSMENT STUDY QUESTIONS AND ANSWERS

Questions

1. When the measured pressure in a compartment is 45 mmHg and the diastolic pressure is 55 mmHg, what is the most appropriate action?
   A. Observation
   B. Elevation
   C. Application of ice
   D. Decompression

2. Normal resting compartmental pressure in adults is typically:
   A. 0 mmHg–10 mmHg
   B. 10 mmHg–20 mmHg
   C. 20 mmHg–30 mmHg
   D. 30 mmHg–40 mmHg

3. Pulses in compartment syndrome are:
   A. Usually absent
   B. Definitely absent
   C. Always weak
   D. Could be normal

4. Which nerve would be involved with an increase in pressure in the anterior compartment of the leg?
   A. Saphenous nerve
   B. Superficial peroneal nerve
   C. Deep peroneal nerve
   D. Sural nerve

5. While performing decompression of the lateral leg, which structure needs to be watched?
   A. Sural nerve
   B. Superficial peroneal nerve
   C. Saphenous vein
   D. Deep peroneal nerve

6. In the case of compartment syndrome of the lower leg, how many compartments are released to insure complete decompression?
   A. One compartment
   B. Two compartments
   C. Three compartments
   D. Four compartments

7. The thigh has how many fascial compartments?
   A. Three compartments
   B. Two compartments
   C. Five compartments
   D. One compartment

8. Claw toes and equinus deformity of the foot can result from compartment syndrome of the leg in which compartment?
   A. Superficial posterior compartment
   B. Deep posterior compartment
   C. Anterior compartment
   D. Lateral compartment

9. Volkmann's ischemic contracture results from:
   A. Disuse atrophy of the muscles
   B. Increased pressure in the thigh
   C. Neglected compartment syndrome of the forearm
   D. Claudication secondary to peripheral vascular disease of lower extremities

10. The sciatic nerve is located in which compartment of the thigh?
    A. Anterior
    B. Lateral
    C. Medial
    D. Posterior

SELF-ASSESSMENT STUDY QUESTIONS AND ANSWERS

Answers

1. D.
2. A.
3. D.
4. C.
5. B.
6. D.
7. A.
8. B.
9. C.
10. D.

CHAPTER

48 Native Arterial Infections

Lindsey M. Korepta and Carlos F. Bechara

OUTLINE

INTRODUCTION
Epidemiology
Pathogenesis
DIAGNOSTIC EVALUATION
Clinical Exam
Radiology
Labs
TREATMENT
Medical Treatment
Surgical Treatment

INTRODUCTION

EPIDEMIOLOGY

Native arterial infections are a condition that implies destruction of the native arterial wall by an infectious process. This may result in sepsis, compression, erosion, embolization, thrombosis, hemorrhage, or pseudoaneurysm formation. Osler et al. first presented the relationship between arterial infections and aneurysm formation in 1885, where he coined the phrase "mycotic aneurysm" in reference to a young patient who was found to have endocarditis of the aortic valve as well as multiple aneurysms of the thoracic aorta on autopsy.[1] The name mycotic aneurysm was chosen by Osler for aneurysms associated with bacterial endocarditis for its similar appearance to fresh fungal vegetations. The term has come to be associated with both true and false aneurysms that are associated with infection of the arterial wall. Mycotic aneurysms carry a high rupture rate and should be considered an urgent medical condition.

PATHOGENESIS

Five basic mechanisms of primary arterial infections have been designated.[2] These mechanisms can be summarized as:

1. **Oslerian mycotic aneurysms:** Unique clinical condition characterized by bacterial endocarditis with septic embolization from valvular vegetations. A primary mycotic aneurysm is not associated with septic emboli from cardiac valve vegetations, but instead is associated with bacteremia that can cause seeding of normal artery or already established aneurysm. Additionally, the arterial wall can be contaminated with bacteria from direct trauma or a contiguous site of infection.
2. **Microbial arteritis with aneurysm formation:** Hematogenous microbial seeding of arteries during an episode of bacteremia. The artery can be normal or atherosclerotic and becomes infected, weakening the arterial wall and causing aneurysm formation.
3. **Infected aneurysms:** Infection of a preexisting aneurysm, often by hematogenous spread and seeding of the arterial wall. While predominantly bacterial, they may also be caused by fungal or viral infection, such as in advanced human immunodeficiency virus (HIV) infection.[3]
4. **Arterial injury with contamination:** Mechanical arterial injury caused by infected/

contaminated surgical instruments during radiologic procedures, drug injection, vascular access, or as a result of traumatic injury.

5. **Arteritis from contagious spread:** Spread from surrounding structures such as osteomyelitis, tuberculous lymph nodes, or narcotic injection-associated abscesses.[4]

The organism most commonly associated with microbial aortitis and Oslerian mycotic aneurysms is *Salmonella*, with decreasing frequency of *Streptococcus, Bacteroides, Arizona hinshawii, Escherichia coli,* and *Staphylococcus aureus.*[2] Femoral aneurysms and intravenous (IV) drug abuse-associated aneurysms are more commonly of the gram-positive species *Staphylococci* and *Streptococci*, with *E. coli* and *Pseudomonas* also being common. The presence of rheumatic fever and bacterial endocarditis has decreased over time in the post-antibiotic era. In a review published in 1986, the most common organisms in endocarditis found in patients with a history of IV drug abuse were *S. aureus* (36%), *Pseudomonas* species (16%), polymicrobial organisms (15%), *Streptococcus faecalis* (13%), and *Streptococcus viridans* (11%). In non-IV drug abusers, the most common organisms in endocarditis were *S. viridans* (22%), *S. aureus* (20%), *S. faecalis* (14%), and *S. epidermidis* (11%).[5] The most common site of primary arterial infections tends to be the larger muscular and elastic arteries such as the abdominal aorta, common femoral artery and superior mesenteric artery (SMA). Patients with gram-negative bacterial isolates have a greater rupture rate than those with gram-positive bacterial organisms (84% vs 10%), and thus warrant earlier intervention.[6]

The organisms most commonly associated with microbial arteritis are *Salmonella*, *Staphylococcus*, and *E. coli.*[2] These tend to occur in localization with an atherosclerotic plaque in the distal aorta, femoral, iliac, and popliteal vessels. Infected aneurysms can occur at a preexisting aneurysm in the body. The organisms most commonly associated with these are the same as microbial aortitis, mycotic aneurysms, and microbial arteritis. The organism most commonly associated with arterial injury with contamination is *S. aureus*. Since these are in arteries with easy access, they tend to occur mostly in peripheral vessels such as the femoral and brachial arteries. The organism most commonly associated with arteritis from contagious spread is *Salmonella*, followed by *Staphylococcus*. In patients with immunosuppression, the most common organisms for causing native arterial infections are *Campylobacter* species, *Listeria* species, and *Mycobacterium tuberculosis.*[2]

DIAGNOSTIC EVALUATION

CLINICAL EXAM

Frequently, patients present with tenderness over the affected artery and systemic signs of sepsis including fever, leukocytosis, malaise, chills or sweats, and arthralgia. The signs and symptoms vary by the location of the affected artery. Thromboembolism or thrombosis can occur and elicit accompanying complaints of acute limb pain, cyanosis, or loss of motor/sensation. Arterial rupture can also be a presenting complaint with hemorrhage and hypovolemic shock.

RADIOLOGY

Computed tomography angiogram (CTA, Figure 48-1) and MRI with arterial phase iodinated contrast are a common first step in the work-up of suspected native arterial infections. CTA is considered the reference imaging gold standard; however, MRI may be more sensitive in detecting tissue edema. Tissue edema has become the hallmark of the inflammatory process associated with native arterial infections.[7] On-table angiography is also another imaging modality used in the work-up of native arterial infections; however, the vessel wall and surrounding tissue are unable to be fully evaluated using this technique given its two-dimensional nature. Tagged white blood cell scans can assist in identifying arterial graft infections, but these are not commonly used in native arterial infections. Using fusion imaging to overlay CT and positron emission tomography (PET) images on top of one another can increase the sensitivity and specificity of detecting native arterial infections.[8,9]

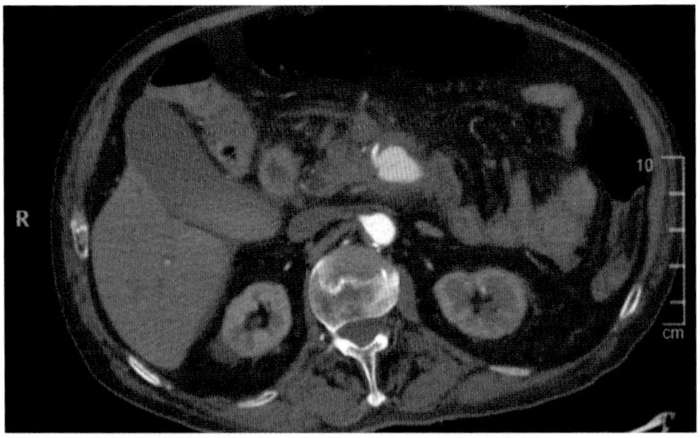

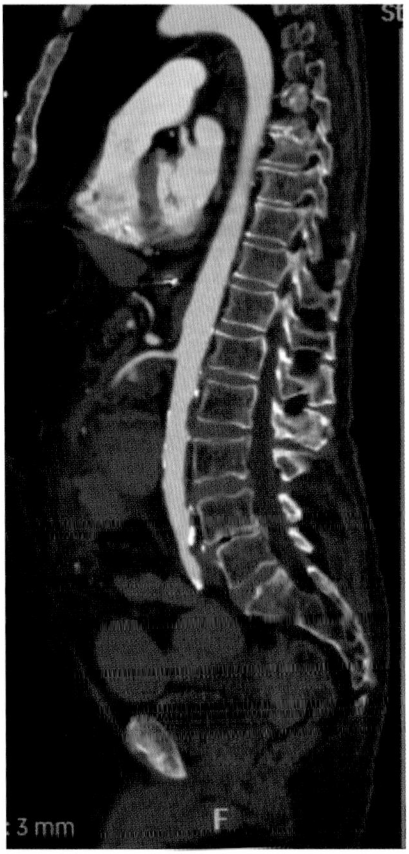

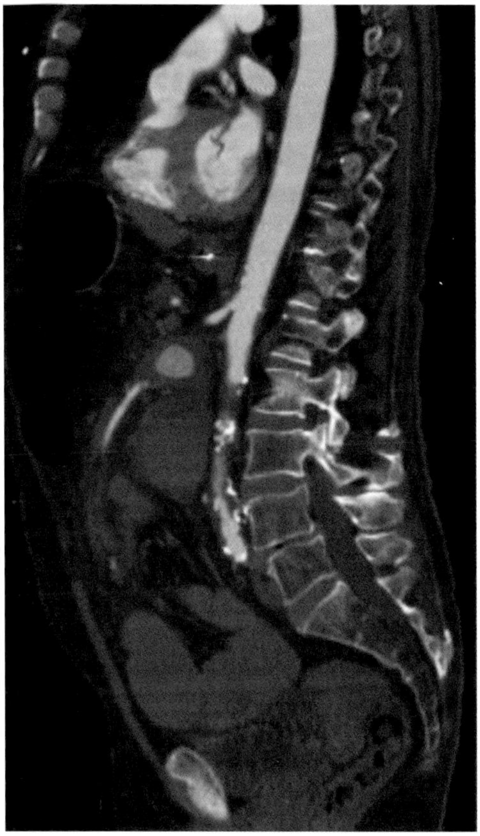

FIGURE 48-1 **A 75-year-old male with multiple skin abscesses and MRSA bacteremia developed a superior mesenteric artery (SMA) pseudoaneurysm.**

LABS

The appropriate laboratory work up includes a complete blood count, basic metabolic panel, two blood cultures from separate peripheral sites, and other markers of sepsis including erythrocyte sediment rate (ESR), C-reactive protein (CRP), and lactic acid. A low suspicion for admission to an intensive care unit can assist with an expedited work-up in these patients.

TREATMENT

MEDICAL TREATMENT

Nonoperative management is focused on antibiotic use to control sepsis and is recommended only for patients at high-risk for surgical reconstruction and those patients who are extremely debilitated. The in-hospital mortality rate in a small series published on solely the medical treatment of infected aortic aneurysms revealed a 50% mortality rate.[10,11] With such a high mortality rate for medical treatment alone, surgical treatment is recommended in all patients who are able to tolerate it.

SURGICAL TREATMENT

Both open and endovascular techniques have been used in the treatment of hemorrhage control and reconstruction of native arterial infections. Open repair consists of debridement of infected tissues with either extra-anatomic bypass or in situ arterial reconstruction. It has become increasingly popular to temporize hemorrhage from infected aneurysm rupture using endovascular techniques, and subsequently bringing the patient back for definitive repair with removal of the infected tissue and/or graft.

The choice of conduit for in-line reconstruction typically includes antibiotic impregnated prosthetic grafts (Dacron or polytetrafluoroethylene), allografts of autologous veins, or human cryopreserved arterial allografts. It has been suggested that rifampin-impregnated grafts are feasible and recommended for low-grade *Staphylococcal* arterial infections.[12] Saphenous and femoral veins have been used as allografts in neoaortoiliac system (NAIS) repair. These surgeries carry high morbidity due to the length of procedure, but have a high 5-year patency rate of 85%.[13] Aneurysmal degeneration of NAIS repairs has been reported; however, a recent publication reported zero incidence of this in a 10-year review.[14,15] Human cryopreserved arterial allografts carry variable 30-day mortality rates reported at 9% to 28% and have variable durability with 89% freedom from reoperation in one study.[16] Early graft-related complication rates are 19%[17] with a reoperation rate of 15.5% and reinfection rate of 4% in other studies.[18] Type 1 diabetes mellitus was noted to be an independent predictor of mortality with this repair.[18] These repairs may also be prone to aneurysmal degeneration over time and warrant close postintervention surveillance for early identification of potential complications. An article published by Hostalrich et al. reviewed the use of xenopericardial grafts as a conduit for in-line repair, but noted that these carry a similarly high 30-day mortality rate of 25% and slightly higher reinfection rate of 5.7%.[19] In situ reconstruction is not recommended in grossly purulent fields or infections with gram-negative species and ligation with extra-anatomic reconstruction should be considered.

Extra-anatomic reconstruction can carry a lower mortality rate than in situ reconstruction and has become an increasingly favored approach to repair over in-line repair. In a review of 51 cases of mycotic aneurysms, the mortality rate of extra-anatomic repair was 18% as compared to in situ reconstruction repair at 32%.[20] While there is no consensus recommendation currently, long-term antibiotics are recommended for a minimum of 6-8 weeks post repair with in-line or extra-anatomic repair. A clinical consult to an infectious disease specialist is warranted for a multidisciplinary approach to antibiotic management in this complex patient population.

A growing series of studies have been published on the use of endovascular in situ reconstruction in native arterial infections (Figure 48-2). This manner of repair can quickly control hemorrhage, which reduces mortality and increases survival at 2 years to 82%, but fatal infection-related complications within the first year can be as high as 19%.[21-24] A study conducted using the Swedish vascular registry reported outcomes on patients presenting with mycotic abdominal aortic aneurysms. There was better short-term survival in Endovascular Aortic Aneurysm Repair (EVAR) patients (74% vs 96% survival at 3 months), without significant difference in long-term survival, infection-related complications, or reoperation as compared to open repair. They concluded that EVAR can be an equally effective way of treating native aortic infections.[25] *Salmonella* infection and leukocytosis were found to increase aneurysm-related morbidity and mortality. Not surprisingly, persistent infection after EVAR was associated with an overall poor prognosis.[26] An important consideration is prolonged antibiotic therapy, as 40% of deaths in a 16-center European study occurred after discontinuation of antibiotic therapy.[24]

Covered vascular stents can also be considered for repair of native arterial infections in extremities such as anastomotic femoral or brachial artery pseudoaneurysms. They can again be used to quickly control hemorrhage but should be followed by surgical debridement with drainage and long-term broad-spectrum antibiotics.[27] Ligation and excision of pseudoaneurysms in peripheral arteries of IV drug abusers has been demonstrated to be a safe and effective treatment without revascularization.[28] Revascularization can be pursued in a staged fashion

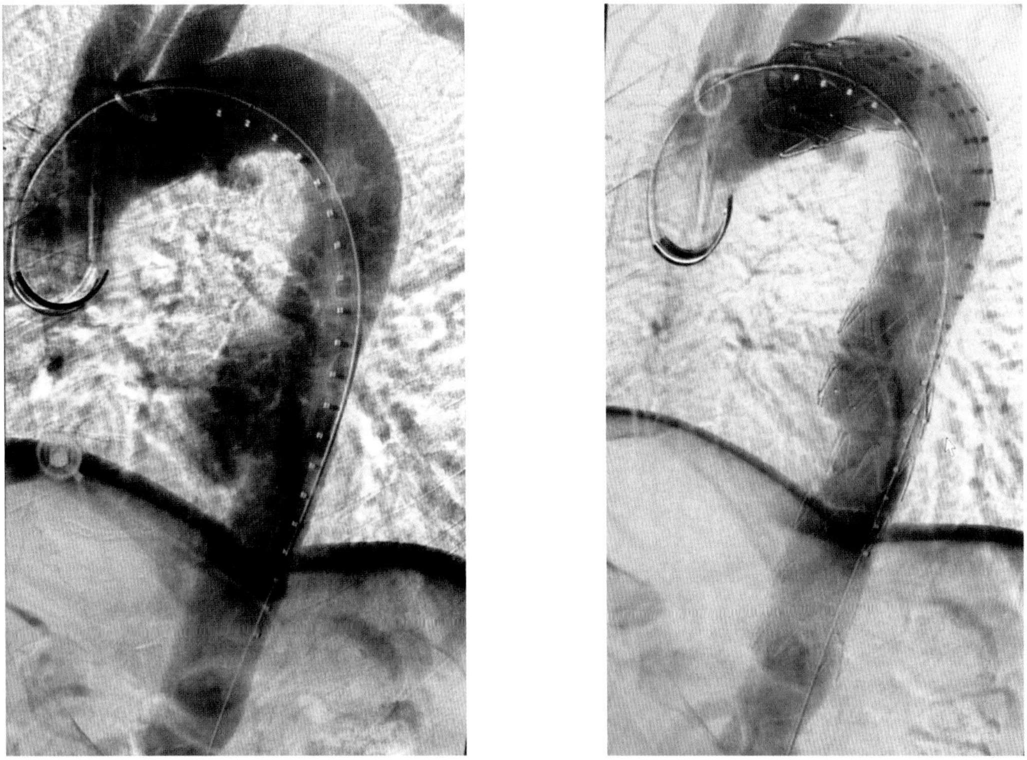

FIGURE 48-2 A 68-year-old male with multiple myeloma and streptococcal meningitis was found to have an expanding thoracic mycotic aneurysm. He was treated with a rifampin-soaked endograft as he was not a candidate for open repair due to his overall fragility and deconditioning.

if the limb becomes ischemic. Adjuvant therapy such as implantation of antibiotic beads into the adjacent field and/or flap closures (sartorius, rectus femoris, gracilis, rectus abdominis, etc.) should be considered at the time of ligation/excision to decrease wound healing complications.

Native arterial infections carry a high rate of morbidity and mortality. As such, they necessitate a thorough and expeditious work-up and careful choice of the best method of repair. Consideration should be given to endovascular repair to temporize life-threatening hemorrhage with further consideration for definitive repair versus long-term antibiotic therapy alone depending on the overall health and life expectancy of the patient. A multidisciplinary team approach involving infectious disease specialists is recommended when approaching patients with this complex condition.

REFERENCES

1. Osler W. The Gulstonian lectures on malignant endocarditis. *BMJ.* 1885;1(1262):467–470.
2. Gelabert HA. Primary arterial infections and antibiotic prophylaxis. In: Moore W, ed. *Vascular and Endovascular and Surgery: A Comprehensive Review.* 8th ed. Philadelphia, PA: Elsevier Saunders; 2013:157–177.
3. Sorelius K, Wanhainen A, Mani K. Infective native aortic aneurysms: call for consensus on definition, terminology, diagnostic criteria, and reporting standards. *Eur J Vasc Endovasc Surg.* 2020;59:333–334.
4. Yellin A. Ruptured mycotic aneurysm, a complication of parenteral drug abuse. *Arch Surg.* 1977,112(8):981–986.
5. Magilligan D, Quinn E. Active infective endocarditis. In: Magilligan DJ, Quinn E, eds. *Endocarditis: Medical and Surgical Management.* New York, NY: Marcel Dekker; 1986:207.

6. Jarrett F, Darling R, Mundth E, Austen WG. Experience with infected aneurysms of the abdominal aorta. *Arch Surg*. 1975;10:1281–1286.
7. Chakfe N, Diener H, Lejay A, et al. European society for vascular surgery (ESVS) 2020 clinical practice guidelines on the management of vascular graft and endograft infections. *Eur J Vasc Endovasc Surg*. 2020; 59:334–384.
8. Fukuchi K, Ishhida Y, Higashi M, et al. Detection of aortic graft infection by fluorodeoxyglucose positron emission tomography: comparison with computed tomographic findings. *J Vasc Surg*. 2005;42(5):919–925.
9. Wook Ryu S, Allman KC. Native aortic and prosthetic vascular stent infection on ^{99m}Tc-labeled white blood cell scintigraphy. *J Nuc Med Technol*. 2014;42:120–121.
10. Kaufman J, Smith R, Capel G, Shah DM, Chang BB, Leather RP. Antibiotic therapy for arterial infection: lessons from the successful treatment of a mycotic femoral artery aneurysm without surgical reconstruction. *Ann Vasc Surg*. 1990;4(6):592–596.
11. Hsu RB, Chang CI, Wu IH, Lin FY. Selective medical treatment of infected aneurysms of the aorta in high risk patients. *J Vasc Surg*. 2009;49(1):66–70.
12. Bandyk DF, Novotney ML, Johnson BL, Back MR, Roth SR. Use of rifampin-soaked gelatin-sealed polyester grafts for in situ treatment of primary aortic and vascular prosthetic infections. *J Surg Res*. 2001;95(1):44–49.
13. Clagett GP, Valentine RJ, Hagino RT. Autogenous aortoiliac/femoral reconstruction from superficial femoral-popliteal veins: feasibility and durability. *J Vasc Surg*. 1997;25(2):255–266.
14. Daenens K, Forneau I, Nevelsteen A. Ten-year experience in autogenous reconstruction with the femoral vein in the treatment of aortofemoral prosthetic infection. *Eur J Vasc Endovasc Surg*. 2003;25:240–245.
15. Savlania A, Tripathi RK. Aortic reconstruction in infected aortic pathology by femoral vein "neo-aorta". *Sem in Vasc Surg*. 2019;32:73–80.
16. Bisdas T, Bredt M, Pichlmaier M, et al. Eight-year experience with cryopreserved arterial homografts for the in-situ reconstruction of abdominal aortic infections. *J Vasc Surg*. 2010;52(2):323–330.
17. Touma J, Cochennec F, Parisot J, Legendre AF, Becquemin J-P, Desgranges P. In situ reconstruction in native and prosthetic aortic infections using cryopreserved arterial allografts. *Eur J of Vasc Endovasc Surg*. 2014;48(3):292–299.
18. Ben Ahmed S, Louvancourt A, Daniel G, et al. Cryopreserved arterial allografts for in situ reconstruction of abdominal aortic native or secondary graft infection. *J Vasc Surg*. 2018;67:468–477.
19. Hostalrich A, Ozdemir BA, Sfeir J, Solovei L, Alric P, Canaud L. Systematic review of native and graft-related aortic infection outcome managed with orthotopic xenopericardial grafts. *J Vasc Surg*. 2019;69:614–618.
20. Brown SL, Busuttil RW, Baker JD, Machleder HI, Moore WS, Barker WF. Bacteriologic and surgical determinants of survival in patients with mycotic aneurysms. *J Vasc Surg*. 1984;1(4):541–547.
21. Berchtold C, Eibl C, Seeling MH, Jakob P, Schonleben K. Endovascular treatment and complete regression of an infected abdominal aortic aneurysm. *J Endovasc ther*. 2002;9(4):543–548.
22. Koeppel TA, Gahlen J, Diehl S, Prosst RL, Dueber C. Mycotic aneurysm of the abdominal aorta with retroperitoneal abscess: successful endovascular repair. *J Vasc Surg*. 2004;40(1):164–166.
23. Kan CD, Lee HL, Yang YJ. Outcome after endovascular stent graft treatment for mycotic aortic aneurysm: a systematic review. *J Vasc Surg*. 2007;46:906–912.
24. Sorelius K, Mani K, Bjorck M, et al. Endovascular treatment of mycotic aortic aneurysms: a European multicenter study. *Circulation*. 2014;130:136–142.
25. Sorelius K, Wanhainen A, Furebring M, et al. Nationwide study of the treatment of mycotic abdominal aortic aneurysms comparing open and endovascular repair. *Circulation*. 2016;134:1822–1823.
26. Kan CD, Lee HL, Luo CY, Yang Y-J. The efficacy of aortic stent grafts in the management of mycotic abdominal aortic aneurysm-institute case management with systemic literature comparison. *Ann Vasc Surg*. 2010; 24:433–440.
27. Kurimoto Y, Tsuchida Y, Saito J, Yama N, Narimatsu E, Asai Y. Emergency endovascular stent-grafting for infected pseudoaneurysm of brachial artery. *Infection*. 2003;31:86–88.
28. Saini NS, Luther A, Mahajan A, Joseph A. Infected pseudoaneurysms in intravenous drug abusers: ligation or reconstruction? *Int J Appl Basic Med Res*. 2014;4:S23–S26.

SELF-ASSESSMENT STUDY QUESTIONS AND ANSWERS

Questions

1. Which is a common method of native arterial infection?
A. Oslerian mycotic aneurysm formation
B. Infected aneurysm formation
C. Arteritis from contagious spread
D. Arterial injury with contamination
E. Microbial arteritis with aneurysm formation
F. All of the above

2. What is the most common bacteria associated with Oslerian mycotic aneurysm formation?
A. *Bacteroides*
B. *Staphylococcus aureus*
C. *Streptococcus*
D. *Salmonella*

3. In patients without a history of IV drug abuse, what is the most common bacteria associated with endocarditis?
A. *Bacteroides*
B. *Staphylococcus aureus*
C. *Streptococcus*
D. *Salmonella*

4. In patients with a femoral aneurysm or history of IV drug abuse, what is the most common bacteria associated with endocarditis?
A. *Bacteroides*
B. *Staphylococcus aureus*
C. *Streptococcus viridans*
D. *Salmonella*

5. What is the most common site of primary arterial infections?
A. Common femoral artery
B. Abdominal aorta
C. Superior mesenteric artery
D. All of the above

6. What is the in-hospital mortality rate for treatment of native arterial infections with antibiotics alone?
A. 25%
B. 50%
C. 75%
D. 90%

7. The choice of conduit for in situ repair of native arterial infections includes all of the following except:
A. Saphenous vein
B. Femoral vein
C. PTFE
D. Cryopreserved artery or vein

8. Covered stents are a viable alternative to open repair in patients with native arterial infections:
A. True
B. False

SELF-ASSESSMENT STUDY QUESTIONS AND ANSWERS

Answers

1. F.
2. D.
3. B.
4. C.
5. D.
6. B.
7. C.
8. A.

CHAPTER

49 Vasculitis and Other Arteriopathies

Erica Leigh Benvenutti and Nezam Altorok

OUTLINE

INTRODUCTION

HISTOPATHOLOGY

IMAGING

LARGE VESSEL VASCULITIS (LVV): TAKAYASU ARTERITIS (TA) AND GIANT CELL ARTERITIS (GCA)

- LVV: Takayasu Arteritis (TA)
- LVV: Giant Cell Arteritis (GCA) Also Known as Temporal Arteritis

MEDIUM VESSEL VASCULITIS: POLYARTERITIS NODOSA (PAN) AND KAWASAKI'S DISEASE (KD)

SMALL VESSEL VASCULITIS (SVV): ANCA-ASSOCIATED VASCULITIS

IMMUNE COMPLEX DEPOSITION VASCULITIS

VARIABLE VASCULITIS (VV): BEHCET'S DISEASE

CONCLUSION

INTRODUCTION

Vasculitis is a group of inflammatory diseases affecting blood vessels of all calibers. Vasculitis is classified based on the involved-vessel size: small, medium, and large vessels vasculitis. The clinical presentation of vasculitis is variable, and it helps to differentiate between the different vasculitis conditions. Also age, race, organ system involvement, histopathology, and serology can facilitate further classification of vasculitis. Management of vasculitis frequently requires a multispecialty approach involving rheumatology, nephrology, neurology, vascular surgery, and cardiology making coordination of care essential. Historically, vasculitis has evolved from an illness with high morbidity and mortality to one of challenging management with recurrent flares and a goal of remission.

For the purposes of this chapter, we will focus on large and medium vasculitis which have surgical applications and means of intervention. Large vessels function as transportation highways delivering oxygen-rich blood and carrying deoxygenated waste to and from vital organs. Medium vessels are utilized in organs where blood flow is a key element to homeostasis and overall function. Small vessel, while acting as part of the delivery system, have few surgical interventions and are best managed with medical therapy via immunosuppression, but it is important for vascular surgery to identify these conditions as often the vasculitis lesions may present with skin ulceration or palpable, nonblanching purpuric skin lesions (Figure 49-1).

It is imperative to differentiate inflammatory conditions of the vascular wall from infectious conditions, as treatment and outcome of management is completely different. For instance, aortic aneurysms have been linked to infections related to syphilis, aspergillus, or rickettsial.[1] Emergent endovascular repairs are more likely to be complicated by graft infection than elective procedures, but similar rates of postoperative graft infection were noted in both thoracic and abdominal aneurysm location.[2] Stenting of infectious aneurysms is controversial and beyond the scope of this chapter. On the other hand, some infection can trigger systemic vasculitis. For instance, hepatitis C infection is often associated

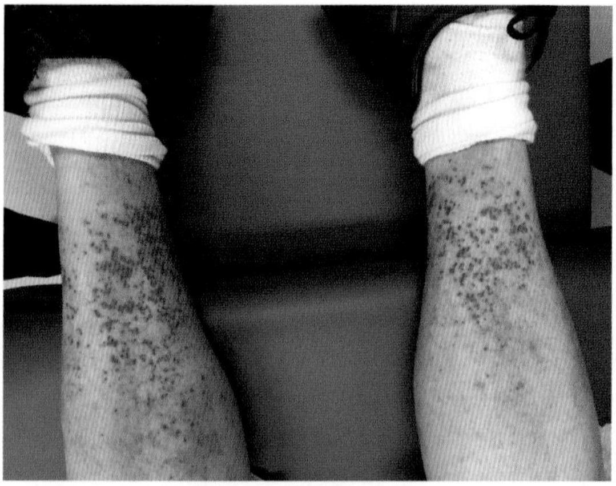

FIGURE 49-1 Palpable purpura in a patient with IgA vasculitis (Henoch-Schönlein purpura).

with cryoglobulinemia. Endocarditis can trigger a leukocytoclastic small vessel vasculitis disease that is similar in histopathology and clinical appearance of systemic vasculitis (Figure 49-2). Identifying these vasculitis mimickers is imperative as it will have significant implications in terms of treatment strategies (antibiotics vs immunosuppressive therapy). Other vasculitis mimickers include drug-induced vasculopathy, such as in the case of cocaine-induced vasculitis, or the result of malignant, atherosclerotic/ischemic, or thromboembolic disease. This should be considered in clinical context based on individual patient risk factors that guide laboratory and differential diagnosis testing to determine the root concern.

HISTOPATHOLOGY

Tissue diagnosis is useful if it is in a location amenable to biopsy, and should always be considered the gold standard test to establish a diagnosis of vasculitis. Skin, renal, or temporal artery biopsies (TABs) are common to diagnose vasculitis. Immunofluorescence is a particularly helpful staining technique for cutaneous and renal biopsy. Pauci-immune, little immunofluorescence staining, in small vessel disease is a distinguishing feature with minimal to no immune complex deposition in ANCA (anti-neutrophilic cytoplasmic antibody)-associated vasculitis (AAV). In contrast, IgA deposition is a key feature in IgA vasculitis (previously known as Henoch-Schönlein Purpura—HSP). Cryoglobulinemia will show immune complex deposition in involved arteries. Skin biopsy should be taken from erythematous, active, or edge of lesions including immunofluorescence and routine pathologic stain with hematoxylin and eosin (H&E). We recommend using Michels solution, or tissue samples should be immediately

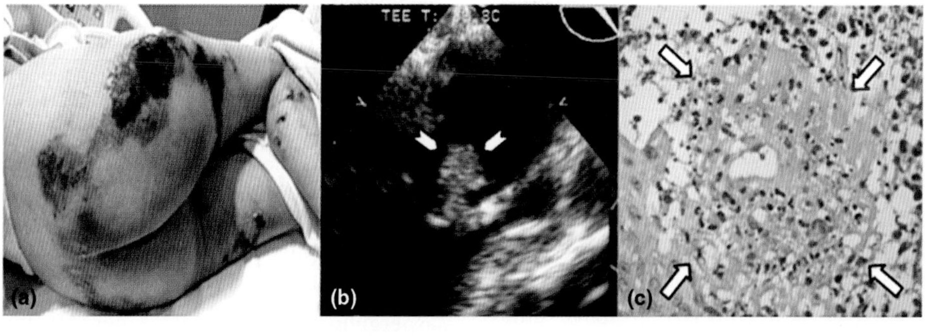

FIGURE 49-2 A 29-year-old female underwent dental extraction 1 month prior to her presentation with painful purpuric skin lesions that progressed to necrotic ulcers over the buttocks and lower extremities (A). Physical examination demonstrated new pansystolic murmur grade IV/VI at the apex of the heart, and splinter hemorrhages. Initial laboratory testing was pertinent for elevated inflammatory markers, low C3 and C4 levels, positive rheumatoid factor (RF), positive p-ANCA (titer 1:5120), and positive antiserine protease 3 (PR-3). Blood cultures grew staphylococcus epidermidis. A trans-esophageal echocardiogram confirmed presence of large vegetation on the mitral valve associated with severe mitral regurgitation (B). Skin biopsy demonstrated small- and medium-sized vessels with reactive endothelium and surrounding acute inflammatory cells as depicted between the arrows (C), on background of fibrinoid necrosis and focal extravasated red blood cells and nuclear dust, all suggestive of leukocytoklastic vasculitis.

frozen in liquid nitrogen before sending the specimens to the pathology laboratory for immunofluorescence studies, and formalin transport media for H&E stain. Old lesions and central ulcer should be avoided when obtaining tissue biopsy because they are less diagnostically useful and may only represent necrotic ischemic tissue.

IMAGING

In contrast to histopathologic diagnosis common for TAB in giant cell arteritis (GCA), some large vessel vasculitis (LVV) utilizes radiographic imaging such as magnetic resonance angiography (MRA) or computed tomography angiography (CTA) for visualization of large vessel, as a biopsy of the aorta and its major branches is problematic. Angiogram can be both diagnostic and therapeutic (e.g., allowing stenting for narrowing/blockages or angioplasty for inflamed areas). Doppler ultrasound (US) of the temporal artery is an emerging tool in the field of GCA. The classical halo sign, which represents hypoechoic wall thickening of the superficial temporal artery, has a sensitivity of 68% and specificity of 81%, compared to positive TAB.[3]

Positron emission tomography (PET) scan uptake can be very useful in establishing diagnosis of LVV, and for evaluating disease activity. PET scan may show areas of activity in blood vessels with active inflammation. FDG (fluorodeoxyglucose)-PET scan activity during clinical remission was associated with future clinical relapse.[4] Essentially, FDG-PET is a radiolabeled sugar molecule that traces uptake during glucose metabolism which aids in the identification of areas of inflammation. It is applicable for LVV but utility decreases in medium mesenteric and small vessel vasculitis such as in the glomeruli. FDG-PET can detect the extent and activity of large-vessel vasculitis in untreated patients but is unreliable in diagnosing vasculitis in patients on steroids.[5] FDG-PET demonstrated excellent accuracy, and contrast-enhanced CT mural thickening showed good accuracy in the diagnosis of LVV.[6] Although even being a useful tool to assist in establishing the diagnosis of vasculitis and for evolution of the disease activity, FDG-PET is not widely available in small, rural hospitals, or hospitals not offering a line of oncologic services. The cost of the test is another factor, adding further limitation in the utilization of PET scan in vasculitis.

LARGE VESSEL VASCULITIS (LVV): TAKAYASU ARTERITIS (TA) AND GIANT CELL ARTERITIS (GCA)

LVV can have several etiologies. In this chapter, we will focus on Takayasu arteritis (TA) and giant cell arteritis (GCA). An atypical presentation of LVV, not meeting diagnostic criteria, requires the provider to consider atypical causes such as infection, IgG-4-related vasculitic disease, malignancy, and other vasculitis mimickers (infective endocarditis, cocaine use, hypercoagulability, etc.).

The 2018 American College of Rheumatology/European League Against Rheumatism guidelines allow for diagnosis of LVV with imaging or histopathology.[7] In general, for LVV anticoagulation is not recommended routinely but can be considered on an individual basis based upon cardiovascular risk factors such as cerebrovascular accidents (CVA), coronary disease, or vascular ischemic end organ damage. Specifically, for vascular surgery, revascularization can be considered on an urgent basis if vessel dissection is imminent or occurring, or if there is critical organ dysfunction because of vasculitis. Current guidelines recommend surgical approaches, including endovascular surgery, using a phased approach or interventions during disease remission.

LVV: TAKAYASU ARTERITIS (TA)

TA is classically seen in women of reproductive age (<40 years), with the highest prevalence in Asian populations. During the course of the disease, two stages predominate: systemic and then pulseless/occlusive disease. It is very common to have constitutional symptoms, which include weight loss, anorexia, fever, fatigue, abdominal pain, arthralgia, and angina as the initial manifestations of TA. Further signs and symptoms are related to branches of the aorta experiencing ischemic disease.

The occlusive phase is characterized by arm or leg claudication, headaches, postural dizziness, and visual disturbances. Occlusion is a spectrum, including reduced/absent pulses or subclavian, aortic, femoral bruits. Inflammation can lead to stenosis or aneurysmal formation in the aorta or in major branches. Surgery should be considered to revascularize stenosed or occluded vessels that cause ischemia with end organ damage. Indications for surgery include cerebral hypoperfusion, renovascular hypertension, or limb claudication with repair of aneurysms or valvular insufficiency.

Pulmonary artery aneurysm or pulseless ischemic limb are well-known complications of TA, and signs and symptoms such as pain, pulselessness, pallor, paresthesia, or paralysis should prompt appropriate vascular radiographic work up with CT-angiogram/MRA or PET-FDG along with appropriate laboratory tests such as erythrocyte sedimentation rate (ESR), C-reactive protein (CRP), and ANCA.

In regard to endovascular interventions, a recent study of 94 vascular interventions were performed in 61 patients. A third of them were of endovascular procedures. The overall mortality was 4.1%, all due to early postoperative complications, which resulted in a rate of surgery-related mortality of 9.8%. All deaths occurred in patients with active disease. Clinical parameters known to be associated with mortality include aneurysm, secondary hypertension, aortic insufficiency, and CVA accident, but were not correlated with mortality in this study.[8] It is recommended to delay elective endovascular interventions or reconstructive surgery till the inflammatory disease is under control. Interventions should be performed in phases of stable remission. However, arterial vessel dissection or critical vascular ischemia of limb or organ requires urgent surgical intervention. Figure 49-3 summarizes our approach to management of TA.

Chen et al. applied endovascular techniques to Type I TA, defined as a progressive inflammatory disease involving the aortic arch and its main branches. This small study examined 11 patients with severe cerebral ischemia undergoing endovascular intervention of the carotid artery. Large ipsilateral cerebral vascular infarcts > 2 weeks duration were enrolled to allow perfusion of the pneumbric area. If clinically indicated, repeat angioplasty with a larger diameter balloon was performed 1–3 months later. Successful revascularization in addition to pre and post immunosuppression provided durable

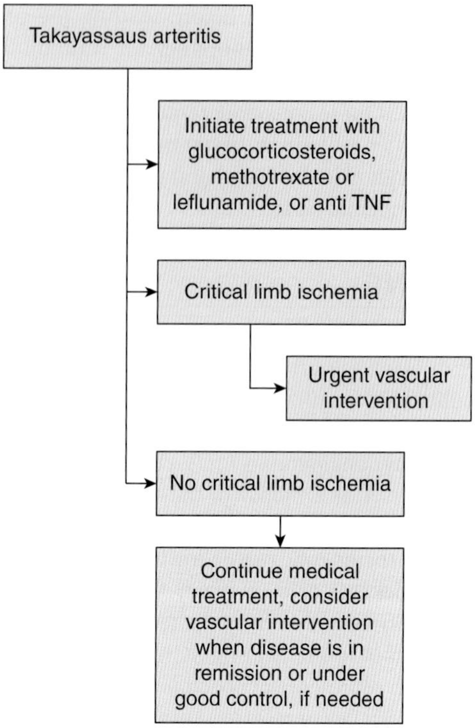

FIGURE 49-3 Suggested approach for management of Takayassaus arteritis.

remission and preserved central nervous system (CNS) functionality in 8/11 patients, the 2 failures resulted from occlusion of a long segment of artery. This study showed safe outcomes in regard to repeat endovascular intervention with pre- and postoperative immunosuppressive therapy used concurrently. This dual approach was beneficial for CNS neurological ischemic deficits caused by occluded carotids.[9] Restenosis is a common complication after treatment with open surgical or endovascular approach, which highlights the importance of multidisciplinary effort from both a surgical and medical perspective.

Both surgical revascularization and endovascular management are safe and effective methods in the treatment of TA. Although the long-term patency of endovascular therapy is low, it can repeatedly be performed and can be used as the preferred approach in treating a short stenosis segment. An endovascular angioplasty should be considered in cases involving organ damage such as renal stenosis causing acute renal failure and renovascular hypertension.

Open surgical repair shows long-term durability and is suitable for complex lesions and failed cases of endovascular management.[10] There is significantly lower risk of restenosis with open surgical intervention than with endovascular intervention, although stroke is generally more common with open surgical intervention than with an endovascular approach. The risk of stroke in open surgery is higher when the supra-aortic branches are involved rather than the renal arteries.[11] A meta-analysis from Jeong et al. found that balloon angioplasty can yield better results than renal artery interventions with stenting. Nonetheless, it is desirable to avoid vessel dissections during balloon angioplasty, which can eventually require stent implantations.[12] Given the rarity of vasculitis, standardized guidelines are lacking, making surgeon experience, location/size of lesion, and patient comorbidities a complex decision.

The cornerstone therapy for TA remains glucocorticosteroids along with other immunosuppressive medications such as methotrexate and leflunamide. Tumor necrosis factor alpha (TNF-α) inhibitors, such as infliximab and adalimumab as well as IL-6 antagonist toclizimub, are used when additional immunosuppression is warranted. In a recent small case study of 56 patients, treatment with leflunomide was associated with complete remission in a significant proportion of patients (68% at 6 months and 55% at 12 months), including patients refractory to previous lines of treatment.[13] Surgery, if indicated, should occur during stable or remission phase of disease. Anticoagulation should be considered on a case to case basis, and guidelines remain sparse in this rare disease.

LVV: GIANT CELL ARTERITIS (GCA) ALSO KNOWN AS TEMPORAL ARTERITIS

GCA has a similar presentation to TA in respect to constitutional symptoms such as weight loss and fever. However, it tends to affect an older population, and the main clinical presentation is headache. The symptom with greatest positive predictive value for GCA is jaw claudication. This can be difficult to differentiate from temporomandibular joint dysfunction, teeth grinding, and other dental infections which can be mimickers. GCA effects predominately a female population over 50 years of age and usually has supporting serology with elevated ESR and/or CRP in 80% of patients with GCA. Patients may present with tenderness over the scalp with swollen temporal artery branches that are not pulsatile (Figure 49-4), or rarely with scalp ischemic necrosis. Clinical criteria most strongly suggestive of GCA in addition to jaw claudication include CRP above 2.45 mg/dl, neck pain, and an ESR of 47 mm/hour or more, in that order.[14] The most common ocular finding is unilateral vision loss known as arteritic anterior ischemic optic neuropathy (AAION). Vision loss in the context of GCA is considered a medical emergency that requires immediate admission and inpatient treatment with intravenous (IV) steroids.

The temporal artery is a readily accessible site on physical exam: pulse can vary from bounding, tender, or painful making patients unable to comb their hair

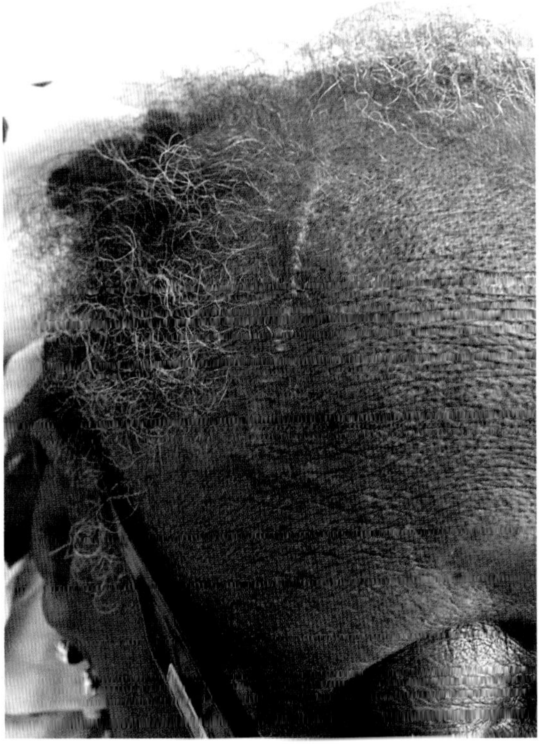

FIGURE 49-4 Markedly dilated temporal arteries in a 76-year-old woman with giant cell arteritis (GCA). The arteries are tender to palpation.

or wear spectacles in the inflammatory infiltration early phase, versus the later ischemic absent or pulseless phase. Studies have shown no classic characteristic nature of the headache to aid physicians, and a temporal location of headache is a more useful clue. We recommend obtaining bilateral TABs in patients suspected to have GCA. TAB is considered the gold standard test for establishing a diagnosis of GCA. However, sensitivity of unilateral TAB is around 80%. The yield of bilateral TAB improves to 90%. A French multicenter study of GCA-related aortitis found negative TABs were characterized by younger age and increased frequency of aortic arch and diffuse arterial involvement compared to those with positive TAB. GCA signs and symptoms on presentation, inflammatory parameters, and glucocorticoid therapy were similar in both TAB positive and TAB negative groups. Aortic wall thickness > 2 mm on CT scan and type of aortic involvement were not significantly different between groups.[15] Imaging modalities such as US, CTA, MRA are gaining acceptance, but TAB still is recommended for diagnostic purposes to date; it remains the gold standard. Recent EULAR guidelines now recognize temporal artery US have first line diagnostic utility. Figure 49-5 demonstrates our suggested immediate-approach to suspected GCA.

Polymyalgia rheumatica (PMR) at diagnosis with inflammation limited to the adventitia in TAB positive specimens appear to identify subsets of patients with more benign disease, but large vessel involvement at diagnosis is associated with reduced survival.[16] An Icelandic study showed high BMI protects against the occurrence of GCA, and smoking may protect against GCA in men.[17]

There is more recent data to support the role of US imaging in GCA. A unilateral halo sign is very suggestive for GCA in the right clinical presentation. The sensitivity of the classical hypo-echoic US comparted to TAB is 52% to 68%, and specificity of 71% to 81%. Furthermore, sequential strategy of US followed by TAB in the case of a negative US had a sensitivity of 78% and specificity of 71%, equivalent to a simultaneous testing strategy. Additionally, male sex was an independent predictive factor for positive US.[3,18]

An in-depth discussion of treatment is beyond the scope of this chapter. Standard therapy includes IV glucocorticoid for vision loss, which requires hospitalization, and oral therapy outpatient for nonvision threatening GCA or PMR. Biopsy is recommended within 1 week of glucocorticosteroids initiation to maximize biopsy yield. In case of no vision loss, typically patients are treated with prednisone 1 mg/kg. Steroid sparing agents such as methotrexate (MTX) have very limited role in treatment of GCA. The IL-6 antagonist, toclizumab, was recently approved for the treatment of GCA, especially in patients with relapse, who are unable to wean off steroids, or who have comorbidities such as diabetes mellitus that prevent the use of steroids.

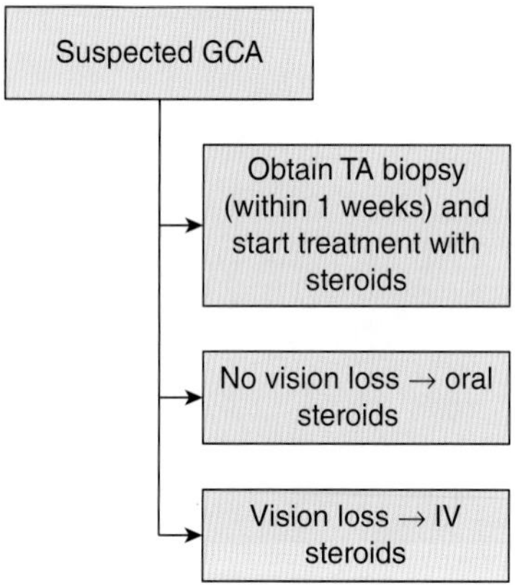

FIGURE 49-5 Immediate management of suspected giant cell arteritis (GCA).

MEDIUM VESSEL VASCULITIS: POLYARTERITIS NODOSA (PAN) AND KAWASAKI'S DISEASE (KD)

Kawasaki disease (KD) typically affects the pediatric population. It is presumed to have a genetic predisposition with infectious insult leading to immune activation. *Streptococcus* is the most common agent; however, recent KD-like presentation in COVID-19 infections are emerging.

Polyarteritis nodosa (PAN) is a medium vessel disorder presenting similar to other ANCA/small vessel vasculitis with renal manifestations evidenced by red cell casts and microscopic hematuria. Typically, ANCA testing is negative in medium vessel vasculitis. PAN is a necrotizing vasculitis which displays

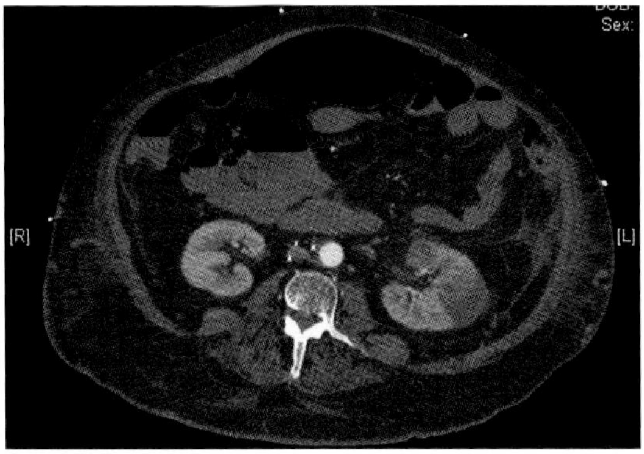

FIGURE 49-6 CT abdomen demonstrating left renal wedge-shaped infarction in a patient with polyarteritis nodosa. Conventional angiogram, rather than CT angiogram, is recommended in these patients.

aneurysmal nodules along the walls of medium-sized muscular arteries, which can lead to ischemia in involved organs such as kidneys (Figure 49-6). Constitutional signs and symptoms include fever, chills, and weight loss. Dermatologic rashes can mimic other diagnoses such as IgA vasculitis, leukocytoclastic vasculitis, erythema multiforme, livedo reticularis, pyoderma gangrenosum, peripheral gangrene, or subcutaneous nodules. Dermatologic lesions are painful and typically nonpruritic with a necrotizing, nongranulomatous involvement of blood vessels. Gastrointestinal (GI) and genitourinary (GU) manifestations include ischemic abdominal and testicular pain. PAN typically spares the lungs, and this is an important feature to differentiate from small vessel vasculitis. Cardiac and neurologic manifestation are rare but are a differentiating feature. Neurologic features include focal defects, hemiplegia/hemiparesis, speech impairment, mononeuritis multiplex, and organic psychosis. Musculoskeletal manifestations include arthralgia, nonerosive arthritis, and myalgia. Familial Mediterranean fever and hepatitis B are associated with PAN. Conversely to small vessel vasculitis generally presenting in adults where renal biopsy is the source of histopathology, skin or muscle biopsy are more frequently performed in children. Frequently CTA or MRA of hepatic, renal, or mesenteric vessels can show cut off, pruning, stenosis, or aneurysm. Biopsy can be helpful, if amenable, but is not necessary for diagnosis. PAN differs from small vessel/ANCA positive vasculitis in that relapses are rare and remission is frequently attained. If a relapse occurs, it commonly involves the skin. Treatment includes glucocorticosteroids along with B cell modulation with rituximab, methotrexate, colchicine, or dapsone if further immunosuppressive therapy is necessary.

KD involves medium and small vessels. Genetic predisposition is a factor with the incidence and prevalence more common in the pediatric Asian population; *staphylococcus* or *streptococcus* infection is a common trigger to the immune system. KD is a mucocutaneous lymph node disease afflicting young children, manifesting as an acute self-limiting systemic vasculitis. KD is the second most common vasculitis in childhood after HSP and the most common cause of childhood-acquired heart disease.[19] Classically nonexudative conjunctivitis, rash of palms/soles that will evolve to desquamation, cervical lymph adenopathy, and erythema of lips/"strawberry" tongue can all be seen. Coronary artery aneurysm is the most feared complication, and it can be seen via coronary angiography, CTA, or MRA on imaging. Delay in diagnosis raises the risk of coronary artery aneurysm formation.

It is recommended to use a combination of warfarin and aspirin (ASA) for treatment of giant aneurysms (>8 mm).[20] This combination of warfarin/ASA reduced myocardial infarction and death in case of aneurysm formation. Stenotic areas at inlet/outlet points of giant aneurysms may require angioplasty, but typically angioplasty should occur after disease stability is attained. However, the risk of myocardial infarction due to uncontrolled inflammation must be considered. Coronary artery aneurysms or ectasia develop in approximately 15% to 25% of untreated children and may lead to ischemic heart disease or sudden death.[21] Myocarditis is common during the acute phase and cytokine storm can cause a KD shock syndrome.

Nonsurgical treatment of KD includes intravenous immunoglobulin (IVIG) and moderate to high dose of aspirin. Less frequently infliximab, a TNF-α inhibitor, or pulse doses of methylprednisolone has been used in refractory cases to IVIG. Alternative therapies such as TNF or glucocorticosteroids are options for patient's unwillingness to accept blood products for religious reasons or for high-risk patients. Refractory disease should be considered in patients who remain febrile and symptomatic. Low-molecular weight heparin (LMWH) or oral warfarin are more common for anticoagulation but abciximab, a platelet aggregation inhibitor, is another option used in KD.

SMALL VESSEL VASCULITIS (SVV): ANCA-ASSOCIATED VASCULITIS

Small vessel vasculitis (SVV) is usually managed with immunosuppressive therapy and little surgical intervention is required but can be indicated in rare circumstances. Typically presenting in middle to late ages with similar constitutional signs and symptoms that include arthralgias, myalgia, fatigue, and occasionally fever. In addition to being systemic disease with multiple organ involvement, skin manifestation of vasculitis is classically a nonblanching palpable purpuric rash in dependent areas. Skin biopsy using 3 millimeter (mm) or 4 mm punch biopsy can be helpful. The majority of patients with SVV will have positive ANCA serology but are differentiated by presentation and the affected organ system.

Granulomatosis polyangiitis (GPA), formerly known as Wegner's disease, is associated with cytoplasmic ANCA (C-ANCA) that is confirmed by testing for anti-proteinase 3 (PR3), and manifests as a cardinal triad of sino-nasal, pulmonary, and renal disease. Epistaxis, hemoptysis, or dark colored urine can be a chief complaint among patients. Pulmonary histology is not required for diagnostic criteria. Pulmonary cavitary lesions, infiltrates, or ground glass opacities on imaging do not require tissue histopathology. Frequently bronchoscopy is used to rule out other etiologies such as infection and can be helpful if it demonstrates classic features of diffuse alveolar hemorrhage such as hemosiderin-laden macrophages. Upper airway disease, including otitis, sinusitis, and rhinitis, is present in >90% of patients with GPA. Nasal perforation and saddle nose can occur in GPA (Figure 49-7). Tracheal stenosis is present in 10% to 30% of patients, and ulcerative or destructive lesions should alert the clinician to the possibility of vasculitis. Tracheobronchial and endobronchial lesions occur in 10% to 50% and nodular or cavitary lesions can be seen in GP. A new movement to label vasculitis as myeloperoxidase (MPO) or proteinase 3 (PR3) AAV has been proposed because this has more bearing on relapse and prognosis. Females, African American patients, or those with severe kidney disease, may be resistant to initial treatment more often than other patients with ANCA-associated small-vessel vasculitis. Increased relapse risk appears to be related to the presence of lung or upper airway disease and anti-PR3 antibody seropositivity.[22]

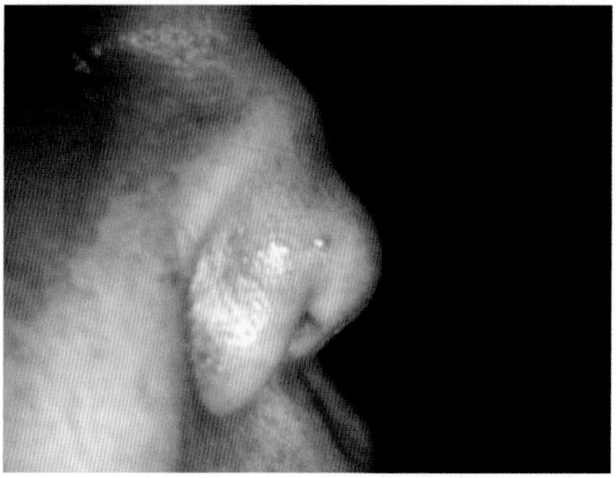

FIGURE 49-7 Saddle nose in a patient with granulomatosis with polyangitis (GPA) due to perforation of the central nasal septum.

Microscopic polyangiitis (MPA) is associated with perinuclear ANCA (P ANCA), which is confirmed by testing for anti-myeloperoxidase (MPO). MPA mainly manifests in renal and pulmonary systems similar to GPA. MPA may present with rapidly progressive glomerulonephritis, which is defined by 50% loss of renal function in less than 3 months and by histopathology revealing crescents in at least 50% of glomeruli. Granulomas seen in GPA are lacking in MPA, and this is an important feature to differentiate between the two conditions. Overall, ANCA serology provides helpful suspicion for SVV but is not diagnostic for a specific disease. For instance, P-ANCA can be positive in inflammatory bowel disease, which is not a vasculitis condition.

Eosinophilic granulomatosis polyangiitis (EGPA), usually P-ANCA positive, manifests with asthma, allergies, eosinophilia, and neuropathic manifestations. Asthma can develop years prior to formal diagnosis. Asthma that is refractory to standard management can prompt a vasculitis workup. Foot drop is a classic example of mononeuritis multiplex with both sensory and motor abnormalities, including paresthesia (numbness, tingling, neuropathic pain) and impedes ambulatory function. Sural nerve biopsy can be helpful with clarifying diagnosis but is not necessary to meet diagnostic criteria. Eosinophilia can be seen on bronchial alveolar lavage and rarely transbronchial biopsy can be utilized. Migratory ground glass lesions on CT are the characteristic lower respiratory tract feature in EGPA. Cardiac involvement is more common in EGPA than the other AAVs occurring in 15% to 50% of patients, and it is disproportionately associated with high mortality. GI involvement with pain, infarction, hemorrhage, and viscus perforation are also more common in EGPA than other AAVs.

Drug-induced vasculitis, commonly occurs with cocaine or heroin that is adulterated with levamisole (Ergamisol), which is a white antiparasitic compound used as a filler that can stimulate the immune system. The clinical presentation of cocaine-induced vasculitis can include ischemic skin lesions especially at the auricles, and positive serology for ANCA, but both MPO and PR-3 are negative in that scenario. A common medication for multiple sclerosis alemtuzumab (Lemtrada) can cause AAV with MPO, P-ANCA positivity.

Other small vessel vasculitides include cryoglobulinemia frequently associated with hepatitis C with necrotic skin lesions, peripheral nerves, and glomeruli involvement. Classically, rheumatoid factor is positive in the majority of patients with cryoglobulinemia and complement 3 and complement 4 levels are low.

Treatment is beyond the scope of this chapter, but providers should be familiar with the more common agents used for induction and remission. Figure 49-8 shows an approach to diagnosis and management of AAV. In addition to high-dose systemic glucocorticosteroids, such as methylprednisolone 1000 mg daily for 3 days followed by oral prednisone 1–2 mg/kg, common induction treatment includes agents such as rituximab or cyclophosphamide. Maintenance agents include azathioprine and mycophenolate mofetil.

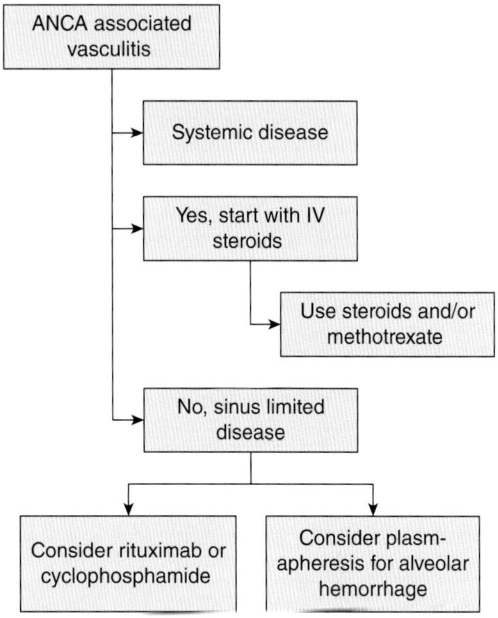

FIGURE 49-8 Approach to ANCA-associated vasculitis.

IMMUNE COMPLEX DEPOSITION VASCULITIS

Immune complex vasculitis, which includes both complement and immunoglobulins, involves small vessels. Therapy is mainly pharmaceutical with glucocorticosteroids or other immunosuppressive agents. Skin or renal biopsy may be required if lab work is nondiagnostic.

Antiglomerular basement membrane (anti-GBM), also known as Goodpasture disease, has a bimodal distribution with pulmonary hemorrhage seen in younger (<30 years old) and/or glomerulonephritis with crescents and necrosis (>50 years old). Nephritic urine shows both proteinuria and hematuria with red blood cells or red blood cell cast with microscopy. Anti-GBM antibodies are usually drawn with ANCA and should be considered in acute renal failure without obvious source of etiology. Dual positive anti-GBM and ANCA serology can occur making renal biopsy crucial to diagnosis, and it carries worse prognosis. Membranous nephropathy is associated with anti-GBM disease. An environmental aspect that is recognized, but not yet understood, is associated with influenza A, viral upper respiratory infection, or previous lung/renal damage. Treatment includes plasma exchange or cycylophosphamide in addition to high-dose glucocorticosteroids.

Cryoglobulinemia is closely associated with viral etiology hepatitis C, cytomegalovirus (CMV), Epstein Barr virus, and Parvovirus 19. Autoimmune associations include systemic lupus erythematosus, mixed connective tissue disease, Sjogren's, and other various cancers such as lymphoma. B cells produce a false positive monoclonal IgM rheumatoid factor. IgG cryoglobulins are associated with monoclonal gammopathy of unknown significance or multiple myeloma. Low complements are a clue to deposition. Skin, renal, and peripheral nerves can be involved. Arthralgia and myalgia are common but frank arthritis or myositis is rare. Membranoproliferative glomerulonephritis is a well-known renal manifestation. Rituximab and plasma exchange are reserved for severe cases.

IgA vasculitis, previously known as Henoch-Schönlein Purpura (HSP), typically affects children but can rarely present in adults, with classical manifestations of arthritis, vasculitic skin rash affecting predominantly gravity-dependent regions (lower extremities, posterior aspects of legs and thighs) (Figure 49-1), hematuria or renal failure, and abdominal pain. It is the most common form of vasculitis in children, particularly boys aged 3–15 years and is self-limited. The typical patient will present after URI and/or abdominal pain along with a characteristic palpable purpuric rash. The differential diagnosis includes another small vessel vasculitis condition. Renal or skin biopsy is utilized to differentiate IgA vasculitis as classically there will be intense IgA deposition in the involved vasculature. Classically, serologies for ANCA, anti-GBM are negative.

Hypo-complement urticarial vasculitis manifest with itchy urticarial rash and low complements (C). Anti-C1q esterase serology is diagnostic with low C1q, C3, and C4. ANA (antinuclear antibody) is frequently positive and ESR is elevated. Histopathology is consistent with leukocytoclastic vasculitis usually post venules. Symptoms and signs include arthralgia or arthritis, chronic obstructive pulmonary disease, asthma, hemoptysis, or dyspnea. GI can manifest as nausea, vomiting, diarrhea, and abdominal pain.

VARIABLE VASCULITIS (VV): BEHCET'S DISEASE

Behcet's disease is one of the variable vasculitis conditions that do not respect traditional vessel caliber as it may involve medium or large arterial or venous circulatory system. A vascular surgeon may participate in the care of Behcet's disease patients if thrombosis causes ischemic end organ damage, formation of arteriovenous fistula, thrombosis threatening extremity, or clot burden requires vascular intervention.

The classical clinical presentation of Behcet's disease includes recurrent oral and genital ulcers in majority of patients, and arthritis, uveitis, and multiorgan systemic involvement can occur. Behcet's disease is more common in Japan, Iran, and Turkey along the old Silk Road. Thrombosis in the venous system can require thrombectomy or thrombolysis, and it can affect the CNS. CNS symptoms can be found in 30% of cases and predominates in European and American rather than the classical Silk Road geographical locations. The most common neuro Behcet's disease (NBD) manifestation is headache. NBD can cause parenchymal lesions affecting brainstem, spinal cord, or cerebellum with cranial nerve involvement. Aneurysm can occur especially in the pulmonary artery, along with arteriovenous fistulas. Dermatologic manifestations including erythema nodosum, pseudofolliculitis, acne form lesion, pustulonodular lesions, or dermatitis. Genital ulcers tend to occur on the scrotum or the penis and, depending on phase of disease, active ulcer versus scar can be diagnostic. *HLA-B51* genetic marker is found in around 60% of Behcet's disease patients. GI ulcers can occur from the mouth to the anus; the most common are oral but those in the lower GI tract visualized on endoscopy can mimic inflammatory bowel disease. Musculoskeletal arthralgia is common with inflammatory arthritis being more uncommon, if it does occur it is nonerosive and nondeforming.

CONCLUSION

In conclusion, vasculitis is a group of conditions caused by inflammation of variable size of blood vessels. There is a role for vascular surgery in management and establishing a diagnosis of these diseases. Table 49-1 summarizes the cardinal manifestations of common vasculitic conditions vascular surgeons may likely encounter. Small vessel vasculitis generally is treated medically. Cases commonly seen by vascular surgeons are in large- to medium-sized vessels that require stenting, grafting, or angioplasty. Vasculitis can threaten limb function requiring thrombectomy or catheter-directed thrombolysis. Behcet's disease, because of its variable nature, may involve vascular surgical application. In general, vascular interventions should be delayed in the setting of active inflammatory vascular disease unless there is an emergent indication such as threatening ischemic injury.

TABLE 49-1 Summary of Common Vasculitis Conditions

Size of Vessel Wall	Disease	Classical Features
Large	Giant cell arteritis	Headache, jaw claudication, age > 50
	Takayasaus arteritis	Pulseless disease, women < 40
Medium	Polyarteritis nodosa	Young adults, multi-systemic disease, associated with hepatitis B.
	Kawasaki's disease	Age < 5, fever, strawberry tongue
Small	Granulomatosis with polyangitis (Wegners disease)	Nasal cavity involvement, cavitary lung lesions, renal dysfunction, positive c-ANCA
	Microscopic polyangiitis	Kidney dysfunction, alveolar hemorrhage, positive p-ANCA
	Allergic granulomatosis with angiitis (Churg Strauss)	History of asthma, eosinophilia, kidney dysfunction, positive ANCA

REFERENCES

1. Deipolyi AR, Czaplicki CD, Oklu R. Inflammatory and infectious aortic diseases. *Cardiovasc Diagn Ther.* 2018;8(suppl 1):S61-S70.
2. Heyer KS, Modi P, Morasch MD, et al. Secondary infections of thoracic and abdominal aortic endografts. *J Vasc Interv Radiol.* 2009;20(2):173-179.
3. Rinagel M, Chatelus E, Jousse-Joulin S, et al. Diagnostic performance of temporal artery ultrasound for the diagnosis of giant cell arteritis: a systematic review and meta-analysis of the literature. *Autoimmun Rev.* 2019; 18(1):56-61.
4. Grayson PC, Alehashemi S, Bagheri AA, et al. (18) F-Fluorodeoxyglucose-Positron emission tomography as an imaging biomarker in a prospective, longitudinal cohort of patients with large vessel vasculitis. *Arthritis Rheumatol.* 2018;70(3):439-449.
5. Papathanasiou ND, Du Y, Menezes LJ, et al. 18F-Fludeoxyglucose PET/CT in the evaluation of large-vessel vasculitis: diagnostic performance and correlation with clinical and laboratory parameters. *Br J Radiol.* 2012;85(1014):e188-e194.
6. Vaidyanathan S, Chattopadhyay A, Mackie SL, Scarsbrook AF. Comparative effectiveness of (18) F-FDG PET-CT and contrast-enhanced CT in the diagnosis of suspected large-vessel vasculitis. *Br J Radiol.* 2018;91(1089):20180247.
7. Hellmich B, Agueda A, Monti S, et al. 2018 Update of the EULAR recommendations for the management of large vessel vasculitis. *Ann Rheum Dis.* 2020;79(1): 19-30.
8. Rosa Neto NS, Shinjo SK, Levy-Neto M, Pereira RMR. Vascular surgery: the main risk factor for mortality in 146 Takayasu arteritis patients. *Rheumatol Int.* 2017; 37(7):1065-1073.
9. Chen B, Yu HX, Zhang J, et al. Endovascular revascularization for carotid artery occlusion in patients with Takayasu arteritis. *Eur J Vasc Endovasc Surg.* 2015; 49(5):498-505.
10. Diao Y, Yan S, Premaratne S, et al. Surgery and endovascular management in patients with takayasu's arteritis: a ten-year retrospective study. *Ann Vasc Surg.* 2020; 63:34-44.
11. Jung JH, Lee YH, Song GG, Jeong HS, Kim JH, Choi SJ. Endovascular versus open surgical intervention in patients with takayasu's arteritis: a meta-analysis. *Eur J Vasc Endovasc Surg.* 2018;55(6):888-899.
12. Jeong HS, Jung JH, Song GG, Choi SJ, Hong SJ. Endovascular balloon angioplasty versus stenting

in patients with Takayasu arteritis: A meta-analysis. *Medicine (Baltimore)*. 2017;96(29):e7558.

13. Cui X, Dai X, Ma L, et al. Efficacy and safety of leflunomide treatment in Takayasu arteritis: case series from the East China cohort. *Semin Arthritis Rheum*. 2020; 50(1):59-65.
14. Hayreh SS, Podhajsky PA, Raman R, Zimmerman B. Giant cell arteritis: validity and reliability of various diagnostic criteria. *Am J Ophthalmol*. 1997;123(3): 285-296.
15. Agard C, Bonnard G, Samson M, et al. Giant cell arteritis-related aortitis with positive or negative temporal artery biopsy: a French multicentre study. *Scand J Rheumatol*. 2019;48(6):474-481.
16. Macchioni P, Boiardi L, Muratore F, et al. Survival predictors in biopsy-proven giant cell arteritis: a northern Italian population-based study. *Rheumatology (Oxford)*. 2019;58(4):609-616.
17. Tomasson G, Bjornsson J, Zhang Y, Gudnason V, Merkel PA. Cardiovascular risk factors and incident giant cell arteritis: a population-based cohort study. *Scand J Rheumatol*. 2019;48(3):213-217.
18. Arida A, Kyprianou M, Kanakis M, Sfikakis PP. The diagnostic value of ultrasonography-derived edema of the temporal artery wall in giant cell arteritis: a second meta-analysis. *BMC Musculoskelet Disord*. 2010;11:44.
19. Dillon MJ, Eleftheriou D, Brogan PA. Medium-size-vessel vasculitis. *Pediatr Nephrol*. 2010;25(9):1641-1652.
20. Levin M, Burns JC, Gordon JB. Warfarin plus aspirin or aspirin alone for patients with giant coronary artery aneurysms secondary to Kawasaki disease? *Cardiology*. 2014;129(3):174-177.
21. Newburger JW, Takahashi M, Gerber MA, et al. Diagnosis, treatment, and long-term management of Kawasaki disease: a statement for health professionals from the committee on rheumatic fever, endocarditis and kawasaki disease, council on cardiovascular disease in the young, American Heart Association. *Circulation*. 2004;110(17):2747-2771.
22. Hogan SL, Falk RJ, Chin H, et al. Predictors of relapse and treatment resistance in antineutrophil cytoplasmic antibody-associated small-vessel vasculitis. *Ann Intern Med*. 2005;143(9):621-631.

SELF-ASSESSMENT STUDY QUESTIONS AND ANSWERS

Questions

1. A 29-year-old male patient presents with fever and joint pain of 1 week duration. He is known to a have history of intravenous drug abuse. On examination, you identified areas of necrotic skin over the upper extremities and systolic murmur over the mitral region. What is the best next management plan for this patient?
   A. Skin biopsy and treat with glucocorticosteroids
   B. Vascular angiogram of upper extremities
   C. Echocardiography and blood cultures
   D. Reassurance and follow up in 1 week

2. A 62-year-old woman presents with bilateral headache and fever along with jaw pain while consuming food for 1 week. She also reported having morning stiffness for an hour. What is the next best management plan for her?
   A. Obtain temporal artery biopsy, then start glucocorticosteroids
   B. Start treatment with systemic glucocorticosteroids, then obtain temporal artery biopsy in 1 week.
   C. Angiogram of the aorta and major branches
   D. Kidney biopsy

3. A 46-year-old man presents with fever, joint pain, and general weakness. On examination, he was found to have elevated blood pressure (190/90 mmHg). Laboratory testing demonstrated creatinine of 3.8 (normal < 1.4), and positive serology for hepatitis B surface antigen. ANCA testing was negative. What is the most likely diagnosis?
   A. Polyarteritis nodosa
   B. ANCA-associated vasculitis
   C. Giant cell arteritis
   D. Bechet's disease

4. A 24-year-old woman presents to her primary care physician (PCP) due to pain in the arms and legs upon repetitive movement and claudication when she is walking more than one block. Her PCP was not able to obtain pulse in the upper extremities. Examination did not demonstrate any features of ischemia in the fingers or toes. What is the best management course for this patient?
   A. Vascular angiogram and stenting of any stenotic lesion identified.
   B. MRI/MRA of the aorta and major branches and immunosuppressive therapy
   C. Intravenous epoprostenol
   D. Hypercoagulability workup

5. Which condition is associated with hepatitis C infection?
   A. ANCA-associated vasculitis
   B. Kawasaki disease
   C. IgA vasculitis
   D. Cryoglobulinemic vasculitis

6. Which organ is not typically involved in polyarteritis nodosa?
   A. Skin
   B. Lungs
   C. Kidneys
   D. Joints

7. Which of the following antibodies is elevated in IgA vasculitis?
   A. IgA
   B. IgG
   C. IgE
   D. None of the above

SELF-ASSESSMENT STUDY QUESTIONS AND ANSWERS

8. A 65-year-old man with insulin dependent diabetes mellitus type II, hypertension, hyperlipidemia, and history of atherosclerotic disease presents with purplish rash on the toes of his left foot. He reports low-grade fever and diffuse myalgia. Seven days ago, he underwent arterial catheterization for recent chest pain and abnormal stress test. On physical examination, he has normal BP, decreased left foot dorsalis pedis pulse, and a blotchy net-like rash on his bilateral feet.

Labs show: ESR of 65 mm/h, C3 and C4 decreased, RF negative, ANA 1:80 weakly positive, serum creatinine of 2.0, hepatitis panel is negative, and anticardiolipin is negative.

Urinalysis shows: 1 + protein, 3 RBC with 1 + blood.

The most likely diagnosis is?

A. Cholesterol emboli syndrome (CES)
B. Polyarteritis nodosa
C. Cryoglobulinemia
D. Thromboangitis obliterans (Buerger's disease)

9. Antineutrophil cytoplasmic antibodies (ANCA) can be positive in the following conditions:

A. Small vessel vasculitis
B. Inflammatory bowel disease
C. Cocaine induced vasculitis
D. All of the above

10. Which of the following presentations are consistent with giant cell arteritis?

A. A 25-year-old woman with headache of 1-week duration
B. A 65-year-old man with headache, scalp tenderness, and jaw claudication
C. A 6-year-old boy with fever and strawberry tongue who was found to have cardiac aneurysm
D. A 30-year-old woman with nasal perforation, alveolar hemorrhage, and acute renal failure

SELF-ASSESSMENT STUDY QUESTIONS AND ANSWERS

Answers

1. C.
2. B.
3. A.
4. B.
5. D.
6. B.
7. D.
8. A.
9. D.
10. B.

CHAPTER

50 Prosthetic Graft Infections

Mohamad A. Chahrour and Jamal J. Hoballah

OUTLINE

INTRODUCTION
ETIOLOGY AND PATHOGENESIS
RISK FACTORS AND PREVENTION
PRESENTATION AND CLASSIFICATION
DIAGNOSIS
MANAGEMENT
General Principles
Carotid Patch Infection
Thoracic Aortic Graft Infection
Abdominal Aortic Graft Infection
Infrainguinal Graft Infections
CONCLUSIONS

INTRODUCTION

Despite all advancements in antimicrobial treatments and surgical infection control, vascular graft infections remain a major cause of morbidity and mortality. Vascular infections can lead to enteric fistulas, pseudoaneurysm formation, ruptures, septic emboli and limb amputation, bacteremia and sepsis, and ultimately death. With the shift in vascular surgery practice from open to less invasive endovascular and percutaneous methods, more stents and stent grafts are being employed to treat vascular patients. In addition, with the advancement of prosthetic material technology, more prosthetic patches and grafts are being used by vascular surgeons in open surgery. This increased utilization of "foreign" material has increased the potential and amplified the complexity of vascular grafts infections. As such, the management of vascular infections usually requires complex strategies involving substantial human and equipment resources, multidisciplinary approaches, as well as prolonged and multiple interventions. In the chapter, we discuss the etiology, classification, presentation, and diagnostic modalities for the different types of vascular graft infections as well as the suggested treatment strategy for each.

ETIOLOGY AND PATHOGENESIS

Vascular graft infections arise from either a contamination at the time of graft insertion or from hematogenous spread or from direct extension of a nearby infection.[1,2] Vascular infections due to contamination at the time of insertion present in the early postoperative period. They are thought to arise due to sterile field contamination in the operating room, from inadequate sterile techniques, contact with patient's skin, iatrogenic bowel injury, or from the transection of lymphatic channels in the presence of remote infected organs.[3,4] Vascular infections due to hematogenous spread usually present later in the postoperative course. Bacteremia from distant infections such as genitourinary, gastrointestinal (GI), foot infections, or periodontal infections can seed the vascular graft. The risk of seeding is highest during the first 2 months but extends for up to 1 year, or until the development of a pseudointimal lining and complete endothelization of the graft.[5] Vascular infections due to extension of a nearby infection occur when a surgical site infection or other nearby infection progresses to the adjacent graft. Examples include a wound infection in the subcutaneous tissue of an infrainguinal bypass that progresses to the deeper planes into the adjacent graft, or a suboptimal coverage of an aortic graft that leads to erosion of the graft into a bowel loop that directly infects the aortic graft.

Gram-positive cocci account for almost two-thirds of vascular graft infections.[6] While historically *Staphylococcus aureus* was the most common isolated organism, recent reports found that coagulase negative staphylococcus have taken the lead.[7] Staphylococcus organisms can establish infection through biofilm and slime production. These biofilms protect the bacteria from the innate immune system and limit the efficacy of antibiotics by preventing them from reaching the bacteria in the biofilm matrix.[8] Other common isolated organisms include gram-negative bacilli such as *Pseudomonas aeruginosa*. These are usually associated with aortoenteric fistulas.[9] Less common organisms include *Candida*, *Cutibacterium*, *Klebsiella*, *Prevotella*, and *Salmonella*.[10] These microorganisms, through the production of various toxins such as elastases and proteases, can cause anastomotic disruption by breaking down arterial wall, leading to pseudoaneurysm formation and bleeding.

RISK FACTORS AND PREVENTION

Risk factors predisposing patients to vascular graft infections include both procedure-specific factors and patient-specific factors. Procedures involving grafts placed in the groin have been found to be more associated with graft vascular infections.[6,11] The superficial location of the graft in the groin and the proximity of the groin to the perineum area have been suggested as explanations to this association. Emergency surgery is another factor associated with vascular graft infections. This is due to the possible insufficient preoperative prepping in such situations.[12] In addition, complex operations, prolonged operative time, redo procedures and procedures involving graft placement in previously infected wound beds have also been associated with increased risk of infections.[13]

Patient specific risk factors include comorbidities leading to immunosuppressive states such as immune disorders, malignancies, chemotherapy, and corticosteroids intake. Conflicting data have been reported on diabetes mellitus, with studies associating diabetes with increased risk of vascular graft infections.[7] Other studies have showed that postoperative hyperglycemia is associated with graft infections, while diabetic patients on insulin have a lower risk of infection due to the anti-inflammatory effect of insulin.[14]

Accordingly, to prevent vascular graft infections from occurring, abiding by surgical site infection prevention recommendations should be emphasized. This includes preoperative antibiotics within 1 hour of skin incision with redosing as needed during the procedure, perioperative glycemic control, and perioperative normothermia.[15] Hair clipping instead of shaving, prepping using alcohol-based antiseptic solutions, and sterile draping along with the use of iodinated skin protective barriers should also be utilized as all have been associated with a lower risk of surgical site infections.[16]

PRESENTATION AND CLASSIFICATION

Infections are generally classified into intra-cavitary when they occur in the chest or abdomen, and extra-cavitary when they occur in the neck, groin, or the extremities. Multiple classification systems have been suggested depending on the time of onset of the infection as well as the extent of the infection with respect to the wound and with respect to the graft itself. These classifications serve to better diagnose, manage, and predict the prognosis of vascular infections.

Early vascular graft infections present within the first 2 months and up to 4 months after the vascular intervention, while infections presenting later are considered late infections.[17] Early infections usually present with clinical findings of surgical site infection (Figure 50-1) including pain, erythema, abscess formation, and sinus tract discharge as well as fever, chills, and leukocytosis. Left untreated, they present with more life threatening presentations including sepsis, hemorrhage from anastomotic rupture as well distal ischemia from graft occlusion and distal septic emboli. The entire graft is usually affected in early infections.

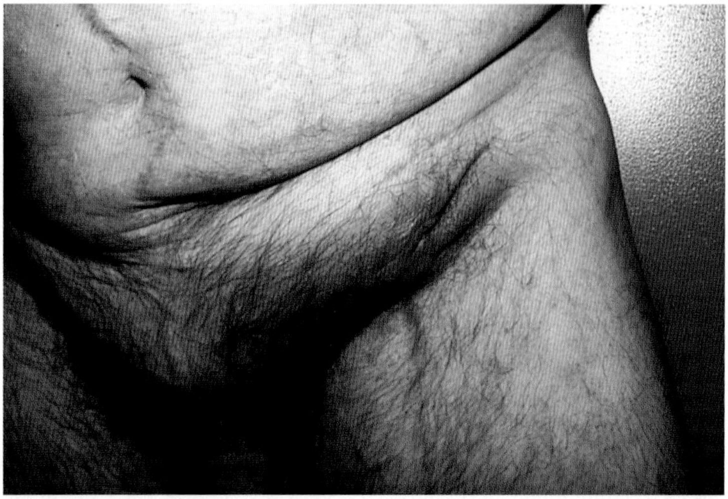

FIGURE 50-1 Groin infection at the level of a femoral anastomosis showing erythema and induration.

Late infections, occurring 4 months after the intervention, are more indolent and present with an insidious onset of fever, sepsis symptoms, an enlarging pulsatile mass in extra-cavitary infections, and GI bleeding in the case of aortoenteric erosion or fistulae. Late infections typically involve either part of or the entirety of the graft.

Regarding the extent of infection, the *Szilagyi* classification was the first suggested classification system categorizing postoperative infections after vascular surgery.[2] According to this classification, infections are categorized into three groups based on their relationship to the wound: Group 1 involves the dermis only; Group 2 extends into the subcutaneous tissue but does not involve the graft; and Group 3 involves the graft. However, since graft involvement can be partial or total, with outcomes and management differences between each type, the *Samson* classification was introduced as a modification to Szilagyi's.[18] This classification categorizes infections into five groups based on the extent of wound and graft involvement: Group 1 involves the dermis only; Group 2 extends into the subcutaneous tissue but does not involve the graft; Group 3 involves the body of the graft but not an anastomotic site; Group 4 involves an exposed anastomosis without bacteremia or bleeding; and Group 5 involves an exposed anastomosis with bacteremia or bleeding.

Another common classification of graft infection is *Bunt's* classification.[19] This classification categorizes infections into seven groups based on both the location of the graft and the extent of graft involvement: Peripheral graft infection which includes four groups: P0 infection of an intracavitary graft; P1 infection of an extracavitary graft; P2 infection of the extracavitary portion of a graft with an intracavitary origin; P3 infection of a prosthetic patch angioplasty; the other three groups include: Graft enteric erosion; graft enteric fistula; and aortic stump sepsis after excision of an infected graft.

DIAGNOSIS

As described above, the presentation of vascular graft infection after surgery can vary from mild local symptoms to severe life-threatening symptoms. In some instances, the only symptom a patient has is fever. Due to the devastating outcomes of untreated vascular graft infections, the clinician should have a high degree of suspicion when symptoms appear in a postoperative vascular surgery patient. As such, and to ease the diagnosis of graft infections, the MAGIC criteria were introduced.[20] Based on these criteria, a vascular graft infection can be diagnosed in the presence of one major criterion and any other major or minor criteria (Table 50-1). Those criteria are established using multiple imaging modalities and sampling techniques as described below.

TABLE 50-1 The MAGIC Classification

Criterion	Clinical/Surgical	Clinical/Surgical	Laboratory
Major			
	Pus (confirmed by microscopy) around graft or in aneurysm sac at surgery	Perigraft fluid on CT scan > 3 months after insertion	Organisms recovered from an explanted graft
	Open wound with exposed graft or communicating sinus	Perigraft gas on CT scan 7 weeks after insertion	Organisms recovered from an intraoperative specimen
	Fistula development, e.g., aortoenteric or aortobronchial	Increase in perigraft gas volume demonstrated on serial imaging	Organisms recovered from a percutaneous, radiologically guided aspirate of perigraft fluid
Minor			
	Localized clinical findings graft infection, e.g., erythema, warmth, swelling, purulent discharge, pain	Other, e.g., suspicious perigraft gas/fluid soft tissue inflammation; aneurysm expansion; pseudoaneurysm formation: focal bowel wall thickening; discitis/osteomyelitis; suspicious metabolic activity on FDG-PET/CT; radiolabeled leukocyte uptake	Blood culture(s) positive and no apparent source except graft infection
	Fever 38 C with graft infection as most likely cause		Abnormally elevated inflammatory markers with graft infection as most likely cause, e.g., erythrocyte sedimentation rate, C reactive protein, white cell count

Reproduced with permission from Chakfé N, Diener H, Lejay A, et al. Editor's Choice - European Society for Vascular Surgery (ESVS) 2020 Clinical Practice Guidelines on the Management of Vascular Graft and Endograft Infections. *Eur J Vasc Endovasc Surg*. 2020;59(3):339-384.

Ultrasound is a very valuable imaging modality in diagnosing vascular graft infections. It is a widespread, low-cost, non-invasive imaging modality that can characterize the presence of fluid collections (hematoma, abscess) under the skin, pseudoaneurysms as well as graft thrombosis. It is an ideal first test in extracavitary infections. However, being operator dependent, its sensitivity in diagnosing vascular graft infections is low, and the absence of findings on ultrasound should not exclude the presence of a vascular graft infection.[21]

CTA is another valuable imaging modality for diagnosing vascular graft infections. CTAs allow for the identification of soft tissue enhancement, gas, infected fluid, pseudoaneurysms, enteric erosions, and enteric fistulas that are all considered signs of vascular graft infections. However, it has been shown that the sensitivity of CTA in diagnosing vascular graft infection ranges between 0.57 and 0.75 while its specificity ranges between 0.48 and 0.76.[22] MRA can also be used when CTA is contraindicated with sensitivity comparable to that of CTA. Accordingly, when a graft infection is highly suspected and US or CTA/MRA are indeterminate, further imaging modalities can be utilized including 18F-fluoro-D-deoxyglucose positron emission tomography/computed tomography (FDG-PET/CT), WBC scintigraphy (Figure 50-2), or single-photon emission computerized tomography (SPECT/CT.)[23,24] These imaging modalities have sensitivities reaching 0.99 when combined.[25] However, they are not first-line modalities as they are

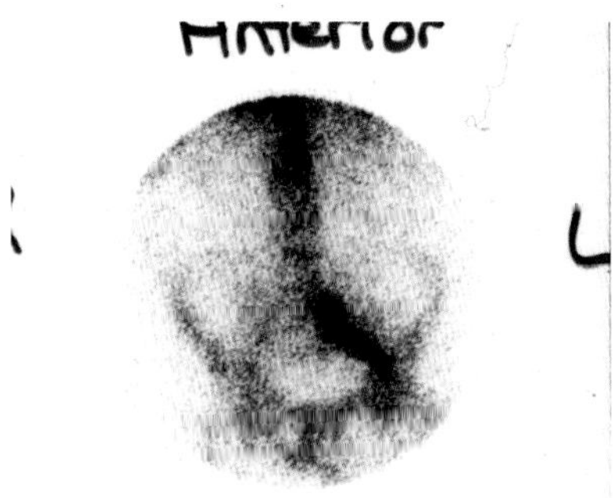

FIGURE 50-2 White cell scan showing increased uptake in the left limb of the graft.

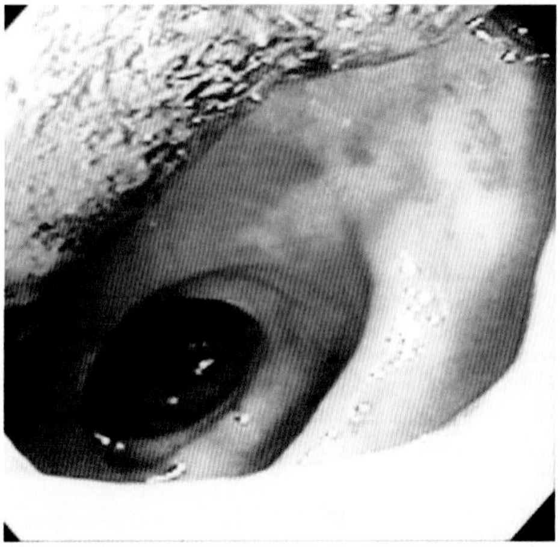

FIGURE 50-3 Endoscopy showing exposed graft.

expensive, not readily available, time consuming, and usually require extensive resources. Finally, in case of GI bleed and suspicion for an enteric-fistula formation, and esophagogastroduodenoscopy (EGD) can demonstrate the presence of a thrombus or an erosion and graft exposure, confirming the diagnosis (Figure 50-3).

MANAGEMENT

GENERAL PRINCIPLES

In general, when a surgical site infection following a vascular surgery is suspected, the first step should be to try to obtain both fluid cultures and blood cultures before starting wide spectrum antibiotics. Long-term antibiotic treatment is needed, tailored to culture results when an organism is identified. In case of Szilagyi I or II infections, 4 weeks of IV antibiotics should be given. In case of Szilagyi III infections, 6 weeks of IV antibiotics followed by 6 months of oral antibiotics is needed.[26] When the isolated organism is Methicillin-resistant Staphylococcus aureus (MRSA), *Pseudomonas*, multidrug resistant or fungi, suppressive lifelong antibiotic therapy is recommended. Surgically, if the graft is not involved, treating the infection follows the general principles of soft tissue infection treatment including drainage of any associated fluid collection, wound debridement, and wound washout. If the graft is involved in the infection, management depends on the type of graft, its incorporation into the adjacent tissue, and the extent of graft involvement. Autogenous grafts are more resistant to infections as compared to prosthetic grafts and accordingly, the preservation of the graft is more tolerated.[27,28] In cases of prosthetic graft involvement, a more aggressive approach is required usually involving the partial or complete excision of the graft.[29] While partial graft excision might be tolerated if only a segment of the graft is infected, a more aggressive approach is required when the anastomosis is involved.[30] Revascularization should be performed preferably prior to the excision to avoid ischemia time.[31] Revascularization should be done through an uninfected field or path. However, in situ graft replacement can still be performed in various circumstances, with a higher risk of re-infection.[32] While these are general principles, specific treatment strategies need to be followed depending on the location of graft infection as detailed below.

Carotid Patch Infection

Surgical site infection following carotid surgery is a rare complication with rates lower than 1% in most large dataset studies.[33] Diabetes mellitus is a common risk factor. Time to infection is bimodal with 50% of infections occurring early and 50% occurring late after the operation. In most of the reported cases, staphylococci were the isolated organisms.[34–36] Management of carotid infections follows the Samson classification with groups I and II managed conservatively, and groups III, IV, and V managed more aggressively. Involvement of the graft requires excision with artery debridement, followed by reconstruction by suturing a new patch (preferably autogenous vein) to healthy artery. In case of extensive infection, reconstruction via interposition vein graft might be required.[37] Using prosthetic material in the reconstruction is associated with a high risk of re-infection and should be avoided whenever possible.[38] The graft should then be covered by a healthy muscle flap using the sternocleidomastoid and long-term antibiotics should be administered.

Thoracic Aortic Graft Infection

Infection of the thoracic aortic graft is a very serious complication with a low estimated incidence rate of 3% but an extremely high mortality rate reaching 75%.[39] Patients with graft infections usually present with sternal wound infection signs, empyema, sepsis, esophageal bleeding, or hemothorax. Management strategies are based on the excision of the infected graft, drainage of any fluid collections, debridement and washout of the infected field, and viable tissue coverage. The infected graft should be replaced by another prosthetic graft or preferably a cryopreserved homograft.[40] In case an aortoesophageal fistula is present, the involved infected material should be excised, and the esophagus should be repaired.

Abdominal Aortic Graft Infection

Aortic graft infection is a devastating complication following Abdominal Aortic Aneurysm repair with a reported incidence rate between 0.5% and 3%.[41] Patients can present with symptoms of sepsis, GI bleeding, or exposed graft in the groin. However, presentation is indolent many times and establishing the diagnosis can be challenging. Accordingly, the use of the more sensitive and specific imaging modalities such as PET/CT or WBC scintigraphy might be required. The mainstay of managing an abdominal aortic graft infection is removal of the infected graft. Otherwise, management strategies depend on the part of graft involved in the infection. If the body of the graft is involved, and the proximal anastomosis is end to end, the graft should be excised. In situ replacement by a cadaveric graft, bovine graft, rifampin impregnated graft, or silver-coated graft is possible, but carries a higher risk of reinfection as the cavity remains infected even after debridement and washout. Extra-anatomic bypass, via an axillofemoral bypass through a lateral approach, is another reconstruction option with a low risk of infection but is associated with a low long-term patency.[42] Such revascularization usually happens in a staged procedure before extracting the infected graft. After extraction, the aortic stump should be sewn in two layers and covered with an omental flap to avoid the complication of aortic stump blow out (Figure 50-4).[43] This can be typically achieved if at least 1-2 cm of healthy infrarenal aorta is present. Neoaortoiliac system (NAIS) reconstruction, originally described by Claggett, has a lower risk of reinfection and a high long-term patency.[44] This is done by creating an in-line reconstruction of a neo-aortic graft using autogenous veins through harvesting the femoral veins while preserving the greater saphenous and deep femoral vein for lower extremity drainage. Patients frequently require fasciotomy after the procedure and suffer from postoperative edema. While the technique is tedious, time and human resource consuming, it has been associated with rewarding outcomes.[45] The use of Bovine grafts has been gaining acceptance as an alternative to using the femoral veins for NAIS reconstruction.[46]

When the body of the graft is involved, and the proximal anastomosis is end to side, the graft should be excised, and the aorta may be primarily closed. Immediate revascularization in such cases is typically not required.

If the infection is limited to the femoral limb of the graft or the groin, other management strategies are suggested. First, an extra-anatomical revascularization to the superficial femoral or profunda should be performed. Then via a retroperitoneal approach,

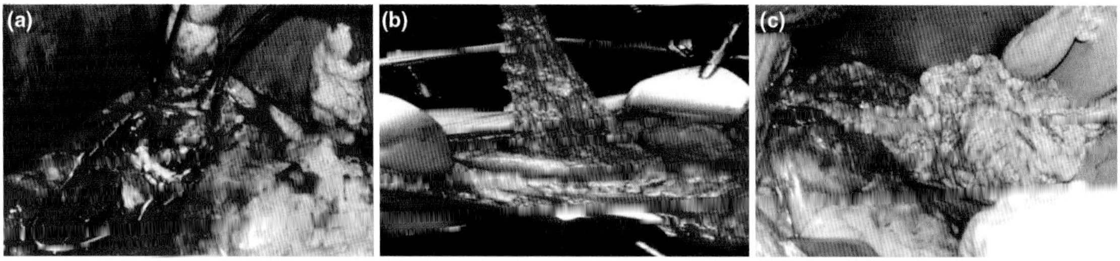

FIGURE 50-4 **Transected aorta oversewn in two layers with omental flap coverage.**

the graft is transected at its origin. Following that, the intact graft is isolated from the infected cavity by closing the peritoneum over the proximal part of the limb. The infected graft is pushed to the groin and via a groin incision, it is dismantled from the artery. The artery is debrided into healthy tissue and primarily closed if possible. Alternatively, the other strategy is transecting the infected limb of the graft through an abdominal incision. This is followed by reconstruction, away from the infected field, using a graft tunneled through the obturator canal to the suprageniculate popliteal artery.

In case an enteric fistula is present, proper closure of the involved duodenal portion should be performed. If not feasible, bowel resection should be done as duodenal leaks are associated with poor outcomes (Figure 50-5).[47]

A similar approach is adopted when dealing with infections after an endovascular aneurysm repair (EVAR). Fenestrated and branched grafts further complicate reconstructions as renal and visceral bypasses will be required after explanting the graft. Percutaneous drainage and antibiotic irrigation of the graft without explanting have also been described but mixed results have been reported on treatment outcomes.[48,49] Such unconventional options are typically reserved to high-risk patients who clearly cannot withstand a definitive graft explanation procedures. While there is no strong evidence supporting the superiority of one reconstruction method over the other, treatment algorithms have been suggested based on single center and retrospective studies (Figure 50-6).

Infrainguinal Graft Infections

Management of infrainguinal graft infections depends on the time of infection, extent of infection, and the type of graft involved. In early infections to autogenous grafts, a conservative strategy can be adopted in management. Along with administering IV antibiotics, dead spaces should be avoided by covering the graft with a muscle flap, evacuating fluid collections, and placing drains or draining catheters. Negative pressure wound therapy with irrigation has also been shown to be effective in such cases.[49] Otherwise, management follows Samson's classification whereby if the suture line of the graft anastomosis is involved (Samson IV or V), the whole graft should be excised. Reconstruction should be performed with an inflow proximal to the proximal anastomosis, an outflow distal to the distal anastomosis, and with tunneling performed through uninvolved areas. The previous anastomoses defects can be primarily repaired. Extraanatomical tunneling can be achieved

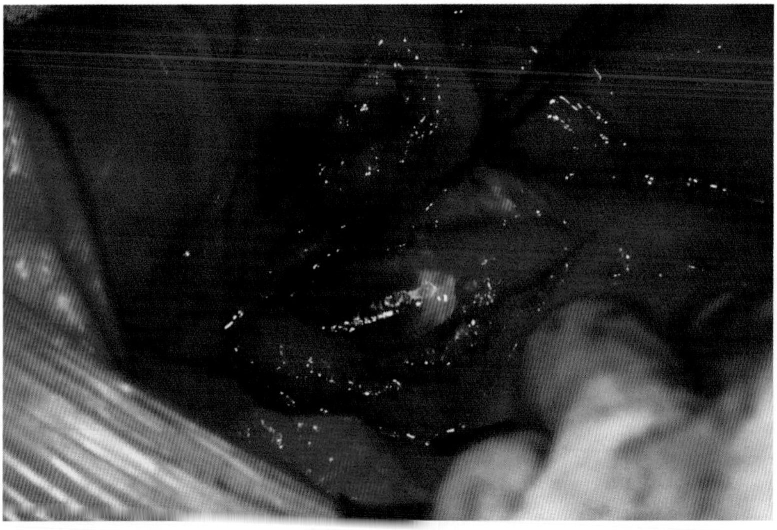

FIGURE 50-5 Stained infected graft with bowel defect.

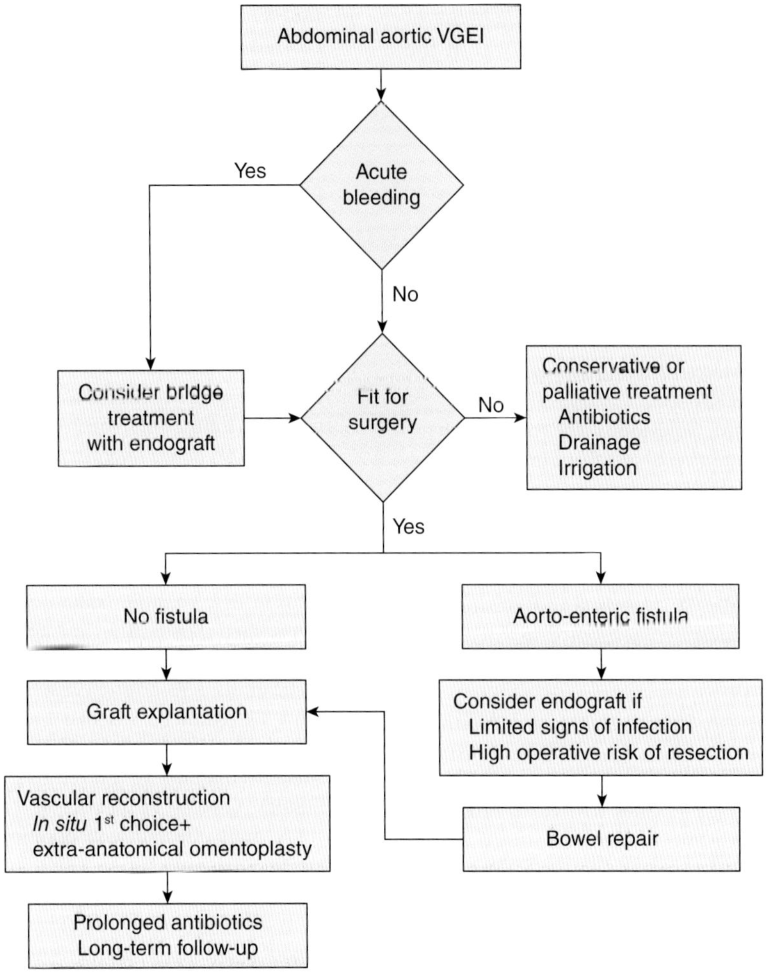

FIGURE 50-6 Proposed algorithm for the management of aortic vascular graft/endograft infection.

via a lateral approach to expose the inflow and outflow arterial segments.[50] Finally, suture lines should be covered by muscle flap or healthy vascularized tissue. In cases of Samson III infections, separate incisions should be performed for exploring the graft proximal and distal to the infected portion. An interposition graft is then reconstructed. The incisions are then closed, and a new incision is made to expose and extract the infected part of the graft. In situ reconstruction might be possible in such cases but tunneling through an area uninvolved by the infection is required in case the infection involves MRSA, *Pseudomonas*, or multidrug-resistant organisms.[26] The wound is left open to close either by secondary intention or by negative pressure wound therapy.

CONCLUSIONS

Prosthetic graft infection is an infrequent condition that is associated with significant morbidity and potentially high mortality. Prosthetic graft infections are challenging for both diagnosis and treatment with very few validated data on the best medical and surgical treatment. The diagnosis should be considered in patients with prosthetic grafts who present with leukocytosis, fever, and specifically in patients with evidence of bacteremia. The management of prosthetic graft infection consists of removal of the infected graft with extraanatomical or in situ graft (anatomical) replacement in addition to antibiotic therapy for a varying period of time.

REFERENCES

1. O'Brien T, Collin J. Prosthetic vascular graft infection. *Br J Surg.* 1992;79:1262-1267.
2. Szilagyi DE, Smith RF, Elliott JP, Vrandecic MP. Infection in arterial reconstruction with synthetic grafts. *Ann Surg.* 1972;176:321-333.
3. Rubin JR, Malone JM, Goldstone J. The role of the lymphatic system in acute arterial prosthetic graft infections. *J Vasc Surg.* 1985;2:92-98.
4. Bandyk DF, Berni GA, Thiele BL, Towne JB. Aortofemoral graft infection due to Staphylococcus epidermidis. *Arch Surg.* 1984;119:102-108.
5. Birinyi LK, Douville EC, Lewis SA, Bjornson HS, Kempczinski RF. Increased resistance to bacteremic graft infection after endothelial cell seeding. *J Vasc Surg.* 1987;5:193-197.
6. Antonios VS, Noel AA, Steckelberg JM, et al. Prosthetic vascular graft infection: a risk factor analysis using a case-control study. *J Infect.* 2006;53:49-55.
7. Siracuse JJ, Nandivada P, Giles KA, et al. Prosthetic graft infections involving the femoral artery. *J Vasc Surg.* 2013;57:700-705.
8. Costerton JW, Stewart PS, Greenberg EP. Bacterial biofilms: a common cause of persistent infections. *Science.* 1999;284:1318-1322.
9. Armstrong PA, Back MR, Wilson JS, Shames ML, Johnson BL, Bandyk DF. Improved outcomes in the recent management of secondary aortoenteric fistula. *J Vasc Surg.* 2005;42:660-666.
10. Legout L, Sarraz-Bournet B, D'Elia PV, et al. Characteristics and prognosis in patients with prosthetic vascular graft infection: a prospective observational cohort study. *Clin Microbiol Infect.* 2012;18: 352-358.
11. Engin C, Posacioglu H, Ayik F, Apaydin AZ. Management of vascular infection in the groin. *Tex Heart Inst J.* 2005;32:529-534.
12. Anagnostopoulos A, Ledergerber B, Kuster SP, et al. Inadequate perioperative prophylaxis and postsurgical complications after graft implantation are important risk factors for subsequent vascular graft infections: prospective results from the vascular graft infection cohort study. *Clin Infect Dis.* 2019;69:621-630.
13. Inui T, Bandyk DF. Vascular surgical site infection: risk factors and preventive measures. *Semin Vasc Surg.* 2015;28:201-207.
14. Vriesendorp TM, Morélis QJ, Devries JH, Legemate DA, Hoekstra JBL. Early post-operative glucose levels are an independent risk factor for infection after peripheral vascular surgery. A retrospective study. *Eur J Vasc Endovasc Surg.* 2004;28:520-525.
15. Berríos-Torres SI, Umscheid CA, Bratzler DW, et al. Centers for disease control and prevention guideline for the prevention of surgical site infection, 2017. *JAMA Surg.* 2017;152:784-791.
16. Kramer A, Assadian O, Lademann J. Prevention of postoperative wound infections by covering the surgical field with iodine-impregnated incision drape (Ioban 2). *GMS Krankenhhyg Interdiszip.* 2010;5(2):Doc08.
17. Calligaro KD, Veith FJ, Schwartz ML, Dougherty MJ, DeLaurentis DA. Differences in early versus late extracavitary arterial graft infections. *J Vasc Surg.* 1995;22: 680-685; discussion 685-688.
18. Samson RH, Veith FJ, Janko GS, Gupta SK, Scher LA. A modified classification and approach to the management of infections involving peripheral arterial prosthetic grafts. *J Vasc Surg.* 1988;8:147-153.
19. Bunt TJ. Synthetic vascular graft infections. I. Graft infections. *Surgery.* 1983;93:733-746.
20. Anagnostopoulos A, Mayer F, Ledergerber B, et al. Editor's choice—validation of the management of aortic graft infection collaboration (MAGIC) criteria for the diagnosis of vascular graft/endograft infection: results from the prospective vascular graft cohort study. *Eur J Vasc Endovasc Surg.* 2021;62:251-257.
21. Legout L, D'Elia PV, Sarraz-Bournet B, et al. Diagnosis and management of prosthetic vascular graft infections. *Medecine et maladies infectieuses.* 2012;42:102-109.
22. Bruggink JL, Slart RH, Pol JA, Reijnen MMPJ, Zeebregts CJ. Current role of imaging in diagnosing aortic graft infections. *Semin Vasc Surg.* 2011;24:182-190.
23. Bruggink JL, Glaudemans AW, Saleem BR, et al. Accuracy of FDG-PET-CT in the diagnostic work-up of vascular prosthetic graft infection. *Eur J Vasc Endovasc Surg.* 2010;40:348-354.
24. de la Rubia-Marcos M, García-Alonso P, Mena-Melgar C, et al. ^{99m}TC-white blood cell scintigraphy with SPECT/CT in the diagnosis of vascular graft infection. *Revista espanola de medicina nuclear e imagen molecular.* 2020;39:347-352.
25. Reinders Folmer EI, Von Meijenfeldt GCI, Van der Laan MJ, et al. Diagnostic imaging in vascular graft infection: a systematic review and meta-analysis. *Eur J Vasc Endovasc Surg.* 2018;56:719-729.

26. Wilson WR, Bower TC, Creager MA, et al. Vascular graft infections, mycotic aneurysms, and endovascular infections: a scientific statement from the American heart association. *Circulation*. 2016;134:e412-e460.
27. Perler BA. The case for conservative management of infected prosthetic grafts. *Adv Surg*. 1996;29:17-32.
28. Treiman GS, Copland S, Yellin AE, Lawrence PF, McNamara RM, Treiman RL. Wound infections involving infrainguinal autogenous vein grafts: a current evaluation of factors determining successful graft preservation. *J Vasc Surg*. 2001;33:948-954.
29. Liu RH, Fraser CD III, Zhou X, Beaulieu RJ, Reifsnyder T. Complete versus partial excision of infected arteriovenous grafts: does remnant graft material impact outcomes? *J Vasc Surg*. 2020;71:174-179.
30. Zetrenne E, Wirth GA, McIntosh BC, Evans GRD, Narayan D. Managing extracavitary prosthetic vascular graft infections: a pathway to success. *Ann Plast Surg*. 2006;57:677-682.
31. Reilly LM, Stoney RJ, Goldstone J, Ehrenfeld WK. Improved management of aortic graft infection: the influence of operation sequence and staging. *J Vasc Surg*. 1987;5:421-431.
32. Lai CH, Luo CY, Lin PY, et al. Surgical consideration of in situ prosthetic replacement for primary infected abdominal aortic aneurysms. *Eur J Vasc Endovasc Surg*. 2011;42:617-624.
33. Knight BC, Tait WF. Dacron patch infection following carotid endarterectomy: a systematic review of the literature. *Eur J Vasc Endovasc Surg*. 2009;37:140-148.
34. Asciutto G, Geier B, Marpe B, Hummel T, Mumme A. Dacron patch infection after carotid angioplasty. A report of 6 cases. *Eur J Vasc Endovasc Surg*. 2007;33:55-57.
35. Naylor AR, Payne D, London NJ, et al. Prosthetic patch infection after carotid endarterectomy. *Eur J Vasc Endovasc Surg*. 2002;23:11-16.
36. Rizzo A, Hertzer NR, O'Hara PJ, Krajewski LP, Beven EG. Dacron carotid patch infection: a report of eight cases. *J Vasc Surg*. 2000;32:602-606.
37. Fatima J, Federico VP, Scali ST, et al. Management of patch infections after carotid endarterectomy and utility of femoral vein interposition bypass graft. *J Vasc Surg*. 2019;69:1815-1823.e1811.
38. Stone PA, Srivastava M, Campbell JE, et al. A 10-year experience of infection following carotid endarterectomy with patch angioplasty. *J Vasc Surg*. 2011;53:1473-1477.
39. Fujii T, Watanabe Y. Multidisciplinary treatment approach for prosthetic vascular graft infection in the thoracic aortic area. *Ann Thorac Cardiovasc Surg*. 2015;21:418-427.
40. Coselli JS, Köksoy C, LeMaire SA. Management of thoracic aortic graft infections. *Ann Thorac Surg*. 1999;67:1990-1993; discussion 1997-1998.
41. Vogel TR, Symons R, Flum DR. The incidence and factors associated with graft infection after aortic aneurysm repair. *J Vasc Surg*. 2008;47:264-269.
42. Samson RH, Showalter DP, Lepore MR Jr, Nair DG, Dorsay DA, Morales RE. Improved patency after axillofemoral bypass for aortoiliac occlusive disease. *J Vasc Surg*. 2018;68:1430-1437.
43. Jamieson RW, Burns PJ, Dawson AR, Fraser SCA. Aortic graft preservation by debridement and omental wrapping. *Ann Vasc Surg*. 2012;26:423.e421-424.
44. Clagett GP, Bowers BL, Lopez-Viego MA, et al. Creation of a neo-aortoiliac system from lower extremity deep and superficial veins. *Ann Surg*. 1993;218:239-248; discussion 248-239.
45. Chung J, Clagett GP. Neoaortoiliac system (NAIS) procedure for the treatment of the infected aortic graft. *Semin Vasc Surg*. 2011;24:220-226.
46. Lutz B, Reeps C, Biro G, Knappich C, Zimmermann A, Eckstein H-H. Bovine pericardium as new technical option for in situ reconstruction of aortic graft infection. *Ann Vasc Surg*. 2017;41:118-126.
47. Valentine RJ, Timaran CH, Modrall GJ, Smith ST, Arko FR, Clagett GP. Secondary aortoenteric fistulas versus paraprosthetic erosions: is bleeding associated with a worse outcome? *J Am Coll Surg*. 2008;207:922-927.
48. Igari K, Kudo T, Toyofuku T, Jibiki M, Sugano N, Inoue Y. Treatment strategies for aortic and peripheral prosthetic graft infection. *Surg Today*. 2014;44:466-471.
49. Batt M, Jean-Baptiste E, O'Connor S, et al. Contemporary management of infrarenal aortic graft infection: early and late results in 82 patients. *Vascular*. 2012;20:129-137.
50. Hoballah JJ, Chalmers RT, Sharp WJ, Kresowik TF, Martinasevic MM, Corson JD. Lateral approach to the popliteal and crural vessels for limb salvage. *Cardiovasc Surg*. 1996;4:165-168.

SELF-ASSESSMENT STUDY QUESTIONS AND ANSWERS

Questions

1. What is the most common isolated organism in vascular graft infections?
   A. Staphylococcus aureus
   B. Staphylococcus epidermidis
   C. Pseudomonas aeruginosa
   D. Candida albicans

2. What is the extent of infection in Samson IV classification?
   A. Epidermis
   B. Subcutaneous tissue
   C. Body of the graft
   D. Graft anastomosis

3. In Bunt's classification, what does a P2 infection involve?
   A. Infection of an intracavitary graft
   B. Infection of an extracavitary graft
   C. Infection of the extracavitary portion of a graft with an intracavitary origin
   D. Infection of a prosthetic patch angioplasty

4. Which of the following strategies decreases the risk of vascular graft infections?
   A. Prepping with aqueous iodophore solutions
   B. Shaving hair
   C. Maintaining normoglycemia in the perioperative period
   D. Maintaining hypothermia in the perioperative period

5. How many weeks of IV antibiotics treatment is required for Samson IV infections?
   A. 2 weeks
   B. 6 weeks
   C. 8 weeks
   D. 12 weeks

6. What aortic reconstruction option is associated with the lowest reinfection rate and highest patency rate?
   A. Extra-anatomic reconstruction
   B. Silver-coated grafts
   C. NAIS
   D. Rifampin-impregnated grafts

7. Infections with which organism require lifelong suppressive antibiotic therapy?
   A. MRSA infection
   B. Pseudomonas infection
   C. Fungal infection
   D. All of the above

8. What is the first-line imaging modality to diagnose extracavitary graft infections?
   A. Ultrasound
   B. CTA
   C. PET/CT
   D. WBC Scintigraphy

9. What is the most sensitive imaging modality to diagnose vascular graft infections?
   A. Ultrasound
   B. CTA
   C. MRI
   D. PET/CT

10. What strategy decreases the risk of aortic stump blowout after graft extraction?
    A. Creating a stump with at least 1-2 cm of healthy infrarenal aorta
    B. Coverage with healthy omentum
    C. Coverage with latissimus dorsi flap
    D. All the above

SELF-ASSESSMENT STUDY QUESTIONS AND ANSWERS

Answers

1. B.
2. D.
3. C.
4. C.
5. B.
6. C.
7. D.
8. A.
9. D.
10. D.

CHAPTER

51 Vascular Tumors and Vascular Oncosurgery

Mamoun A. Al-Basheer and Samer Alharthi

OUTLINE

INTRODUCTION
BENIGN VASCULAR TUMORS
Infantile Hemangioma (IH)
Incidence and Epidemiology
Biology
Clinical Presentation
Diagnostic
Treatment of Infantile Hemangioma
Prognosis
Congenital Hemangiomas (CH)
Kaposiform Hemangioendothelioma (KHE)
Incidence
Etiology and Pathology
Clinical Presentation
Diagnosis
Treatment
MALIGNANT VASCULAR TUMORS
Angiosarcoma
Epithelioid Hemangioendothelioma
VASCULAR ONCOSURGERY
Introduction
Extra-adrenal Paragangliomas
Mediastinal Tumors
Retroperitoneal Tumors
Neurogenic Tumors
Germ Cell, Sex Cord, and Stromal Tumors
Lymphoid and Hematologic Neoplasms
Renal Cell Carcinoma
Pediatric Malignancies
Limb Tumors
CONCLUSION

INTRODUCTION

Vascular tumors describe tumors that encompass a vascular origin that reflect at soft-tissue growth formed from blood vessels. The tumors can develop on any part of the body; they are classified into benign and malignant. Vascular anomalies represent a group of disorders with a wide spectrum entity from a simple "birthmark" to life-threatening conditions. The International Society for the Study of Vascular Anomalies (ISSVA) classified these anomalies into two main categories: vascular tumors and vascular malformation.[1] The main difference between the two types is the proliferation of endothelium, which is observed in the vascular tumor but not in malformation. This section will outline benign (mainly infantile hemangioma [HI], congenital hemangioma, and kaposiform hemangioendothelioma KHE) and malignant vascular tumors by tumor types, diagnosis, and surgical management.

ISSVA classified the vascular tumors into three main categories: benign, locally aggressive or borderline, and malignant. Table 51-1 represents the subtypes for each category.[2]

Vascular oncosurgery describes the discipline of surgical therapy for tumors of or closely involving vascular structures. It is an area of interest and challenge to many in the field due to the multidisciplinary

TABLE 51-1 ISSVA Classification for Vascular Tumors

Vascular Tumor Category	Types
Benign tumors	Infantile hemangioma
	Congenital hemangioma
	Tufted angioma
	Spindle-cell hemangioma
	Epithelioid hemangioma
	Pyogenic granuloma
	Hobnail hemangioma
	Microvenular hemangioma
	Anastomosing hemangioma
	Glomeruloid hemangioma
	Papillary hemangioma
	Intravascular papillary endothelial hyperplasia
	Cutaneous epithelioid angiomatous nodule
	Acquired elastotic hemangioma
	Littoral cell hemangioma of the spleen
Locally aggressive/borderline tumor	Kaposiform hemangioendothelioma
	Retiform hemangioendothelioma
	Papillary intralymphatic angioendothelioma (PILA), Dabska tumor
	Composite hemangioendothelioma
	Pseudomyogenic hemangioendothelioma
	Polymorphous hemangioendothelioma
	Hemangioendothelioma not otherwise specified
	Kaposi sarcoma
Malignant tumor	Angiosarcoma
	Epithelioid hemangioendothelioma

Data from ISSVA classification for vascular anomalies. 2018. https://www.issva.org/UserFiles/file/ISSVA-Classification-2018.pdf.

nature of the practice and the developing referral circles of cases that essentially involve vascular therapists.

BENIGN VASCULAR TUMORS

Benign vascular tumors account for noncancerous tumors, with hemangiomas expounding on the most common form of the tumor.

INFANTILE HEMANGIOMA (IH)

Incidence and Epidemiology

Infantile hemangiomas (IHs) are the most common benign vascular tumors, estimated to occur in 4% to 5% of newborns.[3] They are more common in females, non-Hispanic white patients, and premature infants.[4] Up to this date, there is no genetic mutations on the X chromosome have been reported. However, the increased incidence among females is thought to be related to early parents seeking medical advice in the dermatology clinic for cosmetic concerns when female newborns are affected. Finally, the early withdrawal of placental antiangiogenic factors is strongly related to IH's high incidence among premature infants.[5]

Biology

Although the exact mechanism that causes the initial proliferation of blood vessels followed by involution of the vascular component of hemangioma is unknown, it is believed that proliferation of endothelium most likely occurs when activated T cells and endothelial growth factor A interact with vascular endothelial growth factor receptor (VEGFR) and VEGFR-2 receptors, respectively; this interaction is even more potent in the presence of hypoxia.[6] Furthermore, this proliferation is believed to occur during vasculogenesis which is supported by isolating cells like progenitor/stem cells (HemSC), endothelial cells (HemEC), and pericytes (HemPericytes) from the hemangioma which is expressed during this phase and has the ability for self renewal and differentiation.[7] Additionally, immunostaining IH with monoclonal antibodies against microvascular markers like merosin, GLUT-1 (glucose transporter isoform 1), Lewis Y, and FcgRII (a placental endothelial antigen) are uniquely coexpressed in the more well-differentiated placental microvasculature.[8]

Clinical Presentation

An infantile hemangioma's clinical presentation usually starts as precursor lesions at birth like telangiectasia, pale erythematous macule, or bruise-like patches that are most often mistaken as birth trauma. Then several weeks later, it becomes more clinically apparent.[9] Infantile hemangiomas can be superficial involving the superficial dermis, deep arises from the reticular dermis, or combined.[10]

The natural history of infantile hemangioma has a triphasic evolution: *Early proliferative or growth phase,* which occurs during the first 8 months of life with evidence of rapid growth in the first 3 months, followed by gradual growth thereafter. *Plateau phase,* up to 1 year of life, during this phase the lesion remains stable. Finally, *the involution phase,* when evidence of color changes from bright red to purple can be observed and it becomes more compressible and softer with an average age to complete involution at 3.5 years.[9,11]

Permanent sequelae of IH can occur up to 55% of the time with telangiectasia be the most commonly observed. Others like anetodermal skin, redundant skin, and a persistent superficial component are less observed. Combined hemangiomas leave significantly more sequelae than superficial or deep hemangiomas.[11]

When an infant present with large face or scalp hemangioma, other association like carotid or eye abnormalities should also be evaluated which can be part of *PHACE syndrome* that includes **P**osterior fossa abnormalities (Dandy–Walker complex, cerebellar hypoplasia, atrophy, and dysgenesis/agenesis of the vermis), **H**emangioma (large segmental hemangioma over the face or scalp with a surface area of 22 cm^2), **A**rterial abnormality (carotid aneurysm or stenosis), **C**ardiac abnormality (aortic arch anomalies), and **E**ye abnormalities (microphthalmos, retinal vascular abnormalities, persistent fetal retinal vessels, exophthalmos, coloboma, and optic nerve atrophy).[12] Another syndrome that can have an association with IH is the LUMBAR/PELVIS/SACRAL syndrome which is described in Table 51-2.[10]

TABLE 51-2 LUMBAR/PELVIS/SACRAL Syndrome

LUMBAR	**L**ower body hemangioma and other cutaneous defects
	Urogenital anomalies or ulceration
	Myelopathy
	Bony deformities
	Anorectal malformations or arterial anomalies
	Renal anomalies
PELVIS	**P**erineal hemangioma
	External genital malformations
	Lipomyelomeningocele
	Vesicorenal abnormalities
	Imperforate anus
	Skin tag
SACRAL	**S**pinal dysraphism
	Anogenital
	Cutaneous
	Renal and urologic anomalies **A**ssociated with an angioma of **L**umbosacral localization

Data from PDQ Pediatric Treatment Editorial Board. Childhood Vascular Tumors Treatment (PDQ®): Health Professional Version. 2022 Jun 8. In: PDQ Cancer Information Summaries [Internet]. Bethesda (MD): National Cancer Institute (US); 2002.

Diagnostic

The majority of infantile hemangiomas are diagnosed clinically. Invasive investigation is not usually necessary, however, with atypical appearance or presentation of IH skin biopsy with GLUT-1 staining can be helpful. Furthermore, when there is a deeper lesion without a cutaneous component, imaging studies like computed tomography (CT) and magnetic resonance imaging (MRI) are indicated to confirm the diagnosis and the extension of IH.[9] Additionally, when there are five or more cutaneous hemangiomas, the infant should undergo liver ultrasonography scan to check for hepatic hemangioma.[13]

Treatment of Infantile Hemangioma

The majority of IHs are small and localized. Observation is usually sufficient until spontaneous resolution is achieved. However, a crucial step in the management of IH is to identify the high-risk lesions and initiate early treatment for these lesions (Figure 51-1). The American Academy of Pediatrics (AAP) published a practice guideline for the management of infantile hemangioma.[14] The following are considered high-risk IH by AAP:

1. Life-threatening complications: IH that arises at the "beard-area" where there is airway obstruction risk, >5 cutaneous IH where there is a high risk of association of liver hemangioma or cardiac failure.

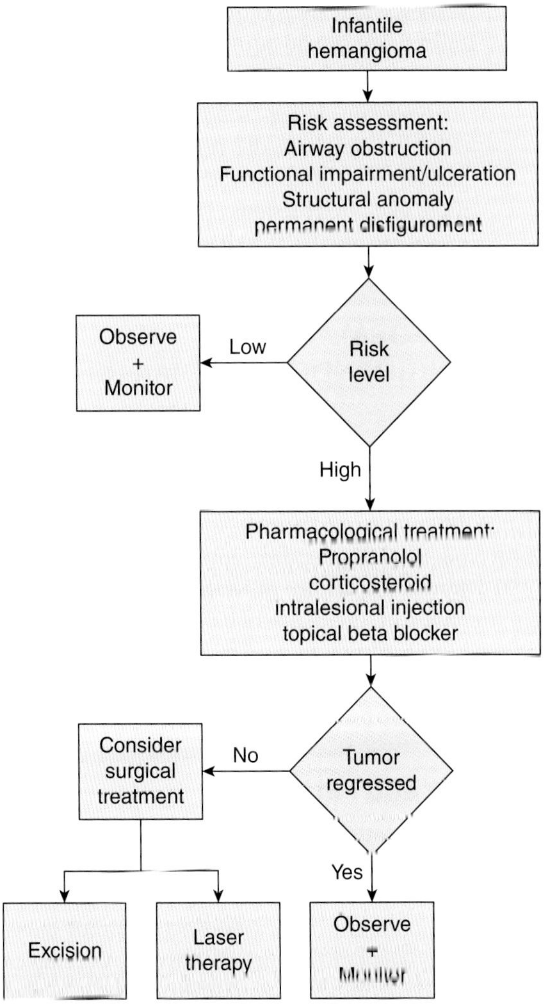

FIGURE 51-1 Approach to infantile hemangioma management. (Reproduced with permission from Abdullah Nasif, MD.)

2. Functional impairment or ulceration: IH involving the lips, oral, or periocular areas.
3. Structural anomalies: When IH is part of one of the known associated syndromes like PHACE LUMBAR syndromes.
4. Permanent disfigurement: Facial IH at the nasal tip or lip (any size), any facial location ≥2 cm, or scalp IH >2 cm.

Pharmacological treatment options for infantile hemangioma include the following[14]:

- *Propranolol:* Oral propranolol is the current first line treatment of choice for IHs requiring systemic therapy. It is believed to cause regression of the IH secondary to vasoconstriction, angiogenesis inhibition, and induction of apoptosis. The recommended dose is 2 mg/kg/day for 3-13 months. Clinician should be aware of possible side effects of propranolol like bradycardia, hypotension, bronchospasm, and hypoglycemia.
- *Corticosteroid:* Oral prednisolone or prednisone is considered to treat IH when there are contraindications or an inadequate response to oral propranolol. A dose of 2-4 mg/kg/day is usually recommended. The high dose of prednisone would have to be slowly tapered over weeks to months. Prednisone's adverse reactions would include irritability, sleep disturbance, hypertension, bone demineralization, cardiomyopathy, and growth retardation.
- *Intralesional injection:* Intralesional injection of triamcinolone and/or betamethasone to treat focal, bulky IHs during proliferation, or in certain critical anatomic locations (e.g., the lip). Adrenal suppression can be observed with large doses (e.g., >4 mg/kg).
- *Topical beta-blocker:* Topical timolol can be used in treating thin and/or superficial IH. It can be applied up to 2-3 times per day for 6-9 months.

Surgical intervention is not commonly performed during infancy due to increased anesthetic risks and blood loss secondary to highly vascular lesions. Surgical treatment options for infantile hemangioma and their applications include the following[14]:

- *Laser therapy:* Although the use of pulsed dye laser therapy (PDL) as an initial treatment is controversial, it is very effective in treating the pain associated with ulcerative IH. Therefore, currently, it is reserved for ulcerated IH and residual lesions such as telangiectasia. In selected patients (with lip and nasal tip lesions) laser therapy has a superior cosmetic result.
- *Excision:* Surgical excision involves removing the residual fibrofatty tissue. It is considered to prevent complications seen with ulcerated lesions, residual lesions, large periocular lesions that interfere with vision, or lesions that do not respond to medical therapy.

Prognosis

For uncomplicated IH, the prognosis is very good. Only less than 10% of IH will leave cosmetic disfigurement and require some intervention. The majority of patients will have complete involution. At 5 and 9 years, 50% and 90% of IH will resolve, respectively.[9]

CONGENITAL HEMANGIOMAS (CH)

Congenital hemangiomas are benign vascular tumors that are extremely rare; the exact prevalence however is unknown. Although clinically they can resemble IH, they are biologically different. Typically, they are fully formed at birth and do not illustrate the postnatal growth seen with IH. Furthermore, they stain negative for GLUT-1 in comparison to infantile hemangioma.[15,16] *GNAQ* and *GNA11* somatic activating mutations have been reported with CH.[15] Congenital hemangiomas are usually solitary and can be found on different parts of the body such as the head, limbs, or neck. They appear rather bluish-red lesions with a *halo* around or "pale-rim" that represent the adjacent less well-perfused skin due to a steal effect noted on ultrasound imaging.[16,17]

There are three subtypes of congenital hemangioma[18]:

1. *Rapidly involuting congenital hemangiomas (RICHs):* They completely regress after birth usually in the first year of life and atrophic scarring can be observed afterward which can be reconstructed and best done before 4 years of age. Although they regress after birth, they can present with thrombocytopenia and coagulopathy soon after birth as in the Kasabach-Merritt phenomenon (KMP). In addition, high-output heart failure can occur and may require ligation of the feeding arteries although not yet well described.[19]
2. *Noninvoluting congenital hemangiomas (NICH):* They persist as coarse telangiectasias over the years without signs of regression.[20] Early surgical excision should be offered to achieve the best cosmetic and functional results in adult life.[21]
3. *Partially involuting congenital hemangiomas (PICH):* They basically regress like RICH but partially after birth and then stabilize and persist more like NICH lesions. Therefore, surgical removal can also be offered to treat these lesions.

KAPOSIFORM HEMANGIOENDOTHELIOMA (KHE)

Incidence

Zukerberg and coworkers first described KHE in 1993 as a vascular tumor of infancy and childhood that is different from IH by its locally aggressive features and focal Kaposi-like appearance.[22] The estimated annual prevalence of KHE is 0.91 per 100,000 children with an incidence of 0.071 per 100,000 children per year. Although until recently it was believed KHE has equal gender distribution, male predominance started to be noted.[23]

Etiology and Pathology

Although the pathogenesis of KHE is poorly understood, it is most likely multifactorial. Sporadic genetic mutations (e.g., activating *GNA14 gene*) are found in about a third of cases of KHE tumor but it is unknown whether they are causative or develop as a result of developing the tumor. At the histological level, dermis, subcutaneous fat, and muscle infiltration with sheets of spindle cells and thin-wall vessels are usually seen with positive immunohistochemical staining for vascular endothelial markers CD31 and CD34, lymphatic endothelial marker VEGFR-3, D2–40, lymphatic endothelial hyaluronan receptor-1 and Prox-1, but negative for glucose transporter-1 (Glut-1) and human herpes virus-8. The predominant feature of the pathology of KHE is the dysregulation of angiogenesis and lymphangiogenesis.[10,23]

Clinical Presentation

KHE has a wide spectrum of manifestations from cutaneous lesions to deep tumors (retroperitoneum, thoracic cavity, and muscle) with or without cutaneous signs (up to 12% are without cutaneous signs). It appears as firm, purpuric lesions when it is superficial and often mistaken for ecchymosis. With deeper lesions, it appears as a bluish-purpuric hue with an ill-defined border. Extremities are more frequently involved in comparison to the trunk or head and neck area. Interestingly, these lesions can be very painful when the patient manifests clinical evidence of KMP which is observed in up to 70% of the patients.[10,23]

Diagnosis

Unlike other hemangiomas, KHE diagnosis often requires a combination of clinical presentation in addition to imaging and histological and laboratory studies. Laboratory evaluation is essential for the diagnosis of KMP. For small and superficial lesions, ultrasound can be sufficient. Yet, MRI is still considered as the first-line assessment imaging tool to determine lesion extension and treatment response. Furthermore, an MRI of the chest and abdomen should be considered in any patient with cutaneous purpura and severe unexplained thrombocytopenia to look for deep KHE associated with KMP. Despite the aggressive investigation recommended, the diagnosis can be delayed in certain cases like in the case of deep KHE without KMP (bone and/or joint). The gold standard for diagnosis of KHE is a biopsy that should be performed whenever possible and safe. However, in the setting of severe KMP, it is often not possible.

Treatment

Expert opinions and clinical experiences are the main driving forces in the recommended management of KHE as no validated scores have been established to assess disease severity. There is no definite treatment guideline for patients with KHE. However, the two factors that determine the treatment strategy for KHE are the size of the lesion and the presence of KMP.[10]

- *Medical treatment:* A combined regimen (e.g., vincristine plus corticosteroids) is recommended for patients with KMP. Platelet transfusion should be avoided except in the presence of active bleeding or preoperatively in preparation for surgery. Transfused platelets can get trapped in the lesion causing worsening swelling and pain. Weaning off corticosteroid treatment is advisable as undesirable side effects are often observed with long-term daily treatment in children. Patients who either relapsed once, the dose was tapered, or did not respond to the initial therapy, showed a high response rate up to 94% to sirolimus therapy (low dose of 2 ng/ml–3 ng/ml). Patients with high serum levels of Ang-2 have less response to sirolimus. Although rare, the side effect of sirolimus like interstitial pneumonitis and *pneumocystis carinii* pneumonia can occur and can be life-threatening in children.[10,23]
- *Surgical treatment:* Localized and uncomplicated KHE can be treated with elective surgical excision. Patients who failed pharmacological therapy can be offered surgical excision. In addition, surgical excision indicated for cosmetic or functional reasons. Surgical excision during the active phase of KMP should be avoided. Arterial embolization may be used to control the disease.[10,23]

MALIGNANT VASCULAR TUMORS

ANGIOSARCOMA

Angiosarcoma is a malignant tumor that rapidly proliferates through the infiltration of anaplastic cells derived from endothelial cells from any part of an individual's body. It mostly affects the adult population and rarely affects children. Risk factors of angiosarcoma tumors include carcinogens such as vinyl chloride, genetic predispositions, radiotherapy, and chronic lymphedema. Furthermore, liver metastasis from angiosarcoma may have a similar clinical presentation to other liver tumors including liver metastasis that can be differentiated by lesion biopsy.

EPITHELIOID HEMANGIOENDOTHELIOMA

Epithelioid hemangioendothelioma describes a vascular type of tumor that is rare and arises from the endothelium thus affecting epithelial cells. The tumor can also develop in soft tissues of extremities, the liver, lymphatic tissue, bone, spleen, and lungs. Females, especially those on contraceptives, seem to have a higher prevalence of the tumor. Compared to angiosarcoma, epithelioid hemangioendothelioma is less common with indolent nature. Moreover, the tumor has distinctive features from other vascular tumors which include encasing surrounding structures and encompassing infiltrative growth patterns, that lack the lobular pattern that hemangioma portrays. The treatment of the epithelioid hemangioendothelioma varies based on its location and the severity stage of the tumor.

VASCULAR ONCOSURGERY

INTRODUCTION

Surgery remains the main stay of treatment for most solid tumors and the main hope of cure for many patients. The relationship between vessels and cancer has been the subject of many studies. Growth of new vessels induced by tumors, a phenomenon called "angiogenesis" has been recognized since 1787. The growth of new capillaries into tumor implants in animal models was described only in 1939. During the same time, it was published that only preexisting vessels could be identified inside some neoplastic lesions. During the 1970s, Folkman started to systematically investigate the role of newly formed vessels in cancer and the angiogenesis theory, i.e., the complete reliance of cancers on new vessels in order to grow and become predominant. Eventually, recent work has demonstrated that some tumors can truly grow without inducing angiogenesis as the neoplastic cells exploit the preexisting vessels by co-opting them.[24]

Primary tumors of blood vessels have been discussed above; however, the importance of these in clinical practice is dwarfed by tumors from different origins invading vessels. A vascular therapist is much more likely to be consulted about vessel involvement by tumors and have to deal with them surgically than come across a primary tumor of blood vessels. Because of the paucity of primary vascular tumor cases worldwide, knowledge of their diagnosis and management is limited.[25] In this section, we will briefly discuss the most encountered solid tumors invading vessels and their surgical management with cases from one of the author's own series (Figure 51-2).

In clinical practice, the following are the most common tumors that encroach on or invade vessels and require vascular expertise for their safe removal:

EXTRA-ADRENAL PARAGANGLIOMAS

These are neoplasms of the paraganglia located within the paravertebral sympathetic and parasympathetic chains. Thus, paragangliomas may arise anywhere along these tracts. Common sites of occurrence include abdomen, retroperitoneum, chest, mediastinum, and various head and neck locations such as jugulotympanic membrane, orbit, nasopharynx, larynx, vagal body, and carotid body.[26,27,28]

MEDIASTINAL TUMORS

The wide variety of tissues within the mediastinum is reflected in the many forms of neoplastic, developmental, and inflammatory masses that can be seen as a localized mass in the mediastinum.

Thymoma, neurogenic tumors. and benign cysts taken together represent 60% of patients with mediastinal masses. Significant differences exist between adults and children concerning the respective frequency of various histological types. Neurogenic tumors, germ cell neoplasms, and foregut cysts represent 80% of childhood lesions whereas primary thymic neoplasms, thyroid masses, and lymphomas are the most frequent in adults. In a large series from the Mayo clinic, tumors were malignant in 25% of cases and 75% were resectable.[29,30]

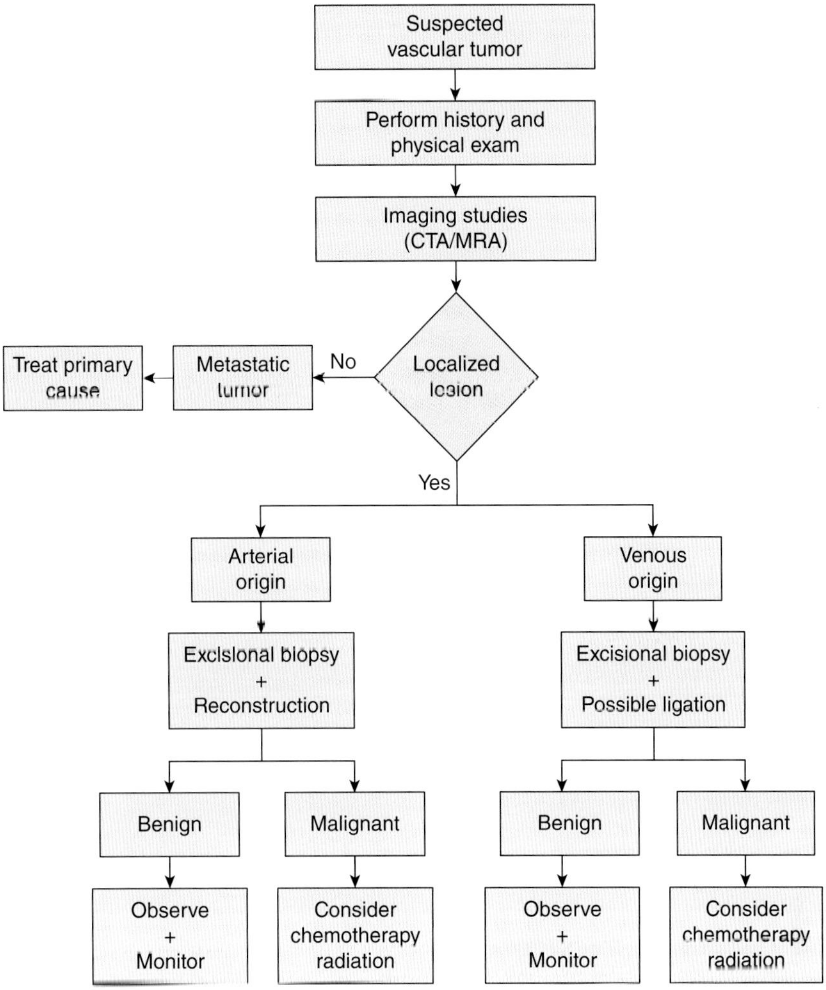

FIGURE 51-2 Approach to vascular tumors management. (Reproduced with permission from Abdullah Nasif, MD.)

Most patients with mediastinal lesions are usually chronically asymptomatic and 83% of incidentally discovered masses are benign. Approximately one-third of mediastinal masses are malignant and are more often symptomatic. Symptoms relate to invasion or obstruction of nearby structures that can include dyspnea, dysphagia, cough from airway compression, superior vena cava (SVC) syndrome, hoarseness from laryngeal nerve involvement or symptoms resulting from spinal cord compression.[30,31]

Obstruction of the SVC produces a characteristic clinical syndrome that can be severe and life threatening. Patients can experience gradual onset of symptoms from incomplete obstruction or can have acute clinical deterioration secondary to complete obstruction from thrombosis. SVC obstruction caused by benign disease typically follows a more gradual course but can present as an aggressive fibrosing process that obliterates the large veins of the mediastinum.[31]

Surgical therapy of these patients includes removal of the tumor and relief of major vascular obstruction. An effective procedure for relief of SVC syndrome is bypass or reconstruction of SVC using vein conduits. The bypass is usually done between

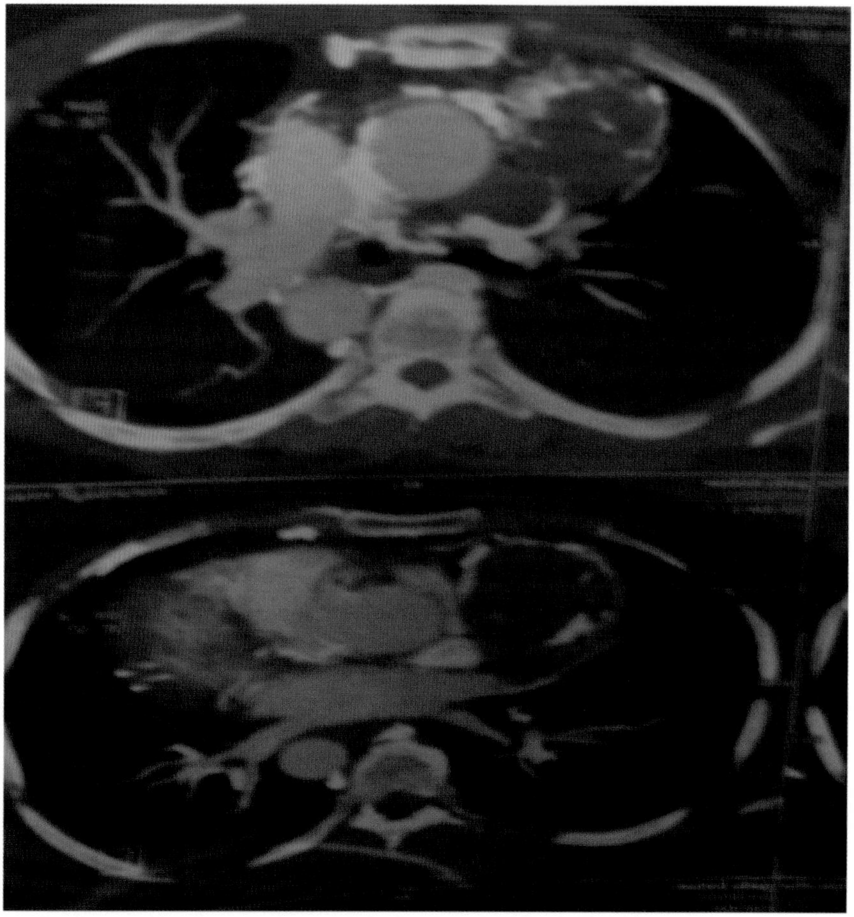

FIGURE 51-3 CT of benign mass causing SVC syndrome.

a patent internal jugular vein and the right cardiac auricle through a partial sternetomy. The conduit can be either a spiral vein made from the long saphenous or a femoral vein (Figures 51-3 and 51-4). The outcome of such procedures is excellent especially when the pathology is benign.

RETROPERITONEAL TUMORS

Solid retroperitoneal neoplasms can grow into a large size that compresses or invades intra a bdominal structures including major vessels. Retroperitoneal neoplasms are predominantly of mesodermal origin, the most frequent tumors located in the retroperitoneum being liposarcomas, leiomyosarcomas, and malignant fibrous histiocytoma. Retroperitoneal sarcomas represent approximately 0.2% of all malignancies being more frequently discovered during the sixth decade of life. Quite often these retroperitoneal masses are found incidentally during imaging investigations especially in early disease stages when the patient has no alarming signs, nor symptoms that could alert the patient. Otherwise, a great percentage of retroperitoneal tumors are detected in advanced stages, when the tumor are large, often being associated with symptoms related to the nearby organ compression or invasion and therefore being less possible to achieve a complete and oncological surgical resection. Complete surgical resection

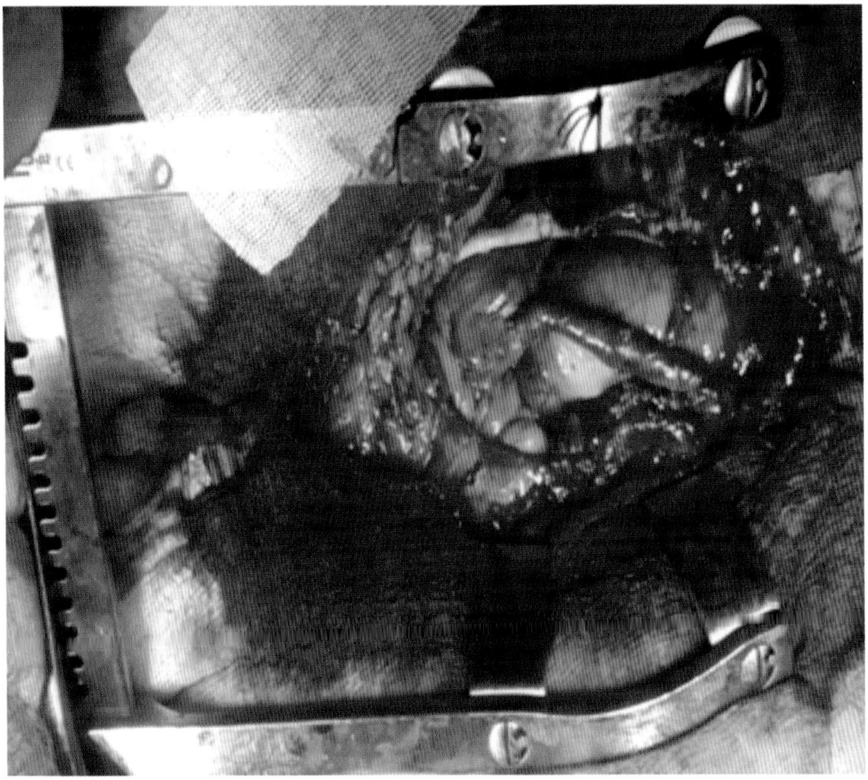

FIGURE 51-4 **Left internal jugular to right cardiac auricle bypass using femoral vein.**

should be attempted as long as there is no metastasis and the patient is fit enough for the surgery.[32,33] Separation of involved organs from tumor should not be attempted; the best results are obtained when involved tissue is removed enbloc with tumor (Figures 51-5 through 51-7).

Neurogenic Tumors

These tumors can be classified as:

(a) Ganglion cell origin (ganglioneuromas, ganglioneuroblastomas, neuroblastomas [NBLs]),

(b) Paraganglionic system origin (pheochromocytomas, paragangliomas), and

(c) Nerve sheath origin (neurilemmomas, neurofibromas, neurofibromatosis, malignant nerve sheath tumors).

Abdominal neurogenic tumors are most commonly located in the retroperitoneum, especially in the paraspinal areas and adrenal glands.[33–35]

Germ Cell, Sex Cord, and Stromal Tumors

Even though germ cell tumors are commonly present in the testes or ovaries, a slight percent of germ cell tumors arise from an extragonadal location. These tumors are supposed to appear from abnormal primordial germ cell remnants that are the cause of germ cells distributed physiologically to liver, bone marrow, and brain or faulty migration of germ cells from the yolk sac or endoderm to the urogenital ridge.[33] Before an analysis of primary extragonadal germ cell tumor is made, a metastasis should be excluded. This type of tumor is more frequently found in men. From the

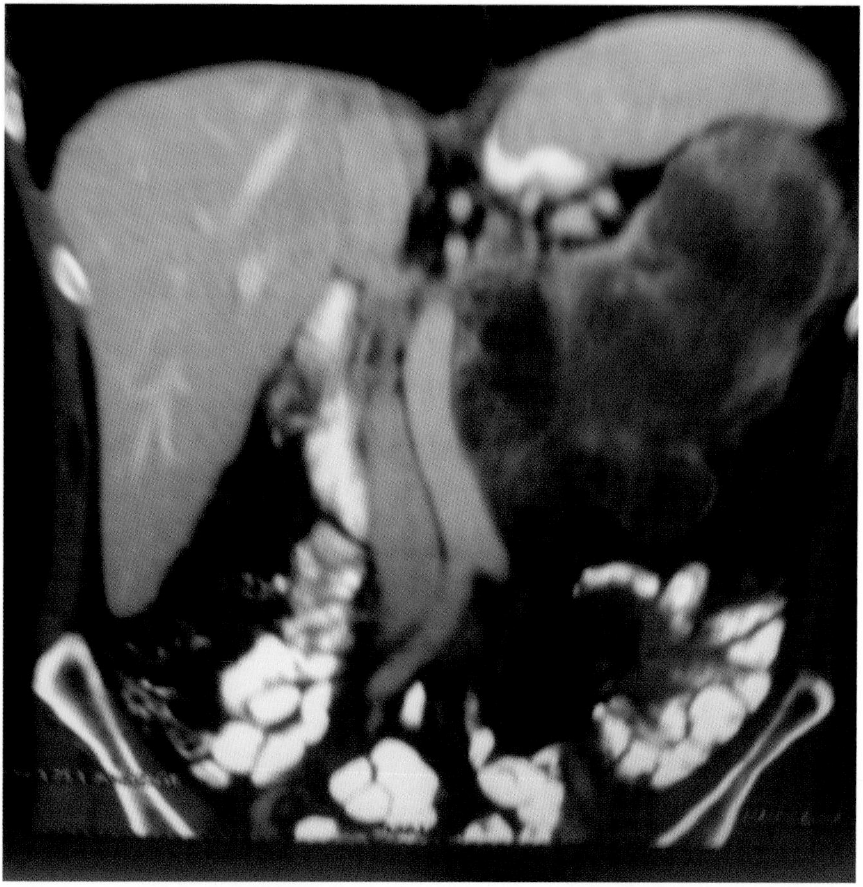

FIGURE 51-5 **CT scan of retroperitoneal sarcoma involving the infrarenal aorta, the left kidney, and descending colon.**

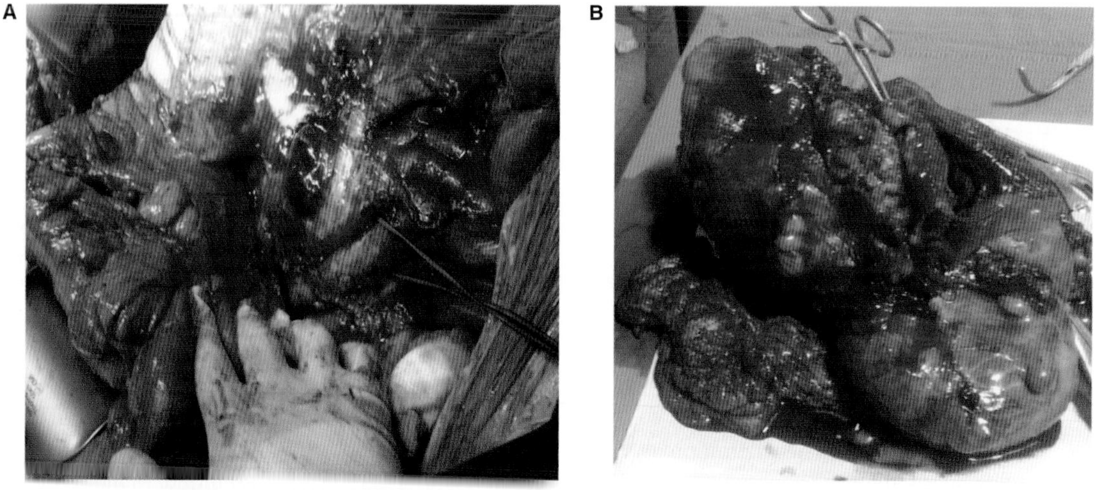

FIGURE 51-6 **A.** Removal of tumor with involved organs. **B.** Resected specimen.

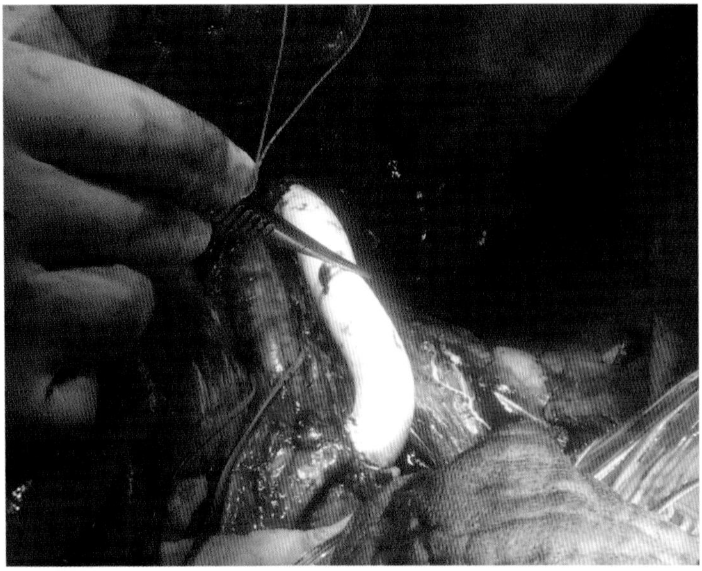

FIGURE 51-7 **Aortic replacement following tumor removal.**

histopathological point of view, these tumors are classified in nonseminomatous germ cell tumors or seminomas, which involve teratoma, yolk sac tumor, choriocarcinoma, mixed germ cell tumors, and embryonal carcinoma. Increased levels of the beta subunit of human chorionic gonadotropin (choriocarcinoma) and of alpha-fetoprotein (yolk sac tumors, embryonal carcinoma) may be found with laboratory tests.[34–36] Some can reach challenging sizes which makes resection especially in young patients the only option (Figures 51-8 throug 51-11).

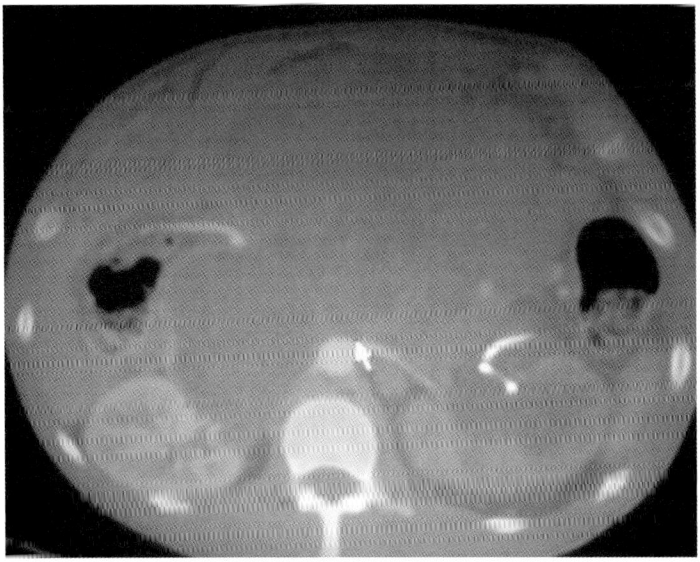

FIGURE 51-8 **Massive germ cell tumor in a young man.**

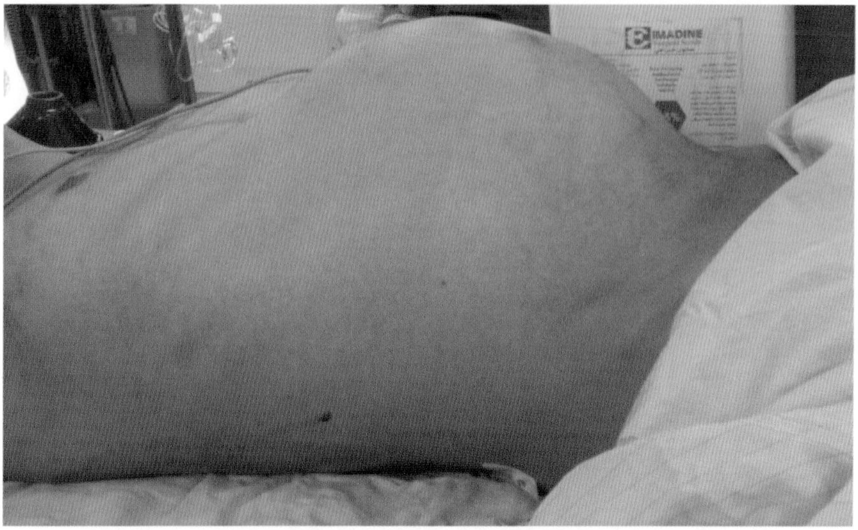

FIGURE 51-9 Massive germ cell tumor causing compressive symptoms.

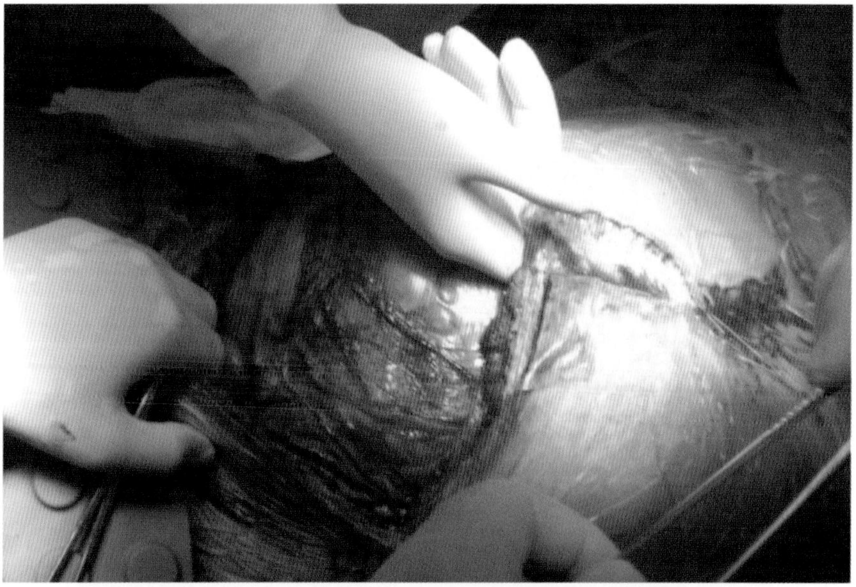

FIGURE 51-10 Mercedes sign laparotomy incision for maximal safe exposure.

Lymphoid and Hematologic Neoplasms

The most common retroperitoneal malignancy is represented by lymphoma that accounts for approximately 33% of the retroperitoneal malignancies.[34,36] Lymphoma is treated with chemotherapy or radiation therapy. Soft-tissue masses can persist after treatment due to fibrosis and cannot be differentiated from viable tumors.[35,37]

Renal Cell Carcinoma

Renal cell carcinoma (RCC) accounts for 2% to 3% of all adult malignancies, representing the seventh most

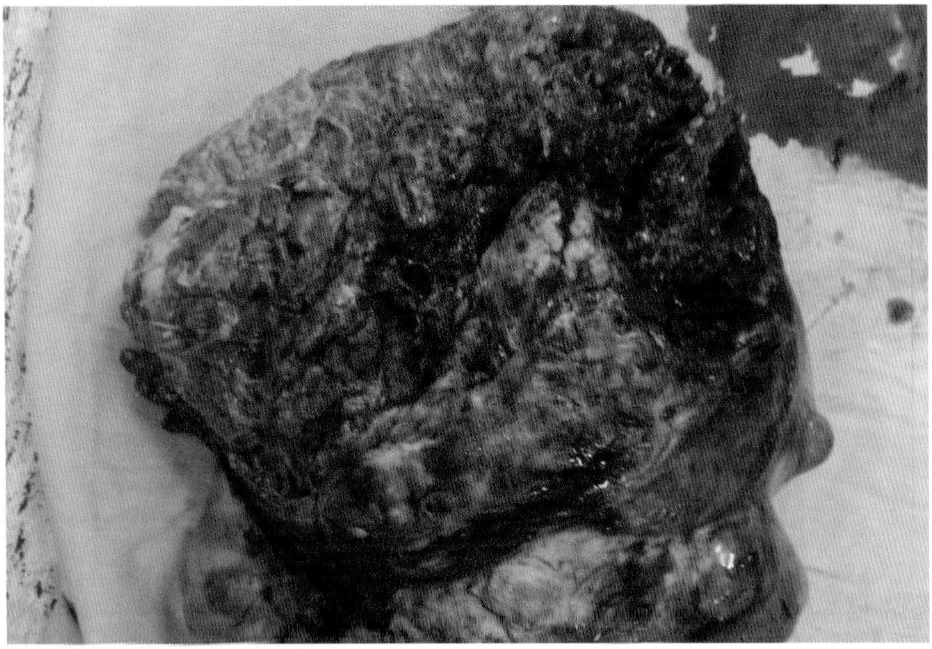

FIGURE 51-11 **Resected tumor with preservation of mesenteric vessels.**

common cancer in men and the ninth most common cancer in women.[38]

The proportion of small and incidental renal tumors has significantly increased owing to the widespread use of abdominal imaging, e.g., ultrasonography, CT, and MRI. More than 50% of RCCs are currently detected incidentally. However, some patients with RCC still present with clinical symptoms such as flank pain, gross hematuria, and palpable abdominal mass (the classical triad); metastatic symptoms like bone pain or lung nodules; or paraneoplastic syndromes such as hypercalcemia, unexplained fever, erythrocytosis, or wasting syndromes.[39–41] RCC, which has a tendency for vascular invasion, extends into the IVC in 4% to 25% of all patients. In patients with nonmetastatic RCC who underwent radical nephrectomy and complete thrombectomy, 5-year survival rates of 30% to 72% have been reported.[39–41]

The surgical technique to resect RCC tumors invading the cava depends on the level of extension of the tumor thrombus; in most cases, a median laparotomy is enough to obtain control of the IVC below hepatic veins following appropriate hepatic mobilization. Transesophageal echocardiogram, control of the contralateral renal vein, and appropriate volume replacement are usually enough to maintain hemodynamics and prevent pulmonary embolization during the longitudinal cavatomy to remove the tumor thrombus. Extension of exposure to lower median sternotomy is sometimes needed for supradiaphragmatic IVC clamping. Invasion of caval wall requires partial caval excision and caval patch or replacement[39–42] (Figures 51-12 through 51-15.)

PEDIATRIC MALIGNANCIES

Two intra-abdominal pediatric tumors can invade or displace vascular structures and might require vascular team involvement. These are neuroblastoma and nephroblastoma (Wilms tumor). The latter is a common malignant childhood neoplasm with a mean age of occurrence of 3 years. It is a complex mass that originates from the kidney and most commonly invades the vascular system by way of the renal vein and IVC, which differentiates it from neuroblastoma.[10] Although there have been reports of vascular invasion from NBL, it is a rare occurrence.

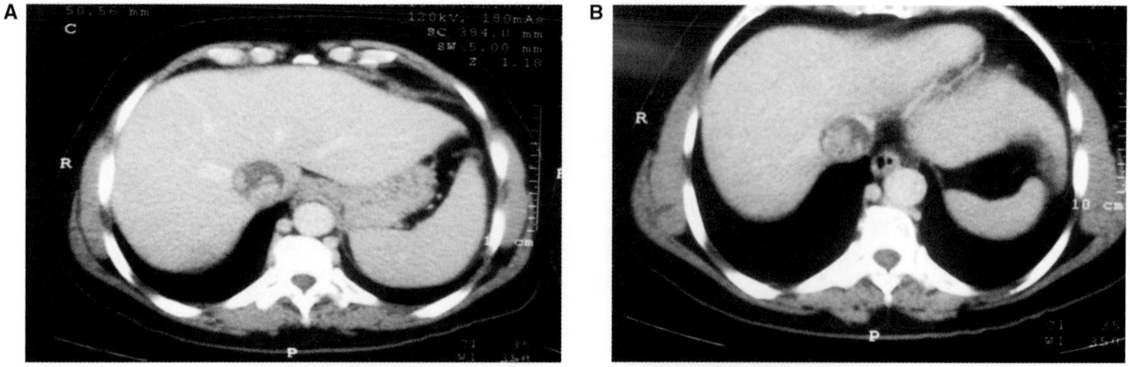

FIGURE 51-12 (A and B) CT of renal cell carcinoma extension to infra diaphragmatic IVC.

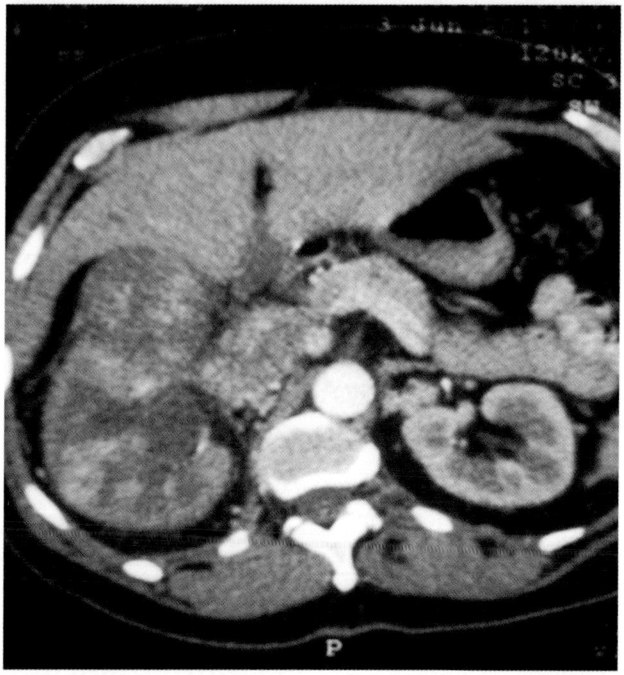

FIGURE 51-13 **CT of renal cell carcinoma invading cava.**

Adrenal NBLs more commonly encase and displace the regional blood vessels.[43–45]

NBL is the most common extracranial tumor in childhood and commonly presents as an abdominal mass. Nephroblastoma is the most common renal tumor in childhood and similarly presents as an abdominal pathology. The natural histories and typical clinical courses of these tumors are very different; thus, early distinction is important. Both occur in early childhood, with Wilms' having a slightly older peak incidence at between 3 and 4 years. Histologically, they are different diseases with NBLs arising from primordial neural crest cells and Wilms' being undifferentiated mesodermal tumors.[44–46] Diagnostic tools include ultrasonography, CT, and MRI.

Treatment of Wilms tumor includes chemotherapy and surgical removal of the tumor. Patients with a Wilms tumor in only one kidney (unilateral

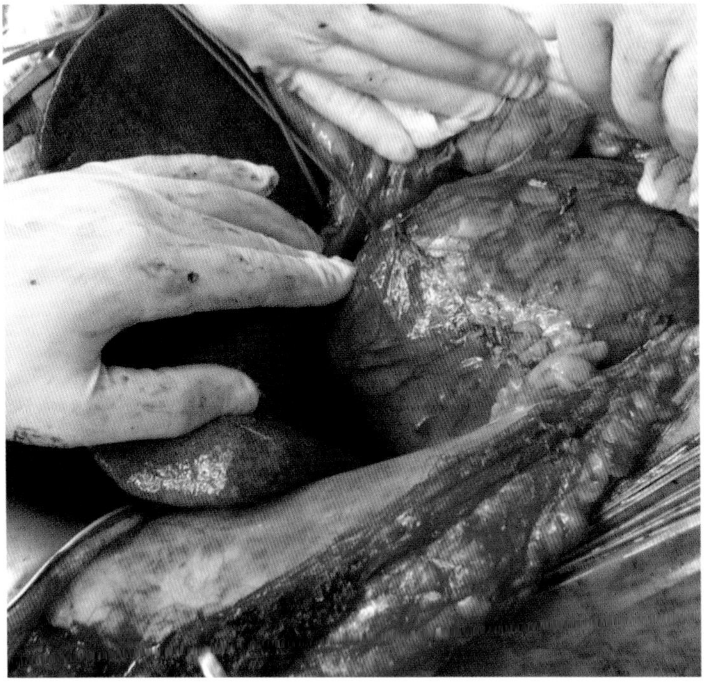

FIGURE 51-14 **Surgical exposure of tumor with vascular controls.**

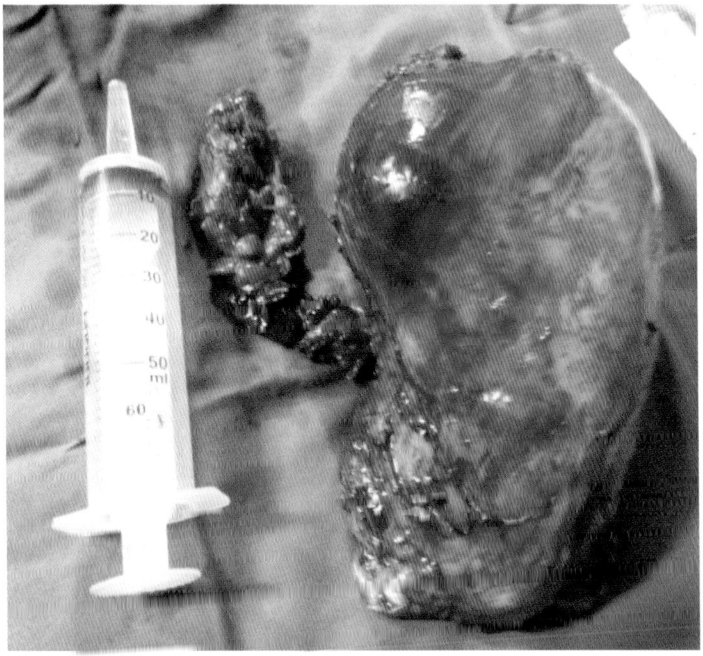

FIGURE 51-15 **Resected specimen with IVC extension.**

tumor) usually undergo removal of the kidney with the tumor. Accordingly, this method is called tumor nephrectomy. As a result, the remaining kidney will enlarge over the following weeks and months, thereby becoming capable of fully taking over the removed one's function. Therefore, it is important to protect the remaining kidney from any damage later in life (Figures 51-16 and 51-17).

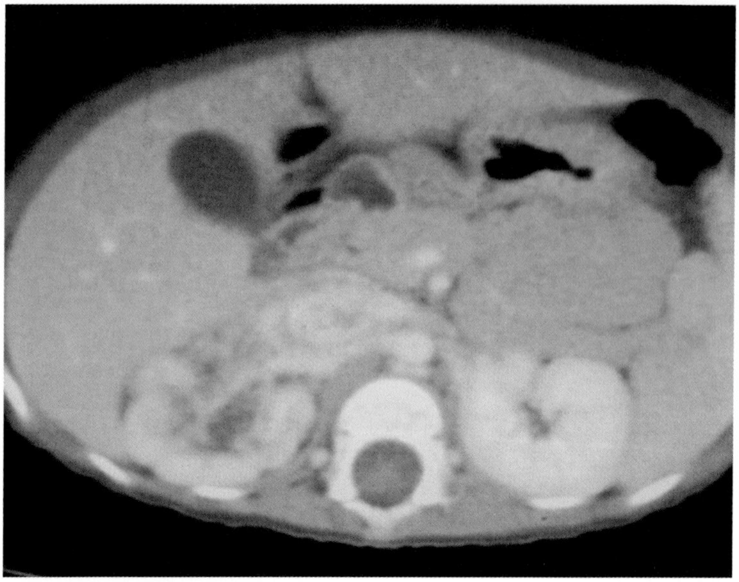

FIGURE 51-16 **Wilms tumor with caval extension.**

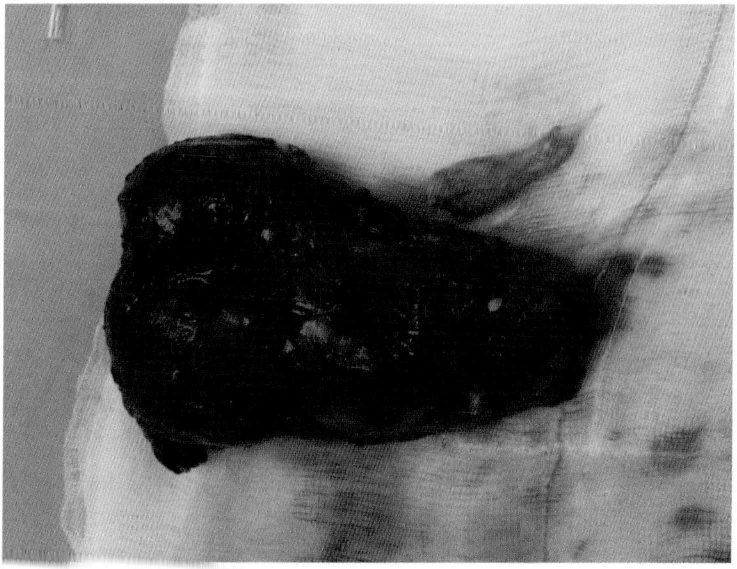

FIGURE 51-17 **Resected (Wilms tumor) specimen.**

If a patient has tumors in both kidneys (bilateral Wilms tumor), treatment options will be assessed individually with the goal to at least save one of the affected organs.[4,46] Chemotherapy, radiation, and surgery are used in NBL therapy depending on the stage with less favorable outcomes than Wilms tumor.[46–48]

LIMB TUMORS

Amputation had been the standard method of treatment for most bone sarcomas, but in the last three decades, there have been several developments of limb-sparing surgery for most malignant bone tumors. Today, limb-sparing surgery is considered safe and routine for approximately 90% of patients with malignant bone tumors of the extremity. Advances in orthopedics, bioengineering, radiographic imaging, radiotherapy, and chemotherapy have contributed to safer, more reliable surgical procedures. Currently, the three most popular options are using an endoprosthesis, allograft prosthetic composite, and biological reconstructions.[49,50]

Selection of the joint-preserving limb salvage operative procedure should be based on tumor origin, site, and bone strength.[50]

Many of these complex cases require the involvement of vascular surgeons to optimize the outcome. Arterial and venous bypass procedures are best performed with natural conduits from the unaffected limb especially where joints are replaced with endoprosthesis.[49-51]

A detailed discussion of revascularization in tumor limb salvage surgery is beyond the scope of this chapter (Figures 51-18 through 51-22).

CONCLUSION

Vascular tumors can be any tumor that originates from the vascular structure at any part of the body. Tumors can be benign or malignant. Vascular hemangioma is the most common benign tumor. During patient evaluation for a possible vascular tumor, physician needs to obtain medical history and perform physical examination to form a differential diagnosis. Imaging study such as CT scan is critical to determine the surgical anatomy. Tumors with the arterial origin are more difficult to manage when it comes to surgical intervention. Arterial reconstruction usually needs to restore the blood supply to the involved organ.

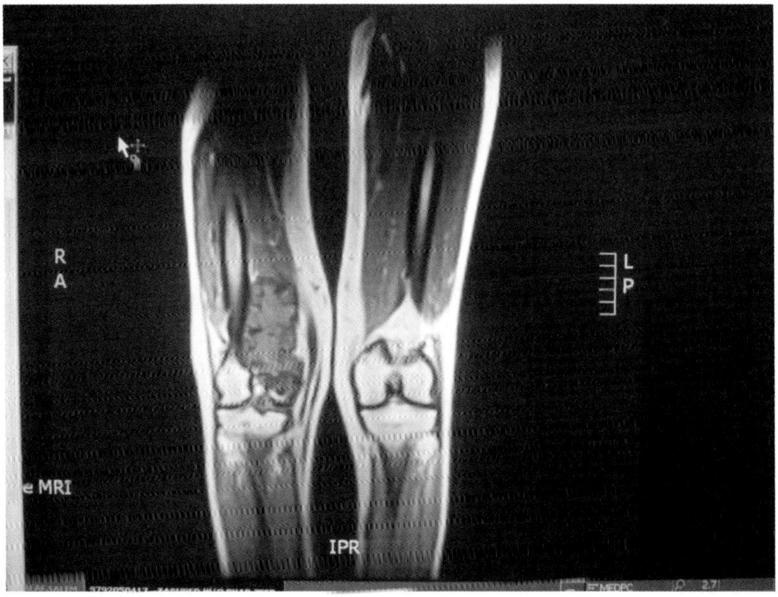

FIGURE 51-18 MRI of knee sarcoma.

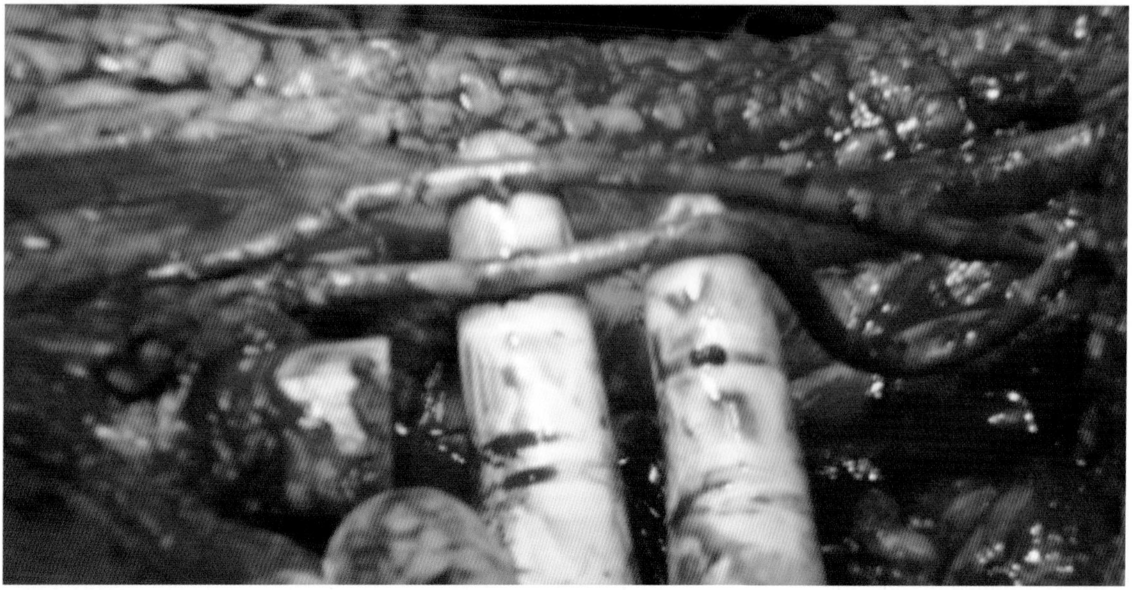

FIGURE 51-19 Arterial and venous bypasses to enable total knee excision.

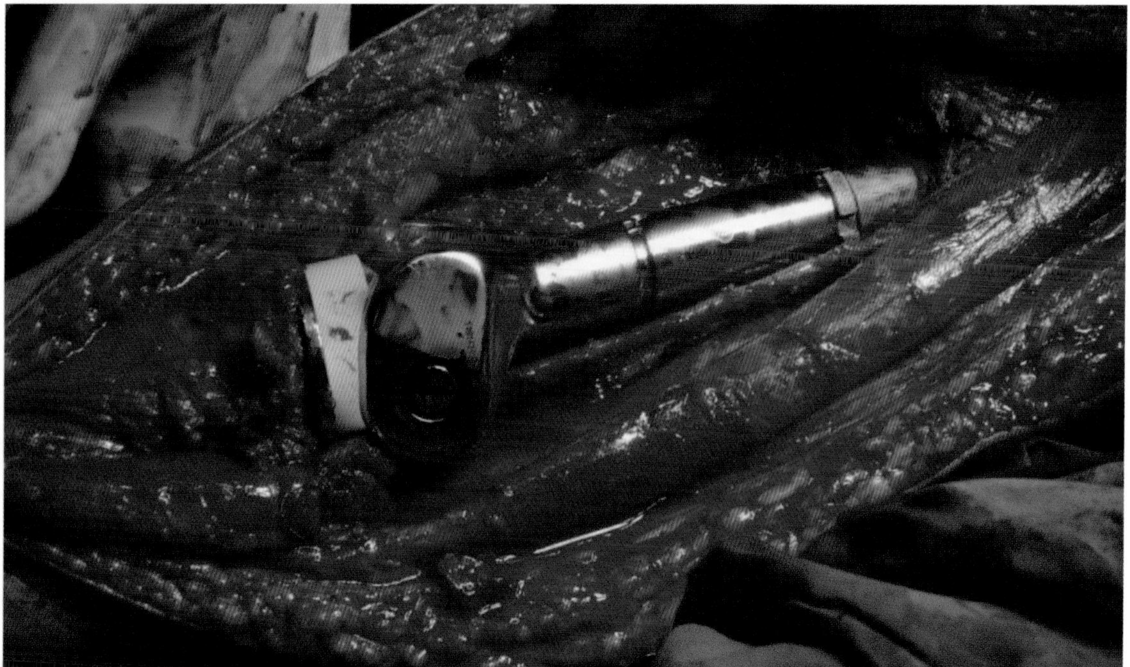

FIGURE 51-20 Endoprosthesis.

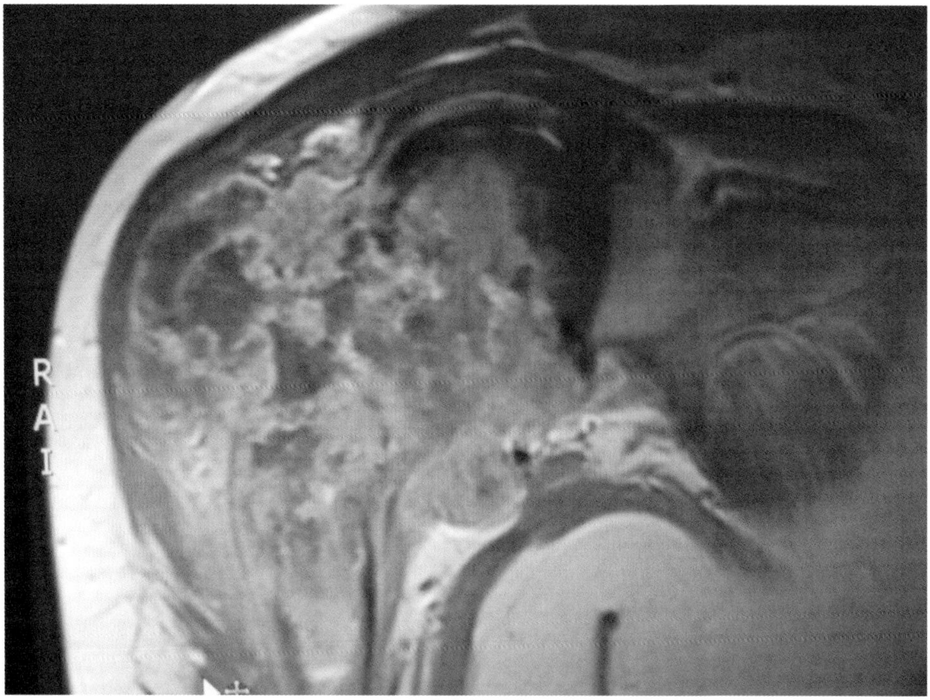

FIGURE 51-21 Humoral chondrosarcoma.

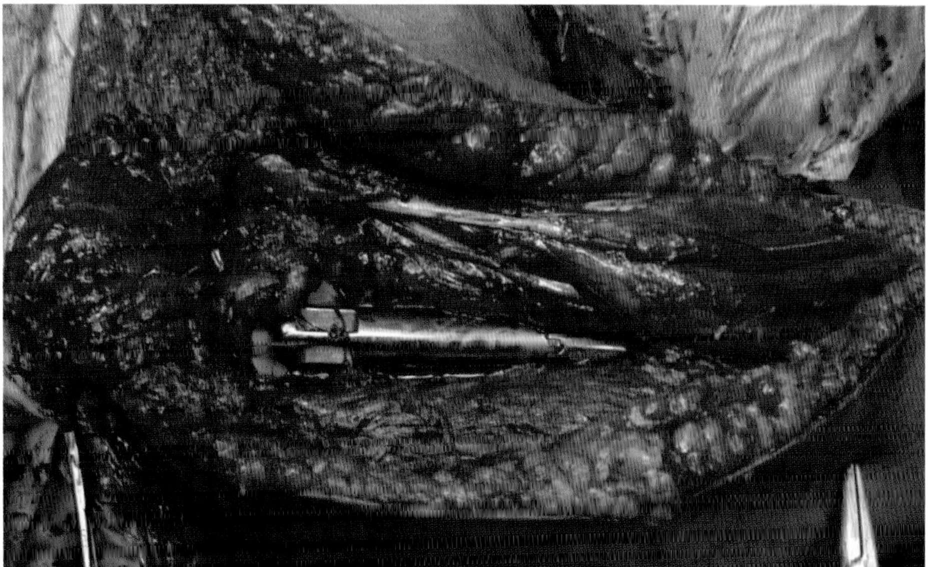

FIGURE 51-22 Tumor removal and joint replacement with endoprosthesis.

It is more challenging to rectify tumors from different origins that invade vascular structures, and it is more common than primary vascular tumors. The ability of vascular reconstruction usually determines the resectability of these tumors.

REFERENCES

1. Wassef M, Blei F, Adams D, et al. Vascular anomalies classification: recommendations from the international society for the study of vascular anomalies. *Pediatrics*. 2015;136:e203-e214.
2. ISSVA classification for vascular anomalies. 2018. Available at https://www.issva.org/UserFiles/file/ISSVA-Classification-2018.pdf.
3. Kilcline C, Frieden IJ. Infantile hemangiomas: how common are they? A systematic review of the medical literature. *Pediatr Dermatol*. 2008;25:168-173.
4. Hemangioma Investigator G, Haggstrom AN, Drolet BA, et al. Prospective study of infantile hemangiomas: demographic, prenatal, and perinatal characteristics. *J Pediatr*. 2007;150:291-294.
5. Bree AF, Siegfried E, Sotelo-Avila C, Nahass G. Infantile hemangiomas: speculation on placental trophoblastic origin. *Arch Dermatol*. 2001;137:573-577.
6. Drolet BA, Frieden IJ. Characteristics of infantile hemangiomas as clues to pathogenesis: does hypoxia connect the dots? *Arch Dermatol*. 2010;146:1295-1299.
7. Greenberger S, Bischoff J. Pathogenesis of infantile haemangioma. *Br J Dermatol*. 2013;169:12-19.
8. North PE, Waner M, Mizeracki A, et al. A unique microvascular phenotype shared by juvenile hemangiomas and human placenta. *Arch Dermatol*. 2001;137:559-70.
9. Chamli A, Aggarwal P, Jamil RT, Litaiem N. *Hemangioma*. Treasure Island, FL: StatPearls; 2020.
10. Childhood Vascular Tumors Treatment (PDQ(R)): Health Professional Version. PDQ Cancer Information Summaries. Bethesda (MD) 2002.
11. Baselga E, Roe E, Coulie J, et al. Risk factors for degree and type of sequelae after involution of untreated hemangiomas of infancy. *JAMA Dermatol*. 2016;152:1239-1243.
12. Garzon MC, Epstein LG, Heyer GL, et al. PHACE syndrome: consensus-derived diagnosis and care recommendations. *J Pediatr*. 2016;178:24-33e2.
13. Horii KA, Drolet BA, Frieden IJ, et al. Prospective study of the frequency of hepatic hemangiomas in infants with multiple cutaneous infantile hemangiomas. *Pediatr Dermatol*. 2011;28:245-253.
14. Krowchuk DP, Frieden IJ, Mancini AJ, et al. Clinical practice guideline for the management of infantile hemangiomas. *Pediatrics*. 2019;143(1):e20183475.
15. Ayturk UM, Couto JA, Hann S, et al. Somatic activating mutations in GNAQ and GNA11 are associated with congenital hemangioma. *Am J Hum Genet*. 2016;98:789-795.
16. Wildgruber M, Sadick M, Muller-Wille R, Wohlgemuth WA. Vascular tumors in infants and adolescents. *Insights Imaging*. 2019;10:30.
17. Ramphul K, Mejias SG, Ramphul-Sicharam Y, Sonaye R. Congenital hemangioma: a case report of a finding every physician should know. *Cureus*. 2018;10:e2485.
18. El Zein S, Boccara O, Soupre V, et al. The histopathology of congenital hemangioma and its clinical correlations: a long-term follow-up study of 55 cases. *Histopathology*. 2020;77(2):275-283.
19. Ren Z, Sun S, Ye Z, Yang J. Congenital hemangioma causing heart failure. *Intensive Care Med*. 2019;45:889-891.
20. Knopfel N, Walchli R, Luchsinger I, Theiler M, Weibel L, Schwieger-Briel A. Congenital hemangioma exhibiting postnatal growth. *Pediatr Dermatol*. 2019;36:548-549.
21. Moreno-Ramirez D, Toledo-Pastrana T, Rios-Martin JJ, Ferrandiz L. Surgical removal of a noninvoluting congenital hemangioma using a modified sub-brow flap. *JAAD Case Rep*. 2016;2:199-201.
22. Zukerberg LR, Nickoloff BJ, Weiss SW. Kaposiform hemangioendothelioma of infancy and childhood. an aggressive neoplasm associated with Kasabach-Merritt syndrome and lymphangiomatosis. *Am J Surg Pathol*. 1993;17:321-328.
23. Ji Y, Chen S, Yang K, Xia C, Li L. Kaposiform hemangioendothelioma: current knowledge and future perspectives. *Orphanet J Rare Dis*. 2020;15:39.
24. Voutouri C, Kirkpatrick ND, Chung E, et al. Experimental and computational analyses reveal dynamics of tumor vessel cooption and optimal treatment strategies. *Proc Natl Acad Sci U S A*. 2019;116(7):2662-2671.
25. Hall AP. The role of angiogenesis in cancer. *Comp Clin Pathol*. 2005;13:95-99.
26. Coldwell DM, Baron RL, Charnsangavej C. Angiosarcoma. Diagnosis and clinical course. *Acta Radiol*. 1989;30(6):627-631.
27. Wieneke JA, Smith A. Paraganglioma: carotid body tumor. *Head Neck Pathol*. 2009;3(4):303-306.
28. Hunt J. Diseases of the paraganglia system. In: Thompson LDR, ed. *Endocrine Pathology, Foundations in Diagnostic Pathology*. Philadelphia: Churchill Livingstone/Elsevier; 2006:157-164.

29. Carter BW, Benveniste MF, Madan R, et al. ITMIG classification of mediastinal compartments and multidisciplinary approach to mediastinal masses. *Radiographics.* 2017;37(2):413-436.
30. Moran CA, Suster S, Koss MN. Primary germ cell tumours of the mediastinum: III. Yolk sac tumour, embryonal carcinoma, choriocarcinoma, and combined nonteratomatous germ cell tumours of the mediastinum–a clinicopathologic and immunohistochemical study of 64 cases. *Cancer.* 1997;80:699-707.
31. Doty JR, Flores JH, Doty DB. Superior vena cava obstruction: bypass using spiral vein graft. *Ann Thorac Surg.* 1999;67(4):1111-1116.
32. Kuehnl A, Schmidt M, Hornung HM, Graser A, Jauch KW, Kopp R. Resection of malignant tumors invading the vena cava: perioperative complications and long-term follow-up. *J Vasc Surg.* 2007;46(3):533-540.
33. Shinagare AB, Jagannathan JP, Ramaiya NH, Hall MN, Van den Abbeele AD. Adult extragonadal germ cell tumors. *AJR: Am J Roentgenol.* 2010;195(4):W274-W280.
34. Rha SE, Byun JY, Jung SE, Chun HJ, Lee HG, Lee JM. Neurogenic tumors in the abdomen: tumor types and imaging characteristics. *Radiographics.* 2003;23(1): 29-43.
35. Parada D, Peña KB, Moreira O, Cohen I, Parada AM, Mejías LD. Extragonadal retroperitoneal germ cell tumor: primary versus metastases? *Arch Esp Urol.* 2007; 60(6):713-719.
36. Mota MMDS, Bezerra ROF, Garcia MRT. Practical approach to primary retroperitoneal masses in adults. *Radiol Bras.* 2018;51(6):391-400.
37. Scholz M, Zehender M, Thalmann GN, Borner M, Thöni H, Studer UE. Extragonadal retroperitoneal germ cell tumor: evidence of origin in the testis. *Ann Oncol.* 2002;13(1):121-124.
38. Ng CS, Wood CG, Silverman PM, Tannir NM, Tamboli P, Sandler CM. Renal cell carcinoma: diagnosis, staging, and surveillance. *AJR: Am J Roentgenol.* 2008;191(4):1220-1232.
39. Wotkowicz C, Wszolek MF, Libertino JA. Resection of renal tumors invading the vena cava. *Urol Clin North Am.* 2008;35(4):657-671; viii.
40. Topaktaş R, Ürkmez A, Tokuç E, Kayar R, Kanberoğlu H, Öztürk Mİ. Surgical management of renal cell carcinoma with associated tumor thrombus extending into the inferior vena cava: a 10-year single-center experience. *Turk J Urol.* 2019;45(5):345-350.
41. Tsuji Y, Goto A, Hara I, et al. Renal cell carcinoma with extension of tumor thrombus into the vena cava: surgical strategy and prognosis. *J Vasc Surg.* 2001;33(4): 789-796.
42. Escudier B, Porta C, Schmidinger M, et al. Renal cell carcinoma: ESMO Clinical Practice Guidelines for diagnosis, treatment and follow-up†. *Ann Oncol.* 2019; 30(5):706-720.
43. Irwin MS, Park JR. Neuroblastoma: paradigm for precision medicine. *Pediatr Clin North Am.* 2015;62(1): 225-256.
44. Swift CC, Eklund MJ, Kraveka JM, Alazraki AL. Updates in diagnosis, management, and treatment of neuroblastoma. *Radiographics.* 2018;38(2):566-580.
45. Emir S. Wilms tumor with intravascular tumor thrombus. *Transl Pediatr.* 2014;3(1):29-33. doi:10.3978/j.issn.2224-4336.2014.01.03.
46. Maris JM, Hogarty MD, Bagatell R, Cohn SL. Neuroblastoma. *Lancet.* 2007;369(9579):2106-2120.
47. Davidoff AM. Wilms' tumor. *Adv Pediatr.* 2012;59(1): 247-267.
48. Xu S, Sun N, Zhang WP, Song HC, Huang CR. Management of Wilms tumor with intravenous thrombus in children: a single center experience. *World J Pediatr.* 2019;15(5):476-482.
49. Zhao J, Xu M, Zheng K, Yu X. Limb salvage surgery with joint preservation for malignant humeral bone tumors: operative procedures and clinical application. *BMC Surg.* 2019;19(1):57.
50. Grimer R, Athanasou N, Gerrand C, et al. UK Guidelines for the management of bone sarcomas. *Sarcoma.* 2010; 2010:317462.
51. Chauhan A, Joshi GR, Chopra BK, Ganguly M, Reddy GR. Limb salvage surgery in bone tumors: a retrospective study of 50 cases in a single center. *Indian J Surg Oncol.* 2013;4(3):248-254.

SELF-ASSESSMENT STUDY QUESTIONS AND ANSWERS

Questions

1. Infantile hemangioma:
A. More common in male
B. More common in female
C. More common in African American
D. Imaging study never indicated

2. Which of the following vascular tumors stain positive with GLUT-1:
A. Infantile hemangioma
B. Congenital hemangioma
C. Kaposiform hemangioendothelioma
D. Epithelioid hemangioma

3. The gold standard in the diagnosis of Kaposiform hemangioendothelioma is:
A. History and physical
B. CT scan
C. Duplex ultrasound
D. Biopsy

4. An 18-month-old female patient was found to have a solaitary bluish-red lesion on her face. Parents stated that it was first noted at birth then it regressed in the first few months; however, it has been stable in size since then. What is the most probable diagnosis and the best next step.
A. Infantile hemangioma; observation as most of these lesions spontaneously resolve.
B. Noninvoluting congenital hemangiomas (NICH); offer surgical excision.
C. Kaposiform hemangioendothelioma; start sirolimus therapy and obtain blood test to rule out Kasabach-Merritt phenomenon.
D. Partially involuting congenital hemangiomas (PICH); suergical exicion is recommned for cosmotic reason.

5. Regarding SVC obstruction the following is true except:
A. It can cause cerebral edema.
B. The gold standard investigation is venography.
C. SVC surgical reconstruction for malignant etiology is contraindicated.
D. Malignant etiologies account for most SVC obstructions

6. Surgical principles in dealing with arteriovenous malformations and vascular tumors include:
A. Take a safe margin of tissue with the glue-filled AVM
B. Use aggressive cautery homeostasis for subdermal and subcutaneous bleeding points to case thrombosis of superficial spread of the AVM
C. It is preferable to attempt enbloc excision technique for lesions containing soft tissue elements
D. Avoid split-thickness grafts for coverage

7. The following are possible etiologies of angiosarcoma arising from vascular endothelium except:
A. Radiation therapy
B. Chemotherapy
C. Lymphedema
D. Vinyl chloride

8. Angiosarcoma:
A. Anaplastic cell derived from endothelial cell
B. Affects only upper extremity
C. Mostly in children
D. Biopsy always not indicated

9. Mediastinal tumors:
A. Mostly symptomatic
B. Incidentally discovered masses are malignant
C. 25% are benign
D. Symptoms usually related to invasion or obstruction of nearby structures

10. LUMBAR syndrome include the following except:
A. L→ **L**ower-body hemangioma
B. M→ Myocardial infarction
C. B→ Bone deformities
D. U→ **U**rogenital anomalies or ulceration

SELF-ASSESSMENT STUDY QUESTIONS AND ANSWERS

Answers

1. B.
2. B.
3. D.
4. D.
5. C.
6. D.
7. C.
8. A.
9. D
10. B.

CHAPTER

52 Erectile Dysfunction

Jonathan H. Demeter and Ahmed El-Zawahry

OUTLINE

GENERAL CONSIDERATIONS AND HISTORY OF ERECTILE DYSFUNCTION

CAUSES OF ERECTILE DYSFUNCTION

- Vascular Causes
- Medication Causes
- Surgical Causes
- Neurological Causes
- Endocrine Causes
- Metabolic and Lifestyle Factors
- Urological Conditions

ANATOMY AND PHYSIOLOGY OF ERECTIONS

- Penile Vascular and Neurological Anatomy
- Phases of Erection
- Neurotransmitters Involved in Erections and Detumescence
- Physiology of Cavernosal Smooth Muscle

CLINICAL FINDINGS

- Differential Diagnosis
- Clinical Staging
- Diagnosis and Evaluation
  - Vascular Testing
    - *Penile duplex Doppler ultrasound*
    - *Cavernosometry*
    - *Pudendal angiography*

MANAGEMENT OF THE CLINICAL PROBLEM

- Medical Treatment
- Surgical Treatment
- Pathway of Treatment

GENERAL CONSIDERATIONS AND HISTORY OF ERECTILE DYSFUNCTION

Erectile dysfunction (ED) is a common problem in men as they age. Generally described as the inability to acquire or sustain a penile erection that is firm enough for satisfactory sexual performance. Over 20% of men may suffer from moderate to severe ED by the age of 40 years.[1] ED can be considered organic, psychogenic, or mixed. Organic ED is due to physical defects either in the relevant neurologic or vascular anatomy and can result from various etiologies including vasculogenic, neurogenic, or hormonal. Psychogenic ED is resultant from various factors and psychologic conflicts inhibit neuropathways responsible for erections including anxiety about the sexual experience, guilt, anger, lack of confidence, depression, or psychosis, among others.[2] A leading cause of organic ED is from diabetes mellitus with hyperglycemia causing damage to the cavernosal nerve and small vessel and ultimately neuropathy and arteriogenic insufficiency.[3] As a marker for small vessel arteriosclerosis, ED is a marker of vascular disease and will precede and predict the development of arterial blood vessel disease in other vessels, classically coronary artery disease. This may occur months to years prior to patients becoming symptomatic from the vascular pathology in other organs. For this reason, the American Urologic Association (AUA)

TABLE 52-1 The Independent Risk Factors for Erectile Dysfunction

Risk Factors for Erectile Dysfunction	
Increased age	Dyslipidemia (elevated total cholesterol and low-density lipoprotein)
Smoking	Depression
Diabetes mellitus	Obesity
Hypertension	Sedentary lifestyle
Lower urinary tract symptoms secondary to benign prostatic hyperplasia	Premature ejaculation

recommends an evaluation for dyslipidemia, diabetes, and possible consultation to a cardiologist in patients with ED that is gradual in onset. A list of risk factors mentioned in the AUA Guidelines for ED is listed in Table 52-1.

CAUSES OF ERECTILE DYSFUNCTION

There are multiple etiologies of ED in men which include from most to least common: vascular, diabetes, medication induced, surgical or radiation changes, neurological, endocrinopathy, and others.[4,5] ED can also be categorized as a psychogenic, organic (without a psychological component), or mixed, a list of causes detailed in Table 52-2.

VASCULAR CAUSES

Vascular causes for ED can originate from an arterial deficiency or a venous pathology.

Diseases and risk factors that impair arterial sufficiency such as hyperlipidemia, tobacco use, lack of exercise and diabetes mellitus (hemoglobin A1C > 6.5) can lead to ED.[6] Hyperglycemia and diabetes mellitus have been directly implicated in the inactivation of endothelial nitric oxide (NO) synthase via glycosylation of the enzyme which is responsible for arterial smooth muscle relaxation and subsequent development and maintenance of an erection.[7]

TABLE 52-2 Causes of Erectile Dysfunction

Causes of Erectile Dysfunction	
Medications	**Neurological Causes**
5-Alpha reductase inhibitors	Injury to peripheral nervous system (pelvic ganglia and lower motor neuron lesions)
Antihypertensive medications (spironolactone, ACE inhibitors/ARB, thiazide diuretics [hydrochlorothiazide])	Stroke or spinal cord injury (upper motor neuron): direct trauma, bone fragment compression, hematoma, tumor, disc compression, ischemia, etc.
Finasteride and Dutasteride	
Antiandrogens, LH-RH antagonist or agonists (leuprolide, degarelix)	Neuropathy (from diabetes mellitus or other etiology)
Cimetidine (H2 blockers)	Trauma (e.g., surgical injury to cavernous nerve)
Psychiatric drugs: selective serotonine reuptake inhibitors (fluoxetine), tricyclic antidepressants, benzodiazepines, phenytoin, antipsychotics (risperidone), etc.	
Vascular Causes	**Endocrine Causes**
Venous leak from cavernosal emissary veins	Hypogonadism (testosterone deficiency)
Arteriosclerosis	Hyperprolactinemia
Arterial insufficiency (from hypertension, hypertriglyceridemia, diabetes, obesity, tobacco use, lack of exercise)	Hyperthyroidism (associated with elevated estrogens)
Surgical Causes	
Radical (cysto)prostatectomy	
Proctectomy	
Pelvic or neurologic/spinal surgeries	

MEDICATION CAUSES

Up to a quarter of ED may be attributed to undesired effects of medications.[8] Many commonly used medications have ED listed as a side effect such as those on Table 52-2. Commonly implicated include 5 alpha-reductase inhibitors, antiandrogens, luteinizing hormone (LH)-releasing hormone analogs and antagonists, antihypertensives, H2 antihistamines, psychiatric medications, and digoxin. Antiandrogens include medications such as bicalutamide and flutamide that are used to treat prostate cancer. Antihypertensives of many classes have been associated with ED including thiazide diuretics, beta-blockers, spironolactone, methyldopa, and clonidine. Multiple classes of psychiatric medications interfere with neurologic and cellular pathways involved in erections such as selective serotonin reuptake inhibitors (sertraline, fluoxetine, etc.), tricyclic antidepressants (e.g., imipramine), benzodiazepines, antipsychotics, and phenytoin.

The total number of medications a man takes including nonprescription medications is correlated with ED even when adjusting for comorbid conditions.[9] Dietary supplements with claims of improving "weight loss," "muscle building," or "sexual enhancement," have unapproved and unlabeled pharmaceutical ingredients including anabolic steroids which may adversely affect erections and alter the hypothalamic-pituitary-testicular axis leading to sexual and reproductive dysfunction.[10] Illicit and recreational substances such as marijuana have been implicated in both endothelial injury and subsequent ED.[11]

SURGICAL CAUSES

Surgeries which interrupt the vascular or neurological supply to the penis can cause ED. Specifically, surgeries that damage the sacral S2 to S4 spinal roots or cavernous nerve, which arises from the inferior hypogastric plexus will result in ED. Nonurologic surgeries such as total proctectomy may precipitate ED. Radical prostatectomy has been implicated in ED and patients undergoing radical prostatectomy should be counselled about the risks of ED as up to 85% of patients may experience some form of postsurgical ED depending on tumor size and extent of nerve-sparing.[4,12] Radiation to the pelvis for treatment of prostate cancer can over time impact autonomic nerves and within 5 years, over half of the men will suffer from ED after radiotherapy.[13]

NEUROLOGICAL CAUSES

As cavernous nerve function is essential to erectile function. Neurologic conditions affecting the parasympathetic pathway will adversely impact erections. Autonomic neuropathy is a common cause of ED especially among diabetic patients via progressive demyelination of peripheral nerves.[3] Diabetic men are at a threefold risk to develop ED, demonstrate worse erectile function than nondiabetic men with ED and a greater impact on their emotional life.[14,15]

ENDOCRINE CAUSES

Endocrine abnormalities can have adverse effects on the cavernosal tissue and sexual response predominantly: hypogonadism (testosterone deficiency), hyperprolactinemia, hypothyroidism, hyperthyroidism, and as previously mentioned diabetes mellitus. Testosterone is responsible for libido and a deficiency may decrease the number of spontaneous nocturnal erections.[16] Hyperprolactinemia, often from prolactin-secreting adenomas or medications (antipsychotics, dopamine receptor blockers such as antiemetics, selective serotoninergic reuptake inhibitor, etc.), and hypothyroidism both suppress LH secretion leading to decreased circulating androgens.[17] Hyperthyroidism alternatively is associated with relatively increased levels of estrogens due to increases in sex hormone binding globulin.[17]

METABOLIC AND LIFESTYLE FACTORS

Lifestyles that negatively impact cardiovascular disease or one's health in general also contribute to ED. This includes stress, sedentary lifestyle, tobacco use, heavy alcohol use especially if causing hepatic insufficiency, renal insufficiency, and illicit drug use.[18]

UROLOGICAL CONDITIONS

Many urological conditions may also affect ED including benign prostatic hyperplasia, chronic prostatitis, pelvic fractures especially if there has been a disruption of the urethra, pelvic surgeries including radical prostatectomy, cystectomy or proctectomy, prior history of penile fracture or priapism, and Peyronie's disease.[18,19] The relationship between benign prostatic hyperplasia and ED may stem from an imbalance in the autonomic control of smooth muscle contraction and relaxation especially with excessive stimulation of alpha1 adrenergic receptors.[20]

ANATOMY AND PHYSIOLOGY OF ERECTIONS

PENILE VASCULAR AND NEUROLOGICAL ANATOMY

The anatomy of the penis including the arrangement of vessels and sinusoids to the fascial and connective tissue location is critical to understand the various etiologies. The arterial supply originates from the anterior branch of the internal iliac artery. This gives rise to the internal pudendal artery then the common penile artery that splits to become the bulbourethral artery, the dorsal artery of the penis, and the deep cavernosal artery. Venous drainage of the corporal bodies occurs via emissary veins which are between the spongy corporal tissue and the tunica albuginea which drain into the deep dorsal vein of the penis. The glans penis is drained by the superficial dorsal penile vein.

The penile erection mechanism occurs via compression of emissary veins as the sinusoids become engorged with blood as the arterioles relax. An erection occurs as blood fills the corpora cavernosa which are two of three corporal bodies which are located on the dorsal aspect of the penis whereas the corpora spongiosum is on the ventral aspect and contains the urethra. The occlusive mechanism is found in the corpora cavernosa whereas the spongiosum does become engorged but does not have as thick **tunica albuginea,** a bilayered connective tissue structure with outer longitudinal and inner circular fibers. The tunica albuginea is relaxed in the flaccid state and stretched in the erect state. The corporal bodies are surrounded by other connective tissue layers, the deeper Buck's fascia, and the more superficial Dartos fascia and most superficial skin. The corpora spongiosum and corpora cavernosum are surrounded by the bulbospongiosus and ischiocaveronosus muscles, respectively, within the pelvis and aid in the rigidity of the erection.[21]

The innervation of the penis includes both autonomic and somatic inputs from pelvic parasympathetic, hypogastric sympathetic, and somatic pudendal nerves. The pelvic ganglion or inferior hypogastric plexus just medial to the internal iliac artery on the posterior-lateral pelvic sidewall houses the autonomic nerves for the penis, including the parasympathetic nerve fibers from sacral nerves derived from S2 to S4 nerve roots and noradrenergic sympathetic nerves from nerve roots T11 to L2.[22] As sympathetic and parasympathetic nerve fibers from the inferior hypogastric plexus near the penis, they coalesce to form the cavernous nerve which innervates the corporal tissues. The parasympathetic nerves are responsible for vasodilation and the stimulation of an erection.[23] Onuf's nucleus which is in the ventral horn of the spinal cord at levels S2 to S4 is responsible for muscular contraction during orgasm and ejaculation.

PHASES OF ERECTION

An erection is divided into four phases: the flaccid, filling, full erection, and rigid erection phases.[24] The arterial smooth muscle contraction maintains a **flaccid state** in which the partial pressure of oxygen is around 35 mmHg.[25] Smooth muscle contraction is maintained by sympathetic nerve inputs whereas sexual stimulation activates the release of neurotransmitters from the nerve terminals beginning the **filling phase**. The relaxation of smooth muscles and dilation of arterioles and arteries increases blood flow as well as blood pressure during systole and diastole. The incoming blood expands the sinusoids and becomes trapped as the venous outflow is reduced when the subtunical venous plexuses are compressed between the tunica albuginea and the peripheral sinusoids. As the tunica are stretches to the capacity, the emissary veins are occluded between the inner and outer layers of the tunica albuginea which further decreases the venous outflow to a minimum. At this point the **full-erection** state occurs and the intracavernous pressure is around 100 mmHg which brings the penis from a dependent position to an erect state. Finally, the rigid erection phase occurs as the ischiocavernousus muscles contract which increases the pressure to several hundred mmHg.[24]

In contrast, penile detumescence occurs in a sequential fashion with a transient rise in intracorporal pressure during the **first phase** which is related to constriction of the cavernous arteries against engorged corpora cavernosa tissue. During the **second phase**, venous drainage begins to occur with a slow pressure decrease, and in the third phase, there is complete restoration to the venous drainage and rapid detumescence.[26]

Erections occur in response to three different pathways: psychogenic, reflexogenic, and nocturnal. The **psychogenic erection** occurs in response to audiovisual stimuli or fantasies and is not maintained in upper spinal cord injuries as it requires input from the forebrain and periaqueductal gray in the midbrain. In contrast, **reflexogenic erections** are preserved in upper spinal cord injuries and occur from tactile stimulation of the genital organs via the ascending pathway and reflex to the cavernous nerves. Finally, **nocturnal erections** occur during rapid eye movement phase of sleep.

NEUROTRANSMITTERS INVOLVED IN ERECTIONS AND DETUMESCENCE

Sympathetic neurotransmitters that are responsible for smooth muscle contraction inhibit erection and promote a flaccid state. **Norepinephrine** is the principal neurotransmitter that contributes to the tonic contraction of the corpora smooth muscle and arterioles by stimulating the alpha-adrenergic receptors in the penile vessels. Endothelin 1, angiotensin II, and intracellular inositol-triphosphate are potent vasoconstrictors and mediate penile flaccidity and detumescence.[27] The neurotransmitters that promote erections include **acetylcholine** via parasympathetic nerves which inhibit adrenergic neurons and stimulate NO synthesis and release stimulating relaxation of the cavernosal smooth muscle. **Nitric oxide** is synthesized by both neuronal and endothelial NO synthase, nNOS, and eNOS, respectively.[28]

After an erection, detumescence is promoted by the cessation of NO synthesis and the breakdown of cyclic guanosine monophosphate (cGMP) via **phosphodiesterase (PDE)** type 5 and this is further promoted via the sympathetic discharges during ejaculation.[29]

PHYSIOLOGY OF CAVERNOSAL SMOOTH MUSCLE

Physiologic mechanisms and molecular pathways resultant in an erection are complex. The smooth muscle of the corpora cavernosa is contracted the majority of the time, unlikely most smooth muscle throughout the body. There are two major molecular mechanisms that promote this contraction: (1) Cytosolic calcium concentration increases and (2) Rho-kinase signaling which is the calcium sensitization pathway. Both mechanisms lead to phosphorylation of Myosin light chain and enable cross bridging with actin and subsequent smooth muscle contraction.[30] The muscle function is coordinated as a functional syncytium because of the presence of ion channels and gap junctions. This facilitates the integrated activity of the muscle and rapid transmission of the neurovascular signals through the corpora.[27]

An erection occurs via parasympathetic noncholinergic nonadrenergic nerve endings activating NO synthase which releases NO, the principal neurotransmitter of penile erection. A wide variety of other molecules, neurotransmitters, and hormones may also be released within the erectile tissue that also effect the erection. The substrates required for NO synthesis (NOS) include L arginine and oxygen, at a level above 55 mmHg partial pressure.[31] The NO diffuses to the adjacent cavernosal or arterial smooth muscle cells and stimulates guanylate cyclase to form cGMP from guanosine triphosphate. Through a cascade of pathways, the cGMP promotes protein kinase-G dependent relaxation through many cellular processes including intracellular calcium decreases and subsequent relaxation of smooth muscle results in an erection.[31] In a separate pathway, prostaglandins such as **prostaglandin E1**, or the medication **alprostadil** (Caverject, Edex) may stimulate adenylate cyclase to convert adenosine triphosphate (ATP) to cyclic adenosine monophosphate (cAMP) signaling, which similarly alters calcium homeostasis and as a result smooth muscle relaxation occurs.[32] PDEs are enzymes responsible for the breakdown of cGMP and cAMP in the penis which opposes the NO pathway, especially PDE type 5 which is primarily responsible for cGMP degradation. Other molecules involved in promoting erections include vasoactive intestinal polypeptide, carbon monoxide, monoamines, amino acids, neuropeptides, and gaseous molecules have also been linked to erection.[32,33] Any disorders, gene, or enzymatic mutation or defects that interfere with the vascular or neuronal pathways has the potential to contribute to ED in men.

CLINICAL FINDINGS

The main clinical finding with ED is the inability to obtain and maintain an erection. As discussed, other clinical findings may include previously undetected cardiovascular disease which may increase a young man's risk of cardiovascular disease up to 50-fold, while ED precedes angina or acute myocardial infarction by 38 months.[34,35] The staging of the disease is discussed later in the section.

DIFFERENTIAL DIAGNOSIS

When evaluating a patient for sexual dysfunction which may be confused with ED, other diagnoses should be considered in the differential or as contributing factors. Some men may report problems with erections when their main complaint is low libido or sexual desire. Ejaculatory disorders such as premature ejaculation or painful ejaculation (dysorgasmia) are also considerations. Some men may have painful erections or penile deformities such as from Peyronie's disease. These conditions and others should be considered as they may be mistaken by the patient or physician as ED or may exacerbate ED symptoms.[18]

Other disorders such as those detailed previously should be explored when taking a history including the libido, problems with ejaculation or orgasm, and any penile deformities or curvatures. Additionally, it is important to be cognizant of other psychosocial factors that may be related to sexual desire and function including social considerations, cultural, religious, educational, the status of the partner(s), and other.[36]

CLINICAL STAGING

Various rigidity scales can be used such as a 0 to 10 scale with 0 being completely flaccid and a 10 being fully rigid. Whereas a 6 may be rigid enough for penetration. Other surveys or physicians use an erection hardness score which grades erection hardness on a 4 point with a score of 4 equates with the penis completely hard and fully rigid.[37]

Validated questionnaires may be used to assess the degree of ED. Many urologists use the International Index of Erectile Function (IIEF) shortened version known as the Sexual Health Inventory of Men (SHIM or IIEF-5), which is a five-question assessment for the severity of ED with each of five questions scored 1-5 with 5 being associated with the best rated sexual function. The questions are specific for erectile function and quantify the severity.[38] A SHIM score of 1-7 indicates severe ED, 8-11 indicates moderate ED, 12-16 is mild/moderate ED, 17-21 is mild ED, and 22-25 is no ED.

DIAGNOSIS AND EVALUATION

When investigating ED clinically, it is important to perform a thorough history and physical examination. The history should include relevant medical, surgical, psychologic, social, medications, and history of pelvic or genital trauma. As with the history of presenting illness for many complaints, the onset, severity, acuity, duration, if it is worsening or stable and situational occurrences (rigidity during partnered relations versus masturbation) should be described or quantified. Acute onset of ED may often be correlated with a psychogenic or new interpersonal conflict or coincide with the addition of a recent change to the patient such as a new medication. Physicians should enquire as to the patient's ability to attain an erection sufficient for penetration and the sustainability until a satisfactory sexual experience is complete. The presence and rigidity of nocturnal erections will provide insight as to a possible psychogenic or organic etiology. Previous erectogenic therapies should be elucidated.

Factors and conditions that are associated with ED include psychological conditions, lifestyle factors, vascular diseases, metabolic disorders, respiratory diseases, urologic conditions, and neurological diseases.

The physical exam should be extensive and include a body mass index, signs of sex characteristics such as beard growth and pubic hair, an absence of which may raise concern for testosterone deficiency. The chest should be examined for gynecomastia. The penis exam should include assessment of the flaccid stretched length, skin lesions, plaque, and the location of the urethra meatus.[36] Palpating and applying pressure on the lateral aspects and also on the dorso-ventral pressure is a method for outlining plaque and septal anatomy. The testicles should be examined for their size, consistency, location, and for the presence of any mass. A digital rectal exam should be considered to assess the prostate for size and possible masses or nodules especially if testosterone replacement is considered.

As patients presenting with ED often have a component of vascular insufficiency, cardiovascular health should be explored. Those patients that can perform three metabolic equivalents are acceptable to proceed with sexual activity. A metabolic equivalent task (MET) is the basal metabolic energy requirement of a person sitting quietly at rest, whereas a sexual activity in long-term couples has been found to range between 2.5 and 3.3 METs.[39] Sexual activity that is energetic or with a new sexual partner may be higher up to 7 in men.[40] An example of 3 METs would be walking along a flat surface for 20 minutes at a brisk pace or climbing two flights of stairs in 10 seconds or less. Those who report dyspnea or angina with a 3 MET equivalent activity should be referred to a cardiologist prior to medical or surgical treatment for ED. Similarly, men with ED have twice the incidence of cardiovascular events compared to the general population and this was even more striking for patients less than 40 years of age who were 7 times more likely to have a cardiovascular event.[41] Thus, younger patients who present with ED, especially at a younger age should be considered to refer to a primary physician or cardiologist with a work-up that includes at a minimum a lipid profile and hemoglobin A1c or fasting glucose test.

AUA guidelines recommend testing total testosterone in all men with ED with testosterone deficiency defined as a level less than 300 ng/dL.[36] Also consider checking thyroid stimulating hormone, complete blood count, hemoglobin A1C, cholesterol panel, and prolactin which may identify abnormalities which are negatively impacting the patients' overall health and erectile function.[16,17,36] If testosterone replacement therapy is planned, a prostate-specific antigen may be beneficial to evaluate for the possibility of prostate cancer which could be exacerbated in such treatment in the work-up for ED.[36]

Vascular Testing

Vascular testing can be performed in a variety of ways. An in-office intracavernous injection with prostaglandin E1 (alprastadil), papaverine, phentolamine, or other vasodilator that can be used to assess for response of an erection. This is performed in the office setting by the physician by injecting the medication with a small needle into the lateral aspect of the corpora cavernosa which avoids the dorsal neurovascular bundle and the ventral urethra. If there is a maintenance of a rigid erection, this would rule out venous leak and confirm adequate veno-occlusive function. However, failure to obtain a rigid erection with this test does not confirm the etiology of the ED.[42]

Penile duplex Doppler ultrasound: It can be performed to assess the arterial integrity and the veno-occlusive mechanism. The AUA guideline suggest such testing may be beneficial to patients with a suspected psychogenic ED to rule out a vascular or organic etiology or in men with previous pelvic trauma or lifelong ED who may be candidates for surgical intervention, in men who have Peyronie's disease who are candidates for penile reconstruction and for identification of men with veno-occlusive dysfunction who are unlikely to benefit from medical therapy.[36] This sonography method uses a 7.5–12 MHz transducer to image the penis after intracavernous injection and audiovisual stimulation. The arterial flow is examined in each of the cavernous arteries with the peak systolic velocity (PSV) of greater than 30 cm per second considered normal and $<$ 25 cm/sec as evidence of severe arterial insufficiency. The PSV is measured with the probe and vessel doppler angle at 60°. Cavernous artery end-diastolic velocity should be identified with a velocity $<$ 3 cm/s normal and greater than 5 cm/s as evidence of venous leak.[43]

Cavernosometry: Cavernosometry is a more sensitive test to detect veno-occlusive dysfunction which is performed by placing two needles into the corpora. One needle measures the pressure while the other is used to infuse heparinized saline into the corpora. The saline is infused to generate an intracavernosal pressure of 30, 60, 90, 120, and 150 mmHg. The flow rate of the saline is measured and should be linear indicating maximal cavernosal artery dilation and often an erectogenic intracavernosal injection (ICI) is given. The flow that is required to maintain the pressure of 150 mmHg is noted and then the infusion is stopped. The pressure decay is measured and veno-occlusion is present when the intracavernosal pressure declines by more than 45 mmHg in 30 seconds. Whereas the flow rate of saline, required to, maintain a rigid erection at 150 mmHg pressure as blood flows out of the corpora, is known as the "flow to maintain". Venous leak is present when the flow to maintain is greater than 5 mL per minute.[44] Cavernosography can be used as an adjunct to visualize the area of leakage during a cavernosometry by adding contrast to the infusion solution. Isolated or primary venous leakage as the cause for ED is rare, but some authors have advocated for penile venous surgery with crural ligation. In a case series of 26 men at a mean follow up of 42.9 months, 73% of men had partial or complete resolution (42.3%) of their ED.[45]

The AUA guidelines do not recommend ligation of the venous channels as a treatment for ED as the heterogeneous body of literature does not offer favorable outcomes. This is likely due to difficulty diagnosing the appropriate subpopulation for which veno-occlusive dysfunction is the main etiology of ED and the most effective surgical techniques for correction.[36]

Pudendal angiography: Pudendal angiography is another vascular test which can delineate the anatomy of the penile vasculature when there is a suspicion of arteriogenic ED.[46] It is an invasive test to confirm vasculogenic ED and should only be used if considering operative revascularization. It is performed with the patient in the [illegible] with intra arterial vasodilators and may diagnose or rule out stenotic internal pudendal or cavernosal arteries as an etiology for ED.

MANAGEMENT OF THE CLINICAL PROBLEM

MEDICAL TREATMENT

Medical treatment for ED should include a medical evaluation as described in the previous section. Initial guidance and management should include improving lifestyle factors which can cause or exacerbate ED including smoking cessation, exercise, stress reduction, control of metabolic disease, and treatment to improve other comorbidities such as hypertension and diabetes mellitus. This may involve referral to an internist or other subspecialists.[47–49] There is evidence that eliminating or minimizing risk factors for cardiovascular disease may improve erectile health in function. Lifestyle changes are more effective when started at an earlier age. Furthermore, improving one's diet to include healthier foods such as the **Mediterranean diet**, which is high in fruits and vegetables as well as nuts, whole grains, fish, and polyunsaturated oils while minimizing processed foods, saturated fats processed meat, and refined grains, leads to improvement in erectile function.[50] Patients should be counseled to avoid tobacco products as there is a dose-related association between tobacco use and ED.[51] Alcohol consumed in moderation defined as 1–2 servings per day or less may improve erectile function due to inhibition on anti-erectogenic sympathetic tone, whereas more than 3 per day or 14 drinks per week can worsen ED via central nervous system sedation, associated decreased libido and potential of alcoholic polyneuropathy, liver dysfunction, estrogen, and testosterone derangements.[52,53]

Adjustments to avoid **antihypertensive** medications which are more likely to interfere with ED should be discussed with the patient and prescribing physician. Nonspecific beta-blockers such as metoprolol and thiazide diuretic which increase angiotensin and therefore sympathetic tone.[54,55] Other medications include antiandrogens, cannabis, anti-[illegible] inhibitors (e.g., fluoxetine(Prozac)), opioids, and other and should be avoided after a shared decision-making process with the patient.[11,56–58]

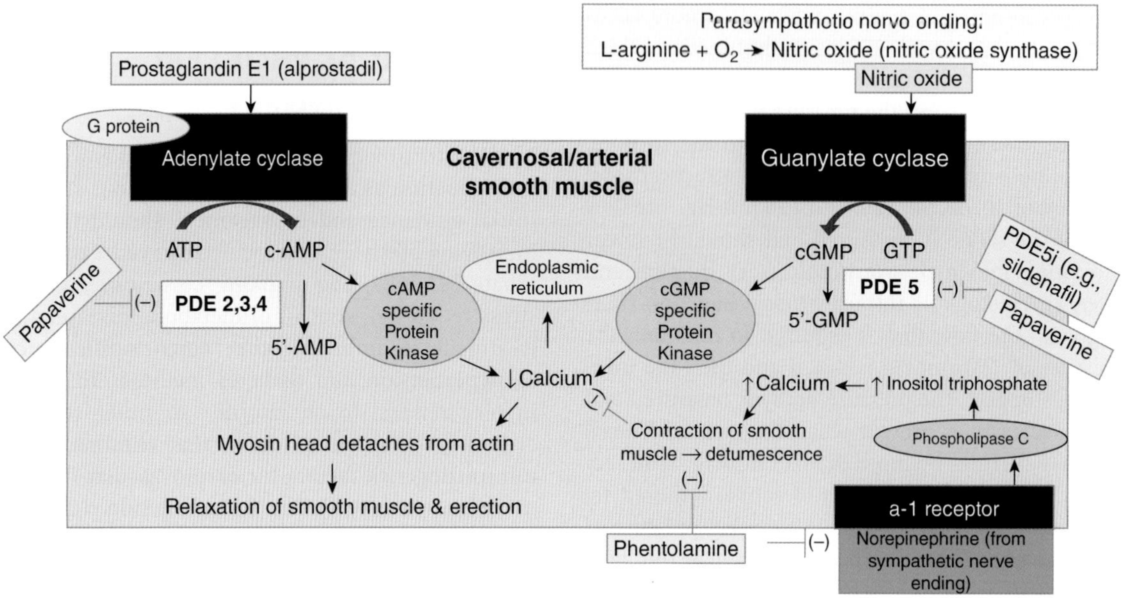

FIGURE 52-1 **Mechanism of penile erection by smooth muscle relaxation and site of action of erectogenic agents.**

Herbal supplements for the treatment of ED have variable success and studies are of low quality. Some common agents used include dehydroepiandrosterone, yohimbine, ginkgo biloba, L-arginine, and ginsengs.[59] These over the counter products in many instances are contaminated with other medications such as PDE inhibitors or toxins including heavy metals.[60]

The AUA recommends discussing lifestyle measures that can improve ED and overall health. Using shared decision making, based on the values of the patient and his partner, all treatment options should be discussed and offer except for those which are contraindicated. The five main treatments that can be considered and re-evaluated for satisfaction and success after implementation are: PDE inhibitors, vacuum devices, intraurethral alprostadil, ICIs, and penile prosthesis surgery.[36]

PDE type-5 is the predominant PDE enzyme in the penis. PDE5 hydrolyzes cGMP to the inactive form of GMP and as previously mentioned cGMP is a key regulator of calcium hemostasis which reduces cytoplasmic calcium and promotes erectogenic vasodilation.[61,62] Some common **PDE type-5 inhibitors** which promote erections are: sildenafil (Viagra, Revatio), vardenafile (Levitra, Staxyn), tadalafil (Cialis), and avanafil (Stendra, Auxillium). The mechanism of these medications and other erectogenic medications is illustrated in Figure 52-1. PDE5 inhibitors have demonstrated superior erectile response rate compared to placebo but do require intact cavernous nerves which stimulate the production of cGMP. Thus, those with cavernous nerve injury such as patients who have undergone radical prostatectomy (without nerve-sparing) or who have severe autonomic neuropathy from diabetes mellitus will likely fail PDE5 inhibitors.[63]

Contraindications to PDE5 inhibitors should be noted as serious side effects and can be seen such as life-threatening hypotension if taken with nitrates. Other common reactions include headache, flushing, sinusitis, rhinitis, and visual disturbances such as impaired color vision. Caution should be used in men who take alpha blockers for blood pressure or lower urinary tract dysfunction due to the risk of hypotension. Alpha blockers should be at least 4 hours apart from PDE5 inhibitors.[64] Vardenafil can increase the risk for torsade de points in men with congenital long QT syndrome and should be avoided in patients which take medications that my increase the QT interval including some antiarrhythmics such as amiodarone, sotalol, and quinidine.

A PDE5 inhibitor should not be used for the treatment of ED if the patient has suffered a myocardial infarction within the past 90 days or has unstable angina especially angina with sexual activity. These medications should be avoided if the patient has New York Heart Association class II (or greater) heart failure within 6 months, or the patient has had a stroke within 6 months, or the patient reports uncontrolled hypertension (>170/100 mmHg) or hypotension (<90/50 mmHg), or hereditary generative retinal disorders such as retinitis pigmentosa, or the patient has uncontrolled arrhythmias, or risk factors for priapism such as sickle cell or leukemia.[65]

Mechanical or vacuum erection devices are effective treatments for ED which create a negative pressure environment around the penis that produces an erection, with up to 93% success rate.[66] Prescription vacuum erection devices are available which have a safety "pop off" valve which limits the risk of overpressurization injury. The device via negative pressure help dilate the cavernous space which pulls blood into the penis and a constriction device or band near the base of the penis can prevent venous outflow. These devices can lead to petechiae formation or hematoma if the device is overpressurized. With excessively long use (greater than 30 minutes) or if the band is left too long on skin, necrosis can occur.[67] These devices may be contraindicated in patients on anticoagulants.

Intra urethral suppositories are another option for the treatment of ED in men which are administered via the urethral meatus. Medicated Urethral System for Erections (MUSE™) is a commercially available system in which alprostadil is the active ingredient. The response rate for patients with mild ED was >90%.[68] The prostaglandin diffuses across the urethra into the corpora spongiosum and then into the corpora cavernosa through collateral vessels. This increases intracellular levels of cAMP in the smooth muscle causing the erection. It is recommended that the first dose be administered in the office to monitor for efficacy or adverse effects such as hypotension. Other adverse effects include penile pain which can occur in up to one-third of patients, urethral burning or minor urethral bleeding, irritation, testicular pain, and pain in the female partner's vagina.[68] If the female partner is pregnant, a barrier condom should be used to avoid induction of labor.

As discussed in the diagnostic section, ICI therapy can be utilized to administer an erectogenic medication which can be diagnostic and therapeutic. Around 90% of patients with ED will respond to these medications.[69] Patients can be taught in the office setting how to perform self-injections which can be performed immediately prior to sexual activity. The agents or combination of medications are injected via a 29-31 gauge needle directly into the cavernosa. A common formulation is alprostadil (Caverject, Edex) which is prostaglandin E1 a direct cAMP stimulator and relaxant of arterial smooth muscle. Another common formulation is Trimix, which is a combination of alprostadil, papaverine, and phenotolamine. Papaverine is a nonspecific PDE inhibitor which increases intracellular cAMP and cGMP by inhibiting their degradation.[70] Phentolamine is a reversible alpha-adrenergic receptor antagonist which blocks sympathetic neuronal input to the smooth muscle. A test dose of these medications should be given in the office by a medical professional and the provider must ensure the patient is flaccid prior to leaving the office as the most serious common adverse event of ICI is priapism, occurring in less than 1% of patients.[71] Other adverse events of ICI including ecchymosis, hematoma, headache, and dizziness which are rare. Men who are unable to perform the injection (with partners unable to perform the injection) are not candidates for ICI. Other contraindications include patients with increased risk of priapism such as sickle cell anemia, leukemia, or history of priapism. Altered anatomy such as scarring from Pyeronie's disease, a short or concealed penis, patients with a large panniculus, poor vision, or poor manual dexterity are poor candidates for ICI. Patients who take monoamine oxidase inhibitors medications should not take alpha-adrenergic medications such as phenylephrine, that may cause the patient to develop priapism.

For patients who do not have satisfactory erections on one therapy may combine therapies. For example, a man who does not achieve erections firm enough with one PDE5 inhibitors may try a combination of PDE5 inhibitor and ICIs, where up to half of the patients may respond to this combination over sildenafil alone.[72] This may be particularly useful in men who have had radical prostatectomies.[73]

Other patients may benefit from sexual stimulation where penetrative intercourse is not performed as a firm erection is not a requirement for sensation, orgasm, or ejaculation. The degree of bother is important as some patients may have meaningful sexual experiences without erections firm enough for penetration or prioritize sexual function as a vital aspect of their relationship with their partner while others have satisfactory romantic and interpersonal relationships without a sexual component. For patients who are not interested in additional medical or surgical therapies, or patients experiencing psychogenic ED, a sex therapist or psychological counselor is beneficial.

SURGICAL TREATMENT

Surgical options for ED can be offered to patients who do not wish to attempt medical therapies or fail them. Crural ligation or venous ligation for venous insufficiency is not recommended any more by the AUA due to low cure rates and difficulty determining which techniques and patient selection are optimal for acceptable outcomes.[36]

Penile revascularization has been reported as restoring ED in young men without diabetes and other comorbid conditions who present with arterial lesions, perhaps secondary to previous blunt pelvic trauma and pelvic vasculature injury or other etiology. Because of the widespread prevalence of ED and only a small subset of patients who would benefit, revascularization surgery is often omitted from most urologists' repertoire in favor of penile prosthesis. There are different techniques described for penile revascularization. Hauri's technique for revascularization uses isolation of the inferior epigastric artery and anastomosis to the dorsal penile artery and deep dorsal penile vein with 7-0 nonabsorbable suture.[74] Another technique described is the Furlow–Fisher modified Virag V technique of deep dorsal vein arterialization in which the epigastric artery is anastomosed to the deep dorsal vein with ligation of the dorsal vein proximal to the anastomosis and a ligature of the most distal aspect of the vein just proximal to the glans.[75,76] Currently, surgeons perform penile revascularization most commonly by anastomosing the inferior epigastric artery to the dorsal penile vein, artery, or both in various arrangements.[77] In one study, patients underwent the either the Hauri procedure when there where communicating branches between the dorsal and cavernosal arteries on doppler ultrasound and digital subtraction angiography or the Furlow–Fisher modification of the Virag V if there was an obstruction in the proximal common penile artery and thus no communicating branches; 85.9% of patients having an erectile function at 3 years and 67.5% of patients having an erectile function at 5 years.[78]

The mainstay of surgical treatment is penile prosthesis in which a device is surgically implanted into the corpora cavernosa. Surgical treatment is for patients who have failed nonsurgical management for ED or patients who cannot withstand nonsurgical management. The two main types of prostheses are inflatable and noninflatable (malleable). The **noninflatable prostheses** are the most mechanically simple with two flexible rods that are inserted into each corporal body. Inflatable prosthesis come in two piece or three-piece inflatable prosthesis. The **two-piece inflatable prothesis** (Ambicor®, Boston Scientific) allows for a fully rigid erection but in the flaccid state will have partial tumescence as the device is pre-filled without a reservoir for which the cylinders can completely empty.[79] A **three-piece inflatable prosthesis** (Boston Scientific 700-CX®, 700-CXR® or Coloplast Titan®) has a reservoir where fluid cycles into the cylinders to produce rigidity and erection.[80] A pump is placed in the scrotum which can be squeezed multiple times to inflate the implant and a button to deflate when sexual activity is complete. The reservoir is usually placed in the pre-vesical space through the inguinal ring or via a counter suprapubic incision, or alternatively in a subcutaneous, subfascial, or submuscular between the peritoneum and transversalis fascia or just deep to the rectus abdominus locations in the abdominal wall.[81] It is important to counsel the patient appropriately for expectations with the prosthesis including postoperative penile length, appearance, and sexual function. As the procedure is done electively adequate glucose control should be maintained prior to surgery with a hemoglobin A1c of less than 8.5% and the patients should stop smoking tobacco.[82] The incision for placement of the prosthesis can be sub-coronal, penoscrotal, or infrapubic. Once the tunica albuginea is exposed, a longitudinal corporotomy is made into the corporal bodies providing access into the cavernous sinuses. To dilate the instrument such as a Hegar, dilator should be aimed slightly laterally and dorsally to minimize the risk of urethral perforation.[83] For patients who have concomitant Pyronine's disease, there may be difficulty with dilation because of corporal fibrosis. The surgeon can straighten the penis with modeling, which is forceful bending of the penis in the opposite direction of the plaque with the implant partial inflated, with plication or with incision and/or grafting.[84] Complications can occur with placement of the penile prosthesis including infection, malfunction, urethral, or crural perforation. Despite perioperative antibiotics, extensive prepping of the surgical site with antimicrobials and infection retardant coating, and surgical site infections occur in approximately 1% to 2% of cases.[82,85] If infected, the patient can present with fever, pain, erythema, purulent drainage from the incision, or crepitus in the penis or scrotum with fixation of the scrotal pump to the skin. Patients can be counseled that the device has a 28.5% chance of mechanical failure and may be in need for replacement over a 10 year period.[86]

PATHWAY OF TREATMENT

Patients should be evaluated and then offered all treatments which are not indicated. Patients willing to undergo medical and lifestyle changes should be offered these less invasive treatments when their clinical situation favors success with such therapies. Figure 52-2 demonstrates the workup including history, physical examination, and appropriate laboratory testing as described previously in the chapter. After counseling and implementing lifestyle changes, a patient can choose appropriate medical and surgical management to which there are no contraindications. The flow chart walks the provider through various surgical and medical therapies and if the patient is not satisfied, the various options are explored again.

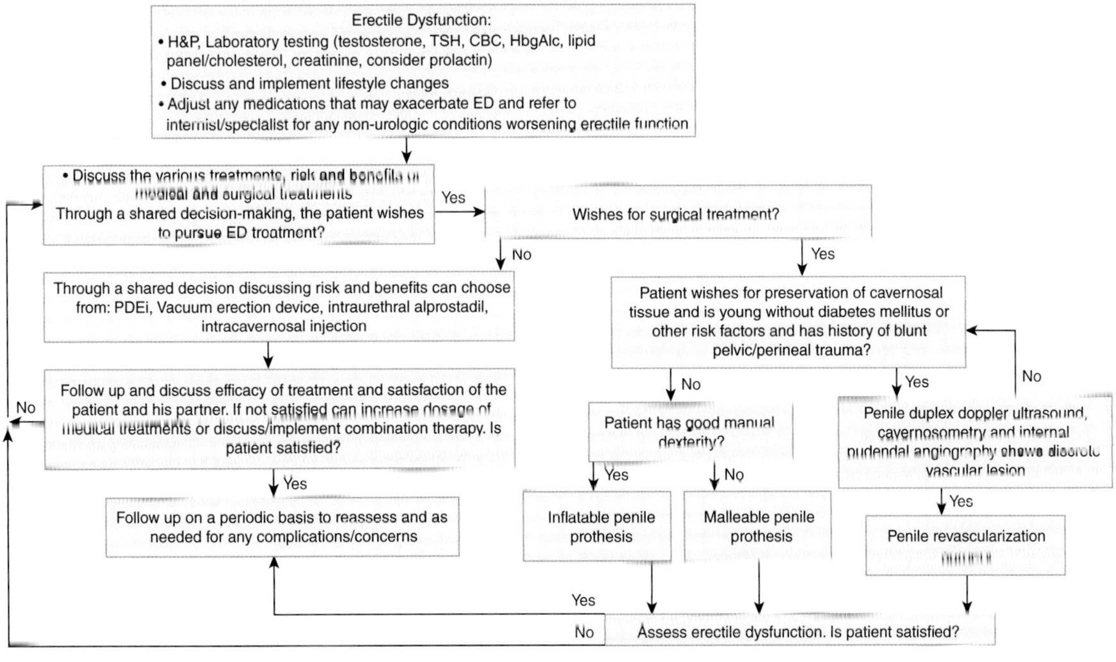

FIGURE 52-2 **Flow chart for the diagnosis, evaluation, and management of erectile dysfunction.**

REFERENCES

1. Laumann EO, West S, Glasser D, Carson C, Rosen R, Kang JH. Prevalence and correlates of erectile dysfunction by race and ethnicity among men aged 40 or older in the United States: from the male attitudes regarding sexual health survey. *J Sex Med.* 2007;4(1):57-65.
2. Melman A, Gingell JC. The epidemiology and pathophysiology of erectile dysfunction. *J Urol.* 1999;161(1):5-11.
3. Ziegler D. Diagnosis and treatment of diabetic autonomic neuropathy. *Curr Diab Rep.* 2001;1(3):216-227.
4. Nelson CJ, Scardino PT, Eastham JA, Mulhall JP. Back to baseline: erectile function recovery after radical prostatectomy from the patients' perspective. *J Sex Med.* 2013;10(6):1636-1643.
5. Ghanem H, Porst H. Etiology and risk factors of erectile dysfunction. *Standard Practice in Sexual Medicine/H Ghanem, H Porst—Blackwell Publishing.* 2006:49-58.
6. Bacon CG, Mittleman MA, Kawachi I, Giovannucci E, Glasser DB, Rimm EB. A prospective study of risk factors for erectile dysfunction. *J Urol.* 2006;176(1):217-221.
7. Musicki B, Kramer MF, Becker RE, Burnett AL. Inactivation of phosphorylated endothelial nitric oxide synthase (Ser-1177) by O-GlcNAc in diabetes-associated erectile dysfunction. *Proc Natl Acad Sci USA.* 2005;102(33):11870-11875.
8. Francis ME, Kusek JW, Nyberg LM, Eggers PW. The contribution of common medical conditions and drug exposures to erectile dysfunction in adult males. *J Urol.* 2007;178(2):591-596; discussion 596.
9. Londoño DC, Slezak JM, Quinn VP, Van Den Eeden SK, Loo RK, Jacobsen SJ. Population-based study of erectile dysfunction and polypharmacy. *BJU Int.* 2012;110(2):254-259.
10. Tucker J, Fischer T, Upjohn L, Mazzera D, Kumar M. Unapproved pharmaceutical ingredients included in dietary supplements associated with US Food and Drug Administration warnings. *JAMA Netw Open.* 2018;1(6):e183337-e183337.
11. Aversa A, Rossi F, Francomano D, et al. Early endothelial dysfunction as a marker of vasculogenic erectile dysfunction in young habitual cannabis users. *Int J Impot Res.* 2008;20(6):566-573.
12. Emanu JC, Avildsen IK, Nelson CJ. Erectile dysfunction after radical prostatectomy: prevalence, medical treatments, and psychosocial interventions. *Curr Opin Support Palliat Care.* 2016;10(1):102-107.
13. Gaither TW, Awad MA, Osterberg EC, et al. The natural history of erectile dysfunction after prostatic radiotherapy: a systematic review and meta-analysis. *J Sex Med.* 2017;14(9):1071-1078.
14. Penson DF, Latini DM, Lubeck DP, Wallace KL, Henning JM, Lue TF. Do impotent men with diabetes have more severe erectile dysfunction and worse quality of life than the general population of impotent patients? Results from the exploratory comprehensive evaluation of erectile dysfunction (ExCEED) database. *Diabetes Care.* 2003;26(4):1093-1099.
15. Hakim LS, Goldstein I. Diabetic sexual dysfunction. *Endocrinol Metab Clin North Am.* 1996;25(2):379-400.
16. Bhasin S, Enzlin P, Coviello A, Basson R. Sexual dysfunction in men and women with endocrine disorders. *Lancet.* 2007;369(9561):597-611.
17. Maggi M, Buvat J, Corona G, Guay A, Torres LO. Hormonal causes of male sexual dysfunctions and their management (hyperprolactinemia, thyroid disorders, GH disorders, and DHEA). *J Sex Med.* 2013;10(3):661-677.
18. Althof SE, Rosen RC, Perelman MA, Rubio-Aurioles E. Standard operating procedures for taking a sexual history. *J Sex Med.* 2013;10(1):26-35.
19. De Nunzio C, Roehrborn CG, Andersson KE, McVary KT. Erectile dysfunction and lower urinary tract symptoms. *Eur Urol Focus.* 2017;3(4-5):352-363.
20. Rosen RC, Giuliano F, Carson CC. Sexual dysfunction and lower urinary tract symptoms (LUTS) associated with benign prostatic hyperplasia (BPH). *Eur Urol.* 2005;47(6):824-837.
21. Claes H, Bijnens B, Baert L. The hemodynamic influence of the ischiocavernosus muscles on erectile function. *J Urol.* 1996;156(3):986-990.
22. Yang CC, Jiang X. Clinical autonomic neurophysiology and the male sexual response: an overview. *J Sex Med.* 2009;6 Suppl 3(suppl 3):221-228.
23. Oakley SH, Mutema GK, Crisp CC, et al. Innervation and histology of the clitoral–urethal complex: a cross-sectional cadaver study. *J Sex Med.* 2013;10(9):2211-2218.
24. Dean RC, Lue TF. Physiology of penile erection and pathophysiology of erectile dysfunction. *Urol Clin North Am.* 2005;32(4):379-395, v.
25. Sattar AA, Salpigides G, Vanderhaeghen JJ, Schulman CC, Wespes E. Cavernous oxygen tension and smooth muscle fibers: relation and function. *J Urol.* 1995;154(5):1736-1739.
26. Bosch RJ, Benard F, Aboseif SR, Stief CG, Lue TF, Tanagho EA. Penile detumescence: characterization of three phases. *J Urol.* 1991;146(3):867-871.
27. Christ GJ, Richards S, Winkler A. Integrative erectile biology: the role of signal transduction and cell-to-cell

communication in coordinating corporal smooth muscle tone and penile erection. *Int J Impot Res*. 1997; 9(2):69-84.

28. Toda N, Ayajiki K, Okamura T. Nitric oxide and penile erectile function. *Pharmacol Ther*. 2005;106(2):233-266.
29. Corbin JD, Beasley A, Turko IV, et al. A photoaffinity probe covalently modifies the catalytic site of the cGMP-binding cGMP-specific phosphodiesterase (PDE-5). *Cell Biochem Biophys*. 1998;29(1-2):145-157.
30. Chitaley K, Wingard CJ, Clinton Webb R, et al. Antagonism of Rho-kinase stimulates rat penile erection via a nitric oxide-independent pathway. *Nat Med*. 2001;7(1):119-122.
31. Burnett AL, Musicki B. The nitric oxide signaling pathway in the penis. *Curr Pharm Des*. 2005; 11(31):3987-3994.
32. Andersson KE. Mechanisms of penile erection and basis for pharmacological treatment of erectile dysfunction. *Pharmacol Rev*. 2011;63(4):811-859.
33. Juenemann KP, Lue TF, Luo JA, Jadallah SA, Nunes LL, Tanagho EA. The role of vasoactive intestinal polypeptide as a neurotransmitter in canine penile erection: a combined in vivo and immunohistochemical study. *J Urol*. 1987;138(4):871-877.
34. Montorsi F, Briganti A, Salonia A, et al. Erectile dysfunction prevalence, time of onset and association with risk factors in 300 consecutive patients with acute chest pain and angiographically documented coronary artery disease. *Eur Urol*. 2003;44(3):360-364; discussion 364-365.
35. Inman BA, Sauver JLS, Jacobson DJ, et al. A population-based, longitudinal study of erectile dysfunction and future coronary artery disease. Paper presented at Mayo Clinic Proceedings 2009.
36. Burnett AL, Nehra A, Breau RH, et al. Erectile dysfunction: AUA guideline. *J Urol*. 2018;200(3):633-641.
37. Mulhall JP, Goldstein I, Bushmakin AG, Cappelleri JC, Hvidsten K. Validation of the erection hardness score. *J Sex Med*. 2007;4(6):1626-1634.
38. Rosen RC, Cappelleri JC, Smith MD, Lipsky J, Peña BM. Development and evaluation of an abridged, 5-item version of the International Index of Erectile Function (IIEF-5) as a diagnostic tool for erectile dysfunction. *Int J Impot Res*. 1999;11(6):319-326.
39. Bohlen JG, Held JP, Sanderson MO, Patterson RP. Heart rate, rate-pressure product, and oxygen uptake during four sexual activities. *Arch Intern Med*. 1984;144(9):1745-1748.
40. Palmeri ST, Kostis JB, Casazza L, et al. Heart rate and blood pressure response in adult men and women during exercise and sexual activity. *Am J Cardiol*. 2007;100(12):1795-1801.
41. Chew K-K, Finn J, Stuckey B, et al. Erectile dysfunction as a predictor for subsequent atherosclerotic cardiovascular events: findings from a linked-data study. *J Sex Med*. 2010;7(1):192-202.
42. Shabsigh R, Padma-Nathan H, Gittleman M, McMurray J, Kaufman J, Goldstein I. Intracavernous alprostadil alfadex (EDEX/VIRIDAL) is effective and safe in patients with erectile dysfunction after failing sildenafil (Viagra). *Urology*. 2000;55(4):477-480.
43. Sikka SC, Hellstrom WJ, Brock G, Morales AM. Standardization of vascular assessment of erectile dysfunction. *J Sex Med*. 2013;10(1):120-129.
44. Teloken PE, Park K, Parker M, Guhring P, Narus J, Mulhall JP. The false diagnosis of venous leak: prevalence and predictors. *J Sex Med*. 2011;8(8): 2344-2349.
45. Çayan S. Primary penile venous leakage surgery with crural ligation in men with erectile dysfunction. *J Urol*. 2008;180(3):1056-1059.
46. Dabaja AA, Teloken P, Mulhall JP. A critical analysis of candidacy for penile revascularization. *J Sex Med*. 2014;11(9):2327-2332.
47. Esposito K, Ciotola M, Giugliano F, et al. Effects of intensive lifestyle changes on erectile dysfunction in men. *J Sex Med*. 2009;6(1):243-250.
48. Derby CA, Mohr BA, Goldstein I, Feldman HA, Johannes CB, McKinlay JB. Modifiable risk factors and erectile dysfunction: can lifestyle changes modify risk? *Urology*. 2000;56(2):302-306.
49. Christensen BS, Grønbaek M, Osler M, Pedersen BV, Graugaard C, Frisch M. Associations between physical and mental health problems and sexual dysfunctions in sexually active Danes. *J Sex Med*. 2011;8(7): 1890-1902.
50. Esposito K, Giugliano F, Maiorino MI, Giugliano D. Dietary factors, mediterranean diet and erectile dysfunction. *J Sex Med*. 2010;7(7):2338-2345.
51. Kupelian V, Link CL, McKinlay JB. Association between smoking, passive smoking, and erectile dysfunction: results from the Boston area community health (BACH) survey. *Eur Urol*. 2007;52(2):416-422.
52. Wang XM, Bai YJ, Yang YB, Li JH, Tang Y, Han P. Alcohol intake and risk of erectile dysfunction: a dose-response meta-analysis of observational studies. *Int J Impot Res*. 2018;30(6):342-351.
53. Pendharkar S, Mattoo SK, Grover S. Sexual dysfunctions in alcohol-dependent men: a study from north India. *Indian J Med Res*. 2016;144(3):393-399.

54. Grimm RH Jr, Grandits GA, Prineas RJ, et al. Long-term effects on sexual function of five antihypertensive drugs and nutritional hygienic treatment in hypertensive men and women. Treatment of mild hypertension study (TOMHS). *Hypertension*. 1997;29(1 Pt 1): 8-14.
55. La Torre A, Giupponi G, Duffy D, Conca A, Catanzariti D. Sexual dysfunction related to drugs: a critical review. Part IV: cardiovascular drugs. *Pharmacopsychiatry*. 2015;48(1):1-6.
56. Rosen RC, Lane RM, Menza M. Effects of SSRIs on sexual function: a critical review. *J Clin Psychopharmacol*. 1999;19(1):67-85.
57. Cioe PA, Friedmann PD, Stein MD. Erectile dysfunction in opioid users: lack of association with serum testosterone. *J Addict Dis*. 2010;29(4):455-460.
58. Ahmadi H, Daneshmand S. Androgen deprivation therapy: evidence-based management of side effects. *BJU Int*. 2013;111(4):543-548.
59. Tamler R, Mechanick JI. Dietary supplements and nutraceuticals in the management of andrologic disorders. *Endocrinol Metab Clin North Am*. 2007;36(2):533-552.
60. Jackson G, Arver S, Banks I, Stecher VJ. Counterfeit phosphodiesterase type 5 inhibitors pose significant safety risks. *Int J Clin Pract*. 2010;64(4):497-504.
61. Goldstein I, Lue TF, Padma-Nathan H, Rosen RC, Steers WD, Wicker PA. Oral sildenafil in the treatment of erectile dysfunction. Sildenafil study group. *N Engl J Med*. 1998;338(20):1397-1404.
62. Sopko NA, Hannan JL, Bivalacqua TJ. Understanding and targeting the Rho kinase pathway in erectile dysfunction. *Nat Rev Urol*. 2014;11(11):622-628.
63. Gontero P, Kirby R. Proerectile pharmacological prophylaxis following nerve-sparing radical prostatectomy (NSRP). *Prostate Cancer Prostatic Dis*. 2004;7(3):223-226.
64. Porst H, Burnett A, Brock G, et al. SOP conservative (medical and mechanical) treatment of erectile dysfunction. *J Sex Med*. 2013;10(1):130-171.
65. Brien JC, Trussell JC. Erectile dysfunction for primary care providers. *Can J Urol*. 2008;15(suppl 1):63-70; discussion 70.
66. Zippe CD, Pahlajani G. Vacuum erection devices to treat erectile dysfunction and early penile rehabilitation following radical prostatectomy. *Curr Urol Rep*. 2008;9(6):506-513.
67. Sidi AA, Lewis JH. Clinical trial of a simplified vacuum erection device for impotence treatment. *Urology*. 1992;39(6):526-528.
68. Lewis R. Combined use of transurethral alprostadil and an adjustable penile constriction band in men with erectile dysfunction: results from a multicenter trial. Paper presented at: Journal of Urology 1998.
69. Glina S, Virag R, Luis Rhoden E, Sharlip ID. Intracavernous injection of papaverine for erectile failure R. Virag. *J Sex Med*. 2010;7(4pt1):1331-1335.
70. Virag R, Shoukry K, Floresco J, Nollet F, Greco E. Intracavernous self-injection of vasoactive drugs in the treatment of impotence: 8-year experience with 615 cases. *J Urol*. 1991;145(2):287-292.
71. Coombs PG, Heck M, Guhring P, Narus J, Mulhall JP. A review of outcomes of an intracavernosal injection therapy programme. *BJU Int*. 2012;110(11):1787-1791.
72. McMahon CG, Samali R, Johnson H. Treatment of intracorporeal injection nonresponse with sildenafil alone or in combination with triple agent intracorporeal injection therapy. *J Urol*. 1999;162(6):1992-1998.
73. Mydlo JH, Viterbo R, Crispen P. Use of combined intracorporal injection and a phosphodiesterase-5 inhibitor therapy for men with a suboptimal response to sildenafil and/or vardenafil monotherapy after radical retropubic prostatectomy. *BJU Int*. 2005;95(6):843-846.
74. Hauri D. A new operative technique in vasculogenic erectile impotence. *World J Urol*. 1986;4(4):237-249.
75. Furlow W, Fisher J, Knoll L, Benson R, Motley R, Lee I. Current status of penile revascularization with deep dorsal vein arterialization: experience with 95 patients. *Int J Impot Res*. 1990;2(suppl 2):348.
76. Virag R, Zwang G, Dermange H, Legman M, Penven J. Investigation and surgical treatment of vasculogenic impotency (author's transl). *Journal des maladies vasculaires*. 1980;5(3):205-209.
77. Zuckerman JM, McCammon KA, Tisdale BE, et al. Outcome of penile revascularization for arteriogenic erectile dysfunction after pelvic fracture urethral injuries. *Urology*. 2012;80(6):1369-1374.
78. Kawanishi Y, Kimura K, Nakanishi R, Kojima K, Numata A. Penile revascularization surgery for arteriogenic erectile dysfunction: the long-term efficacy rate calculated by survival analysis. *BJU Int*. 2004; 94(3):361-368.
79. Gentile G, Franceschelli A, Massenio P, et al. Patient's satisfaction after 2-piece inflatable penile prosthesis implantation: an Italian multicentric study. *Archivio Italiano di Urologia e Andrologia*. 2016:1-3.
80. Montorsi F, Rigatti P, Carmignani G, et al. AMS three-piece inflatable implants for erectile dysfunction: a long-term multi-institutional study in 200 consecutive patients. *Eur Urol*. 2000;37(1):50-55.

81. Henry G, Hsiao W, Karpman E, et al. A guide for inflatable penile prosthesis reservoir placement: pertinent anatomical measurements of the retropubic space. *J Sex Med.* 2014;11(1):273-278.
82. Hebert KJ, Kohler TS. Penile prosthesis infection: myths and realities. *World J Mens Health.* 2019;37(3):276-287.
83. Chung E, Van C, Wilson I, Cartmill R. Penile prosthesis implantation for the treatment for male erectile dysfunction: clinical outcomes and lessons learnt after 955 procedures. *World J Urol.* 2013;31(3):591-595.
84. Nehra A, Alterowitz R, Culkin DJ, et al. Peyronie's disease: AUA guideline. *J Urol.* 2015;194(3):745-753.
85. Mandava SH, Serefoglu EC, Freier MT, Wilson SK, Hellstrom WJ. Infection retardant coated inflatable penile prostheses decrease the incidence of infection: a systematic review and meta-analysis. *J Urol.* 2012;188(5):1855-1860.
86. Carson CC, Mulcahy JJ, Govier FE. Efficacy, safety and patient satisfaction outcomes of the AMS 700CX inflatable penile prosthesis: results of a long-term multicenter study. *J Urol.* 2000;164(2):376-380.

SELF-ASSESSMENT STUDY QUESTIONS AND ANSWERS

Questions

1. Ten weeks after having placement of a two-piece inflatable penile prosthesis, a 66-year-old man reports that he has decreased penis size and is unable to satisfy his partner. On examination, he has a fully functional prosthesis. The next step is:
A. Referral to a psychologist specializing in sex therapy
B. Prescribe sildenafil to be taken at least 60 minutes prior to sexual activity
C. Upsize to a larger two-piece prosthesis
D. Removal and simultaneous placement of a three-piece prosthesis

2. A 41-year-old man with diabetes uses intracavernosal injection to treat his erectile dysfunction and develops a painful erection for over 5 hours. He is seen in the emergency department and a physician administers intracavernosal phenylephrine. This may cause:
A. Hypertension and tachycardia
B. Hypotension and flushing
C. Hypertension and bradycardia
D. Premature ventricular contraction

3. A 59-year-old man has an 80 degree dorsal penile curvature with maximal point of inflection half way from the base of the penile shaft and the glans. His Sexual health Inventory for Men score is 17 with the use of tadalafil. The next step is:
A. Collagenase clostridium histolyticum (Xiaflex)
B. Penile plication
C. Penile prosthesis with modeling
D. Incision and grafting procedure

4. A 58-year-man undergoes a radical prostatectomy for low-risk prostate cancer with nerve sparing. He subsequently fails treatment with sildenafil and attempts the use of alprostadil at a dose of 1000 micrograms. The most likely outcome is
A. Erection not adequate for penetrative intercourse
B. Headaches
C. Urethral burning
D. Tachycardia

5. A 68-year-old man with a history of coronary artery disease with previous coronary angioplasty has been prescribed tadalafil for erectile dysfunction. During sexual activity, he develops substernal chest pain described as "crushing" in nature. The best next step is:
A. Take nitroglycerin if it has been at least 12 hours since his last tadalafil dose
B. Take nitroglycerin if it has been 48 hours since his last tadalafil dose
C. Stop sexual activity and rest
D. Stop sexual activity and seek emergent medical evaluation and treatment

6. A 53-year-old diabetic patient has erectile dysfunction and is given a trial of intraurethral alprostadil in the clinic. He reports penile and scrotal pain with a firm erection. The next best step is:
A. Oral phenylephrine
B. Intracavernosal phenylephrine injection
C. Oral acetaminophen
D. Oral terbutaline

7. A 27-year-old man with medical history including schizophrenia amputated his penis 5 hours ago during a psychotic episode. He presents to the emergency department with a heart rate of 95 and a blood pressure of 135/75 mmHg. The penis has been placed on ice since the injury. Microvascular repair versus macroscopic repair of the penile shaft will result in:
A. Decreased risk for erectile disfunction
B. Equivalent risk for erectile disfunction
C. Similar preservation of penile shaft skin
D. Similar preservation of penile sensation

8. A 61-year-old man sustains a small proximal crural perforation during a penoscrotal incision for a three-piece inflatable penile prosthesis. Appropriate intra-operative management would include:
A. Aborting the placement of the penile prosthesis
B. Place a malleable prosthesis rather than an inflatable
C. Extend the corporotomy and then primarily repair
D. Securing the exit tubing of the ipsilateral cylinder

SELF-ASSESSMENT STUDY QUESTIONS AND ANSWERS

9. A 39-year-old man who does not follow with a primary care physician reports erectile dysfunction with a Sexual Health Inventory Score of 16. He does not take nitrates as needed for chest pain. He should be counseled regarding:

A. His risk of infertility
B. His increased risk for coronary artery disease
C. His risk for penile cancer
D. The need for revascularization of his cavernosal arteries.

10. A 34-year-old man with past medical history of seasonal allergies reports difficulty of erections. In office intracavernosal injection with audiovisual stimulation results in a firm erection. The peak systolic velocity on the right and left cavernosal arteries were 33 and 35 cm/sec, respectively. The end diastolic velocity was 2 cm per second. The most likely cause for his erectile dysfunction is:

A. Psychogenic
B. Arterial insufficiency
C. Arterial insufficiency and venous leak
D. Cavernousal nerve neuropathy

SELF-ASSESSMENT STUDY QUESTIONS AND ANSWERS

Answers

1. A.
2. C.
3. D.
4. A.
5. D.
6. B.
7. B.
8. D.
9. B.
10. A.

CHAPTER 53

Chronic Lower Extremity Ulcers Management and Evaluation

Munier Nazzal and Karen Bauer

OUTLINE

INTRODUCTION
- **Epidemiology**

DIFFERENTIAL DIAGNOSIS

PATHOPHYSIOLOGY OF ULCER BY DISEASE CONDITION
- **Venous Ulcer**
- **Arterial Ulcers**
- **Diabetic/Neuropathic Ulcer**
- **Pyoderma Gangrenosum**
- **Vasculitic Ulcers**
- **Livedo Vasculopathy**
- **Drug-induced Ulcers**
- **Calciphylaxis**

ASSESSMENT AND MANAGEMENT
- **General Principles**
- **Basic Laboratory Evaluation**
- **Advanced Laboratory Evaluation**
- **Tissue Biopsy and Culture**
- **Imaging**
- **Ulcer Infection**
- **Tissue Debridement**
- **Wound Dressing**
  - Moisture Neutral
    - *Films*
    - *Hydrocolloids*
    - *Contact layers*
  - Moisture Additive
    - *Hydrogels*
  - Absorptive
    - *Foams*
    - *Alginates*
    - *Gelling hydrofibers*
    - *Super absorbents and wound fillers*
    - *Composite dressings*
    - *Negative pressure wound therapy*
  - Bioactive
    - *Collagen*
    - *Cellular and tissue-based products (bioengineered skin substitute)*
  - Medicated Dressings
  - Antimicrobial Dressings
    - *Medical-grade Manuka honey*
    - *Silver*
    - *Polyhexamethylene biguanide hydrochloride (PHMB)*
    - *Gentian violet and methylene blue*
    - *Acetic acid*
    - *Diakycarbmoyl chloride (DACC)*
    - *Iodine*
    - *Sodium hypochlorite (Dakin's solution)*
    - *Topical antibiotics*
    - *Topical antifungals*
    - *Enzymatic debriding agents*
    - *Topical corticosteroids*
    - *Wound cleansers*
    - *Growth factors*
    - *Hyperbaric oxygen*

ASSESSMENT AND MANAGEMENT BY ULCER TYPE
- **Venous Ulcers**
- **Arterial Ulcers**
- **Mixed Arterial and Venous Ulcers**

Diabetic Foot Ulcers
Atypical Ulcers
Pyoderma gangrenosum (PG)
Vasculitis ulcers
Livedo vasculopathy (LV)
Drug-induced ulcers
Calciphylaxis
SUMMARY

INTRODUCTION

Ulcers are defined as nonhealing, full-thickness wounds of different etiologies. In most cases, healing failure is related to underlying conditions such as diabetes, lower-extremity arterial or venous disease, or generalized patient health such as in malnutrition and impaired mobility. Skin ulcerations are a common condition that are increasing in prevalence, secondary to the aging population and an increase in chronic health problems. Lower extremity (LE) ulcers are described to be chronic if they do not show tendency to heal after 3 months of appropriate treatment or are still not fully healed at 12 months.[1] The impact of chronic skin ulcers is multifactorial and includes physical symptoms, intractable pain, loss of function, loss of work days, and social stress on the patient, family, and caregivers. There are also significant associated economic implications for the patient, family, and the health-care system as whole.

EPIDEMIOLOGY

Chronic ulcers of the LEs are a common problem affecting about 1% to 2% of the adult population in the United States.[1] Treatment of these ulcers represents a major economic burden, with an annual cost of $23.9 to $27.9 billion.[2,3] Economic impact of chronic ulcers in the United States has been found to be much higher than is recognized based on Medicare data, as a good proportion of expenditure occurs in the outpatient setting. The total Medicare spending estimates in 2014 ranged from $28.1 to $96.8 billion.[4]

Because of differing etiologies and management, LE ulcers are divided into ulcers that affect the legs and ulcers that affect the feet. Leg ulcerations are generally secondary to venous disease or atypical causes, while ulcers on the feet are typically secondary to neuropathy and arterial disease.[5] LE venous disease accounts for more than 70% of leg ulcers, while about 85% of foot ulcers are caused by peripheral neuropathy and commonly associated with peripheral arterial occlusive disease. Presence of neuropathy results in modifying the symptoms that might result from peripheral arterial occlusive disease.[6] In a study of the 2014 Medicare population, the prevalence of wounds of all types increased with age, with surgical wounds being of highest prevalence (4%), followed by diabetic foot infections (3.4%). Among chronic ulcers, the most common type identified in this study were pressure ulcers (1.8%), venous ulcers (0.9%), diabetic foot ulcers (0.7%), and arterial ulcers (0.4%) (Table 53-1).[4]

DIFFERENTIAL DIAGNOSIS

Chronic wounds can be caused by a number of conditions that span many medical disciplines and a multitude of diseases, including but not limited to: trauma, surgery, venous disease, arterial disease, diabetes, neuropathy, connective tissue disease, vasculitis, hypertension, and other rheumatological or autoimmune conditions. Because of this, training of the wound specialist should include all related medical conditions. Although a high proportion of LE ulcers are claimed to be of vascular origin, the reality is that only a small percentage of them can be directly attributed to vascular disease. As explained in Table 53-1, arterial and venous ulcers account for a high percentage of chronic LE ulcers, but overall in the general population they are not the most common causes of ulcerations. The combined prevalence of arterial, venous, and diabetic foot ulcers,

TABLE 53-1 Prevalence of Wounds in the Medical Population in 2014 by the Type of Wound and Beneficiary Demographics

Wound Type	Prevalence (%)	Total Medicare Spending by Wound Type (Primary Dx) ($ M)	Medicare Spending per Beneficiary Mean Value
Surgical infection	4	146.7	2,604
Diabetic infection	3.4	5546.6	2,846
Surgical wound	3	5775.6	3,364
Traumatic wound	2.8	1292.3	830
Skin disorder	2.6	773.3	514
Chronic ulcer	2.3	1420.7	1,104
Venous infection	2.3	146.7	114
Pressure ulcer	1.8	3870.2	3,696
Venous ulcer	0.9	569.0	1,138
Diabetic foot ulcer	0.7	631.4	1,555
Arterial ulcer	0.4	2085.0	9,105
Skin infection	0.1	12.8	346

Note: Highest Medicare spending on surgical wounds, and highest per beneficiary expenditure on arterial ulcers.

Data from Nussbaum SR, Carter MJ, Fife CE, et al. An Economic Evaluation of the Impact, Cost, and Medicare Policy Implications of Chronic Nonhealing Wounds. Value Health. 2018;21(1):27-32 and Singer AJ, Tassiopoulos A, Kirsner RS. Evaluation and Management of Lower-Extremity Ulcers. *N Engl J Med.* 2017;377(16):1559-1567

as shown in Table 53-1, is about 2% compared to 4% of surgical infections alone.[4] The involvement of the vascular specialist in the management of chronic LE ulcers is based on the fact that delayed healing is highly attributable to the presence of vascular disease. As will be shown in the evaluation section of this chapter, it is necessary for all chronic LE ulcers to be evaluated for the presence of a vascular component.

The differential diagnosis of chronic ulcers can be extensive and exhaustive, as shown in Table 53-2. However, when ulcer etiologies are divided into groups of similar pathophysiology and management implications, the proper diagnosis can be efficiently reached.

Accompanying symptoms and anatomic distribution help to identify the potential causes for LE ulcers. For example, ulcers that occur on the medial aspect of the limb (gaiter area) (see Figure 53-1) and are associated with skin color changes (hyperpigmentation or hemosiderin staining) are expected to be of either a pure venous or a mixed arterial and venous disease. Patients that express ulcer pain that is out of proportion to the presence of the ulceration itself raises the probability of a vasculitic or inflammatory etiology (see Figure 53-2). Ulcers associated with violaceous coloration surrounding the ulcerated area increases the probability of pyoderma gangrenosum (PG; see Figure 53-3). Ulcers occurring in patients with chronic kidney disease and associated gangrenous changes increases the possibility of calciphylaxis (see Figure 53-4).

The differential diagnosis favors the most probable LE ulcer etiologies, which in clinical practice, are venous ulcers, arterial ulcers (see Figure 53-5), mixed arterial and venous ulcers, diabetic foot ulcers (see Figure 53-6), and medication-related ulcers (see Figure 53-7). Venous ulcers occur primarily in the gaiter area (the lower part of the calf to one inch below the ankle), and are associated with other signs of venous insufficiency such as edema, skin color changes, eczematous changes and in advanced cases, lipodermatosclerosis. Usually venous ulcers, if pure, are not associated with severe pain, unless accompanied by infection. Conversely, arterial ulcers are, if not associated with neuropathy, severely painful. Arterial ulcers occur as the last stage of chronic LE arterial disease and signify critical limb ischemia.[7] Diabetic foot ulcers are not often associated with significant pain because of neuropathy. Diabetic foot ulcers

TABLE 53-2 Differential Diagnosis of Chronic Ulcers

	Skin Conditions			
Medical Conditions	**Primary Skin Conditions**	**Malignant Skin Conditions**	**Medication/Drug Induced**	**Infections**
• Diabetes mellitus • Venous disease • Arterial disease • Mixed arterial/venous • Trauma • Hypertension • Neuropathy • Nutritional disorders • Pressure • Calciphylaxis • Warfarin-induced necrosis • Cholesterol embolization • Levideo vasculopathy • Nutrition (calorie, protein, vitamin, mineral deficiencies) • Autoimmune and vasculitis: Scleroderma Cutaneous lupus erythromatosis Inflammatory bowel disease Rheumatoid arthritis • Blood disorders: Sickle cell Polycythemia Thrombocytopenia Paraproteinemia	• Sarcoidosis • Ulcerative pyoderma gangrenosum • Necrobiosis lipoidica • Panniculitis • Bullous skin disease (bullous pemphigoid, lichen planus, pemphigus, porphyria cutanea tarda) • Steven Johnson syndrome • Toxic epidermal necrolysis	• Cutaneous malignancy • Squamous cell carcinoma • Basal cell carcinoma • Melanoma • Merkel cell carcinoma • Merkel cell carcinoma • Kaposi sarcoma • Malignant fibrous histiocytoma • Lymphoproliferative malignancy • Internal malignant metastasis	• Hydroxurea • Methotrexate • Chemotherapy • BCG vaccination • Immunosuppresive therapy • Vasoconstrictive cocaine	• Bacterial: necrotizing fasciitis, ecthema gangrenosum, septic emboli, endocarditis, sexually transmitted disease, diphtheria • Atypical mycobacterium: leprosy, buruli ulcer, meningococcemia, others • Viral: herpes, varicella-zoster, cytomegalovirus • Fungal

Data from Morton LM, Phillips TJ. Wound healing and treating wounds: Differential diagnosis and evaluation of chronic wounds. *J Am Acad Dermatol.* 2016;74(4):589-605.

occur in areas of local pressure such as the plantar aspect of the metatarsal heads, the medial malleoli, and the heels, often in the context of Charcot's arthropathy.

In the United States, there is an ongoing controversy about whether foot ulcers are more accurately classified as pressure ulcers or as diabetic ulcers. This dialogue certainly poses medicolegal significance,

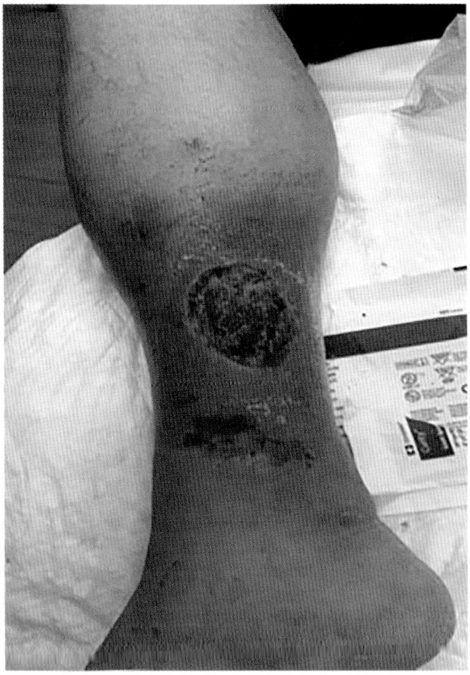

FIGURE 53-1 **Venous ulcer.**

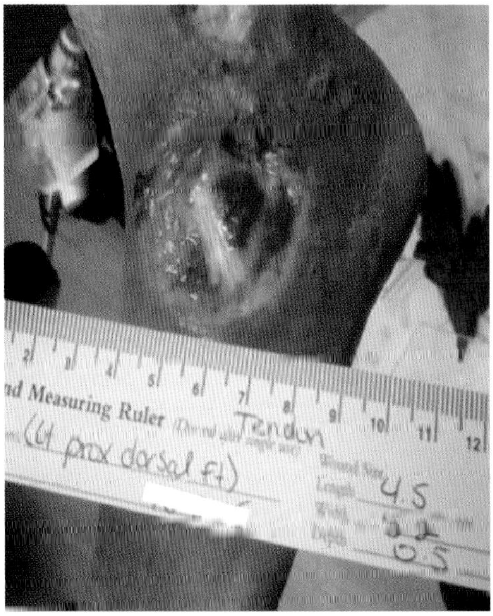

FIGURE 53-2 **Vasculitis.**

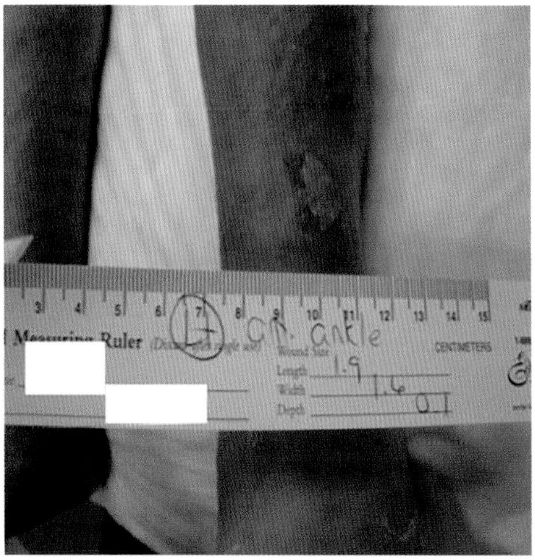

FIGURE 53-3 **Pyoderma gangrenosum.**

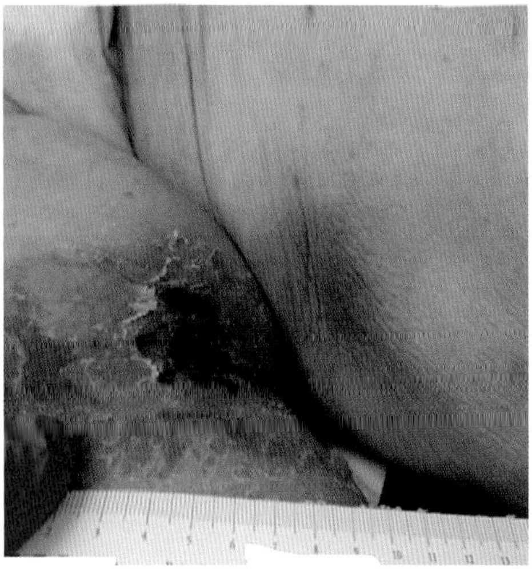

FIGURE 53-4 **Calciphylaxis.**

as CMS rules that management of pressure ulcers acquired within a healthcare facility will not be financially covered by Medicare. A comparison between venous, arterial and diabetic foot ulcers is detailed in Table 53-3.

Pressure ulcers are common in older patients and represent a management challenge because they usually occur in patients who have other significant comorbid conditions (see Figure 53-8). Pressure

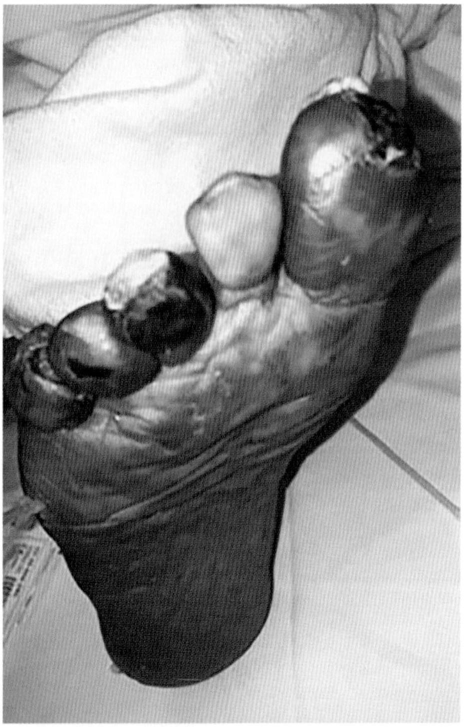

FIGURE 53-5 Arterial ulcer.

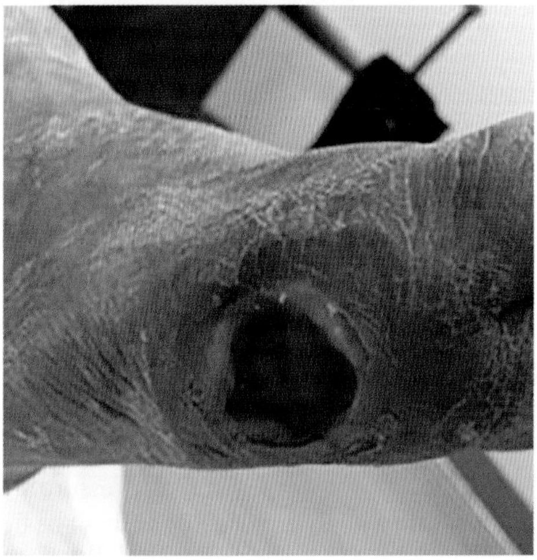

FIGURE 53-6 Diabetic ulcer.

ulcers typically present on the heels, sacrum, ischial tuberosities, greater trochanters, lateral malleoli, and less commonly on the shoulders, scapulae, and elbows.

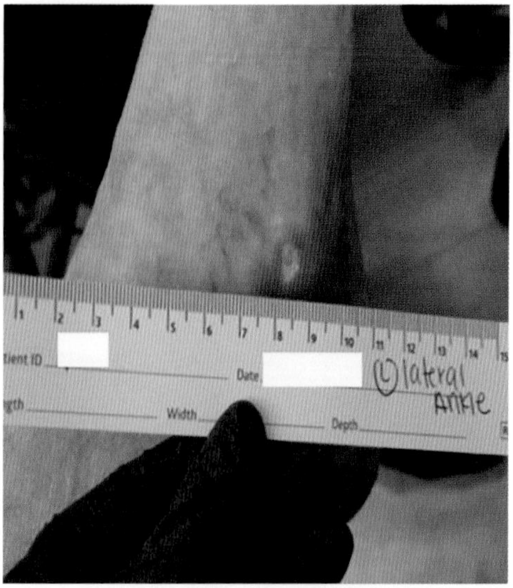

FIGURE 53-7 Hydroxyurea-related ulcer.

Patients with vasculitis can present with cutaneous nodules, skin color changes, and ulcers with scalloped borders. Usually, the ulcers are smaller in size as compared with other types of ulcers and they are exquisitely tender and painful. Vasculitic ulcers can result from medium vessel disease and large vessel disease. In some cases, such as in cryoglobulinemia, the presence of ulcerations carries a poor prognosis.[8,9]

PATHOPHYSIOLOGY OF ULCER BY DISEASE CONDITION

The pathophysiology of chronic ulcers is as variable as the differential diagnosis of chronic ulcers. Generally, the direct cause of ulceration is related to a trauma (even minor) or skin necrosis in an areas of the skin that is associated with delayed healing for different reasons. The skin area with chronic ulcer is usually an abnormal area secondary to either abnormal skin (e.g., venous disease, stasis, vasculitis, diabetes), abnormal circulation (ischemic ulcers, diabetes, vasculitis, calciphylaxis, drug associated ulcers) abnormal skin structure (skin disease, malignancy, connective tissue disease, radiation) or a combination of these factors.

TABLE 53-3 Venous, Arterial, Diabetic and Pressure Ulcers

Ulcer Type	Location	Clinical Morphology	Symptoms	Treatment
Venous	Gaiter area in the lower calf down to the around malleolar area	Ulcer irregular, shallow, fibrinous base with granulation tissue and occasional scattered necrotic areas, skin color changes around the ulcer such as dark discoloration, hemosiderin, thickened skin, swollen leg with inverted champagne bottle appearance of the leg	Heaviness in the leg swelling, pain might be significant but not necessarily. Pain and swelling might improve by laying flat and may worsen by standing and sitting. Pruritus	Compression Leg elevation Surgical treatment: high ligation, stripping, ablation, injection sclerotherapy
Arterial	Most distal part of the extremities including toes, heels, malleoli, areas of bone prominence, areas of amputated stumps	Ulcer with sharply demarcated edges, punched-out appearance on possibly granulation tissue but minimal, significant necrotic tissue, pale, and dry ulcer, leg showing signs of chronic ischemia such as loss of hair, atrophic skin, pale leg possible dependent rubor, delayed capillary filling	History of claudication possible, severe pain around the ulcer, pain is worse laying flat or elevation and better with dependency. Tenderness around ulcer area	Risk factor modification, antiplatelet therapy, statins, revascularization (open and endo)
Diabetic	Areas of repetitive trauma, plantar surface, bony prominences, areas of pressure	Punched out borders of the ulcer, elevated edges with callus formation, foot showing Charcot changes and deformities, limited movement around toes and ankles, skin color changes, and skin breaks. Dry skin, pink extremity, ulcer might have granulation, usually with necrotic base	Deformity of the foot, decreased sensation, capillary circulation might be decreased, edema, and deformed toes	Debridement Offloading Corrective surgery of the bone and joints Others: topical growth factors, hyperbaric oxygen therapy, and skin and connective tissue therapy (CTT)
Pressure ulcer	Bony prominence, heels, tibia, gluteal, sacral, ischial tuberosity, scalp, elbow	Atrophic skin changes and loss of muscles	Might be painful, wastes tissue, necrotic base, infection, minimal granulation tissue, escar Deep, macerated	Debridement Control of infection Control of soiling Offloading Nursing assistance Moist control Nutrition

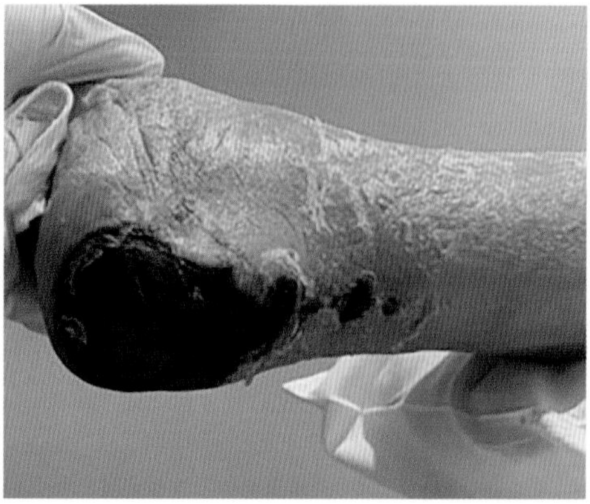

FIGURE 53-8 Pressure ulcer.

VENOUS ULCER

Venous ulcers might be singular or multiple and usually occur in the gaiter area. The most common causes are related to venous hypertension, either from venous occlusive disease or reflux in the deep and/or superficial veins. Venous hypertension can also be part of arteriovenous malformations such as Klippel-Trenaunay syndrome. Varicose veins might be present and manifested either as small varicosities or large tortuous veins. Additional findings in the LE might include hemosiderin deposits in the subcutaneous tissue, stasis dermatitis, thickening of the skin such as in dermatosclerosis, or lipodermatosclerosis. A venous ulcer represents the latest stage of venous hypertension. Based on the Clinical Etiological Anatomical Pathological classification, clinical class 6 is the presence of active venous ulcer, class 5 is a history of prior ulceration that is closed at that time of evaluation, class 4 displays pigmentation, eczematous changes, and skin thickening, class 3 represents venous-related edema, class 2 represents patients with varicose veins, class 1 represent patients with telangiectasia or reticular veins, and class 0 represents no clinical findings or symptoms.[10]

Although most pure venous ulcers are located on the medial aspect of the leg, they can occur on the posterior aspect of the leg or the lateral aspect of the leg or ankle. Ulcerations may also be present near incompetent perforators.

Venous reflux, venous obstruction, or a mixture of both can lead to the development of LE ulcerations because of venous hypertension which causes increased capillary permeability and lymphatic damage leading to edema of the LE. Pathologic skin changes and reduced capillary blood flow, together with increased edema, result in tissue damage and leads to ulceration.[10] In chronic venous disease, the clinical condition is expected to worsen to ulceration in about 50% of affected patients, while about 30% of patients with varicose veins alone develop skin changes over time. This progression occurs faster in those with history of deep venous thrombosis, which causes higher degrees of venous obstruction, thus increasing venous hypertension.[11–13]

The mechanisms underlying venous ulcerations are a combination of microscopic and macroscopic pathological processes. Destruction of vein wall architecture and cellular abnormalities lead to venous dysfunction and venous hypertension. Venous hypertension then leads to chronic inflammatory responses. Chronic inflammation leads to white blood cell extravasation into the dermis which in turn secrete a number of pro-inflammatory cytokines. These cytokines change the phenotype of fibroblasts to a contractile phenotype which causes an increase in the tension in the dermis. These factors combined lead to skin ulceration. Chronic extravasation of macromolecules, red blood cell degradation products, and iron overload cause the skin changes seen in patients with venous hypertension. The chronic inflammation lead to white blood cell extravasation into the dermis which in turn secrete a number of pro-inflammatory cytokines. These cytokines change the phenotype of fibroblasts to a contractile phenotype which will cause an increase in the tension of the dermis. The presence of iron causes the macrophages to change to an active stage leading to tissue destruction rather than repair.[14]

ARTERIAL ULCERS

Arterial ulcers are often markers for generalized arteriosclerosis and are caused by chronic peripheral occlusive arterial disease, which leads to reduced perfusion of the LEs. Some arterial ulcers are secondary to minor trauma, which causes an increase in oxygen and nutrient demand that cannot be met in the presence of arterial occlusive disease. Arterial ulcers typically occur on the most distal part of the

LE, including the forefoot, malleolar areas, or the tibial areas. Usually, patients with arterial ulcers manifest symptoms of arterial occlusive disease such as claudication or rest pain, and suffer from other risk factors such as hypertension, diabetes, hyperlipidemia, and smoking. Amputation risk is high in arterial ulceration, with nearly one-third of amputations being attributed to arterial disease.[15] Reduced blood flow to the LEs, like any organ, leads to decreased perfusion and subsequent tissue necrosis. If ischemia is profound, gangrenous changes result and might lead to minor or major amputations. Infection can complicate many arterial ulcers, although it often goes undetected as the classic inflammatory signs are masked by the lack of perfusion.

DIABETIC/ NEUROPATHIC ULCER

Foot ulcers are among the most significant complication affecting people with diabetes. In patients with diabetes, the prevalence of ulcer formation ranges from 4% to 10%, with a lifetime incidence of about 25%. Amputations from diabetic foot ulcers account for more than half of nontraumatic LE amputations.[16] Ulcer development in diabetes mellitus is a multifactorial process. Contributing factors include ischemia, foot deformities, and infection. Chronic hyperglycemia results in vascular complications including endothelial injury, elevated production of reactive oxygen species, and abnormal stimulation of the hemodynamic regulation system, all of which leads to microvascular and macrovascular changes that affect various organs including the skin, muscle, kidneys, and heart. Even in the presence of acceptable macrovascular circulation, the microvascular perfusion is impaired in diabetic foot ulcers.[17]

The angiosome principle is important to discuss in association with diabetic foot ulcers. This concept was first published in 1987 as an explanation for arterial blood flow to the foot being supplied in blocks and segments. The foot can be divided into five distinct angiosome segments (angiosomes) that originate from the three calf arteries, with one angiosome supplied by the anterior tibial artery, another one supplied by the peroneal artery, and three angiosomes supplied by the posterior tibial artery.[18] The angiosomes are connected with each other by what is called "the choke vessels," which ensure blood flow to different parts of the foot if a specific artery is occluded. These choke vessels are believed to be incompetent in diabetic patients, which leads to localized ischemia in certain segments of the foot, in the presence of a patent artery but occlusion of the others.

PYODERMA GANGRENOSUM

PG is believed to be an autoimmune process with an associated inflammatory component. Its diagnosis is often based on the presence of comorbid conditions such as inflammatory bowel disease, rheumatoid arthritis, and others. It is associated with a rapid progression from a small skin lesion to larger lesions in a short period of time. These ulcers often begin after minor trauma. The pathognomonic sign is an ulcer that worsens when subjected to sharp debridement, biopsy, or other harsh contact. These ulcerations often have violaceous borders. The exact etiology of PG is not clear; however, it is associated with systemic disease in about 50% to 70% of the time.[19,20]

VASCULITIC ULCERS

Vasculitic ulcers occur as a result of a number of inflammatory conditions affecting vessels of different sizes. The classification of such diseases are based on the size of the vessels affected as well as the presence or lack of medial complex deep ulceration. Inflammatory conditions lead to blood vessels occlusion, which in effect causes ischemia of the affected area and results in ulceration secondary to skin and subcutaneous tissue destruction. Not all vasculitic conditions are associated with skin ulcerations. The most common type of vasculitis occurs following an infection, related to certain drugs such as beta-blockers and thiazide diuretics, or in association with malignancies and collagen-related diseases. Some cases have been reported after hepatitis C and HIV infection. The common factor between all vasculitic conditions is the occlusion of the arteries supplying tissue that results in tissue destruction. The lesion usually starts as a small purpura like area that then expands and ulcerates. Systemic vasculitic disease should be ruled out in these conditions.[20] The LEs are usually involved, showing ulcers and vasculitic lesions.[21]

LIVEDO VASCULOPATHY

Livedo vasculopathy (LV) is characterized by painful, recurrent perimaleolar ulcerations. It has predilection for women over men (3:1). Ulceration is the acute manifestation of LV. It is believed that ulceration is secondary to reduced cutaneous perfusion which leads to disruption of the skin and subcutaneous tissue in the affected area. It has been postulated that this is related to excessive coagulation activity, which contributes to reduced perfusion of the middle and upper dermis. It produces painful ischemia of the affected area (angina cutis) leading to cutaneous infarction, necrosis, and ulceration.

DRUG-INDUCED ULCERS

Drug-induced ulcers are typically immunological and toxic reactions. They result from immune-complex diseases as well as microcirculation disturbances. Hydroxyurea, a drug used in the treatment of chronic myeloid leukemia, polycythemia, sickle cell anemia, or essential thrombocytopenia is an example of a drug that can cause LE ulceration and is the most well-known drug for skin ulcerations.[22] Typically, these ulcers are very painful with sharp borders, and occur on the ankle or heel after prolonged treatment with hydroxyurea. In these patients, vascular causes should be ruled out to prevent focusing only on the probable drug as a causative factor. Both the effect of hydroxyurea on the red blood cells as well as the hyperviscosity of the underlying condition contribute to arterial occlusion and destruction of the skin and subcutaneous tissue in the affected area, which leads to ulceration.

Warfarin is another drug that can cause necrosis of the skin and subcutaneous tissue.[23] In this case, the ulceration can occur on any part of the body, but usually presents in areas with high subcutaneous adipose tissue, such as the breasts, thighs, abdomen, and the gluteal region. Warfarin-induced skin necrosis does not commonly occur on the LEs. Warfarin-induced ischemic changes are associated with protein C and S deficiency, which contributes to cutaneous thrombosis. Heparin can also cause thrombosis and necrosis secondary to heparin-induced thrombocytopenia (HIT) which results from heparin/platelet factor for complex antibody formation. The newer direct oral anticoagulant medications have a rare incidence of documented skin necrosis, although future implications remains to be seen.[24]

CALCIPHYLAXIS

Calcific uremic arteriolopathy, or calciphylaxis, is not a common condition encountered by the wound specialist. However, once encountered, it becomes a challenge to manage. The incidence is likely underestimated because of misdiagnosis. It is estimated to occur in uremic patients who are on hemodialysis at a rate of 35 cases per 10,000 patients in the United States.[25] Risk factors include diabetes mellitus, obesity, warfarin therapy, and poorly controlled secondary hyperparathyroidism. Calciphylaxis is primarily linked to hyperphosphatemia and hyperparathyroidism, but low parathyroid hormone levels is associated with an increased risk of calciphylaxis. The exact mechanism of developing calciphylaxis is not well known.[26,27]

ASSESSMENT AND MANAGEMENT

GENERAL PRINCIPLES

The assessment and management of LE ulcers should follow specific guidelines and is multidisciplinary in nature. A full medical history including wound specific history, comorbid conditions, nutritional assessment, circulation assessment, infection evaluation, and evaluation of socioeconomic factors of the patient should be obtained. The wound etiology should be determined, which can be done primarily utilizing clinical data such as anatomic location, appearance, type and amount of exudate, and associated regional and systemic characteristics. Bone or deep tissue involvement should be determined.

A multidisciplinary approach to ulcer management is needed, especially in ulcers that are difficult to heal, present themselves with recurrent infection, or are atypical. Correction of regional underlying abnormalities such as inadequate circulation, infection, or bone involvement should be achieved to minimize recurrence. Underlying systemic diseases such as diabetes, and cardiac disease must be optimally managed as well, which may involve inclusion of other specialties such as endocrinologists, rheumatologists, cardiologists, and infectious disease specialists. General principles of local ulcer management include debridement, control of bioburden, appropriate dressings, compression in venous ulcers, offloading of diabetic and pressure ulcers, revascularization of arterial ulcers, medical management when needed, and referral to the appropriate specialist when needed.

Because of the multiplicity of causes of LE ulcers, evaluation should follow a well-organized, comprehensive scheme to ensure adequate data for inclusion and exclusion of differential factors. Ulcer evaluation should focus on identifying both primary and contributory causes and contributors to determine projected ulcer healing; the key top ulcer management is accurately identifying ulcer causes. The evaluation should follow a step-up plan, starting with the most common causes and advancing to more unusual causes if basic clinical evaluation and diagnostic tests do not identify a cause, or if the ulcer fails to heal in spite of appropriate management.

All patients with LE ulcers should be evaluated for the presence of infection, arterial occlusive disease, comorbid conditions, altered nutrition, and socioeconomic factors that might interfere with proper medical management. Patients with skin changes that are associated with chronic venous insufficiency or suspected venous ulcerations should undergo venous duplex imaging. Patients with exposed bone or close bone proximity should undergo plain radiographic imaging to rule out the presence of osteomyelitis. In case of high suspicion and in the absence of radiological evidence of osteomyelitis further evaluation should be done including MRI or nuclear studies to document or rule out the presence of osteomyelitis. Deep tissue cultures, bone cultures, and bone biopsy might be needed for definitive diagnosis and to guide antibiotic and treatment when needed, but routine swab culturing is not recommended. In a systemic review of about 45 randomizes studies of more than 4000 patients, the authors showed no benefit of prophylactic systemic antibiotics for LE ulcers.[11]

BASIC LABORATORY EVALUATION

Patients with chronic cutaneous ulcers should be evaluated by obtaining blood chemistry tests including a kidney function panel, electrolytes, blood sugar, hemoglobin A1c, homocysteine, and complete blood count with differential. Additionally, sedimentation rate and C-reactive protein should be obtained specially if suspecting underlying chronic infection or osteomyelitis.

ADVANCED LABORATORY EVALUATION

In patients with chronic, nonhealing ulcers, or when atypical causes are suspected, parathormone levels, calcium level, albumin and prealbumin, phosphorus, magnesium, folate, and vitamin levels should be considered. Patients who are suspected to have autoimmune disease or an element of vasculitis can be evaluated by obtaining rheumatoid factor, antinuclear antibodies, antiphospholipid antibodies including lupus anticoagulant, immunoglobulin G, and immunoglobin M.

TISSUE BIOPSY AND CULTURE

In many conditions in which the ulcer is not closing in the expected timeframe or the exact underlying cause cannot be identified, tissue biopsy should be taken, and should include skin edges. Tissue biopsy assists in diagnosis of a number of clinical conditions such as malignancies, autoimmune bullous disorders, neuropathic ulcers, and nonatherosclerotic ischemic ulcers such as vasculitis. In patients with suspected infection, fungal, anaerobic, and aerobic cultures can be taken to identify causative organisms. Clinicians should check with laboratory teams to ensure biopsy and culture specimen are submitted in the proper format

IMAGING

Patients who present with skin or LE changes that are consistent with venous disease should undergo a venous duplex ultrasound for the presence of deep vein occlusion, large vein reflux, or perforator reflux. If venous duplex is negative for occlusive disease or reflux, more advanced imaging such as magnetic resonance or computerized tomographic venous imaging should be obtained to evaluate the more proximal segments (iliac veins and the inferior vena cava). In some cases, a venographic study, with or without intravascular ultrasound, might be needed.

In patients with LE ulceration or gangrenous changes where arterial occlusive disease is suspected, the presence of an arterial occlusive element should be ruled out. Diagnostic studies include the ankle-brachial index, segmental pressure/pulse volume recording, real-time arterial duplex ultrasound, and perfusion studies including transcutaneous oxygen saturation, laser doppler flow, or other perfusion evaluation methods such as infrared spectroscopy.[28,29]

ULCER INFECTION

Infection is one of the most common factors that delays healing. Most, if not all ulcers, are colonized with bacteria. A critical threshold of 10^5 bacteria per gram of tissue is considered infection that might interfere with healing.[30] Deep tissue culture is the standard of care to identify causative organism, although it is considered controversial as culture technique may affect results.[31] Targeted antibiotic therapy based on culture and sensitivity is preferred over empiric therapy based on most probable bacterial infection and current literature suggests consideration of local antimicrobials or antispectics, which will be discussed later in this chapter, in the absence of regional or systemic signs or symptoms of infection.[32]

TISSUE DEBRIDEMENT

Although no one debridement method has been shown to be more effective in achieving healing, sharp debridement remains the standard therapy and should be considered in any ulcer with necrotic tissue, hypertrophic tissue, or suspected biofilm. Sharp debridement removes necrotic, infected tissue and callous, reduces pressure and edema in the affected area, allows the drainage, helps optimize topical therapy, and stimulates healing.[33] Other debridement methods include larval debridement in conjunction with a moist dressing, which can cause maceration of the ulcer, but may remove necrotic tissue and organisms from the ulcer bed. It is especially used in diabetic foot ulcers. This method of debridement cannot be used for thickened and hard issues such as callus.[34] Enzymatic debridement using collagenase can be used in some cases but the process is slow and might not replace sharp debridement.

WOUND DRESSING

The primary goal of wound dressings is to maintain or restore a physiologic wound milieu to support the biochemical processes needed to achieve wound closure. The concept of moist wound healing has been accepted since the 1960s, with knowledge that traditional dressings such as gauze are suboptimal.[35] Clinicians must recognize the physiologic factors in wound healing to optimize the local wound healing environment. Factors that must be considered are wear time of the dressing, underlying etiology, size, location, drainage type and amount, periwound condition, type of exposed underlying structure, and severity of the wound. To optimize topical therapy, dead space must be adequately filled to ensure that all tissue is in contact with the treatment regimen. Compatibility must be considered, especially when utilizing multiple dressing types on the same wound or when adjunctive modalities are being used, such as hyperbaric oxygen therapy (HBOT) or electrical stimulation. Financial and insurance issues, access to home health, and patient or caregiver ability, are paramount.[36] There is no one "best" dressing, as dressings must be chosen based on a number of constantly evolving factors throughout the life of the wound.[35] Adequate topical management compliments systemic management of the wounded patient and can accelerate wound healing time, decrease wound-related pain, minimize drainage and odor, decrease wound infection risk, and improve quality of life. Still, evidence in favor of a specific dressing for any wound etiology is lacking, with available studies being low powered, biased, imprecise, or sparse.[37,38] Dressings are divided into categories based primarily on moisture levels as follows.

Moisture Neutral

Films: Transparent polyurethane or other polymer membranes that are impermeable to liquid, water, and bacteria.[39] Film dressings play a limited role in advanced wound healing.

Hydrocolloids: Hydrocolloids are one of the most widely used dressings. They are made of gelatin, pectin, polysaccharides, or sodium carboxymethylcellulose, and usually have a water-impermeable outer layer and a colloid inner layer.[36,39]

Contact layers: These dressings aremade of woven or perforated material and are used to line a wound bed, to protect a graft site, to hold hydrogels, collagens, or cellular/tissue based products to the wound bed, or to protect fragile epithelium.[36,40]

Moisture Additive

Hydrogels: Hydrogels are water soluble polymers, usually glycerin and water, and are available in gauzes, gels, and sheets.[39,40]

Absorptive

Foams: Foam dressings have a hydrophobic outer layer that protects the wound from contaminate but still allows gas exchange. Foams are not ideal for dry or low-exudative wounds, as they can further dry the wound bed.[39]

Alginates: Alginates are made from sodium and calcium salts, and consist of fibers derived from brown seaweed or kelp. They are absorptive, nonocclusive, and may form a protective film over the wound.[36,39]

Gelling hydrofibers: Gelling hydrofibers are different from alginates and are composed of sodium carboxymethylcellulose or blended super absorbents. Gelling hydrofibers are available in pads, ropes, and bordered composite dressings.[36]

Super absorbents and wound fillers: These are highly absorptive dressings made from fibers such as cellulose, cotton, or rayon. Wound fillers are supplied as beads, creams, foams, pillows, gels, ointments, pastes, pads, powders, strands, or other formulations to maintain a moist wound healing environment.

Composite dressings: Composite dressings are combination dressings that contain two or three layers of distinct dressing materials, such as an alginate and a foam.

Negative pressure wound therapy: Negative pressure wound therapy is available as a foam that is plain, antimicrobial, or a higher density for tunneling and undermining. Instillation systems that can be used with antiseptics or other solutions are now available and often utilized for patients who do not tolerate sharp debridement or have a need for recurrent debridement.[40]

Bioactive

Collagen: Collagen is a major structural protein that may stimulate fibroblast formation, decrease protease activity, and facilitate endothelial migration.[36,39] Most collagen dressings are derived from bovine, equine, porcine, and/or avian sources. Collagen decreases protease levels.[36]

Cellular and tissue-based products (bioengineered skin substitute): These products may be acellular or cellular and are chemotactic for necessary growth factors and cytokines. They are derived from a number of substrates that include but are not limited to: human amniotic tissue, fetal bovine dermal tissue, human foreskin, porcine bladder tissue, shark cartilage, and others. A systematic review showed promise for hyaluronic acid derivatives in improving wound healing times, specifically in venous leg ulcers (VLUs), diabetic foot ulcers, and burns.[41]

Medicated Dressings

Of recent attention is the concept of biofilm and its contribution to nonhealing wounds. Antimicrobial wound management is a challenge, as systemic antibiotics do not adequately penetrate wound biofilm and local antibiotics have led to tolerance and resistance.[32,42] Topical antimicrobial therapy duration should be determined by frequent wound assessment, at least every two weeks.[32]

Antimicrobial Dressings

Medical-grade Manuka honey: Medical-grade honey is reported to have activity against over 60 bacteria species that include anaerobes and aerobes.[40]

Silver: Silver dressings come in many types: salts (silver nitrate, silver sulphadiazine), metallic (nanocrystalline), or ionic silver combined with ethylenediamine tetraacetate and benzethonium chloride (antibiofilm agents).[32,40] Silver sulfadizine is supplied as a cream (1%). It has broad spectrum against *Candida*; used to prevent and treat serious burn and wound infections.

Polyhexamethylene biguanide hydrochloride (PHMB): PHMB is another antimicrobial with a molecular structure similar to chlorhexidine.[40]

Gentian violet and methylene blue: These are antiseptic dyes and weak antibacterials used to treat fungal infections of skin, abrasions, ringworm, or athlete's foot.[43]

Acetic acid: Acetic acid is compounded to 0.25%, 0.5%, and 1% solutions. It has shown activity against gram-positive and gram-negative bacteria, including *Pseudomonas aeruginosa.*

Diakycarbmoyl chloride (DACC): DACC is available in different shapes and sizes. It irreversibly binds bacteria and removes it when the dressing is changed.

Iodine: Iodine compounds are formulated in solutions and are microbicidal against bacteria, fungi, viruses, spores, protozoa, and yeasts. Research supports the use of cadexemer iodine, especially in the treatment of venous leg ulcerations.[44]

Sodium hypochlorite (Dakin's solution): Dakin's and other chlorine-releasing solutions (0.0125%, 0.125%, 0.25%, and 0.5%) are active against vegetative bacteria, viruses, and some spores and fungi, but have a high risk of cytotoxicity.

Topical antibiotics: Antibiotic creams and/or ointments may promote resistance, have no known efficacy, and should only be used in rare cases and by experienced wound clinicians.[32] Topical metronidazole may be used in fungating wounds, but is used for odor control more than wound healing. Mupirocin is used in unique cases.

Topical antifungals: Antifungal creams, powders, liquids, or sprays should be reserved for unique cases where fungal overgrowth is either confirmed by deep tissue or highly suspected clinically. Appropriate wound care must occur concurrently, such as management of wound exudate and other moisture sources.[32]

Enzymatic debriding agents: Enzymatic debriding agents allow for removal, softening, or loosening of necrotic tissue without harming healthy tissue. Collagenase is currently the only enzymatic debriding agent available in the United States. Low-powered studies support the use of collagenase in pressure ulcers, diabetic foot ulcers, and burns.[45]

Topical corticosteroids: In atypical ulcers with an exaggerated inflammatory response, topical steroids may benefit.[46]

Wound cleansers: It has been accepted that 0.9% normal saline is adequate for wound cleansing, however with the focused attention on biofilm and its role in delayed wound healing, newer cleansing agents are being studied. One study with 308 participants suggests consideration of wound cleansing with hypochlorite/hypochlorous acid solutions, polyhexanides, octenidine, or povidone-iodine.[47] The optimal cleansing agent has not been identified, especially in infected wounds, irrigation with an antiseptic solution may be beneficial and wounds should be thoroughly cleansed with each dressing change.[32]

Growth factors: Growth factors are component of the physiologic wound mileu. Certain cytokine growth factors, such as platelet-derived growth factor (PDGF), fibroblast growth factor, vascular endothelial growth factor (VEGF), IGF, and others are proven to accelerate and augment wound healing. Cytokines, when balanced in normal wound healing, accelerate proliferation, stimulate endothelial cell, promote angiogenesis, and are chemotactic for fibroblasts and other inflammatory cells. Deficiencies in these growth factors will interfere with wound healing and may lead to ulcer chronicity. Chronic wounds are generally stalled in an inflammatory state with high levels of metalloproteinases and proteolytic enzymes.[48] Recombinant growth factors have been used to replicate the role of growth factors in normal wound healing including cell migration, proliferation, and differentiation. They are thought to allow modulation of wound healing through applying external factors to mimic the internal growth factors in healing. The growth factor half-life is short, but extrinsic growth factor application has shown to have a significant impact on healing in animal studies and small sized clinical studies.[47] Among these growth factors are: topically applied PDGF, VEGF, and epidermal growth factor (EGF). These growth factors are indicated primarily in diabetic foot ulcers; however, none show conclusive evidence and thus further research is needed.[48]

Hyperbaric oxygen: HBOT has been used in the treatment of a number of conditions. In wound management, the primary FDA-approved indications for HBOT include chronic Wagner grade 3 or higher diabetic foot ulcers, chronic refractory osteomyelitis, soft tissue radionecrosis, necrotizing fasciitis, and conditions such acute ischemia. In spite of being present for a long period of time, the efficacy and safety profile of HBOT remains controversial in many conditions and certainly in the management of LE ulcerations.

HBOT is the administration of 100% oxygen in a high-pressure chamber. The chamber pressure is usually between 2 and 3 atm absolute. For wound healing indications, treatment generally consists of daily sessions lasting about 2 hours for a total of 30-90 sessions. The mechanism of action of HBOT is multifactorial. Perhaps the most obvious mechanism is the increased oxygen concentration at the site of the ulcer. Many ulcers, in spite of varied etiologies, display a component of local hypoxia and ischemia. It is expected that provision of high oxygen concentration at the ulcerated site improves healing partially by promoting angiogenesis. In addition to this, other mechanisms has been implicated to explain the action of HBOT, including improved fibroblast proliferation, increased collagen synthesis, augmented bactericidal activity of leukocytes, decreased inflammation via vasoconstriction, and decreased pro-inflammatory cytokines.[49]

HBOT is absolutely contraindicated in patients with a pneumothorax or potential for developing pneumothorax, and relatively contraindicated in history of optic neuritis, febrile state (fever decreases seizure threshold), active upper respiratory or sinus infection, and hypoglycemia. Medications should also be considered, such as some chemotherapeutic agents. All host factors such as optimization of circulation, offloading, glycemic control, and infection management should occur prior to initiation of HBOT.

Studies solidifying the use of HBOT in wound healing are limited, and in case of diabetic foot ulcers there is no agreement on its efficacy. In a metanalysis of randomized clinical trials, it was found that HBOT was associated with a greater reduction in wound surface area than standard therapy alone but there was no difference between both groups with respect to the incidence of healed ulcers, risk of minor or major amputations, or adverse events.[50]

ASSESSMENT AND MANAGEMENT BY ULCER TYPE

Management of ulcers follow the same principles outlined in the previous section including ulcer evaluation, vascular evaluation, debridement, dressing, and control of infection. In addition, different types of ulcers requires certain treatments that does not apply to other types as will be discussed in the following sections (Figures 53-9 and 53-10).

VENOUS ULCERS

Evaluation of patients with a VLU should include venous anatomy evaluation for reflux including deep vein, perforator, greater saphenous vein, and small saphenous vein reflux. In addition, ultrasound should be performed to rule out presence of occlusive or thrombotic disease. This can be done by duplex ultrasound. If duplex ultrasound is inconclusive or suggestive of more proximal involvement, either venous magnetic resonance or CT venogram should be performed to rule out iliac vein or inferior vena cava involvement. The presence of venous reflux or occlusive disease should be corrected to improve ulcer healing.

The medical management of venous ulcers must include compression therapy as its mainstay, but arterial disease should be ruled out prior to application of compression wraps.[51] Studies show that multilayer bandages perform better than single layer bandages in VLU management. Compression stocking might not be adequate in the VLU management phase. Intermittent pneumatic compression has been reported to improve healing when used in conjunction with compression garments and standard therapy.[52] Weight loss in obese patients is recommended to help control venous hypertension and is linked to immobility and venous ulceration.[53] Calf muscle activity is important, thus making referral to a physical therapist is a consideration in patients with a compromised gait, limited mobility, or ankle immobility. Elevation of the legs remain important as well, even when aggressive compression modalities are utilized.

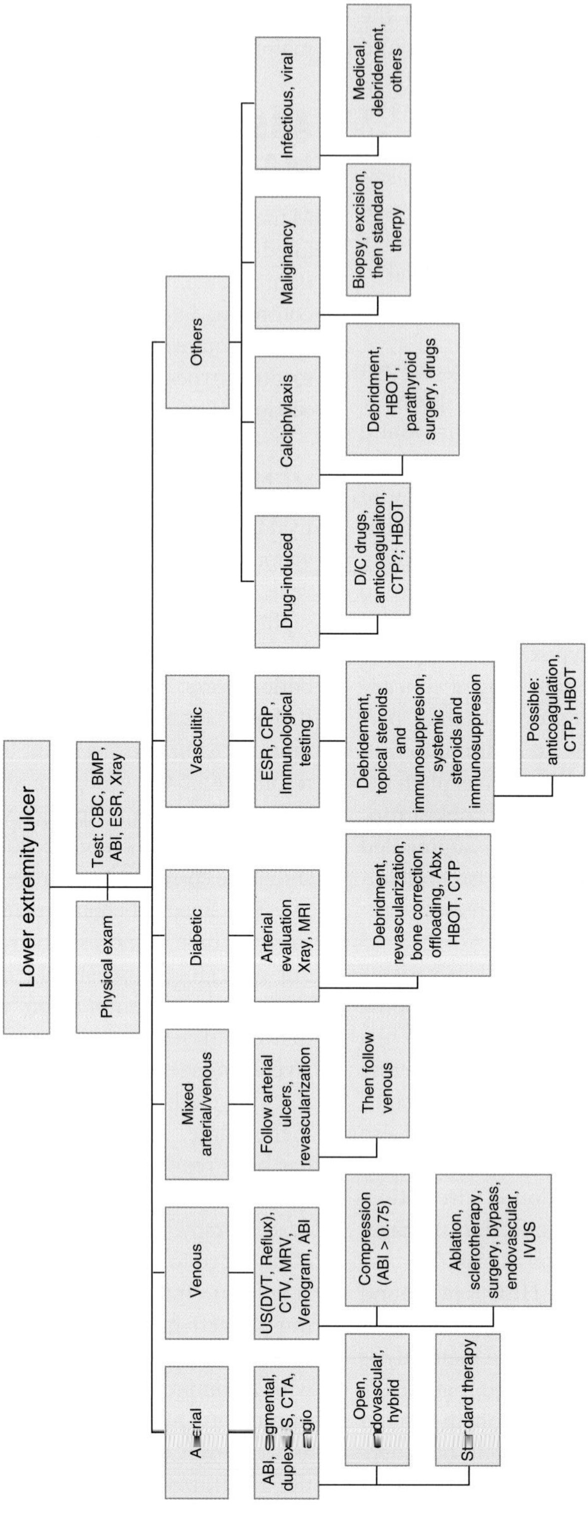

FIGURE 53-9 Algorithm for lower extremity ulcer evaluation.

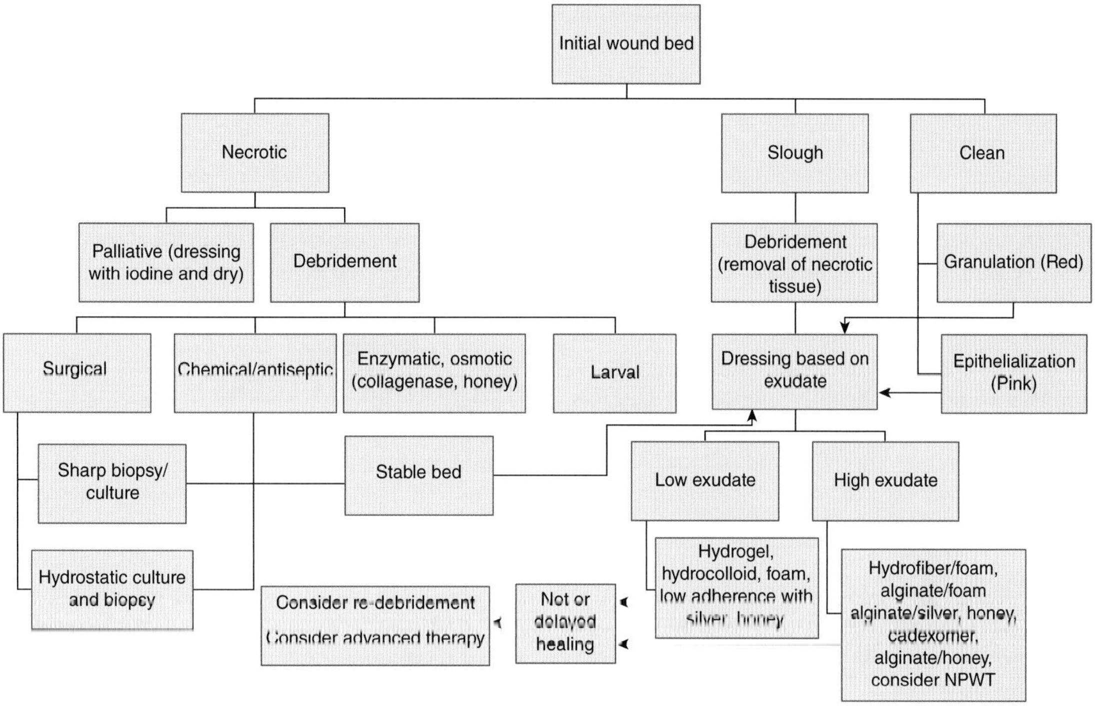

FIGURE 53-10 **Wound bed preparation and dressing.**

Nutrition evaluation for zinc deficiency, folic acid, and vitamin D might be of benefit in patients with refractory venous ulcers. Venous ulcer healing was reported to improve with supplemental vitamin D, folic acid, and flavonoids in low powered studies, but other dietary supplements were not shown to have any beneficial effect.[54] Venoactive drugs such as micronized purified flavonoid fraction (MPFF) have been reported to improve the healing rates of venous ulcers by controlling inflammation.[10,51] Other drugs, such as pentoxifylline and sulodexide, have been associated with improved venous ulcer healing when supplemented with compression therapy.[51] Pentoxifylline, a methylated xanthine derivative, is a phosphodiesterase inhibitor with antioxidant properties that reduces inflammation. It has been known to reduce blood viscosity and potentially decrease platelet aggregation and clotting. On the other hand, sulodexide is a combination of heparin and dermatan sulfate, and has antithrombotic and pro fibrinolytic properties in addition to its anti-inflammatory effects. Both pentoxifylline and sulodexide were found to have improved ulcer healing compared to placebo and better results when combined with compression therapy.[55,56] Based on the 2018 European cardiovascular disease management guidelines, pentoxifylline, sulodexide and MPFF were granted grade A evidence in the treatment of venous ulcers.[51]

Debridement of venous ulcer is recommended to remove necrotic tissue, biofilm, and to remove any surface debris. Repetitive debridement might be needed. Recommended debridement forms include surgical debridement, and hydrosurgical debridement. Enzymatic debridement is recommended only in the absence of a trained surgical specialist. Biological debridement using larval therapy can be an alternative to surgical debridement.[48]

Surgical treatment of venous reflux has been shown to improve venous ulcer healing. In a randomized trial of early endovenous ablation and venous ulceration, the authors found that early ablation resulted in improved healing of venous ulcers and more ulcer free time than in patients who had deferred endovenous ablation. The median time to ulcer healing was 56 days in the early intervention group compared to 82 days in the deferred intervention group. While the median ulcer free time during the first year was 306 days in the early intervention group, compared to 278 days in the deferred intervention group.[57] In a comparative study of compression therapy alone to surgery with high ligation, endovenous laser ablation, and foam sclerotherapy for active venous ulcers, it was found that the ulcer healing time was shorter in patients with compression therapy plus surgical intervention versus compression therapy alone. Ulcer recurrence at 12 months was also significantly reduced in patients with compression therapy and intervention group. Both calf perforator vein reflux and isolated superficial vein reflux were risk factor for ulcer recurrence.[58]

Recently, biologic/cellular and tissue-based products (CTP) have been implicated in the treatment of different types of LE ulcers, including venous ulcers. There are many acellular and cellular products that have FDA approval, some of them specifically for venous ulcerations. These products are numerous and vary in composition, including allografts, human-derived cellular products, dehydrated human amniotic membrane, animal-derived extracellular matrix products, and others. Application of these products must follow local Medicare guidelines and most cannot be applied until documenting nonhealing for four weeks and host factors have been optimized. In comparison with compression alone, these agents have not generated solid recommendations about routine use in the treatment of venous ulcers.

ARTERIAL ULCERS

The only effective treatment for arterial ulcers is revascularization. This includes endovascular interventions as well as open surgical procedures with the goal of treatment is to improve perfusion to the affected extremity. Sometimes, a hybrid procedure of both open and endovascular intervention might be needed. In addition to surgical/endovascular interventions, platelet aggregation inhibition, statin therapy, cessation of the smoking and other risk factor modification are needed to maintain patency of revascularized segments. Certain medications such as cilostazol (Pletal) may benefit in some cases. In cases where revascularization is not possible, prostacyclin derivatives can be employed. In certain cases, HBOT might help heal ulcerated areas but such effect might not be durable and this may present an insurance coverage challenge. Overall, arterial ulcers that are dry and stable should be left dry and stable until revascularization is performed. Debridement should only be considered in arterial ulcers in the absence of prior revascularization if there is wet gangrene or infection.

MIXED ARTERIAL AND VENOUS ULCERS

In cases of mixed venous and arterial ulcerations, treatment should be directed at improving the perfusion and reducing edema as both contribute to delayed healing. Mild compression, calf muscle exercises, supervised walking programs, and leg elevation can be utilized to help manage the venous pathology until revascularization is performed. The frequency of mixed ulcerations are reported to be as high as 14% with moderate peripheral arterial occlusive disease and about 2.2% with severe arterial occlusive disease.[59]

DIABETIC FOOT ULCERS

Diabetic foot ulcers are traditionally classified using the Wagner grading system, which was described in 1987. The Wagner ulcer classification is divided into six grades: Grade 0 with no open lesions but with deformity or cellulitis; grade 1 with superficial diabetic ulcer, partial or full-thickness, grade 2 ulcer with extension to ligaments, tendon, joint capsule, or deep fascia without abscess or osteomyelitis; grade 3 with deep ulcer with abscess, osteomyelitis, or joint sepsis; grade 4 with gangrene localized to portion of the forefoot or heel; grade 5 with extensive gangrenous involvement of the entire foot.[60] The limitations of the Wagner classification system is that it is only descriptive, without addressing the presence of ischemia, deformity, and the full scope of infection. Because of these limitations, newer classifications are being described. The latest is the wound, ischemia, and foot infection (WIfI) system, which was described in 2014. According to the WIfI scale, risk stratification is based on a score from 0 to 3, which includes assessment and extent of ischemia, infection, and ulcer severity.[61] There are other classification systems, which will not be discussed in this chapter.

The management of diabetic foot ulcers is undoubtedly multifactorial and multidisciplinary. Because of the multiplicity of factors contributing to diabetic foot ulcers including circulation, infection, and bone deformities, specialists from many different disciplines need to work closely together. Generally, the main principles in management of diabetic foot ulcers include: revascularization in patients with arterial occlusive disease, control of infection including osteomyelitis, offloading to relieve the pressure on ulcerated areas, and proper dressings to help manage bacterial burden and ulcer moisture. Glycemic control cannot be over emphasized, and both self-reported blood glucose levels and HbA1C should be closely monitored. All patients, regardless of clinical pulse examination, should undergo at least basic arterial testing in the form of ABIs and should undergo more comprehensive arterial imaging if disease is suspected.

Knowledge of offloading devices is important; total contact casting is the gold standard of offloading the diabetic forefoot ulcer and can be utilized in mid and hindfoot ulcers also. Total contact casting should always be applied by trained licensed professionals, which may include medical assistants, nurses, or advanced practice providers, and should ideally be evaluated by a healthcare provider once applied. Referral to orthotic professionals and physiotherapy is often of great benefit.

Other emerging therapies with controversial effects include electrotherapy, ultrasound therapy, and application of CTP. HBOT is approved for advanced stages of diabetic foot ulcers. Cellular/tissue-based products are being increasingly used in the treatment of diabetic foot ulcers. In one systematic review of 17 trials of about 1655 patients, the authors showed that CTP can increase the likelihood of complete ulcer healing when used with standard treatment as compared to standard treatment alone. However, there is no conclusive evidence that such products decrease the recurrence of ulceration or improves limb salvage on the long term.[19] Local therapy in DFU should also include sharp debridement and topical therapy that targets biofilm, moisture management, and promotion of granulation tissue.

ATYPICAL ULCERS

Pyoderma gangrenosum (PG): Although the diagnosis of PG is mostly clinical, biopsy may reveal the presence of nonspecific neutrophilic or leukocytic infiltration. Laboratory findings include leukocytosis and elevated CRP.[20] As previously discussed, a classic sign of PG is ulcer worsening after sharp debridement or similar procedure. These lesions may follow minor trauma and often appear inflamed. Even when PG is suspected, venous and arterial contribution should be considered and either ruled out or treated, and conditions such as diabetes still need optimization.

The treatment of PG includes topical application of products containing immunosuppressive agents such as tacrolimus, corticosteroids, or cyclosporine. On occasions, a short course of systemic steroids might work given. For recalcitrant cases, long-term immunosuppression may be needed, and input from rheumatology is important. Other products that may be used include TNF antagonists, azathioprine, cyclophosphamide and mycophenolate mofetil. While immunosuppression is paramount in the management of PG, it can also interfere with wound healing.

Vasculitis ulcers: Vasculitic ulcers occur secondary to a group of inflammatory vascular processes that are heterogeneous in both nature and distribution. These changes affect different vessel size range from small vessel disease to large vessel disease. The classification of vasculitis is based on the size of the vessel affected as well as the presence or lack of immune complex depositions. Again, even when vasculitis is suspected or confirmed, other contributory factors should be acknowledged and managed.

Once an ulcer is diagnosed to be vasculitic in origin, histological evaluation is indicated to prove the diagnosis. A deep spindle-shaped biopsy should be taken, involving part of the skin and part of the ulcerated area. Deposits of immunoglobin M and immunoglobulin G complexes are found under immunofluorescence microscopy. Cryoglobulins can be detected in the serum. Elevation of inflammatory parameters such as ESR, CRP, and leukocytosis might be found.

Patients with systemic vasculitis can be treated by immunosuppression with corticosteroids or cyclophosphamide. Plasmapheresis might be indicated in severe conditions. Other medications that might be prescribed include colchicine, dapsone, or other immunosuppressants. Other rare conditions, include TB-associated vasculitic ulcers. In such conditions culture or PCR sequencing can be performed and if proven, should initiate treatment for TB.

Patients with vasculitic ulcers can develop worsening of their ulcerations after debridement of biopsy with an increase in ulcer size.[21] Compression therapy might help in some vasculitic ulcerations.

Livedo vasculopathy (LV): Ulcerations secondary to LV should be differentiated from other types of vasculitis. This differentiation has an implication in ulcer management, as LV does not respond to steroid therapy. It has been reported that administration of low molecular weight heparin at a dosage of 1 mg/kg can produce an acceptable response. If patient complains of significant pain, or extensive ulcerations are present, full systemic treatment with low molecular weight heparin twice per day can be helpful.[20]

Drug-induced ulcers: A number of medications have been implicated in ulcer development including hydroxyurea, warfarin, nifedipine, barbiturates, hydroxychlorothiazole, diltiazem, amezinium metisuplfate, and erythropoietin.[21] A balance between the severity of the medical condition necessitating the drug therapy and the condition of the ulcer needs to be taken into consideration. In some cases, the option of another therapeutic regimen and discontinuing the drug is causing the ulcer should be considered.

Treatment of drug-induced ulcers varies, based on the underlying medical condition associated with the drugs as well as with the drugs themselves. In warfarin-induced skin necrosis, the treatment is to stop warfarin anticoagulation and start the patient on heparin followed by consideration of direct anticoagulant medication or a slow reintroduction of warfarin at lower doses. In cases of hydroxyurea ulceration, some conditions (such as polycythemia) mandate continuance of the drug, alternative medication should be considered. Antiplatelet therapy has also been advised. In case of HIT, other anticoagulation medications need to be considered to replace heparin therapy. As always, management of the ulcers should include management of contributory factors and basic topical therapy techniques as well as compression therapy if indicated.

Calciphylaxis: There are no current, evidence-based recommendations for the management of calciphylaxis. Most of the treatment modalities are focused management of the lesions themselves and includes surgical debridement, antibiotic therapy as indicated, and moist wound healing. Sodium thiosulfate can be used as an adjunctive treatment. Its mechanism of action is thought to be related to calcium chelation, or through a vasodilatory effect and a stabilizing effect on the endothelium. Vitamin D analogs and calcium-based phosphates should be avoided. Other treatment modalities used include apheresis and tissue plasminogen activator. However, these treatments are not supported by conclusive evidence. In a meta-analysis evaluating sodium thiosulfate, surgical parathyroidectomy, HBOT, and bisphosphophonates for calciphylaxis treatment in patients with chronic renal disease including patients with end-stage renal disease, the authors found no significant clinical benefits of these five most frequently used treatment modalities for calciphylaxis.

SUMMARY

LE ulcers are a growing problem with high patient, societal, and healthcare system ramifications. The management of LE ulcers follow the same principles in all types including ulcer evaluation, bed preparation, dressing, correcting of underlying conditions, surgical debridement and correction of deformities, and management of nutrition. In all types, the goal is to heal the ulcer in the shortest period of time and to restore the function of the organ involved. In many cases, ulcer management goes beyond the patient to the family and surrounding environment. Because of the multiplicity of causes of nonhealing ulcers, management is in many cases multidisciplinary and involves different specialties. Because of that chronic ulcers of the LEs are best managed in a center where different specialist interact and help in evaluation and management of such ulcers.

REFERENCES

1. Alavi A, Sibbald RG, Phillips TJ, et al. What's new: management of venous leg ulcers: approach to venous leg ulcers. *J Am Acad Dermatol.* 2016;74:627-640.

2. Rice JB, Desai U, Cummings AK, Birnbaum HG, Skornicki M, Parsons N. Burden of venous leg ulcers in the United States. *J Med Econ*. 2014;17:347-356.
3. Rice JB, Desai U, Cummings AKG, Birnbaum HG, Skornicki M, Parsons NB. Burden of diabetic foot ulcers for Medicare and private insurers. *Diabetes Care*. 2014; 37:651-658.
4. Morton LM, Phillips TJ. Wound healing and treating wounds: differential diagnosis and evaluation of chronic wounds. *J Am Acad Dermatol*. 2016;(74) 4:589-605.
5. Agale SV. Chronic leg ulcers: epidemiology, aetiopathogenesis, and management. Ulcers 2013. Available at https://www.hindawi.com/journals/ulcers/2013/413604/.
6. Springer AJ, Tassiopoulos A, Kirsner R. Evaluation and management of lower extremities lower extremity ulcers. *N Engl J Med*. 2017;377:1559-67.
7. Gerhard-Herman MD, Gornik HL, et al. 2016 AHA/ACC guideline on the management of patients with lower extremity peripheral artery disease: executive summary: a report of the American college of Cardiology/American Heart Association Task Force on clinical practice guidelines. *Circulation*. 2017;135: e686-e725.
8. Stone JH, Nousari HC. "Essential" cutaneous vasculitis: what every rheumatologist should know about vasculitis of the skin. *Curr Opin Rheumatol*. 2001;13:23-34.
9. Ramos-Casals M, Stone JH, Cid MC, Bosch X. The cryoglobulinaemias. *Lancet*. 2012;379:348-360.
10. Nicolaides AN. The most severe the stage of a chronic venous disease: an update on the management of patients with venous leg ulcers. *Adv Ther*. 2020; 37(Suppl 1):19-24.
11. Lee AJ, Robertson LA, Boghossian SM, et al. Progression of varicose veins and chronic venous insufficiency in the general population in the Edinburgh Vein study. *J Vasc Surg Venous Lymphat Disord*. 2015;3(1):18-26.
12. Robertson LA, Evans CJ, Lee AJ, Allan PL, Ruckley CV, Fowkes FG. Incidence and risk factors for venous reflux in the general population: Edinburgh Vein study. *Eur J Vasc Endovasc Surg*. 2014;48(2):208-214.
13. Lozano Sanchez FS, Gonzalez-Porras JR, Diaz Sanchez S, et al. Negative impact of deep venous thrombosis on chronic venous disease. *Thromb Res*. 2013;131(4): e123-e126.
14. Meulendijks A, Franssen W, Schoonhoven L, Neumann H. A scoping review on chronic venous disease and the development of a venous ulcer: the role of obesity and mobility. *J Tissue Viability*. 2020;29(3):190-196.
15. Shu J, Santulli G. Update on peripheral arterial disease: epidemiology and evidence based facts. *Atherosclerosis*. 2018;275:379-381.
16. Lung C, Wu F, Liao F, Pu F, Fan Y, Jan Y-K. Emerging technologies for the prevention and management of diabetic foot ulcers. *J Tissue Viability*. 2020;29:61-68.
17. Frykberg R. Diabetic foot ulcers: pathogenesis and management. *Am Fam Phys*. 2002;66(9):1655-1662.
18. Ching YH, Sutton TL, Pierpont YN, Robson MC, Payne WG. The use of growth factors and other humoral agents to accelerate and enhance burn wound healing. *Eplasty*. 2011;11:e41.
19. Todhunter J. Understanding the differential diagnosis of leg ulcers: focus on atypical ulcers. *JCN*. 2019, 33(1):29-37.
20. Meyer V, Kerk, Meyer S, Goerge T. Differential diagnosis and therapy of leg ulcers. *JDDG*. 2011;9:1035-1052.
21. Sirieix ME, Debure C, Baudot N, et al. Leg ulcers and hydroxyurea: forty-one cases. *Arch Dermatol*. 1999; 135:818-820.
22. Trautmann A, Seitz CS. The complex clinical picture of side effects to anticoagulation. *Med Clin North Am*. 2010;94:821-834, xii-iii.
23. Nigwekar SU, Zhao S, Wenger J, et al. A nationally representative study of calcific uremic arteriolopathy risk factors. *J Am Soc Nephrol*. 2016;27:3421-3429.
24. Vu T, Gooderham M. Adverse drug reactions and cutaneous manifestations associated with anticoagulation. *J Cutan Med Surg*. 2017;21(6):540-550.
25. Rogers NM, Teubner DJO, Coates PTH. Calcific uremic arteriolopathy: advances in pathogenesis and treatment. *Semin Dial*. 2007;20(2):150-157.
26. Nigwekar SU, Kroshinsky D, Nazarian RM, et al. Calciphylaxis: risk factors, diagnosis, and treatment. *Am J Kidney Dis*. 2015;66:133-146.
27. Udomkarnjananun S, Kongnatthasate K, Praditpornsilpa K, Eiam-Ong S, Jaber BL, Susantitaphong P. Treatment of calciphylaxis in CKD: a systematic review and meta-analysis. *Kidney Int Rep*. 2019;4: 231-244.
28. Santeneam TB, Poyck PP, Ubbink DT. Systematic review and meta-analysis of skin substitutes in the treatment of diabetic foot ulcers: highlights of a Cochrane systematic review. *Wound Rep Reg*. 2016;24:737-744.
29. Nicolaides A, Kakkos S, Baekgaard N, et al. Management of chronic venous disorders of the lower limbs. Guidelines according to scientific evidence part I. *Int Angiol*. 2018;37(3):181-254.
30. Han G, Ceilley R. Chronic wound healing: a review of current management and treatments. *Adv Ther*. 2017; 34:599-610.
31. Steed DL, Donohoe D, Webster MW, Lindsley L. Effect of extensive debridement and treatment on healing of diabetic foot ulcers. *J Am Coll Surg*. 1996;183:61-64.

32. International Wound Infection Institute (IWII). Wound infection in clinical practice. Wounds International. 2016.
33. Wounds UK. Effective debridement in a changing NHS: a UK consensus. London: Wounds UK; 2013. Available at www.wounds-uk.com. Accessed March 2013.
34. O'Meara S, Al-Kurdi D, Ologun Y, Ovington LG, Martyn-St James M, Richardson R. Antibiotics and antiseptics for venous leg ulcers. *Cochrane Database Rev*. 2014;1:CD003557.
35. Jones A, San Miguel L.Are modern wound dressings a clinical and cost-effective alternative to the use of gauze? *J Wound Care*. 2006;15(2):65-69.
36. Principles of wound healing and topical management. In: Bryant RA, Nix DP, eds. *Acute & Chronic Wounds: Current Management Concepts*. St. Louis: Elsevier; 2016:306-24.
37. Norman G, Westby MJ, Rithalia AD, Stubbs N, Soares MO, Dumville JC. Dressings and topical agents for treating venous leg ulcers. *Cochrane Database Syst Rev*. 2018;6(6):CD012583.
38. Westby MJ, Dumville JC, Soares MO, Stubbs N, Norman G. Dressings and topical agents for treating pressure ulcers. *Cochrane Database Syst Rev*. 2017;6(6): CD011947.
39. Dhivya S, Padma VV, Santhini E. Wound dressings- a review. *Biomedicine*. 2015;5 (4):e49.
40. Boateng J, Catanzano O. Advanced therapeutic dressings for effective wound healing: a review. *J Pharm Sci*. 2015;104:3653-3680.
41. Voigt J, Driver VR. Hyaluronic acid derivatives and their healing effect on burns, epithelial surgical wounds, and chronic wounds: a systematic review and meta-analysis of randomized controlled trials. *Wound Repair Regen*. 2012;20:317-331.
42. Daeschlein G. Antimicrobial and antiseptic strategies in wound management. *Int Wound J*. 2013;10(suppl1):9-14.
43. Woo KY, Heil J. A prospective evaluation of methylene blue and gentian violet dressing for management of chronic wounds with local infection. *Int. Wound J*. 2017;14:1029-1035.
44. O'Donnell TF, Passman MA, Marston WA, et al. Management of venous leg ulcers: clinical practice guidelines of the society for vascular surgery and the American Venous Forum. *J Vasc Surg*. 2014;60(2 supp):3S-59S.
45. Patry J, Blanchette V. Enzymatic debridement with collagenase in wounds and ulcers: a systematic review and meta-analysis. *Int Wound J*. 2017;14:1055-1065.
46. Bosanquet DC, Rangaraj A, Richards AJ, Riddell A, Saravolac VM, Harding KG. Topical steroids for chronic wounds displaying abnormal inflammation. *Ann R Coll Surg Engl*. 2013;95:291-296.
47. Assadian O, Kammerlander G, Geyrhofer C, et al. Use of wet-to-moist cleansing with different irrigation solutions to reduce bacterial burden in chronic wounds. *J Wound Care*. 2018;27(10):S10-S16.
48. Tamakawa S, Hyashida K. Advances in surgical applications of the growth factors for wound healing. *Burns Trauma*. 2019;7:10.
49. Zhao D, Luo S, Xu W, Hu J, Lin S, Wang N. Efficacy and safety of hyperbaric oxygen therapy used in patients with diabetic foot: a meta-analysis of randomized clinical trials. *Clin Ther*. 2017;39:2088-2094.
50. Taylor G, Palmer J. The vascular terrirories (angiosomes) of the body: experimental study and clinical applications. *Br J Plast Surg*. 1987;40:113-141.
51. Nelson EA, Hillman A, Thomas K. Intermittent pneumatic compression for treating venous leg ulcers. *Cochrane Database Syst Rev*. 2014(5):CD001899.
52. Barber GA, Weller CD, Gibson SJ. Effects and associations of nutrition in patients with venous leg ulcers: a systematic review. *J Adv Nurs*. 2018;74(4):774-87.
53. Liu X, Zheng G, Chen B, Xie H, Zhang T. Compression and surgery with high ligation–endovenous laser ablation–foam sclerotherapy with compression alone for active venous ulcers. *Sci Rep*. 2019;9:14021.
54. Wu B, Lu J, Yang M, Xu T. Sulodexide for treating venous leg ulcers. *Cochrane Database Syst Rev*. 2016(6):CD010694.
55. Coccheri S, Bignamini AA. Pharmacological adjuncts for chronic venous ulcer healing. *Phlebology*. 2016;31(5): 366-367.
56. Gohel M, Heatley F, Liu L, et al. A randomized trial of early endovenous ablation and venous ulceration. *N Eng J Med*. 2018;378(22):2105-2114.
57. Crawford J, Lal B, Duran W, Pappas P. Pathophysiology of venous ulceration. *J Vasc Surg Venous Lymphat Dis*. 2017;5:596-605.
58. Humphreys ML, Stewart AH, Gohel MS, Taylor M, Whyman MR, Poskitt KR. Management of mixed arterial and venous leg ulcers. *Br J Surg*. 2007;94:1104-1107.
59. Singh N, Armstrong DG, Lipsky BA. Preventing foot ulcers in patients with diabetes. *J Am Med Assoc*. 2005;293:217-228.
60. Mills JL, Conte MS, Armstrong DG, et al. The Society for Vascular Surgery Lower Extremity Threatened Limb Classification System: risk stratification based on wound, ischemia, and foot infection (WIfI). *J Vasc Surg*. 2014;59(1):220-234.e1-2.
61. Trengove NJ, Stacey MC, McGechie DF, Mata S. Qualitative bacteriology and leg ulcer healing. *J Wound Care*. 1996;5(6):277-280.

SELF-ASSESSMENT STUDY QUESTIONS AND ANSWERS

Questions

1. Ulcers of the lower extremities are considered chronic if they are not healing for a period of:
   A. 6 weeks
   B. 8 weeks
   C. 12 weeks
   D. 6 months

2. The prevalence of wounds in all Medicare patients is highest for:
   A. Surgical wounds
   B. Diabetic ulcers
   C. Pressure ulcers
   D. Arterial ulcers

3. Venous ulcers are secondary to:
   A. Inflammatory changes causing WBC activation
   B. Increase in fibroblast contractile phenotype
   C. Increase tension in the dermis leading to skin destruction
   D. All of the above

4. Diabetic foot ulcers are associated with:
   A. Incidence of amputation 10%
   B. Arterial occlusive disease is the main cause of amputatiuon
   C. Angiosome principle is least applicable to diabetic patients
   D. Choke vessels are vessels are less functional in diabetic patients

5. In patients with pyoderma gagrenosum:
   A. Initial debridement improves healing
   B. Is associated with systemic disease in 50% to 60% of patients
   C. Might be associated with inflammatory conditions such as rheumatoid arthritis
   D. Drug induced in most cases

6. Skin ulceration is associated with the following drugs:
   A. Cocaine
   B. Methotrexate
   C. Hydroxyurea
   D. All of the above

7. Calciphylaxis is typically associated with all of the following except:
   A. Arterial occlusive disease
   B. Hyperphosphatemia
   C. Hyperparathyroidism
   D. Low parathyroid levels

8. The following is considered an absorptive dressing except:
   A. Collagen
   B. Foam
   C. Alginate
   D. Gelling hydrofibers

9. Iodine solutions can be used in dressing as microbicidal against:
   A. Fungi, bacteria, spores, protozoa and viruses
   B. Only bacteria
   C. Only yeasts and bacterial
   D. Spores and bacterial only

10. Growth factors improving wound healing include:
    A. PDGF, FGF but not IGF
    B. IGF, PDGF, but not FGF
    C. PDGF, VEGF, IGF and FGF
    D. Only VEGF

SELF-ASSESSMENT STUDY QUESTIONS AND ANSWERS

Answers

1. C.
2. A.
3. D.
4. D.
5. C.
6. D.
7. A.
8. A.
9. A.
10. C.

CHAPTER

54 Business Aspects of a Cardiovascular Center

Bhagwan Satiani and Christopher McQuinn

OUTLINE

INTRODUCTION
MANAGEMENT & DEVELOPMENT
GOVERNANCE
OPERATIONS & EFFICIENCY
PATIENT ACCESS
- Wait Times
- No Shows

FINANCIAL MANAGEMENT
- Financial Statements
- Using Financial Statements to Make Decisions
- Cost Volume Profit (CVP) Analysis

BUSINESS MANAGER ROLE
MANAGING THE REVENUE CYCLE
COMPENSATION METHODS FOR PHYSICIANS
- Legal Constraints
- Value-based and Newer Models for Reimbursement
- Future of Payments
- Quality of Care-based Payments

RECOVERING FROM COVID-19

INTRODUCTION

To streamline care, improve quality, and reduce inefficiencies, development of disease-specific service lines has often been employed by medical centers and physician groups. Often cited examples of this can be seen with neuroscience centers, wound care, cancer, and other specialties. The concept of developing a multidisciplinary cardiovascular center (CVC) has been around for some time but is not without challenges. The care of the cardiovascular patient is often split between many subspecialties with many of them vying for market share for similar disease processes. Furthermore, parochial silos often hamper productive integration between specialties especially within academic medical centers.

The development of a CVC and in particular the streamlining of care for vascular disease remain a priority for many health systems given the projected growth in the demand for cardiovascular disease-specific service as well as the rapid growth and development of new technologies targeted at vascular disease.

CVCs, like all centers of excellence, bring together a variety of healthcare professionals and in some cases institutions, to provide better value based upon healthcare outcomes and business efficiencies.[1]

In this chapter, we will discuss not only the management but operational and financial considerations important for institutions and medical groups in forming and operating a successful multidisciplinary CVC.

MANAGEMENT & DEVELOPMENT

The development of a multispecialty CVC by its essence requires the integration and collaboration of multiple groups of physicians focused on the cardiovascular health of the patient. This practice group may include vascular surgeons, cardiologists, vascular medicine physicians, radiologists, and cardiothoracic surgeons all of whom need to seamlessly integrate to provide coordinated, efficient, and quality care. To provide this care requires ensuring access to the "appropriate" specialist at the right time. This in turn needs to be balanced with distribution of care from high volume, central, critical access locations to smaller outreach same day surgery or clinics. Accomplishing this requires among other tasks, efficient patient access, scheduling, minimizing wait times to be seen, reducing no shows, and offering convenient clinic hours.

It is essential that there is a strong leadership team to ensure an effective, integrated CVC that can balance the varying tasks and responsibilities involved with coordinating multiple specialties and providers (Figure 54-1). A "dyad" of a physician leader with an administrator may provide the best value and balance to create an environment of trust and shared values. The leadership team must also integrate several essential skills to provide management oversight finances, daily operations as well as long-term project management and strategic awareness. Most importantly the leadership team must create shared values and goals to achieve buy in from the entire staff and organizational structure. All members must therefore agree upon ideals and be fully invested in the mission of the CVC.

Integration of specialized centers of care can be difficult in academic medical centers where issues such as departmental silos, line of authority, reporting of outcomes, and separate departmental finances may be a major stumbling block in a united focus on the CVC.

Also, to consider is the significant overlap in the care provided by specialties in a CVC. Internal competition can be fierce for referrals and procedural volumes with specialty overlap. Especially given that competence and procedural volume standards can vary significantly as determined by specialty organizations. To effectively moderate these potential conflicts, agreements must be set ahead of time by setting

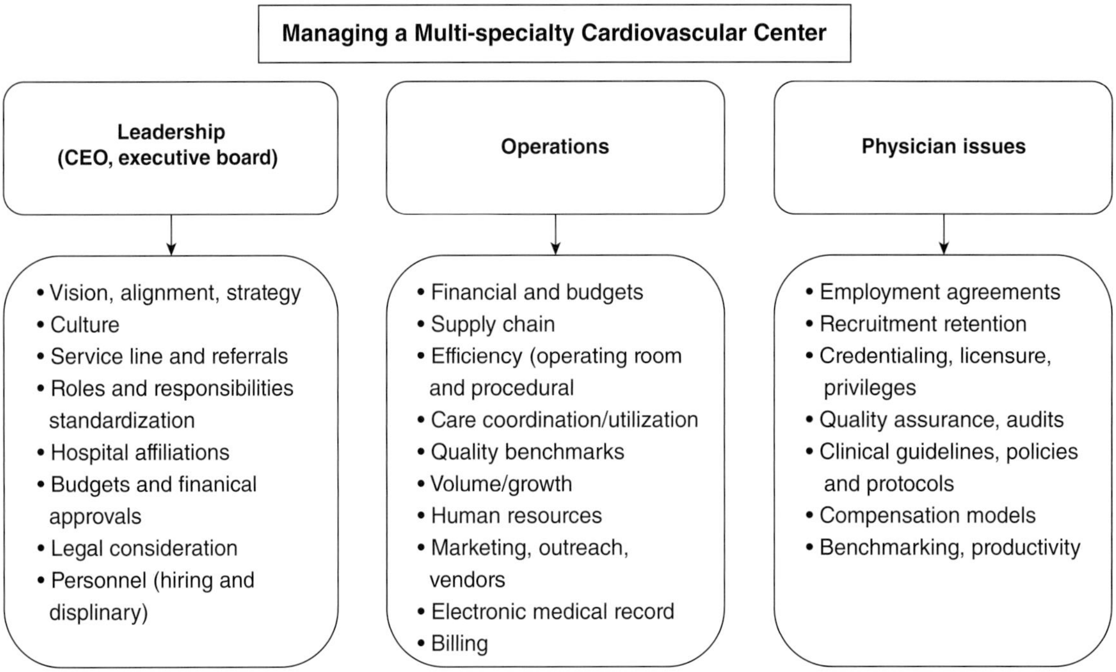

FIGURE 54-1 Management of a cardiovascular center is shown with details of tasks shown under three main management objectives.

a high bar tied to privileges for specific procedures. In addition, there must be complete transparency regarding compensation and financial incentives and unanimous agreement among all the specialty groups.

GOVERNANCE

The development of a governance structure for a CVC has significantly different considerations than governance models used by hospital systems. Traditional models of governance used by hospitals and academic medical centers typically consist of multiple levels of vertical leadership and bureaucracy. These models are ill equipped for managing CVCs given the need for quick execution of strategic plans and expedited decision making. One option is a matrixed governance structure though this model requires cooperation among all departments which may cause delays in execution of time-sensitive decisions. Another option is an integrated operating structure in which all reports occur directly to leaders of a service line or subservice line within a CVC (Figure 54-1). This structure lends itself to more efficient communication and decision-making yet can be more complex because of the number of personnel and functions reporting to very few individuals. Overall, the governance and management structure need to be tailored to organizational and cultural needs as not all models are suited for all environments and at times a hybrid or entirely new approach may need to be taken.

OPERATIONS & EFFICIENCY

There must be a multi-pronged effort to promote efficiency throughout the enterprise to achieve the highest productivity. In healthcare, efficiency can be described as providing a quality service using the fewest resources possible. The traditional definition of productivity is "the ratio of a measure of total outputs to a measure of inputs used in the production of goods and services."[2] In simple terms, inputs are assumed to be labor, capital invested in the business, and the goods available to workers. Outputs in the CVC include all the units or subunits such as the number of procedures or diagnostic tests, number of visits, or the revenue generated. So outputs must exceed inputs.

In the business of healthcare, productivity can be increased, for instance, by technology such as faster Internet service to allow workers to finish their tasks quicker. In the vascular imaging area, for instance, it can be better imaging technology with faster processors to allow sonographers to compete the test quicker. Management can contribute significantly to improve productivity and hence the bottom line. A strategic planning and management system that is utilized by many organizations is called the balanced scorecard (BSC).[3] The BSC is based on four legs of a stool and includes: financial, stakeholder, internal, and organizational capacity. The BSC then links strategic goals related to each leg with the programs and the metrics that the CVC may be working on (Table 54-1).

In diagnostic noninvasive vascular testing, for example, these could include: minimizing appointment access time, wait times to see a physician or schedule a test, reducing no show rates, increase procedure room utilization rate, aim for staff productivity exceeding a benchmark all to achieve the best throughput in noninvasive procedures (Figure 54-2).[4,5]

PATIENT ACCESS

WAIT TIMES

As patients, all of us have experienced the frustration of having to either access the health system or the wait time in a physician office. Unfortunately, wait times have increased by 30% in large US cities since 2014.[6] The pressure to increase physician productivity metrics is a major reason for the increase in wait times. It is important to note that patient satisfaction and their inclination to recommend a practice goes down with wait times greater than 20 minutes.[6] Some reasons for excessive wait times are unavoidable such as the physician being stuck in a procedure or a family emergency. It takes a skilled front-line worker to handle this with reassurance and calmness.

NO SHOWS

No shows are a major source of loss of revenue in every practice. This is especially true of vascular

TABLE 54-1 Operational Key Performance Indicators to Monitor

Metric	Monitoring
Volumes & growth	Outpatient volume % growth
	Growth in market share
	New referring physicians/ Advanced Practice Nurse (APN) added
	Referring physicians, APN complaints
	New technology budget
	Referral rate by zip code
	Case-mix index
Efficiency	Appointment access time
	Wait time to see physician or test
	No show rates
	Operating room or procedure room utilization rate
	Staff productivity
	Throughput in invasive, non-invasive procedures
Employees retention	Physician, nurses, and employee retention/attrition rate
	Employees satisfaction
	Absenteeism
	Recognition programs
	Complaint resolution audits
Patient outcomes/ satisfaction	In-hospital and outpatient adjusted mortality and morbidity for index procedures by specialty and physician
	Re-admissions % emergency department visits
	Proportion of patients not meeting CMS quality indicators for each specialty
	Healthcare Consumer Assessment of Healthcare Providers and Systems (HCAHPS) score

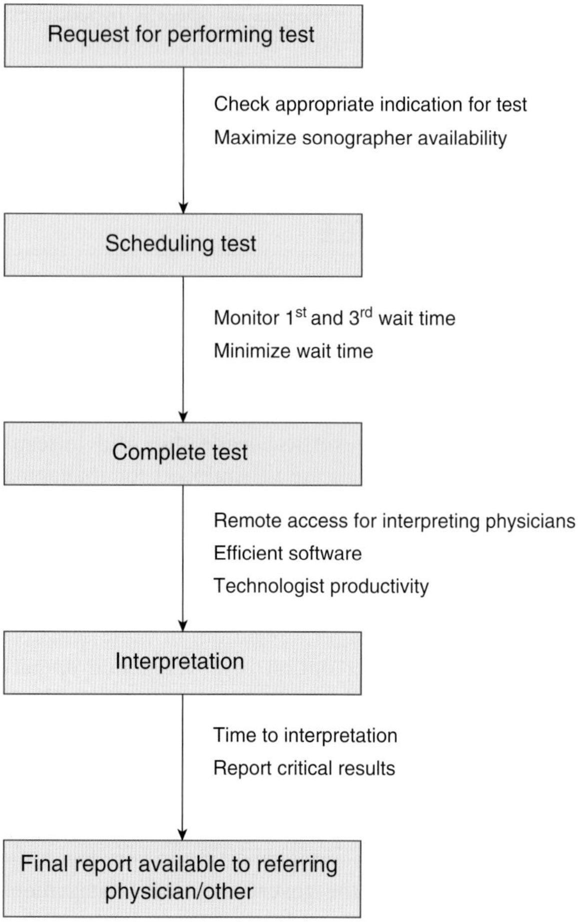

FIGURE 54-2 Steps to improving efficiency in the noninvasive vascular laboratory.

invasive procedures or even noninvasive tests due to high fixed costs and highly compensated employees working in those areas. Many strategies such as overbooking or even penalties for not canceling ahead of time have been tried without much success.[7] Many studies have identified sociodemographic factors and history as predictive factors, but the options are limited.[8] Most (>90%) practices rely on technology-related reminders to reduce the number ideally down to <5%.[9] Most practices also send reminders 2 days prior to an appointment. The no show rate doubles to 10% if there is no response to a reminder and is down to 3% if the patient confirms the appointment reminder. Some practices use more than one method such as a "my chart" type program-generated email reminder in addition to a text message.

FINANCIAL MANAGEMENT

Ideally, the financial management of the CVC must be fully integrated into the center itself. By creating a singular budget as well as a unified profit and loss statement, it allows for financial pressures to be dispersed among all service lines. Financial pressures such as decreasing payments, increasing costs, or changing payor demographic that may be disproportionately affecting one specialty can then be dispersed among the center allowing for continued unified strategic development. Although for most centers and systems compensation is still primarily tied to physician work volume, measured by relative value units (RVUs), progressively increasing share of this is likely going to be related to quality performance. When considering a compensation system for a CVC, broadly based and shared quality and performance metrics are essential. Shared metrics in relation to compensation ensure that overall system performance and service line integration is a priority. Transparency of the financial compensation plan, incentives, bonuses, and quality- or performance-related at-risk payments is critical to ensure multispecialty collaboration and integration.

FINANCIAL STATEMENTS

Physicians in executive leadership roles in the CVC do not have to be financial experts.

They have an accounting professional who constructs financial statements for the group to peruse. However, it is critical that they have enough working knowledge to spot inconsistencies and ask the right questions instead of voting on and approving financial reports routinely. In a supervisory and leadership role, physicians on the executive committee also have a fiduciary responsibility to act conscientiously.

There are three basic financial statements that must be provided to users of the financial information: the balance sheet, the income statement, and the statement of cash flows.[10] The balance sheet presents a picture of the entity at a specific point in time. It is called a balance sheet because the assets (the resources the entity has to support its operations) must be equal to the liabilities (what it owes its suppliers and creditors) plus owners' equity (what the owners have contributed to the entity and what is available for them).

The income statement is also called the "profit and loss" statement or "P&L" or "statement of income and expense." This statement basically includes net income, which is calculated by subtracting expenses from net revenue. Revenue is shown as all medical charges with contractual adjustments resulting in net revenue. The income statement and the statement of cash flows cover a period of time and provide the link between balance sheets.

The statement of cash flows tells the reader of the financial statements how cash was generated during the period and how it was spent.

USING FINANCIAL STATEMENTS TO MAKE DECISIONS

A useful tool for physicians and managers involved in managing the finances of the CVC is ratio analysis. Information necessary to perform ratio analysis can be found in the financial statement. It must be remembered that ratios in and of themselves are just numbers. It is important to compare ratios to the ratios of similar practices, historical ratios for the practice, or budgeted or expected ratios for the current year.

The four common ratios used and a brief example of each is seen in Table 54-2.

COST VOLUME PROFIT (CVP) ANALYSIS

CVP is used to gauge the consequences of changes in the company's volume of activity on costs, revenue, and profits. Profit is of course revenue minus expenses. In a not for profit organization and tax exempt instead of profit the term "revenue over expenses" may be used. Profits may be a function of many factors including volume, price, fixed cost, variable cost, and the payer mix. Fixed costs such as building expenses are usually but not always related to a time period rather than variation in volume. Variable costs such as supplies change proportionally with an increase or decrease in volume. CVP analysis is useful when the center is considering expansion of

TABLE 54-2 List of Some Ratios to Monitor Based upon Financial Statements

Type of Ratio	Measures	Examples of Use
Liquidity	Short-term ability to pay maturing obligations	Current ratio Quick or acid ratio
Activity	Effectiveness in using assets employed	Receivables turnover Days outstanding Asset turnover
Profitability	Degree of success or failure for a given period	Return on assets Return on revenue Return on equity
Coverage	Degree of protection for long-term creditors and investors	Debt to total assets Debt to equity Times interest earned

a test or procedure, adding a service, or possibly raising prices on a service.

Contribution margin—a term commonly used in break-even analysis and often misunderstood—is simply the difference between the total sales revenue and the variable costs assigned to it. In other words, contribution margin is what remains from revenues to cover fixed costs when all variable costs are covered.

BUSINESS MANAGER ROLE

Good business managers are worth their weight in gold. Excellent managers are five times more likely to be engaged with their staff compared to those who are rated as poor. They have great impact on the work environment and financial and human resource viability of the enterprise. Their ability to communicate with others, care for others, stay calm in a crisis, and retain good workers can be the difference between success and failure of the CVC.

A proper job description specific to the CVC must be written encompassing all the responsibilities entrusted to them. A 4-year college degree is preferred with an associate's or bachelor's degree in business administration to enable handling business operations. Licensure is not required although membership in The Professional Association of Health Care Office Management (PAHCOM) and Medical Group Management Association (MGMA) is helpful.

Managers have multitude responsibilities, which should be part of their written job description and some examples are listed as follows:

- Human resources: Hiring, firing, evaluation, training, orientation, complaints, the legal aspects, customer service, and scheduling.
- Financial & budgeting: Responsibility for budgets, coding, billing, accounting, budgets, revenue cycle, accounts payable, the payroll system, insurances, audits, and reporting responsibility to the board or the executive committee of the CVC.
- Legal: Familiarity with federal, state, and municipal laws, confidentiality, and proper storage of information for patients, health, and safety regulations; compliance of staff with licensure and certification so they can practice legally; professional liability basics.
- Marketing: Branding, advertising, patient surveys, working with agencies
- Information technology: Supervise selection of information technology
- Others: Communication, interpersonal, and leadership skills.

MANAGING THE REVENUE CYCLE

The revenue cycle consists of all clinical and administrative processes related to processing of claims, payment's, and collection of revenue. Managing the revenue cycle will be one of the most critical parts of the CVC. With the increasing complexity of billing and reimbursement, policies, and procedures for collecting all revenue due the practice need to be organized and efficient so that the components follow the patients' journey from the initial visit to full recovery of funds (Figure 54-3). If contracted to

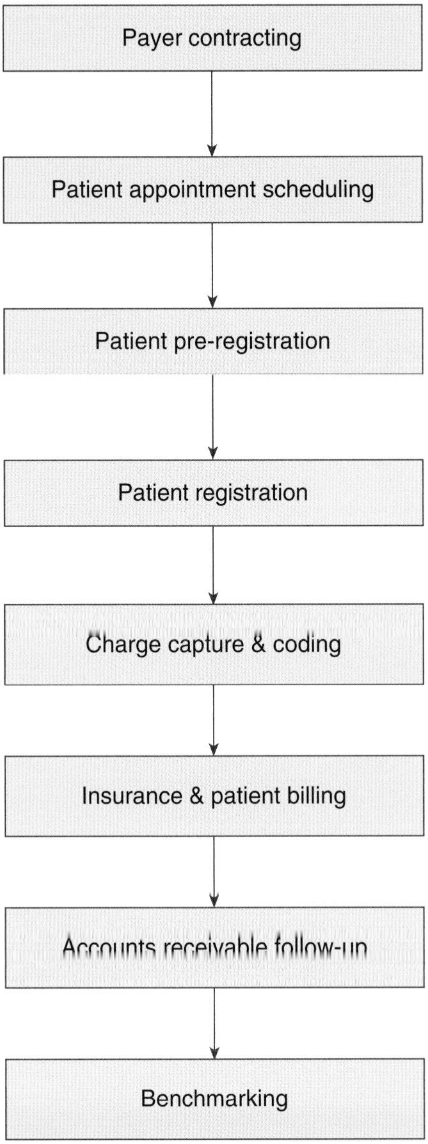

FIGURE 54-3 Components of the revenue cycle from the first patient contact to final collection of funds.

outside firms the fees may vary from 2% to 10% or more depending on the volume and dollar amount per charge.[11] Even if an external company is hired to manage the cycle, the front office being the first contact with the patient must be well trained to start the process competently. Some common metrics of revenue performance and financial key performance Indicators are indicated in Table 54-3.

COMPENSATION METHODS FOR PHYSICIANS

The increasing shift to value-based payment, pressure on physicians to contain costs, and to align their incentives with the CVC leads to constant evolution of compensation models. A compensation plan is a "method of allocating revenues and expenses in a medical practice and determining payment to the practice's surgeons for their services."[12]

The ideal plan should be fair, transparent, market driven (tied to an acceptable benchmark), legally compliant, and easy to comprehend as well as to implement (Figure 54-4). Although there is constant change in incentives, salary plus incentive and productivity-based compensation models are the most common compensation structures with a prevalence of 40% and 34%, respectively.[13] As shown in Table 54-5, the two extremes are guaranteed salary and a 100% productivity model with most hybrid plans being somewhere in between.

The employer desires a surgeon satisfied with their work environment and tools of the profession, is productive, and delivers high quality and safe care. The surgeon in turn wants transparency, fairness, stability of income, and incentives suited for their type of practice and age. Younger vascular specialists with debt or young children may want income security whereas the senior surgeon with an established practice may prefer more incentives to maximize compensation. Older surgeons may want limited call, stable income, and administrative duties.

Compensation plans in a CVC will depend on whether the VS are truly a single entity, both legally with single tax identification number (TIN) and functionality or separate entities. Regardless, compensation must fit within the regulatory structure in terms of both, being commercially reasonable and at fair market value (FMV). The Internal Revenue Service (IRS) provides a vague definition of FMV as "the price of a service between a willing buyer and a willing seller, neither being under any compulsion to buy or sell and both having a reasonable knowledge of the relevant facts."[14] What makes meeting the FMV requirement challenging is that there is no clear-cut definition of FMV nor is there well-defined guidance from the government on how the employer

TABLE 54-3 Revenue Performance and Financial Key Performance Indicators

	Metric	Explanation	Formula	Target	Comments
Cash management	Gross collection % rate	Total payments received during the period—refunds/ total amount of charges billed	Total payments—refunds/total charges	Median about 41% but varies by specialty	
	Net collection % rate	Total charges- adjustments/ net fees or total collected	Total receipts—refunds/ total charges—contractual adjustments	Median 94%	Measures efficiency in collecting contracted reimbursement amounts due, amount of revenue lost due to uncollectible debt, late filing, or noncontractual adjustments
	Total charge lag days	Measures charge capture workflow efficiency and identifies delays in cash	Total number of days from the revenue recognition date less the date of service by CPT code and the total number of CPT unit of service codes billed	7 days	Generally average monthly
	Collected versus collectable ratio		Payments received in May/June/July (90 days) in May allowable charges/allowable charges generated in May		
	Copayments collected	Point of service collection		> 85% of expected	***Core KPI***
	Self-Pay			With increase in high deductible plans, collection will vary based on the amount of the balance. A/R estimates should be adjusted depending on the HDP in the practice	
Billing	Lag charges from date of service	Average number of days from date of service or discharge to posting date		<2 days ideal	

	Denial rate on first time "clean" claim submission (First Pass)	Denials Ratio Percentage of claims denied by payer	% clean claims/number of claims	95%	***Core KPI:*** Overall denial rate of 15% affects profitability
Accounts receivables & collections	Days in accounts receivables or average collection period	Average number of days for an account to be paid	Net patient Accounts Receivable (from balance sheet/net patient service revenue/365	20–35 days depending on payer mix (surgical specialties higher range); ideally < 30 days	Should be part of "aging" report
	Posting of cash and any contractual adjustments			Ideally one business day	
	Accounts receivables > 90 days	Claims over 90 days unpaid	Total receivables > 90 days/total A/R	<15% of total	Should be part of "aging" report; ***Core KPI***
	Bad Debts write off		Bad debt as a percentage of revenue		Should be part of "aging" report
	Practice operating margin ratio	It determines net income from operations and operating revenue annually. Operating income includes revenue from patient care services, other operations, and government appropriations			***Core KPI***; Gives practice of overall operations; measures financial performance of a physician entity on an accrual basis
Patient Access	% of patients with complete and accurate pre-registration information		Complete pre-registrations/total registrations		
	Compliance with physician authorization requirement		Benchmark: 96%–98% compliance		
	Patient schedule occupied		"no show" rate		***Core KPI***
	Work relative value units (WRVUS)				

NOTE: Core Key Performance Indicator (**KPIs**) are the most important.

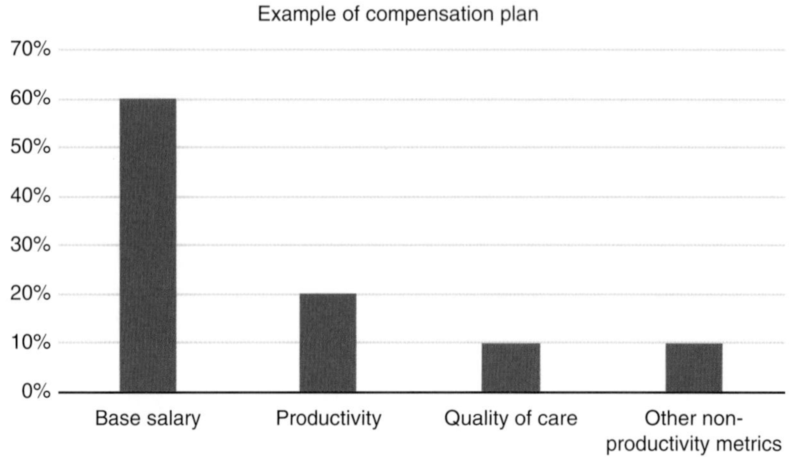

FIGURE 54-4 Example of parts of one type of compensation plan.

should calculate FMV. The best the CVC can do is to make the process fair, consistent, and transparent. Often the best path is to use market information, national benchmarks such as MGMA, Faculty Practice Solutions Center (associated with Association of American Medical Colleges), local survey by specialty or hire an expert in the compensation area (Table 54-4).

Medicare, the largest payer for vascular diseases, drives surgeon and hospital behavior in healthcare services. The prices for surgeon services for the 38 million Medicare beneficiaries in the traditional fee-for-service program are set by the federal government. For instance, Medicare currently withholds 1% of Medicare payments, 30% tied to HCAHPS (Hospital Consumer Assessment of Healthcare Providers and Systems) survey.[15] However, surveys show that for specialists, only 2.3% of compensation is tied to patient satisfaction scores.[16] There are also indications that health systems are starting to shift toward rewarding quality metrics. In their recent search assignments, Merritt Hawkins has observed an increase in offers to physicians in which a production bonus associated with quality metrics was involved (from 7% in 2011 to 39% in 2013).[17]

Since productivity is part of many compensation plans, measurement and benchmarking is important. Productivity can be measured by RVUs, net collections or similar measures. Individualistic plans emphasize productivity, net collections, work RVUs (WRVUs), or some combination thereof (Figure 54-3). Group-oriented plans as in a hospital or multispecialty group in a CVC, rewards may partly be based on the success of the unit, the hospital, or the health system. As an example, in a CVC a 60/20/20 plan would consist of individual productivity accounting for 60%, subspecialty for 20%, and the rest dependent on overall CVC profitability. Advantages and disadvantages of various type of plans are shown in Table 54-5.

In a CVC owned by an academic medical center, the compensation plan may be part of a holistic "XYZ" plan.[10] The largest component of this plan is the base salary (X) tied to academic rank, historical salary and/or market factors. The (Y) component is tied to teaching, research, and/or service efforts plus compensation for administrative work like a directorship. The Faculty Practice Solution Center, part of the Association of American Medical Colleges, is used as the benchmark for appointments such as a directorship. The (Z) portion represents the clinical or nonclinical incentives. The chief component (Y) meets the 90% threshold of median income.

The trend has been for increasing use of WRVU-based compensation in both private and academic practices. In a recent survey of vascular surgeons, almost 70% of those responding stated that productivity metrics were a part of their compensation plan.[18]

TABLE 54-4 Common Compensation Benchmarking Sources for Vascular Specialists

Firm	Details	Website
Medical Group Management Association (MGMA)	Represents 5,800 organization managers; Costs to access 140 physician specialties and provide "Datadive" Provider Compensation Data (Including total pay, bonus/incentives, retirement), Productivity (work RVUs, total RVUs, professional collections and charges), and Benefit metrics (hours worked per week/year and weeks of vacation)	www.mgma.com
Clinical Practice Solutions Center (CPSC)	Collaboration between the Association of American Medical Colleges (AAMC) and Vizient; 90+ participating organizations (mostly academic), over 140,000 providers, 126 specialties benchmarked, more than 5,000 users nationwide	https://www.clinicalpracticesolutionscenter.org/
Sullivan Cotter	Workforce compensation and performance improvement resources; compensation and rewards, Governance and compliance, Workforce analytics, Business and practice valuations, Tools and technology solutions, Mergers and acquisitions, and Clinical workforce optimization	https://sullivancotter.com/
AMGA (American Medical Group Association)	More than 175,000 physicians' practice in member organizations; Discounted prices for members; data from a record 272 medical groups representing more than 117,000 practicing clinicians, 143 specialties, 27 other healthcare provider positions, and 39 executive and leadership positions	https://www.amga.org/
Jackson	Established physician recruiting firm	https://www.jacksonphysiciansearch.com
Modern Healthcare	Annual Physician Compensation Survey includes several large firms	https://www.modernhealthcare.com/
Doximity	Doximity Physician Compensation Report draws on the responses of more than 65,000 licensed U.S. doctors in 40 medical specialties	https://www.doximity.com
Merritt Hawkins	Mostly a recruiting firm; compensation data available for physicians recruited by their firm	https://www.merritthawkins.com/
Medscape	Popular Physicians Compensation Report: More than 20,000 physicians in 29 specialties responded to the last online survey, results were weighted to the American Medical Association's physician distribution by specialty	https://www.medscape.org/

TABLE 54-5 Advantages and Disadvantages of Various Compensation Plans

Type of Plan	Advantages	Disadvantages
Pure productivity	1. Easier to understand 2. Incentive to work harder 3. Perceived as fair unless disparate pay 4. Easier to satisfy group and individuals 5. Can be legally compliant to award productivity bonuses 6. And adjusted for payer	1. May cause friction in multispecialty groups with overhead attribution 2. Friction because of internal competition 3. Overtreatment is a possibility unless steps taken to audit 4. Seen as unfair if disparate pay or production/referrals disparities
Straight salary	1. Easy to understand 2. Simple accounting 3. Works well if equal productivity 4. Team unity if no significant disparities 5. Apparently less legal risk (Stark) 6. Adjustment to payer mix easier 7. Avoids incentive to over treat	1. No incentive to work harder 2. Friction if low productivity or laziness by some members 3. Possible friction about overhead between high producers and low producers 4. Hard to institute incentive measures
Base guaranteed salary and incentive	1. Easy to comprehend and implement 2. Stark violations uncommon 3. Income predictability and stability 4. Better success in single specialty with essentially equal productivity 5. Perception of team effort	1. Benchmark used for base pay/incentives may be disagreed about 2. May allow slacking off laziness by some members 3. Motivation to produce may be a problem if incentives are not large
Equal share salary and production incentive combination	1. Easy to comprehend 2. Relatively easy to execute (half guaranteed, half incentive) 3. Group effort involved in measuring both production and incentive measures 4. Can also include quality/patient satisfaction and other measures as incentives 5. Works better in single specialties but cam work in some multispecialty practices	1. Financial expertise acumen required to monitor finances 2. Disputes may occur about exact definition of overhead and what is shared 3. Disputes may also occur about inequal work relative work units, collections, and benchmarks for the formula to divide revenue

Compensation at risk for nonproduction incentives may reach 15% to 20% of the bonus "pool" amount, although a < 10% number is likely the reasonable range for specialists. These activities may include population management measures, Healthcare Effectiveness Data and Information Set (HEDIS) or the Medicare Access and CHIP Reauthorization Act of 2015 (MACRA) metrics, patient experience surveys, good citizenship, or ease of access to care. On-call compensation is usually a daily stipend that is negotiated between parties and varies by specialty and demand. Because of the regulatory environment, director compensation is generally set in a formal contract. The stipend for this also depends on the specialty, the demand, and the number of hours worked.

LEGAL CONSTRAINTS

Compensation and incentive plans offered by physician-owned surgery groups are different than those offered by hospital affiliated/owned entities. Surgeon compensation plans are always under scrutiny and influenced by federal and state laws, which are confusing and continue to change. The IRS only provides guidance related to the federal tax code, particularly when a surgeon is employed by a tax-exempt entity, without any specific laws that dictate FMV compensation. As an example, the Stark law prohibits a surgeon from referring a Medicare or Medicaid patient to a designated health service (DHS) if the surgeon or the surgeon's immediate family has any financial relationship with the healthcare entity that provides the DHS.[19] Relevant to a surgical practice, at least one of the exemptions to the Stark regulations must apply for a practice to legally generate income from these sources. Many surgery groups and hospitals use the "bonafide" group practice exemption to avoid violating the federal statute.

VALUE-BASED AND NEWER MODELS FOR REIMBURSEMENT

Although, payment for "value" was predicted to make up for an increasing share of payments for healthcare, adaptation has been slow. This is partly because there is no consensus on the definition of value or its metrics. Centers for Medicare & Medicaid Services (CMS) is still pushing such programs so it will continue to be a part of future. Ms. Seema Verma, CMS administrator, has stated, "Value-based payment … is the future. So make no mistake: If your business model is focused merely on increasing volume rather than improving health outcomes, coordinating care, and cutting waste, you will not succeed under the new paradigm."[20]

CMS has been active in creating "Alternative Payment Model (APM)" and introduced several variations each with a different focus. These models are designed to replace existing fee-for-service payments with reimbursement incentives designed for "value" care (i.e., high-quality and cost-effective care). In 2018, 35.8% of US healthcare payments flowed through APMs

Employers in the United States spent about $700 billion in 2019 to pay for their employee's healthcare services. Lately, the trend has been for employers to keep the "middleman" out and contract directly with health systems or physician groups. Major employers like Walmart, General Electric, Boeing, and Lowe's have started to bundle services and contract with them and apparently saved billions of dollars. Other companies have partnered to form National Alliance of Healthcare Purchaser Coalitions.[21] The CVC must be continually aware of not only trends but regulations and legislation being proposed that will affect it.

FUTURE OF PAYMENTS

With the change in payment systems, surgeon-hospital alignment, accountable care organizations (ACOs), and the shortage of surgeons, it is likely that there will be not only be upward pressure on surgeon compensation, but a demand for compensation for nonpatient care related responsibilities. However, although compensation may rise, the work relative units stay flat, unless the shortage of vascular surgeons leads to more work per surgeon. If compensation rises, this could put more pressure on the organization to cut costs or look for other ways to increase revenue. Value-based care, if implemented strategically, may be an alternative. A generational change will also put pressure on employers to offer part-time and flexible employment opportunities.

The CVC must be tuned into future innovative payment models such as ACOs, bundle- and episode-based payments, population-based payments, and balance the downside financial risk with the financial rewards.

QUALITY OF CARE-BASED PAYMENTS

As entities such a Medicare transition from fee-for-service models to pay-for-performance models, the quality of the care provided, outcomes will be progressively more important in compensation and reimbursement. The prevailing thought being that higher quality of care up front will in turn lead to lower costs overall. As such, CVC must be proactive in developing internal quality metrics in line with expectations from major payers. Quality audits performed by a dedicated quality assurance department serve a multifunctional role; to ensure safe, value-based patient care, and to preserve quality-based reimbursements and overall center financial solvency.

Also, to consider is the push to create transparency with the public regarding physician financial data, quality performance, and overall value estimation. To accomplish these objectives, Medicare in 2008 began the Physician Feedback Program which collects data on quality, cost, and resource use on a hospital and provider level and provides participants with their data in comparison to their peers. Although this transition to quality payment programs is ongoing, it has not yet reached a peak.[22] As such CVC must be aware that their quality and performance metrics will not only be evaluated in relation to the potential payments but also shared with their patients and referrers.

RECOVERING FROM COVID-19

Management must be proactive in planning for returning to a full schedule and re-starting all the facets of the CVC as the COVID-19 crisis abates. Considering the uncertainty associated with the recovery, by necessity this must be a phased procedure over time depending on the demand and then adjusting personnel and supplies accordingly. This means that management must have a solid handle on the number of patients/tests/procedures seen prior to the crisis and a weekly trend line showing recovery. Protocols must be in place that deal with screening staff and physicians, classification of the urgency of visits/tests or procedures, and an assured supply chain to provide PPE. Wearing masks, cleaning hands and objects, and physical distancing are going to be with us for the near future.

Billing software must all be kept up to date as CMS announces new International Classification of Disease (ICD) and Current Procedural Terminology (CPT) codes associated with tele-visits and procedures. Staff must be educated along with physicians on a regular basis. Collection activity will need to be altered due to the crisis.

Financial managers must be integrated into the executive structure so the need for extra capital is evident ahead of time to allow meeting with banks or other sources. Budgets will need to be revised considering the historical volumes, revenues, write-offs, and collection ratios. Contracts with suppliers and vendors must be contacted for payback deferments for supplies, rent, and utilities. By this time, most practices must have Paycheck Protection Program (PPP) loans, forgivable, and unforgivable, on the books. Financial forecasts will be needed to allow planning of return of loans if necessary.[23] Human resources staff will probably be the most stressed during the COVID-19 crisis because decisions will have to be made about furloughing or termination, depending on whether the crisis is fading or recurring. Depending on financial viability, furloughing of valued employees may allow the CVC to fund their benefits such as health insurance to support them. Physician compensation may have to be frozen or decreased if there is a shortfall in revenue for a prolonged period of time.

REFERENCES

1. George MO. *The Lean Six Sigma Guide to Doing More with Less*. Hoboken, NJ: John Wiley and Sons; 2010.
2. What is productivity and how is it measured? Available at https://www.pc.gov.au/news-media/pc-news/previous-editions/pc-news-may-2015/productivity-and-how-measured#:~:text=Measured%20productivity%20is%20the%20ratio,output%20%E2%80%94%20it%20is%20the%20residual. Accessed July 7, 2020.
3. Balanced Scorecard Basics. Available at https://balancedscorecard.org/bsc-basics-overview/
4. Satiani B, Kiser D, Mason T. Turnaround time and timeliness of physician interpretation in the vascular laboratory. *Vasc Endovasc Surg*. 2012; 46(2) 167-171.
5. Haurani J. Kiser D, Satiani B. Improving efficiency measures is a necessary part of the vascular lab and can be used to satisfy requirements of future accreditation and payment models. *J Vasc Surg Venous Lymphat Disord*. 2019;7:325-332.
6. Gritters J. The cost of long wait times. Available at https://www.athenahealth.com/knowledge-hub/financial-performance/cost-long-wait-times. Accessed July 1, 2020.
7. Satiani B, Miller S, Patel D. No-show rates in the vascular laboratory: analysis and possible solutions. *J Vasc Interv Radiol*. 2009;20:87-91.
8. Harvey BH, Liu C, Ai J, et al. Predicting no-shows in radiology using regression modeling of data available

in the electronic medical record. *J Am Coll Radiol.* 2017; 14:1303-1309.

9. Finnegan J. 4 ways to cut down on no-show patients at your practice. Available at https://www.fiercehealthcare.com/practices/4-steps-to-cut-down-no-show-appointments-elmont-teaching-health-center. Accessed July 7, 2020.
10. Satiani B. The Smarter Physician: conquering your practice's billing and reimbursement. Available at https://payhip.com/b/ET8q. Accessed July 8, 2020.
11. Manley R, Satiani B. Revenue cycle management. *J Vasc Surg.* 2009;50:1232-1238.
12. Johnson BA, Keegan DW. *Physician Compensation Plans.* Englewood, CO: Medical Group Management Association; 2006.
13. Kane CK. New data on physician compensation methods: One size does not fit all. American Medical Association. Available at https://www.ama-assn.org/sites/ama-assn.org/files/corp/media-browser/premium/health-policy/prp-phys-comp-methods-2014_0.pdf. Accessed July 7, 2020.
14. Internal Revenue Service. National office technical advice memorandum. Available at https://www.irs.gov/pub/irs-wd/0303010.pdf. Accessed July 7, 2020.
15. Strate C. How does patient satisfaction impact reimbursement? Available at https://www.accessefm.com/blog/how-does-patient-satisfaction-impact-reimbursement. Accessed June 26, 2020.
16. Gordon D. MGMA: Gradual shift toward provider pay tied to quality metrics. Becker's Hospital Review. Available at https://www.beckershospitalreview.com/compensation-issues/mgma-gradual-shift-toward-provider-pay-tied-to-quality-metrics.html. Accessed 7/7/2020.
17. Beauliue D. Building compensation plans in a pay-for-performance era. Medical Economics. Available at https://www.medicaleconomics.com/view/building-compensation-plans-pay-performance-era. Accessed July 7, 2020.
18. Satiani B, Matthews MA, Gable D. Work effort, productivity, and compensation trends in members of the Society for Vascular Surgery. *Vasc Endovascular Surg.* 2002;46:509-514.
19. Satiani B Exceptions to the Stark law: practical considerations for surgeons. *Plast Reconstr Surg.* 2006; 117:1012-1022.
20. Brandy M, "Americans 'fed up' with high healthcare costs, surprise billing, Verma says," *Modern Healthcare*, September 10, 2019.
21. National Alliance of Healthcare Purchaser Coalitions. Available at https://www.nationalalliancehealth.org/about/coalition-members. Accessed July 1, 2020.
22. Medicare FFS Physician Feedback Program/Value-Based Payment Modifier. Available at https://www.cms.gov/Medicare/Medicare Fee for Service-Payment/PhysicianFeedbackProgram. Accessed July 7, 2020.
23. Satiani B, Zigrang TA, Bailey-Wheaton JL. COVID-19 Financial resources for physicians. *J Vasc Surg.* 2020;72(4):1161-1165.

SELF-ASSESSMENT STUDY QUESTIONS AND ANSWERS

Questions

1. Traditional models of governance used by hospitals and academic medical centers are typically ill equipped to manage CVCs given the need for quick execution of plan and decisive decision-making.
   A. True
   B. False

2. Which of the following are governance/leadership models that are well suited for integrated CVCs?
   A. Matrixed governance
   B. Integrated operating structure
   C. Dyad leadership model
   D. All of the above

3. An often used definition of productivity is the ratio of a measure of total outputs to a measure of inputs used in the production of goods and services.
   A. True
   B. False

4. Which of the following are components of a strategic planning management system in a cardiovascular center?
   A. Financial
   B. Stakeholder
   C. Internal
   D. Organizational capacity
   E. All of the above

5. Which of the following Federal Laws is important in regulating physician compensation?
   A. HIPPAA
   B. Stark
   C. Anti-Kickback Statute
   D. PATH regulations

SELF-ASSESSMENT STUDY QUESTIONS AND ANSWERS

Answers

1. A.
2. D.
3. A.
4. E.
5. B.

CHAPTER

55 Leadership and Physicians as Leaders in Health Care Organizations

Jack W. Sample and Charles Brunicardi

OUTLINE

INTRODUCTION
WHAT MAKES A LEADER?
FUNDAMENTAL PRINCIPLES OF LEADERSHIP IN MEDICINE
- Lead with Values
- Establish a Clear Vision
- Developing Self-awareness
- Lead by Action, Not by Position
- Balance

THE ROLE OF THE PHYSICIAN LEADER IN THE MODERN HEALTH CARE SYSTEM
THE SURGEON LEADER OR THE SERVANT LEADER: EXAMINING DIFFERENT STYLES OF LEADERSHIP
COERCIVE
AUTHORITATIVE
AFFILIATIVE
DEMOCRATIC
PACESETTING
COACHING
CONCLUSION

INTRODUCTION

The field of surgery continues to evolve at an astonishing pace. Briefly visiting the history of surgery, we can marvel at the leaps and bounds this field has made in a relatively short period of time. Joseph Lister's theory of antisepsis did not take prominence in practice until the early twentieth century, yet at the end of the century, we witnessed the revolution of minimally invasive surgery championed by the laparoscopic approach. Only time will tell the next momentous innovation within the field of surgery. The evolution of surgery expands beyond technological advancement and the ability to successfully complete surgical procedures once thought to be impossible. Surgical culture has also undergone immense change. Historically, surgery was a field dominated by surgeons who led with a command-and-control style of practice.[1] This was, in part, secondary to the nature of the specialty at that time. Surgeons were once tasked with being the sole caretaker of their patients, being highly specialized in the ability to treat pathology with surgical technique. In the operating room, surgeons acted as sole decision-makers in the oversight of patient care. Recent decades have brought forth a transformation toward a more dynamic and interdisciplinary health care system that places increasing focus on the patient experience.[2] In recent years, policymakers and scholars have taken interest in better understanding how the role of leadership has changed in today's health care system, and what qualities will make an effective leader in today's health care landscape.[3] This new dynamic approach to medicine has disrupted the old norms of many health care specialties, particularly the field of surgery. The old norms of the commanding surgeon have been disrupted as the evolution of our health care system brings forth new standards of multidisciplinary care. As the single-provider style of care phases out, a new era of surgical culture is ushered in placing greater emphasis on team dynamics and leadership abilities.

What can be done to ensure future generations of surgeons are capable of filling new demands for strong surgeon leaders? Medicine is a perpetually evolving field, constantly being disrupted by technological advancement. To stay up to date with emerging evidence, medical professionals commit to being lifelong learners within their field. This same precedent should be applied equally to all areas of medical training, including leadership development for medical trainees. Leadership is fluid, and our understanding of its principles changes over time. It is imperative for surgical training programs to acknowledge the value of quality leadership development for their trainees. How important is the interplay of leadership and surgery? The National Residency Match Program's (NRMP) data for the 2018 match cycle showed leadership qualities were a citing factor 61% of the time when considering surgery applicants.[4] In their program requirements for graduate medical education in general surgery, the Accreditation Council for Graduate Medical Education (ACGME) stated "the surgeon must effectively function in interprofessional and, often, multidisciplinary teams, frequently in a leadership role."[5] Despite seemingly increasing acknowledgment of leadership development and its integral role within medical education, trainees appear to lack leadership competency. A study investigating resident perception about the importance of leadership surveyed 43 general surgery residents at a program. Of the 23 residents who responded, 93% identified leadership skills as important for career development, but over half rated their own leadership skills as low competency.[6] This raises many questions regarding the current state of leadership development training in medical education. It is worthwhile for surgical programs to consider potential barriers or reasons for why some trainees believe they lack competency in leadership abilities.

Behind any successful organization is a successful leader. Today's health care system faces new challenges which must be addressed through the guidance of quality leadership. James Stoller discussed factors that may have contributed to the emerging demand we are seeing for physician-based leaders. "Taken together, the current challenges facing health care, organizational challenges of health care organizations, the features of physicians and their training that conspire against collaboration and followership, the perceived needs of trainees, and the extra mandate for resonant leadership in health care underscore the need for developing excellent physician-leaders."[7] The ushering in of the modern health care system has created avenues of opportunity for physician leaders to enter the arena of higher-level leadership positions. The increasing demand for high-quality leadership abilities in surgical trainees and physicians is met by an emerging body of literature discussing the prospect of physician leaders in health care systems.[7] History has proven the field of surgery to be committed to extraordinary adaptation and innovation. A new spotlight falls on the role of the surgeon leader in our modern health care system. Leadership principles are intertwined within the field of surgery, as surgeons inherently assume tremendous responsibility when treating patients within the operating theater. To ensure future success within health care organizations, prioritizing quality leadership development should be high on the agenda. Likewise, surgical training programs should reflect on what resources they offer to promote leadership development for surgical trainees. Investing resources into leadership development is an investment in organizational success. This chapter discusses the fundamentals of leadership and how they relate to surgeon leaders, the role of the surgeon leader in modern health care organizations, and various styles of leadership.

WHAT MAKES A LEADER?

Leadership is a topic that has surmounted in seemingly endless discussions, publications, and debates over its intricacies. Yet, it is easy to recognize high-quality leadership when we see it. What are these characteristics that appear to be so foundational to quality leadership? The Chinese philosopher and founder of Taoism, Lao Tzu, eloquently defined leadership by saying "a leader is best when people barely know he exists, when his work is done, his aim fulfilled, they will say: we did it ourselves." The words of Loa Tzu encapsulate the idea of leadership in a refined and understandable manner. One interpretation of Lao Tzu's written word is that a leader's

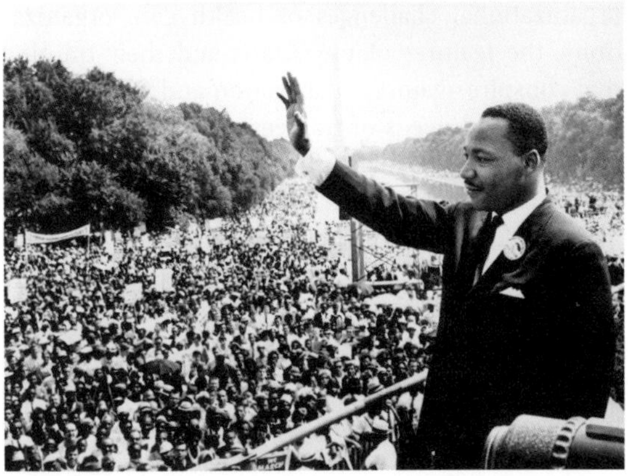

FIGURE 55-1 Reverend Dr Martin Luther King, Jr, March on Washington. (Agence France Presse, Contributor/ Getty Images.)

success is measured by their ability to engage others and collectively inspire action toward a shared vision, ultimately resulting in followers becoming their own leaders. This style of selfless leadership is exemplified in the workings of Reverend Dr Martin Luther King, Jr (Figure 55-1), a champion of the twentieth century civil rights movement. King was an extraordinarily educated man whose admirable determination became the framework for quintessential leadership for decades after his passing. King was a visionary who did not waiver from his values and beliefs. He acted selflessly in his pursuit of justice, displaying incredible determinationand willingness to lead. King is an exemplar of leadership, and his actions have inspired generations of rising leaders, including surgeons.[8]

FUNDAMENTAL PRINCIPLES OF LEADERSHIP IN MEDICINE

Leadership comes in many flavors. For decades, differing theories and models of leadership have been proposed, accepted, and even rejected. Leadership concepts are not static either, rather, they are fluid concepts that adapt to an ever-changing landscape of organizational design. To discuss every component and style of leadership would be overambitious; however, there are several boiled down components of successful leadership that seem to be foundational to many leadership theories. When applied diligently, these principles can act as a recipe for successful leadership development. Strong leaders are not created in one day, and the skills and experiences required to develop into a successful leader cannot all be learned from the pages of a book. This does not, however, undermine the importance of what we can learn through studying differing leadership styles and the actions of some of history's greatest leaders.

LEAD WITH VALUES

Imagine a beautiful sports car driving slowly down the road as the sun's rays bounce off its sleek exterior. Attractive from afar, but closer inspection reveals a lawn mower engine below the hood. A leader without a set of core values is like a sports car with a lawnmower engine. A well-understood set of values is integral to the success of a strong leader. *How,* and for *what,* will you lead, if you do not know *why* you lead? This is a question any leader should ask themselves to challenge their abilities and gain a better understanding of their aim. The German philosopher Friedrich Nietzsche is credited with saying "he who has a why to live for can bear almost any how." When applied to leadership, a leader who knows *why* he or she leads is better equipped to handle challenges and resolve conflict. Our values guide our decision-making process and help us navigate through obstacles. The "leader" who lacks values is blinded to their vision, simply occupying a position of assumed power, and not truly fulfilling the role of a leader. Personality traits such as charisma or persuasiveness may allow someone to rise into a leadership position, but without values to guide their action, they may struggle to inspire others to work toward a shared vision.

A core set of values is the compass a leader uses to navigate through challenges. The values of a leader are two-fold. It is paramount for a leader to understand their own core values, as well as the values of the organization they represent. Values give purpose to action. Imagine a CEO who is not aligned with the core values of their organization. How effective can this leader be in their attempts to inspire collaborative change within their organization? This is

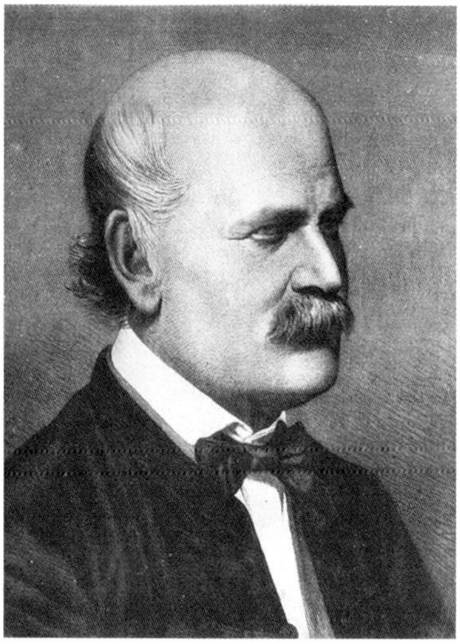

FIGURE 55-2 Dr Ignaz Semmelweis. (Brandstaetter images/Contributor, Getty images.)

exceptionally important for leaders in medicine, a field built on foundational values, such as empathy, justice, and honesty. Many great innovators of medicine led with their values, sacrificing themselves to harsh public criticisms in the pursuit of improving public health, and our modern health care system is forever in debt to their resilience. Hungarian physician Ignaz Philipp Semmelweis (Figure 55-2), described as the "savior of mothers," pioneered antiseptic practice years before the famous works of Louis Pasteur and Joseph Lister. Semmelweis postulated why puerperal fever was so rampant in some obstetric clinics but not in others close in proximity. After collecting data showing a significant reduction in puerperal fever at clinics that employed routine handwashing measures, he was ridiculed by colleagues for his "outlandish" theory. Despite heavy criticism, Semmelweis was resilient, standing by his evidence and urging practitioners to improve hygiene. Semmelweis's theory resulted in greatly reduced postpartum mortality rates at obstetric clinics that adopted his practices. His adherence to his values combined with his persistence ultimately resulted in observations that went on to inspire germ theory and save an innumerable number of lives around the world.

Semmelweis is an exemplar of the value-based leader in medicine. He stood resolute by his findings, challenging the status quo for what he believed was for the greater good of others. Surely the expectation is not for every medical leader to revolutionize our contemporary understanding of medicine. These great innovators of medicine serve as inspiration, impacting generations of future physician leaders. When developing your *why*, ask "why do I lead?" or "for what purpose do I serve through leading?" The ability to honestly answer these questions is an important step in establishing your core leadership values.

ESTABLISH A CLEAR VISION

Leadership is not a position; it is an action. This action is guided by a set of values and requires a vision to lead toward. A clear vision is the destination a leader sets out to reach. Imagine leading an expedition to sea, setting sail with no clear vision as to where your ship will sail. Will this plan result in success for you and your team members? Therefore, it is the essence of a leader to establish and inspire a unifying vision and take ownership of that vision until completion. Surgery is a field of visionaries. Surgeons set a vision for how they will improve the patient's condition each time they enter the operating theater. Practicing surgery without a clear vision would be a risky game. By nature, surgeons are required to be well-calculated planners, but it is imperative for them to effectively communicate their vision to team members. Proficiently inspiring a shared vision helps create a vested interest among team members. Additionally, a clear vision in surgery may help team members foresee obstacles and take a more preventative approach.

A vision can be set for the near future or for years to come. When Martin Luther King delivered his historical "I Have a Dream" speech at the March on Washington, he described his vision for the future of our country. He spoke clearly about his mission for equality to reign across our country, and for children to be born into a land in which people were judged by the content of character rather than the color of their skin. King was a visionary; his vision was clear, understandable, and obtainable. His ability to create a unifying vision for the country to rally behind is one of his most defining qualities as a leader. Likewise, pioneers of surgery had clear visions in mind when they set out to revolutionize this field. In the 1940s,

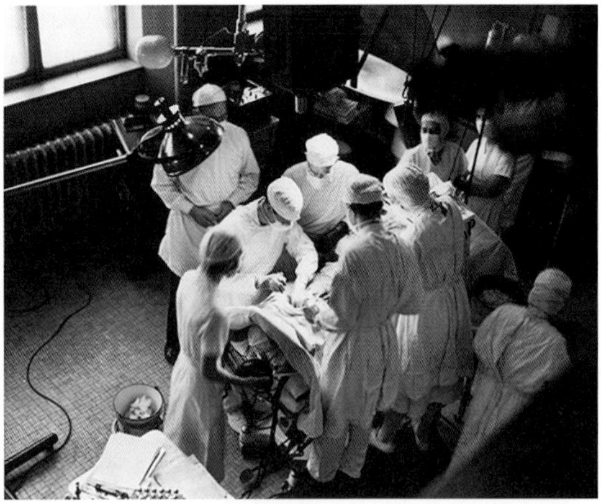

FIGURE 55-3 Dr Alfred Blalock performing surgery, assisted by Vivien Thomas (top left). (Image courtesy of the Chesney Archives, Johns Hopkins Medicine, Nursing, and Public Health.)

revered surgeons Alfred Blalock and Vivien Thomas (Figure 55-3) conjured a vision of shattering the taboo surrounding performing surgery on the human heart, pioneering the field of cardiac surgery. Their vision was daring, and quite frankly, unheard of at the time. Still, they persisted. Their clear and common vision to offer a permanent surgical treatment option for "blue baby syndrome" guided their efforts which culminated in one of the most historic surgical success stories of the twentieth century. Their work, along with the contributions of pediatric cardiologist Helen Taussig, ushered in a new era of surgery and expanded the horizons for what was thought to be possible at that time.

A clear and well-established vision is integral to a successful leader, and this vision will permeate through an organization and enable others to act purposefully. This is particularly relevant in the field of surgery. A surgeon enters the operating theater with a clear vision of how they will use operative technique to improve the health of a patient. The success of a surgical team depends on the leader's ability to establish a clear and unifying vision, and their ability to convey that vision to all team members. Consider the following questions when determining your team's vision: "How will we know we successfully reached our vision? Is the vision clearly understood by all members of the team? What obstacles stand in the way of the shared vision?"

DEVELOPING SELF-AWARENESS

Surgery is a constantly evolving field, with advances in technology and shifts in culture challenging old norms. Surgeons and aspiring trainees commit to be lifelong learners in their field. Remaining up to date in a rapidly advancing field can be difficult and anxiety provoking at times. Therefore, a great skillset for surgeon leaders is to develop a high degree of self-awareness. This is advantageous for a multitude of reasons. Firstly, an honest and accurate self-assessment of one's strengths and weaknesses are of paramount importance in medical practice. Self-awareness is a conduit for self-introspection, granting a truthful look into one's abilities and limitations. In the operation theater, mistakes can be catastrophic; surgeon's who display a high degree of self-awareness regarding their abilities can minimize complications before they occur. Secondly, self-awareness allows leaders the ability to recognize how they are perceived by others. Team members may equate a leader's self-awareness with approachability, or on the contrary, a lack thereof. Good team dynamics will ultimately help a procedure run smoothly. Can you think of a situation in which a team-member could not pick up on cue that was noticeably irritating to other team members?

Harvard Business Review described two types of self-awareness in leadership, internal and external self-awareness. Internal self-awareness is the ability of a leader to understand their own values and the impact they have on others. External self-awareness is the ability of a leader to understand how others perceive them.[9] Both are paramount to the success of a leader when working toward a shared vision within an organization. Daniel Goleman described self-awareness as one of five components constituting emotional intelligence. Goleman describes emotional intelligence as a critical component observed in nearly all highly successful leaders.[10] In a study conducting randomly interviewing 10 internal medicine department chairs, emotional intelligence was identified as a fundamental principle that is essential to leadership ability within health care organizations.[11] Emotional intelligence and its associations with self-awareness and communication skills are paramount to successful leadership within an organization.

The importance of developing self-awareness in surgical trainees is gaining more traction in recent times, but more research should be performed investigating the interplay of emotional intelligence within the field of surgery. One study investigating self-awareness of learning styles among general surgery residents at an academic hospital was performed by comparing self-identified learned styles with a results of a standard learned style assessment. This study demonstrated that nearly half of the residents surveyed had major discrepancies in their self-identified learning styles when compared to the results of their standard assessment scores,[12] highlighting a demand for improved self-awareness development within surgical training programs.

Self-awareness is a means of self-calibration. The ability to recognize strengths and weaknesses is an asset to surgeons and surgical trainees. It is imperative for medical training to dedicate time and effort toward developing self-awareness in trainees. Being self-aware starts with being honest and adopting an open mindset. It is difficult to solve a problem when you do not recognize one exists. Self-awareness within the operating room can strengthen individual performance as well as foster a stronger team dynamic and result in greater organizational success. No matter the amount of rigorous training, a surgeon is still prone to human error. There is no shame in recognizing personal weakness and reaching out for a colleague's advice, especially when it is for the benefit of a patient's health. Developing self-awareness in surgical training is achievable when an environment is created that is conducive to learning.

LEAD BY ACTION, NOT BY POSITION

Successful leaders share a strong willingness to act. These actions, and their purpose, define a leader's success. What good is a leader who does not act? Initiating action, bringing about progressive change, and challenging the status quo are all responsibilities of a successful leader. Highly sought-after leadership qualities are rendered useless if a leader cannot translate ideas into shared action. Purposeful action then becomes a measure of success in a leader.

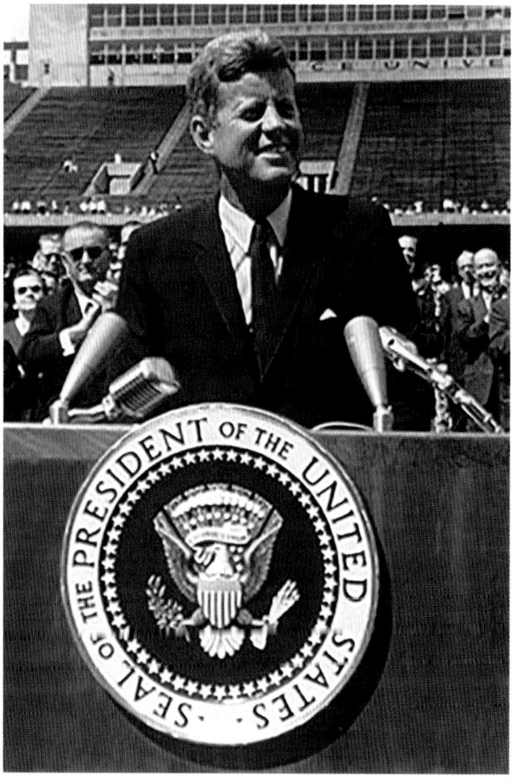

FIGURE 55-4 The 35th President, John Fitzgerald Kennedy, speech at Rice University. (Reproduced with permission from National Aeronautics and Space Administration [NASA].)

The 35th president of the United States of America, John Fitzgerald Kennedy (Figure 55-4) is renowned for his poise and resolute character during his service as commander in chief. His unwavering nature in the face of international crisis remains one of his most admirable leadership qualities. However, it was his action and willingness to lead, despite being the youngest sitting president in history, which defines Kennedy's leadership legacy. In his 1961 special message to Congress,[13] Kennedy displayed a willingness to act, breaking the political status quo for what he believed was in the best interest of humanity.

"The Constitution imposes upon me the obligation to 'from time to time give to the Congress information of the State of the Union.' While this has traditionally been interpreted as an annual affair, this tradition has been broken in extraordinary times.

These are extraordinary times. And we face an extraordinary challenge. Our strength as well as our convictions have imposed upon this nation the role of leader in freedom's cause." – President Kennedy, May 25, 1961

A health care team can benefit greatly from a leader who actively identifies gaps that need to be filled and institutes a plan of action to achieve a vision. This lends into the discussion of leadership versus management. What defines a quality leader as opposed to an individual occupying a managerial position? Both titles may be successful in guiding a group of subordinates toward some desired goal, so what exactly delineates the two? A manager is responsible for the completion of a task in which they use their position to guide subordinates in a systematic-like fashion. Managers occupy a position, and their actions are a responsibility, often set by an organization, and is less often tied to values. On the other hand, leaders act in accordance with a set of values, and empower subordinates to work toward a shared vision. Leaders are fluid, and act to inspire.[14] Surgeon leaders are thrust into a unique paradigm where they are required to fulfill their clinical duties of treating pathology by surgical technique, but also to function as a leader within the operating room. Unlike other industries in which one individual may be elected as the organization leader with separate day-to-day responsibilities as the other works, the surgeon leader has duality of duty. The University of Michigan Institute for Social Research found that supervisors with better productivity served a more differentiated role when compared to supervisors of low productivity. It was found that supervisors with a higher degree of differentiation of their role from other workers spent more time building interpersonal relationships, had higher worker morale, and higher employee satisfaction.[15] The degree of differentiation required for surgeon leaders to create the most ideal work environment for others within the operating room is unknown, but it is important for surgeon leaders to be cognizant of the duality of their role within practice: the healer and the team leader.

Surgery is a result-driven field, and a surgeon who can provide the actions required to achieve desired results will be successful. It is a necessity for a surgeon to display confidence and willingness to act. More so than any other medical specialty, surgery is a fast-paced practice with actions that can result in life or death. A surgeon will largely be respected by their willingness to act, and the result of their actions, above all else. The value of willing surgeon extends outside the operating theater as well. Surgeon leaders can benefit from a willingness to learn, adapt, mentor, and challenge the status quo.

BALANCE

Being a physician is not easy. Years of dedicated training are burdened by increasing costs of education. Young practitioners enter a field of increasing expectations, rising costs of care, higher patient volumes, and little time for personal wellness. This is not a new problem, but it has garnered increasing attention over the past few decades. This emerging outcry in the medical community to shed light on physician burnout is long overdue. With nearly one-half of practicing physicians experiencing some degree of burnout, the evidence is clear.[16] Successful surgeon leaders are required to be masters of balance, considered to be a jack of all trades within the operating room and on the hospital floor. The high expectations and demanding structure of a surgeon's career are undoubtably taxing, and surgeons are just as vulnerable to mental, physical, and emotion erosion. There is much to say about the importance of wellness and the obstacles physicians face which make it increasingly difficult. In concluding the fundamental principles of leadership, let us not forget to find our own happy balance in life. Although not a medical doctor by trade, the beloved author, Theodor "Dr Seuss" Geisel eloquently captured the essence of balance in his book *Oh, the Places You'll Go!*, writing, "Step with care and great tact, and remember that life's a great balancing act."

THE ROLE OF THE PHYSICIAN LEADER IN THE MODERN HEALTH CARE SYSTEM

What is the role of the surgeon leader in today's health care system? A growing body of literature discussing physician-based leader has attracted significant attention. There are several factors which likely contributed to this leadership trend gaining traction. Modern health care organizations are becoming conglomerates, bogged down by increasing volumes, shifting cultures, rapidly evolving technology, and a growing patient dissatisfaction with the current system. Prophet and GE Healthcare Camden Group performed a study which demonstrated 81% of consumers are unsatisfied with their health care experience.[11] Patient satisfaction is an important and useful measure of quality health care.[17,18] Patient satisfaction also appears to be associated with hospital profitability, as shown by a study conducted by Deloitte which demonstrated a strong correlation between patient experience and profitability at hospitals.[13] Despite this, hospital CEOs surveyed in 2014 did not rank patient satisfaction within their top five issues confronting hospitals for that year.[14] What factors are driving this emerging gap? Perhaps the complexities of modern health care organizations have caused our health care system to drift away from its roots. The gap between the priorities of hospital leaders and the wishes of patients is seemingly paradoxical, and the factors contributing to this gap likely span well beyond the scope of this chapter. An ideal health care system prioritizes quality care, increased access to care, affordability, and patient satisfaction. In practice, this balance is extremely difficult to maintain as the equilibrium appears to sometimes tilt too far in one direction. Although not an absolute antidote, increasing physician leadership in hospitals may be part of the remedy for this problem.

Physicians and health care providers have a unique understanding of the patient interaction. Health care providers are accustomed to serving the best interest of the patient as a top priority as this is fundamental to their years of training. They have an insider perspective that can be an asset to upper-level leadership. Trastek described the value of physician-based leadership saying "Health care providers can identify gaps in technology and medical procedures to lead change that increases the value of health care. Last and most importantly, health care providers should always be aligned with the best interests of the patient. Although the constant and rapid changes in the current health care landscape may be putting pressure on this bedrock concept of health care, it remains the primary value of the entire profession."[15,19] A cross-sectional study identified CEOs at top 100 US hospitals, comparing how hospital ranking varied depending on if leadership was head by physician or nonphysician CEOs. Using Index of Hospital Quality (IHQ) as an empiric measure across three specialty fields, the average hospital quality score was higher for hospitals led by physician CEOs.[16,19] The results of this study have limitations and does not prove physician CEOs are more effective hospital leaders, but it does open the door for discussion as to what role physicians may play in modern health care organizations. Physicians, by nature, are servant leaders who possess a unique insider-perspective of patient interactions. How can the views and opinions of an experienced clinician empower hospital leadership to realign its priorities with the values of medicine? There are many questions to be asked about the role of physician leaders within modern health care. Perhaps the value of physician-based leadership within our health care system has not been recognized until recently. Future studies will be necessary to determine the differences of physician leaders and their effect on organization management. For the time being, we should continue to offer our surgical trainees avenue to expand their horizons of leadership and continue to invest resources to leadership development in practicing surgeons. Additionally, education and training in hospital and health care business might be the way to allow physicians get involved in the business of health care at an early stage of their career.

Does this imply modern health care systems should phase out business-minded leaders? Absolutely not. Hospitals would almost certainly fail without the unique perspective business savvy leaders have to offer. The business of health care defies the contemporary business model of supply and demand. The most important "product" our modern health care systems are offering is certainly quality patient care, measured by hospital outcomes and patient satisfaction. While health care professionals may be masters of patient interactions, business leaders have a unique understanding of how to market that understanding to the "consumers," that is, the patient. Interestingly, research from Boston University's School of Hospitality Administration showed patients surveyed were willing to pay 38%

more for a hospital room that offered certain amenities similar to those found in a hotel.[18,20] This alludes to complexities involved in producing patient satisfaction. Patient satisfaction is multifactorial, with factors other than quality of medical care are highly valued by patients. The amalgam of diverse mindsets between health care professionals and business minded leaders likely offers higher quality of care for patients. Perhaps a "health administration" degree and/or fellowship training leading to "Boards" in health care administration should be the answer to produce the hybrid physician / health care administrators that will lead health care systems in the future.

THE SURGEON LEADER OR THE SERVANT LEADER: EXAMINING DIFFERENT STYLES OF LEADERSHIP

Almost unrecognizable when compared to its former self, the modern system of health care has transformed over time. Massive technological advancement, cultural shifts, cost of care, and the concept of patient-centered care are just a few of the driving forces behind this health care transformation. Conklin described the transformation of our health care system to a system of "managed care" that perpetually evolves and is influenced by culture, values, and economics.[21] As our healthcare system continues to transform, physician-based leadership has emerged as an integral component. Despite our understanding of organizational leadership in non-healthcare industries, our healthcare system continues to be dominated by outdated styles of leadership[22]. Modern major industries remain dominated by a transactional style of leadership,[24,25] in which the system operates through mutual dependence between parties, incentivized by set goals and rewards. In the transactional leadership system, authority is often set by hierarchal structures, and leaders are followed as it is in best interest of the followers to do so.[23]

First introduced by James Downton, and later expanded upon by James Burn, transformational leadership behavior and its implication in organizational leadership has explored for decades. The concepts of transformational leadership have been further expanded upon in a large body of work, notably by the works of Bass and others.[24,25] The transformational leadership model encourages leadership through action, inspiring others to follow suit. A transformational leader is increasingly self-aware and can cultivate an energetic culture that better supports the individual needs of employees.[26] Sfantou et al. captured the essence of transformational leaders by stating "Transformational leaders typically have the ability to inspire confidence, staff respect and they communicate loyalty through a shared vision, resulting in increased productivity, strengthen employee morale, and job satisfaction."[27] Often viewed as the counterpart to transformational leadership, transactional leadership behavior is more of a managerial style, focused on the supervision of an organization using reward and punishment to motivate employees. In times of crisis, transactional leaders may find more success to achieve rapid short-term goals; however, this style falls short to its counterpart when aiming to achieve long-term organizational success. Although the styles of transformational and transactional leadership are often viewed as opposites, other studies have shown them to be complimentary, with highly functioning leaderships displaying components of both styles.[27] Transformational physician leaders have been shown to correlate with transactional physician leaders, and this correlation is accentuated in the top quartile of transformational physician leaders.[28] This empiric evidence is likely derived from the idea of transformational and transactional leadership being additive, rather than opposite. Highly effective transformational leaders may originate as transactional leaders, gaining the trust of their subordinates through goal-oriented success before transitioning to a dominantly transformational style of leadership.

Does the transformational-transactional leadership model exist within the field of surgery? Recent studies have demonstrated that constructs of transformational and transactional leadership models are applicable to surgeons.[29] The Multifactorial Leadership Questionnaire (MLQ) is a well-established system used to score transformational and transactional leadership styles.[30] It has been empirically demonstrated that surgeons vary widely in their transformational leadership scores and less so in their transactional leadership scores.[29] This again lends credence to the idea of transformational and transactional leadership concepts being additive to each other. Now understanding the basic principles of transformational and transactional leadership behavior, and that this model of leadership does exist within surgery, how may these leadership behaviors influence operating room dynamics? The transformational leaders value their subordinates and work to gain their trust through their own meaningful actions. Transformational leaders inspire others to work toward a shared vision for their organization, but also inspire others to achieve new personal heights. They are stimulating and constantly challenge the status quo of their organization and of those around them. It may be easy to envision how transformational surgeon leaders would have great success in strengthening operating room team dynamics.[30] On the other hand, transactional leaders are more goal-oriented and may delineate clear expectations and roles for team members. These leaders are more focused on achieving the task at hand. Again, it is easy to envision how transactional leadership characteristics are essential in the operating room.

Introduced decades ago, the concept of transformational-transactional leaders has persevered as one of the best understood leadership models. Prior to its conception by leadership scholars, the principles of transformational leadership can be observed within the works of historical leaders. Martin Luther King Jr epitomized transformational leadership ideals as he led a cultural transformation within the United States. Through his shared vision, he collectively inspired Americans of all colors to challenge the status quo of inequality. King was a role model for his followers, and he embodied every word that he preached. Transitioning away from the aforementioned leadership model, there are several other models of leadership worth exploring. Many of the leadership ideas and examples discussed thus far have a common denominator: the concept of servant-based leadership. Loa Tzu summated the virtues of leadership by defining a leader as an individual who enables others to succeed. The Reverend Dr Martin Luther King Jr displayed quintessential aspects of a true servant leader, selflessly giving himself for the prosperity of a nation and generations to come. Surgeon leaders dedicate years of their lives to scholarly pursuit and the acquisition of knowledge to provide the highest quality of surgical care to patients, a sacrifice that is not unsubstantial by any means. Robert Greenleaf coined the term "servant leader" and described the nature of a servant leader. "The servant-leader is servant first. It begins with the natural feeling that one wants to serve. Then conscious choice brings one to aspire to lead.[31] The best test is: do those served grow as persons: do they, while being served, become healthier, wiser, freer, more autonomous, more likely themselves to become servants? And, what is the effect on the least privileged in society; will they benefit, or, at least, not be further deprived?"[32] Greenleaf's idea of the servant leader opened the door for new styles of leadership to enter the arena of organizational management. The paradox of a leader who is also a servant tilted the paradigm of hierarchical leadership structures that dominated organizations. This new style of leadership was focused on quality relationships, values, and promoting positive behavior, which ultimately will better the work of an organization.[32]

But what constitutes a servant leadership? Are there certain qualities that qualify an individual as a "servant leader," or is this style defined solely by action? Spearman described his own interpretation of 10 characteristics that are fundamental to the development of a servant leader. These 10 characteristics are as follows:

- Listening
- Empathy
- Healing
- Awareness
- Persuasion
- Conceptualization
- Foresight
- Stewardship
- Commitment to growth of people
- Building community

Spearman wrote these 10 characteristics not as an exhaustive list to identify servant leaders, but as a roadmap of how to develop qualities of servant leadership.[33] Is not the physician's primary value to serve first? The roles of a physician are seemingly endless and differ greatly between specialties. However, the bedrock of all medicine is resolute; to always put the patient first. One can argue that the practice of medicine inherently adopts principles of servant leadership. Even without intention, physicians are almost always serving others as leaders in their respective fields. Servant leadership in medicine transcends the day-to-day practices of physicians and can be found at all levels of our health care systems. The management of our health care industry can benefit from the powers of physician-based servant leadership. Physician leaders who are deeply motivated to serve the patient first may be better equipped to identify breaks in the chain of care that outside leaders may not recognize.

The fundamentals of leadership and their interplay within medicine are not limited to the servant leadership style. There are many different styles of leadership through which the principles discussed in this chapter can be practiced. Daniel Goleman described six styles of leadership, each stemming from different components of emotional intelligence.[34] Emotional intelligence, as discussed earlier, is integral to the foundation of leadership development. The six styles of leadership identified by Goleman are: *Coercive, Authoritative, Affiliative, Democratic, Pacesetting,* and *Coaching*. Each of these six styles have their own strengths, limitations, and effectiveness depending on circumstance.

COERCIVE

A coercive leader rules with an iron fist, disrupting the organizational climate by effectively delivering a desired result in an undesirable manner. Using a "get onboard or get out" approach, this style erodes team dynamics. The utility of the coercive leadership style is limited. It is apparent why this style is only appropriate in rare circumstances, such as an organization catastrophe when rapid decision making is necessitated. This rigid style of leadership was likely dominant in the early years of surgery, when surgeons took absolute control of decision making. As our health care system evolved to prioritize interdisciplinary practice, the coercive leader grew out of favor.

AUTHORITATIVE

The authoritative leader "rallies the troops" to achieve a shared vision energetically and effectively. Goleman defines the authoritative leader as powerful, proficient, and vision oriented. This style of leadership has great practical utility within surgery, for instance, when inspiring the staff of an operating room to work in harmony during a surgical procedure to achieve a desired outcome, which is the vision.

AFFILIATIVE

"People come first." Affiliative leaders value individuals. This style of leadership creates an environment that bolsters team dynamics, promotes flexibility, and allows for risk taking. Affiliative leaders are never complacent and adapt to the needs of those around them. These individuals demonstrate a high degree of self-awareness. An affiliative leader is effective in providing feedback, which is of importance in surgical training. However, an affiliative leader may allow undesired work to go uncorrected.

DEMOCRATIC

A democratic leader is in the business of building respect. This style of leader is inclusive and encourages participation by all members. The democratic style of leadership is effective in generating ideas, quelling conflict, and in discussing a vision. This style may be ineffective when time is of the essence, requiring rapid decision making.

PACESETTING

The pacesetting leader is obsessive over standards of excellence. These lofty expectations are met with a high level of performance from the leader himself. This leader seeks out members who are willing to take self-initiative and would rather replace than teach. This fast-paced style of leadership can deliver desired results in a timely manner, but it is not effective in most situations. Pacesetting leadership can promote higher rates of burnout and demoralize team members who do not meet expectations. This style of leadership, like coercive, has sparing utility in certain circumstances.

COACHING

A coaching leader is future-minded. These leaders act almost as counselors in their approach to leadership and work diligently to motivate and develop others. This style of leadership has obvious benefits, such as the emphasis it places on creating an environment that fosters personal development. Drawbacks of this coaching style are its difficult practicality in a fast-paced work environment. Mentorship is paramount in surgery. Coaching leadership may be difficult to exemplify during the day-to-day hustle of surgery, but when possible, has tremendous importance in the education of surgical trainees.

Leaders come in many styles. A successful leader does not simply master one single style of leadership. Successful leaders are flexible and able to blend multiple leadership styles when they see fit. Each of the styles mentioned above has its own unique strengths and weaknesses, and an experienced leader possesses the knowledge of when to apply components to each respective style. For these reasons, learning about different styles of leadership is critically important to leadership development. With time comes mastery, and these varying styles provide a framework for which to lead by. Training programs can use fundamental principles of leadership and different styles of leadership to effectively teach leadership development to trainees.

CONCLUSION

Leadership is difficult to describe in words but easy to recognize in practice. If asked to summarize what defines a strong leader in a few words, what would you say? It may be challenging to capture the vast intricacies of leadership in a few words. Yet, we almost instinctually recognize the tremendous leadership qualities of Martin Luther King Jr or Loa Tzu. Perhaps it is the intangibles of leadership that matter most; those characteristics that are difficult to put in words or on paper.

Leadership exists in many styles, but there are several commonalities that can be drawn between them. Successful leaders have a well-established set of core values. They create a shared and unified vision to work toward. Strong leadership necessitates a willingness to act and a high degree of self-awareness, culminating in a well-balanced individual. These principles of leadership, when effectively employed through various leadership styles, create proficient leaders. The modern health care system has disrupted old norms, and there is a new demand for the physician leader. It is imperative for medical training programs to dedicate resources toward leadership development. Throughout history, the world has been wowed by the great achievements within the field of surgery, and the future generations of surgeons will carry this torch of excellence as leaders in surgery.

REFERENCES

1. Awad SS, Hayley B, Fagan SP, Berger DH, Brunicardi FC. The impact of a novel resident leadership training curriculum. *Am J Surg*. 2004;188(5):481-484.
2. Wolf JA. Patient experience: the new heart of healthcare leadership. *Front Health Serv Manage*. 2017;33(3):3-16.
3. WHO-AHPSR. *Open Mindsets: Participatory Leadership for Health*. Geneva, Switzerland. World Health Organization, Alliance for Health Policy and System Research; 2016.
4. National Resident Matching Program, Data Release and Research Committee. Results of the 2018 NRMP Program Director Survey. National Resident Matching Program, Washington, DC. 2018. Available at https://www.nrmp.org/wp-content/uploads/2018/07/NRMP-2018-Program-Director-Survey-for-WWW.pdf. Accessed November 1, 2020.
5. Accreditation Council for Graduate Medical Education. ACGME Program Requirements for Graduate Medical Education in General Surgery. 2020. Available at https://www.acgme.org/Portals/0/PFAssets/ProgramRequirements/440_GeneralSurgery_2020.pdf?ver=2020-06-22-085958-260. Accessed November 28, 2020.
6. Itani KM, Liscum K, Brunicardi FC. Physician leadership is a new mandate in surgical training. *Am J Surg*. 2004;187(3):328-331.
7. Stoller JK. Developing physician-leaders: a call to action. *J Gen Intern Med*. 2009;24(7):876-878.

8. Brunicardi FC, Cotton RT, Cole GW, Martinez G. The leadership principles of Dr Martin Luther King, Jr and their relevance to surgery. *J Natl Med Assoc*. 2007; 99(1):7-14.
9. Eurich T. What self-awareness really is (and how to cultivate it). *Har Bus Rev*. 2019. Available at https://hbr.org/2018/01/what-self-awareness-really-is-and-how-to-cultivate-it. Accessed October 2020.
10. Goleman D. What makes a leader? *Har Bus Rev*. 1998; 76(6):93-102.
11. Lobas JG. Leadership in academic medicine: capabilities and conditions for organizational success. *Am J Med*. 2006;119(7):617-621.
12. Pang JHY, Goetz A, Hook L, et al. Self-awareness of learning styles among surgical trainees. *J Am Coll Surg*. 2015;S56.
13. Papers of John F. Kennedy. Presidential Papers. President's Office Files. Speech Files. Special message to Congress on urgent national needs, 25 May 1961. Available at https://www.jfklibrary.org/asset-viewer/archives/JFKPOF/034/JFKPOF-034-030. Accessed April 11, 2021.
14. Gavin, M. Leadership vs. management: what's the difference? *Har Bus Rev*. 2019 October. Available at https://online.hbs.edu/blog/post/leadership-vs-management. Accessed April 10, 2021.
15. Kahn, RL, Daniel K. *Leadership Practices in Relation to Productivity and Morale*. Ann Arbor, MI: Institute for Social Research, University of Michigan; 1952.
16. Yates SW. Physician stress and burnout. *Am J Med*. 2020;133(2):160-164.
17. Prakash B. Patient satisfaction. *J Cutan Aesthet Surg*. 2010;3(3):151-155.
18. Prophet GE: Healthcare Camden Group. The current state of the patient experience. 2016. Available at https://www.prophet.com/patient experience/the-current-state-of-the-patient-experience.html. Accessed November 1, 2020.
19. Goodall AH. Physician-leaders and hospital performance: is there an association? *Soc Sci Med*. 2011; 73(4):535-539.
20. Suess C, Mody M, Guarracino G. Hospitality Healthscapes: The new standard for making hospitals more hospitable. *Boston Hospitality Review*. 2017. Available at http://www.bu.edu/bhr/2017/06/07/hospitality-healthscapes/. Accessed November 5, 2020.
21. Deloitte. The value of patient experience. Hospitals with better patient-reported experience perform better financially. Available at https://www2.deloitte.com/content/dam/Deloitte/us/Documents/life-sciences-health-care/us-dchs-the-value-of-patient-experience.pdf. Accessed November 5, 2020.
22. Top Issues Confronting Hospitals: 2014. *Health Exec*. 2015;30(2):90.
23. Conklin TP. Health care in the united states: an evolving system. *Michigan Family Review*. 2002; 7(1):5-17.
24. Burns JM. *Leadership*. New York: Harper & Row; 1978.
25. Bass BM. *Leadership and Performance*. New York: Free Press; 1985.
26. Schwartz RW, Tumblin TF. The power of servant leadership to transform health care organizations for the 21st-century economy. *Arch Surg*. 2002;137(12):1419-1427.
27. Sfantou DF, Laliotis A, Patelarou AE, Sifaki-Pistolla D, Matalliotakis M, Patelarou E. Importance of leadership style towards quality of care measures in healthcare settings: a systematic review. *Healthcare (Basel)*. 2017;5(4):73.
28. Xirasagar S, Samuels ME, Stoskopf CH. Physician leadership styles and effectiveness: an empirical study. *Med Care Res Rev*. 2015;62(6):720-740.
29. Hu YY, Parker SH, Lipsitz SR, et al. Surgeons' leadership styles and team behavior in the operating room. *J Am Coll Surg*. 2016;222(1):41-51.
30. Bass BM, Avolio BJ. *Full Range Leadership Development: Manual for the Multifactor Leadership Questionnaire*. Palo Alto, CA: Mindgarden; 1997.
31. Trastek VF, Hamilton NW, Niles WW. Leadership models in health care: a case for servant leadership. *Mayo Clin Proc*. 2014;89(3):374-381.
32. Greenleaf RK. *Servant-Leadership: A Journey into the Nature of Legitimate Power and Greatness*. New York: Paulist Press; 1977.
33. Spears LC. Character and servant leadership: ten characteristics of effective, Caring Leaders. *The Journal of Virtues & Leadership*. 2010;1(1):25-30.
34. Goleman D. Leadership that gets results. *Harv Bus Rev*. 2000;78:78-93.

SELF-ASSESSMENT STUDY QUESTIONS AND ANSWERS

Questions

1. While in the operating room, you work alongside a surgeon who displays a keen sense of awareness of the needs of others in the room. This surgeon provides excellent feedback to the surgical resident, creating a healthy team dynamic within the operating room. According to Goleman's styles of leadership, what style best describes this surgeon?
A. Coercive
B. Authoritative
C. Affiliative
D. Democratic
E. Pacesetting
F. Coaching

2. Civil Rights leader, Martin Luther King Jr, would best be described displaying which style of leadership?
A. Democratic
B. Transformational
C. Transactional
D. Affiliative
E. Servant leader

3. Transactional surgeon leaders have been shown to strengthen team dynamics within the operating room compared to transformational surgeon leaders.
A. True
B. False

4. Which leadership style is best described as a managerial system of mutual dependence between parties in which goals are set and behavior is reinforced by reward and punishment?
A. Democratic leadership style
B. Servant leadership
C. Transactional leadership
D. Transformational leadership

5. Which characteristic would best describe a transformational leader?
A. Passiveness
B. Inspires a vision
C. Resistant to change
D. Rewards performance

6. Which of the following would be an example of a transactional surgeon leader?
A. A surgeon calls a preoperative interdisciplinary team debriefing to discuss the goals of the complicated case ahead.
B. A surgeon intellectually engages the medical student during a case, asking appropriate questions related to the case.
C. A surgeon seeks the perspective of the anesthesiologist regarding the patient's preoperative INR level.
D. A surgeon confronts the surgical technician regarding an instrument that was dropped during the case.

7. Which style of leadership, according to Goleman's styles of leadership, would best fit a disaster scenario when quick and effective decision-making is of the essence?
A. Coercive
B. Authoritative
C. Affiliative
D. Democratic
E. Pacesetting
F. Coaching

SELF-ASSESSMENT STUDY QUESTIONS AND ANSWERS

8. According to the University of Michigan Institute for Social Research, which of the following is NOT a class of variable consistently associated with productivity of an organization?

A. Supervisors serving a differentiated role from workers
B. Degree of delegation of authority
C. Employee-oriented supervision
D. A system of consistent employee feedback
E. Healthy group relationships

9. Which of the following characteristics best describes a leader rather than a manager?

A. Policy and procedure
B. Position
C. Task oriented
D. Vision
E. Coordinates action

10. A leader's ability to understand how others perceive them is best described as which of the following?

A. Interpersonal communication
B. Motivational interviewing
C. Internal self-awareness
D. External self-awareness

SELF-ASSESSMENT STUDY QUESTIONS AND ANSWERS

Answers

1. C.
2. B.
3. B.
4. C.
5. B.
6. A.
7. C.
8. D.
9. D.
10. D.

CHAPTER

56 Pediatric Vascular Surgery

Heitham Albeshri and Alexandre d'Audiffret

OUTLINE

GENERAL CONSIDERATIONS
ACUTE EXTREMITY ARTERIAL OCCLUSIONS
- Etiology and Risk Factors
- Clinical Presentation and Evaluation
- Management
  - Iatrogenic Arterial Occlusion
  - Noniatrogenic Arterial Occlusion

CHRONIC ARTERIAL OCCLUSIVE DISEASES
- Clinical Presentation and Evaluation
- Management

ARTERIAL ANEURYSMS
- Aortic Aneurysms
- Peripheral Aneurysms

RENOVASCULAR HYPERTENTION
- Introduction and Etiology
- Clinical Presentation & Diagnosis
- Laboratory and Radiological Evaluation
- Management
  - Medical Therapy
  - Surgical and Endovascular Interventions

VENOUS DISORDERS
- Venous Malformations
- Klippel-Trenaunay Syndrome
- Venous Thrombosis and Postphlebitic Syndrome

GENERAL CONSIDERATIONS

Vascular pathologies in the pediatric population, specifically in children less than 5 years old, are rare but remain a challenge for vascular surgeons who are commonly consulted after failed conservative measures. The management of arterial disease in the pediatric population is unfortunately poorly outlined in the literature, consisting mostly of small series and case reports. Furthermore, surgical strategies need to contemplate patient size, conduit availability, and future patient growth. While the etiologies of vascular diseases in this population are wide-ranging, we will focus, in this chapter, on the most likely encountered ones in an academic medical center.

ACUTE EXTREMITY ARTERIAL OCCLUSIONS

ETIOLOGY AND RISK FACTORS

Acute arterial occlusions in the pediatric population are rare and commonly require immediate attention to avoid catastrophic consequences (Table 56-1). A retrospective analysis of the KID database involving more than 4 million inpatients aged from less than 12 months to 20 years of age revealed that the most common causes of extremity arterial thrombosis in the neonate and infant populations were arterial cannulations and cardiac catheterizations while in children older than 5 years, noniatrogenic traumatic injuries were responsible for the vast majority

TABLE 56-1 Compiled Prevalence of Acute Extremity Arterial Occlusions, Mechanisms, and Site of Injury among Various Age Groups[1,2,20]

	Neonate	Infants	<5 years old	>5 years old
Prevalence (per 10,000 discharges)	1.67	7.09	2.02	3.86
Etiology				
Cardiac cath	29.5%	28.2%	9%	13.3
Arterial cannulation	29.1%	17.6%	22.5%	27%
Penetrating trauma	0%	0%	0.9%	22%
Non iatrogenic	0%	0%		1%
Involved Extremity				
Upper extremity	6%	6%	6%	6%
Lower extremity	94%	94%	94%	94%

of acute extremity ischemic events. Similar findings have been described by Kayssi et al. in a retrospective analysis at The Hospital for Sick Children in Toronto. Other less common contributing factors to acute arterial occlusions include primary hypercoagulability, prothrombin gene mutation, and congenital popliteal entrapment.[1,2]

The exact mechanism leading to arterial thrombosis following access for diagnostic, intervention, or monitoring remains ill-defined. Two commonly accepted theories are (1) femoral arterial spasm leading to thrombosis, and (2) intimal damage and associated platelet aggregation.[3,4] Interestingly, Alexander et al. reported that besides the patient's age, a femoral artery diameter of less than 3 mm was an independent predictor of postcatheterization loss of distal pulse. Also, a ratio between the outer sheath diameter and the cannulated artery less than 0.5 has been described as a predictor of femoral artery vasospasm.[5,6]

Noniatrogenic arterial occlusions, which are more commonly seen in children older than 2 years, are often the result of mechanical compression, intimal flap with localized dissection, or penetrating trauma with transection. The most commonly affected vessels are the brachial artery, femoral artery, and popliteal artery.

CLINICAL PRESENTATION AND EVALUATION

Symptoms and clinical presentations vary depending on the etiology of the inciting event, the location of the affected artery, and the age of the patient. As most of these events occur in patients less than 5 years of age who undergo diagnostic studies or interventions under general anesthesia, diagnosis can be challenging. Femoral arterial palpation postcatheterization is suboptimal as a soft thrombus will allow for pulsatility to be detected despite the loss of flow. Some authors have recommended performing a routine duplex ultrasound study of the access site postprocedure and reported a 5% overall prevalence of femoral artery thrombosis and 19% for patients less than one year of age.[7] A careful examination of the involved extremity will include documentation of the capillary refill, temperature, and the presence of Doppler signals. While the diagnosis of acute occlusion is made clinically, it is confirmed using an arterial duplex ultrasound. Diagnostic angiography is rarely indicated and should be avoided, especially in neonates and infants.

Assessment of patients with a traumatic arterial injury can be equally challenging. Commonly the vascular surgeon is consulted in the operating room to assess a pulseless hand associated with a supracondylar humeral fracture, or a cold foot following a tibial fracture of knee dislocation. As mentioned above, a thorough physical examination should be performed and include intraoperative ultrasonography. In most cases, the distinction between severe vasospasm and thrombosis can be difficult intraoperatively following an orthopedic reduction. This has led to us to frequently explore the artery for direct Doppler insonation following adventitial bathing with 30 to 60 mg of papaverine. In cases where a combined orthopedic and vascular injury are suspected, proceeding to a hybrid surgical room remains the best option and offers the most flexibility in management for this older pediatric population.

MANAGEMENT

Iatrogenic Arterial Occlusion

- **Anticoagulation** – The first line of therapy remains unfractionated heparin or low-molecular-weight heparin when a thrombus has been detected in the femoral artery with loss of distal pulses. Both drugs are doses based on weight and age and titrated to therapeutic levels (Partial Thromboplastin Time [PTT]: 60–85 seconds, anti-Xa: 0.5-1 units/mL). Anticoagulation is continued until the restoration of a distal pulse, up to 24 hours. A repeat duplex is performed to document the absence of a thrombus. If the thrombus remains present but the limb is not threatened, the patient is discharged on anticoagulation with duplex follow-up at 2, 6, and 12 weeks.[8]
- **Thrombolysis** – systemic tissue plasminogen activator (tPA) is indicated when the patient fails to respond to conventional anticoagulation or experiences worsening symptoms. More than 90% of patients respond to this therapeutic approach; however, bleeding complications occur at the access site in up to 50% of patients with more than 15% requiring blood transfusion.[9] Dosage recommendations range from 0.25 to 0.5 mg/kg/hr until distal perfusion returns. Lower doses are preferred in patients less than 1 week to minimize the risks of intracerebral bleeding.
- **Surgical thrombectomy** – Surgical thrombectomy is rarely required as the majority of patients will respond to medical management. A surgical approach is reserved for patients who remain at risk of limb loss with no arterial flow and no distal Doppler signals.[10] The thrombectomy is performed with a #2 Fogarty catheter via a transverse arteriotomy, which is closed primarily with interrupted 7.0 or 8.0 polypropylene sutures. In the case of arterial dissection with a subadventitial hematoma, we perform a longitudinal arteriotomy that is closed using a segment of the ipsilateral greater saphenous vein. Intra-arterial or peri adventitial papaverine can be used before the Doppler insonation of the distal arteries in the operating room.
- **Long-term anticoagulation** – Patients with persistent arterial thrombosis by ultrasonography without symptoms should receive anticoagulation for 3 months before reevaluation with a repeat duplex. Failed recanalization should be monitored during the child's growth to prevent potential limb length discrepancies.

Noniatrogenic Arterial Occlusion

- **Anticoagulation** – Primary arterial thrombosis associated with sepsis, congenital hypercoagulability disorders, and autoimmune vasculitis are primarily treated with systemic anticoagulation. Surgical thrombectomy is reserved for failure to respond.
- **Surgical Exploration and Repair** – Successful management of vascular trauma in pediatric patients follows standard principles, including prompt surgical intervention with exploration and reconstruction. This may prove to be challenging due to the paucity of available conduit, vessel diameters, and predisposition to severe vasospasm. The greater saphenous vein is readily available in children including neonates and has proved to be valuable provided microvascular anastomotic techniques

are used. Alternative may be longitudinally spliced saphenous veins, jugular veins, and cryopreserved conduits.[11,12] In case of brachial artery injury following a supracondylar humeral fracture in patients as young as 4 years old, these authors have had success with the use of a reversed ipsilateral basilic vein using interrupted 8.0 polypropylene sutures.

CHRONIC ARTERIAL OCCLUSIVE DISEASES

CLINICAL PRESENTATION AND EVALUATION

Pediatric chronic arterial occlusive diseases are uncommon. Various causes have been recognized, including iatrogenic injury, blunt or penetrating trauma, vasculitis, and congenital anomalies.[13,14] In this author's experience, the most common presentations have been claudication following multiple common femoral artery accesses for cardiac catheterization or post–blunt trauma. In contrast to the adult population, untreated chronic occlusive disease in the pediatric population may lead to limb length discrepancy, and growth retardation and, as a result, require proper attention.[15] A limb length discrepancy greater than 2 cm has been shown to be associated with gait deviations and spinal deformities.[16] Unfortunately a correlation with the ankle-brachial index (ABI) remains ill-defined. Accepted recommendations are to proceed with revascularization in growing children with greater than 1-cm limb length discrepancy and exercise ABIs consistent with claudication.

Preoperative angiography may be required when the pathology is located below the inguinal ligament as CT angiography and magnetic resonance arteriography are unreliable. However, CT angiography is helpful for more proximal occlusions.

MANAGEMENT

Surgical revascularization remains the mainstay of therapy regardless of age. The greater saphenous vein remains the conduit of choice in this older pediatric patient population and has proven to be a durable conduit despite evidence of stable aneurysmal degeneration being reported in up to 14% of patients and stable ectasia in 50%.[17] Other useful conduits for revascularization include the hypogastric artery or cryopreserved veins or arteries.

ARTERIAL ANEURYSMS

AORTIC ANEURYSMS

Primary congenital aortic aneurysms are extremely rare and currently only 16 cases have been reported in the literature since Howorth first reported in 1967.[18] Secondary or acquired aneurysms associated with congenital and aortic malformations, systemic diseases, connective tissue disorders, and umbilical artery catheterization are far more frequent.

PERIPHERAL ANEURYSMS

A recent retrospective review of 41 cases from the University of Michigan categorizes nonaortic aneurysms as traumatic, dysplastic, or congenital. Aneurysmal degeneration was observed most commonly in the renal arteries (36%), followed by the lower extremity arteries (29%), upper extremity arteries (17%), and finally aortic mesenteric vessels (14%) and extracranial carotid artery and its branches (7%). Currently, there are clear recommendations; however, the experiences described in the literature overwhelmingly favor early conventional surgical repair using the hypogastric artery as the conduit of choice as venous conduits are prone to aneurysmal degeneration in end artery low resistance arterial beds.[19]

RENOVASCULAR HYPERTENTION

INTRODUCTION AND ETIOLOGY

The US Department of Health and Human Services published *The Fourth Report on the Diagnosis, Evaluation, and Treatment of High Blood Pressure in Children and Adolescents* where hypertension is defined as an average systolic or diastolic blood pressure that is greater than the 95th percentile for sex, age, and height on at least three separate occasions.[20]

With an overall prevalence in the pediatric population of 1% to 3%, essential hypertension is rarely diagnosed in children younger than 10 years old and 70% of the cases in this age group are secondary to renal parenchymal disease associated with renal artery stenosis. In contrast, the progressive increase in the prevalence of childhood obesity over the past decade has enabled primary or essential hypertension to evolve to an epidemic proportion in the adolescent population.[1,2]

Renal artery stenosis accounts for up to 10% of renal parenchymal causes of secondary HTN in children. At a histological level, intimal and medial fibrodysplasia are responsible for 30% to 50% of renal artery stenosis in the pediatric population in contrast to 5% to 10% in the adult population.[3,5] Interestingly, this is not the case in Asia and South Africa where inflammatory causes like Takayasu arteritis (TA) are more common and have a higher association with renal artery stenosis.[6,13]

Lastly, renal artery stenosis may also be associated with genetic diseases including type 1 neurofibromatosis, Marfan syndrome, Williams' syndrome, or rubella syndrome.[7,8,14,15]

Other causes of pediatric hypertension include coarctation of the aorta, neoplasms, and endocrine etiologies.

CLINICAL PRESENTATION & DIAGNOSIS

The diagnosis of renovascular hypertension (RVHTN) can be elusive as children may present with ill-defined complaints including irritability, behavioral changes, or failure to thrive. In contrast, older children may complain of headache, lethargy, or epistaxis. Symptoms related to end-organ effects manifesting as renal insufficiency, hypertensive encephalopathy, or left ventricular hypertrophy can be observed later in life.[9,10] Finally, a family history of early onset of hypertension, a history of umbilical catheterization, recurrent urinary tract infections, or a history of abdominal irradiation should raise a high index of suspicion for RVHTN.[9]

Standardized procedures for the accurate measurement of the blood pressure (BP) is essential in a patient with suspected RVHTN, which include the following: (a) the child should be seated for 3 to 5 minutes with uncrossed legs in a quiet room, (b) blood pressure should be measured in the right arm at the heart level, (c) the length of the cuff should be 80% to 100% of the arm. When the blood pressure is found to be elevated, it is advisable to obtain a blood pressure measurement in all four extremities to evaluate for coarctation of the aorta and middle aortic syndrome.[3,12]

LABORATORY AND RADIOLOGICAL EVALUATION

There is no single screening study that can effectively exclude all the causes of renovascular hypertension in the patient population. A step-wise approach is required to make a conclusive diagnosis.

- *Basic Metabolic Panel and Urinalysis:* The basic metabolic panel is simple and helps to identify renal dysfunction. *Hypertensive hyponatremic syndrome* is the result of the activation of the renin-angiotensin-aldosterone system with unilateral renal artery stenosis resulting in pressure natriuresis from the contralateral normal kidney. Although rare but *secondary hyperaldosteronism* may also develop in case of unilateral stenosis leading to excessive urinary potassium loss and subsequently hypokalemia. However, when the serum creatinine is elevated, bilateral RAS disease should be suspected as normal serum creatinine is often observed with unilateral RAS. Finally, prolonged hypoperfusion in the setting of unilateral renal artery stenosis may lead to glomerular hyperfiltration in the contralateral kidney and compensatory hypertrophy associated with proteinuria and glycosuria.[3]
- *Plasma Renin Activity:* Numerous studies have attempted to utilize measurements of the plasma renin activity routinely to identify renovascular hypertension. However, most children with bilateral stenosis and up to 40% unilateral disease are likely to have normal renin levels.[12,16]
- *Noninvasive Imaging:* Doppler Duplex ultrasonography is the recommended first-line study

to evaluate children suspected of renovascular hypertension to assess arterial velocities and kidney sizes. Magnetic resonance angiography has a high sensitivity (92%–98%) and specificity (70%–96%) and provides a good quality image without exposure to radiation but it lacks intraparenchymal vessel visualization. On the other hand, computed tomography angiography, with low radiation protocols, has proven to be the best and fastest alternative to angiography with a sensitivity as high as 85%.

- *Invasive imaging studies:* Digital subtraction angiography is the most invasive modality but remains the "gold standard" for the diagnosis of renal artery stenosis and allows for therapeutic intervention. Renal vein venin sampling is usually performed in conjunction with angiography and requires taking a blood sample from inferior vena cava and each renal vein. Renal vein renin ratios of >1.5:1 between the affected and the contralateral kidney are considered significant and predict a satisfactory response to revascularization. However, it has low sensitivity (74%) and specificity (59%). Finally, evaluation for end-organ damage sequelae resulting from severe hypertension using echocardiography and ophthalmological examination is also performed as part of the evaluation.[3,17]

MANAGEMENT

Medical Therapy

Restoring renal flow is the goal to cure but many of these children awaiting revascularization need an effective method for blood pressure control. Although evidence that supports the efficacy of weight reduction, regular physical activity, or DASH diet (more of fruits, vegetables, low-fat milk products, and low salt content) for pressure reduction in children and adolescents is limited, such intervention is advisable and strongly supported as the first step.[12]

Different antihypertension medication classes are available. It is recommended that a single agent be initiated until target blood pressure is reached or until maximum dose or a side effect of the drug is encountered at which time an additional agent should be added. When renal artery stenosis is suspected, a vasodilator (e.g., hydralazine, minoxidil) and/or a beta-blocker (atenolol, metoprolol, propranolol) should be the first option to control the BP, as worsening of renal function with ACE inhibitors in the setting of RAS is very likely. Glucocorticoids and/or cytotoxic medications (e.g., methotrexate) are used for the treatment of renal artery stenosis resulting from Takayasu arteritis and need to be continued for at least 2 to 3 years followed by gradual tapering.[3,9,12,20]

Surgical and Endovascular Interventions

The choice of invasive therapy is influenced by the renal anatomy, disease etiology, and clinical expertize of the institution.

- *Percutaneous transluminal angioplasty:* Balloon angioplasty is the first-line therapy for lesions ≤10-mm-long, mid to distal lesions, segmental renal artery stenosis, or renal artery stenosis associated with neurofibromatosis. Renal artery stenting tends to increase the risk of neointimal hyperplasia and subsequently restenosis and is generally avoided.[3,14,18] Typically, 25% cure and 50% improvement have been reported with endovascular interventions.
- *Surgical Revascularization:* Surgical revascularization is indicated for refractory hypertension after angioplasty, longer lesion (>10 mm), multiple or bilateral stenosis and is curative in up to 70% of the cases. While technically challenging in children less than 3 years old, careful preoperative reconstructive configurations planning is critical to minimize kidney ischemic times and to facilitate better renal artery patency. Renal artery reimplantation remains the favored procedure, followed by aorto-renal bypass using the harvested internal iliac artery
- *Nephrectomy:* In patients with nonreconstructable disease including (a) multiple intrarenal

stenosis that is not feasible to either open or endovascular option, (b) nonfunctioning atrophied kidneys, and (c) in the presence of sufficient contralateral kidney, nephrectomy remains an acceptable option.

The blood pressure postoperatively often takes some time to reduce. This is true with either endovascular angioplasty or surgical revascularization and most commonly is due to postoperative edema or vasospasm of the renal artery. To date, no randomized trials comparing medical management to surgical revascularization for pediatric renovascular hypertension have been published.

VENOUS DISORDERS

VENOUS MALFORMATIONS

Among all vascular anomalies, venous malformations are the most common with a prevalence of 1% to 4% where slightly less than half are located in the extremities. These lesions may range from superficial varicosities with little symptoms to deep complex lesions associated with significant dysfunction and aesthetic complications.

Venous malformations are most effectively evaluated by MRI. Indications for intervention are usually guided by the patient's disabling symptoms or appearance. Initially, an endovascular approach is preferred using sclerotherapy and embolization. Commonly used agents include ethanol, sodium tetradecyl, and bleomycin. Surgical intervention is reserved for lesions resistant to sclerotherapy.[21]

KLIPPEL-TRENAUNAY SYNDROME

Klippel-Trenaunay syndrome (KTS) is a congenital disorder defined by the presence of lower extremity port wine stains, bony and soft tissue hypertrophic lesions, and venous malformation with or without lymphatic abnormalities. No specific radiological, genetic, or laboratory study is required to confirm the diagnosis. Patient commonly presents with chronic venous insufficiency, cellulitis, superficial thrombophlebitis, deep venous thrombosis, calcified venous malformations, and intraosseous vascular malformations.delis et al.[22] In order to properly delineate the anatomy, patient with KTS should undergo an MRI which will highlight the persistent embryonic veins (the lateral marginal vein, and the persistent sciatic vein).

Initial management is conservative with compression stocking until the age of 4, at which time limb length is monitored. Closure of the PEV may be considered, as well as surgical debulking and sclerotherapy. A multidisciplinary approach has had the best success in managing this difficult patient population.[23]

VENOUS THROMBOSIS AND POSTPHLEBITIC SYNDROME

The overall incidence of venous thrombosis in children is estimated at 0.49 per 10,000 per year. More than 90% of these events are provoked, most commonly (1) presence of indwelling central catheter, (2) sepsis, (3) trauma, (4) inherited coagulopathy, and (5) malignancies. Therapeutic guidelines are similar to adult recommendations. However, a lower incidence of thrombotic events has been observed in the pediatric population compared to adult.

The postphlebitic syndrome is seen with equal frequency in the pediatric population estimated between 9% and 24%. Bleeding complications from the anticoagulation regimens vary between 0% and 9%.[24]

REFERENCES

1. Kayssi A, Metias M, Langer JC, et al. The spectrum and management of noniatrogenic vascular trauma in the pediatric population. *J Pediatr Surg*. 2018;53:771-774.
2. Kayssi A, Shaikh F, Roche-Nagle G, Brandao LR, Williams SA, Rubin BB. Management of acute limb ischemia in the pediatric population. *J Vasc Surg*. 2014; 60:106-110.
3. Alexander J, Yohannan T, Abutineh I, et al. Ultrasound-guided femoral arterial access in pediatric cardiac catheterizations: a prospective evaluation of the prevalence, risk factors, and mechanism for acute loss of arterial pulse. *Catheter Cardiovasc Interv*. 2016;88:1098-1107.
4. Mortensson W, Hallbook T, Lundstrom NR. Percutaneous catheterization of the femoral vessels in children. II. Thrombotic occlusion of the catheterized

artery: frequency and causes. *Pediatr Radiol.* 1975; 4:1-9.

5. Franken EA Jr., Girod D, Sequeira FW, Smith WL, Hurwitz R, Smith JA. Femoral artery spasm in children: catheter size is the principal cause. *AJR Am J Roentgenol.* 1982;138:295-298.
6. Sahn DJ, Goldberg SJ, Allen HD, et al. A new technique for noninvasive evaluation of femoral arterial and venous anatomy before and after percutaneous cardiac catheterization in children and infants. *Am J Cardiol.* 1982;49:349-355.
7. Glatz AC, Keashen R, Chang J, et al. Outcomes using a clinical practice pathway for the management of pulse loss following pediatric cardiac catheterization. *Catheter Cardiovasc Interv.* 2015;85:111-117.
8. Gupta AA, Leaker M, Andrew M, et al. Safety and outcomes of thrombolysis with tissue plasminogen activator for treatment of intravascular thrombosis in children. *J Pediatr.* 2001;139:682-688.
9. Zenz W, Muntean W, Beitzke A, Zobel G, Riccabona M, Gamillscheg A. Tissue plasminogen activator (alteplase) treatment for femoral artery thrombosis after cardiac catheterisation in infants and children. *Br Heart J.* 1993;70:382-385.
10. Lin PH, Dodson TF, Bush RL, et al. Surgical intervention for complications caused by femoral artery catheterization in pediatric patients. *J Vasc Surg.* 2001;34: 1071-1078.
11. LaQuaglia MP, Upton J, May JW Jr. Microvascular reconstruction of major arteries in neonates and small children. *J Pediatr Surg.* 1991;26:1136-1140.
12. Bonasso PC, d'Audiffret A, Vaughan R, Pillai L. Feasibility of cryopreserved conduits for complex vascular reconstruction in the pediatric population: the case of a 3-year-old with femoral vessels transections. *Vasc Endovascular Surg.* 2018;52:553-555.
13. Richardson JD, Fallat M, Nagaraj HS, Groff DB, Flint LM. Arterial injuries in children. *Arch Surg.* 1981;116: 685-690.
14. Flanigan DP, Keifer TJ, Schuler JJ, Ryan TJ, Castronuovo JJ. Experience with latrogenic pediatric vascular injuries. Incidence, etiology, management, and results. *Ann Surg.* 1983;198:430-442.
15. Eliason JL, Coleman DM, Gumushian A, Stanley JC. Arterial reconstructions for chronic lower extremity ischemia in preadolescent and adolescent children. *J Vasc Surg.* 2018;67:1207-1216.
16. Gordon JE, Davis LE. Leg length discrepancy: the natural history (and what do we really know). *J Pediatr Orthop.* 2019;39:S10-S13.
17. Cardneau JD, Henke PK, Upchurch GR Jr, et al. Efficacy and durability of autogenous saphenous vein conduits for lower extremity arterial reconstructions in preadolescent children. *J Vasc Surg.* 2001;34:34-40.
18. Howorth MB Jr. Aneurysm of abdominal aorta in the newborn infant. Report of case. *N Engl J Med.* 1967; 276:1133-1134.
19. Davis FM, Eliason JL, Ganesh SK, Blatt NB, Stanley JC, Coleman DM. Pediatric nonaortic arterial aneurysms. *J Vasc Surg.* 2016;63:466-476.e1.
20. Totapally BR, Raszynski A, Khan D, Amjad I, Biehler J. Extremity arterial thromboses in hospitalized children: a national database analysis of prevalence and therapeutic interventions. *Pediatr Crit Care Med.* 2019;20:e154-e159.
21. Cox JA, Bartlett E, Lee EI. Vascular malformations: a review. *Semin Plast Surg.* 2014;28:58-63.
22. Delis KT, Gloviczki P, Wennberg PW, Rooke TW, Driscoll DJ. Hemodynamic impairment, venous segmental disease, and clinical severity scoring in limbs with Klippel-Trenaunay syndrome. *J Vasc Surg.* 2007; 45(3):561-567.
23. John PR. Klippel-Trenaunay syndrome. *Tech Vasc Interv Radiol*, 2019;22:100634.
24. Goldenberg NA, Bernard TJ. Venous thromboembolism in children. *Hematol Oncol Clin North Am.* 2010; 24:151-166.

SELF-ASSESSMENT STUDY QUESTIONS AND ANSWERS

Questions

1. A 3-year-old female patient was brought to the emergency department by her parents with a concern of right groin pain and coolness of her right leg. After further history taking you found that the patient underwent cardiac catheterization to evaluate possible congenital heart anomaly via right femoral artery access few days ago. On examination, her right femoral pulse is faint and weaker than the left side. Duplex ultrasound of the right groin showed no pseudoaneurysm but it confirmed a soft nonobstructed thrombus in the right common femoral artery. What is your next step in managing this patient?

A. Take the patient emergently to the cath lab for thrombolysis initiation.
B. Reassure the parents that the thrombus is not obstructive and discharge home with ultrasound in 2 weeks.
C. Admit the patient and start weight-based IV heparin and close vascular monitoring.
D. Take the patient within 6 hours for open thrombectomy.
E. Admit for observation and if the symptoms worsen in the next 24 hours, procced with anticoagulation.

2. The most common peripheral aneurysm in pediatric population is:

A. Renal artery aneurysm
B. Popliteal artery aneurysm
C. Brachial artery aneurysm
D. Splenic artery aneurysm
E. Extracranial carotid artery aneurysm

3. A 10-year-old male patient who is known to have hypertension that was diagnosed last year was referred to you by his pediatrician with a concern of renal artery stenosis. You confirmed 7-mm stenosis in the main left renal artery by angiogram. His parents are concerned that his BP is not controlled despite having him on three antihypertensive medications. What is the best treatment option for him at this point?

A. Continue medical treatment and refer him for weight reduction surgery.
B. Offer percutaneous transluminal angioplasty as the next treatment.
C. The patient will need open aorto-renal bypass using a harvested internal iliac artery.
D. Given his age, the best surgical treatment for him will be open revascularization with reimplantation of his renal artery.
E. This patient failed treatment and he will need an early nephrectomy.

SELF-ASSESSMENT STUDY QUESTIONS AND ANSWERS

Answers

1. C.
2. A.
3. B.

CHAPTER

57 Artificial Intelligence and Vascular Surgery

Qiong Qiu and Munier Nazzal

OUTLINE

INTRODUCTION
FUNDAMENTALS OF ARTIFICIAL INTELLIGENCE
ARTIFICIAL INTELLIGENCE IN MEDICINE
ARTIFICIAL INTELLIGENCE IN VASCULAR SURGERY
MACHINE LEARNING ALGORITHM DEVELOPMENT FRAMEWORK
THE ROLE OF THE SURGEON
CURRENT LIMITATIONS
FUTURE DIRECTIONS
SUMMARY

INTRODUCTION

First introduced in 1956 at a Dartmouth College conference, the concept of artificial intelligence (AI) is not new. However, with the recent advances in computing power and data storage, artificial intelligence has been integrated into our daily lives. From autocomplete to Amazon recommendations, AI algorithms have influenced how we search, shop, and get around. With the transition to electronic medical records, whole-genome sequences, and high-resolution images, medicine has also entered the era of big data and has the potential benefit from the promise of AI. In medicine, AI promises not only increased convenience but also provides comprehensive and personalized care. Although hoping to achieve no human error, the accuracy depends on data entry as a source of potential error.

The earliest work of AI in medicine occurred in the 1970s. The first NIH-sponsored AI in Medicine workshop occurred in 1975 at Rutgers University.[1] In 1976, the first AI prototype in medicine, the CASNET model, was presented at the Academy of Ophthalmology meeting. This model can process patient and disease-specific inputs and produce treatment recommendations for those with glaucoma.[2] In the late 2000s, the growth of AI is fueled by significant advances in the field of computer science, such as increased processing speed and power. With the development of the convolutional neural network (CNN), a type of deep learning network, the application of AI in high-resolution medical images became possible. For example, after training on 14,884 3D optical coherence tomography scans, AI applications can make referral recommendations for a range of sight-threatening retinal diseases better than the experts.[3] In nephrology, 700,000 medical records were used to create an AI algorithm that can predict the development of acute kidney injury 48 hours before traditional clinical care.[4]

Although the application of machine learning (ML) to clinical medicine is in its infancy, many algorithms have been developed to predict clinical outcomes such as sepsis, dementia, readmission, and mortality postchemotherapy.[5–8] Dr Topol, a cardiologist and an expert in translational research, has predicated that AI technology will be incorporated into every clinical practice.[9] However, despite its seemly unlimited potential, the current clinical application of AI is still a work in progress.

FUNDAMENTALS OF ARTIFICIAL INTELLIGENCE

By definition, AI describes any design system that demonstrates the properties of human intelligence, such as reasoning, learning, adaptation, or sensory understanding. In its most basic form, an AI algorithm is a set of algorithms that produces output based on input data without human interference between both these points. The human role is during the input stage and in creating the algorithms that help analyze the data for the needed output. There are many subfields under the AI umbrella, including ML, deep learning, and CNN (Figure 57-1). The field of AI can also be subdivided into a physical branch which consists of physical assistive robots for care, surgery, or drug delivery, and a visual branch focusing more on the analysis of medical images. **Natural language processing** is another specialized subset of AI algorithms designed to process and "understand" speech or written language. This algorithm is best suited to process large sets of text, such as analyzing clinical notes to produce a condensed clinical summary.

Machine learning (ML), often used interchangeably with AI, is technically a subset of AI. A ML algorithm independently identifies patterns within large datasets without being explicitly programed. The machine develops a process based on the models within a set of known input and output data (Figure 57-2A). The resulting pattern recognition algorithm is then used to predict outcomes based on known input data. Traditional ML algorithms include data analysis tools such as logistic regression, Bayesian networks, Random Forest, and support vector machines. ML is especially useful in identifying patterns that are maybe indiscernible during manual analysis. Furthermore, compared to traditional statistical analysis, ML permits more complex nonlinear relationships and multivariate effects in its analysis.

Supervised learning is an optimization of the trial-and-error learning process based on the labeled data set. Under this system, labeled inputs and outputs are provided to train the program. The resulting algorithm generalizes from the prelabeled training data set to analyze unknown input data. This type of learning is best suited to predict or classify known future outcomes.

Unsupervised learning is an optimization of the trial-and-error learning process of unlabeled data. Under this system, unlabeled inputs and outputs are provided to train the program. The goal of the program is to identify hidden patterns and natural structures within the data sets. This type of learning is best

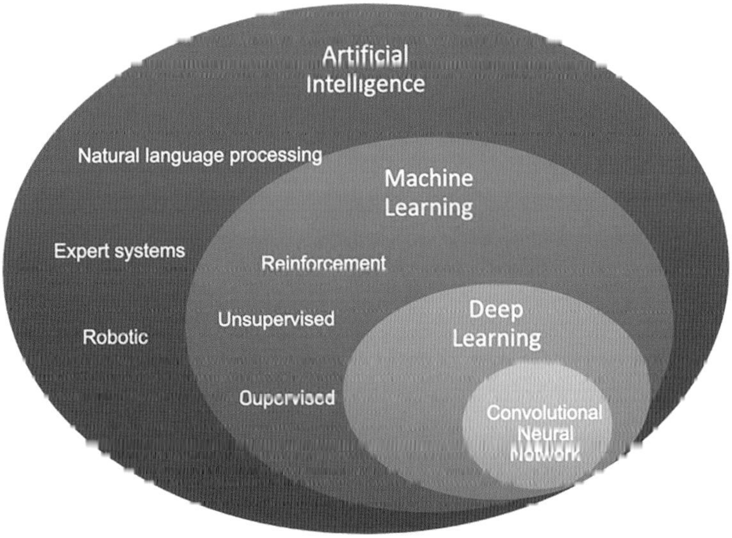

FIGURE 57-1 Graphic representation of the subtypes of artificial intelligence methods.

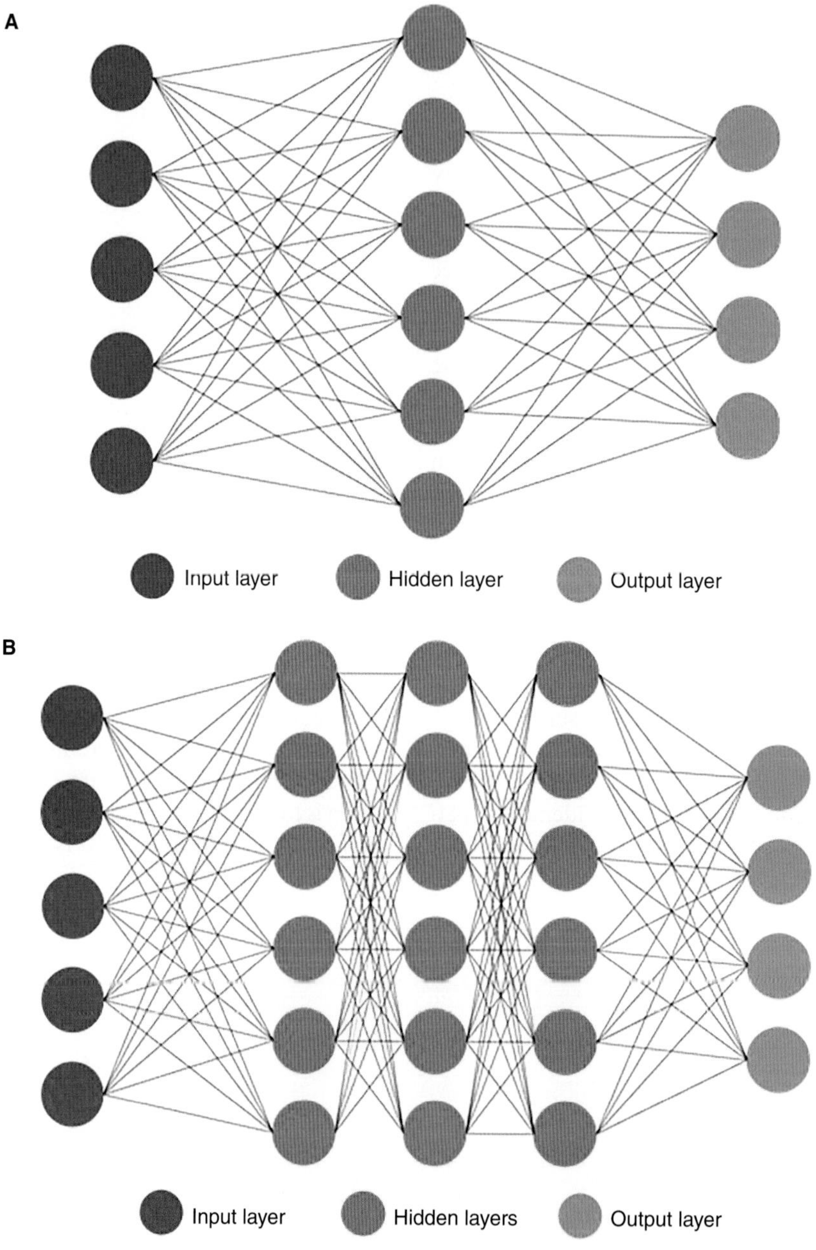

FIGURE 57-2 Architecture of machine learning networks. A) Simple machine learning network consisting of an input layer, a single hidden layer, and an output layer. **B**) A deep machine learning network consists of an input layer, many hidden layers, and an output layer.

suited to analyze complex relationships among the variables without any prior assumptions.

Reinforcement learning is a training program that makes decisions based on the ability to maximize a predefined reward. Like unsupervised learning, it does not require a prelabeled input dataset. However, unlike simple unsupervised learning, reinforcement learning can learn from its successes and failures. The length of reinforcement learning training must balance between the cost of exploration and reward of exploitation of current knowledge (dataset).

An artificial neural network (ANN) is a subset of ML. This system is inspired by the biological nervous system where each neuron is connected to multiple other neurons and organized in layers. These neurons also process inputs to produce outputs. The first layer within the system is known as the "input layer." The last layer is the "output layer." In between these two layers are the "hidden layers." These inner layers are also known as the "black box" because the exact strength of the connections between the neurons is unknown. Only those who design the hidden data algorithms have knowledge of the secrets of the black box. Based on that it is difficult to validate the accuracy of such algorithms by others. The black box is like the trade secrets that cannot be exposed to competition.

Deep learning (DL), a subset of ANN, uses unlabeled input and output dataset to identify the underlying patterns and structures. However, it differs from simple unsupervised learning in that the algorithms use multiple layers to extract multiple levels of features (Figure 57-2B). These layers allow the algorithm to amplify variables that are important for classification while suppressing the irrelevant ones. The development of DL-fueled advancements in multiple fields, such as speech recognition, visual object recognition, and genomics. Among the numerous DL algorithms, artificial neural network (ANN) and CNN are the most commonly used.

Convolutional neural network (CNN), a subset of DL, is also a multiple layers network based on the principle of convolution, a mathematical operation that produces a third function based on two other functions. This system is inspired by the properties of the visual cortex, where each neuron processes only a portion of the input image. Each neuron also filters the original image before passing the information to the next layer of neurons. The same process is repeated in each layer until all of the input images are processed. Overall this process breaks down the dataset into overlapping portions processed by smaller neural networks and pools the results, which is especially useful for processing images.

ARTIFICIAL INTELLIGENCE IN MEDICINE

Since the 1970s, there has been growing interest in the potential application of AI in both medical research and clinical practice. With the emergence of "big data" within health care, the interest in applying AI algorithms to clinical programs has gained new momentum. Interest in AI has skyrocketed in the past decade. Confidence in the potential usefulness of AI in health care is shared by many ventral capitalists and it has fueled the growth of venture capital-backed AI health care startups. The global AI health market is predicted by Frost & Sullivan to grow from $600 million in 2014 to $6.6 billion by 2021.[10] The 10 leading disease types studied in AI literature in 2016 were oncology, neurology, cardiovascular, urogenital, pregnancy, gastrointestinal, respiratory, skin, endocrine, and nutrition. The number of AI-related clinical trials has also increased over the past few years.[11] Interestingly, most of the projects from high-income countries tend to focus on a specific disease such as cancer or cardiovascular disease, while those from low- and middle-income countries tend to target public health care.[12,13] Furthermore, not all areas of medicine benefit equally from ML. Based on the review of recently published studies within PubMed, deep learning is used highest in diagnostic imaging, electrodiagnosis, genetic diagnosis, clinical laboratory, and mass screening, respectively.

Given the more robust nature of AI-based imaging processing algorithms, many of the health-related AI-based diagnostic models have proliferated in medical specialties that depend heavily on visual inspection and imaging process. In dermatology, skin cancer classification algorithm based on deep-learning networks has resulted in similar cancer detection rates as dermatologists. For example, Esteva et al. used a single CNN trained on 129,450 clinical images has demonstrated similar cancer detection rates as 21 board-certified dermatologists with an AUC of 0.96 for carcinoma and an AUC of 0.94 for melanoma.[14] In ophthalmology, deep CNNs trained on 130,000 retinal fundus photographs were able to diagnose age related macular degeneration with an accuracy of 88% to 92% with an AUC between 0.94 and 0.96, which is nearly as high as that for expert human graders.[15] Lastly, in gastroenterology, a ML algorithm was used to identify diminutive polyps (≤5 mm) on real-time colonoscopy images with 94% accuracy and a negative predictive value of 96%.[16] This algorithm was further validated on 27,113 colonoscopy images from 1,138 patients with 94% sensitivity and an AUC of 0.98. These studies demonstrated the value and potential of machine-aided diagnosis in the not-too-distant future.

In addition, given the health care system's financial incentives and the increased prevalence of electronic health records (EHR), it is not surprising that many AI models have been developed to predict financially significant events such as surgical site infection, prolonged length of stay, and 30-day readmission. Prediction model trained on EHR of 216,221 adult patients was able to predict unplanned 30-day readmission with an AUC of 0.75 and prolonged length of stay with an AUC of 0.85.[17] Similarly, Soguero-Ruiz et al. used a ML algorithm trained on the EHR of over 1,000 patients to predict the risk of postoperative surgical site infections in patients undergoing gastrointestinal surgery.[18] Shameer et al. also used a ML model trained on the EHR of 1,068 patients with 4,205 variables to predict 30-day readmission rate with an accuracy of 83% and ACU of 0.78.[5] These are only a small sample of the vast amount of AI-related research within medicine, and they represent the beginning of the era of machine-aided medicine.

Overall, clinical, translational, and public health are some of the fields with the highest potential in the future. In clinical fields, ML is well suited to perform disease prediction and diagnosis, treatment effectiveness, and outcome prediction. Within translational medicine, ML application can aid in drug discovery or repurposing of drugs based on mechanism of action and large clinical trials. Public health benefits from ML-powered prediction of the epidemic outbreak and precision health, exemplified by the AI prediction models of COVID-19 epidemic.[19]

ARTIFICIAL INTELLIGENCE IN VASCULAR SURGERY

In contrast, there are fewer AI-related publications for vascular diseases compared to other medical specialties such as ophthalmology, dermatology, neurology, oncology, and cardiology.[20] As Dr Raffort, an expert in ML in vascular surgery, categorized, most of the AI research within vascular surgery falls into two categories—image analysis and risk prediction and prognostication.[21]

Given the importance of imaging in the diagnosis and treatment of vascular disease, it is unsurprising that multiple groups applied ML technology to automate the interpretation of vascular images such as aortic aneurysm segmentation.[22,23] Many of these studies utilize image segmentation, which is the process of sorting digital images into multiple sets of pixels. These sets of pixels then replace the individual pixels as the unit of analysis. Zhug et al. developed a process to segment abdominal aortic aneurysm (AAA) on CT angiograms. Using a database of 20 CT angiograms, the system was able to reduce the mean segmentation time per patient to 7.4 ±3.8 minus from the 20 to 30 minutes per patient with the human excerpt methods.[22] Because multiple imaging modalities are often used together to support clinic decisions, other groups have worked to perform multimodal image segmentation. Wang et al., for instance, developed a neuro network that can be used on both CT and MR images to analyze and identify aortic aneurysms.[24] Lareyre et al. further extended image segmentation by developing an automatic process for detecting aortic lumen, AAA, and the associated thrombus and calcification, based on a database of CT images from 40 patients with AAA.[23] Other researchers also trained deep learning algorithms on CT angiograms to detect and measure aortic vascular calcifications.[25,26] Lastly, ML algorithms have also been used to classify the geometry and fluid dynamic of AAA. Shum et al. used a decision-tree algorithm trained on 70 CT images of aortic aneurysms to predict rupture with an accuracy of 87%.[27]

Image analyses also aid in risk-stratifying patients and can aid in prognostication. In patients with carotid artery stenosis, models trained on carotid ultrasound and MRI can perform both carotid artery segmentation and risk stratify patients.[28–30] Such models produce results that are comparable to expert interpretations; however, only a few of these models are cross-validated on large standardized datasets. For patients with AAA, Turto et al. developed a four-variable ANN network trained on 102 patients with ruptured AAA requiring operation that can predict survival with 83% sensitivity and 86% specificity.[31] For those who underwent endovascular aneurysm repair (EVAR), Karthikesalingam et al. trained an ANN model on 761 patients to classify patients into low-risk and high-risk groups for post-EVAR complications such as limb complications within 5 years (1% vs, 8%) and 5-year mortality (12% vs 21%).[32] Similarly, Attallah and Ma used a Bayesian network and back-propagation neuronal network to classify patients who underwent EVAR into low- and high-risk groups for reintervention.[33] Most of the existing prognostication models in vascular surgery remain rooted in image analysis.

In comparison, there are fewer ML algorithms predicting patient's risks based on a broader set of health information. Our group recently developed a five-variable decision-tree model trained on data from 326,853 patients to predict the risk of amputation in patients with diabetes with a sensitivity of 76% and a specificity of 79% with an AUC of 0.84 (data to be published). This predicational model can be accessed at https://grenut.shinyapps.io/amputation/. Lastly, Chang et al. recently published a DL predictive model trained on a national database of 72,435 patients who underwent infra-inguinal vascular surgeries with upper thigh incisions. This model was able to divide patients into low- and high-risk groups, which formed the basis in determining the usage of closed incision negative pressure therapy. The authors concluded that the model-based risk stratification resulted in more efficient utilization of resources to reduce surgical site infection and resulted in an estimated saving of $231 to $458 per patient.[34] This last study highlights the potential of how machine-assisted medicine can improve not only patient outcomes but also reduce health care spending.

MACHINE LEARNING ALGORITHM DEVELOPMENT FRAMEWORK

The development of AI or ML algorithms can be divided into two stages: training and predicting (Figure 57-3). The raw data is initially processed either manually or automatically to identify the

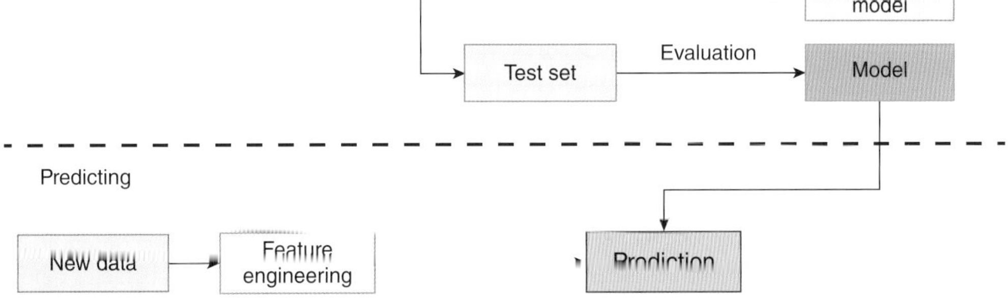

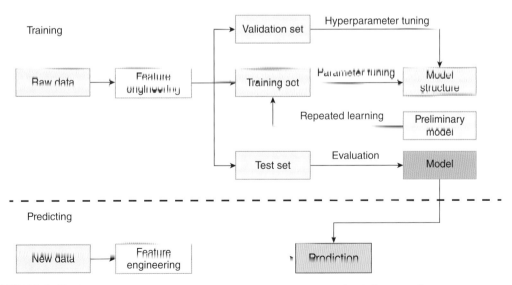

FIGURE 57-3 Machine learning algorithm development framework. The raw data is first manually processed to highlight the studied features and reduce noise. The dataset is then divided into a validation set, a training set, and a test set. The validation set is used to select the model structure. The training set is used to train the model and to fine-tune the model structure. After repeated learning, the test set is used to validate the preliminary model to produce the final model. The final model is then tested on new data to evaluate the model's prediction ability.

salient features. The resulting dataset is then divided into three sets: validation set, training set, and test set. The validation set is used to tune the hyperparameter of the model structure. The training set is then used to fine-tune both the hyperparameter and the parameter of the preliminary model. This process can be repeated as many times as necessary to produce the final ML model. The test set is used to evaluate the accuracy, sensitivity, and specificity of the final model. Lastly, the resulting ML model can be used to process a new dataset to produce the desired predictions.

The final output from these ML neural networks is often compared with physicians' assessments. This comparison is quantified using receiver operating characteristic (ROC), a plot of true-positive versus false-positive rates. The accuracy of the ML algorithm is expressed by the area under the curve (AUC). Most of the published ML-based prediction models have an AUC between 0.67 and 0.94.[5–8,35] The accuracy of the network can be increased through parameter adjustments and increasing the size of the training database.

Exposing the ML model to a new dataset is also an important step to evaluate the model's generalizability and overcome **Overfitting**. When the initial dataset used for training does not accurately reflect the underlying population, then the resulting classification algorithm will be biased toward the distribution within the dataset.[36] One effective method to reduce bias and improve the classification's accuracy is to introduce new data into the training set. The gold standard for assessing the generalizability of the model, the test dataset used for validation, should be collected independently from the training dataset.[37]

THE ROLE OF THE SURGEON

Surgeons also play an essential role in developing AI applications by identifying the relevant clinical questions for the database to answer.[38] Furthermore, clinical experience and medical knowledge are necessary to determine if a particular database is suitable to answer the clinical question. For instance, although inpatient databases are more readily available, outpatient data with social-economic information may be more effective at training risk-stratification algorithms for many vascular diseases such as aortic aneurysm and venous stasis.

Surgeons are also critical to the development and maintenance of medical databases, such as large clinical data registries. Collaborations with data scientists would improve the efficiency and accuracy of health information collection. These resulting databases can facilitate international cooperation and data sharing to improve the quality and safety of care. Such movement is already underway with Vascunet as one such international patient registry endorsed by the European Society for Vascular Surgery.[39] These curated medical databases are better suited for training AI algorithms than traditional EMRs because of the standardization of information entry. Thus, these curated medical databases provide a more uniform, reliable, and comprehensive patient information to train predictive models.

Lastly, surgeons' and other clinicians' experience and expertize are needed to evaluate AI applications for clinical usage. With the increasing number of AI algorithms flooding the health care market, surgeons and other clinicians must be prepared to assess these emerging technologies' clinical value. Surgeons must determine if an AI algorithm can provide accurate results and whether the algorithm is relevant for their patient population. Thus, a basic understanding of computer science, mathematics, and statistics are critical for surgeons to adequately assess the benefits, risks, and limitations of new AI technologies. Surgeons need to understand the benefit and limitation of AI applications ourselves, but we must also explain these concepts to our patients and guide them toward the most appropriate tool.

CURRENT LIMITATIONS

AI technology promises many potential benefits; however, it faces formidable obstacles before it can be fully integrated into clinical settings. One of the major impediments of widespread adaptation of AI algorithms in medicine is the lack of standardized algorithm validation process. Despite the proliferation of medical AI algorithms, there are few standardized validation datasets which place the burden of evaluating individual algorithms on the physicians and health systems. Unfortunately, few clinicians and health systems are equipped to validate AI algorithms internally. Moreover, because the health systems that are equipped to conduct internal validation tend to be larger and more financially well-off, the pattern of AI adaption would likely exacerbate existing health disparities. Therefore, a robust and standardized validation process of algorithms is necessary before the general public can benefit from AI algorithms in medicine.

With the transition to EHR and the corresponding increase in health care data, there has been a considerable interest in leveraging the power of AI algorithms to health care. However, unlike the uniformed data autogenerated through technology companies such as Facebook or Google, medical data is both structured (such as coded diagnosis and laboratory tests) and unstructured (such as free-text clinic notes).[40] Given the diversity in EHR systems and medical practices, these medical data are usually heterogeneous and manually entered into the medical record. Therefore, there are often missing or erroneous data within many raw medical databases. These inaccuracies within the datasets limit the ability of AI algorithms to be clinically useful or universally acceptable.

Furthermore, because AI is trained on preexisting datasets, the resulting algorithms will reflect and amplify the preexisting biases, including racial bias. Many medical datasets contain patient demographic imbalances, and patients enrolled in medical studies often do not reflect the underlying population, which are biased toward the majority within the sample and can exacerbate the preexisting racial disparities. For example, most AI algorithms for skin cancer detection are trained on datasets with few patients of color.[41]

Moreover, the optimization of AI algorithms depends on the availability of a large set of medical data. The proper storage and de-identification of these medical data are especially important in the age of hacking. In addition, there is a greater concern for the privacy and security of patient information. The recent Google health data scandal highlights the concern for privacy in the era of medical data research. The Nightingale project granted Google access to health information with identifiable data of tens of millions of patients treated within the Ascension healthcare network without the knowledge of the patients.[42]

Although we have accepted many black box therapies such as hydralazine for hypertension and electroconvulsive therapy for severe depression, the same standard does not extend to AI algorithms. The majority of AI algorithms, such as ANN, have a "black box" design, with limited information regarding how the computer identified the patterns.[38] The lack of explanation for their results can lead unintended consequences for high-stake fields like criminal justice and healthcare.[43] The negative risks of opaqueness has led to governing organizations such as the European Union's General Data Protection Regulation require transparency of algorithm before it can be used in patient care.[44] Within high stake fields such as medicine, a mistake within an AI algorithm can lead to hundreds if not thousands of deaths. Furthermore, under the current judicial system, the doctors and hospital systems utilizing the AI algorithm would be held responsible for the algorithm's mistake. Thus, there has been a movement to produce explainable AI, which would explain why an algorithm reaches its conclusion. Unfortunately, such a reverse engineering process is challenging and remains a work in process.

Lastly, there are some unique concerns with AI algorithms in vascular surgery. Most current AI research focuses on only one type of data, either image or categorical data. However, much of the diagnosis of vascular diseases depends on a combination of high-resolution medical imaging and patient factors, which increases the difficulty of producing a comprehensive prediction algorithm. Furthermore, the severity of vascular diseases is often heavily influenced by patients' lifestyles, which are more challenging to collect and quantify. These lifestyle factors and social determinants of health indices are often missing within existing medical databases. To capture a complete picture of the diseases, researchers may need to collect social media or mobile data. Thus, more comprehensive databases are needed to train algorithms to predict health outcomes of vascular diseases.

FUTURE DIRECTIONS

In the short term, the most significant potential of AI lies in its ability to analyze medical images because of their consistent and reliable data compared to EHR databases. Applying ML algorithms to medical images before and after diagnosis of diseases can build an algorithm that can lead to earlier diagnosis and treatment of diseases in the future. In the long term, AI has great potential to improve all aspects of medicine, from risk stratification, direct patient care, education, and surgeons training to postcare surveillance systems. In vascular surgery, specifically, combining AI imaging algorithms with robotic surgery can lead to machine-assisted surgery, which has important implications for surgical training and practice. AI models can be used to predict potential for predicting progression of disease such as carotid stenosis and abdominal aortic aneurysm with potential future complications such stroke or rupture respectively. Adding to that the inclusion of genetic analysis to the clinical data, the potential of AI to guide vascular disease management is monumental. Lastly, surgical education presents a new frontier for AI research in vascular surgery.

Simulation models of open operations and endovascular operations built through ML have been used in the training of surgical residents. In the era of COVID-19, these simulation models can serve as essential adjuncts for residency and fellowship training. The power of AI lies in its ability to identify and learn from patterns within large databases. Thus, medical AI's predictive potential will only increase as the field of medicine generates more medical data.

Furthermore, although much of the current AI research has been focused on leveraging existing medical databases to predict health outcomes, AI, particularly natural language processing, can also be used to improve the overall health care workflow and, in turn, physician well-being. The ever-increasing documentation requirement has long been cited as one of the contributing factors for increased physician burnout. The power of natural language processing can be used to improve health care processes, such as producing AI-assisted discharge summaries. Much of the discussion around physician burnout has been centered around the increasing burden of documentation. Thus, by improving the efficiency of documentation, AI has the potential not only to increase the efficiency of the documentation process but also to improve physical well-being.

SUMMARY

As medicine enters the era of big data, AI offers the potential to usher in a new era of personalized precision medicine and transform health care as we know it. With their ability to process large volumes of data and self-learn, AI systems can enhance patients' risk-stratification, diagnostic accuracy, and workflow efficiency. Nevertheless, most of the available AI models must overcome many obstacles before they can be seamlessly integrated into daily clinical practice. Successful adaptation of novel algorithms into clinical practice requires the clinicians to have the ability to differentiate the actual capability of the AI algorithms from the hype. A basic understanding of the AI systems enables surgeons to prepare themselves and their patients for the era of machine-assisted medicine. Finally, the appropriate application of medicine-assisted medicine will improve clinical outcomes and free surgeons to spend more time caring for our patients and restore compassion to health care.

REFERENCES

1. Kulikowski CA. Beginnings of artificial intelligence in medicine (AIM): computational artifice assisting scientific inquiry and clinical art with reflections on present AIM challenges. *Yearb Med Inform.* 2019;28(1):249-256.
2. Weiss SM, Kulikowski CA, Amarel S, Safir A. A model-based method for computer-aided medical decision-making. *Artif Intell.* 1978;11(1-2):145-172.
3. De Fauw J, Ledsam JR, Romera-Paredes B, et al. Clinically applicable deep learning for diagnosis and referral in retinal disease. *Nat Med.* 2018;24:1342-1350.
4. Tomašev N, Glorot X, Rae JW, et al. A clinically applicable approach to continuous prediction of future acute kidney injury. *Nature (London).* 2019;572(7767):116-119.
5. Shameer K, Johnson KW, Yahi A, et al. Predictive modeling of hospital readmission rates using electronic

medical record-wide machine learning: a case-study using Mount Sinai heart failure cohort. *Pac Symp Biocomput*. 2017;22:276-287.

6. Horng S, Sontag DA, Halpern Y, Jernite Y, Shapiro NI, Nathanson LA. Creating an automated trigger for sepsis clinical decision support at emergency department triage using machine learning. *PLoS One*. 2017;12(4):e0174708.
7. Ben Miled Z, Haas K, Black CM, et al. Predicting dementia with routine care EMR data. *Artif Intell Med*. 2020;102:101771.
8. Elfiky AA, Pany MJ, Parikh RB, Obermeyer Z. Development and application of a machine learning approach to assess short-term mortality risk among patients with cancer starting chemotherapy. *JAMA Netw Open*. 2018;1(3):e180926.
9. Topol EJ. High-performance medicine: the convergence of human and artificial intelligence. *Nat Med*. 2019;25(1):44-56.
10. Frost & Sullivan. From $600 M to $6 Billion, artificial intelligence systems poised for dramatic market expansion in healthcare. Robotics & Machine Learning. Available at https://www.frost.com/news/press-releases/600-m-6-billion-artificial-intelligence-systems-poised-dramatic-market-expansion-healthcare/. Accessed on January 18, 2016.
11. Kolachalama VB, Garg PS. Machine learning and medical education. *NPJ Digit Med*. 2018;1(1):54.
12. Vuong QH, Ho MT, Vuong TT, et al. Artificial intelligence vs. natural stupidity: evaluating AI readiness for the Vietnamese medical information system. *J Clin Med*. 2019;8(2):160.
13. Raffort J, Adam C, Carrier M, Lareyre F. Fundamentals in artificial intelligence for vascular surgeons. *Ann Vasc Surg*. 2020;65:254-260.
14. Esteva A, Kuprel B, Novoa RA, et al. Dermatologist-level classification of skin cancer with deep neural networks. *Nature*. 2017;542(7639):115-118.
15. Burlina PM, Joshi N, Pekala M, Pacheco KD, Freund DE, Bressler NM. Automated grading of age-related macular degeneration from color fundus images using deep convolutional neural networks. *JAMA Ophthalmol*. 2017;135(11):1170-1176.
16. Mori Y, Kudo SE, Misawa M, et al. Real-time use of artificial intelligence in identification of diminutive polyps during colonoscopy: a prospective study. *Ann Intern Med*. 2018;169(6):357-366.
17. Rajkomar A, Oren E, Chen K, et al. Scalable and accurate deep learning with electronic health records. *NPJ Digit Med*. 2018;1(1):18.
18. Soguero-Ruiz C, Fei WM, Jenssen R, et al. Data-driven temporal prediction of surgical site infection. *AMIA Annu Symp Proc*. 2015;2015:1164-1173.
19. Noorbakhsh-Sabet N, Zand R, Zhang Y, Abedi V. Artificial intelligence transforms the future of health care. *Am J Med*. 2019;132(7):795-801.
20. Rajasinghe HA, Miller LE, Chahwan SH, Zamora AJ. Underutilization of artificial intelligence by vascular specialists. *Ann Vasc Surg*. 2019;61:2-3.
21. Raffort J, Adam C, Carrier M, et al. Artificial intelligence in abdominal aortic aneurysm. *J Vasc Surg*. 2020;72(1):321-333.e321.
22. Zhuge F, Rubin GD, Sun S, Napel S. An abdominal aortic aneurysm segmentation method: level set with region and statistical information. *Med Phys*. 2006;33(5):1440-1453.
23. Lareyre F, Adam C, Carrier M, Dommerc C, Mialhe C, Raffort J. A fully automated pipeline for mining abdominal aortic aneurysm using image segmentation. *Sci Rep*. 2019;9(1):13750.
24. Wang D, Zhang R, Zhu J, et al. Neural network fusion: a novel CT-MR aortic aneurysm image segmentation method. *Proc SPIE Int Soc Opt Eng*. 2018;10574:1057424.
25. Kurugol S, Come CE, Diaz AA, et al. Automated quantitative 3D analysis of aorta size, morphology, and mural calcification distributions. *Med Phys*. 2015;42(9):5467-5478.
26. Graffy PM, Liu J, O'Connor S, Summers RM, Pickhardt PJ. Automated segmentation and quantification of aortic calcification at abdominal CT: application of a deep learning-based algorithm to a longitudinal screening cohort. *Abdom Radiol*. 2019;44(8):2921-2928.
27. Shum J, Martufi G, Di Martino E, et al. Quantitative assessment of abdominal aortic aneurysm geometry. *Ann Biomed Eng*. 2011;39(1):277-286.
28. Gastounioti A, Kolias V, Golemati S, et al. CAROTID: a web-based platform for optimal personalized management of atherosclerotic patients. *Comput Methods Programs Biomed*. 2014;114(2):183-193.
29. Kumar PK, Araki T, Rajan J, Laird JR, Nicolaides A, Suri JS. State of the art review on automated lumen and adventitial border delineation and its measurements in carotid ultrasound. *Comput Methods Programs Biomed*. 2018;163:155-168.
30. Gao S, van 't Klooster R, Kitslaar PH, et al. Learning-based automated segmentation of the carotid artery vessel wall in dual-sequence MRI using subdivision surface fitting. *Med Phys*. 2017;44(10):5244-5259.
31. Turton EPL, Scott DJA, Delbridge M, Snowden S, Kester RC. Ruptured abdominal aortic aneurysm:

a novel method of outcome prediction using neural network technology. *Eur J Vasc Endovasc Surg.* 2000;19(2):184-189.

32. Karthikesalingam A, Attallah O, Ma X, et al. An artificial neural network stratifies the risks of reintervention and mortality after endovascular aneurysm repair; a retrospective observational study. *PLoS One.* 2015;10(7):e0129024.
33. Attallah O, Ma X. Bayesian neural network approach for determining the risk of re-intervention after endovascular aortic aneurysm repair. *Proc Inst Mech Eng H.* 2014;228(9):857-866.
34. Chang B, Sun Z, Peiris P, Huang ES, Benrashid E, Dillavou ED. Deep learning–based risk model for best management of closed groin incisions after vascular surgery. *J Surg Res.* 2020;254:408-416.
35. Lau L, Kankanige Y, Rubinstein B, et al. Machine-learning algorithms predict graft failure after liver transplantation. *Transplantation.* 2017;101(4):e125-e132.
36. Krittanawong C, Johnson KW, Rosenson RS, et al. Deep learning for cardiovascular medicine: a practical primer. *Eur Heart J.* 2019;40(25):2058-2073.
37. Park SH, Han K. Methodologic guide for evaluating clinical performance and effect of artificial intelligence technology for medical diagnosis and prediction. *Radiology.* 2018;286(3):800-809.
38. Cabitza F, Rasoini R, Gensini GF. Unintended consequences of machine learning in medicine. *JAMA.* 2017;318(6):517-518.
39. Lareyre F, Adam C, Carrier M, Chakfé N, Raffort J. Artificial intelligence for education of vascular surgeons. *Eur J Vasc Endovasc Surg.* 2020;59(6):870-871.
40. Miotto R, Wang F, Wang S, Jiang X, Dudley JT. Deep learning for healthcare: review, opportunities and challenges. *Brief Bioinform.* 2017;19(6):1236-1246.
41. Adamson AS, Smith A. Machine learning and health care disparities in dermatology. *JAMA Dermatol.* 2018; 154(11):1247-1248.
42. Ledford H. Google health-data scandal spooks researchers. *Nature.* 2019. doi:10.1038/d41586-019-03574-5
43. Wexler R. Computers are harming justice. *New York Times.* 2017:A27.
44. Yuan B, Li J. The policy effect of the general data protection regulation (GDPR) on the digital public health sector in the European union: an empirical investigation. *Int J Environ Res Public Health.* 2019;16(6):1070.

SELF-ASSESSMENT STUDY QUESTIONS AND ANSWERS

Questions

1. Which of the following is NOT a class of machine learning models?
   A. Structured learning
   B. Reinforcement learning
   C. Supervised learning
   D. None of the above

2. What is the role of the validation dataset in developing a machine learning model?
   A. Accelerating the convergence of the training algorithm
   B. Evaluating how well the model performs
   C. Finding the optimal hyperparameter values for the model
   D. Comparing the model performance to pre-existing benchmarks

3. In which of the following ways is AI currently being used for vascular surgery?
   A. Augmenting the interpretation of vascular images
   B. Recommending language for explaining treatment options to patients
   C. Comparing the significance of a patient's risk factors for adverse outcomes
   D. None of the above

4. What are some current limitations of AI in medicine?
   A. Reliance on the existence of a "good" training dataset with all relevant information
   B. Difficulty in interpreting and understanding AI algorithm recommendations
   C. Lack of standardized evaluation processes
   D. All of the above

5. Which of the following is NOT a type of machine learning model?
   A. Convolutional neural network
   B. Clustered neural network
   C. Deep neural network
   D. Artificial neural network

SELF-ASSESSMENT STUDY QUESTIONS AND ANSWERS

Answers

1. A.
2. C.
3. A.
4. D.
5. B.

Index

Note: Page numbers followed by *f* denote figures; those followed by *t* denote tables.

A

abdominal aortic aneurysmal (AAA) disease, 391–399
  clinical findings, 393
    signs and symptoms, 393
  diagnosis, 394
  differential diagnosis, 393, 394*t*, 395*f*
  general consideration and history, 391–393
    anatomy of aortic aneurysm disease, 391–392
    history of aortic aneurysm disease, 391
    pathophysiology of aortic aneurysm disease, 392–393
  management, 393–399
    indications for repair, 395–396
    methods of repair of AAA, 396–398
    open *versus* endovascular repair of AAA, 398–399
    postoperative surveillance, 399
acute limb ischemia, 487–499
  classification, 491, 492*t*
  clinical presentation, 488–490
    medical history, 489
    physical examination, 489–490
  conclusions, 499
  diagnosis and differentials, 491–492
    aortic occlusion, 491
    femoropopliteal occlusion, 492
    iliac occlusion, 492
    infragenicular occlusion, 492
  etiology, 488
    embolism, 488
    thrombosis, 488
  evaluation and investigation, 492
    catheter-based angiography, 492
    computed tomography angiography, 492
    noninvasive physiologic tests, 492
    ultrasound, 492
  initial management and treatment, 493
    anticoagulation, 493
    treatment selection, 493
  management options, 493–499
    comparing open *versus* endovascular options, 496–497
    endovascular approaches, 495–496
    fasciotomy, 497–499
    open revascularization, 493–495
acute mesenteric ischemia (AMI), 578–590
  clinical findings, 583
  diagnosis, 584–585
    abdominal x-ray, 584
    CT angiogram, 584–585
    diagnostic laparoscopy, 585
    laboratory values, 584–585
    magnetic resonance angiogram (MRA), 585
    ultrasound, 584
  differential diagnosis, 583–584
  general considerations and history, 579–583
    embolic causes, 579–582
    history of AMI, 579
    introduction, 579
    mesenteric venous thrombosis (MVT), 583
  management, 585–590
    bowel evaluation, 588–589
    complications and follow up, 589–590
    endovascular therapies, 585–586
    hybrid procedure: retrograde open mesenteric stenting (ROMS), 587
    medical therapies, 585
    open surgery, 587–588
    treatment for mesenteric venous thrombosis, 588

AI (artificial intelligence). *See* artificial intelligence (AI)
ALARA (as low as reasonably achievable) principle, 47
AMI (acute mesenteric ischemia). *see* acute mesenteric ischemia (AMI)
amputation techniques in vascular disease, 170–193
  anatomic variants, 171–172
  clinical findings, 172
  diagnosis and preoperative considerations, 172–176
    ambulation energy, 175–176
    ambulation rate, 175
    angiography, 174
    ankle-brachial index (ABI), 173
    fluorescence imaging, 174
    preoperative planning, 174–175
    skin perfusion pressure (SPP), 173–174
    staged amputation, 174–175
    tissue evaluation methods, 172–174
    toe pressures (TBP), 173
    transcutaneous oximetry ($TcPO_2$), 173
  epidemiology, 172
  general considerations and history, 171–172, 171*f*
  management and surgical technique, 176–191
    anesthesia, 176
    antibiotics, 176–177
    blood vessels, 177
    bone, 179–181, 179*f*
    cryoamputation (physiologic amputation), 190–191
    digit/ray resection, 181–182
    Gritti-Stokes amputation, 188
    hindfoot (Chopart, Boyd, and Pirigoff), 183–184
    knee disarticulation (KD), 187–188
    Lisfranc, 182–183
    muscles, 177–179
    nerves, 177
    Syme (ankle disarticulation), 184–185
    transfemoral (TFA), 189–190
    transmetatarsal (TMA), 182
    transtibial (TTA), 185–187
  postoperative management, 191–193
    complications, 192–193
    contracture, 193
    infection, 193
    mortality, 192
    pain, 193
    routine care, 191–192
    thrombolytic events, 192–193
antiplatelet therapy, 96
aortic dissection, 404–422
  chronic, 420–422
    branched and fenestrated endovascular aortic repair (B/FEVAR), 420–422
    open thoracoabdominal aneurysm repair, 420
    TEVAR, 420
  clinical findings, 408–409
    signs and symptoms of acute aortic dissection, 408–409
    signs and symptoms of malperfusion, 409
  complicated type B aortic dissection—malperfusion, 416
  complicated type B aortic dissection—ruptured, 416
  diagnosis, 409–412
    chest radiography (CXR), 412
    computed tomography angiography (CTA), 409–410
    intravascular ultrasound (IVUS), 410
    limitations, 412
    magnetic resonance angiography (MRA), 410
    transesophageal echocardiography (TEE), 410–411
    transthoracic echocardiography, 410
  differential diagnosis, 409
  endovascular management, 416–418
    emerging endovascular techniques
      STABLE (Petticoat) and STABILISE, 418
    mesenteric/renal/iliac stenting, 417
    percutaneous fenestration, 417–418
    TEVAR, 416–417
  general considerations and history, 405–408
    anatomy and classification, 405–406
    epidemiology, 406–407
    genetic and molecular basis, 407–408
    historical background, 405
    pathophysiology of malperfusion, 408
    risk factors, 407
  management, 412–416
    general techniques, 414–415
    postoperative complications, 415–416
    uncomplicated aortic dissection: endovascular management, 413–414
    uncomplicated aortic dissection: medical management, 412–413
  open management, 418–420
    open bypass, 420
    open fenestration, 418–420

aortic dissection, open management (*Cont.*):
open surgical management, 416
aortic occlusion, 491
arterial anatomy and pathophysiology, 380–386
arterial anatomy, 380–381
arterial pathophysiology, 381–386
aneurysmal disease, 383–384
atherosclerotic disease, 381–383
dissections, 384–386
intimal hyperplasia, 386
overview, 380
arterial ulcers, 846–847
arterioles, 4
arteriovenous access-related VTOS, 327–329
arteriovenous malformations (AVMs), 337–349
classification, 340–341, 340*t*, 341*f*
conclusion, 347
definition, 337
diagnostic evaluation, 341–342
etiology: genetic aspect, 338–339
pathophysiology, 339
follow-up, 347
incidence, 337–338, 338*t*
treatment, 342–347
endovascular/embolosclerotherapy, 343–347
surgical/excisional therapy, 343
artificial intelligence (AI) and vascular surgery, 122, 906–914
artificial intelligence in medicine, 909–910
artificial intelligence in vascular surgery, 910–911
current limitations, 912–913
fundamentals of artificial intelligence, 907–909
future directions, 914
introduction, 906
machine learning algorithm development framework, 911–912, 911*f*
Aselli, Gasparo, 353
atherosclerotic carotid disease, 526–541
background and history, 526–527
clinical findings, 527–528
diagnosis, 528–530
differential diagnosis, 528, 529*t*
diseases affecting the extracranial carotid territory, 528
management, 531–541
asymptomatic carotid stenosis, 532
carotid endarterectomy (CEA), 532–535
conclusion, 541
diagnosis, 528–531
symptomatic carotid stenosis, 531–532
transcarotid artery revascularization (TCAR), 538–541
transfemoral carotid stenting (TFCAS), 535–538
atrial fibrillation, 100
atrioventricular block, 101–102
AVMs (arteriovenous malformations). *see* arteriovenous malformations (AVMs)

B

banding, 660
Beaussier, 439
Bernoulli's principle, 145
beta-adrenergic blockade therapy, 96–97
Blalock, Alfred, 884, 884*f*
blunt trauma, 704
bruits and poststenotic dilatation, 151
business aspects of a cardiovascular center, 863–876
business manager role, 868
compensation methods for physicians, 869–874
future of payments, 875
legal constraints, 875
quality of care-based payments, 875–876
value-based and newer models for reimbursement, 875
financial management, 867–868
cost volume profit (CVP) analysis, 867–868
financial statements, 867
using financial statements to make decisions, 867
governance, 865
introduction, 863
management and development, 863–865
managing the revenue cycle, 868–869
operations and efficiency, 865
patient access, 865–866
no shows, 865–866
wait times, 865
recovering from COVID-19, 876

C

calciphylaxis, 848
capillaries, 4–5, 4*f*
cardiac arrhythmias and conduction abnormalities, 100–102
cardiac evaluation of the vascular patient, 92–102
atrial fibrillation, 100
atrioventricular block, 101–102
cardiac arrhythmias and conduction abnormalities, 100–102
cardiac sources of arterial embolism, 98–100
atrial thrombi, 98–99
cardiac tumors, 99–100
infective endocarditis (IE), 99

cardiac evaluation of the vascular patient (*Cont.*):
left ventricular thrombi, 99
myxoma, 99–100
papillary fibroelastoma (PFE), 100
perioperative medical management, 96–97
antiplatelet therapy, 96
beta-adrenergic blockade therapy, 96–97
statin therapy, 96
perioperative myocardial injury and infarction, 97–98
preoperative risk assessment, 92–96
coronary angiography, 95
noninvasive cardiac evaluation, 94–95
risk assessment tools, 92–94, 93*t*–94*t*
surgical timing after percutaneous coronary intervention, 95–96
torsades des pointes, 100–101
ventricular arrhythmias, 101
carotid endarterectomy (CEA), 532–535
Carrel, Alexis, 651
central vascular trauma, 703–715
blunt trauma, 704
diagnosis, 704–705
computed tomography of the abdomen, 704–705
exploratory laparotomy, 705
focused assessment with sonography in trauma (FAST), 705
physical examination, 704
endovascular management of renal trauma, 713–714
penetrating injuries, 713–714
epidemiology, 703
general principles of management of abdominal vascular trauma, 705–710
damage control principles, 705–706
operative management, 706–710
management of blunt traumatic abdominal vascular injury, 713
Zone II abdominal vascular injuries, 713
management of penetrating abdominal vascular injuries, 710–713
Zone I vascular injuries (central abdominal hematoma), 710–713
Zone III abdominal vascular injuries, 714–715
iliac artery, 714
iliac vein, 714–715
cephalic arch stenosis, 328
chronic lower extremity ischemia, 504–510
clinical findings, 504–505
diagnosis, 505–507
differential diagnosis, 505
general consideration and history, 504
management, 507–510
chronic lower extremity ulcers management and evaluation, 839–858
assessment and management, 848–853
advanced laboratory evaluation, 849
basic laboratory evaluation, 849
general principles, 848–849
imaging, 849–850
tissue biopsy and culture, 849
tissue debridement, 580
ulcer infection, 850
by ulcer type, 853–858
wound dressing, 850–853
differential diagnosis, 840–844
introduction, 840
epidemiology, 840, 841*t*
pathophysiology of ulcer by disease condition, 844–848
arterial ulcers, 846–847
calciphylaxis, 848
diabeteic/neuropathic ulcers, 847
drug-induced ulcers, 848
livedo vasculopathy, 848
pyoderma gangrenosum, 847
vasculitic ulcers, 847
venous ulcers, 846
summary, 858
chronic mesenteric ischemia, 568–574
clinical findings, 569
considerations, 573–574
aortic reconstruction and mesenteric revascularization, 573
mesenteric infarction, 573
nonatherosclerotic causes of chronic mesenteric ischemia, 573–574
remedial procedures after open surgical mesenteric revascularization, 573
diagnosis, 569–570
invasive modalities, 570–
noninvasive modalities, 570
differential diagnosis, 569
general considerations and history, 568–569
management, 570–573
antegrade aortoceliac to superior mesenteric artery bypass, 572
endovascular intervention, 571–572
retrograde aorta to superior mesenteric artery bypass, 572–573
surgical management, 572
outcomes, 574

chronic upper extremity ischemia, 516–521
conclusion, 521
differential diagnosis, 517
introduction, 516
outcomes, 520–521
pathology, 516–517
presentation and symptoms, 517
treatment, 518–520, 518*f*–519*f*
workup, 517–518
chronic venous disease, 285–293
clinical findings, 286–287
conclusions, 293
diagnosis/differential diagnosis, 287–288
management, 289–293
overview, 285
pathophysiology, 285–286
testing, 288–289
chronic venous disease of the upper extremities and central veins, 321–331
algorithm for care, 330–331
anatomy, 322–325
costoclavicular junction (CCJ) and subclavian vein, 323–324
deltopectoral groove/triangle and the cephalic vein, 323
intrathoracic venous problems, 324–325
notable upper arm relationships, 323–325
overview, 322–323
clinical presentation, 325
conclusion, 331
introduction, 321–322
specific problems, 326–330
arteriovenous access-related VTOS, 327–329
cephalic arch stenosis, 328
costoclavicular junction stenosis, 328
HeRO graft, 329
intermittent positional stenosis (McCleery's syndrome), 326
intrathoracic venous stenosis, 328–329
obstruction secondary to malignancy, 329–330
pacemaker and catheter-induced obstruction, 329
peripheral stenoses, 327–328
postphebitic obstruction (chronic Paget-Schroetter syndrome), 326–327
venous thoracic outlet syndrome (VTOS), 326–327
coagulation cascade, 34–35, 37*f*
compartment syndrome, 740–757
basic anatomy, 741–745
chronic exertional compartment syndrome, 756–757
clinical findings, 746–747
complications, 754
diagnosis, 747–748
differential diagnosis, 747
general considerations/history, 740–741
management, 748
endovascular options, 748
open surgery: fasciotomies, 749–754
pathophysiology/associated molecular problems, 745–746
Volkmann's ischemic contracture, 754–756
Complex regional pain syndrome (CRPS), 226–230
clinical findings, 227
diagnosis, 228
differential diagnosis, 227–228
management, 228–230
overview and history, 226
pathophysiology, 226–227
summary, 230
Cooley, Denton, 391
Cooper, Astley, 391
costoclavicular junction stenosis, 328
COVID-19, recovering from, 876
Creech technique, 164, 164*f*
cryoamputation (physiologic amputation), 190–191

D

DeBakey, Michael, 391, 405, 439
deep venous thromboembolism (DVT), 258–266
case presentation, 266
clinical findings, 259
diagnosis, 260–262
imaging, 260–262
rationale, 260
differential diagnosis, 259–260
general considerations, 258–259
epidemiology and risk factors for DVT, 258–259
pathophysiology, 259
management, 262–266
acute LE DVT with large central vein thrombosis, 265
distal (calf) DVT, 265–266
interventional, 264–265
lower extremity DVT (LE DVT), 265–266
modalities of treatment, 262–265
pharmacologic—anticoagulation, 262–263
severe obstructive proximal (iliofemoral) DVT, 265
treatment of DVT based on anatomical location, 265–266
upper extremity DVT (UE DVT), 265
Dejerine syndrome, 557

De Vinci, Leonardo, 623
diabeteic/neuropathic ulcers, 847
dose area product (DAP), 46
Dotter, Charles, 487
drug-induced ulcers, 848
Dubost, Charles, 391
DVT (deep venous thromboembolism). *see* deep venous thromboembolism (DVT)

E

endovascular diagnosis and treatment, 202–215
- access, 202–205
  - axillary artery, 204
  - brachial artery, 204–205
  - femoral artery, 202–203
  - popliteal artery, 203–204
  - radial artery, 205
  - superficial femoral artery, 203
  - tibial access, 204
- equipment, 207–209
  - catheters, 208–209
  - guidewires, 207–208
  - guiding catheters, 208
  - needles, 207
  - sheaths, 208
- hemostasis, 205–207
  - closure devices, 205–207
  - compression devices, 207
  - manual pressure, 205
- liquid agents, 214–215
- mechanical, 212–213
- overview, 202
- particles, 213–214
- scarred groins, 205
- treatment devices, 209–213
  - balloon angioplasty, 209–210
  - embolization tools, 212
  - stents, 210–212
- of visceral aneurysms, 445–446

erectile dysfunction, 820–831
- anatomy and physiology of erections, 823–825
  - neurotransmitters involved in erections and detumescence, 824
  - penile vascular and neurological anatomy, 823
  - phases of erection, 823–824
  - physiology of cavernosal smooth muscle, 824–825
- causes, 821–823, 821*t*
  - endocrine causes, 822
  - medication causes, 822
  - metabolic and lifestyle factors, 822
  - neurological causes, 822
  - surgical causes, 822
  - urological conditions, 822–823
  - vascular causes, 821
- clinical findings, 825–827
  - clinical staging, 825
  - diagnosis and evaluation, 825–827
  - differential diagnosis, 825
- general considerations and history, 820–821
- management of the clinical problem, 827–831
  - medical treatment, 827–830
  - pathway of treatment, 831
  - surgical treatment, 830–831

F

fasciotomy, 497–499
femoropopliteal occlusion, 492
FemoStop device, 207
first rib resection, 616–617

G

giant cell arteritis (GCA), 773–774
Gigli saw blade, 179, 179*f*
Gilbert, Augustine, 623
Greenleaf, Robert, 889, 889*f*
Gritti-Stokes amputation, 188

H

Hamburg Classification of congenital vascular malformations (VCMs), 337, 338*t*
Harvey, William, 18
hemodialysis access, 650–668
- follow-up monitoring of established dialysis access, 664–665
- history and general considerations of dialysis therapy, 651–652
- indwelling dialysis catheters, 665–668
  - complex long-term indwelling catheters, 666–667
  - complications of catheter insertion, 667–668
  - technique for insertion of temporary dialysis access, 666
- long-term outcomes of dialysis access, 665
- overview of common permanent dialysis access approaches, 652–653
  - autogenous access, 653
  - prosthetic access, 654
- overview of complex permanent dialysis access approaches, 656–659
  - complex autogenous tissue dialysis access creation, 657–658
  - complex prosthetic dialysis access creation, 658–659
- postoperative complications, 659–664
  - aneurysm and pseudoaneurysm, 662
  - banding, 660
  - bleeding and hematoma, 661–662
  - cardiopulmonary complications, 663
  - graft thrombosis and failure, 663–664

postoperative complications, graft thrombosis and failure (*Cont.*):
- infection, 662
- neuropathy, 662
- preoperative workup of patients, 652
- procedure details, 654–655
  - autogenous venous constructs, 654–655
  - prosthetic arm access, 655

HeRO graft, 329
Hunter, John, 391

I

iliac occlusion, 492
infragenicular occlusion, 492
intermittent pneumatic compression (IPC), 359
intermittent positional stenosis (McCleery's syndrome), 326
intramural hematoma (IMH), 430
intrathoracic venous stenosis, 328–329

J

Jepson, Paul, 740

K

Kaposiform hemangioendothelioma (KHE), 900–901
Kennedy, John Fitzgerald, 885–886, 885*f*
King, Reverend Martin Luther, 89, 882, 882*f*
Klippel-Trenaunay syndrome, 119–120, 120*f*, 902

L

Laennec, 405
laminar flow, 21–22, 21*f*
Lao Tzu, 881, 889
Laplace, Pierre, 19
large vessel vasculitis (LVV), 771–774
- giant cell arteritis (GCA), 773–774
- Takayasu arteritis (TA), 771–772

leadership and physicians as leaders in health care organizations, 880–891
- conclusion, 891
- fundamental principles of leadership in medicine, 882–886
  - balance, 886
  - developing self-awareness, 884–885
  - establish a clear vision, 883–884
  - lead by action, not by position, 885–886
  - lead with values, 882–883
- introduction, 880–881
- leadership styles, 888–891
  - affiliative, 890
  - authoritative, 890
  - coaching, 891
  - coercive, 890
  - democratic, 890–891
  - pacesetting, 891
- role of the physician leader in the modern health care system, 886–888
- what makes a leader?, 881–882

Lisfranc, 182–183
Lister, Joseph, 883
livedo vasculopathy, 848
lower extremity swelling and differential diagnosis, 364–374
- clinical diagnosis, 365, 369–374
  - diagnostic testing, 374
  - duplex ultrasound, 373–374
  - history, 365, 371
  - patient reported symptoms, 371
  - physical examination, 365, 371
  - treatment and surveillance, 365, 374
- epidemiology, 365, 369
- introduction, 364, 365–366
- pathophysiology, 364–365, 366–368
  - causes of increased capillary filtration, 365, 368–369
  - causes of reduced lymphatic drainage, 365, 369
  - deleterious effects of fluid stasis, 365, 366. 368
  - increased capillary hydrostatic pressure, 368
  - increased capillary permeability, 368–369
  - obesity as a cause of edema, 369
  - reduced plasma oncotic pressure, 368
  - Starling principle and its revision, 365–366

lower extremity ulcers, chronic, management and evaluation. *see* chronic lower extremity ulcers management and evaluation
LVV (large vessel vasculitis), 771–774
- giant cell arteritis (GCA), 773–774
- Takayasu arteritis (TA), 771–772

lymphedema, 353–360
- clinical findings, 355–356
- diagnosis, 357–358
  - computed tomography (CT), 358
  - direct contrast lymphangiography, 358
  - lymphoscintigraphy, 358
  - magnetic resonance lymphography, 358
- differential diagnosis, 356–357
- general considerations and history, 353–355
  - lymphatic anatomy and physiology, 353–354

lymphedema, general considerations and history (*Cont.*):
- lymphedema causes and prevalence, 354–355
- management, 358–360
  - anastomotic microsurgical techniques, 359–360
  - intermittent pneumatic compression (IPC), 359
  - medical management, 358–359
  - suction-assisted lipectomy, 359
  - surgical management, 359–360

M

machine learning algorithm development framework, 911–912, 911*f*
MAGIC classification, 786, 787*t*
mangled extremity, 687
Matas, Rudolph, 391
Maunoir, 405
McCleery's syndrome, 326
McDonald, Donald A., 19
mesenteric venous thrombosis (MVT), 583
Mitchell, Silas Weir, 228

N

native arterial infections, 761–765
- diagnostic evaluation, 762–763
  - clinical exam, 762
  - labs, 763
  - radiology, 762
- introduction, 761–762
  - epidemiology, 761
  - pathogenesis, 761–762
- treatment, 763–765
  - medical treatment, 763
  - surgical treatment, 764–765

neck vascular trauma, 693–698
- blunt cerebrovascular injuries (BCVI), 696–697
- carotid artery injury, 695–696
- clinical anatomy, 693–694
- internal jugular vein injury, 696
- introduction, 693
- management of specific injuries, 695–697
- operative approach to vascular injuries in the neck, 697–698
- penetrating cervical vascular injuries, 694–695
- subclavian vessel injuries, 696
- thyroidal vessel injuries, 696
- vertebral artery injuries, 696

Nietzsche, Friedrich, 882
noninvasive evaluation of arterial disease, 126–139
- conclusion, 138
- extracranial carotid evaluation, 127–129
  - indication, 127
  - interpretation, 129
  - surveillance, 129
  - technical, 127–129
- lower extremity evaluation, 134–138
  - indication, 134
  - interpretation, 135–137
  - surveillance, 138
  - technical, 134–135
- mesenteric evaluation, 132–134
  - indication, 132
  - interpretation, 132–134
  - surveillance, 134
  - technical, 132
- overview, 126–127, 139*f*
- renal evaluation, 129–132
  - indication, 129–130
  - interpretation, 130–131
  - surveillance, 131–132
  - technical, 130

noninvasive evaluation of venous disease, 109–122
- classification system (CEAP), 111–115
- history and physical examination, 109–111, 110*t*
- introduction, 109
- laboratory tests, 117
- noninvasive imaging modalities, 117–122
  - CT venography, 119
  - MR venography, 119–120, 120*f*
  - new diagnostic methods (artificial intelligence), 122
  - plethysmography, 120–122
  - venous duplex ultrasound (DUS), 117–119
- revised venous clinical severity score (VCSS), 115–117, 116*t*

nonocclusive mesenteric ischemia (NOMI), 582–583
no shows, 865–866

O

Ohm's law, 19–20

P

pacemaker and catheter-induced obstruction, 329
Palmaz, Julio, 391
Parodi, Juan, 391
Pasteur, Louis, 883
pediatric malignancies, 809–813
pediatric vascular surgery, 896–902
- acute extremity arterial occlusions, 896–899
  - clinical presentation and evaluation, 897–898
  - etiology and risk factors, 896–897
  - management, 898–899
- arterial aneurysms, 899
  - aortic aneurysms, 899
  - peripheral aneurysms, 899
- chronic arterial occlusive diseases, 899
  - clinical presentation and evaluation, 899
  - management, 899

pediatric vascular surgery (*Cont.*):
  general considerations, 896
  renovascular hypertension, 899–902
    clinical presentation and diagnosis, 900
    introduction and etiology, 899–900
    laboratory and radiological evaluation, 900–901
    management, 901–902
  venous disorders, 902
    Klippel-Trenaunay syndrome, 902
    venous malformations, 902
    venous thrombosis and postphlebitic syndrome, 902
penetrating aortic ulcerations and intramural hematomas, 430–434
  background, 430
  clinical findings, 431
  intramural hematoma (IMH), 430
  laboratory evaluation, 431–432
    imaging, 431–432
  natural history and disease progression, 432
  penetrating aortic ulcer (PAU), 430
  summary, 434
  treatment, 432–434
    ascending aorta, 433
    descending aorta, 433–434
    medical management, 432–433
    surgical management, 433–434
peripheral arterial aneurysms, 461–481
  lower extremity aneurysms, 463–477
    common femoral aneurysm, 463–466
    femoral artery false aneurysm, 467–469
    infrapopliteal aneurysm, 477
    popliteal aneurysm, 471–477
    profunda femoral artery aneurysm, 471
    superficial femoral artery aneurysm, 469–471
  upper extremity aneurysms, 477–480
    axillary artery aneurysms, 477–478
    brachial artery aneurysm, 478
    infected peripheral arterial aneurysms, 478–480
peripheral stenoses, 327–328
peripheral vascular trauma, 673–688
  diagnoses, 675–676
  epidemiology, 674
  introduction, 673–674
  operative management, 679–685
    arterial repair, 679–682
    medical exposure of the popliteal vessels, 684–685
    operative exposure and vascular control, 679
    specific injuries, 682–684
    tibial injuries, 685
    venous repair, 682
  postoperative complications, 685–687
    early, 685–686
    late, 687
  preoperative trauma management, 674–675
    airway and breathing management, 674
    circulation management, 674–675
    disability management, 675
    extremity tourniquete management, 675
  special scenarios, 687–688
    injuries with poor functional outcomes, 688
    mangled extremity, 687
    postoperative management, 688
    stenting, 688
    vascular damage control approach, 687–688
  types of vessel injuries, 676–679
peripheral venous aneurysm, 480
  popliteal venous aneurysm, 480
physics for the vascular specialist, 144–154
  aneurysms and arterial wall stress, 153–154
  arterial hemodynamics, 144–145
    fluid energy losses (Bernoulli's principle), 145
    fluid pressure and energy, 144–145
  blood flow patterns, 147–149
    bifurcations and branches, 149
    boundary layer separation, 147–148
    laminar flow, 147
    pulsatile flow, 149
    turbulent flow, 147
  hemodynamic principles in the treatment of arterial disease, 152–153
  hemodynamics of arterial stenosis, 149–152
    abnormal pressure and flow, 151
    bruits and poststenotic dilatation, 151
    collateral circulation, 151, 151*f*
    critical stenosis, 150–151, 150*f*
    distribution of vascular resistance and blood flow, 152
    energy losses, 149–150
    stenosis length and multiple stenoses, 151
    vascular steal, 152

physics for the vascular specialist (*Cont.*):
  normal pressure and flow, 146–147
  overview, 144, 153–154
  Poiseuille's law and vascular resistance, 145–146
plug flow, 21*f*, 22
Poiseuille, J.L.M., 18
Poiseuille's law, 20, 23, 145–146
portal hypertension, 622–644
  anatomy, 623–625
  clinical findings, 629–630
    encephalopathy, 629
    hepatorenal syndrome, 630
    variceal formation, 629
  diagnosis and evaluation, 630–632
    angiography, computed tomography angiography (CTA), and magnetic resonance angiography (MRA), 632
    noninvasive evaluation, 631
    serum markers, 631–632
  differential diagnosis, 625–629
    arteriovenous fistulas, 628–629
    extrahepatic postsinusoidal obstruction, 628
    extrahepatic presinusoidal obstruction, 627
    intrahepatic presinusoidal obstruction, 628
    intrahepatic sinusoidal and postsinusoidal obstruction, 628
  general consideration and history, 623
  invasive evaluation, 632–644
    endoscopic exam, 632–634
    endoscopic treatment of esophageal variceal bleeding, 636–637
    liver biopsy, 631
    liver transplantation, 642–643
    nonselective shunts, 641
    nonshunting procedures, 642
    pharmacotherapy, 635–636
    selective shunts, 641–642
    tamponade therapy, 637
    transjugular intrahepatic portosystemic shunt, 637–640
    treatment of portal hypertension and its complications, 634
postphebitic obstruction (chronic Paget-Schroetter syndrome), 326–327
prosthetic graft infections, 784–792
  conclusions, 791–792
  diagnosis, 786–788
  etiology and pathogenesis, 784–785
  introduction, 784
  management, 788–791
    general principles, 788–791
  presentation and classification, 785–786
  risk factors and prevention, 785
pulmonary embolism (PE), 270–279
  diagnosis, 271–273, 272*f*
  differential diagnosis, 271, 271*t*
  general consideration and history, 270–273
  management, 273–279
pyoderna gangrenosum, 847

R

radiation safety and the vascular specialist, 44–61
  conclusions, 61
  importance of radiation safety education and occupational exposure, 47–50
    as low as reasonably achievable (ALARA) principle, 47
    occupational exposure and health risk, 49–50
    radiation safety variation, 47
    vascular procedures and radiation exposure, 47–49
  overview of radiation dangers, risks, and exposure, 44–47
    absorbed dose, 45
    basic definitions of radiation, 45–46
    dose area product (DAP), 46
    effective dose, 45
    exposure, 45
    radiation exposure and biologic effects, 46
    radiation exposure types, 46–47
    reference air kerma (RAK), 45
    substantial radiation dose level (SRDL), 45–46
    x-ray production, 45
  radiation exposure and vascular surgery patients, 50–51
  radiation exposure during endovascular procedures, 51–52
  radiation exposure guidelines, 59–61
  special considerations, 58–59
    alternative imaging, 59
    carbon dioxide (CO_2) angiography, 58–59
    patient radiation education and consent, 59
    pregnancy, 58
  techniques to lower radiation exposure during procedures, 52–57
    checklist, 57*t*
    fluoroscopy time and dosimeters, 57
    imaging equipment techniques to lower radiation exposure, 53–56

radiation safety and the vascular specialist (*Cont.*):
  limiting radiation exposure to patient, 53
  protective equipment and garments, 56–57
  skin damage to patient, 53
reference air kerma (RAK), 45
renal artery stenosis (RAS), 595–606
  clinical findings, 598
    screening, 598
    signs and symptoms, 598
  diagnosis, 599–601
    computed tomograpic angiography (CTA), 600
    invasive imaging, 601
    laboratory evaluation, 599
    magnetic resonance angiography (MRA), 600–601
    renal duplex ultrasonography, 599–600
  differential diagnosis, 599, 599*t*
  general consideration and history, 595–598
    anatomy, 597
    causes, 595–597
    history, 595
    pathophysiology of renovascular hypertension, 597–598
  management, 601–606
    aortorenal bypass, 605–606
    aortorenal endarterectomy, 605
    complications, 604, 606
    endovascular stenting, 603–604
    endovascular therapy, 603
    extra-anatomic bypass, 606
    indications for intervention, 602–603
    medical therapy, 601–602
    open surgery, 605
    percutaneous transluminal angioplasty (PTA), 603
    renal artery re-implantation, 606
    surveillance and follow-up, 604, 606
resistance, 20–21, 21*f*
resuscitative endovascular balloon occlusion of the aorta for vascular trauma, 729–736
  complications and pitfalls, 735–736
  conclusions and outcomes, 736
  contraindications, 731
  devices, 731–732
  historical perspective of aortic control for torso hemorrhage, 729–730
  indications, 730–731
  introduction, 729
  preparation and equipment, 731
  technique, 732–735
    accessing the femoral artery, 732–733
    balloon catheter selection and insertion, 733–734
    balloon deflation, 734–735
    balloon inflation, 734
    operative definitive hemostasis, 734
    sheath removal, 735
Reynolds number, 22–23
role of the surgeon, 912

S
scalenectomy, 616
Semmelweis, Ignaz, 883, 883*f*
shear, 22
STABLE (Petticoat) and STABI-LISE, 418
Starling principle, 365–366
statin therapy, 96
steal syndrome, 660
Stemmer's sign, 356, 356*f*
Stoller, James, 881
Strandness, Eugene, 126
stroke, 526–527
substantial radiation dose level (SRDL), 45–46
suction-assisted lipectomy, 359
superficial venous insufficiency and varicose veins, 298–314
  anatomy and physiology, 299–300
  definitions, 298
  diagnosis, 303–305
    differential diagnosis, 304
    symptoms, 303–304
  duplex ultrasound, 306–307
  epidemiology, 298
  etiology and pathophysiology, 302–303
  future directions, 314
  history, 298–299
  management, 307–314
    comparison of interventional methods, 313–314
    indications for treatment, 307
    nontumescent nonthermal (NTNT) methods, 311–313
    thermal tumescent methods, 308–311
    treatment, 307–314
  risk factors, 302
  types of veins, 300–302
Syme (ankle disarticulation), 184–185, 185*f*

T
Takayasu arteritis (TA), 771–772
TCAR (transcarotid artery revascularization), 538–541
TFCAS (transfemoral carotid stenting), 535–538
Thomas, Vivien, 884, 884*f*
thoracic endovascular aortic repair (TEVAR), 416–417, 721–723
thoracic outlet syndrome (TOS) and supraclavicular decompression, 612–619
  cause, 612

thoracic outlet syndrome (TOS) (*Cont.*):
- definition, 612
- operative strategy, 614–615
  - anatomy of the thoracic outlet, 614–615
- operative technique, 615–618
  - brachial plexus neurolysis, 617
  - drain placement and closure, 618
  - first rib resection, 616–617
  - management of subclavian vein occlusion, stenosis, or other pathologies, 618
  - positioning and incision, 615–616
  - scalenectomy, 616
  - subclavian artery aneurysm or pathology management, 617
- postoperative management, 618–619
- presentation and physical findings, 613–614
- types, 612–613
  - arterial TOS, 613
  - neurogenic TOS, 612–613
  - venous TOS, 613

thoracic vascular trauma, 719–726
- blunt trauma, 720
- descending thoracic aorta, 721, 725
  - azygous vein, 726
  - internal mammary artery, 726
  - left carotid artery, 725–726
  - pulmonary artery, 726
  - pulmonary veins, 726
  - subclavian artery, 725
  - subclavian vein, 725
  - thoracic endovascular aortic repair (TEVAR), 721–723
  - thoracic vena cava, 725
- introduction, 719
- management of specific injuries, 720–721, 724–725
  - ascending aorta, 724
  - blunt cardiac trauma, 721
  - cardiac injuries, 724
  - innominate artery, 725
  - preoperative management and decision making, 720–721
  - transverse aortic arch, 724–725
- nonoperative management, 723
- penetrating trauma, 723–724
- TEVAR *versus* open management, 723
- thoracic cavity anatomy, 719–720

thoracoabdominal aortic aneurysms, 453–458
- clinical findings, 453–454
- diagnosis, 455
- differential diagnosis, 454–455
- general considerations and history, 453
- management, 455–458

thrombosis and hemostasis, 34–40
- approach to a patient with bleeding, 35–38
  - factor XIII deficiency, 38
  - PFA-100, 37
  - PT and aPTT, 35–36
  - PT and aPTT mixing study, 36
  - thrombin time, 36
  - vWD profile, 37–38
- approach to a patient with thrombosis, 38–40
  - antiphospholipid syndrome, 39
  - antithrombin deficiency, 39
  - Factor V Leiden, 38
  - protein C deficiency, 39
  - protein S deficiency, 39
  - prothrombin G20210A mutation or Factor II mutation, 38–39
  - thrombophilia testing, 39–40
  - treatment, 40
- hemostasis, 34–35
- introduction, 34

torsades des pointes, 100–101
transcarotid artery revascularization (TCAR), 538–541
transfemoral carotid stenting (TFCAS), 535–538
transitional flow, 22
treadmill exercise testing, 29
turbulent flow, 21*f*, 22

V

VAAs (visceral aneurysms). *see* Visceral aneurysms (VAAs)
Van Volkmann, Richard, 740
van Wesel, Andreas, 623
varicose veins. *see* superficial venous insufficiency and varicose veins
vascular biology, 2–14
- adventitia and perivascular adipose tissue (tunica externa), 6–12
  - capillaries, 9–10
  - pericytes, 11
  - venous system, 11–12
- basic principles of circulatory function, 12–14
- blood vessel structure and function, 5–6
  - endothelium (tunica intima), 5
  - smooth muscle layer (tunica media), 5–6
- overview of blood vessels, 2–5

vascular graft conduits: types and patency, 217–222
- autogenous vein grafts, 217–219
  - lower extremity veins, 217–218, 219*f*
  - upper extremity veins, 218
  - vein graft configuration, 219
  - vein graft preparation, 218–219

vascular graft conduits: types and patency (*Cont.*):
- graft patency, 221–222
- graft surveillance, 222
- introduction, 217
- prosthetic graft, 219–221

vascular hemodynamics, 18–30
- clinical case, 29–30
- clinical twist: ABI and segmental pressures, 27–30
  - clinical correlate of ABI, 28
  - definition and measurement of ABI, 27–28, 28*t*
  - peripheral artery disease (PAD), 27
  - physiology of ABI, 28
  - segmental pressures, 28–29
  - treadmill exercise testing, 29
- overview and historical background, 18–19
- physics, 19–24
  - compliance, 23–24, 24*f*
  - laminar flow, 21–22, 21*f*
  - Ohm's law, 19–20
  - plug flow, 21*f*, 22
  - Poiseuille's law, 20
  - Reynolds number, 22–23
  - shear, 22
  - transitional flow, 22
  - turbulent flow, 21*f*, 22
  - type of flow, 21–23
  - types of resistance, 20–21, 21*f*
  - velocity of blood flow, 19, 19*f*
  - wall tension, 23, 23*f*
- vascular circulation, 24–27
  - arteries, 24
  - cardiac output, 26–27
  - flow regulation, 25
  - mean arterial pressure, 26
  - microcirculation, 25
  - pressures in the cardiovascular system, 25–27, 26*f*
  - pulse pressure, 26, 27*f*
  - types and characteristics of blood vessels, 24–25
  - veins, 24–25

vascular steal, 152

vascular surgical techniques: open surgical exposure of arteries, veins, and other open techniques for occlusive disease and anterior spine exposure, 159–169
- anterior spine exposure, 166–169
- arteriotomy and endarterectomy, 163–166
  - endarterectomy, 163
  - vessel reconstruction, 164–166
- overview, 159
- vessel exposure and control, 160–163
  - anatomy, 160
  - balloon occlusion, 162
  - dissection, 160–161
  - incision, 160
  - redo dissection, 161
  - retractors, 160
  - tourniquet, 162–163
  - vascular clamping, 161–162
  - vessel control, 161

vascular tumors and vascular oncosurgery, 796–816
- benign vascular tumors, 797–801
  - congenital hemangiomas (CH), 800
  - infantile hemangioma (IH), 797–800
  - Kaposiform hemangioendothelioma (KHE), 800–901
- conclusion, 813–816
- introduction, 796–797, 797*t*
- malignant vascular tumors, 801–802
  - angiosarcoma, 801–802
  - epithelioid hemangioendothelioma, 802

vascular oncosurgery, 802–813
- extra-adrenal paragangliomas, 802
- limb tumors, 813
- mediastinal tumors, 802–804
- pediatric malignancies, 809–813
- retroperitoneal tumors, 804–809

vasculitic ulcers, 847

vasculitis and other arteriopathies, 769–779
- conclusion, 778–779
- histopathology, 770–771
- imaging, 771
- immune complex deposition vasculitis, 777–778
- introduction, 769–770
- large vessel vasculitis (LVV), 771–774
  - giant cell arteritis (GCA), 773–774
  - Takayasu arteritis (TA), 771–772
- medium vessel vasculitis: polyarteritis nodosa (PAN) and Kawasaki's disease (KD), 774–776
- small vessel vasculitis (SVV): ANCA-associated vasculitis, 776–777
- variable vasculitis (VV): Behcet's disease, 778

velocity of blood flow, 19, 19*f*

venous anatomy and physiology, 238–253
- anatomy of mature venous system, 243–247
  - abdomen/pelvis, 245–247
  - lower extremity, 244–245
  - thorax/neck, 245
  - upper extremity, 245
- anomalies of mature venous system, 248–250
  - inferior vena cava anomalies, 250
  - renal vein anomalies, 250

venous anatomy and physiology (*Cont.*):
  superior vena cava anomalies, 248–249
 embryology of the venous system, 238–242
  cardinal system, 241–242
  umbilical system, 241
  vitelline system, 239–240
 hemodynamic role of perforating veins, 253
 histology of venous system, 242–243
 overview, 238
 physiology of venous system, 250–253
  muscle pump, 252
  venous resistance, 252–253
  venous return, 251–252
  venous valve cycle, 252–253
  venous volume, 250–251
venous insufficiency, superficial. *see* superficial venous insufficiency and varicose veins
venous thoracic outlet syndrome (VTOS), 326–327
venous ulcers, 846
ventricular arrhythmias, 101
venules, 5
vertebrobasilar insufficiency, 547–563
 anatomy and pathophysiology, 548–556
  anatomy of the vertebrobasilar system, 548–550
  mechanisms of vertebrobasilar insufficiency, 550–556
  vascular supply to the brainstem and cerebellum, 550
 clinical features, 556–557
  neurologic symptoms, 556
  physical exam findings, 556–557
 diagnostic measures, 558–559
  catheter-based angiography, 559
  computed tomography, 558–559
  magnetic resonance imaging, 559
  ultrasound, 559
 differential diagnosis, 558
  dizziness, nausea, and vomiting, 558
  double vision or diplopia, 558
  syncope and coma, 558
 management, 559–563
  acute thrombotic occlusion, 559–561
  chronic high-grade stenosis or occlusion, 561–562
  vertebrobasilar dolichoctasia, 562–563
 vertebrobasilar syndromes, 557–558
  lateral medullary (Wallenburg) syndrome, 557
  lateral pontine syndrome, 557
  medial medullary (Dejerine) syndrome, 557
  top of the basilar syndrome, 558
  ventral pontine (locked-in) syndrome, 557–558
visceral aneurysms (VAAs), 438–448
 clinical findings, 440–442
  celiac artery aneurysms, 441
  gastroduodenal/pancreaticoduodenal artery aneurysms, 441
  hepatic artery aneurysms, 441
  jejunal, ilial, colic, and inferior mesenteric artery aneurysms, 441–442
  splenic artery aneurysms, 441
  superior mesenteric artery aneurysms, 441
 diagnosis, 442
 differential diagnosis, 442
 general consideration and history, 438–440
  celiac artery aneurysms (CAAs), 440
  gastric, gastroepiploic arteries, pancreaticoduodenal, and gastroduodenal artery aneurysms, 440
  hepatic artery aneurysms, 439–440
  ileal, jejunal, and colic artery aneurysms, 440
  inferior mesenteric artery aneurysms, 440
  splenic artery aneurysms, 439
  superior mesenteric artery aneurysms, 440
 management, 442–446, 443*f*
  endovascular treatment of celiac artery aneurysms, 445
  endovascular treatment of gastric, gasteoepiploic, gastroduodenal, and pancreaticoduodenal aneurysms, 446
  endovascular treatment of hepatic artery aneurysms, 445
  endovascular treatment of jejunal, ileal, and colic artery aneurysms, 446
  endovascular treatment of splenic artery aneurysms, 445
  endovascular treatment of superior mesenteric artery aneurysms, 445
  general considerations of endovascular management, 442–445

visceral aneurysms (VAAs) (*Cont.*):
open repair, 446–448
general considerations, 446
open repair of celiac artery aneurysms, 447
open repair of gastric, gastroepiploic, gastroduodenal, and pancreaticoduodenal artery aneurysms, 447
open repair of hepatic artery aneurysms, 447
open repair of jejunal, ileal, and colic artery aneurysms, 447–448
open repair of splenic artery aneurysms, 446
open repair of superior mesenteric artery aneurysms, 447
Volkmann's ischemic contracture, 754–756

W
wait times, 865
Wallenburg syndrome, 557
wall tension, 23, 23*f*
wound healing for the vascular specialist, 68–85
classification of wounds, 76
factors affecting wound healing, 76–83
advanced age, 77–78
diabetes mellitus, 80
drugs, steroids, and chemotherapeutic drugs, 79–80
hypoxia, hypoperfusion, and anemia, 78
metabolic disorders, 80–81
nutrition, 81–83
uremia, 80–81
historical methods of wound healing, 76
phases of wound healing, 69–74
epithelialization, 73–74, 74*f*
hemostasis and inflammation, 69–71
matrix synthesis, 72–73
maturation and remodeling, 73
proliferation, 71–72
role of growth factors in wound healing, 74–76, 74*t*–75*t*
summary, 85
wound contraction, 76
wound infection, 83–85

Y
Young, Thomas, 18

Z
Zone I vascular injuries (central abdominal hematoma), 710–713
Zone II abdominal vascular injuries, 713
Zone III abdominal vascular injuries, 714–715
iliac artery, 714
iliac vein, 714–715